Thieme

Endoscopic Lateral Skull Base Surgery

Principles, Anatomy, Approaches

Daniele Marchioni, MD
Professor of Otorhinolaryngology and Head & Neck Surgery
Head, Department of Otorhinolaryngology
University Hospital Polyclinic
Modena, Italy

Livio Presutti, MD
Professor of Otorhinolaryngology and Head & Neck Surgery
Department of Otorhinolaryngology
Sant'orsola Malpighi Polyclinic IRCCS
Azienda Ospedaliera University
Bologna, Italy

2005 illustrations

Thieme
Stuttgart • New York • Delhi • Rio de Janeiro

Library of Congress Cataloging-in-Publication Data
is available from the publisher.

Important note: Medicine is an ever-changing science undergoing continual development. Research and clinical experience are continually expanding our knowledge, in particular our knowledge of proper treatment and drug therapy. Insofar as this book mentions any dosage or application, readers may rest assured that the authors, editors, and publishers have made every effort to ensure that such references are in accordance with **the state of knowledge at the time of production of the book.**
Nevertheless, this does not involve, imply, or express any guarantee or responsibility on the part of the publishers in respect to any dosage instructions and forms of applications stated in the book. **Every user is requested to examine carefully** the manufacturers' leaflets accompanying each drug and to check, if necessary in consultation with a physician or specialist, whether the dosage schedules mentioned therein or the contraindications stated by the manufacturers differ from the statements made in the present book. Such examination is particularly important with drugs that are either rarely used or have been newly released on the market. Every dosage schedule or every form of application used is entirely at the user's own risk and responsibility. The authors and publishers request every user to report to the publishers any discrepancies or inaccuracies noticed. If errors in this work are found after publication, errata will be posted at www.thieme.com on the product description page.

Some of the product names, patents, and registered designs referred to in this book are in fact registered trademarks or proprietary names even though specific reference to this fact is not always made in the text. Therefore, the appearance of a name without designation as proprietary is not to be construed as a representation by the publisher that it is in the public domain.
Thieme addresses people of all gender identities equally. We encourage our authors to use gender-neutral or gender-equal expressions wherever the context allows.

Georg Thieme Verlag KG
Rüdigerstraße 14, 70469 Stuttgart Germany
www.thieme.de
+49 [0]711 8931 421, customerservice@thieme.de

Cover design: © Thieme
Cover image source: © Daniele Marchioni
Typesetting by DiTech, India

Printed in Germany by Westermann Druck Zwickau GmbH   5 4 3 2 1

ISBN 978-3-13-241277-4

Also available as an e-book:
eISBN (PDF): 978-3-13-241435-8
eISBN (epub): 978-3-13-258236-1

Contents

Videos

Foreword

The use of endoscopes in ear surgery has become a great tool in the arsenal of the ear and skull base surgeon. This big leap toward accepting this technology is twofold: on one hand, it is mainly due to the advancement of the quality of the images; on the other hand, it is due to the innovation by the pioneers of this field.

Professors Marchioni and Presutti edited a state-of-the-art book entitled *Endoscopic Lateral Skull Base Surgery*. Their book includes 14 chapters that thoroughly cover all aspects of skull base surgery, including anatomy, principles, and approaches.

The editors feel fortunate to have assembled a cadre of world-renowned experts to share their clinical insights and expertise in several areas that are vital to endoscopic skull base surgery. This book is substantively edited by two pioneers of endoscopic ear surgery who continue to push the boundaries by using the endoscope beyond its traditional use in middle ear surgery. They continue to expand the use of the endoscope by applying their endoscopic techniques to inner ear and skull base surgeries. In my opinion, this book is the holy grail of endoscopic skull base surgery. Each chapter elucidates a great deal of information for novices, as well as experts in the field of skull base surgery.

On behalf of the editors, I would like to extend sincere gratitude to each contributing author for dedicating a significant amount of time and effort toward the completion of this comprehensive book.

George Wanna, MD, FACS
Site Chair
Department of Otolaryngology
New York Eye and Ear Infirmary of Mount Sinai
Mount Sinai Hospital
New York, New York, USA

Preface

After finishing our book *Endoscopic Ear Surgery* (Thieme, 2015), we realized the need for a book that would extend the description of endoscopic anatomy and endoscopic techniques to the inner ear and lateral skull base.

In the last decade, endoscopic ear surgery has taken a step further: The discovery of new approaches and anatomical structures made it possible to treat pathologies of the inner ear and the petrous apex. Although surgery of the lateral cranial base relies mainly on microscopic approaches, the introduction of endoscopic surgery to the otological community has enabled the surgeon to use the endoscope in combination with the microscope to produce more effective approaches to the lateral skull base, with a lower morbidity.

In 2011, we started to investigate a possible transcanal treatment for lesions located in the lateral skull base. Our aim was exploring the possibility of using the external auditory canal as a natural surgical corridor to reach some anatomical areas located in the lateral skull base. We began to develop anatomical and surgical concepts by following the same rationale that was used for the development of the transnasal endoscopic approaches to the anterior skull base. The principle was to develop the surgical possibility of directly and endoscopically reaching the tumors located in the lateral cranial base in order to avoid dural, cerebral, and vascular manipulation and to work only on the tumor itself, through a minimally invasive procedure. These surgical principles led to the first scientific publication on the topic, centering on the endoscopic transcanal dissection to reach the internal auditory canal. At the end of 2012, this technique was for the first time successfully applied in a patient suffering from cochlear schwannoma. Following this, the first transcanal approaches using the external auditory canal as a surgical corridor to the lateral cranial base were performed.

This book contains our latest experiences on lateral skull base surgery. We are describing traditional surgical approaches combined with endoscopic steps but have also included the most up-to-date fully endoscopic transcanal approaches to the lateral skull base, with a focus on the anatomical details and surgical strategies.

We created the illustrations in this book by ourselves. We also used the collection of images from our surgical procedures to share our recent experiences with the readers.

We hope that this book will be a starting point to develop endoscopic lateral skull base surgery in the future and that it will help the next generation of surgeons to improve the anatomical and surgical knowledge of the lateral skull base for the benefit of our patients.

Daniele Marchioni, MD
Livio Presutti, MD

Contributors

Lukas Anschütz, MD
Department of Otorhinolaryngology – Head and Neck Surgery
Inselspital, Bern University Hospital
University of Bern
Bern, Switzerland

Mohamed Badr-El-Dine, MD
Senior Consultant Otology Neurotology & Skull Base Surgery
Sultan Qaboos University Hospital Muscat, Oman;
Professor of Otolaryngology Faculty of Medicine
University of Alexandria
Alexandria, Egypt

Daniele Bernardeschi, MD, PhD
Otolaryngologist
ENT Department
Pitié-Salpêtrière Hospital
Paris, France

Luca Bianconi, MD
Otolaryngologist
Polyclinic Hospital of Borgo Trento
University of Verona
Verona, Italy

Nicola Bisi, MD
Department of Otorhinolaryngology
University Hospital of Verona
Verona, Italy

Marco Bonali, MD
ENT specialist
Department of Otorhinolarynogology – Head and Neck surgery
University Hospital of Modena
Modena, Italy

Marco Carner, MD
Professor
University of Verona
Verona, Italy

Raphaelle A. Chemtob, MD
Resident Physician
Cleveland Clinic Foundation
Cleveland, Ohio, USA

Elisa Ciceri, MD
Department of Neuroradiology
IRCCS Fondazione Istitute Neurologico "C.Besta"
Milan, Italy

Matteo Alicandri Ciufelli, MD
Associate Professor
Department of Maternal-Child and Adult Medical and Surgical Sciences
University of Modena and Reggio Emilia
Modena, Italy

Matteo Fermi, MD
Otorhinolaryngologist
Research Assistant
IRCCS Policlinico Sant'Orsola Malpighi
Alma Mater Studiorum – University of Bologna
Bologna, Emilia-Romagna, Italy

Antonio Gulino, MD
ENT Surgeon
Department of Otolaryngology
Verona University Hospital
Syracuse, Sicily, Italy

Brandon Isaacson, MD
Professor
Department of Otolaryngology – Head and Neck Surgery
UT Southwestern Medical Center
Dallas, Texas, USA

Nicholas Jufas, FRACS, MBBS (Hons), MS, BSc (Med)
Clinical Associate Professor
Department of Otolaryngology,
Head and Neck Surgery
Sydney University;
Macquarie University;
Sydney Endoscopic Ear Surgery Research Group
Royal North Shore Hospital
Sydney, Australia

Seiji Kakeatha, MD
Professor of Otolaryngology – Head and Neck Surgery
Faculty of Medicine
Yamagata University
Yamagata, Japan

Mustafa Kapadia MD
ENT Specialist;
Director of Education
Tarabichi Stammberger Ear Sinus Institute
Dubai, UAE

Noritaka Komune, MD, PhD
Assistant Professor
Department of Otorhinolaryngology – Head and Neck Surgery
Kyushu University Hospital
Fukuoka, Japan

Jonathan H.K. Kong, FRACS, FRCS, MS, MBBS (Syd), AMusA
Clinical Associate Professor
Department of Otolaryngology,
Head and Neck Surgery
Sydney University;
Macquarie University;
Sydney Endoscopic Ear Surgery Research Group
Royal Prince Alfred Hospital
Sydney, Australia

Elliott D. Kozin, MD
Assistant Professor
Harvard Medical School
Massachusetts Eye and Ear
Boston, Massachusetts, USA

Daniel J. Lee, MD, FACS
Associate Professor
Harvard Medical School
Massachusetts Eye and Ear
Boston, Massachusetts, USA

Daniele Marchioni, MD
Professor of Otorhinolaryngology and Head & Neck Surgery
Head, Department of Otorhinolaryngology
University Hospital Polyclinic
Modena, Italy

Andrea Martone, MD
Resident Physician
Department of Otorhinolaryngology – Head and Neck surgery
University Hospital Policlinico Modena
Modena, Italy

Barbara Masotto, MD
Head of Posterior Cranial Fossa Unit
Department of Neurosurgery
University Hospital of Verona
Verona, Italy

Gabriele Molteni, MD, PhD, FEBORL-HNS
Associate Professor of Otolaryngology
Section of Otorhinolaryngology – Head and Neck Surgery
Deparment of Surgery, Odontosomatology, and Pediatrics
University of Verona
Verona, Italy

Joao Flavio Nogueira, MD
Professor
Department of Otolaryngology – Head and Neck Surgery
Sinus & Oto Center
Hospital São Carlos
Fortaleza, Brazil

Nirmal Patel MBBS (Hons) FRACS (OHNS) MS (Research)
Clinical Professor of Surgery, Macquarie University;
Clinical Associate Professor,
Department of Otolaryngology,
Head and Neck Surgery
University of Sydney
Royal North Shore Hospital
Sydney Endoscopic Ear Surgery Research Group
Sydney, Australia

Giacomo Pavesi, MD
Head
Department of Neurosurgery
Modena Polyclinic University Hospital
Modena, Italy

Giampietro Pinna, MD
Head
Department of Neurosurgery
University Hospital of Verona
Verona, Italy

Livio Presutti, MD
Professor of Otorhinolaryngology and Head & Neck Surgery
Department of Otorhinolaryngology
Sant'orsola Malpighi Polyclinic IRCCS
Azienda Ospedaliera University
Bologna, Italy

Alejandro Rivas, MD
Division Chief of Otology/Neurotology
Department of Otolaryngology – Head and Neck Surgery
Vanderbilt University Medical Center
Nashville, Tennessee, USA

Stefano De Rossi, MD
Department of Otorhinolaryngology and Head & Neck surgery
Mater Salutis Hospital
Legnago, Verona, Italy

Alessia Rubini, MD
Consultant ENT Surgeon
Section of Otorhinolaryngology
Head and Neck Surgery
Deparment of Surgery, Odontosomatology, and Pediatrics
University of Verona
Verona, Italy

Alexander J. Saxby, MB, BChir, MA (Cantab.) FRACS
Clinical Associate Professor
Department of Otolaryngology,
Head and Neck Surgery
University of Sydney;
Royal Prince Alfred Hospital
Sydney Endoscopic Ear Surgery Research Group
Sydney, Australia

Davide Soloperto, MD PhD
Consultant
Azienda Ospedaliera Universitaria Integrata
Verona Italy

Muaz Tarabichi, MD
Co-Founder
Tarabichi Stammberger Ear and Sinus Institute
Dubai, United Arab Emirates

Domenico Villari, MD
ENT Specialist
University Hospital Policlinico di Modena
Modena, Emilia Romagna, Italy

George Wanna, MD, FACS
Professor of Otolaryngology – Head and Neck Surgery;
Professor of Neurosurgery
Icahn School of Medicine at Mount Sinai;
Chair, Department of Otolaryngology
New York Eye and Ear Infirmary
of Mount Sinai and Mount Sinai Beth Israel
New York, New York, USA

Chapter 1

Anatomy of the Lateral Skull Base

1 Anatomy of the Lateral Skull Base

Mustafa Kapadia, Livio Presutti, Alejandro Rivas, and Daniele Marchioni

Abstract

The lateral skull base is a very complex anatomical region separating the brain from the ear and the upper neck. It is composed by the temporal, sphenoid, and occipital bones, and contains vital neurovascular structures. An advanced understanding of its three-dimensional architecture is therefore mandatory for the surgeon approaching this area. In particular, a detailed knowledge of the anatomy of the temporal bone is the cornerstone to correctly perform lateral skull base surgery. In fact, it occupies a central position in the lateral skull base and contains several noble structures having a winding course such as the internal carotid artery, the sigmoid sinus with the internal jugular vein, the internal auditory canal with the acoustic-facial bundle, and the facial nerve. In the same way, the knowledge of the anatomical entities located in close relationship with the temporal bone plays a key role: (1) the jugular foramen, anterolaterally bounded by the petrous temporal bone and posteromedially by the basioccipital bone, transmitting the sigmoid sinus, the jugular bulb, the inferior petrosal sinus, the lower cranial nerves (IX, X, XI) with their ganglia, and the meningeal branches of the occipital artery and the ascending pharyngeal artery; (2) the infratemporal fossa, a complex three-dimensional nonfascial bound space located inferomedial to the zygomatic arch and the ramus of the mandible, acting as a conduit for the neurovascular structure entering and leaving the skull base; and (3) the cerebellopontine angle, the anatomic space between the petrous bone and the petrosal cerebellar surface folding around the pons and the middle cerebellar peduncle, containing the posterior cranial fossa nerves.

Keywords: lateral skull base anatomy, temporal bone, jugular foramen, infratemporal fossa, cerebellopontine angle, petrous apex

1.1 Introduction

The skull base forms the floor of the cranial cavity and separates the brain from the ear, the paranasal sinuses, and the upper neck. This anatomic region is complex and poses surgical challenges for otolaryngologists and neurosurgeons alike. In the skull base, there are numerous foramina that transmit cranial nerves, blood vessels, and other structures. The skull base foramina are openings located in the inferior portion of the cranium. They allow for the passage of several vascular and nervous structures. From an inferior view, there are 10 conventionally described skull base foramina: the greater palatine, lesser palatine, lacerum, ovale, spinosum, external opening of the carotid canal, stylomastoid, jugular, mastoid, and the external opening of the hypoglossal canal (see ▶ Fig. 1.1, ▶ Fig. 1.2, ▶ Fig. 1.3, ▶ Fig. 1.4). Working knowledge of the anatomy of the skull base is essential for effective surgical treatment of diseases in this area.

The five bones that make up the skull base are the ethmoid, sphenoid, occipital, frontal, and temporal bones. The skull base can be subdivided into three regions: the anterior, middle, and posterior cranial fossae (see ▶ Fig. 1.1).

The anterior cranial fossa is formed by the anterior and cribriform plate of the ethmoid bone, the lesser wings of the sphenoid, and the jugum sphenoidale. The middle cranial fossa is composed of the body and the greater wing of the sphenoid, the anterior surface of the temporal pyramid, and parts of the temporal squama. The posterior cranial fossa is bordered by the clivus, the pyramid of the temporal bone, and the occipital bone.

Irish and coworkers in 1994 reviewed 77 skull base malignancies from a clinical point of view. From this work, they developed a classification system of three regions based upon anatomic boundaries and tumor growth patterns. Region I is composed of the anterior cranial fossa. Tumors of this region are commonly resected via an anterior approach. Region II includes the infratemporal and pterygopalatine fossae, with a possible tumor extension into the middle cranial fossa. Region III involves the temporal bone with a possible tumor extension into the posterior or middle cranial fossa. From a clinical point of view, the "lateral skull base" is defined as the anatomical compartments resulting from the combination of Regions II and III. Anatomically, Region II

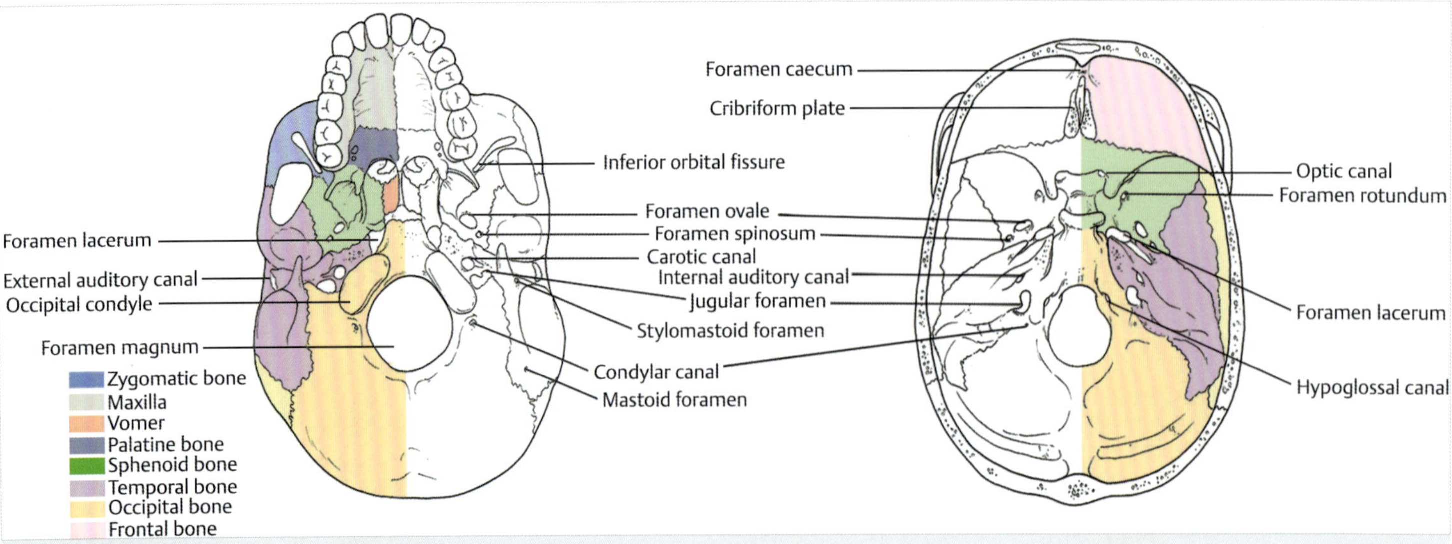

Fig. 1.1 Skull base foramina: exocranial and endocranial surfaces.

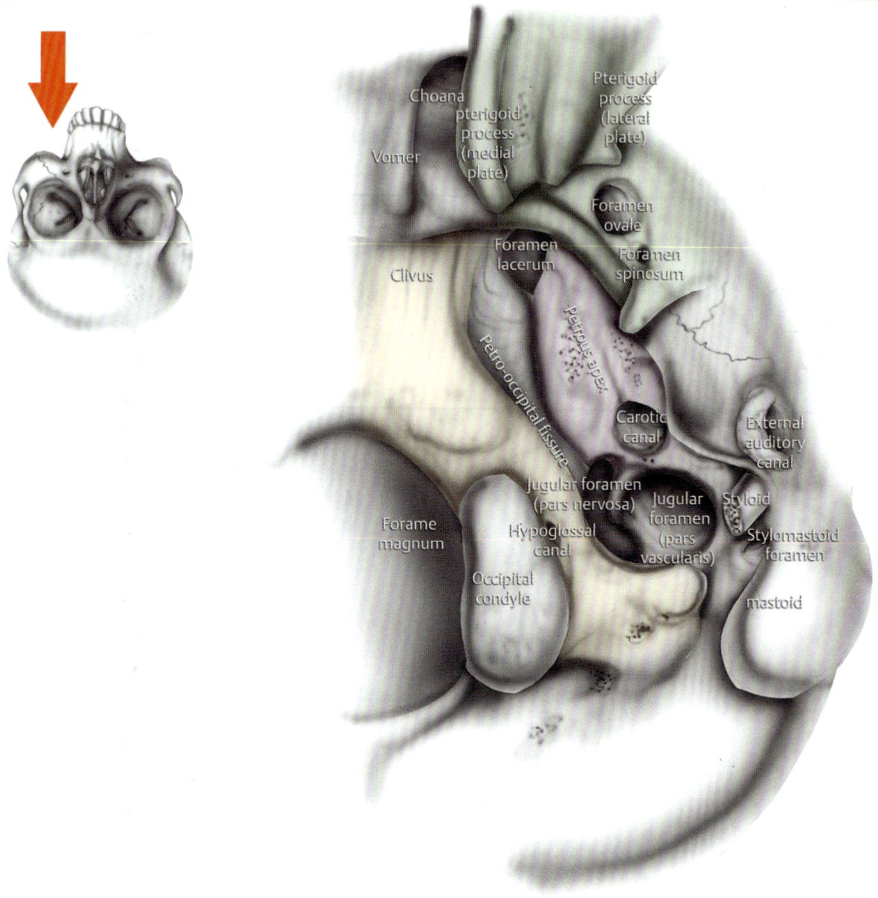

Fig. 1.2 Left exocranial surfaces of the skull base: the skull foramina are shown.

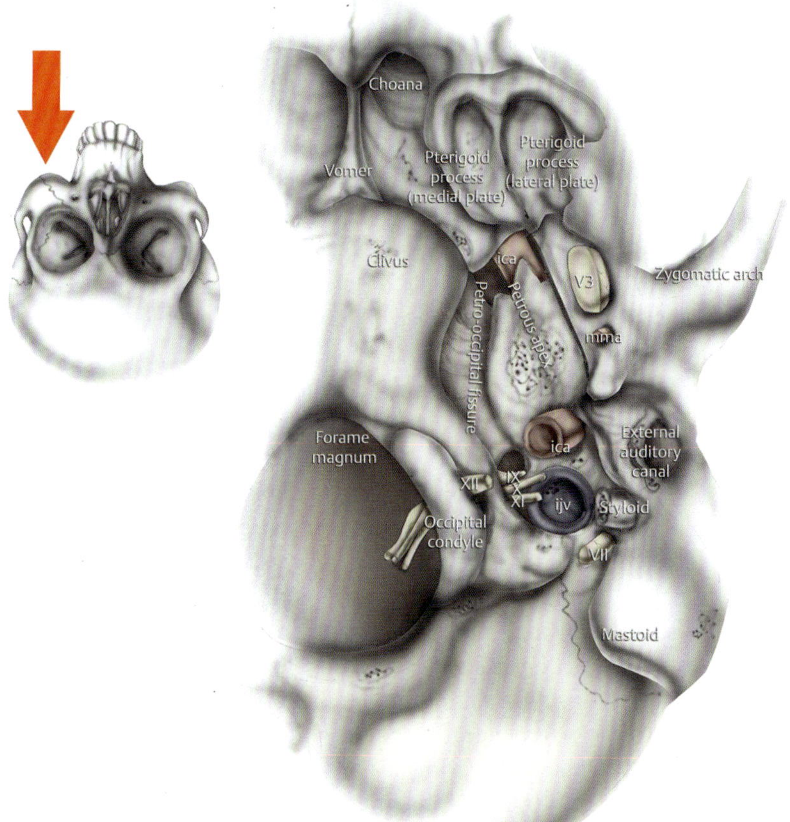

Fig. 1.3 Cranial nerves and vascular structures in the left exocranial surfaces of the skull base. *ica: internal carotid artery; ijv: internal jugular vein; mma: middle meningeal artery.*

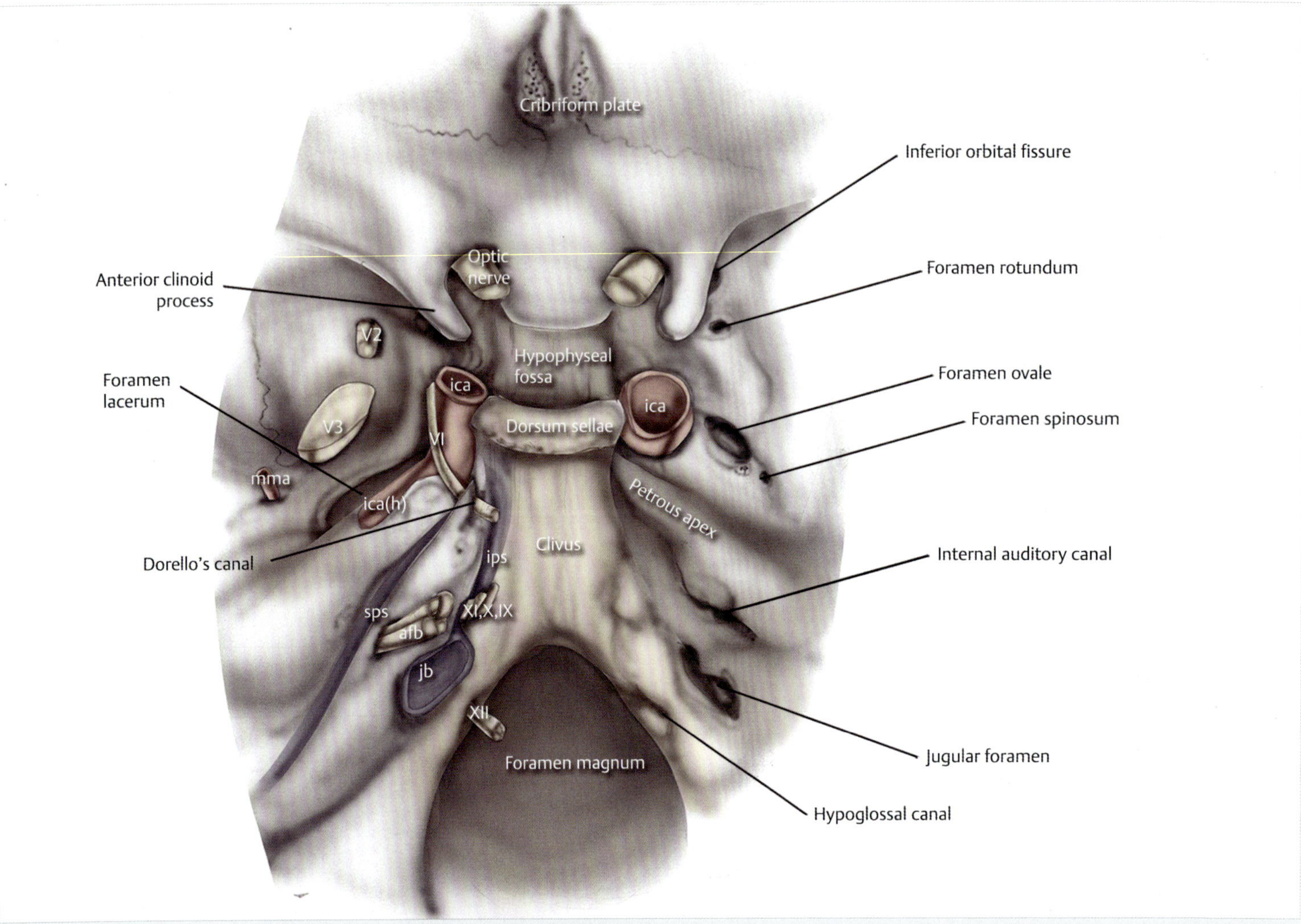

Fig. 1.4 Cranial nerves and vascular structures in the endocranial surfaces of the skull base. *afb: acoustic-facial bundle; ica(h): horizontal portion of internal carotid artery; ica: internal carotid artery; ips: inferior petrosal sinus; jb: jugular bulb; mma: middle meningeal artery; sps: superior petrosal sinus.*

extends from the posterior wall of the orbit to the petrous temporal bone and it is formed by the infratemporal and pterygopalatine fossae and the overlying part of the middle cranial fossa. In this region, there are several important neurovascular structures which include the internal carotid artery (ICA), the facial nerve, the vestibulocochlear nerve, and the maxillary (V2) and the mandibular (V3) divisions of the trigeminal nerve. Region III is located mainly in the posterior cranial fossa and also includes the posterior segment of the middle cranial fossa. Vital structures located in this region include the internal jugular vein and the vagus, the glossopharyngeal, the spinal accessory, and the hypoglossal nerves.

The lateral skull base has very noble and complex anatomical structures (see ▸ Fig. 1.5 and ▸ Fig. 1.6). Lateral skull base surgery demands an advanced anatomical knowledge of the temporal bone and a three-dimensional animated perception of the related surrounding structures. The surgical procedures are technically challenging because the pathological site is concealed deep within, which requires extensive bone drilling and tissue retraction, and because vital neurovascular structures are located in a relatively small area.

1.2 The Temporal Bone

The temporal bone occupies the central position in the lateral skull base and is anteriorly bounded by the zygomatic bone, and the greater wing and pterygoid plate of the sphenoid bone, superiorly by the parietal bone, posteriorly and posteromedially by the occipital bone, and medially by the clivus (see ▸ Fig. 1.7). There are various vital structures related to the lateral skull base like the acoustic-facial bundle, trigeminal nerve, cochlea, semicircular canals, ICA, sigmoid sinus, internal jugular vein, lower cranial nerves, and brain parenchyma. Most of the times diseases in this area are benign, so we have to protect and preserve most of the vital structures.

The temporal bone has five different parts: the squamous, mastoid, tympanic, petrous, and styloid process (see ▸ Fig. 1.8). These parts are arranged around the external auditory canal and the tympanic cavity so that the tympanic part is directed downwards, the squamous part upwards and forwards, the mastoid part backwards, and the petrous part directed medially and inwards. The petrous temporal bone is a three-cornered pyramid with the base directed laterally and its long axis directed anteriorly and medially forming an angle of about 45 degrees with the median plane of the skull. The petrous apex is rough and uneven, having an anterior opening for the carotid canal, and it forms the posterolateral boundary of the foramen lacerum along with the greater wing of the sphenoid and the basioccipital bone. The labyrinth and the internal auditory canal (IAC) are located within the petrous temporal part. The petrous part of the ICA enters temporal bone through the carotid canal situated on its inferior surface. The other important structure related to the temporal bone is the jugular foramen (JF), which is located in the petro-occipital region.

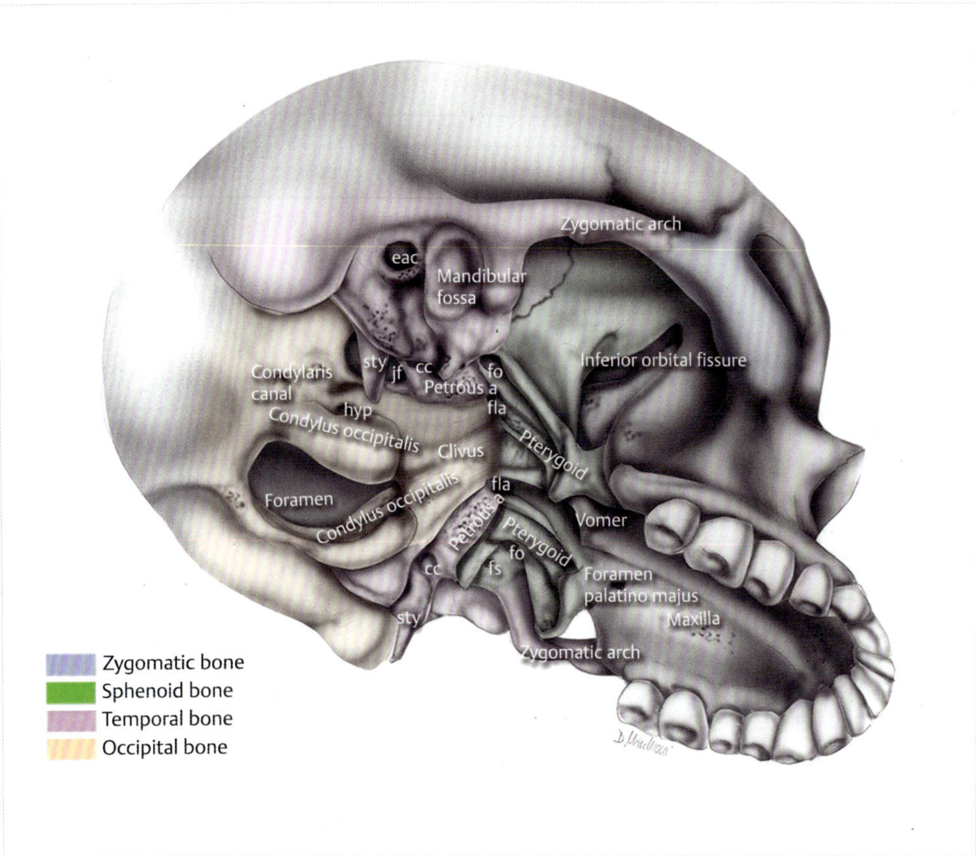

Fig. 1.5 Skull base bones. *cc: carotid canal; eac: external auditory canal; fla: foramen lacerum; fo: foramen ovale; fs: foramen spinosum; hyp: hypoglossal canal; jf: jugular foramen; petrous a: petrous apex; sty: styloid process.*

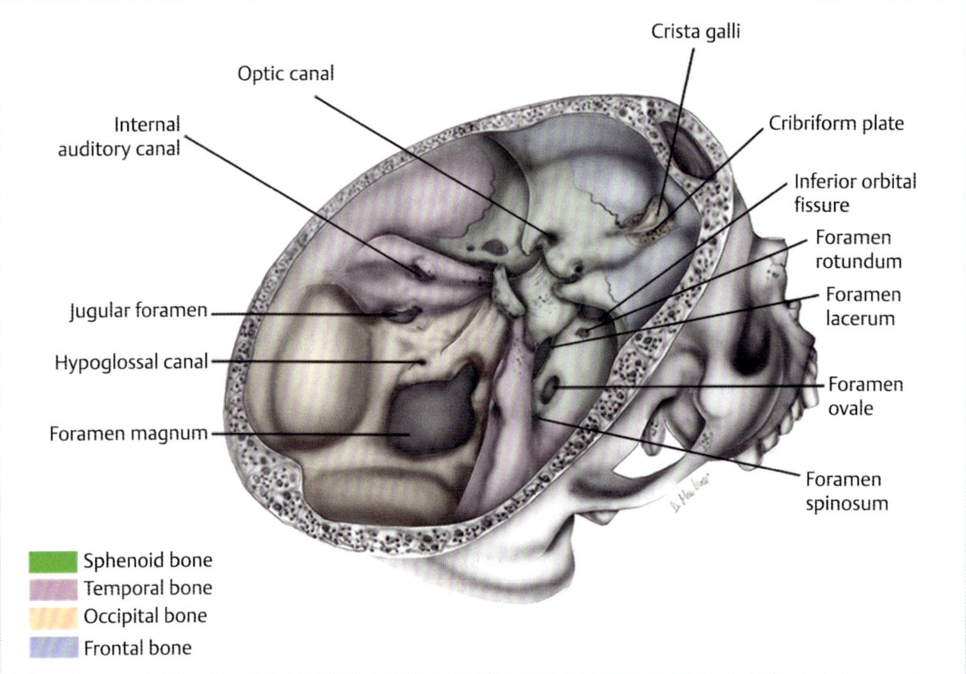

Fig. 1.6 Endocranial view of skull base bones.

1.3 Internal Auditory Canal

The IAC is a bony, 8 to 10 mm long neurovascular channel which runs from the posterior cranial fossa to the petrous temporal bone. It transmits the facial nerve, the cochlear-vestibular nerve, the nervus intermedius, and the labyrinthine artery (see ▶ Fig. 1.9 and ▶ Fig. 1.10). It has three distinguishable parts, namely, the porus (medial end) located on the posterior surface of the petrous bone, the canal itself and the fundus (lateral end), which is formed by a thin cribriform plate of bone separating the cochlea and the vestibule from the IAC. The fundus also constitutes the medial wall of the vestibule and its height and width are 2.5 to 4.0 mm and 2 to 3 mm, respectively. The fundus is divided by a transverse crest into a superior and an inferior quadrant. The superior quadrant is further divided into an antero-superior area for the facial nerve and a posterosuperior area for the superior vestibular nerve by a vertical crest/Bill's bar. The inferior quadrant contains the cochlear nerve anteriorly, and the inferior vestibular nerve and the singular nerve posteriorly (see ▶ Fig. 1.11). The dura and arachnoid membranes extend up to the fundus and are attached to the transverse crest.

The petrous ICA enters the temporal bone through the carotid canal anterior to the JF, being separated from it by the carotid ridge. It ascends upward and laterally as a vertical segment, then it turns medially under the bony eustachian tube acutely bending and continuing forward and medially as a horizontal segment. It gets out of the temporal bone through the petrous apex, passes through the foramen lacerum, and it becomes the cavernous segment of the ICA. The average length of the petrous ICA is 30 mm; the horizontal segment is twice the length of the vertical segment (see ▶ Fig. 1.12). The petrous part is often covered by very thick periosteum and its average diameter ranges between 3 and 5 mm. The first intrapetrous bend under the eustachian tube is an acute bend measuring approximately between 80 and 85 degrees. The petrous carotid is separated from the most anterior basal turn of the cochlea by a 2- to 3-mm-thick bone. The greater superficial petrosal nerve (GSPN) serves as an important landmark to identify the petrous carotid during a middle fossa approach as it runs superior and parallel to it (see ▶ Fig. 1.13). The carotid artery is surrounded in its canal by a venous plexus and by the pericarotid sympathetic plexus derived from the ascending branch of the superior cervical ganglion of the sympathetic trunk.

1.4 Facial Nerve

The facial nerve is one of the most important structures to be encountered during lateral skull base surgery, and its damage leads to significant functional and psycho-social morbidity for the patient. The facial nerve is a mixed nerve (motor root and sensory root/nervus intermedius) which innervates the second branchial arch derivatives. It contains five different populations of fibers (see ▶ Fig. 1.14):

- Special sensory fibers for taste sensation from anterior two-thirds of the tongue via the chorda tympani nerve (see ▶ Fig. 1.15).
- Somatic sensory fibers supplying the skin of the external auditory canal and the adjacent conchal region along with the auricular branch of the vagus nerve.
- Special visceral efferent fibers supplying the stapedius muscle, the posterior belly of digastric, the stylohyoid, and the muscles connected to the facial expression (see ▶ Fig. 1.14).
- General visceral efferent fibers for the lacrimal gland and the mucous secreting glands of the nasal cavity via the GSPN and for the submandibular and sublingual glands via the chorda tympani nerve (see ▶ Fig. 1.15 and ▶ Fig. 1.16).
- Visceral afferent fibers supplying the mucosa of the palate, pharynx, and nose.

The facial nerve nucleus is located in the pons, ventrolateral to the abducens nucleus, and it is represented in the precentral gyrus of the cerebral cortex. The facial nerve course is broadly divided into three parts: intracranial (cisternal), intratemporal, and extratemporal part. The facial nerve emerges from the lower border of the pons between the olive and the restiform body as a motor and sensory root (nervus intermedius) and continues as an intracranial segment till the porus of the IAC (see ▶ Fig. 1.17). The total length of the intracranial segment is around 22 to 25 mm. It is cradled in a groove on the superior surface of the cochlear nerve. The sensory root runs parallel to it and joins it in spiraling fashion in the fundus of the IAC.

The intratemporal part is further subdivided into four segments (see ▶ Fig. 1.18):

- The IAC segment is about 7 to 9 mm long and it extends from the porus till the fundus of IAC. It runs slightly anterior and superior to the cochlear nerve and it occupies the anterosuperior quadrant at the level of the fundus of the IAC.
- The labyrinthine segment is the smallest and the narrowest segment measuring around 3 to 5 mm in length and 0.68 mm in diameter. It extends from the fundus of the IAC heading anteriorly and laterally, running superior to the cochlea and vestibule until it reaches the geniculate ganglion. This segment is usually surrounded by very thick periosteum and can act as a strangulating tunnel in the presence of facial nerve edema leading to facial nerve palsy. At the level of the geniculate ganglion, it takes an acute bend of 75 degrees to form the first genu and

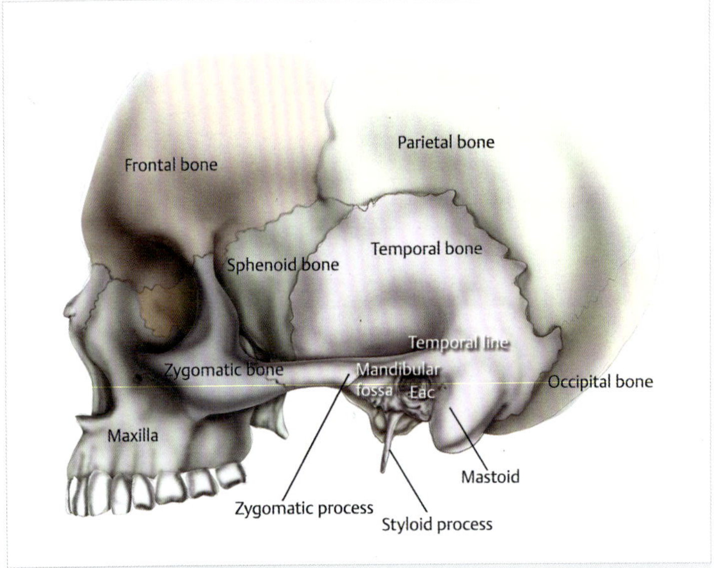

Fig. 1.7 Temporal bone in the skull. Lateral view. *Eac: external auditory canal.*

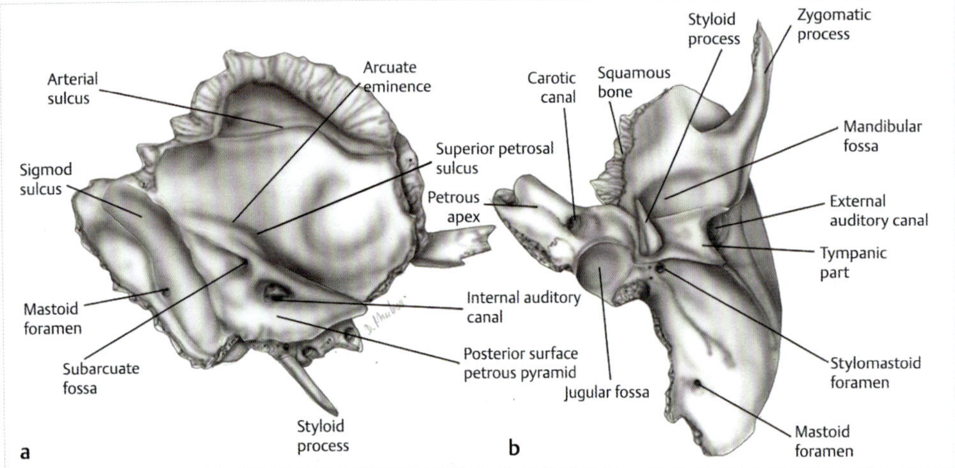

Fig. 1.8 Temporal bone: **(a)** posterior fossa surface of the temporal bone; **(b)** base view of the temporal bone.

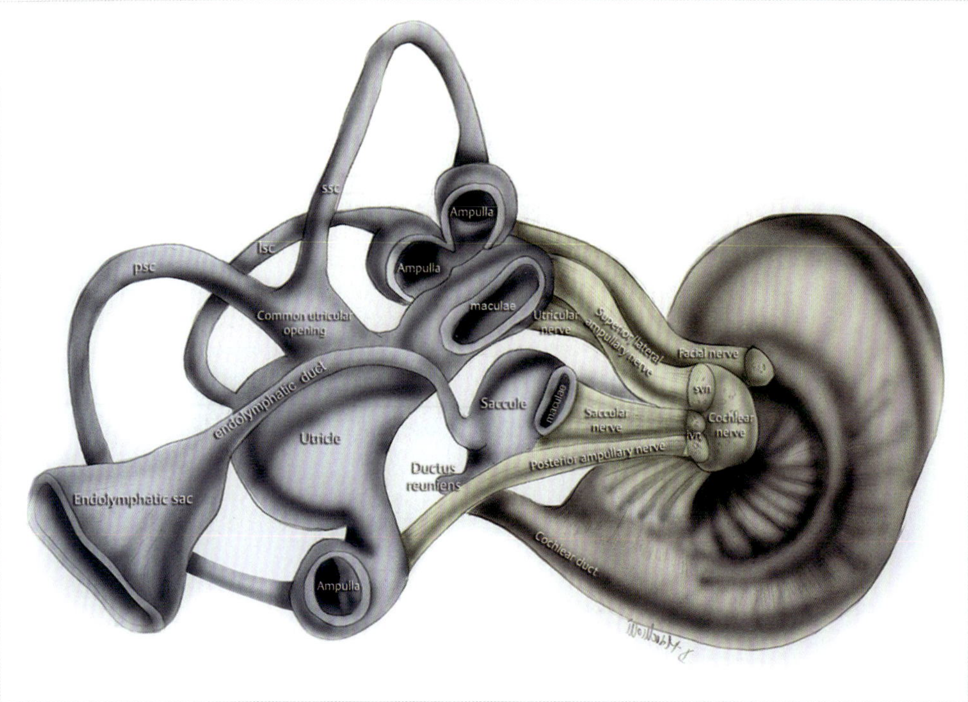

Fig. 1.9 Left ear. Drawing showing the acoustic-facial nerves from behind inside the internal auditory canal (IAC). The eighth nerve, upon passing into the IAC under the facial nerve, divides into two branches: the cochlear nerve and the vestibular nerve. The cochlear nerve runs into the fundus of the IAC, attaching to the foraminous tract of the fundus, forming the tractus spiralis foraminosus. The vestibular nerve divides into two branches: the upper branch which divides into the utricular nerve (which attaches on the elliptical recess) and the superior ampullary nerve (for the superior membranous ampulla), and the lower branch which divides into the saccular nerve (which attaches on the spherical recess) and the posterior ampullary nerve, which passes into the singular foramen. *ivn: inferior vestibular nerve; lsc: lateral semicircular canal; psc: posterior semicircular canal; ssc: superior semicircular canal; svn: superior vestibular nerve.*

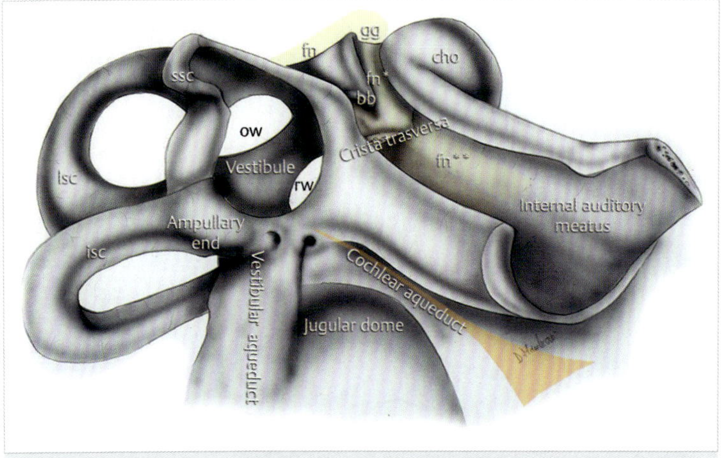

Fig. 1.10 Left ear. Anatomical relationships between the vestibule and the fundus of the internal auditory canal (IAC) from behind. The inner facial nerve is represented in yellow; the labyrinthine facial nerve is descending from the geniculate ganglion to the fundus of the IAC; the intrameatal facial nerve runs from laterally to medially, from anteriorly to posteriorly. *bb: Bill's bar; cho: cochlea; fn: facial nerve; fn*: labyrinthine facial nerve; fn**: intrameatal facial nerve; gg: geniculate ganglion; lsc: lateral semicircular canal; ow: oval window; psc: posterior semicircular canal; rw: round window; ssc: superior semicircular canal.*

then it continues as the tympanic segment. The first branch, the GSPN, arises from the anterior portion of the geniculate ganglion. It leaves the tympanic cavity and enters the middle cranial fossa through the facial hiatus and it runs forward to the foramen lacerum. At the level of the foramen lacerum, it is joined by the sympathetic fibers of the deep petrosal nerve and it forms the vidian nerve (nerve of the pterygoid canal). The vidian nerve passes through the pterygopalatine fossa to enter the sphenopalatine ganglion.

- The tympanic segment runs parallel to the long axis of the petrous pyramid and it is around 11 to 13 mm long. It passes posteriorly and laterally on the medial wall of the tympanic cavity between the oval window inferiorly and the lateral semicircular canal superiorly. At the level of the posterior wall of the tympanic cavity near the pyramidal eminence it turns 95 to 125 degrees forming the second genu and continuing as the mastoid segment. The tympanic segment doesn't give any branches.
- The mastoid segment extends from the second genu to the stylomastoid foramen measuring 15 to 18 mm in length. It runs vertically downwards and slightly laterally on the posterior wall of the tympanic cavity in such a way that the nerve is more superficial at the stylomastoid foramen than at the level of the second genu. This segment gives off two branches, the nerve to the stapedius muscle and the chorda tympani nerve. The chorda tympani nerve usually arises about 4 mm superior to the stylomastoid foramen, but very rarely it may arise distal to it. During a posterior tympanotomy approach, the mastoid segment forms the medial limit and the chorda tympani the lateral limit for bone removal (see ▸ Fig. 1.19, ▸ Fig. 1.20, ▸ Fig. 1.21).

The facial nerve emerges from the stylomastoid foramen and it continues as the extratemporal segment running anteriorly through the parotid gland. It divides at the posterior border of the ramus of the mandible into two main branches, namely, the superior temporofacial branch and the inferior cervicofacial branch. From this, a plexiform arrangement of nerves forms known as the pes anserinus, which is eventually distributed over the muscles of the head, face, and upper part of neck (see ▸ Fig. 1.14).

Blood supply of the facial nerve:

- Intracranial part: anterior inferior cerebellar artery (AICA).
- IAC segment: labyrinthine artery (branch of AICA).
- Intratemporal segment: anastomosing branches of the superficial petrosal artery (branch of middle meningeal artery) and the stylomastoid artery (branch of posterior auricular artery). These branches form a rich arterial plexus between the fallopian canal periosteum and the epineurium of the facial nerve.

1.5 Jugular Foramen

The JF is a deeply located bony channel that transmits neurovascular structures from the posterior cranial fossa to the superior laterocervical area. A safe surgical access to this foramen is hindered by the important surrounding structures (see ▸ Fig. 1.22, ▸ Fig. 1.23).

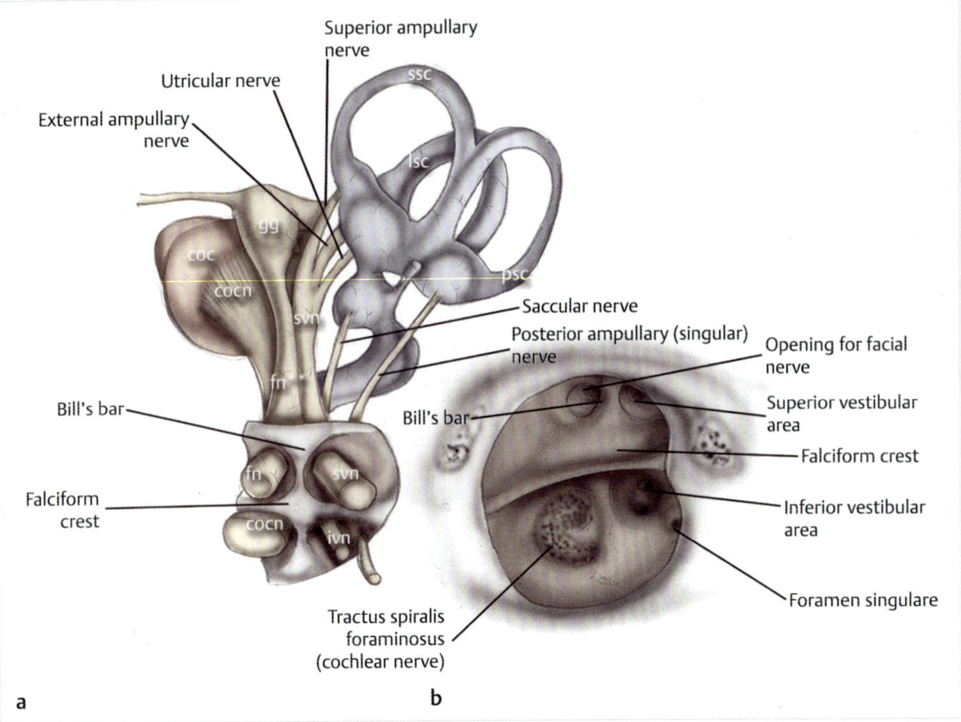

Fig. 1.11 Left side. **(a, b)** Anatomy of the fundus of the internal auditory canal (IAC); the nerves are separated by a transverse crest into a lower and an upper compartment. In the lower compartment, the inferior vestibular nerve and the singular nerve lie posteriorly while the cochlear nerve lies anteriorly. In the upper compartment, a vertical crest separates two nerves: the facial nerve lying anteriorly and the superior vestibular nerve lying posteriorly. *coc: cochlea; cocn: cochlear nerve; fn**: labyrinthine segment of facial nerve; gg: geniculate ganglion; ivn: inferior vestibular nerve; lsc: lateral semicircular canal; psc: posterior semicircular canal; ssc: superior semicircular canal; svn: superior vestibular nerve.*

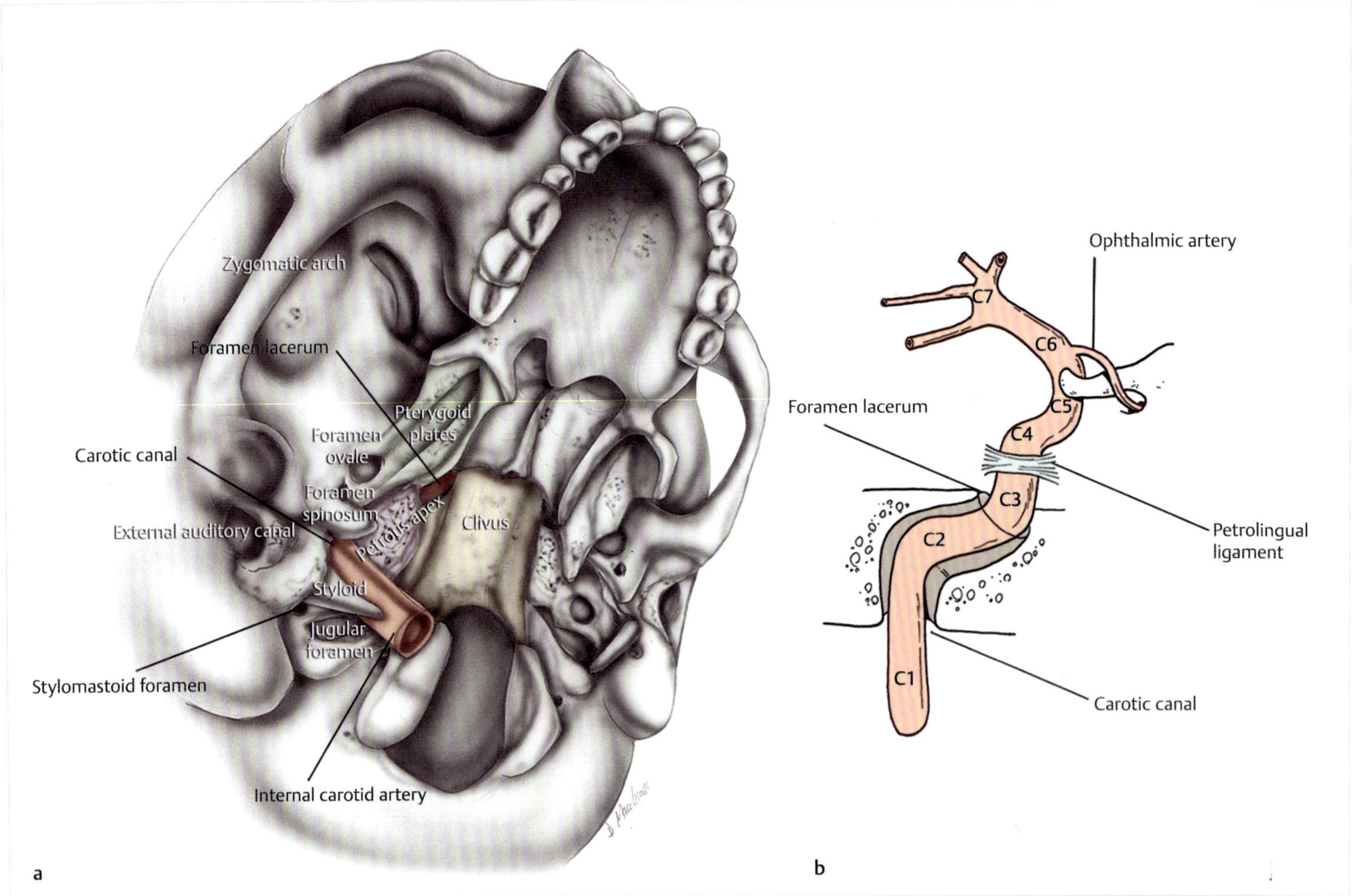

Fig. 1.12 Right side. The internal carotid artery at the base of the skull **(a)** and its subdivision (Bouthillier classification) **(b)**.

It is located in the posterior portion of the petro-occipital fissure, it is bounded anterolaterally by the petrous temporal bone and posteromedially by the basioccipital bone. In about 68% of the cases, the right foramen is larger than the left one, equal to the left in 12%, and smaller than the left in 20% of the patients.

The long axis of the JF is directed from the posterolateral wide part to the anteromedial narrow part. The structures passing through the JF are the sigmoid sinus, jugular bulb, inferior petrosal sinus, lower cranial nerves (IX, X, XI) with their ganglia, and meningeal branches of the occipital artery and ascending pharyngeal artery.

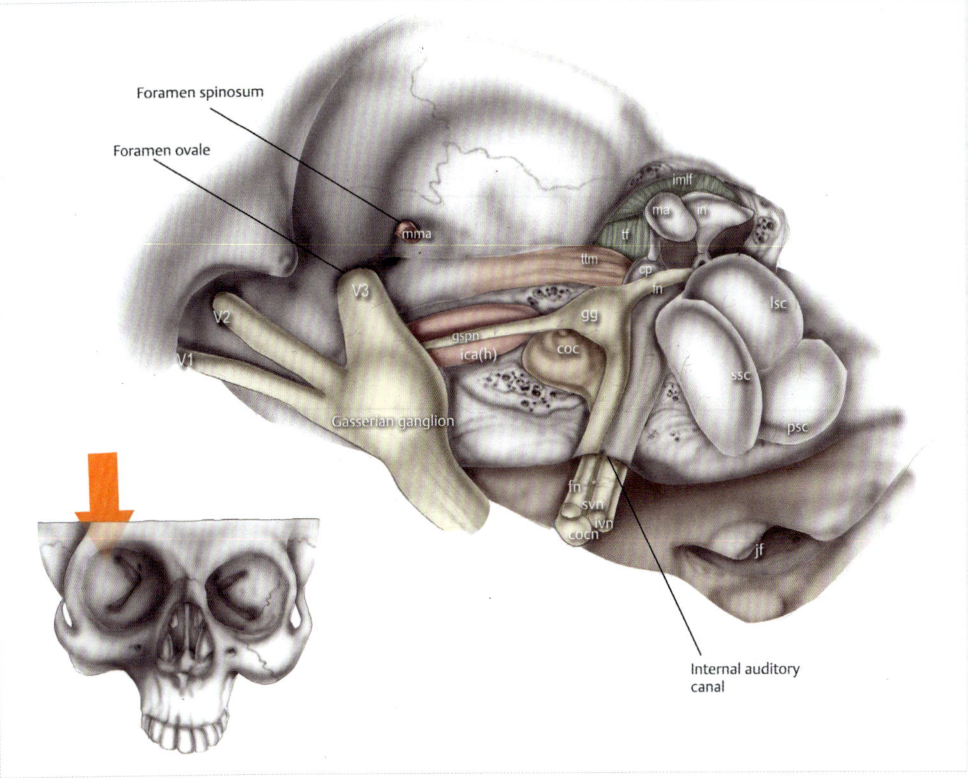

Fig. 1.13 Right side. Anatomy of the facial nerve, in relation to the surrounding anatomical structures, from a middle fossa approach. *coc: cochlea; cocn: cochlear nerve; cp: cochleariform process; fn**: intrameatal facial nerve; gg: geniculate ganglion; gspn: greater superficial petrosal nerve; ica(h): horizontal portion of internal carotid artery; imlf: incudomalleolar lateral fold; in: incus; ivn: inferior vestibular nerve; jf: jugular foramen; lsc: lateral semicircular canal; ma: malleus; mma: middle meningeal artery; psc: posterior semicircular canal; ssc: superior semicircular canal; svn: superior vestibular nerve; tf: tensor fold; ttm: tensor tympani muscle.*

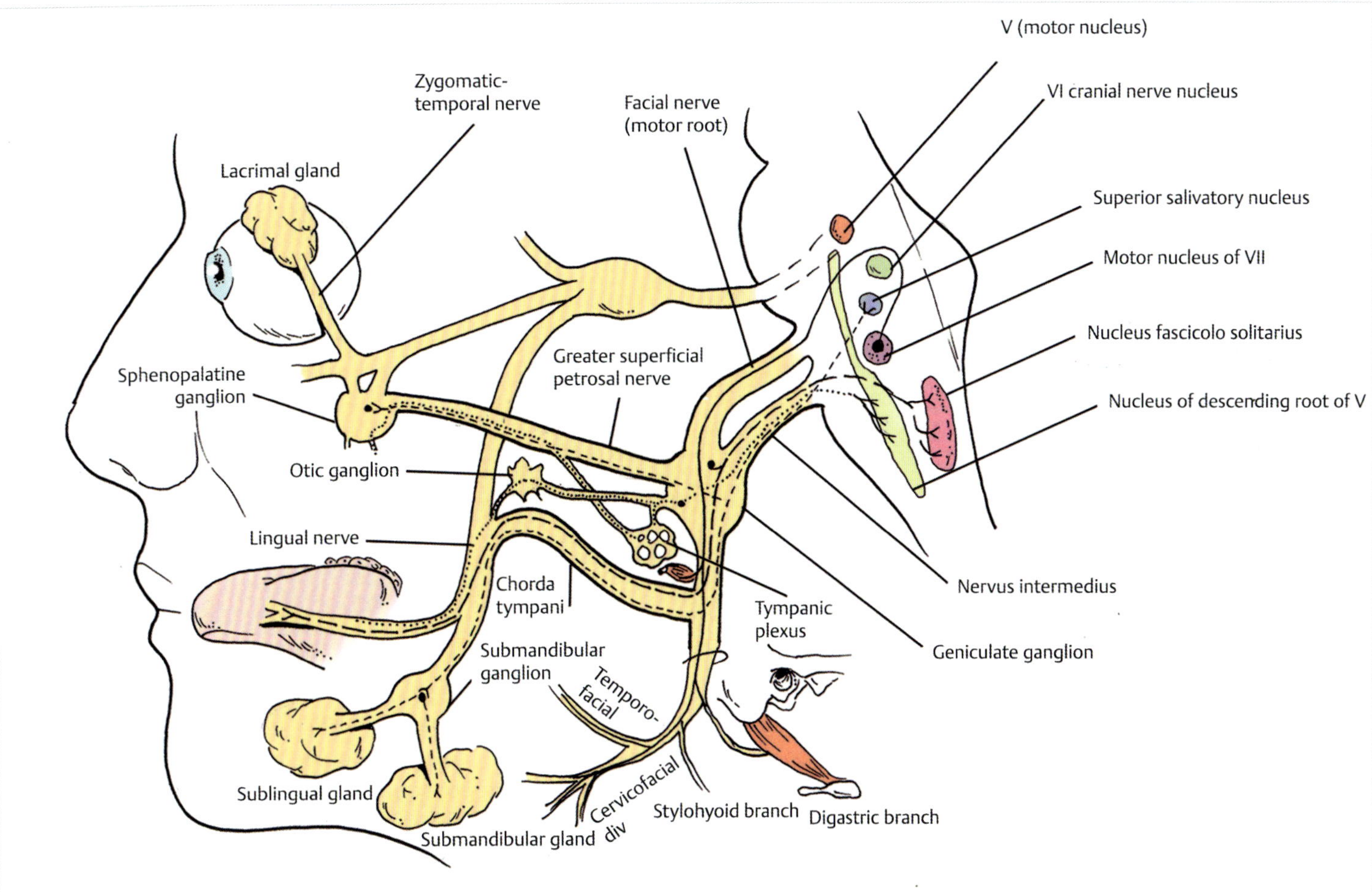

Fig. 1.14 Left side. Fibers and nucleus of the facial nerve.

There are two different ways of dividing the JF into an anatomical compartments. The first classification system divides the JF into an anteromedial (pars nervosa) smaller compartment containing the inferior petrosal sinus and the glossopharyngeal nerve and a posterolateral (pars vascularis) larger compartment containing the superior section of the jugular bulb, the vagus nerve, the spinal accessory nerve, and the meningeal branches of the occipital and the ascending pharyngeal artery (see ▶ Fig. 1.24).

In the second description the JF is divided into three compartments by the dura mater, namely, a large posterolateral venous compartment containing the sigmoid sinus, an intermediate neural compartment containing lower cranial nerves IX, X, and XI, and

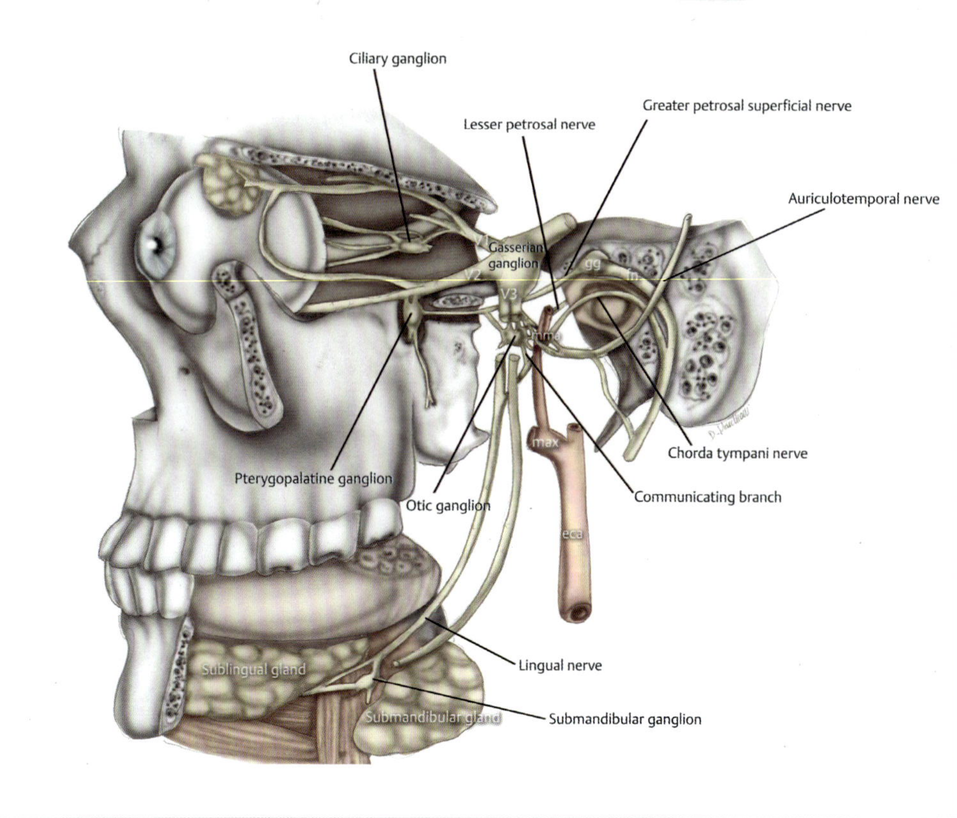

Fig. 1.15 Facial nerve and trigeminal nerve fibers' anastomosis. The anatomical relationship between the chorda tympany and lingual nerve is shown. *eca: external carotid artery; fn: facial nerve; gg: geniculate ganglion; max: maxillary artery; mma: middle meningeal artery.*

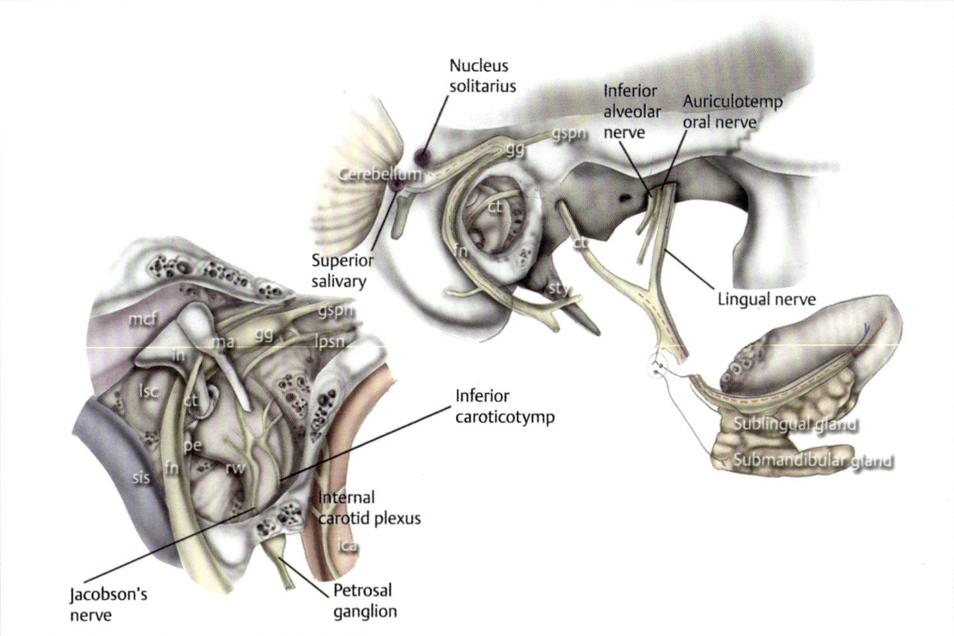

Fig. 1.16 Anatomy of the nerves on the medial wall of the tympanic cavity and anastomosis between the facial nerve and the trigeminal nerve. *ct: chorda tympani; fn: facial nerve; gg: geniculate ganglion; gspn: greater superficial petrosal nerve; ica: internal carotid artery; in: incus; lpsn: lesser petrosal superficial nerve; lsc: lateral semicircular canal; ma: malleus; mcf: middle cranial fossa;*
pe: pyramidal eminence; rw: round window; sis: sigmoid sinus; sty: styloid process.

a small anteromedial venous compartment containing the inferior petrosal sinus. The sigmoid sinus drains into the posterior portion of the jugular bulb. The height of the jugular bulb varies a lot and it can be as high as the IAC. It is very important to note that the wall of the jugular bulb is very thin and fragile as it lacks an adventitia layer. As it gets out of the JF and it becomes the internal jugular vein, it is reinforced by the periosteal ring and it acquires a normal venous structure. Most often the inferior petrosal sinus (IPS) enters the JF passing between cranial nerves IX and X. IPS has a variable course and drainage pattern, terminating into the anterior portion of the jugular bulb in 90% of cases but it might rarely have multiple openings in both the jugular bulb and the internal jugular vein (see ▶ Fig. 1.25).

At the level of the external orifice of the JF, it gives rise to the tympanic branch (Jacobson's nerve), which crosses the tympanic canaliculus to enter the tympanic cavity where it gives rise to the tympanic plexus. The auricular branch (Arnold's nerve) arises at the level of the superior vagal ganglion and it is joined by a branch from the inferior glossopharyngeal ganglion (see ▶ Fig. 1.24). The auricular branch passes laterally in a shallow groove on the anterior wall of the jugular bulb to reach the lateral wall of the jugular fossa, where it enters the mastoid canaliculus and ascends toward the mastoid segment of the facial canal, giving off an ascending branch to the facial nerve as it crosses lateral to it before turning downward to exit the temporal bone through the tympanomastoid fissure (see ▶ Fig. 1.24).

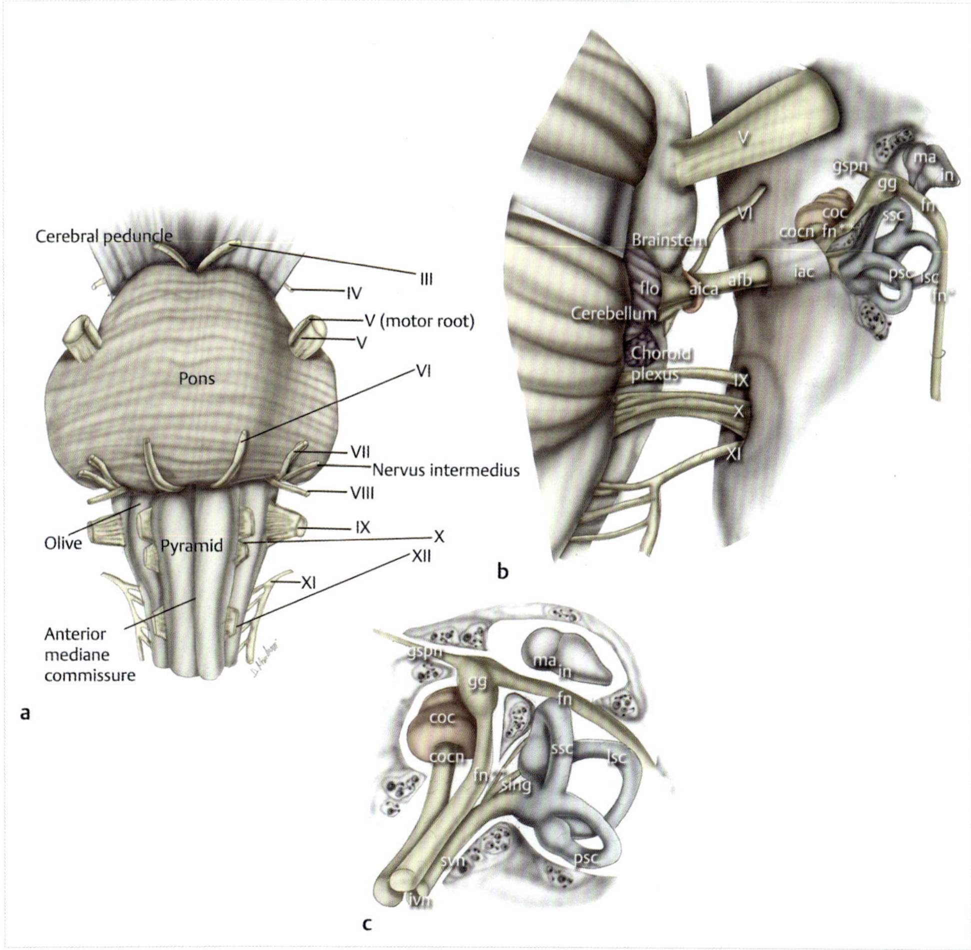

Fig. 1.17 **(a, b)** Topographic anatomy of the cranial nerves on the frontal surface of the brainstem and inside the cerebellopontine angle. **(c)** Acoustic-facial bundle inside the internal auditory canal (IAC). *aica: anterior inferior cerebellar artery; coc: cochlea; cocn: cochlear nerve; flo: floccules; fn: tympanic segment of facial nerve; fn*: mastoid segment of facial nerve; fn**: intrameatal facial nerve; gg: geniculate ganglion; gspn: greater superficial petrosal nerve; iac: internal auditory canal; in: incus; ivn: inferior vestibular nerve; lsc: lateral semicircular canal; ma: malleus; psc: posterior semicircular canal; sing: singular nerve; ssc: superior semicircular canal; svn: superior vestibular nerve.*

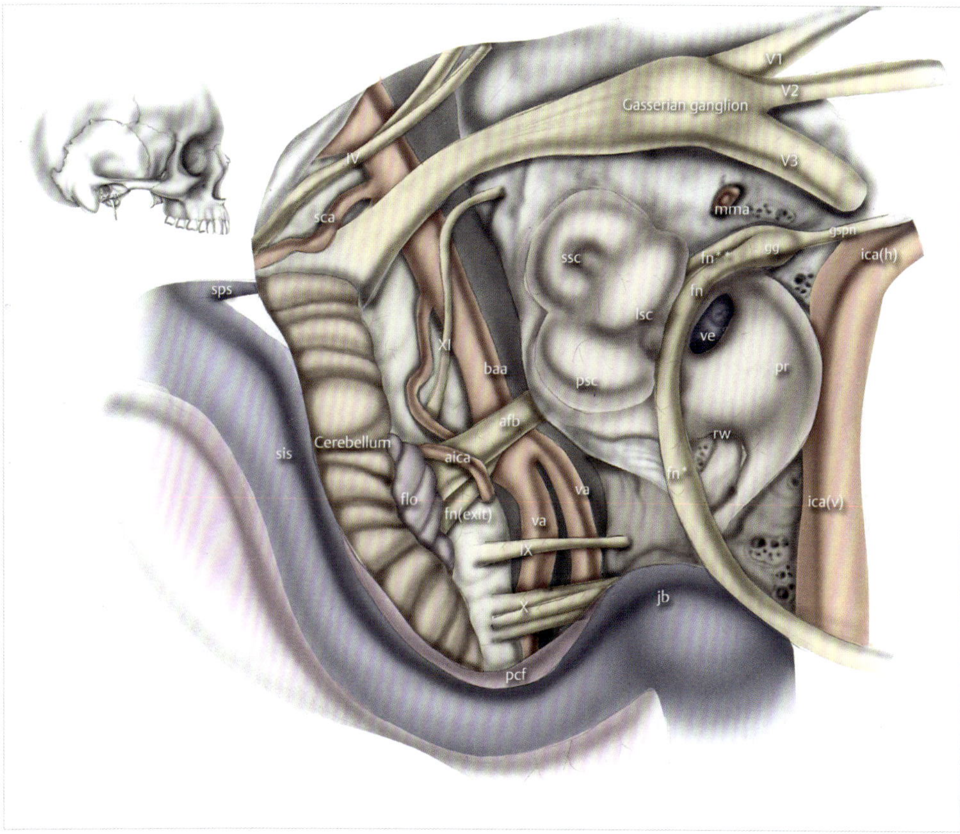

Fig. 1.18 Lateral view of the cerebellopontine angle. The relationship between the cranial nerves and the temporal bone is shown. *afb: acoustic-facial bundle; aica: anterior inferior cerebellar artery; baa: basilar artery; flo: floccules; fn (exit): facial nerve at the exit zone; fn: tympanic segment of facial nerve; fn*: mastoid segment of facial nerve; gg: geniculate ganglion; gspn: greater superficial petrosal nerve; iac: internal auditory canal; ica(h): horizontal segment of internal carotid artery; ica(v): vertical segment of internal carotid artery; jb: jugular bulb; lsc: lateral semicircular canal; mma: middle meningeal artery; pcf: posterior cranial fossa (dura layer); pr: promontory; psc: posterior semicircular canal; rw: round window; sca: superior cerebellar artery; sis: sigmoid sinus; sps: superior petrosal sinus; ssc: superior semicircular canal; va: vertebral artery; ve: vestibule.*

1.6 Infratemporal Fossa

The infratemporal fossa (ITF) is a complex three-dimensional nonfascial bound space inferomedial to the zygomatic arch and the ramus of the mandible. It acts as a conduit for neurovascular structures entering and leaving the skull base (see ▶ Fig. 1.26). Due to its deep-seated location and important neurovascular structures, it is wise for neuro-otologists and skull base surgeons to have a thorough knowledge of its boundaries and adjacent structures. Fisch in 1977 first described different ITF approaches to surgically access and treat various lesions arising in and around this space.

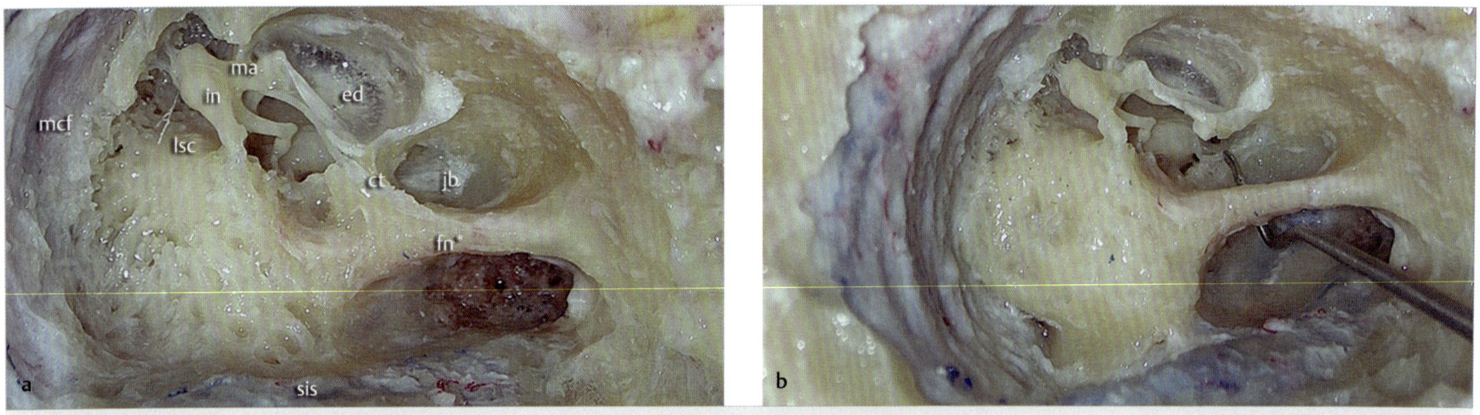

Fig. 1.19 Temporal bone dissection (right side): **(a)** A mastoidectomy with canal wall down procedure is performed exposing the tympanic cavity. The facial nerve is skeletonized in the mastoid. The retrofacial cells are removed connecting the mastoid to the hypotympanum **(b)**. *ct: chorda tympani; ed: eardrum; fn*: mastoid segment of facial nerve; in: incus; jb: jugular bulb; lsc: lateral semicircular canal; ma: malleus; mcf: middle cranial fossa; sis: sigmoid sinus.*

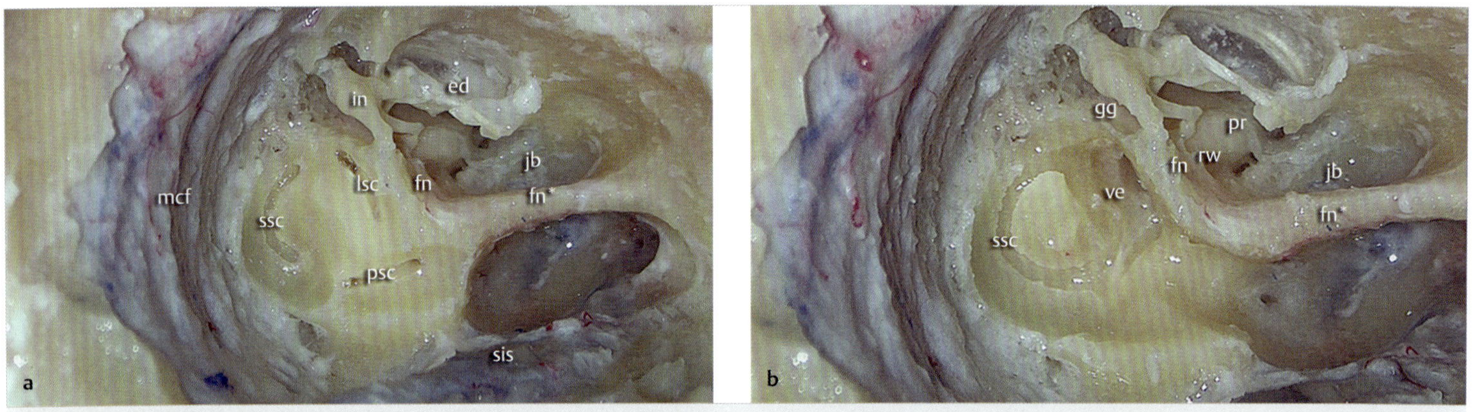

Fig. 1.20 Temporal bone dissection (right side): **(a)** The labyrinthectomy is performed. The semicircular canals are opened. **(b)** The vestibule is exposed. *ed: eardrum; fn: tympanic segment of facial nerve; fn*: mastoid segment of facial nerve; gg: geniculate ganglion; in: incus; jb: jugular bulb; lsc: lateral semicircular canal; ma: malleus; mcf: middle cranial fossa; pr: promontory; psc: posterior semicircular canal; rw: round window; sis: sigmoid sinus; ssc: superior semicircular canal; ve: vestibule.*

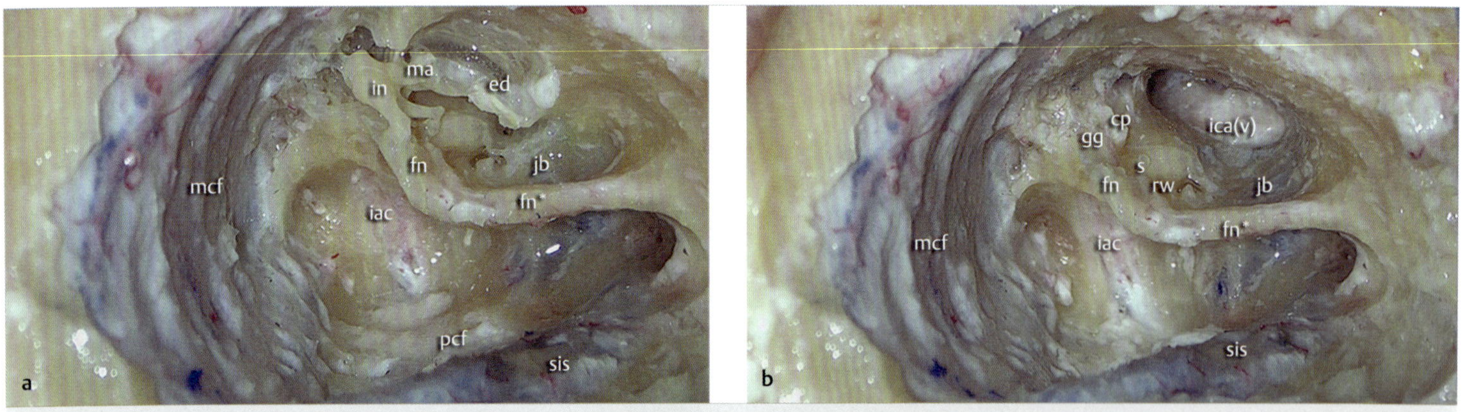

Fig. 1.21 Temporal bone dissection (right side): **(a)** The internal auditory canal (IAC) is skeletonized. **(b)** The transmastoid anatomy of the facial nerve inside the temporal bone is noted after the ossicular chain is removed. *cp: cochleariform process; ed: eardrum; fn: tympanic segment of facial nerve; fn*: mastoid segment of facial nerve; gg: geniculate ganglion; ica(v): vertical portion of internal carotid artery; in: incus; jb: jugular bulb; ma: malleus; mcf: middle cranial fossa; rw: round window; s: stapes; sis: sigmoid sinus.*

The ITF is an irregular space that can be described as an inverted square-shaped pyramid superiorly communicating with the temporal fossa under the zygomatic arch. It communicates medially through the pterygomaxillary fissure with the pterygopalatine fossa (see ▶ Fig. 1.31), anteriorly through the inferior orbital fissure with the orbit, and superomedially through the foramen ovale and spinosum with the middle cranial fossa (see ▶ Fig. 1.27, ▶ Fig. 1.28, ▶ Fig. 1.29, ▶ Fig. 1.30, ▶ Fig. 1.31). Due to the venous connections between the pterygoid venous plexus and the cavernous sinus, potentially life-threatening infections can spread from ITF to the cavernous sinus leading to cavernous sinus thrombosis.

The ITF is anteriorly bounded by the posterolateral surface of the maxillary sinus. Medially, it is bounded by the lateral pterygoid plate, the medial pterygoid and tensor veli palatini muscles, and the ramus of the mandible forms the lateral boundary (see

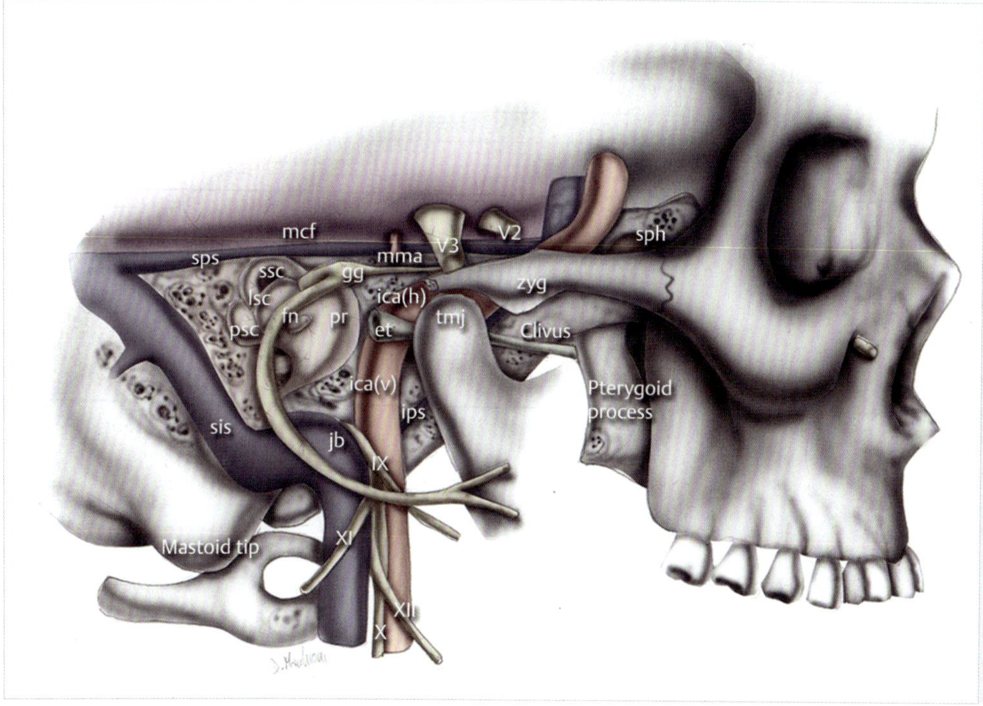

Fig. 1.22 Lateral view of lateral skull base: The anatomical relationship between the vascular and nervous structures is shown. *et: eustachian tube; fn: facial nerve; gg: geniculate ganglion; ica (h): horizontal portion of internal carotid artery; ica(v): vertical portion of internal carotid artery; ips: inferior petrosal sinus; jb: jugular bulb; lsc: lateral semicircular canal; mcf: middle cranial fossa; mma: middle meningeal artery; pr: promontory; psc: posterior semicircular canal; sis: sigmoid sinus; sph: sphenoid; sps: superior petrosal sinus; ssc: superior semicircular canal; tmj: temporal mandibular joint; zyg: zygomatic arch.*

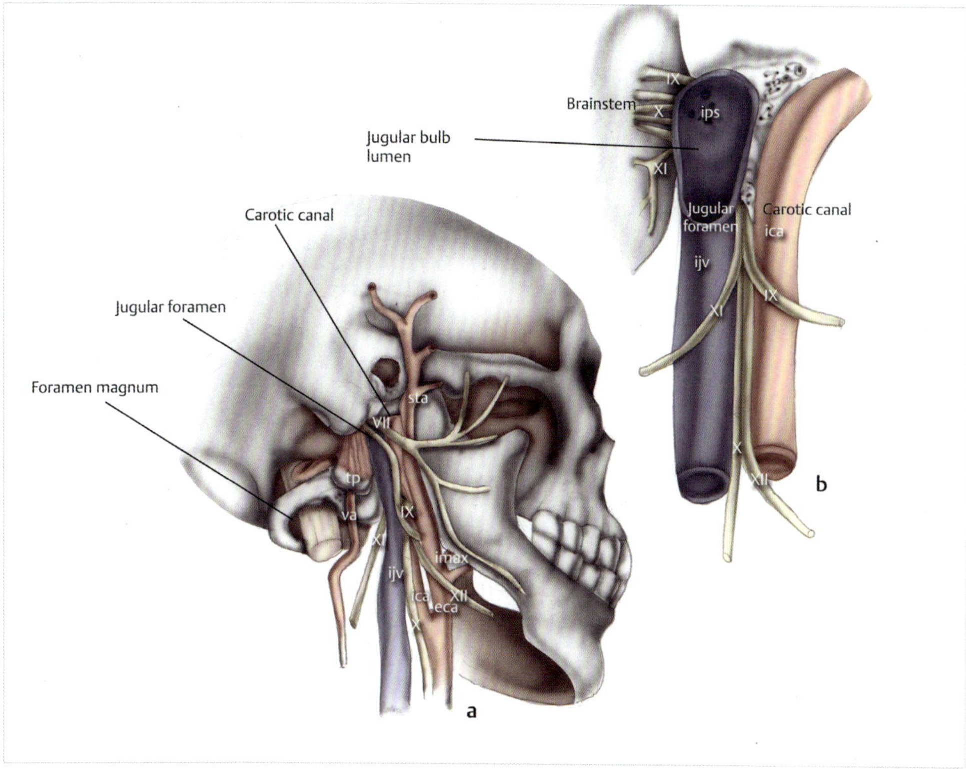

Fig. 1.23 **(a)** The jugular foramen anatomy (right side). **(b)** The lateral wall of the jugular bulb has been removed to expose the lumen of the vein. The opening of the inferior petrosal sinus into the lumen of the jugular bulb is noted. The lower cranial nerve runs from the brainstem to the upper neck through the jugular foramen passing medially to the jugular bulb. *eca: external carotid artery; ica: internal carotid artery; ijv: internal jugular vein; imax: internal maxillary artery; ips: inferior petrosal sinus; sta: superficial temporal artery; tp: transverse process of atlas; va: vertebral artery.*

▶ Fig. 1.30, ▶ Fig. 1.31, ▶ Fig. 1.32). Superiorly, it is bounded by the infratemporal surface and the infratemporal crest of the greater wing of the sphenoid bone and inferiorly, it is closed by the insertion of the medial pterygoid muscle on the ramus of the mandible. The posterior boundary of the ITF is loosely defined and by the carotid sheath and the tympanic plate and the styloid process of the temporal bone.

As mentioned earlier, the ITF acts as a passageway for neurovascular structures passing to and from the orbit, the middle cranial fossa, the pterygopalatine fossa, and the temporal fossa. It contains the following structures:

- Muscles:
  - Medial pterygoid muscle.
  - Lateral pterygoid muscle.
  - Inferior part of temporalis muscle.
- Vascular structures:
  - Maxillary artery and its branches.
  - Maxillary vein.
  - Pterygoid venous plexus.
- Nerves:
  - Mandibular nerve and its branches.
  - Chorda tympani nerve.
  - Otic ganglion.

The muscles of mastication are associated with the ITF; the lateral pterygoid muscle occupies most of the superior ITF while the medial pterygoid muscle forms the inferior boundary. The masseter and temporalis muscles insert and originate from the borders

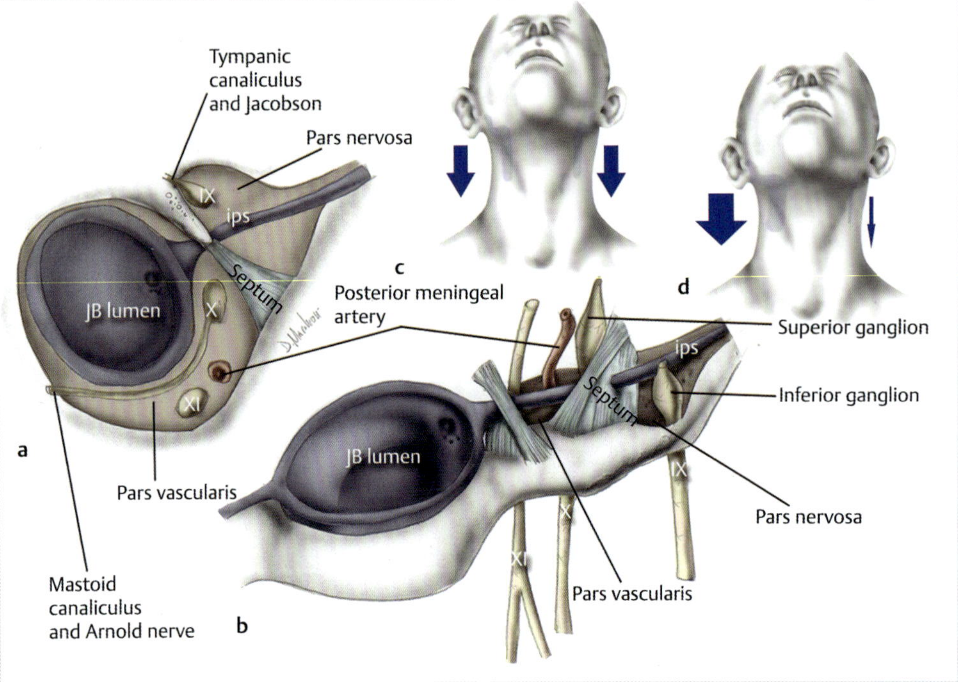

Fig. 1.24 (a, b) Anatomy of the jugular foramen: the anteromedial (pars nervosa) compartment and the posterolateral (pars vascularis) compartment are noted. **(c, d)** Venous drainage through the jugular foramen. In the majority of cases the transverse sinuses are equal in size (**c**); asymmetric size of transverse sinuses with the dominant size and the narrow size in the contralateral portion (**d**). *ips: inferior petrosal sinus; JB: jugular bulb.*

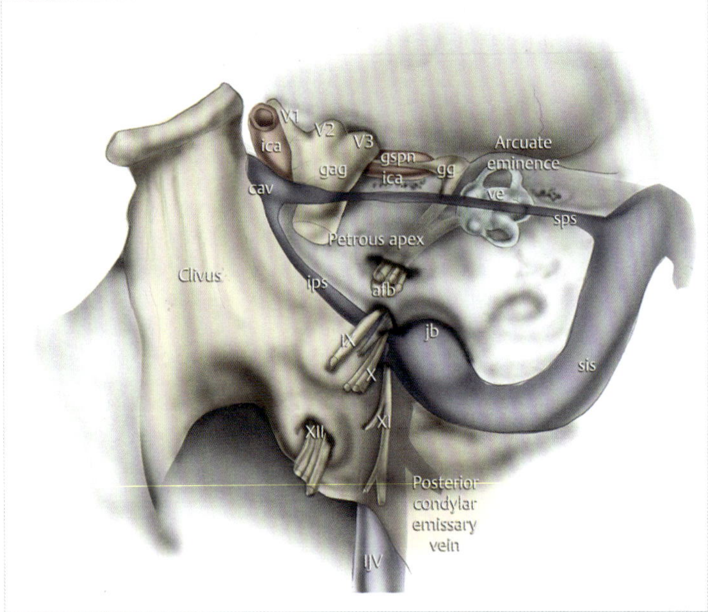

Fig. 1.25 Endocranial anatomy of petrosal sinus (Right side). *afb: acoustic-facial bundle; cav: cavernous sinus; gag: gasserian ganglion; gg: geniculate ganglion; gspn: greater superficial petrosal nerve; i ca: internal carotid artery; IJV: internal jugular vein; ips: inferior petrosal sinus; jb: jugular bulb; sps: superior petrosal sinus; ve: vestibule.*

of the fossa. The lateral pterygoid muscle arises from two heads (upper and lower) from the infratemporal surface of the greater wing of the sphenoid and lateral pterygoid plate, respectively, and inserts into the pterygoid fovea on the mandibular condyle (see ▶ Fig. 1.32). The lateral pterygoid is the only muscle of mastication that depresses the mandible and opens the jaw (see ▶ Fig. 1.32a,b). The medial pterygoid muscle also has two heads of origin (deep and superficial), from the lateral pterygoid plate and the maxillary tuberosity, respectively, and inserts on the medial surface of the ramus of the mandible near its angle. All the muscles of mastication are supplied by the mandibular nerve.

The maxillary artery is the seventh (terminal) branch of the external carotid artery that originates at the neck of the mandible and runs through the ITF between the condylar process of the mandible and the sphenomandibular ligament to enter the pterygopalatine fossa. The maxillary artery is divided into three parts in relation to the lateral pterygoid muscle. The first part (mandibular) lies deep to the condyle of the mandible, the second part (pterygoid) lies on the lateral pterygoid muscle, and the third part (pterygopalatine) lies in the pterygopalatine fossa. All the three parts of the maxillary artery give several branches, described below:

- Branches from the first part:
  - Deep auricular artery.
  - Anterior tympanic artery.
  - Middle meningeal artery.
  - Accessory meningeal artery.
  - Inferior alveolar artery.
- Branches from the second part:
  - Anterior and posterior deep temporal arteries.
  - Pterygoid branch.
  - Masseteric branch.
  - Buccinator branch.
- Branches from the third part:
  - Posterior superior alveolar artery.
  - Infraorbital artery.
  - Descending palatine artery.
  - Pharyngeal branch.
  - Pterygoid canal artery.
  - Sphenopalatine artery.

The pterygoid venous plexus has two parts—a superficial part between the temporalis and the lateral pterygoid muscles and a deep-lying part medial to the lateral pterygoid muscle. Most often, the deep-lying part of the pterygoid plexus is better developed. It receives tributaries corresponding to the branches of the maxillary artery. It mainly drains the orbit and the area in and around the ITF. The pterygoid venous plexus is drained by the maxillary vein which begins at its posterior border and it accompanies only the first part of the maxillary artery. Inside the parotid gland it joins the superficial temporal vein to form the retromandibular vein (see ▶ Fig. 1.33a).

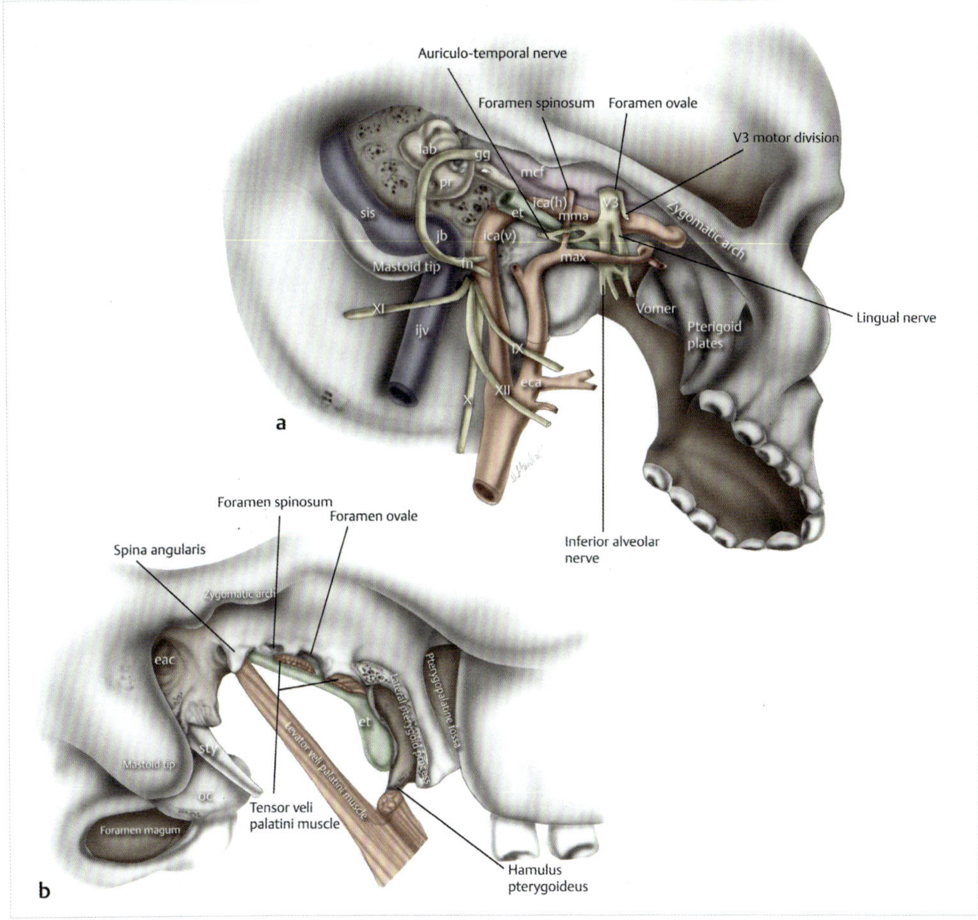

Fig. 1.26 (a, b) Anatomy of the infratemporal fossa (right side). *eac: external auditory canal; eca: external carotid artery; et: eustachian tube; fn: facial nerve; gg: geniculate ganglion; ica(h): horizontal portion of internal carotid artery; ica(v): vertical portion of internal carotid artery; ijv: internal jugular vein; jb: jugular bulb; l ab: labyrinthine block; max: internal maxillary artery; mcf: middle cranial fossa; mma: middle meningeal artery; oc: occipital condyle; pr: promontory; sis: sigmoid sinus; sty: styloid process.*

The ITF is densely innervated and it provides a gateway for the mandibular nerve, the chorda tympani nerve, and the otic ganglion. These nerves grant sensory and motor functions to the lower face, the muscles of mastication, and the dura mater. The mandibular nerve is a mixed nerve which enters the ITF through the foramen ovale. It runs between the lateral pterygoid and the tensor veli palatini muscles and divides into smaller anterior and larger posterior branches. Just before its bifurcation, it gives motor branches to the tensor veli palatini, the tensor tympani, and the medial pterygoid muscles and a sensory meningeal branch to the dura mater (see ▶ Fig. 1.31). The anterior division gives four branches: one sensory buccal branch and three motor branches to the masseter, the temporalis, and the lateral pterygoid muscles. The posterior division is mainly sensory and gives three branches, namely, the auriculotemporal nerve, the lingual nerve, and the inferior alveolar nerve (see ▶ Fig. 1.29).

The chorda tympani nerve enters the ITF through the petrotympanic fissure and joins the lingual nerve. The chorda tympani nerve carries the taste sensation from the anterior two-thirds of the tongue and provides secretomotor fibers to the submandibular and sublingual salivary glands. The otic ganglion is located in the ITF on the medial side of the mandibular nerve inferior to the foramen ovale. The presynaptic parasympathetic fibers mainly stem from the lesser petrosal nerve (formed by the tympanic plexus). The postsynaptic parasympathetic secretomotor fibers supply the parotid gland via the auriculotemporal nerve.

1.7 Cerebellopontine Angle

The cerebellopontine angle (CPA) is the anatomic space between the petrous bone and the petrosal cerebellar surface folding around the pons and the middle cerebellar peduncle, containing the posterior cranial fossa nerves (see ▶ Fig. 1.17 and ▶ Fig. 1.34).

Examining the anatomy of the CPA, we can define three neurovascular complexes:

- The upper complex (including the trigeminal, oculomotor, and trochlear nerves; the midbrain; the cerebellomesencephalic fissure; the superior cerebellar artery [SCA]; the superior cerebellar peduncle; and the tentorial surface of the cerebellum) (see ▶ Fig. 1.35).
- The middle complex (including the acoustic-facial nerve bundle and the abducent nerve; the pons; the cerebellopontine fissure; the AICA; the middle cerebellar peduncle; and the petrosal surface of the cerebellum) (see ▶ Fig. 1.17a,b).
- The lower complex (including the lower mixed cranial nerves; the hypoglossal nerve; the medulla; the cerebellomedullary fissure; the posterior inferior cerebellar artery [PICA]; the inferior cerebellar peduncle; and the suboccipital surface of the cerebellum) (see ▶ Fig. 1.17a,b).

1.7.1 Relevant Nervous Contents

The trigeminal nerve emerges laterally from the pons, in proximity to its superior border, with a larger sensory root and a smaller motor root. The fibers of the sensory root have their somas in the trigeminal ganglion, in a dural duplication approximately 1.5 cm from the apex of the petrous ridge. Three roots arise from the trigeminal ganglion in Meckel's cave: the ophthalmic nerve (V1), the maxillary nerve (V2), and the mandibular nerve (V3).

The acoustic-facial bundle arises from the brainstem close to the pontomedullary sulcus. The facial nerve exits at the level of the pontomedullary junction about 1 to 2 mm anteriorly to the vestibular nerve; after this level the facial nerve immediately meets the vestibulocochlear bundle. The eighth and the

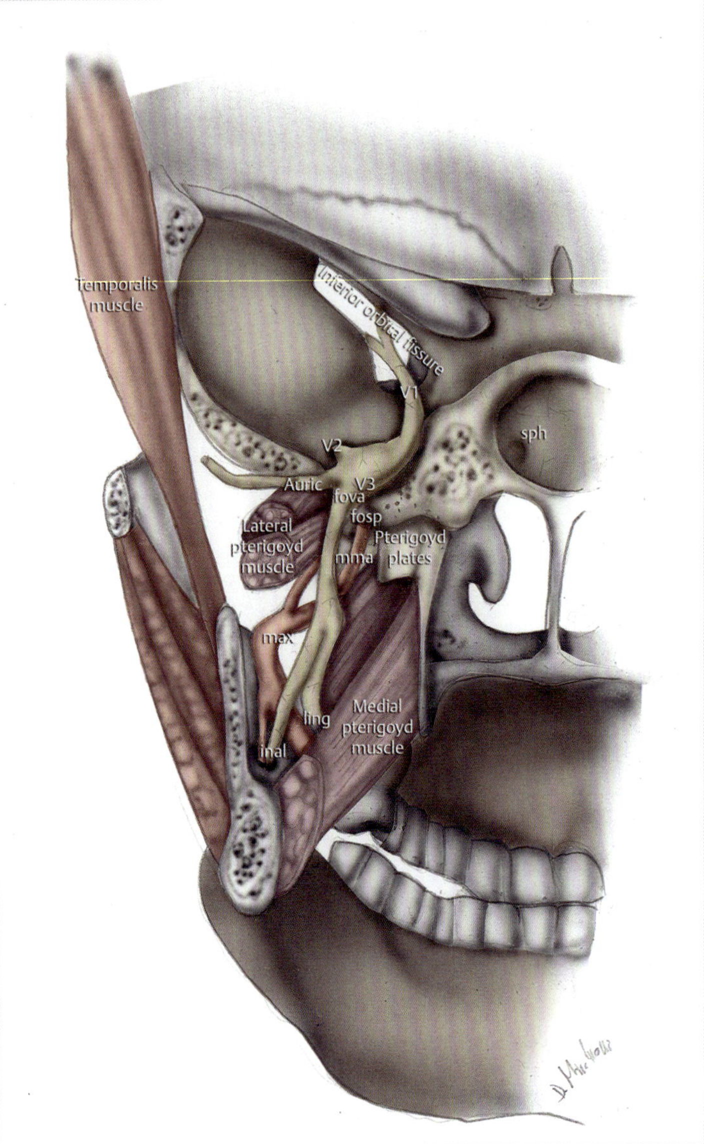

Fig. 1.27 Infratemporal fossa anatomy; posterior view (left side). *auric: auriculotemporal nerve; fosp: foramen spinosum; fova: foramen ovale; inal: inferior alveolar nerve; ling: lingual nerve; max: maxillary artery; mma: middle meningeal artery; sph: sphenoid.*

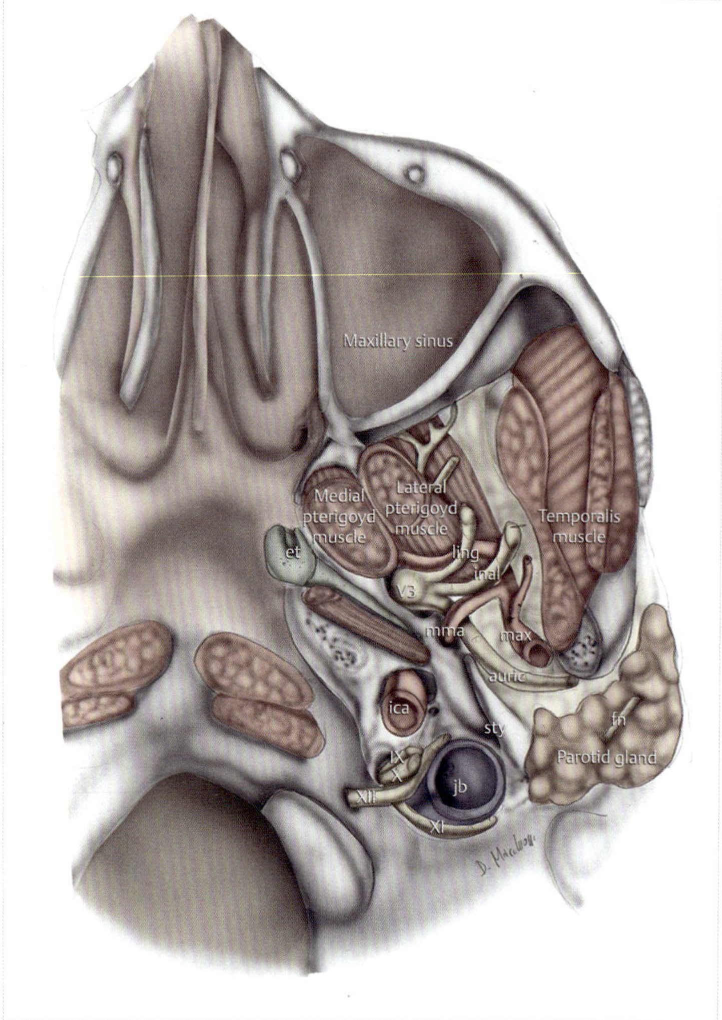

Fig. 1.28 Infratemporal fossa anatomy; axial view (left side). *auric: auriculotemporal nerve; et: eustachian tube; fn: facial nerve; ica: internal carotid artery; inal: inferior alveolar nerve; jb: jugular bulb; ling: lingual nerve; max: maxillary artery; mma: middle meningeal artery; sty: styloid process.*

intermediate nerves join the facial nerve in the CPA. The gap between the vestibulocochlear bundle and the facial nerve is well visible at the level of the pontomedullary sulcus; these nerves get closer as they approach the meatus. The so formed acoustic-facial bundle runs forward and lateral to the posterior surface of the petrous bone, entering the IAC. During its course in the CPA, the position of the facial nerve in relation to the other nerves is anterior and medial until the IAC is reached, while the vestibular nerve is located superiorly and the cochlear nerve inferiorly. In the porus of the IAC, the position of the nerves changes: the facial nerve runs superiorly with the vestibular nerve and the cochlear nerve is inferior.

The lower cranial nerves originate from the medulla oblongata and run superolaterally to enter the JF.

Topdown, the lower cranial nerves are located as follows:

- The glossopharyngeal nerve: This nerve is in the most superior position to the other lower cranial nerves and it is made up of a single root.
- The vagus nerve: Located in the intermediate position, this nerve at the exit zone is close to the glossopharyngeal nerve and it is made up of multiple roots.
- The spinal accessory nerve, located at the most inferior extremity, it is formed by two distinct roots: the cranial root and the spinal root. The exit zone of the cranial root is close to the fibers of the vagus nerve. This nerve is small if compared to the other root. The spinal root is larger and it is made up of multiple roots from the spinal cord; these roots merge into a single trunk that ascends the upper portion of the cervical canal and enters the posterior fossa through the foramen magnum.

The exit zone of the hypoglossal nerve is located medially on the ventral surface of medulla oblongata. The fibers of this nerve are grouped into two main trunks that usually merge inside the hypoglossal canal.

The PICA often runs in between the two roots of hypoglossal nerve.

1.8 Internal Carotid Artery

According to Bouthillier's classification, the ICA is divided into seven segments according to the anatomical relationship of the artery with the adjacent structures and the anatomical compartments it crosses (see ▶ Fig. 1.12):

- Cervical segment (C1).
- Petrous segment (C2).
- Lacerum segment (C3).

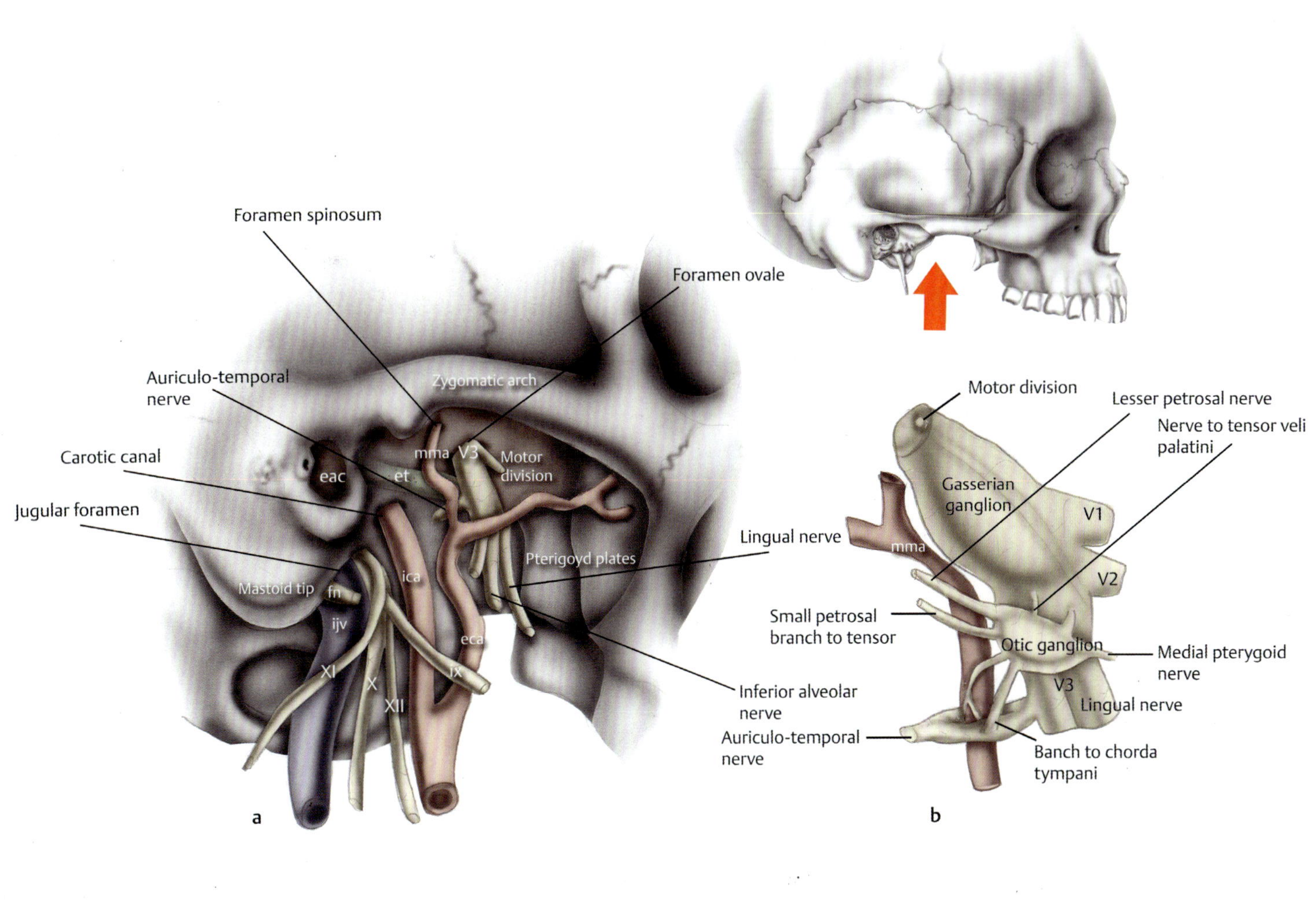

Fig. 1.29 Infratemporal fossa anatomy; lateral view (right side) **(a)**; anatomy of the otic ganglion in relation to trigeminal nerve **(b)**. *eac: external auditory canal; eca: external carotid artery; et: eustachian tube; fn: facial nerve; ica: internal carotid artery; ijv: internal jugular vein; mma: middle meningeal artery.*

- Cavernous segment (C4).
- Clinoid segment (C5).
- Ophthalmic segment (C6).
- Communicating segment (C7).

The C1 segment is the most inferior segment of the ICA, it is located in the neck. It starts from the carotid bulb where an enlargement of the artery is present. From the bulb, the vascular structure ascends at the base of skull, forming the ascending cervical segment. In this area a tortuosity of the artery may be present.

The C2 segment of the ICA enters the skull base inside the temporal bone through the carotid canal. The petrous ICA has two distinct segments: a vertical and a horizontal segment; between the two segments, the ICA forms a genu.

The caroticotympanic artery arises from the vertical portion of the ICA in proximity of the carotid genu. This branch anastomoses with the inferior tympanic branches of the ascending pharyngeal artery. The vidian artery may arise from the horizontal segment of C2, before entering the anterior foramen lacerum.

The C3 segment is a short segment which runs above the foramen lacerum, and ascends in the carotid sulcus, until the petrolingual ligament. The petrolingual ligament is a reflection of the periosteum between the lingual and the petrosal process of the sphenoid bone.

The cavernous segment, or C4, of the ICA begins at the level of the petrolingual ligament and extends to the proximal dural ring, which is formed by the medial and inferior periosteum of the anterior clinoid process. The cavernous segment is surrounded by the cavernous sinus. Bottomup, the artery ascends toward the posterior clinoid process, then it moves forward by the side of the body of the sphenoid bone, and it curves upward on the medial side of the anterior clinoid process forming the carotid siphon until it perforates the dura mater forming the roof of the sinus. The abducent nerve runs lateral to this level. Two arterial branches arise from this segment—the meningohypophyseal artery and the inferolateral trunk.

Once the artery has got out of the cavernous sinus, the ICA begins as the clinoid segment (C5). This is a short segment between the proximal dural ring and the distal dural ring, after which the carotid artery enters the subarachnoid space and it is considered "intradural." The ophthalmic artery may arise from this segment. The C6 (or ophthalmic) segment extends from the distal dural ring to the origin of the posterior communicating artery, running parallel to the optic nerve. The ophthalmic artery and the superior hypophyseal artery arise from this segment.

The C7 segment of the ICA begins just proximal to the origin of the posterior communicating artery and ends as the ICA bifurcates into its terminal branches, the anterior and middle cerebral arteries. Two major branches, the posterior communicating artery and the anterior choroidal artery, arise from the communicating segment. The ICA can receive blood via an important collateral pathway supplying the brain, the cerebral arterial circle,

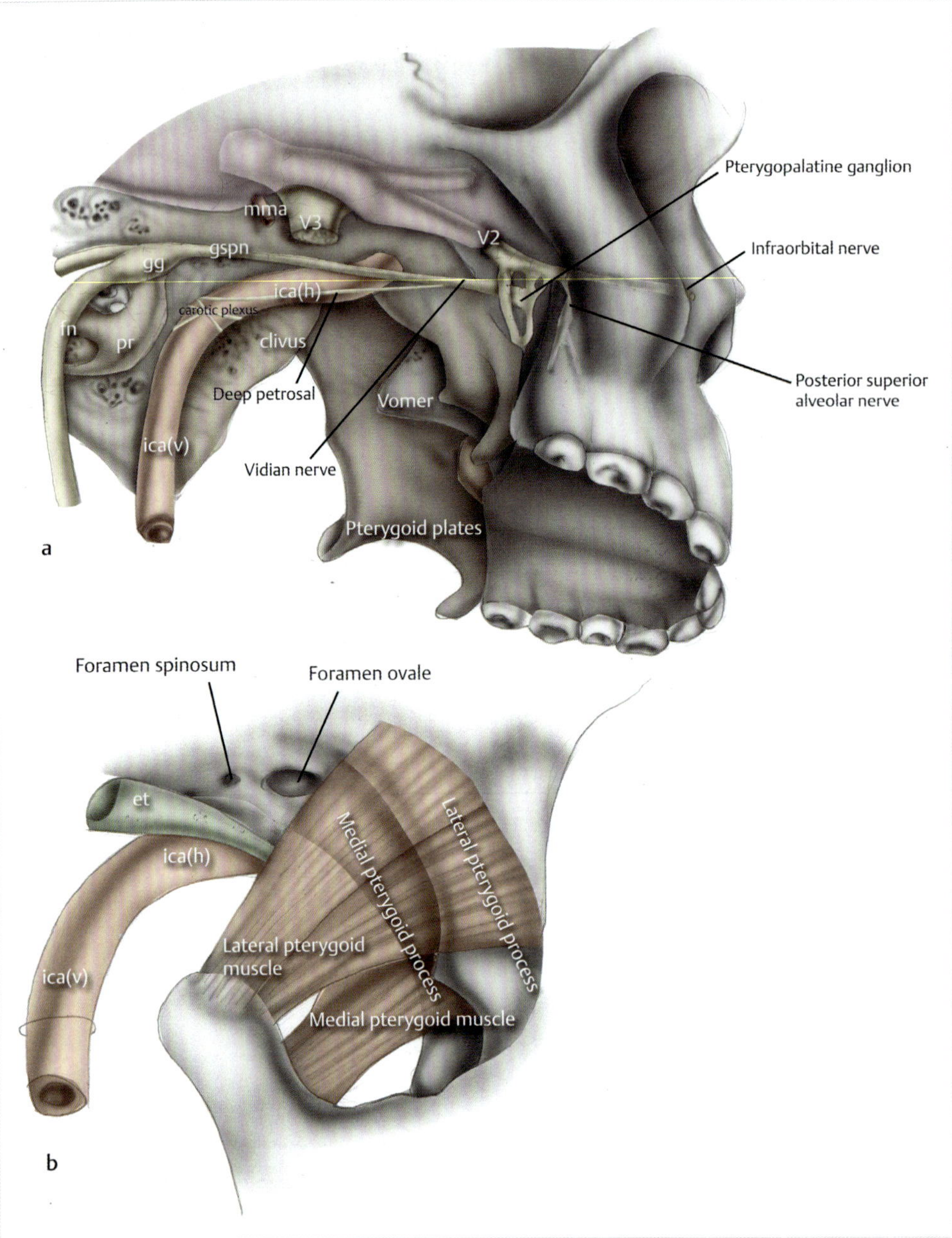

Fig. 1.30 **(a)** Infratemporal fossa and pterygopalatine fossa anatomy (right side). **(b)** Temporomandibular joint and pterygoid muscles insertions. *et: eustachian tube; fn: facial nerve; gg: geniculate ganglion; gspn: greater superficial petrosal nerve; ica(h): horizontal portion of internal carotid artery; ica(v): vertical portion of internal carotid artery; mma: middle meningeal artery; pr: promontory.*

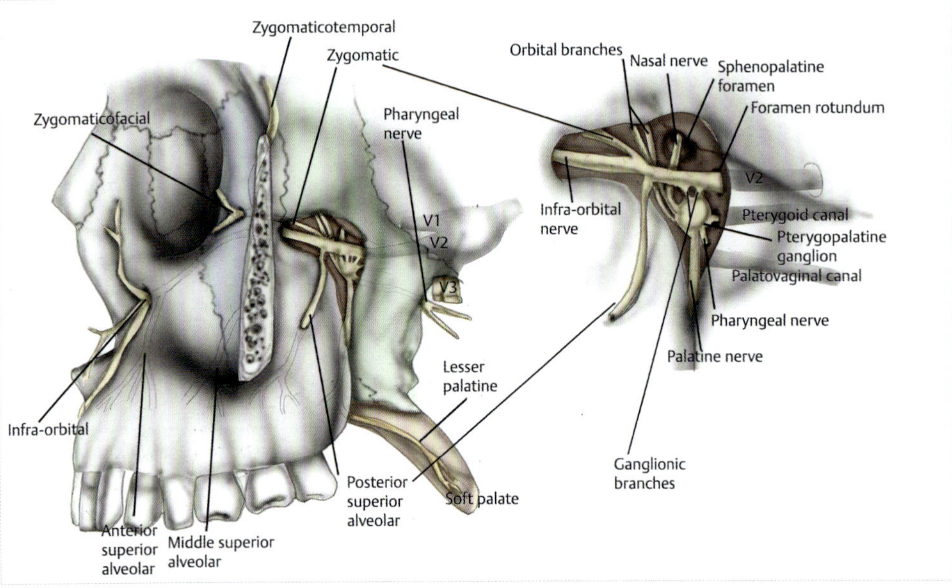

Fig. 1.31 Nervous contents of the pterygopalatine (pterygomaxillary) fossa (lateral view; left side).

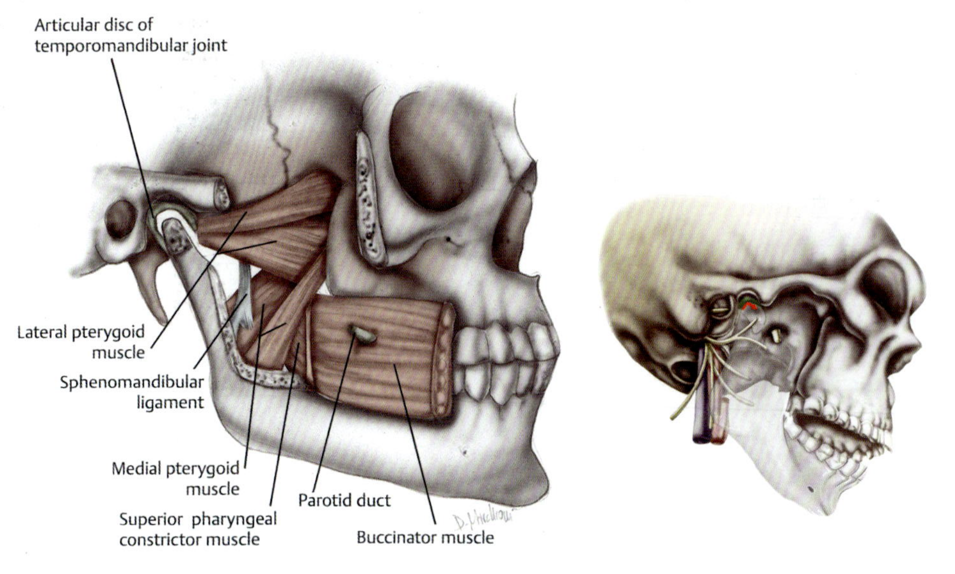

Fig. 1.32 Temporomandibular joint and muscle contents in the infratemporal fossa (right side).

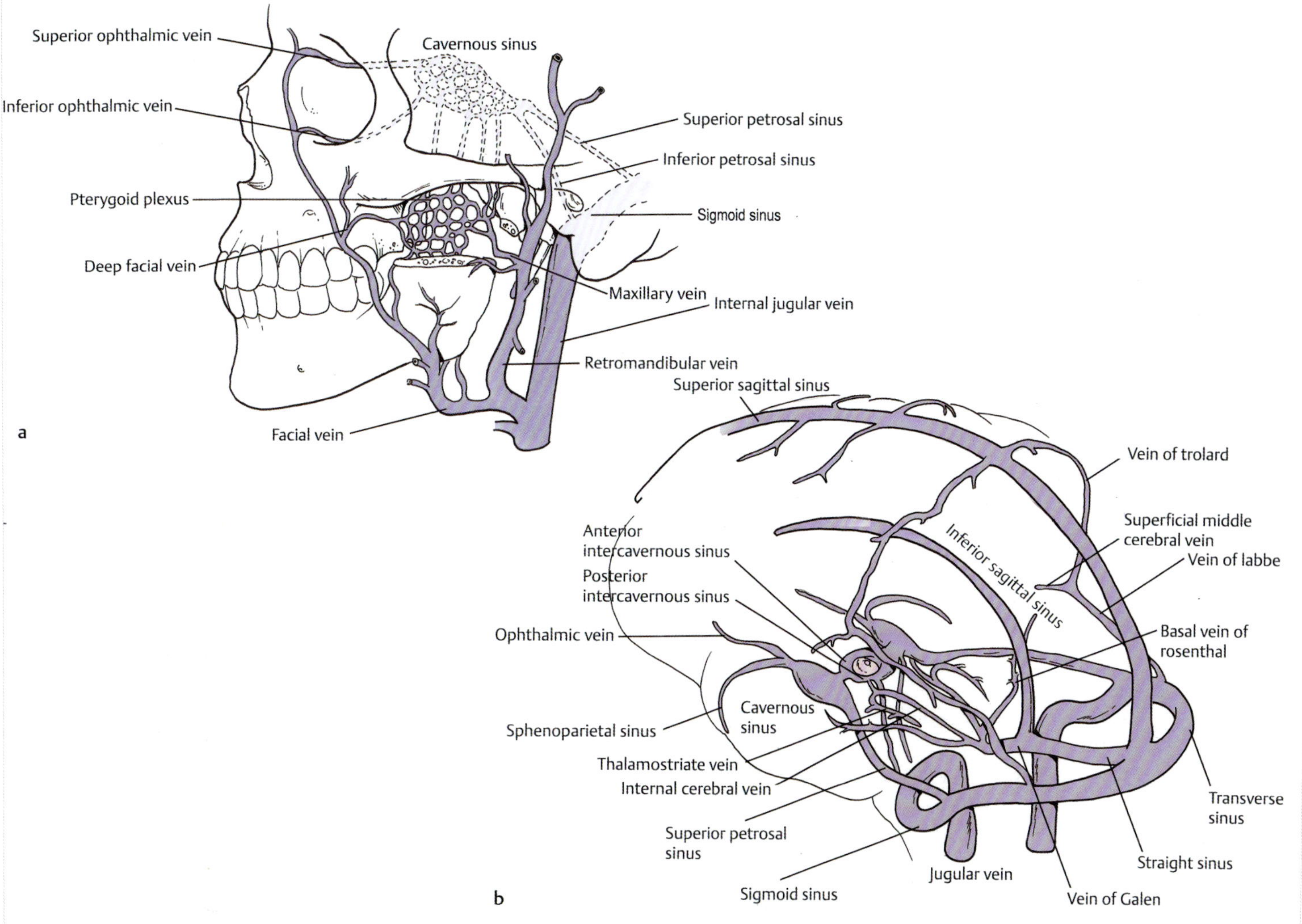

Fig. 1.33 Venous drainage of the head and skull base. **(a)** Venous system of the infratemporal fossa. **(b)** Venous system of the brain.

which is more commonly known as the circle of Willis (see ▶ Fig. 1.36 and ▶ Fig. 1.37).

1.9 Basilar Artery

The basilar artery is a large median vessel arising from the confluence of the two vertebral arteries at the junction between the medulla oblongata and the pons at the exit zone of the sixth cranial nerves (see ▶ Fig. 1.37).

Bottomup, it gives the following branches on either side:

- Pontine branches.
- AICA.
- Internal auditory (labyrinthine) artery.
- SCA.
- Posterior cerebral artery.

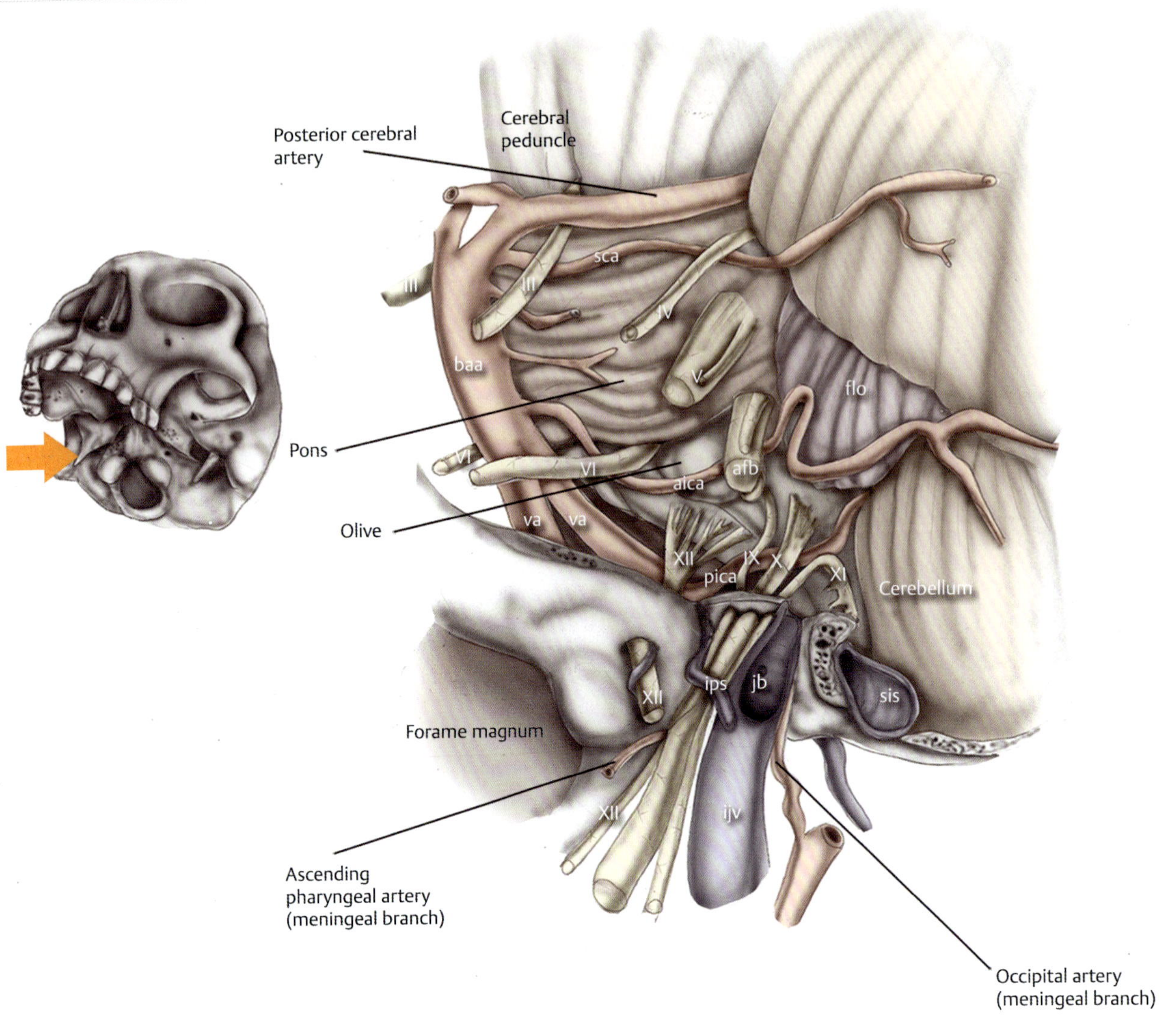

Fig. 1.34 Cerebellopontine angle anatomy (left side). *afb: acoustic-facial bundle; aica: anterior inferior cerebellar artery; baa: basilar artery; flo: flocculus; ijv: internal jugular vein; ips: inferior petrosal sinus; jb: jugular bulb; pica: posterior inferior cerebellar artery; sca: superior cerebellar artery; sis: sigmoid sinus; va: vertebral artery.*

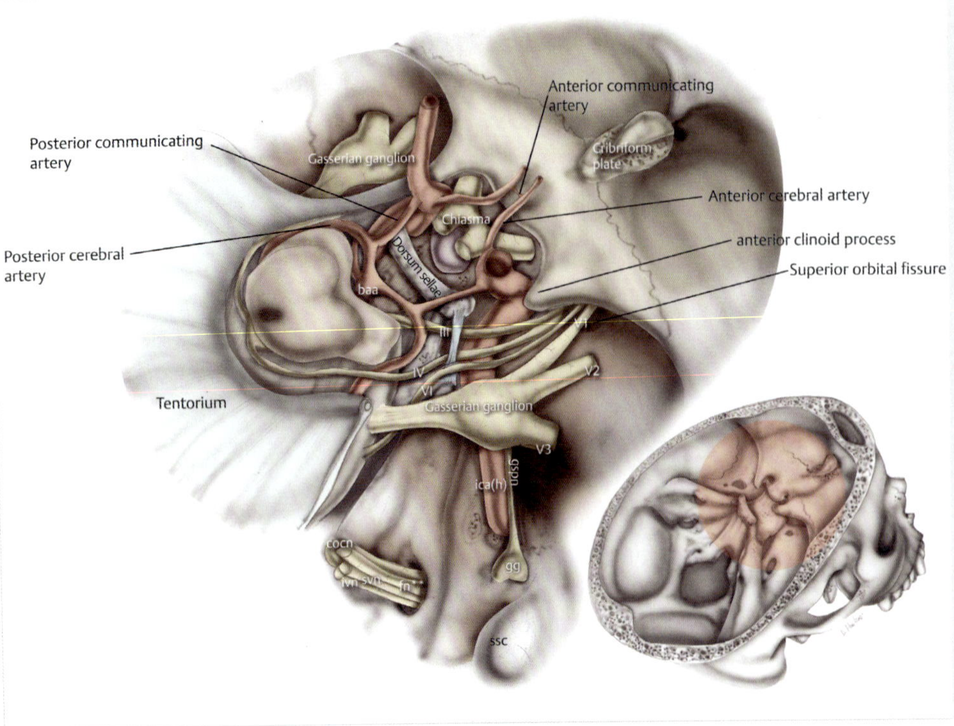

Fig. 1.35 Relationships of the cranial nerves with the endocranial surface of the skull base and brainstem. *baa: basilar artery; cocn: cochlear nerve; fn**: facial nerve in the cerebellopontine angle; gg: geniculate ganglion; gspn: greater superficial petrosal nerve; ica(h): horizontal portion of internal carotid artery; ivn: inferior vestibular nerve; ssc: superior semicircular canal; svn: superior vestibular nerve.*

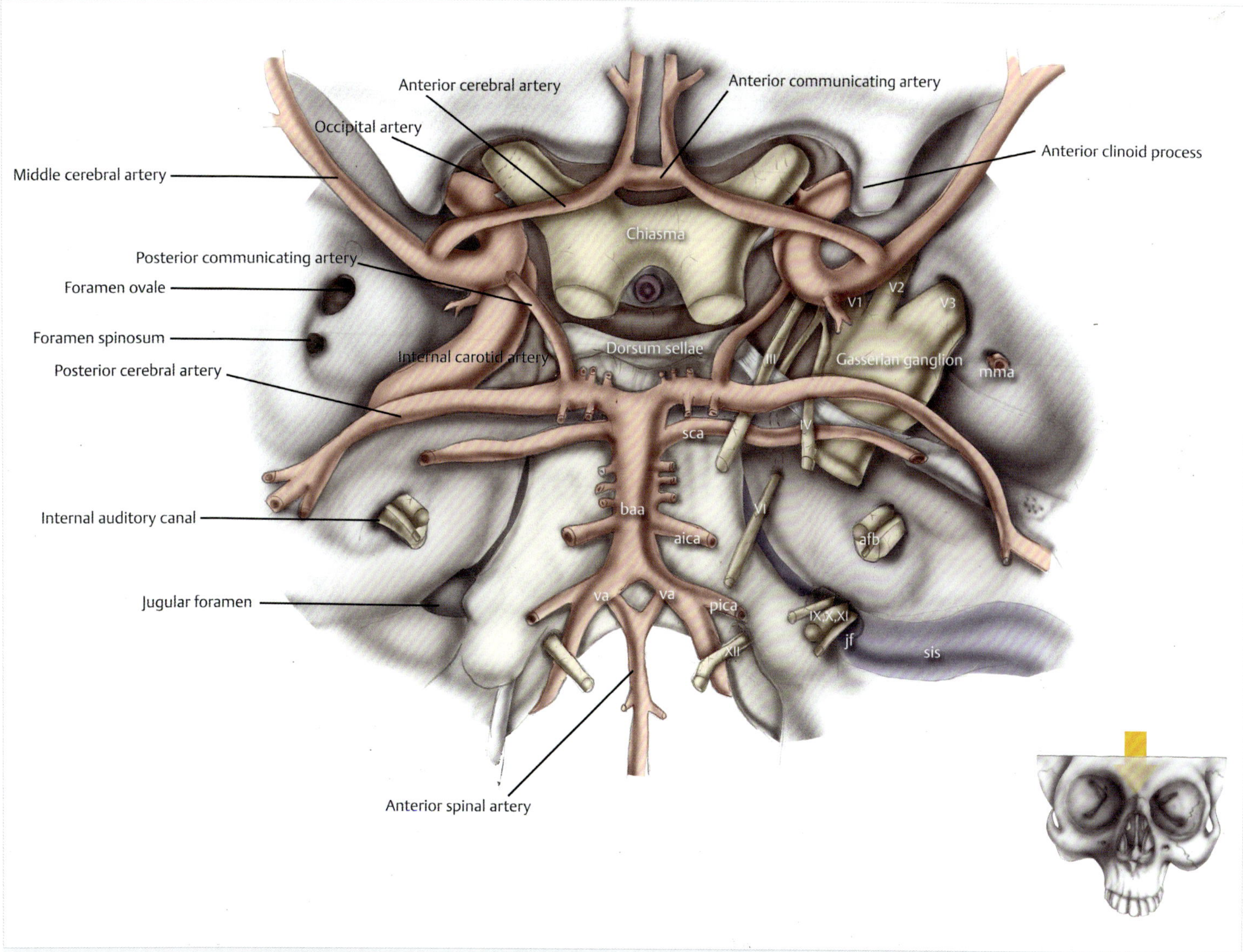

Fig. 1.36 Arterial vascularization of the brainstem and circle of Willis; endocranial view. *afb: acoustic-facial bundle; aica: anterior inferior cerebellar artery; baa: basilar artery; jf: jugular foramen; mma: middle meningeal artery; pica: posterior inferior cerebellar artery; sca: superior cerebellar artery; sis: sigmoid sinus; va: vertebral artery.*

The pontine branches are numerous small branches which arise from the front and sides of the basilar artery along its course and supply the pons.

The internal auditory (labyrinthine) artery, consisting of a long slender branch, has a variable origin. It usually arises from the anterior inferior cerebellar artery.

The AICA arises from the basilar artery and runs posterolaterally ventral to the acoustic-facial bundle. This branch supplies the inferior and middle cerebellar peduncles of the cerebellum and the adjacent hemisphere, from the anterior to the inferior portion.

In most patients, the internal auditory or labyrinthine artery arises from the AICA in proximity to the IAC, entering the IAC and following the acoustic-facial bundle inside the temporal bone, supplying the cochlea and the vestibule.

In the majority of cases, the internal auditory artery runs between the facial nerve and the cochlear nerve, at the level of the porus. Branching and anastomosis of the internal auditory artery are highly variable in the middle to proximal portion of the IAC. We can consider three branches:

- The anterior vestibular artery runs on the anterior surface of the superior vestibular nerve.
- The vestibulocochlear artery runs on the inferior surface of the inferior vestibular nerve.
- The cochlear artery runs at the center of the cochlear nerve near the fundus.

The SCA arises near the distal portion of the basilar artery, immediately before the formation of the posterior cerebral arteries. It passes laterally below the oculomotor nerve, which separates it from the posterior cerebral artery, and curves round the cerebral peduncle below the trochlear nerve to reach the superior cerebellar surface (see ▶ Fig. 1.35). The posterior cerebral artery is a terminal branch of the basilar artery.

The PICA arises directly from the vertebral artery. This artery supplies the cerebellum and part of the brain.

1.10 Venous Drainage from the Skull Base

The skull base dural venous sinuses are the cavernous and intercavernous sinuses, the superior and inferior petrosal sinuses, the occipital sinus, and the lateral sinuses (see ▶ Fig. 1.33).

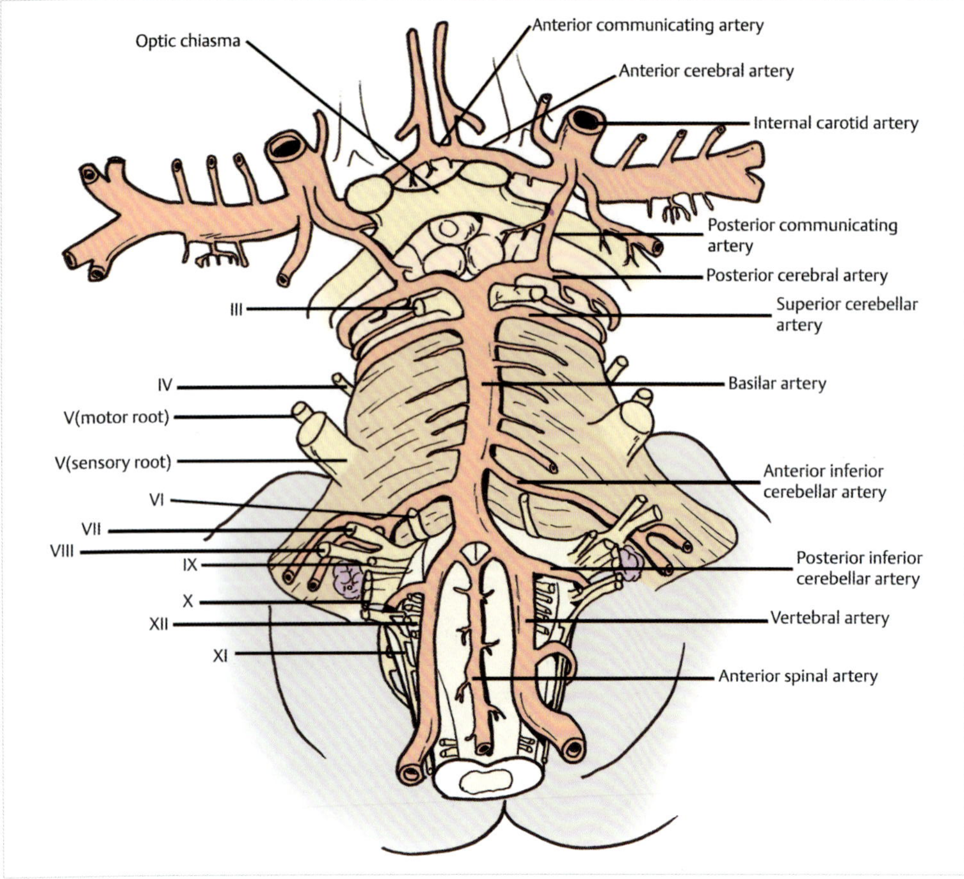

Fig. 1.37 Arterial vascularization of the brainstem in relation to the cranial nerves. Anterior view.

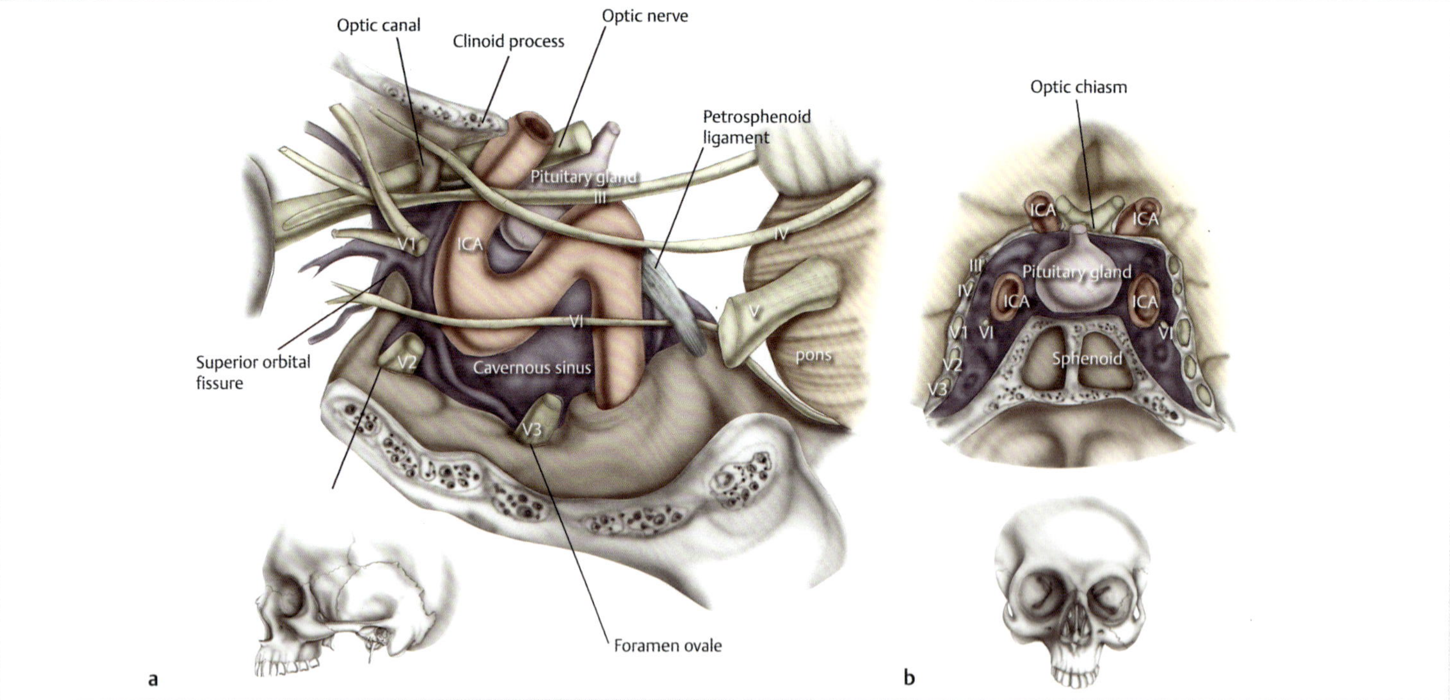

Fig. 1.38 Cavernous sinus anatomy. **(a)** Lateral view on the left side; **(b)** Anterior view. *ica: internal carotid artery.*

1.10.1 Cavernous Sinus

The cavernous sinus is a paired dural venous sinus located in the middle cranial fossa on either side of the body of the sphenoid bone and the pituitary gland. It is present between the two layers of the dura mater, that is, the endosteal layer (forming the medial wall and floor) and the meningeal layer (forming roof and lateral wall). Each cavernous sinus is 2 cm long and 1 cm wide and it antero-posteriorly extends from the medial end of the superior orbital fissure to the apex of the petrous temporal bone.

Each cavernous sinus is separated by multiple septa lined with endothelium, dividing it into small "caverns" and from which it takes its name. It has several tributaries and connections with important surrounding structures, and it is arguably the most clinically important dural venous sinus (see ▶ Fig. 1.38 and ▶ Fig. 1.39). The cavernous sinus is anteriorly related to the anterior clinoid and

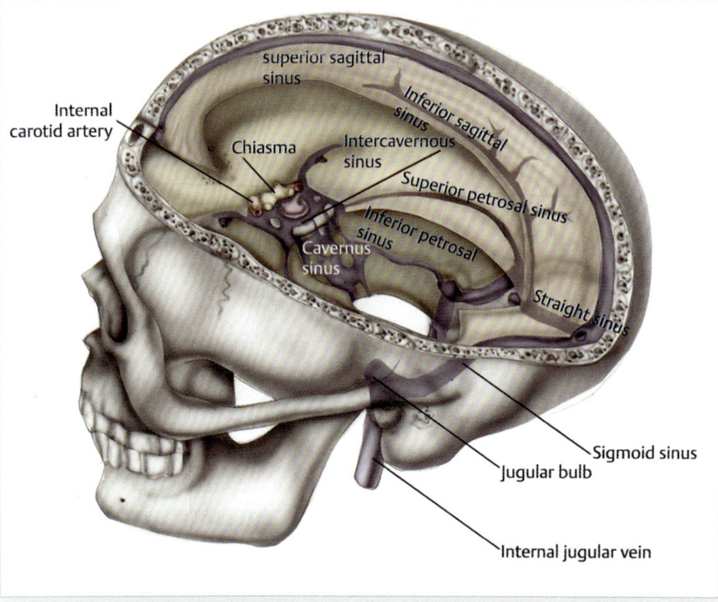

Fig. 1.39 Cavernous sinus anatomy related with inferior and superior petrous sinuses.

the superior orbital fissure. Posteriorly, it is related to the tip of the petrous part of the temporal bone. Medially, it is related to the pituitary gland and sphenoid sinus, and it laterally extends up to the junction of the greater wing of the sphenoid bone.

Several important neurovascular structures cross the sinus and its lateral wall. The lateral wall is a double-layered dural structure with cranial nerves traversing it. The cranial nerves passing through its lateral wall from top to bottom are: the oculomotor nerve, the trochlear nerve, the ophthalmic division (V1), and the maxillary division (V2) of the trigeminal nerve. The ICA along with its sympathetic plexus and the abducent nerve (inferolateral to ICA) passes through the sinus (see ▶ Fig. 1.38).

The cavernous sinus is the site of venous confluences that receive tributaries from the orbit, the anterior and middle cranial fossae, and the sylvian fissure. The cavernous sinus drains via the superior and inferior petrosal sinuses into the internal jugular vein. Both cavernous sinuses are interconnected in the midline by the anterior and posterior intercavernous sinuses (see ▶ Fig. 1.33).

The tributaries of the cavernous sinus are:

- Superior ophthalmic vein.
- Inferior ophthalmic vein.
- Central vein of the retina.
- Sphenoparietal sinus.
- Middle meningeal vein.
- Superficial middle cerebral vein.
- Inferior cerebral vein.

Communications of the cavernous sinus are:

- With the opposite side via intercavernous sinuses.
- With the pterygoid venous plexus via emissary veins.
- With the facial vein via superior ophthalmic vein.
- With the internal vertebral venous plexuses via basilar plexus of veins.

The superior sagittal sinus, the straight sinus, and the right and left transverse sinuses merge, forming the confluence sinus.

The *inferior petrosal sinuses* are two sinuses that drain the cavernous sinus into the internal jugular vein, ending in the superior bulb of the internal jugular vein. These sinuses lie in a groove between the petrous apex and the clivus (see ▶ Fig. 1.25).

A variable junction between the inferior petrosal sinus and the jugular area is anatomically possible. In most cases, the junction is located at the level of the jugular bulb, but it may also be at the level of the anterior condylar vein, or at the level of the lower extracranial jugular vein; multiple junctions are also possible. Also, a direct junction between the inferior petrosal sinus and the vertebral venous plexus, or the absence of inferior petrosal sinus are described in literature.

The *superior petrosal sinus* receives blood from the cavernous sinus and it turns backwards and laterally to drain into the transverse sinus. The sinus runs along the margin of the tentorium cerebelli, in a groove in the petrous part of the temporal bone formed by the sinus itself—the superior petrosal sulcus (see ▶ Fig. 1.25).

The *transverse sinuses or lateral sinuses* (left and right lateral sinus) run laterally in a groove along the interior surface of the occipital bone. They drain from the confluence of sinuses (by the internal occipital protuberance) to the sigmoid sinuses, which ultimately connect to the internal jugular vein. Several veins and sinuses drain into the transverse sinuses like:

- Inferior cerebellar veins.
- Occipital veins.
- Temporal veins.
- Superior petrosal sinus.
- Straight sinus.
- Superior sagittal sinus.

In the majority of the cases, the right transverse sinus is a continuation of the superior sagittal sinus, whereas the left transverse sinus receives most of its supply from the straight sinus. Usually, the transverse sinuses are similar in size but an asymmetric size of transverse sinuses is present in about 15 to 20% of patients with the presence of a narrow size in one transverse sinus and a dominant size in the other (see ▶ Fig. 1.24c,d).

The *sigmoid sinus* represents the anteroinferior continuation of the transverse sinus. This sinus runs inferiorly, forming an S-shaped curve and it drains into the JF. Along its course, the sigmoid sinus also receives blood from the cerebral veins, cerebellar veins, diploic veins, and emissary veins.

1.11 Neck at the Base of Skull

Some surgical approaches to the lateral skull base require the anatomical knowledge of the upper portion of the neck close to the skull. Especially during the infratemporal approaches or the transtemporal approaches, if the isolation of the ICA and the internal jugular vein as lower cranial nerves in the neck is required, then the dissection of the neck is mandatory (see Chapters 2 and 6; also see ▶ Fig. 1.40, ▶ Fig. 1.41, ▶ Fig. 1.42, ▶ Fig. 1.43).

Around the skull base, we recognize some muscles, and vascular and nervous structures:

- Muscles:
  - Superficial layer:
    - Digastric muscle.
    - Stylohyoid muscle.
    - Sternocleidomastoid muscle.
  - Middle layer:
    - Levator scapulae muscle.
    - Splenius capitis muscle.

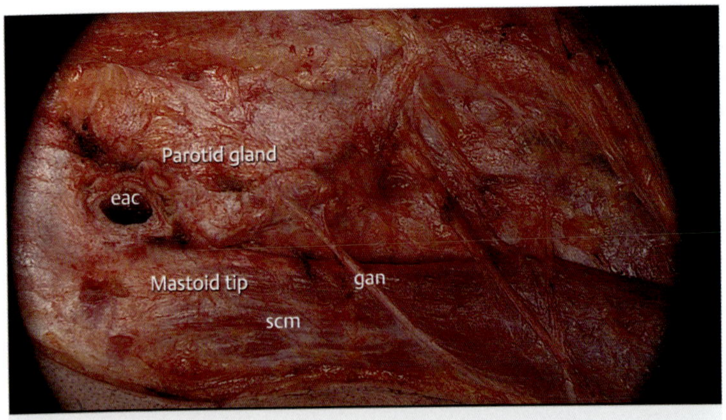

Fig. 1.40 Neck anatomy during an infratemporal approach (right side): The external auditory canal has been transected; the sternocleidomastoid muscle with the greater auricular nerve have been isolated. The parotid gland can be seen. *eac: external auditory canal; gan: greater auricular nerve; scm: sternocleidomastoid muscle.*

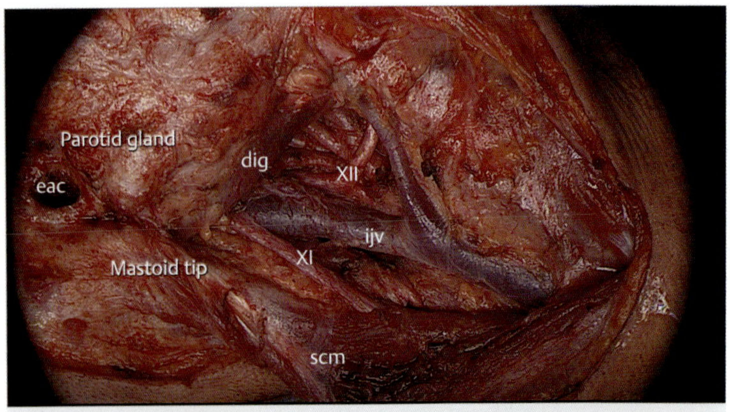

Fig. 1.41 Neck anatomy during an infratemporal approach (right side): The major vascular structures are isolated in the upper neck; the lower cranial nerves are detected. *dig: digastric muscle; eac: external auditory canal; ijv: internal jugular vein; scm: sternocleidomastoid muscle.*

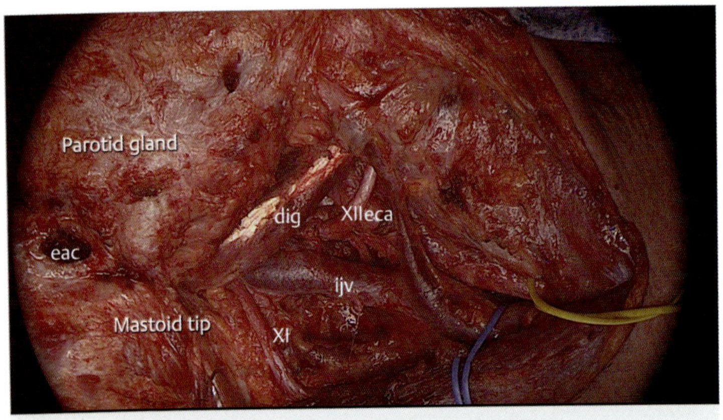

Fig. 1.42 Neck anatomy during an infratemporal approach (right side): The internal jugular vein and the common carotid artery are isolated and marked. *dig: digastric muscle; eac: external auditory canal; eca: external carotid artery; ijv: internal jugular vein.*

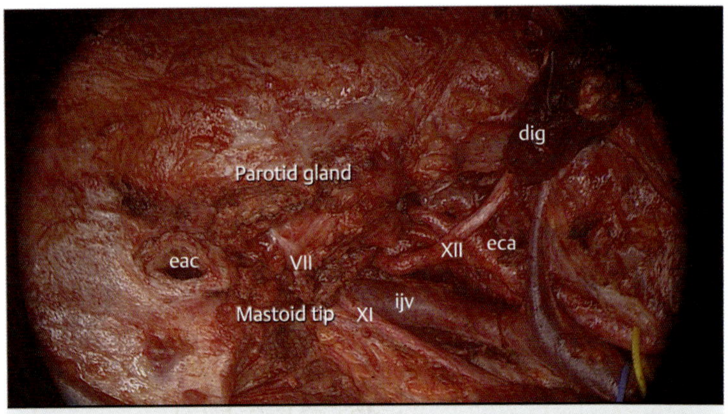

Fig. 1.43 Neck anatomy during an infratemporal approach (right side): The digastric muscle has been cut and the superficial parotid gland partially removed to recognize the extratemporal facial nerve at the level of the stylomastoid foramen. *dig: digastric muscle; eac: external auditory canal; eca: external carotid artery; ijv: internal jugular vein.*

    - Longissimus capitis muscle.
  - The deeper layer:
    - Obliquus capitis superior and inferior muscles attaching to the transverse process of the atlas.
- Vascular structures:
  - ICA.
  - External carotid artery and branches (superior thyroid artery, lingual artery, facial artery, occipital artery, posterior auricular artery, ascending pharyngeal artery, superficial temporal artery, and maxillary artery).
  - Internal jugular vein.
  - External jugular vein and branches.
  - Vertebral artery.
- Nervous structures:
  - Lower cranial nerves (IX, X, XI).
  - Cranial nerve XII.
  - Extratemporal cranial nerve VII running in the parotid gland.

1.12 Medial Wall of Tympanic Cavity: The Transcanal Door to the Fundus of the IAC

The tympanic cavity is an air-filled compartment surrounded by bone that is separated from the external ear by a thin tympanic membrane and it is in direct communication with the pharynx via the eustachian tube.

We recognize six borders located in the tympanic cavity (see ▶ Fig. 1.53):

- The lateral wall is formed by the tympanic membrane and by the scutum (the lateral bony wall of the epitympanum). It separates the tympanic cavity from the external auditory canal.
- The roof is formed by a thin bone from the petrous part of the temporal bone (tegmen tympani). It separates the middle ear from the middle cranial fossa.
- The floor consists of a thin layer of bone, which separates the middle ear from the jugular bulb of the internal jugular vein.
- The posterior wall consists of a bony partition between the tympanic cavity and the mastoid air cells. Superiorly, the aditus ad antrum is formed by a wide cell allowing for the connection between the posterior epitympanum and the mastoid cell system.
- The anterior wall is a thin bony plate with an opening represented by the eustachian tube. A second opening is represented by the canal for the tensor tympani muscle. This wall separates the middle ear from the ICA.
- The medial wall is formed by the lateral wall of the internal ear. It contains a prominent bulge, the promontory, with two openings, the fenestra vestibuli and the fenestra cochleae,

connecting respectively with the labyrinthine block and with the cochlea. The facial nerve runs in this wall.

The tympanic cavity can be divided into five subspaces. The mesotympanum is the space which is possible to visualize through the external auditory canal through the use of an otoscope or a microscope. The retrotympanum lies posteriorly, superiorly the epitympanum, anteriorly the protympanum, and inferiorly the hypotympanum.

Some important anatomical structures in the tympanic cavity are:

the ossicular chain with ligamentous folds; some nervous structures (the facial nerve, the chorda tympani nerve, Jacobson's nerve); a few muscular structures (the stapedius muscle, the tensor tympany muscle); and some major vascular structures (the ICA, the jugular bulb).

The medial wall of the tympanic cavity has a close relationship with the inner ear and with some lateral skull base areas lying in the petrous apex. For this reason, we can consider the tympanic cavity as a surgical door to reach the petrous apex and the IAC.

The removal of the ossicular chain and the stapes allows for the exposition of the medial wall of the vestibule and the spherical recess anteriorly (see ▶ Fig. 1.44, ▶ Fig. 1.45, ▶ Fig. 1.46, ▶ Fig. 1.47, ▶ Fig. 1.48, ▶ Fig. 1.49, ▶ Fig. 1.50, ▶ Fig. 1.51). The labyrinthine tract of the facial nerve as an imaginary line passing from the geniculate ganglion to the spherical recess just above the apical turn of the cochlea in fact shows where the facial nerve runs into the inner ear (see ▶ Fig. 1.52, ▶ Fig. 1.53, ▶ Fig. 1.54).

The vestibule is located between the tympanic cavity laterally and the IAC medially. The medial wall of the vestibule presents important anatomical landmarks—the spherical recess and the elliptical recess (see ▶ Fig. 1.51).

These two anatomical landmarks are two hollows in the medial vestibular wall separated by a bony ridge called the vestibular crest. This crest circumscribes the spherical recess and exhibits an inferior concavity.

The spherical recess is a microperforated bone area where the inferior vestibular nerve enters (it represents the superior cribriform macula). After the removal of the stapes, the most caudal portion of the medial vestibular wall and saccule is visible; the spherical recess is located in the anterior portion of the vestibule. The spherical recess separates the fundus of the IAC from the vestibule: it is a particularly fragile bone wall that is easily removable with a curette. Removing the spherical recess causes

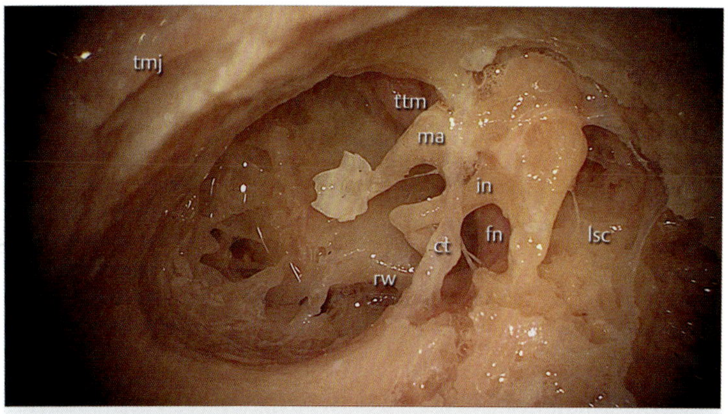

Fig. 1.44 Cadaveric dissection: Transcanal anatomy (left side). Once the skin of the external auditory canal and the eardrum were removed, the bony walls of external auditory canal were drilled exposing the tympanic cavity. *ct: chorda tympani; fn: tympanic segment of facial nerve; in: incus; lsc: lateral semicircular canal; ma: malleus; rw: round window; tmj: temporomandibular joint; ttm: tensor tympani muscle.*

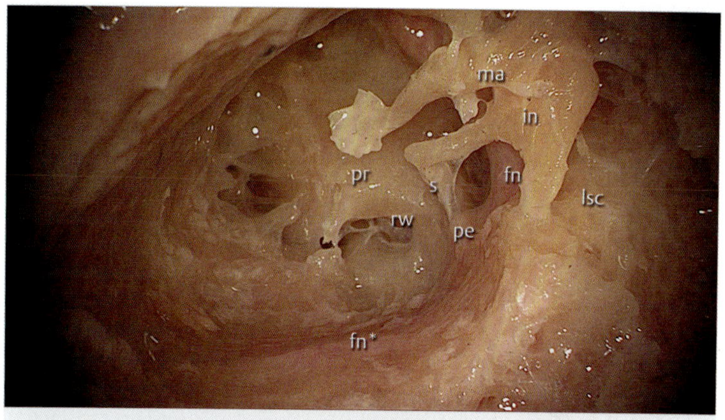

Fig. 1.45 Cadaveric dissection: Transcanal anatomy (left side). The mastoid portion of facial nerve is isolated. *fn*: mastoid segment of facial nerve; fn: tympanic segment of facial nerve; in: incus; lsc: lateral semicircular canal; ma: malleus; pe: pyramidal eminence; pr: promontory; rw: round window; s: stapes.*

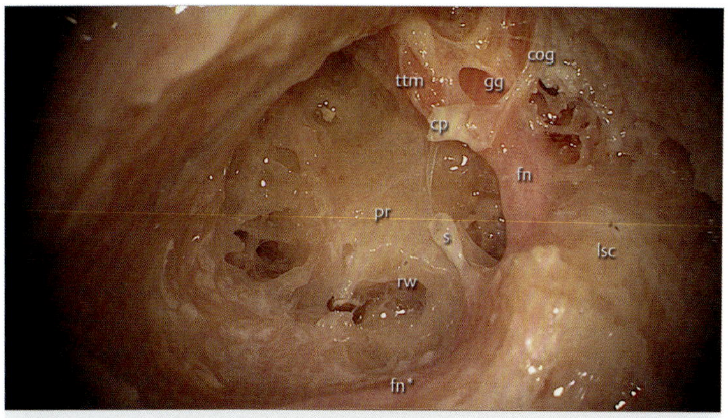

Fig. 1.46 Cadaveric dissection: Transcanal anatomy (left side). The incus and the malleus are removed. The facial nerve anatomy from geniculate ganglion to mastoid segment is visible. *cp: cochleariform process; fn*: mastoid segment of facial nerve; fn: tympanic segment of facial nerve; gg: geniculate ganglion; lsc: lateral semicircular canal; pr: promontory; rw: round window; s: stapes; ttm: tensor tympani muscle.*

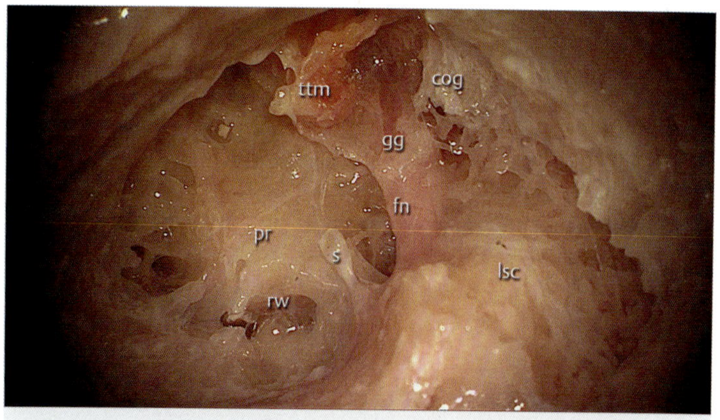

Fig. 1.47 Cadaveric dissection: Transcanal anatomy (left side). The tensor tympani muscle is removed from its canal, exposing the geniculate ganglion. *fn: tympanic segment of facial nerve; gg: geniculate ganglion; lsc: lateral semicircular canal; pr: promontory; rw: round window; s: stapes; ttm: tensor tympani muscle.*

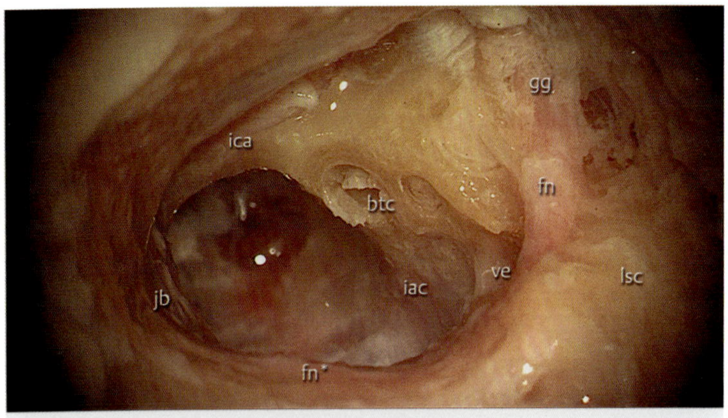

Fig. 1.48 Cadaveric dissection: Transcanal anatomy (left side). Once the stapes has been removed and the vertical internal carotid artery has been detected, the hypotympanic cells and the infracochlear cells are drilled. The basal turn of the cochlea is opened and the internal auditory canal (IAC) is skeletonized. The anatomical relationship between the IAC and the cochlea is noted through the transcanal route. *btc: basal turn of cochlea; fn*: mastoid segment of facial nerve; fn: tympanic segment of facial nerve; gg: geniculate ganglion; iac: internal auditory canal; ica: internal carotid artery; jb: jugular bulb; lsc: lateral semicircular canal; ve: vestibule.*

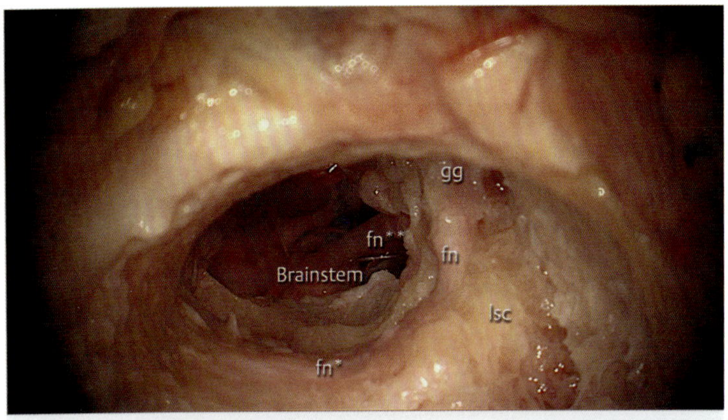

Fig. 1.50 Cadaveric dissection: Transcanal anatomy (left side). The dura of the internal auditory canal (IAC) and of the posterior cranial fossa are opened exposing the facial nerve until its exit zone in the brainstem. *fn: tympanic segment of facial nerve; fn*: mastoid segment of facial nerve; fn**: facial nerve into the cerebellopontine angle; gg: geniculate ganglion; lsc: lateral semicircular canal.*

cerebrospinal fluid (CSF) leakage in the patient because it creates a communication between the IAC and the middle ear and it also interrupts the inferior vestibular nerve.

The elliptical recess is smaller and it is located in a posterosuperior position to the spherical recess. It is an oval hollow on the utricle. This is a cribrose area adherent to the superior vestibular nerve. Viewing the elliptical recess using the endoscope is difficult due to its anatomical position: it is located cephalad to the plane passing through the tympanic portion of the facial nerve. This cribriform area is very thin and separates the superior portion of the IAC from the vestibule. Posteriorly to the elliptical recess, we can find the sulciform gutter (fossula sulciformis), which is a small cleft located in the most cranial portion of the vestibule's medial wall, beyond the elliptical recess and beneath the end of the common crus on the superior portion of the vestibule. The sulciform gutter has a slightly oblique course and it cranially deepens, creating a vestibular opening of the vestibular aqueduct.

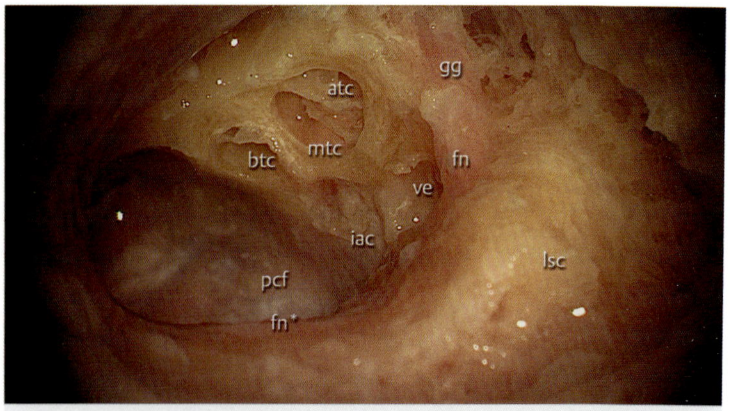

Fig. 1.49 Cadaveric dissection: Transcanal anatomy (left side). The promontory is drilled exposing the cochlear turns. *atc: apical turn of cochlea; btc: basal turn of cochlea; fn: tympanic segment of facial nerve; fn*: mastoid segment of facial nerve; gg: geniculate ganglion; iac: internal auditory canal; lsc: lateral semicircular canal; mtc: middle turn of cochlea; pcf: posterior cranial fossa dura; ve: vestibule.*

The cochlea is cone shaped and it is located almost horizontally in front of the vestibule; its apex (cupula) is directed forward and sideways, with a slight inclination downward, toward the upper and frontal parts of the labyrinthic wall of the tympanic cavity; its base corresponds to the bottom of the internal acoustic meatus, and it is perforated by several openings for the passage of the cochlear division of the acoustic nerve. It measures about 5 mm from its base to its apex, and its breadth across the base is about 9 mm. It consists of a cone-shaped central axis, the modiolus; a canal, the inner wall of which is formed by the central axis, wound spirally around it for 2 and three-fourth turns, from the base to the apex; and a delicate lamina, the osseous spiral lamina, which projects from the modiolus, and, following the windings of the canal, partially subdivides it into two. A membrane, termed the basilar membrane, stretches from the free border of this lamina to the outer wall of the bony cochlea and completely separates the canal into two passages, which, however, communicate with each other at the apex of the modiolus through a small opening named the helicotrema.

The first 3 to 4 mm of the basal turn of the cochlea is called the subvestibular portion of the cochlea because it is located beneath the vestibule under the oval window. Here it is separated from the vestibule by a cleft whose inner wall is formed by the last quarter of the first turn of the cochlea; this is the vestibulocochlear cleft. The next portion of the basal coil is carried anteriorly by the helicoid form of the cochlea. It closely approximates the floor of the fundus of the IAC. The base of the cochlea is in intimate relation with the lower portion of the fundus of the IAC via the tractus spiralis foraminosus. The latter is an opening in the cochlear area of the fundus of the internal acoustic meatus through which the fibers of the cochlear nerve leave the bony labyrinth to enter the IAC. This area is very thin and it is easily removed, thus allowing for the opening of the IAC in its more caudal portion and for the exposure of the cochlear nerve.

To reach the fundus of the IAC, the promontory should be removed, exposing the cochlear turns. A bony area between the cochlea and the vestibule is detected (the cochlear/vestibular bone). This bone separates the tympanic cavity from the fundus of the IAC. The cochlear vestibular bone is carefully removed to expose the fundus of the IAC (see ► Fig. 1.48, ► Fig. 1.49, ► Fig. 1.50). The removal of the cochlear-vestibular bone enables

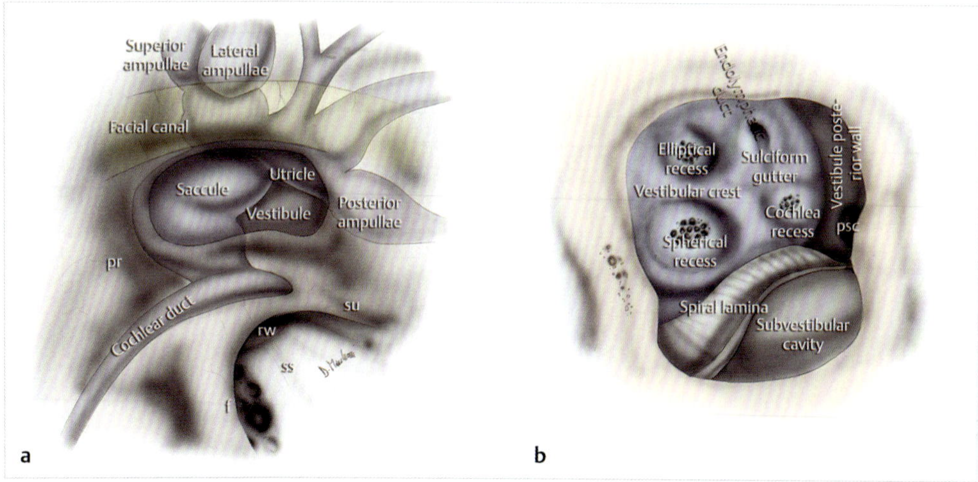

Fig. 1.51 **(a, b)** Left-side view of the oval window after stapes removal. Drawing showing the position of the saccule and the utricle in relation to the oval window. The saccule occupies the major anterior portion visible through the oval window in a lateral to medial direction. *f: finiculus; pr: promontory; psc: posterior semicircular canal opening; rw: round window; ss: sinus subtympanicus; su: subiculum.*

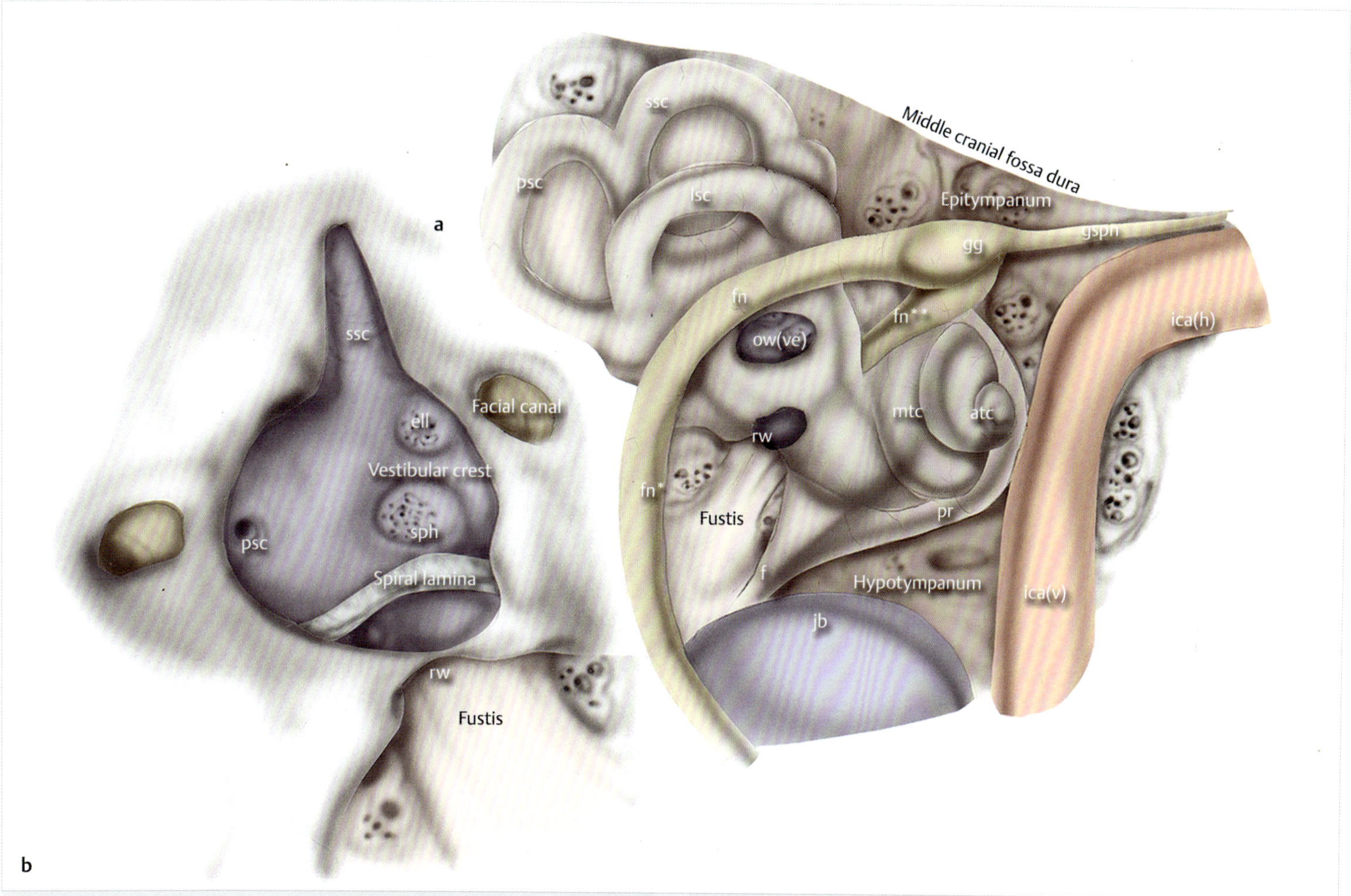

Fig. 1.52 Right side. **(a)** The most important anatomical structures lying on the medial wall of the tympanic cavity. It is important to note the position of labyrinthine facial nerve in the medial wall of the tympanic cavity; this segment of the facial nerve arises from the geniculate ganglion and runs just above the medial turn of cochlea, with an oblique orientation in a lateral to medial direction, inserting into the fundus of the internal auditory canal (IAC). **(b)** The oval window has been enlarged, removing the tympanic facial nerve to see the whole medial wall of the vestibule. We can note the relationship between the spherical and the elliptical recesses. The spherical recess is represented by a cribrose plate where the inferior vestibular nerve is inserted; the elliptical recess looks smaller and it is represented by a cribrose plate where the superior vestibular nerve is inserted. Inferiorly enlarging the oval window allows one to see the osseous spiral lamina. This is the line of separation between the vestibule and the cochlea. *atc: apical turn of cochlea; ell: elliptical recess; f: finiculus; fn: tympanic segment of facial nerve; fn*: mastoid segment of facial nerve; fn**: labyrinthine portion of facial nerve; gg: geniculate ganglion; gspn: greater superficial petrosal nerve; ica(h): horizontal portion of internal carotid artery; ica(v): vertical portion of internal carotid artery; jb: jugular bulb; lsc: lateral semicircular canal; mtc: middle turn of cochlea; ow(ve): oval window, view of the vestibule; pr: promontory; psc: posterior semicircular canal; rw: round window; sph: spherical recess; ssc: superior semicircular canal.*

the surgeon to expose the cochlear nerve in the superficial and anterior position with its insertion to the cochlea easily visible. The inferior vestibular nerve with its insertion to the spherical recess is located in a superficial and posterior position, while the facial nerve runs deep anterosuperiorly. Through the opening of the cochlear-vestibular bone, the facial nerve is seen on a deeper plane between the cochlear and inferior vestibular nerves (see ▶ Fig. 1.55).

The IAC has a slight oblique orientation from an anterior to a posterior and from a superior to an inferior direction, especially

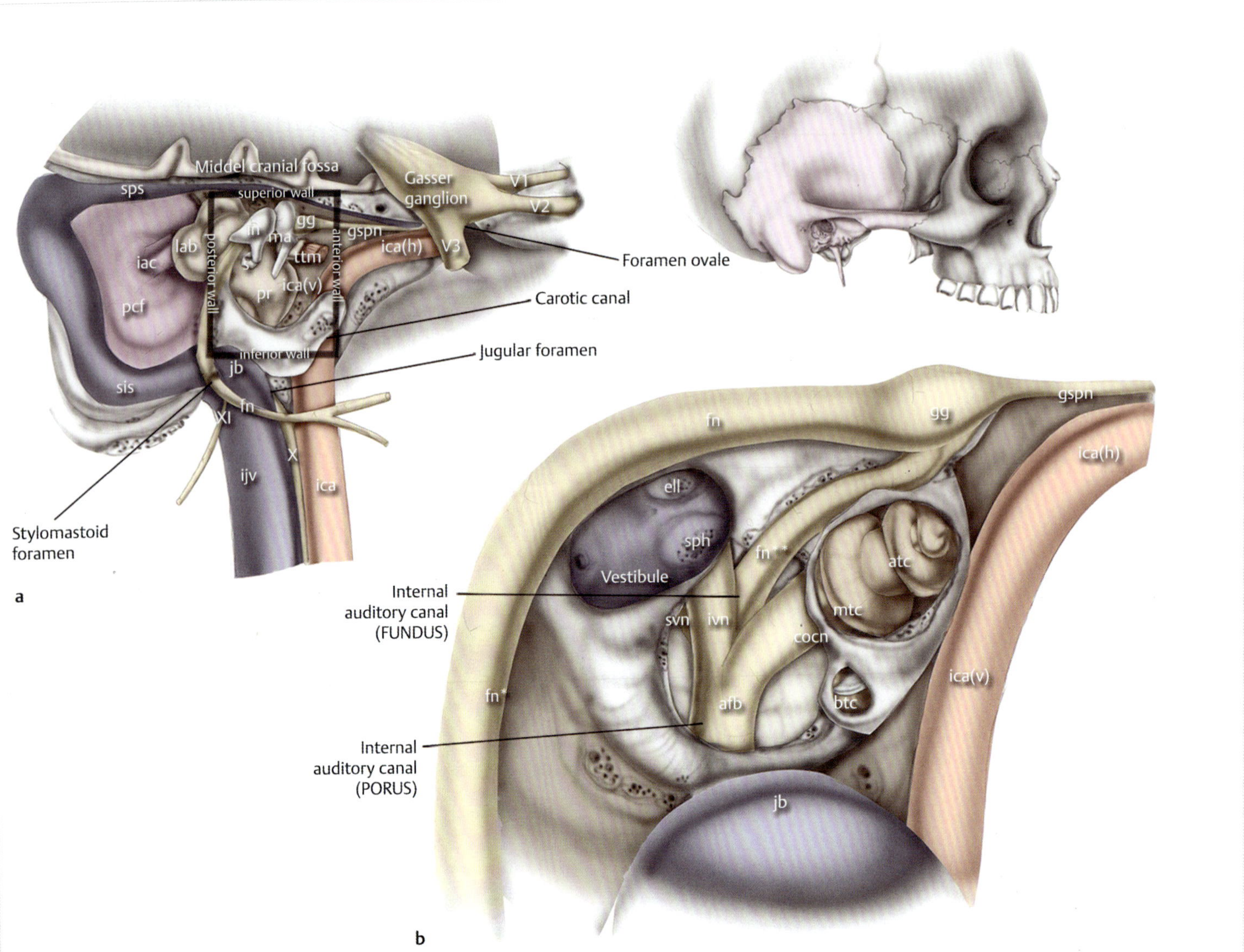

Fig. 1.53 (Right side) **(a)** Walls of the tympanic cavity in relation to the temporal bone and its contents. **(b)** Medial wall of the tympanic cavity after the removal of the promontory. The drawing represents the anatomy of the internal auditory canal (IAC) from the fundus to the porus during a transcanal approach. The anatomical relationship between the facial nerve, the cochlear nerve, and the vestibular nerves and the IAC can be seen. *afb: acoustic-facial bundle; atc: apical turn of cochlea; btc: basal turn of cochlea; cocn: cochlear nerve; ell: elliptical recess; fn: facial nerve; fn*: mastoid segment of facial nerve; fn**: facial nerve into the IAC; gg: geniculate ganglion; gspn: greater superficial petrosal nerve; iac: internal auditory canal; ica: internal carotid artery; ica(h): horizontal portion of internal carotid artery; ica(v): vertical portion of internal carotid artery; ijv: internal jugular vein; in: incus; ivn: inferior vestibular nerve; jb: jugular bulb; lab: labyrinthine block; ma: malleus; mtc: middle turn of cochlea; pcf: posterior cranial fossa; pr: promontory; s: stapes; sis: sigmoid sinus; sph: spherical recess; sps: superior petrosal sinus; svn: superior vestibular nerve; ttm: tensor tympani muscle.*

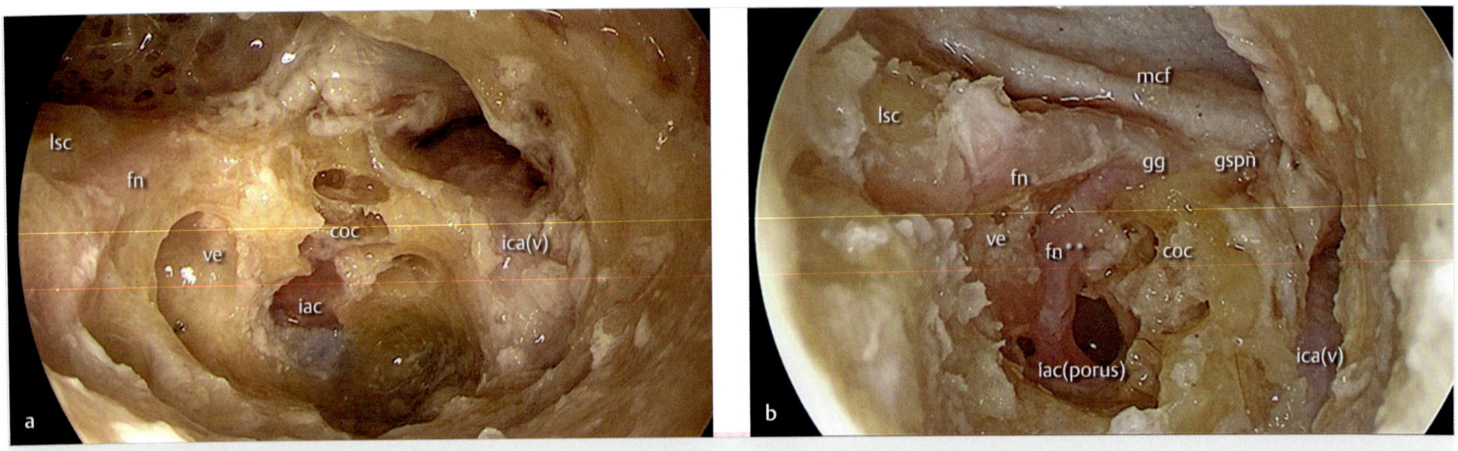

Fig. 1.54 Transcanal transpromontorial approach to the internal auditory canal (IAC) (right side). **(a)** The ossicular chain was removed, the vestibule opening is seen, and the cochlear turns are exposed; the IAC is skeletonized in the fundus. **(b)** The IAC dura is cut, exposing the facial nerve from the tympanic segment to the porus. *coc: cochlea; fn: tympanic segment of facial nerve; fn**: facial nerve into the IAC; gg: geniculate ganglion; gspn: greater superficial petrosal nerve; iac: internal auditory canal; ica(v): vertical portion of internal carotid artery; lsc: lateral semicircular canal; mcf: middle cranial fossa dura; ve: vestibule.*

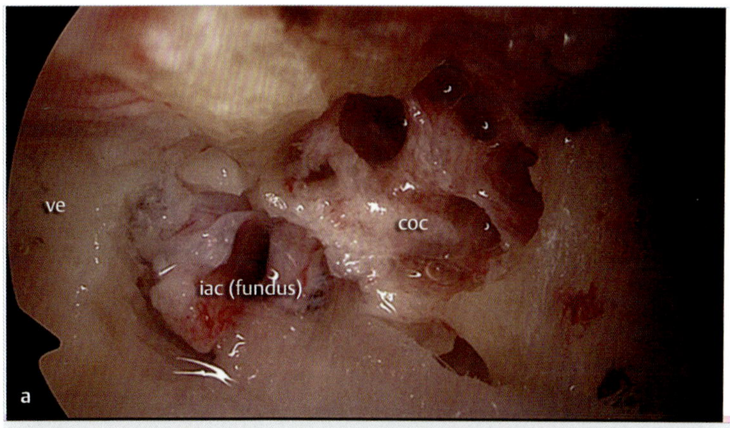

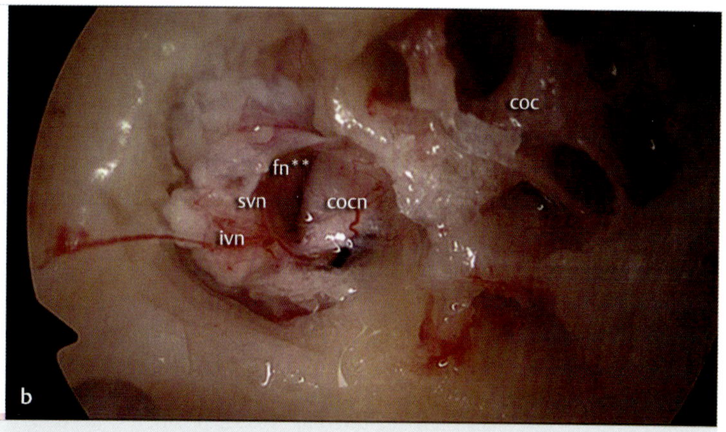

Fig. 1.55 (a, b) Right side: Internal auditory canal (IAC) during a transcanal transpromontorial approach. The anatomical relationship between the facial nerve, the cochlear nerve, and the vestibular nerves can be noticed in the fundus of the IAC through the transpromontorial surgical route. *coc: cochlea; cocn: cochlear nerve; fn**: facial nerve into the IAC; iac: internal auditory canal; ivn: inferior vestibular nerve; svn: superior vestibular nerve; ve: vestibule.*

from the most lateral anterior/superior portion lying close to the cochlear-vestibular bone in the fundus, to the medial posterior inferior portion, lying in the porus, in relation to the dura of the posterior fossa.

The posterior fossa dura may be reached through the medial wall of the tympanic cavity, by drilling the promontory and the skeletonized IAC, from the fundus to the porus. The opening of the dura of the posterior fossa at this level enables the surgeon to gain access to the CPA in front of the exit zone of the acoustic-facial bundle from the brainstem (see ▶ Fig. 1.50).

Suggested Readings

Avci E, Dagtekin A, Akture E, Uluc K, Baskaya MK. Microsurgical anatomy of the vein of Labbé. Surg Radiol Anat. 2011; 33(7):569–573

Belal A, Jr. Retrolabyrinthine surgery: anatomy and pathology. Am J Otol. 1986; 7 (1):29–33

Bouthillier A, van Loveren HR, Keller JT. Segments of the internal carotid artery: a new classification. Neurosurgery. 1996; 38(3):425–432, discussion 432–433

Brackmann DE. The facial nerve in the infratemporal approach. Otolaryngol Head Neck Surg. 1987; 97(1):15–17

Bryant L, Goodmurphy CW, Han JK. Endoscopic and three-dimensional radiographic imaging of the pterygopalatine and infratemporal fossae: improving surgical landmarks. Ann Otol Rhinol Laryngol. 2014; 123(2):111–116

Cokkeser Y, Aristegui M, Naguib MB, Saleh E, Taibah AK, Sanna M. Identification of internal acoustic canal in the middle cranial fossa approach: a safe technique. Otolaryngol Head Neck Surg. 2001; 124(1):94–98

Cruz OLM. Surgical anatomy of the lateral skull base. In: Cummings Otolaryngology Head and Neck Surgery, 5th ed. Philadelphia, PA: Mosby, Elsevier; 2010:2434–2441

Day JD, Kellogg JX, Tschabitscher M, Fukushima T. Surface and superficial surgical anatomy of the posterolateral cranial base: significance for surgical planning and approach. Neurosurgery. 1996; 38(6):1079–1083, discussion 1083–1084

Dew LA, Shelton C, Harnsberger HR, Thompson BG, Jr. Surgical exposure of the petrous internal carotid artery: practical application for skull base surgery. Laryngoscope. 1997; 107(7):967–976

Dichiro G, Fisher RL, Nelson KB. The jugular foramen. J Neurosurg. 1964; 21:447–460

Domb GH, Chole RA. Anatomical studies of the posterior petrous apex with regard to hearing preservation in acoustic neuroma removal. Laryngoscope. 1980; 90(11 Pt 1):1769–1776

Dolenc VV. Microsurgical Anatomy and Surgery of the Central Skull Base. New York, NY: Springer-Verlag; 2003

Donald PJ. Infratemporal fossa-middle cranial fossa approach. In: Donald PJ, ed. Surgery of the Skull Base. Philadelphia, PA: Lippincott Raven; 1998:309-39

Donaldson A, Duckert LG, Lambert PM, Rubel EW. Anson & Donaldson: Surgical Anatomy of the Temporal Bone. New York, NY: Raven Press; 1992

Fisch U, Esslen E. Total intratemporal exposure of the facial nerve: pathologic findings in Bell's palsy. Arch Otolaryngol. 1972; 95(4):335–341

Fisch U, Fagan P, Valavanis A. The infratemporal fossa approach for the lateral skull base. Otolaryngol Clin North Am. 1984; 17(3):513–552

Fisch U, Mattox D. Microsurgery of the Skull Base. New York, NY: Thieme Medical Publishers; 1988

Geurkink NA. Surgical anatomy of the temporal bone posterior to the internal auditory canal: an operative approach. Laryngoscope. 1977; 87(6):975–986

Gibo H, Lenkey C, Rhoton AL, Jr. Microsurgical anatomy of the supraclinoid portion of the internal carotid artery. J Neurosurg. 1981; 55(4):560–574

Hacein-Bey L, Daniels DL, Ulmer JL, et al. The ascending pharyngeal artery: branches, anastomoses, and clinical significance. AJNR Am J Neuroradiol. 2002; 23 (7):1246–1256

Harris FS, Rhoton AL. Anatomy of the cavernous sinus: a microsurgical study. J Neurosurg. 1976; 45(2):169–180

Irish JC, Gullane PJ, Gentili F, et al. Tumors of the skull base: outcome and survival analysis of 77 cases. Head Neck. 1994; 16(1):3–10

Joo W, Yoshioka F, Funaki T, Mizokami K, Rhoton AL, Jr. Microsurgical anatomy of the trigeminal nerve. Clin Anat. 2014; 27(1):61–88

Khonsary SA, Ma Q, Villablanca P, Emerson J, Malkasian D. Clinical functional anatomy of the pterygopalatine ganglion, cephalgia and related dysautonomias: a review. Surg Neurol Int. 2013; 4 Suppl 6:S422–S428

Kveton JF, Cooper MH. Microsurgical anatomy of the jugular foramen region. Am J Otol. 1988; 9(2):109–112

Lang J. Clinical Anatomy of the Posterior Cranial Fossa and Its Foramina. New York, NY: Thieme; 1991

Lang J, Jr, Samii A. Retrosigmoidal approach to the posterior cranial fossa: an anatomical study. Acta Neurochir (Wien). 1991; 111(3–4):147–153

Lang J. Topographical anatomy of the skull base and adjacent tissues. In: Scheunemann H, Schurmann K, Helms J, eds. Tumors of the Skull Base. Berlin, NY: Walter de Gruyter; 1986:3-28

Leonetti JP, Smith PG, Linthicum FH. The petrous carotid artery: anatomic relationships in skull base surgery. Otolaryngol Head Neck Surg. 1990; 102(1):3–12

Marchioni D, Alicandri-Ciufelli M, Mattioli F, et al. From external to internal auditory canal: surgical anatomy by an exclusive endoscopic approach. Eur Arch Otorhinolaryngol. 2013; 270(4):1267–1275

Marchioni D, Alicandri-Ciufelli M, Piccinini A, et al. Surgical anatomy of transcanal endoscopic approach to the tympanic facial nerve. Laryngoscope. 2011; 121 (7):1565–1573

Marchioni D, Alicandri-Ciufelli M, Rubini A, Masotto B, Pavesi G, Presutti L. Exclusive endoscopic transcanal transpromontorial approach: a new perspective for internal auditory canal vestibular schwannoma treatment. J Neurosurg. 2017; 126 (1):98–105

Marchioni D, Alicandri-Ciufelli M, Rubini A, Presutti L. Endoscopic transcanal corridors to the lateral skull base: initial experiences. Laryngoscope. 2015; 125 Suppl 5:S1–S13

Marchioni D, Soloperto D, Rubini A, Nogueira JF, Badr-El-Dine M, Presutti L. Endoscopic facial nerve surgery. Otolaryngol Clin North Am. 2016; 49(5):1173–1187

Maurer J, Pelster H, Amedee RG, Mann WJ. Intraoperative monitoring of motor cranial nerves in skull base surgery. Skull Base Surg. 1995; 5(3):169–175

Parisier SC. The middle cranial fossa approach to the internal auditory canal—an anatomical study stressing critical distances between surgical landmarks. Laryngoscope. 1977; 87(4 Pt 2) Suppl 4:1–20

Perese DM. Superficial veins of the brain from a surgical point of view. J Neurosurg. 1960; 17:402–412

Renn WH, Rhoton AL, Jr. Microsurgical anatomy of the sellar region. J Neurosurg. 1975; 43(3):288–298

Rhoton AL, Jr, Buza R. Microsurgical anatomy of the jugular foramen. J Neurosurg. 1975; 42(5):541–550

Rhoton AL, Jr. Jugular foramen. Neurosurgery. 2000; 47(3) Suppl:S267–S285

Rhoton AL, Jr. Microsurgical anatomy of the brainstem surface facing an acoustic neuroma. Surg Neurol. 1986; 25(4):326–339

Rhoton AL, Jr. The cavernous sinus, the cavernous venous plexus, and the carotid collar. Neurosurgery. 2002; 51(4) Suppl:S375–S410

Rhoton AL, Jr. The cerebellopontine angle and posterior fossa cranial nerves by the retrosigmoid approach. Neurosurgery. 2000; 47(3) Suppl:S93–S129

Rhoton AL, Jr. The cerebral veins. Neurosurgery. 2002; 51(4) Suppl:S159–S205

Rhoton ALJ. Anatomy of the pituitary gland and sellar region. In: Thapar K, Kovacs K, Scheithauer BW, Lloyd RV, eds. Diagnosis and Management of Pituitary Tumors. Totowa, NJ: Humana Press; 2000:13–40

Sanna M, De Donato G, Taibah A, Russo A, Falcioni M, Mancini F. Infratemporal fossa approaches to the lateral skull base. Keio J Med. 1999; 48(4):189–200

Sekhar LN, Estonillo R. Transtemporal approach to the skull base: an anatomical study. Neurosurgery. 1986; 19(5):799–808

Silva PS, Vilarinho A, Carvalho B, Vaz R. Anatomical variations of the vein of Labbé: an angiographic study. Surg Radiol Anat. 2014; 36(8):769–773

Tanriover N, Abe H, Rhoton AL, Jr, Kawashima M, Sanus GZ, Akar Z. Microsurgical anatomy of the superior petrosal venous complex: new classifications and implications for subtemporal transtentorial and retrosigmoid suprameatal approaches. J Neurosurg. 2007; 106(6):1041–1050

Ulm AJ, Quiroga M, Russo A, et al. Normal anatomical variations of the V_3 segment of the vertebral artery: surgical implications. J Neurosurg Spine. 2010; 13 (4):451–460

Watanabe A, Nagaseki Y, Ohkubo S, et al. Anatomical variations of the ten triangles around the cavernous sinus. Clin Anat. 2003; 16(1):9–14

Watanabe T, Igarashi T, Fukushima T, Yoshino A, Katayama Y. Anatomical variation of superior petrosal vein and its management during surgery for cerebellopontine angle meningiomas. Acta Neurochir (Wien). 2013; 155(10):1871–1878

Chapter 2

Microscopic Approaches to Lateral Skull Base: Overview

2

2 Microscopic Approaches to Lateral Skull Base: Overview

Daniele Marchioni, Mohamed Badr El Dine, Luca Bianconi, and Daniele Bernardeschi

Abstract

Recent innovations in the surgical techniques and an improved knowledge of anatomy have led to a safe removal of lateral skull base tumors, with acceptable morbidity and mortality rates. However, the selection of the approach still represents a matter of debate among surgeons, with several pathways being developed through the years. The most widely used approaches used to reach lesions located in the lateral skull base are the transpetrous routes (translabyrinthine, retrolabyrinthine, transotic, transcochlear approaches), the retrosigmoid route, the middle cranial fossa approach, and the infratemporal approaches. The aim of this chapter is to classify these approaches according to their relationship to the otic capsule, and showcase indications for their use focusing on the translabyrinthine approach, retrolabyrinthine approach, and infratemporal approaches. After a thorough description of the surgical technique with the aid of multiple images to aid adequate understanding of the surgical steps, for each approach a "hints and tips" session will offer the experts' insight. Furthermore, indications on the role of the endoscope as an aid in each of the approaches have been added to the chapter.

Keywords: lateral skull base, translabyrinthine approach, retrolabyrinthine approach, infratemporal approach, microscopic approach, cerebellopontine angle surgery

2.1 Introduction

Until recently skull base surgery was considered "no man's land" because of the highly complex anatomy and even more perplexing morphological organization of the contained neurovascular structures coupled with a plethora of pathological conditions encountered in this region.

Because of the continuous exciting and promising innovations in skull base surgery, tumors that were once thought to be most difficult and surgically unapproachable are now becoming safely manageable with reasonable morbidity and mortality rates.

However, the selection of the proper approach is a great challenge for both neurosurgeons and otologists. Approaches must be individualized and tailored according to the patient's clinical condition, the size of the tumor, and the status of the patient's audiometry. The surgeon's skills and preference are paramount in the final choice of the approach. Over the years, several different surgical approaches with many modifications and combinations have been developed. The main requirement of any approach is to ensure total tumor removal with the lowest morbidity rate. The access must be sufficient to allow the surgeon a complete control over any possible bleeding but with minimum trauma to the brain and neural structures.

Advanced tumors involve several anatomic zones that are often surgically approached by various specialties. Therefore, a multidisciplinary surgical team is needed for optimal execution of these technically difficult surgical approaches and to achieve the lowest possible morbidity and the best results.

Lateral skull base approaches have been principally created to address intracranial pathologies involving the posterior and middle cranial fossae. These approaches can provide access inferiorly to the infratemporal fossa and posteriorly to the craniovertebral junction. Also, major extracranial pathology such as diseases of the temporal bone can be reached by lateral skull base approaches.

The lateral skull base constitutes an anatomic boundary between the fields of neurosurgery and otolaryngology. Surgery in this region has always been a challenge for both disciplines owing to the presence of important anatomical structures such as the internal carotid artery, the otic capsule, and the facial nerve. Several approaches have been developed to reach a pathological process located in the lateral skull base and in the fundus of the internal auditory canal (IAC) and petrous apex. Despite the benign nature and limited dimensions of the lesions located in this anatomical region, extensive surgical approaches are often required to reach and remove the disease. The transpetrous routes (translabyrinthine, transotic, and transcochlear approaches), the retrosigmoid route, and the middle cranial fossa approach are the most widely used routes to reach lateral skull base lesions. All of these approaches are open and based on the use of a microscope. More recently, endoscopic surgical procedures for lateral skull base lesions have been introduced. At present, these procedures are indicated just for lesions with limited dimension located in the lateral skull base/inner ear, lying on the same line as the external auditory canal (see Chapter 9).

Considering all the surgical procedures, lateral skull base approaches can be classified according to the surgical route related to the otic capsule. We can distinguish approaches passing through the otic capsule, and approaches with a conservative attitude to the otic capsule.

- ***Approaches passing through the otic capsule***
  The sacrifice of hearing function is necessary with these approaches:
  - Translabyrinthine approach
  - Transcochlear/transotic approaches
  - Transcanal/transpromontorial approaches
- ***Approaches preserving the otic capsule***
  - Middle cranial fossa (passing above the otic capsule)
  - Transcanal suprageniculate approach (passing above the otic capsule)
  - Retrosigmoid approach (passing behind the otic capsule)
  - Retrolabyrinthine approach (passing behind the otic capsule)
  - Transcanal infracochlear approach (passing behind the otic capsule)
  - Infratemporal fossa Type A (passing inferiorly to the otic capsule)
  - Petro-occipital transsigmoid (POTS) (passing inferiorly to the otic capsule)
  - Infratemporal fossa Types B, C, and D (passing anteriorly to the otic capsule)

In this chapter, we will describe the main surgical approaches to the lateral skull base using a microscopic procedure. Transcochlear-transotic approaches and transcanal (transpromontorial, suprageniculate, infracochlear) approaches, such as retrosigmoid and middle cranial fossa approaches, are not included in this chapter since they are described in apposite chapters (see Chapters 6, 7, 8, 10, 11, and 13).

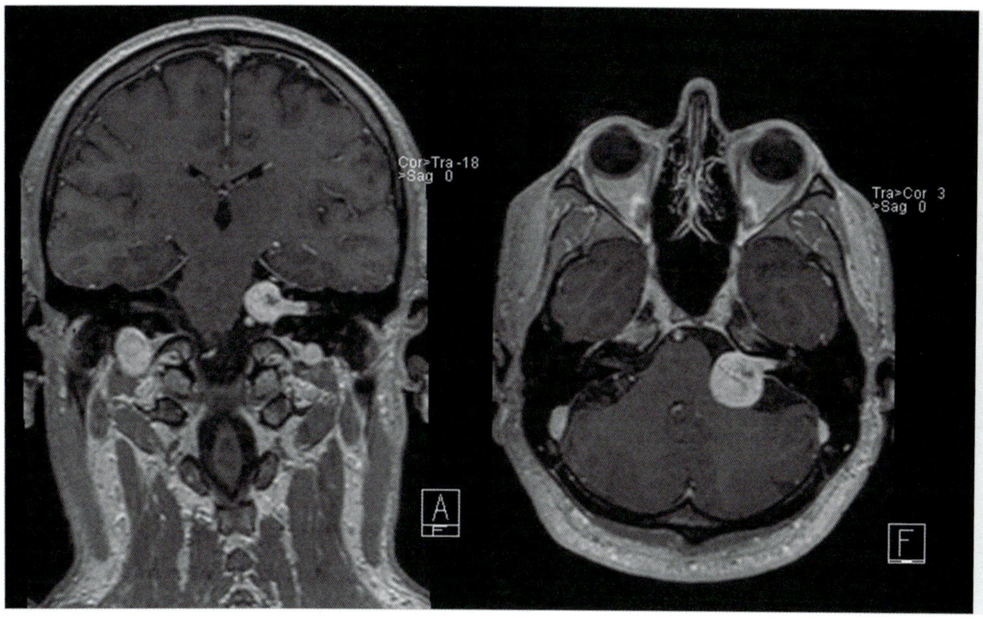

Fig. 2.1 Magnetic resonance imaging (MRI) study: Typical indication for a translabyrinthine approach, acoustic neuroma with internal auditory canal (IAC) and cerebellopontine angle (CPA) involvement.

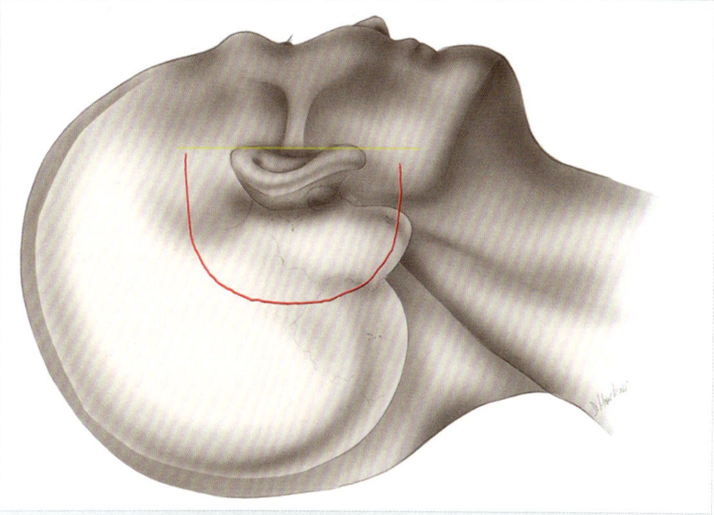

Fig. 2.2 The incision (*red line*) is made approximately 4 cm behind the retroauricular sulcus. An imaginary line (*yellow line*) passing anteriorly to the external auditory canal (EAC) defines the anterior ending of the incision.

2.2 Translabyrinthine Approach

2.2.1 Indications

Cerebellopontine angle (CPA) tumors with or without IAC involvement (acoustic neuroma, meningioma, epidermoid or dermoid tumors) with unserviceable hearing (see ▶ Fig. 2.1).

2.2.2 Advantages

- Direct approach to the IAC and CPA avoiding cerebellar retraction.
- Direct exposure of the facial nerve in the fundus of the IAC.

2.2.3 Limitations

- The middle fossa, sigmoid sinus, and jugular bulb are the anatomical limits of this approach.
- The sacrifice of the hearing function is mandatory since this approach passes through the otic capsule.

2.2.4 The Use of the Endoscope

In this technique, endoscopic-assisted surgery is not necessary because of good control of the CPA and IAC. Only in case of epidermoid lesion is the use of the endoscope at the end of the microscopical resection of the tumor recommended in order to detect any residual disease in the CPA and temporal bone surface.

2.2.5 Surgical Approach (see also Clinical Case 1)

The patient is placed in a supine position with the head turned to the contralateral side; a facial nerve monitoring is always used.

A C-shaped incision is made approximately 4 cm behind the retroauricular sulcus (▶ Fig. 2.2). A muscle and periosteal flap is elevated to uncover the occipitomastoid bone (▶ Fig. 2.3 and ▶ Fig. 2.4). An enlarged mastoidectomy is started detecting the dura of the middle cranial fossa superiorly and the sigmoid sinus posteroinferiorly; the posterior auditory canal is gently skeletonized (▶ Fig. 2.5). The mastoid cells are removed between the middle cranial fossa and the sigmoid sinus exposing the antrum and the short process of the incus. The labyrinthine block is also exposed. Inferiorly, the cells around the sigmoid sinus and the tip of the mastoid with the digastric ridge are also detected. A further drilling anteriorly to the sigmoid sinus allows the exposure of the posterior fossa dura so as to detect the mastoid segment of the facial nerve. The digastric ridge is used as a landmark to detect the most inferior portion of the facial nerve in the mastoid

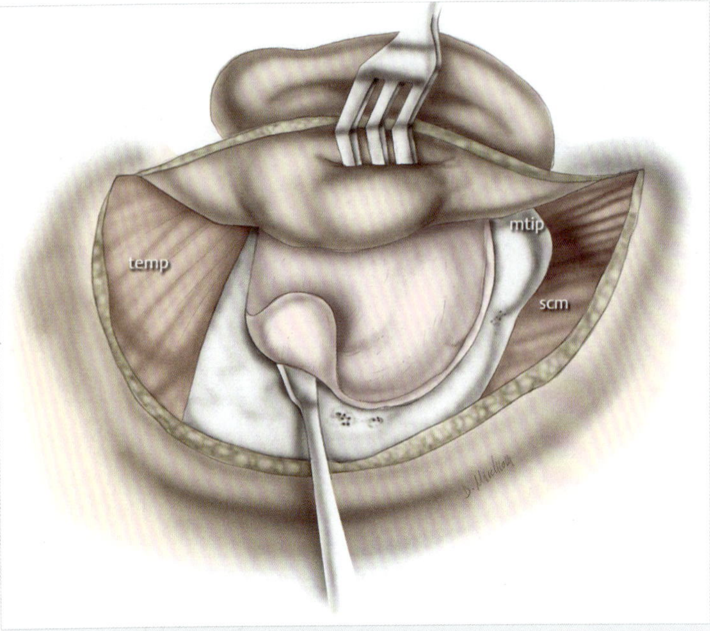

Fig. 2.3 Right side: After skin flap elevation, the periosteal flap is elevated to uncover the occipitomastoid bone. *mtip: mastoid tip; scm: sternocleidomastoid muscle; temp: temporalis muscle.*

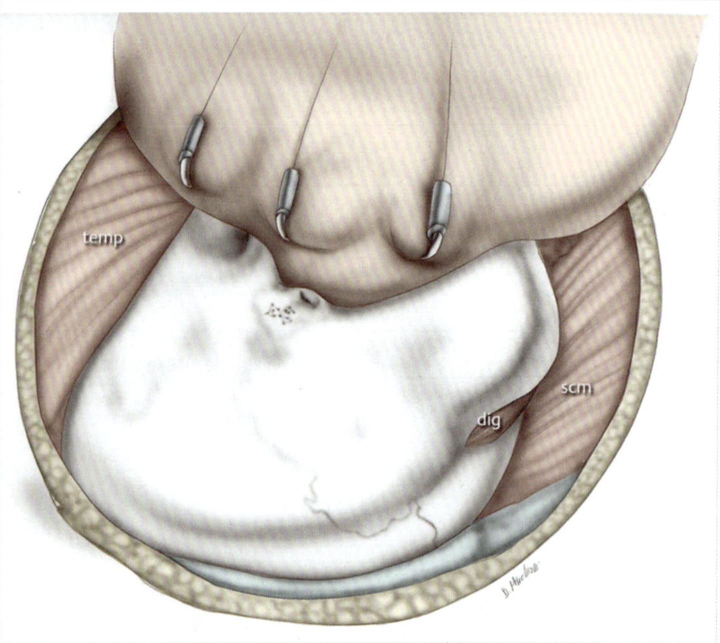

Fig. 2.4 Right side: The occipitomastoid bone is exposed; the posterior wall of the external auditory canal (EAC) is detected with Henle's spine. *dig: digastric muscle; scm: sternocleidomastoid muscle; temp: temporalis muscle.*

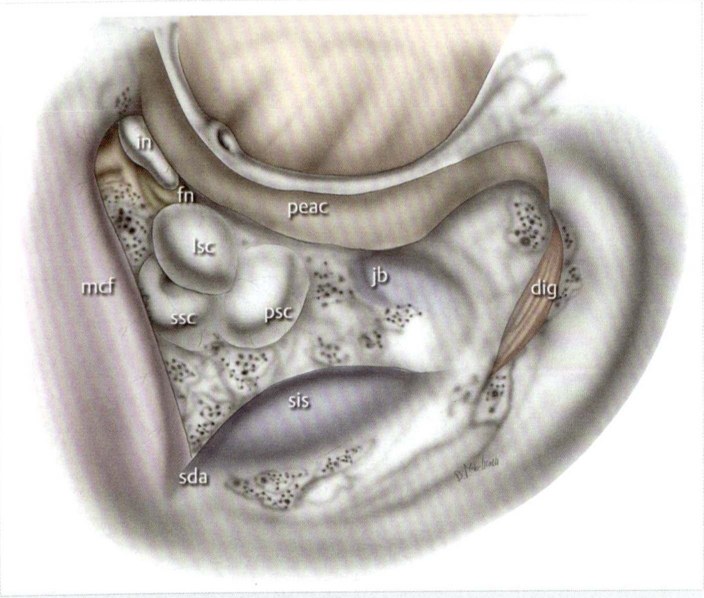

Fig. 2.5 Right side: A wide mastoidectomy is performed exposing the anatomical landmarks. *dig: digastric muscle; fn: facial nerve; in: incus; jb: jugular bulb; lsc: lateral semicircular canal; mcf: middle cranial fossa; peac: posterior wall of external auditory canal; psc: posterior semicircular canal; sda: sinodural angle; sis: sigmoid sinus; ssc: superior semicircular canal.*

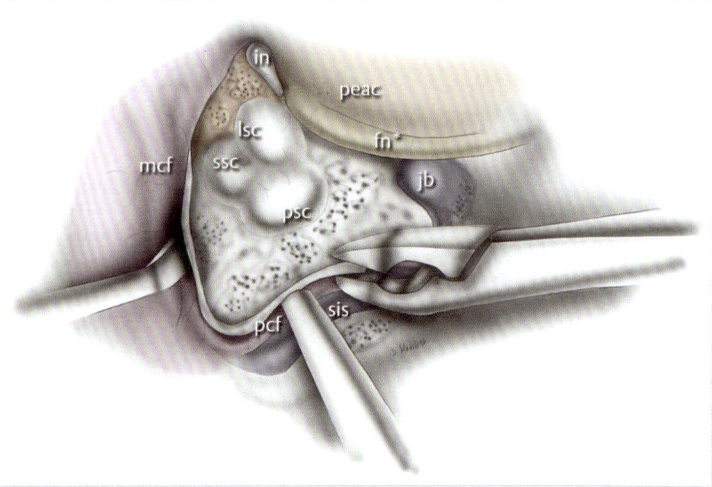

Fig. 2.6 Right side: The dura of posterior and middle cranial fossae is gently detached from the mastoid bone. The bone is removed using a rongeur. *fn*: mastoid segment of facial nerve; in: incus; jb: jugular bulb; lsc: lateral semicircular canal; mcf: middle cranial fossa; pcf: posterior cranial fossa; peac: posterior wall of external auditory canal; psc: posterior semicircular canal; sis: sigmoid sinus; ssc: superior semicircular canal.*

close to the styloid foramen (▶ Fig. 2.6 and ▶ Fig. 2.7). After facial nerve detection, the sigmoid sinus is skeletonized inferiorly and under the facial nerve until the jugular bulb is visible, representing the inferior limit of the transtemporal approach to the IAC and CPA. All the mastoid cells between the sigmoid sinus and the labyrinthine block are removed exposing the endolymphatic sac just behind the posterior semicircular canal (▶ Fig. 2.7). If necessary, the second genu of the facial nerve and the chorda timpani are skeletonized (see Clinical Case 1 ▶ Fig. 2.33 and ▶ Fig. 2.34) and a posterior tympanotomy is performed between the corda tympani and the facial nerve, detecting the incudostapedial joint and the round window niche (see Clinical Case 1 ▶ Fig. 2.34). This procedure is not necessary during a traditional translabyrinthine approach but it is mandatory if a cochlear implant is simultaneously required (see Clinical Case 2), the tympanic segment of the facial nerve is exposed until the geniculate ganglion and the anatomical relationship between the labyrinthine and the facial nerve is clearly visible (see Clinical Case 1 ▶ Fig. 2.36). A labyrinthectomy is then performed and the lateral, superior, and posterior canals are opened exposing the ampullas (▶ Fig. 2.8 and ▶ Fig. 2.9). Further drilling on the canals allows a deeper exposition of the vestibule which is an important landmark for the fundus of the IAC (▶ Fig. 2.10, ▶ Fig. 2.11, ▶ Fig. 2.12). The drilling of the vestibule starts under the control of the facial nerve in order

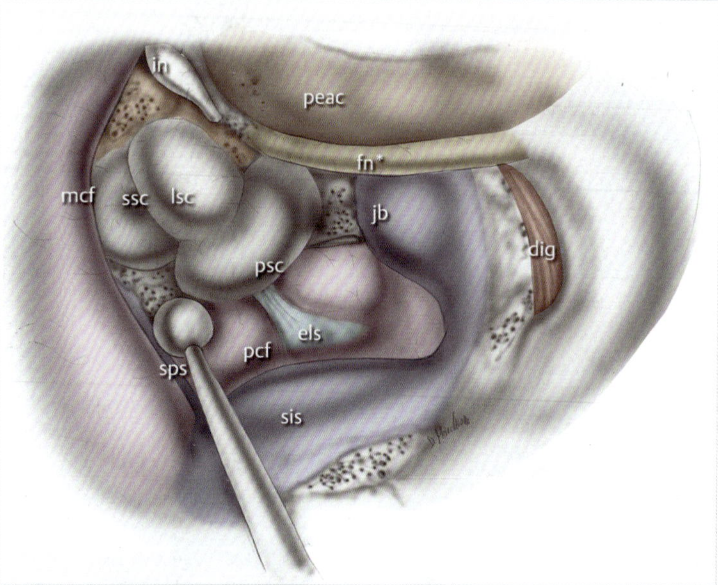

Fig. 2.7 Right side: A diamond bur is used to remove the mastoid bone uncovering the dura of the posterior fossa and the superior petrosal sinus, exposing the endolymphatic sac. *dig: digastric ridge; els: endolymphatic sac; fn*: mastoid segment of facial nerve; in: incus; jb: jugular bulb; lsc: lateral semicircular canal; mcf: middle cranial fossa; pcf: posterior cranial fossa; peac: posterior wall of external auditory canal; psc: posterior semicircular canal; sis: sigmoid sinus; sps: superior petrosal sinus; ssc: superior semicircular canal.*

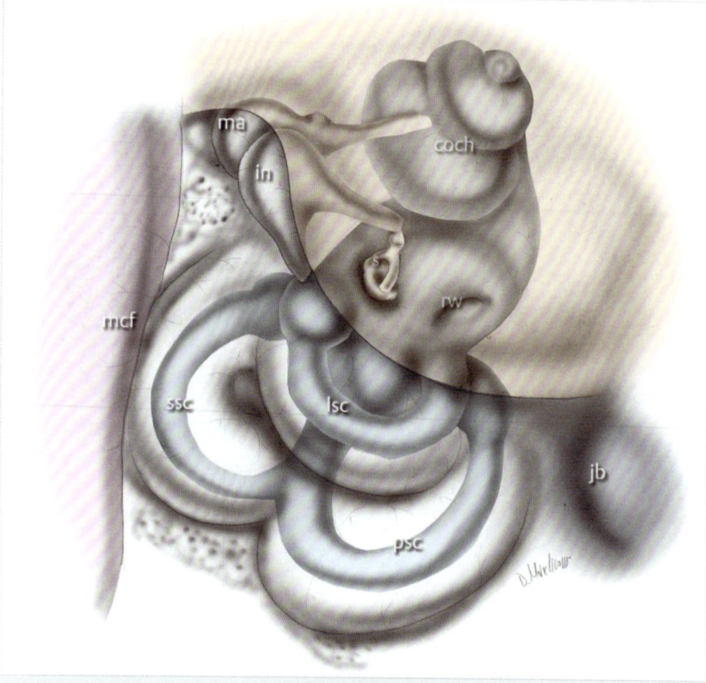

Fig. 2.8 Right side: Anatomical position of the semicircular canals in relation to the vestibule and the cochlea during the translabyrinthine approach. *coch: cochlea; in: incus; jb: jugular bulb; lsc: lateral semicircular canal; ma: malleus; mcf: middle cranial fossa; psc: posterior semicircular canal; rw: round window; s: stapes; sis: sigmoid sinus; ssc: superior semicircular canal.*

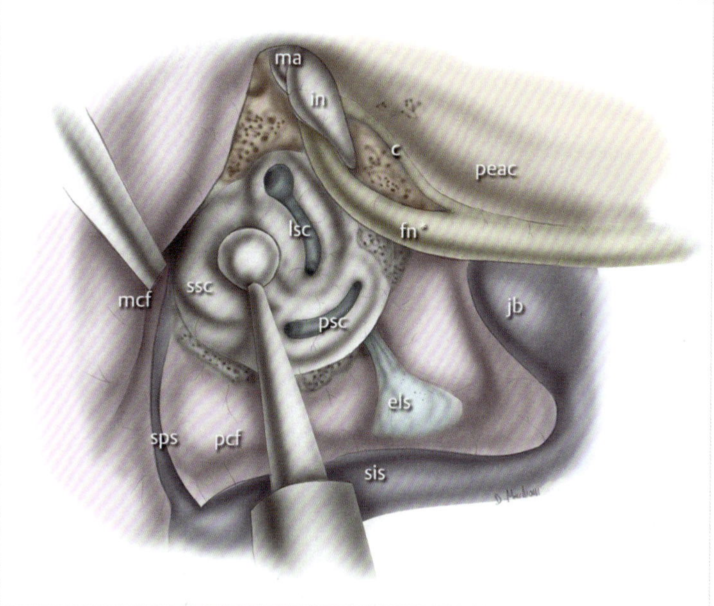

Fig. 2.9 Right side: The labyrinthectomy is started; the semicircular canals are opened. *c: chorda tympani; els: endolymphatic sac; fn*: mastoid segment of facial nerve; in: incus; jb: jugular bulb; lsc: lateral semicircular canal; ma: malleus; mcf: middle cranial fossa; pcf: posterior cranial fossa; peac: posterior wall of external auditory canal; psc: posterior semicircular canal; sis: sigmoid sinus; sps: superior petrosal sinus; ssc: superior semicircular canal.*

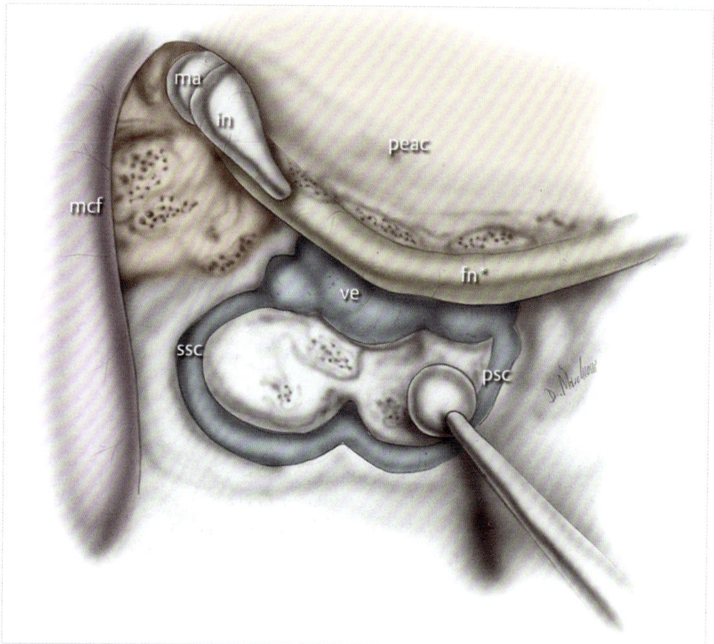

Fig. 2.10 Right side: The vestibule is opened. *fn*: mastoid segment of facial nerve; in: incus; ma: malleus; mcf: middle cranial fossa; peac: posterior wall of external auditory canal; psc: posterior semicircular canal; ssc: superior semicircular canal; ve: vestibule.*

to expose the dura of the IAC and the falciform crest (▶ Fig. 2.13). The last bone is removed in order to expose the IAC inside the petrous bone. The jugular bulb is the inferior limit of the drilling, the porus with the posterior cranial fossa is the posterior one, and the middle cranial fossa with the superior petrosal sinus is the superior one. Drilling in this anatomical area allows the exposure of the lateral portion of the IAC. The IAC is further exposed detecting the superior and inferior limits of this canal until the porus, creating two deep troughs, superiorly and inferiorly (▶ Fig. 2.14 and ▶ Fig. 2.15). The IAC must be exposed circumferentially, removing the bone between the jugular bulb end and the inferior aspect of the IAC, and the bone between the middle cranial fossa and the superior aspect of the IAC. The falciform crest is exposed and the nerve inside the IAC is also detected (▶ Fig. 2.16). The dura of the IAC is opened and the superior vestibular nerve is cut in order to expose the facial nerve in the IAC

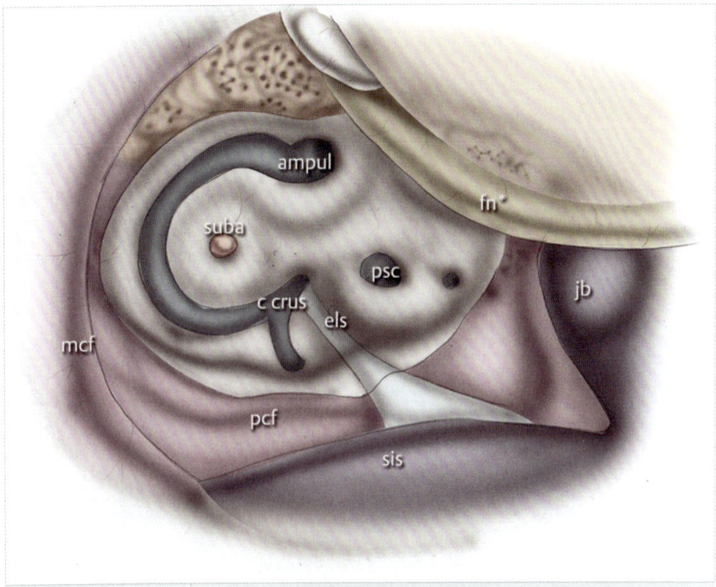

Fig. 2.11 Right side: Schematic drawing showing the anatomical relationship between the subarcuate artery, the semicircular canals, and endolymphatic sac. *ampul: ampulla of semicircular canals; c crus: common crus; els: endolymphatic sac; fn*: mastoid segment of facial nerve; jb: jugular bulb; mcf: middle cranial fossa; psc: posterior semicircular canal; sis: sigmoid sinus; suba: subarcuate artery.*

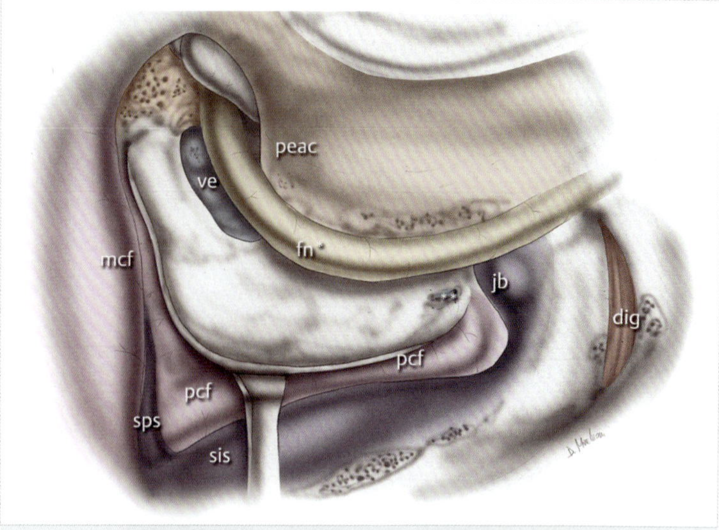

Fig. 2.12 Right side: The temporal bone is detached from the dura of the posterior fossa before starting to isolate the internal auditory canal (IAC). *fn*: mastoid segment of facial nerve; mcf: middle cranial fossa; pcf: posterior cranial fossa; peac: posterior wall of external auditory canal; sis: sigmoid sinus; sps: superior petrosal sinus; ve: vestibule; **: Cochlear aqueduct.*

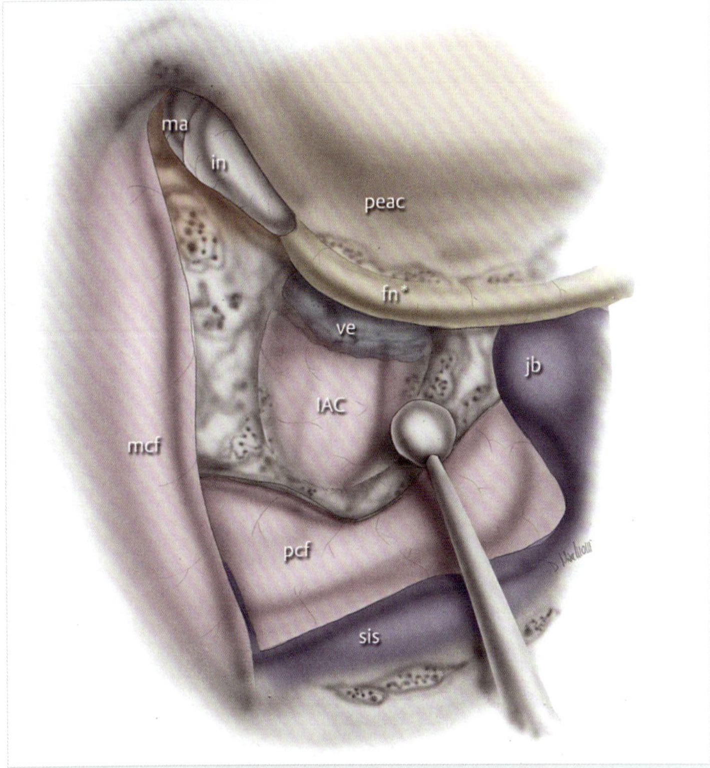

Fig. 2.13 Right side: The drilling of the internal auditory canal (IAC) is started just around the vestibule, using a diamond bur. *fn*: mastoid segment of facial nerve; IAC: internal auditory canal; in: incus; jb: jugular bulb; ma: malleus; mcf: middle cranial fossa; pcf: posterior cranial fossa; peac: posterior wall of external auditory canal; sis: sigmoid sinus; ve: vestibule.*

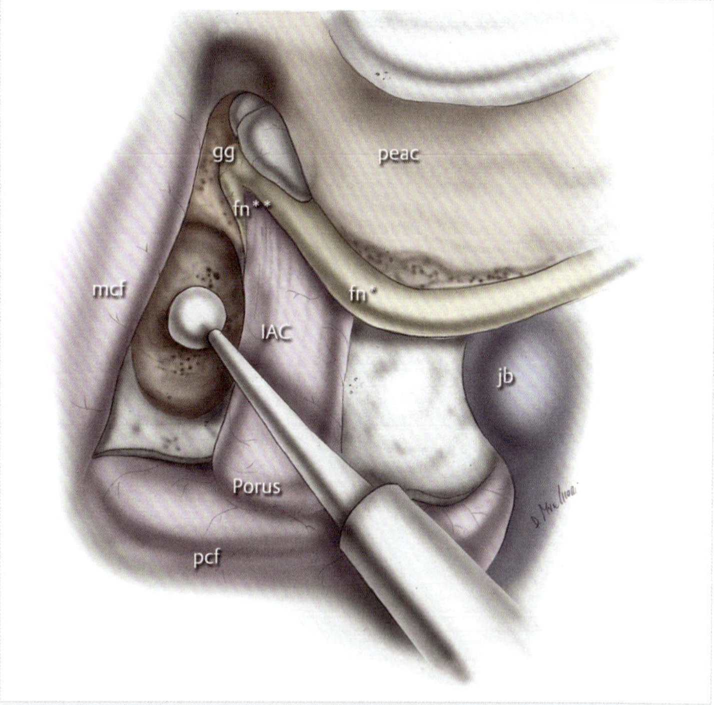

Fig. 2.14 Right side: The internal auditory canal (IAC) is further exposed; a deep trough in the superior portion of the IAC is also performed. *fn*: mastoid segment of facial nerve; fn**: labyrinthine segment of facial nerve; gg: geniculate ganglion; IAC: internal auditory canal; jb: jugular bulb; mcf: middle cranial fossa; pcf: posterior cranial fossa; peac: posterior wall of external auditory canal.*

(see Clinical Case 1). The facial nerve is detected in the superior-medial aspect of the IAC over the falciform crest after the superior vestibular nerve resection (see Clinical Case 1 ▶ Fig. 2.45). The dura of the IAC is further incised exposing the facial nerve until the porus (see Clinical Case 1 ▶ Fig. 2.46 and ▶ Fig. 2.47).

The dura of the posterior fossa is excised along the posterior surface of the temporal bone and along the inferior aspect of the superior petrosal sinus (▶ Fig. 2.17). The acoustic neuroma is exposed inside the CPA, and the inferior limit of the neuroma with respect to the mixed nerves and the anterior inferior cerebellar artery (AICA) is now visible (▶ Fig. 2.18). The superior limit of the neuroma with respect to the trigeminal nerve is also exposed. The dissection of the acoustic neuroma from the brainstem surface is started. Cottonoids are placed on the brainstem

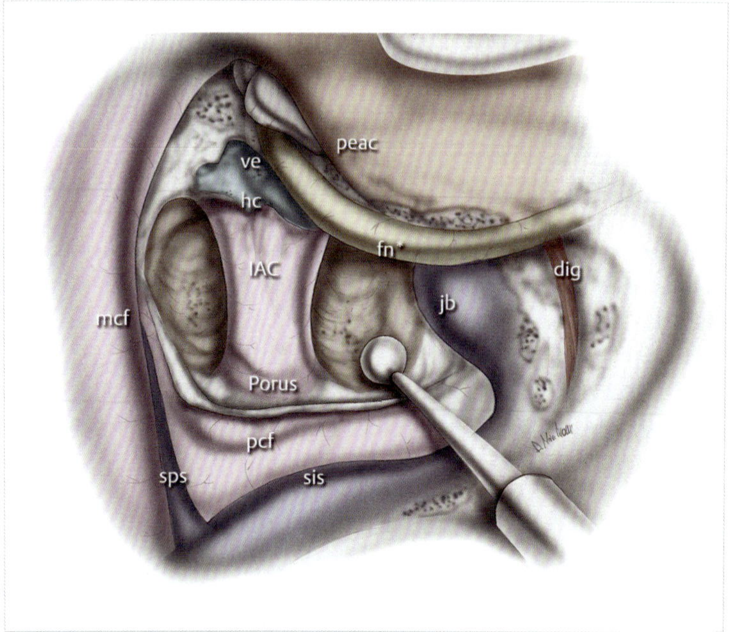

Fig. 2.15 Right side: A deep trough is also performed in the inferior portion of the internal auditory canal (IAC) between the IAC and jugular bulb. *fn*: mastoid segment of facial nerve; hc: horizontal crest; IAC: internal auditory canal; jb: jugular bulb; mcf: middle cranial fossa; pcf: posterior cranial fossa; peac: posterior wall of external auditory canal; sps: superior petrosal sinus; ve: vestibule.*

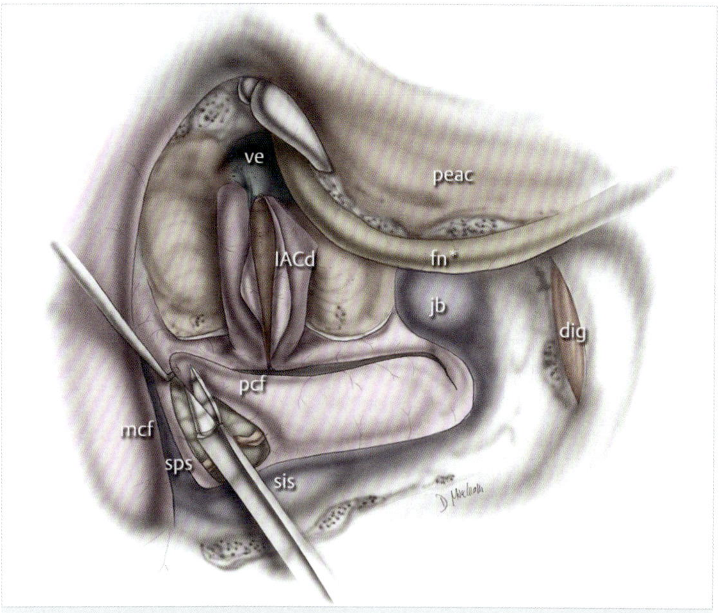

Fig. 2.17 Right side: The dura of the internal auditory canal (IAC) and of the posterior cranial fossa is cut, entering the cerebellopontine angle (CPA). *dig: digastric ridge; fn*: mastoid segment of facial nerve; IAC d: dura of the IAC; jb: jugular bulb; mcf: middle cranial fossa; pcf: posterior cranial fossa; peac: posterior wall of external auditory canal; sps: superior petrosal sinus; ve: vestibule.*

and cerebellum to protect the vascular and nervous structures. The dissection must run around the tumor, carefully detaching the arachnoid layer (▶ Fig. 2.19–2.23). In case of a large tumor, identification and gentle detachment from the surface of the neuroma of lower cranial nerves and trigeminal nerve are mandatory. Cottonoids are used to find the right plane of dissection between these nerves and the tumor (▶ Fig. 2.20). Large vessels

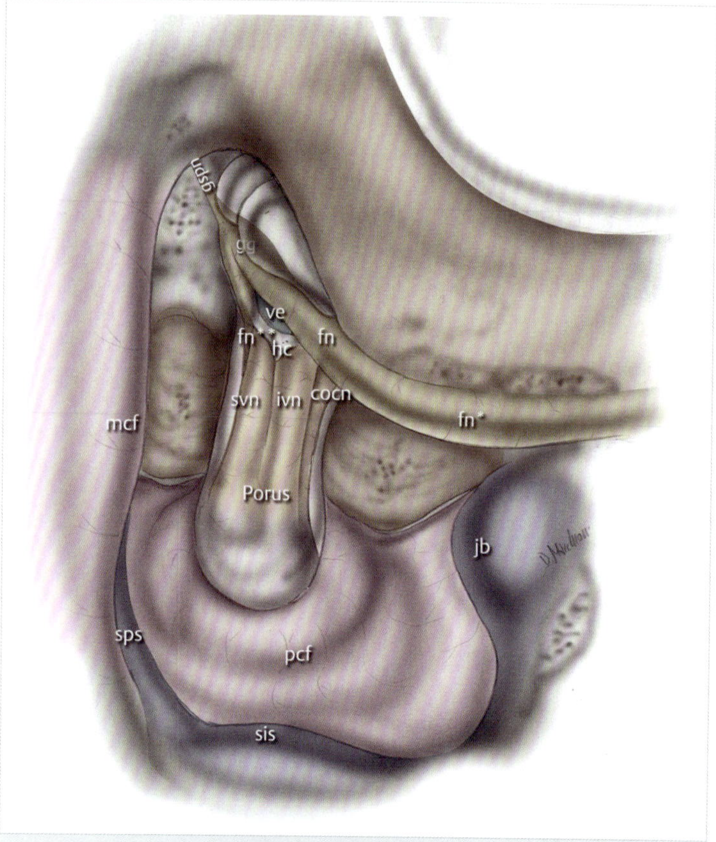

Fig. 2.16 Right side: Anatomy of the internal auditory canal (IAC). *cocn: cochlear nerve; fn*: mastoid segment of facial nerve; fn**: facial nerve into the IAC; gg: geniculate ganglion; gspn: greater superficial petrosal nerve; hc: horizontal crest; ivn: inferior vestibular nerve; jb: jugular bulb; mcf: middle cranial fossa; pcf: posterior cranial fossa; sps: superior petrosal sinus; svn: superior vestibular nerve; ve: vestibule.*

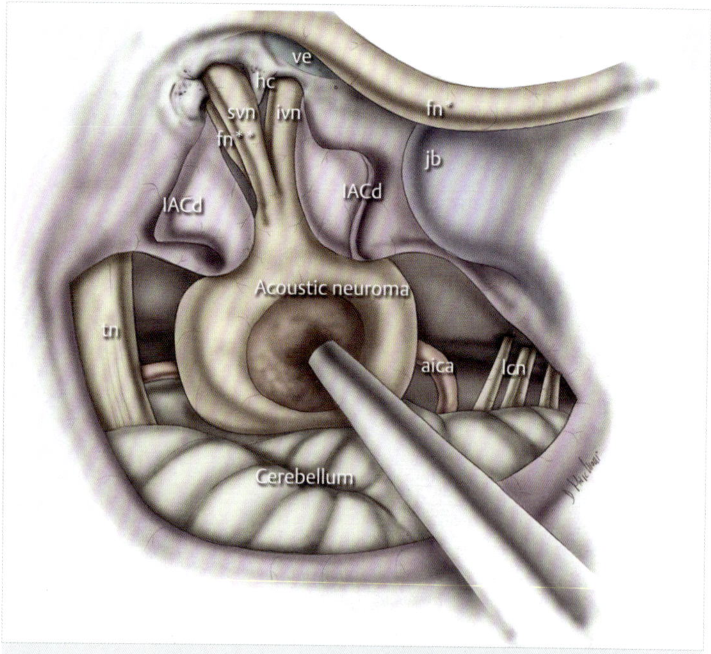

Fig. 2.18 Right side: The acoustic neuroma is exposed in the cerebellopontine angle (CPA). A central debulking of the mass is performed using a Sonopet aspirator. *fn*: mastoid segment of facial nerve; fn**: facial nerve into the internal auditory canal (IAC); hc: horizontal crest; IAC d: dura of the IAC; ivn: inferior vestibular nerve; jb: jugular bulb; lcn: lower cranial nerves; svn: superior vestibular nerve; ve: vestibule.*

may be found around the tumor. Also in this case, a gentle dissection, separating the vascular structures from the tumor, is necessary. A small bipolar instrument is used to coagulate the small perforating vessels extending into the tumor (► Fig. 2.21). In case of a large tumor, a central debulking of the mass should be considered in order to mobilize the whole neuroma, enabling the surgeon to easily detect and detach the facial nerve from the lesion (► Fig. 2.18). A facial nerve stimulator may be useful to find the nerve along the tumor. The neuroma is carefully detached and progressively from the facial nerve. In this way, the whole tumor is devascularized. The acoustic neuroma is removed, preserving the facial nerve (► Fig. 2.24). The CPA is checked under a microscopic view, and the integrity of the facial nerve is observed. The transtemporal approach to the IAC and CPA is now complete (see Clinical Case 1 ► Fig. 2.50 and ► Fig. 2.51). The transtemporal axis entry zone of the facial nerve into the brainstem is exposed. The incus is removed and a muscle pad is used to close the aditus ad antrum (► Fig. 2.25). Bone dust with fibrin glue is used in order to separate the middle ear from the mastoid and the CPA (see Clinical Case 1 ► Fig. 2.53). A long strip of abdominal fat is used to obliterate the surgical cavity (► Fig. 2.26). The muscle and periosteum are replaced and sutured, and a watertight suture of the skin is done. A compressive bandage is used to cover the site of the surgery.

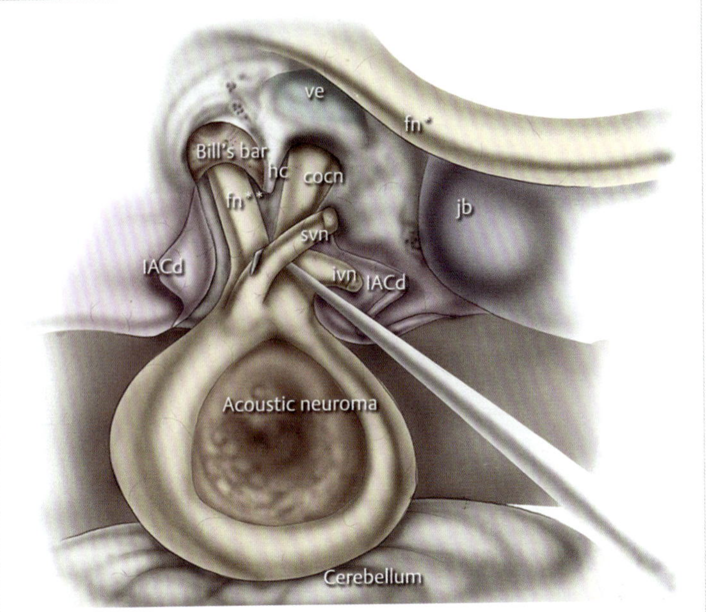

Fig. 2.19 Right side: The vestibular nerves are cut at the level of the fundus of the internal auditory canal (IAC), and the facial nerve is identified. *cocn: cochlear nerve; fn*: mastoid segment of facial nerve; fn**: facial nerve into the IAC; hc: horizontal crest; IAC d: dura of the IAC; ivn: inferior vestibular nerve; jb: jugular bulb; svn: superior vestibular nerve; ve: vestibule.*

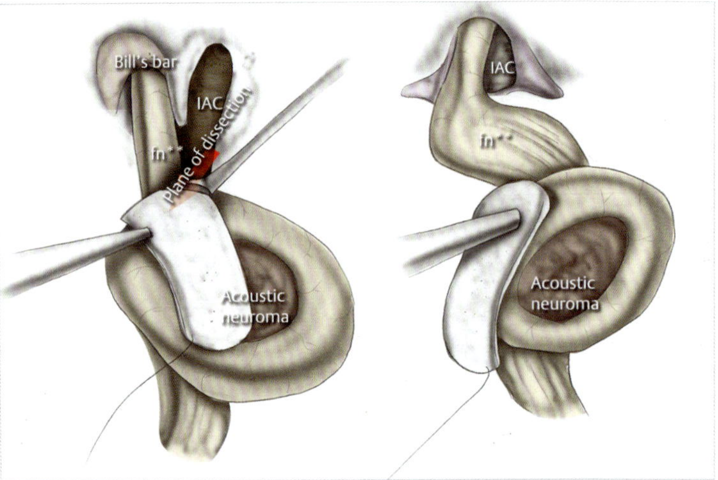

Fig. 2.20 Right side: The tumor is progressively removed from the facial nerve. A cottonoid is used to detach the tumor from the facial nerve, identifying a correct surgical plan of dissection. *fn**: facial nerve into the IAC; IAC: internal auditory canal.*

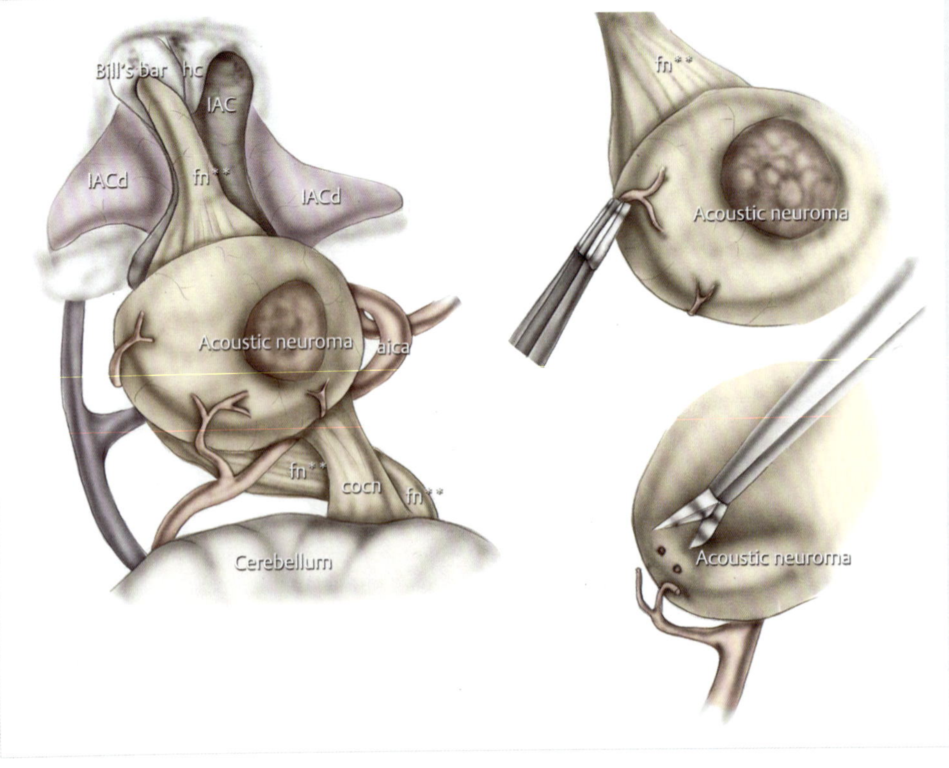

Fig. 2.21 Right side: The tumor is detached from the vascular structures arising from the anterior inferior cerebellar artery (AICA). A small bipolar tool is used to coagulate the small vessels around the tumor. Microscissors are used to cut the vessels in proximity to the tumor. *cocn: cochlear nerve; fn**: facial nerve into the IAC and cerebellopontine angle (CPA); hd: horizontal crest; IAC: internal auditory canal; IACd: dura of IAC.*

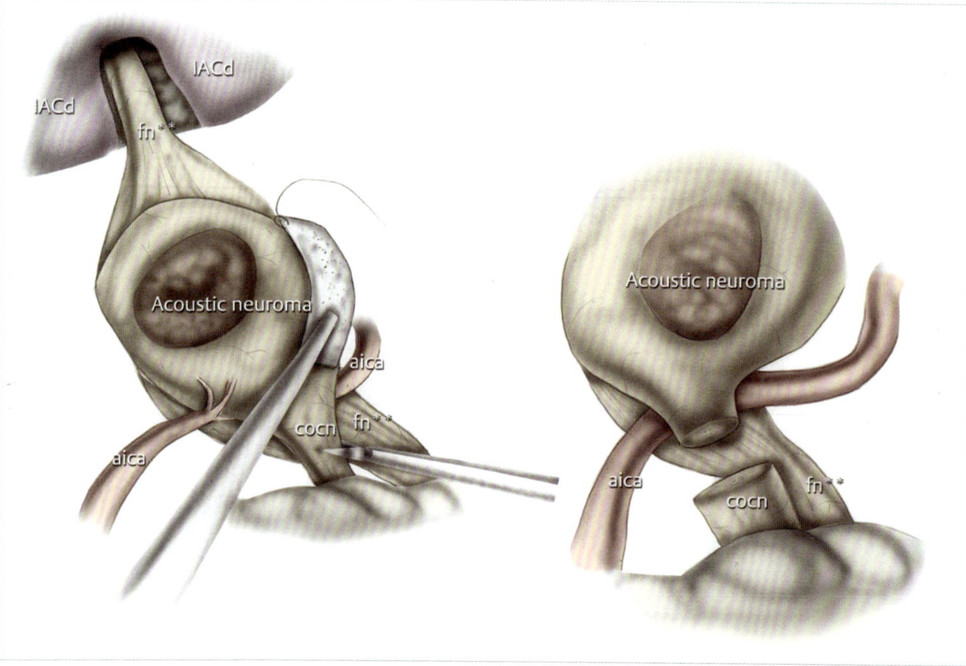

Fig. 2.22 Right side: The cochlear nerve is cut at the entrance close to the brainstem. *cocn: cochlear nerve; fn**: facial nerve in the internal auditory canal (IAC) and cerebellopontine angle (CPA); IACd: dura of IAC.*

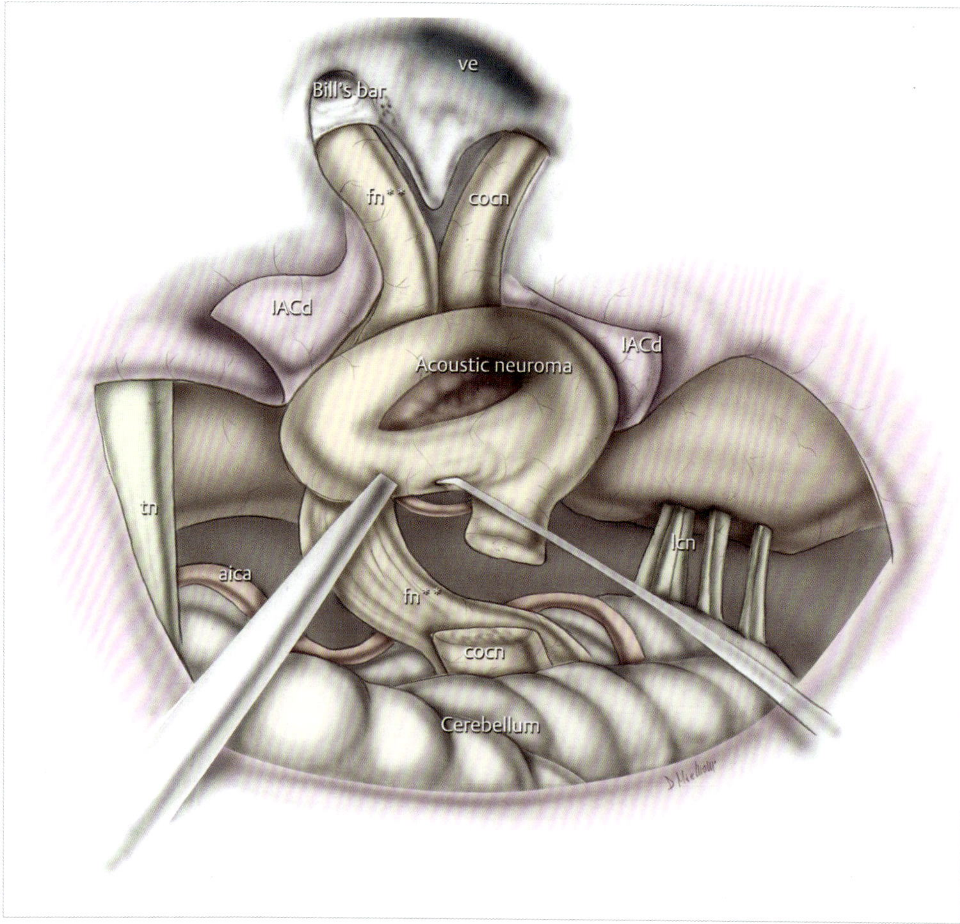

Fig. 2.23 Right side: The tumor is removed from the cerebellopontine angle (CPA). *cocn: cochlear nerve: fn**: facial nerve in the internal auditory canal (IAC) and CPA; IACd: dura of IAC; lcn: lower cranial nerves; tn: trigeminal nerve; ve: vestibule.*

2.2.6 Hints and Pitfalls

- Since there is close relationship between the second genu of the facial nerve and the labyrinthine block, before starting the labyrinthectomy, a diamond bur is used to detect the second genu of the facial nerve, just anteriorly to the lateral semicircular canal. This step is important to avoid damage to the nerve while opening the labyrinth (see Clinical Case 2). During the labyrinthectomy, a large diamond bur is used, and continuous irrigation is necessary to avoid heat dissipation which may damage the nerve (see Clinical Case 2 ▶ Fig. 2.56). Once the labyrinthine is open, the semicircular canals are identified. A bony plane anteriorly to the lateral semicircular canal must be left in place in order to protect the facial nerve during the following steps (see Clinical Case 2 ▶ Fig. 2.57 and ▶ Fig. 2.58). After the identification of the vestibule, the IAC dissection is started. During this operation, a diamond bur is used under continuous irrigation of the surgical field. The surgeon must be careful especially during the bone removal in the most superior and anterior portions of the IAC fundus, since the intralabyrinthine

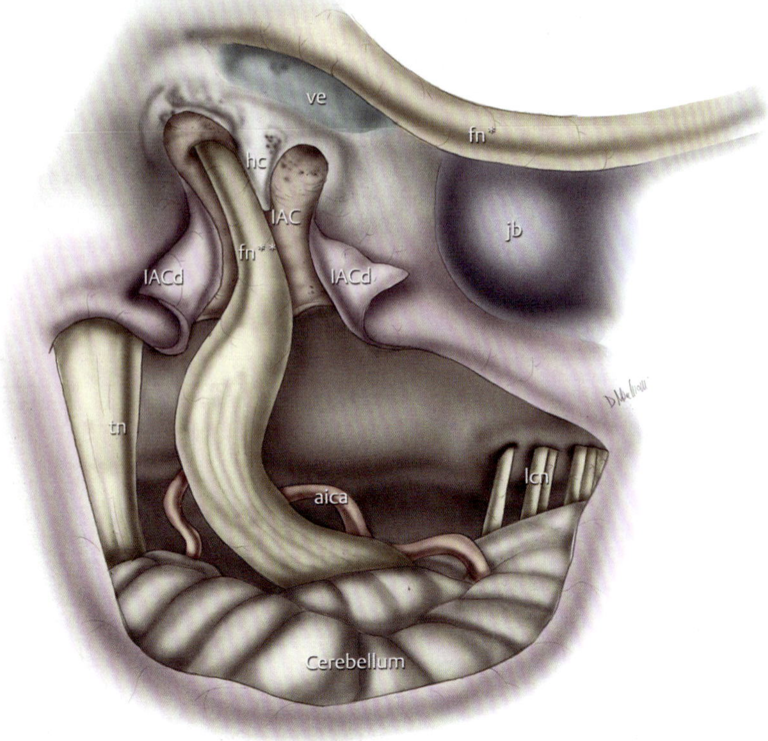

Fig. 2.24 Right side: Microscopic view of the surgical field after tumor removal. The facial nerve is preserved. *fn*: mastoid segment of facial nerve; fn**: facial nerve into the IAC and cerebellopontine angle (CPA); hc: horizontal crest; IAC: internal auditory canal; IACd: dura of IAC; jb: jugular bulb; lcn: lower cranial nerves; tn: trigeminal nerve; ve: vestibule.*

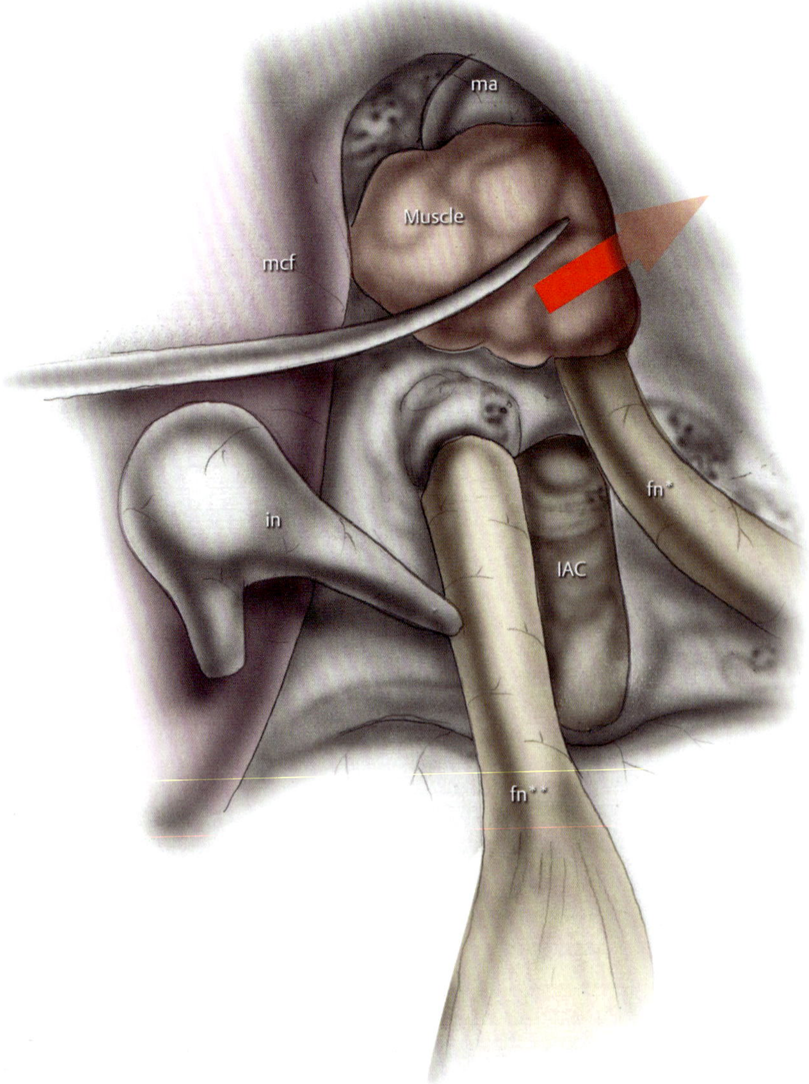

Fig. 2.25 Right side: A muscle is used to obliterate the antrum, excluding the surgical cavity from the middle ear. The muscle is pushed into the antrum (*red arrow*). *fn*: facial nerve mastoid segment; IAC: internal auditory canal; in: incus; ma: malleus; mcf: middle cranial fossa.*

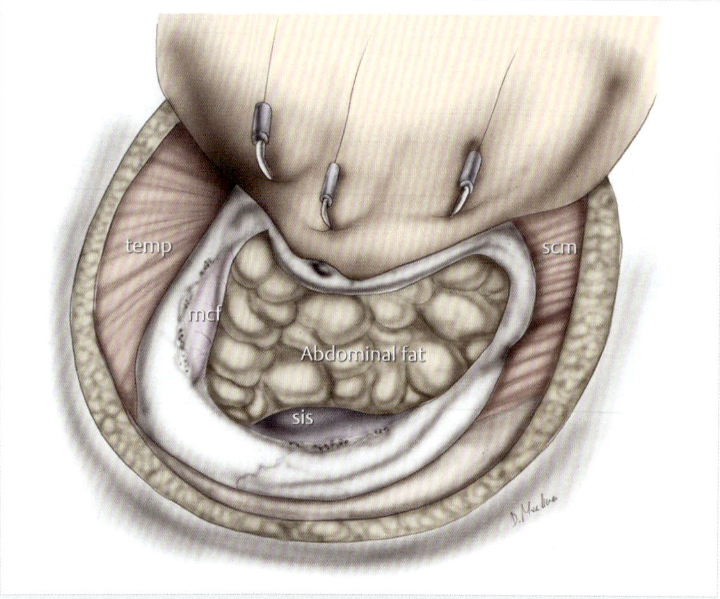

Fig. 2.26 Right side: The surgical cavity is obliterated with abdominal fat. *mcf: middle cranial fossa; scm: sternocleidomastoid muscle; sis: sigmoid sinus; temp: temporalis muscle.*

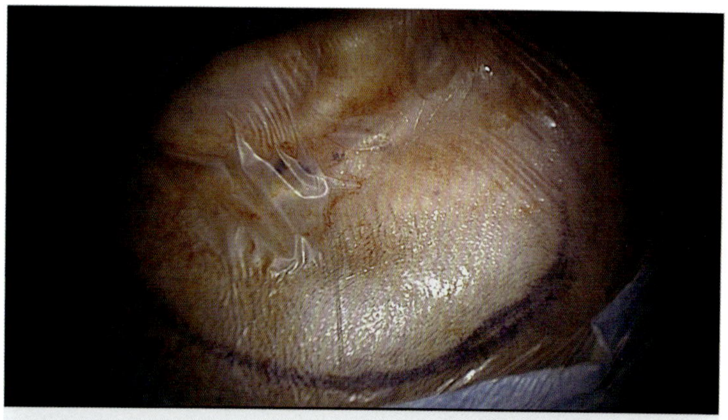

Fig. 2.27 Clinical Case 1, Left side: A C-shaped postauricular incision is made, 4 cm behind the retroauricular sulcus. The anterosuperior part of the incision must be placed over the ear attachment. The anteroinferior portion of the incision must be placed just inferiorly on the tip of the mastoid.

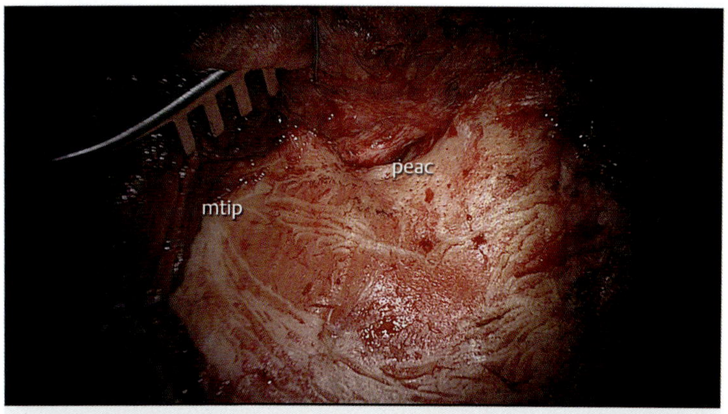

Fig. 2.28 Clinical Case 1, Left side: The mastoid bone is widely exposed after musculoperiosteal layer elevation. The posterior aspect of the external auditory canal (EAC) is detected. *mtip: mastoid tip; peac: posterior wall of external auditory canal.*

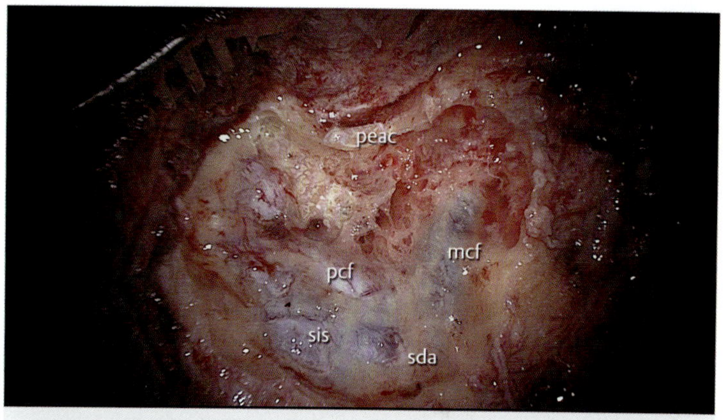

Fig. 2.29 Clinical Case 1, Left side: An extended mastoidectomy is performed, exposing the sinodural angle posteriorly, the middle fossa superiorly, and the lateral sinus. *mcf: middle cranial fossa; pcf: posterior cranial fossa; peac: posterior wall of external auditory canal; sda: sinodural angle; sis: sigmoid sinus.*

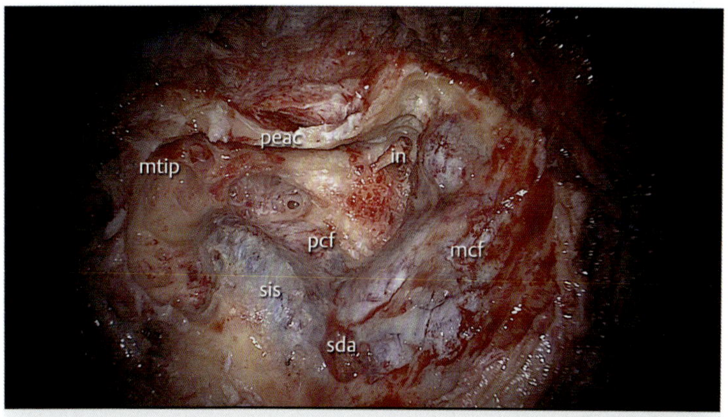

Fig. 2.30 Clinical Case 1, Left side: The middle fossa and the lateral sinus are widely skeletonized. The antrum and the incudomalleolar joint are detected. The posterior fossa dura is exposed just anteriorly to the sigmoid sinus. *in: incus; mcf: middle cranial fossa; mtip: mastoid tip; pcf: posterior cranial fossa; peac: posterior wall of external auditory canal; sda: sinodural angle; sis: sigmoid sinus.*

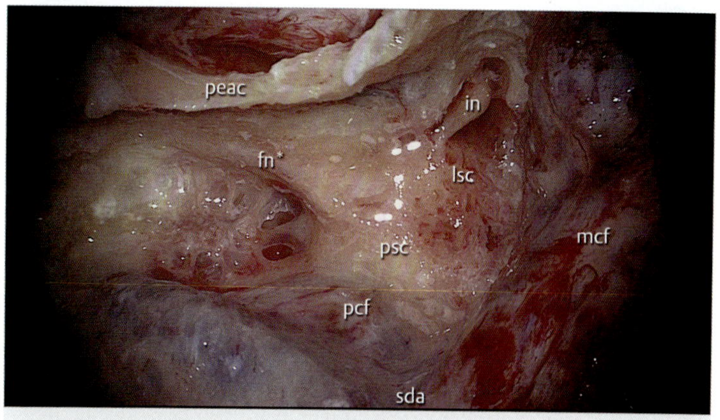

Fig. 2.31 Clinical Case 1, Left side: After digastric ridge exposure, the mastoid segment of the facial nerve is detected. The intersinus facial cells are drilled. *fn*: mastoid segment of facial nerve; in: incus; lsc: lateral semicircular canal; mcf: middle cranial fossa; pcf: posterior cranial fossa; peac: posterior wall of external auditory canal; psc: posterior semicircular canal; sda: sinodural angle; sis: sigmoid sinus.*

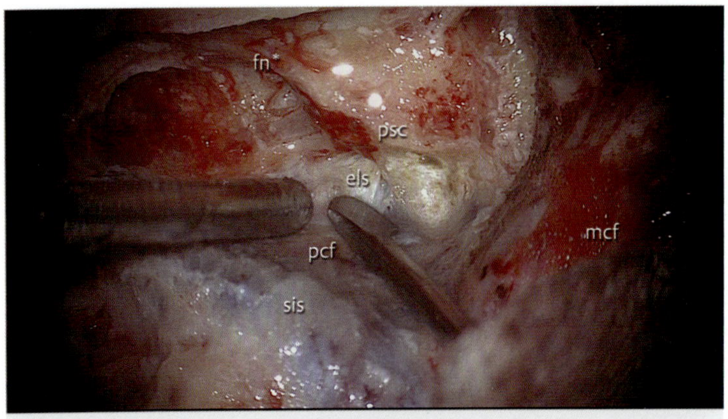

Fig. 2.32 Clinical Case 1, Left side: The posterior fossa is detached from the mastoid bone, and the endolymphatic sac is exposed, dissecting the dura of the posterior fossa just posteriorly to the posterior semicircular canal. *fn*: mastoid segment of facial nerve; mcf: middle cranial fossa; pcf: posterior cranial fossa; psc: posterior semicircular canal; sis: sigmoid sinus.*

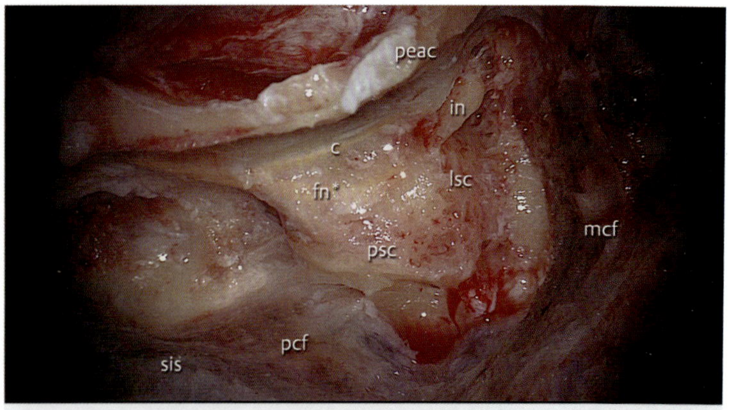

Fig. 2.33 Clinical Case 1, Left side:The second genu of the facial nerve and the corda tympani are exposed. The labyrinthine block is skeletonized. *c: chorda tympani; fn*: mastoid segment of facial nerve; in: incus; lsc: lateral semicircular canal; mcf: middle cranial fossa; pcf: posterior cranial fossa; peac: posterior wall of external auditory canal; psc: posterior semicircular canal; sis: sigmoid sinus.*

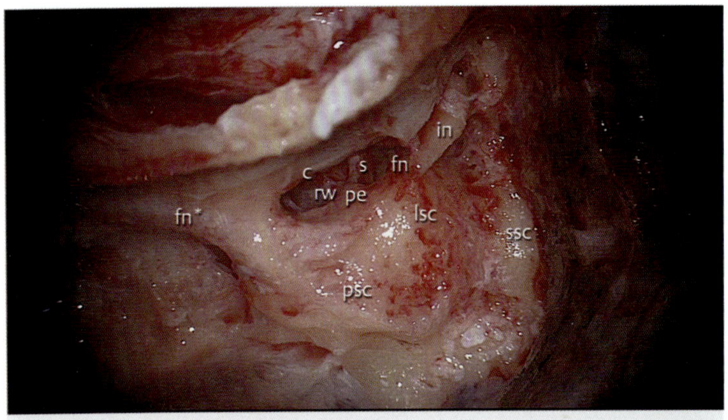

Fig. 2.34 Clinical Case 1, Left side: A posterior tympanotomy is made, exposing the incudostapedial joint. The anatomical relationship between the second genu of the facial nerve and the lateral semicircular canal can be noticed. *c: chorda tympani; fn: tympanic segment of facial nerve; fn*: mastoid segment of facial nerve; in: incus; lsc: lateral semicircular canal; pe: pyramidal eminence; psc: posterior semicircular canal; rw: round window; s: stapes.*

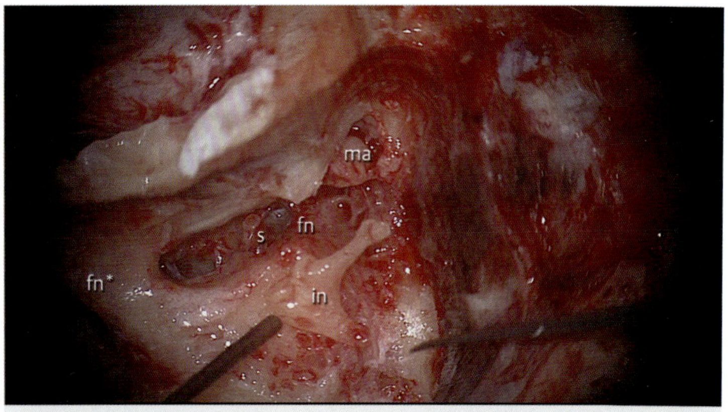

Fig. 2.35 Clinical Case 1, Left side: The incus is removed. The tympanic segment of the facial nerve is now visible. This step is not necessary during a traditional translabyrinthine approach, but in case a better exposure of the facial nerve is required to plan a cochlear implant during this procedure. *fn: tympanic segment of facial nerve; fn*: mastoid segment of facial nerve; in: incus; ma: malleus; s: stapes.*

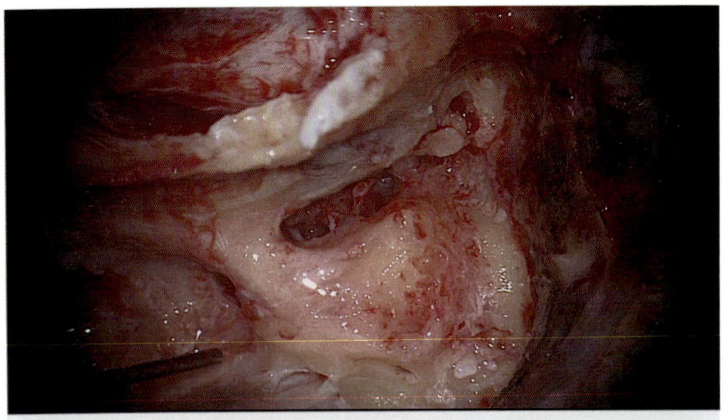

Fig. 2.36 Clinical Case 1, Left side: The anatomical relationship between the facial neve and labyrinthine block can be noticed. The geniculate ganglion is located just superiorly to the cochleariform process.

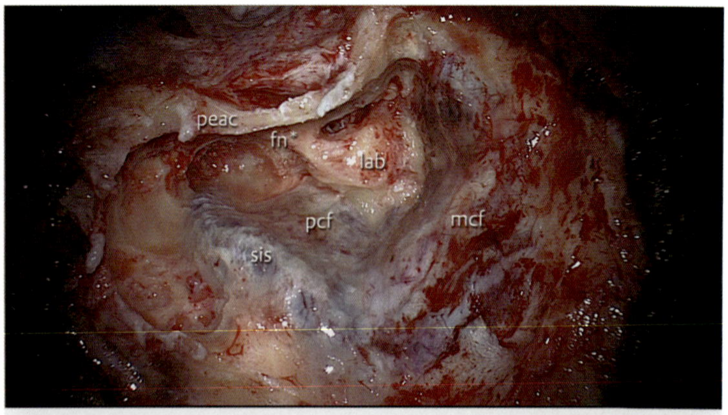

Fig. 2.37 Clinical Case 1, Left side: Panoramic view of the dissection; the posterior fossa dura, the middle fossa dura, and the sigmoid sinus with the sinodural angle are widely exposed. The facial nerve is detected from the stylomastoid foramen to the geniculate ganglion but not uncovered; the labyrinthine block is skeletonized. *fn*: mastoid segment of facial nerve; laboratory: labyrinthine block; mcf: middle cranial fossa; pcf: posterior cranial fossa; peac: posterior wall of external auditory canal; sis: sigmoid sinus.*

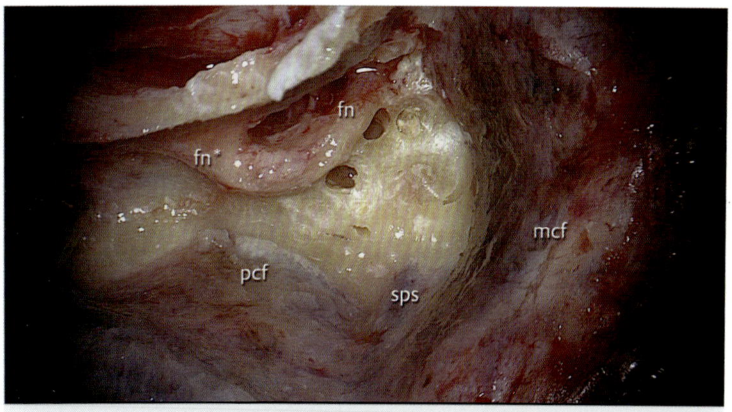

Fig. 2.38 Clinical Case 1, Left side: The labyrinthectomy is performed, opening the superior, posterior, and lateral canals, leaving the most anterior portion of the lateral semicircular canal to protect the tympanic segment of the facial nerve, by detecting the ampullae of the lateral and superior semicircular canals. *fn: tympanic segment of facial nerve; fn**: mastoid segment of facial nerve; mcf: middle cranial fossa; pcf: posterior cranial fossa; sps: superior petrosal sinus.*

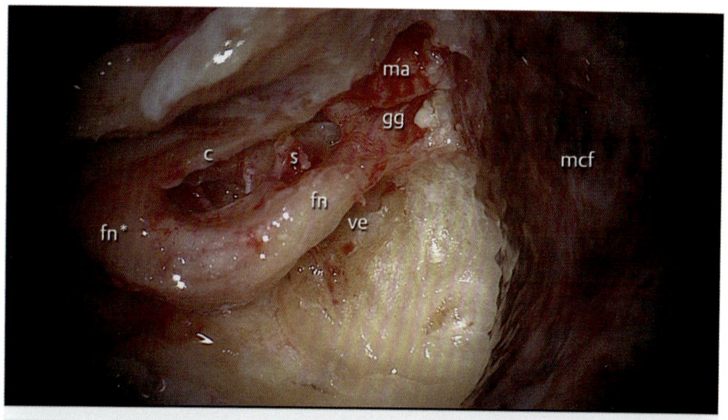

Fig. 2.39 Clinical Case 1, Left side: The vestibule is exposed after a further drilling of the labyrinthine block. *c: chorda tympani; fn: tympanic segment of facial nerve; fn**: mastoid segment of facial nerve; gg: geniculate ganglion; ma: malleus; mcf: middle cranial fossa; s: stapes; ve: vestibule.*

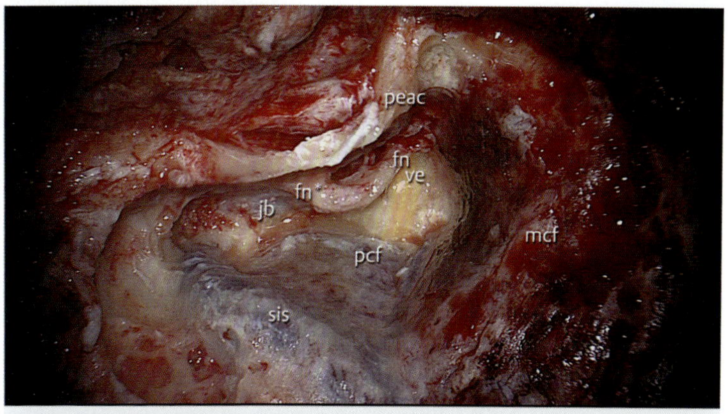

Fig. 2.40 Clinical Case 1, Left side: Temporal bone overview after vestibule opening. The sigmoid sinus is followed until the jugular bulb is detected under the retrofacial cells. After the labyrinthectomy and vestibule opening, the bone of the temporal bone between the dura of the posterior fossa and middle fossa are removed using a large diamond bur, identifying the porus of the internal auditory canal (IAC). *fn: tympanic segment of facial nerve; fn**: mastoid segment of facial nerve; jb: jugular bulb; mcf: middle cranial fossa; pcf: posterior cranial fossa; peac: posterior wall of external auditory canal; sis: sigmoid sinus; ve: vestibule.*

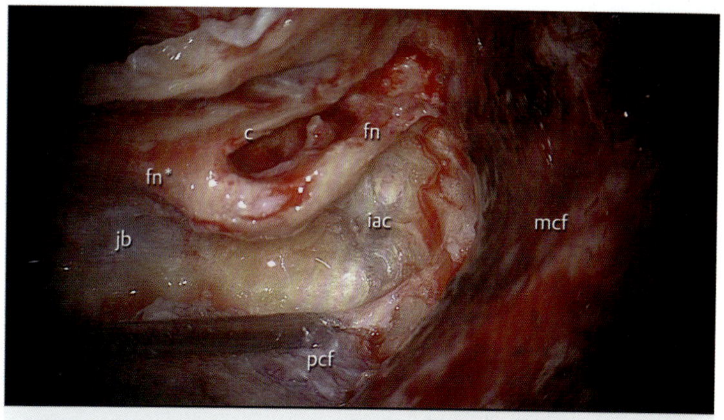

Fig. 2.41 Clinical Case 1, Left side: The dura of the internal auditory canal (IAC) is detected under the vestibule. The inferior and superior limits of the IAC are progressively identified, drilling in parallel to the IAC orientation. *c: chorda tympani; fn: tympanic segment of facial nerve; fn**: mastoid segment of facial nerve; iac: internal auditory canal; jb: jugular bulb; mcf: middle cranial fossa; pcf: posterior cranial fossa.*

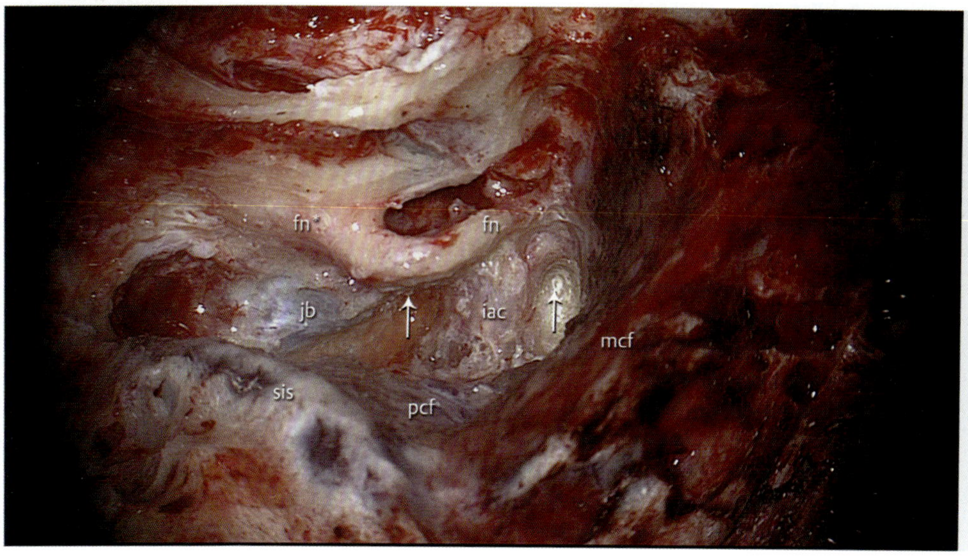

Fig. 2.42 Clinical Case 1, Left side: The bones between the jugular bulb and the inferior limit of the internal auditory canal (IAC), as well as the bone in between the middle fossa dura and the superior limit of the IAC, are deeply drilled, producing a 270° exposure of the dura of the IAC. *fn: tympanic segment of facial nerve; fn**: *mastoid segment of facial nerve; iac: internal auditory canal; jb: jugular bulb; mcf: middle cranial fossa; pcf: posterior cranial fossa; sis: sigmoid sinus; Arrows:* bony removal around the IAC creating two deep toughs, superior and inferior with respect to the dura of the IAC, uncovering for 270 degrees of the IAC.

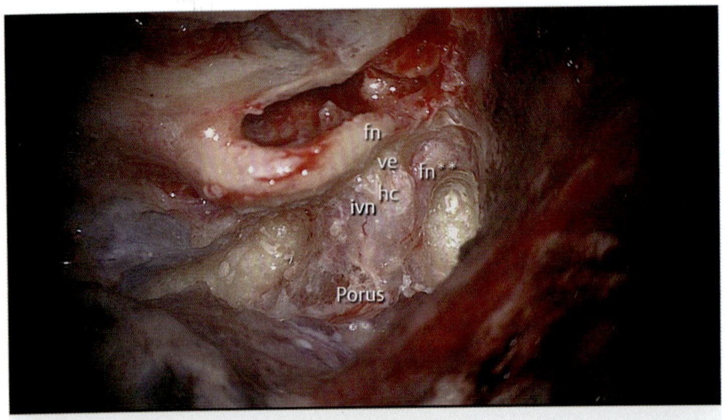

Fig. 2.43 Clinical Case 1, Left side: The transverse crest (horizontal crest) is exposed in the fundus of the internal auditory canal (IAC), separating the superior vestibular nerve superiorly from the inferior vestibular nerve inferiorly. *fn: tympanic segment of facial nerve; fn**: labyrinthine portion of facial nerve; hc: horizontal (transverse) crest; ivn: inferior vestibular nerve; ve: vestibule.*

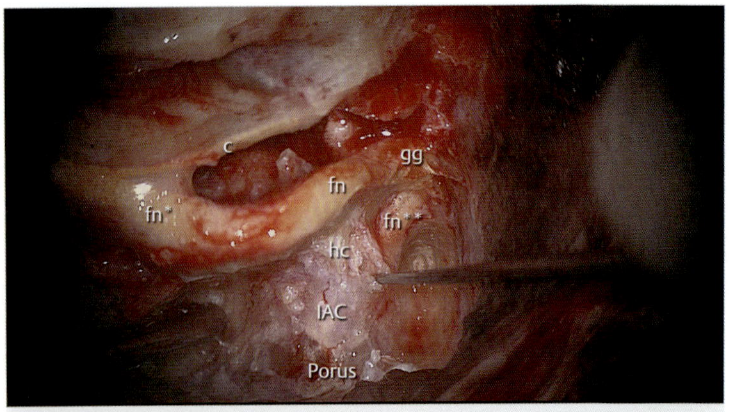

Fig. 2.44 Clinical Case 1, Left side: The dura of the internal auditory canal (IAC) is opened at the fundus; the superior vestibular nerve is identified lying superiorly to the transverse crest. The facial nerve runs medial to the superior vestibular nerve. *c: chorda tympani; fn: tympanic segment of facial nerve; fn*: mastoid segment of facial nerve; fn**: labyrinthine portion of facial nerve; gg: geniculate ganglion; hc: horizontal (transverse) crest; IAC: internal auditory canal.*

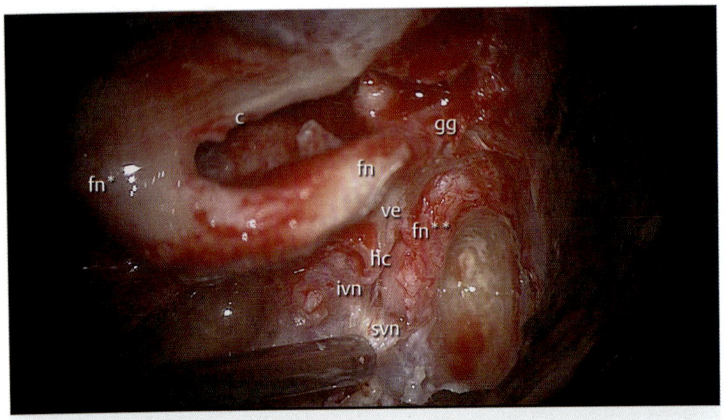

Fig. 2.45 Clinical Case 1, Left side: The superior vestibular nerve is detached; the facial nerve is identified. *c: chorda tympani; fn: tympanic segment of facial nerve; fn*: mastoid segment of facial nerve; fn**: labyrinthine portion of facial nerve; gg: geniculate ganglion; hc: horizontal (transverse) crest; ivn: inferior vestibular nerve; svn: superior vestibular nerve.*

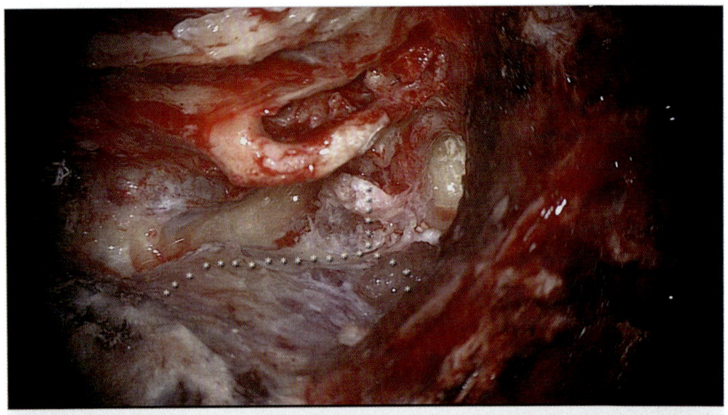

Fig. 2.46 Clinical Case 1, Left side: The dura of the internal auditory canal (IAC) is opened until the porus, and an incision of the posterior cranial dura is made. *See the asterisked line.*

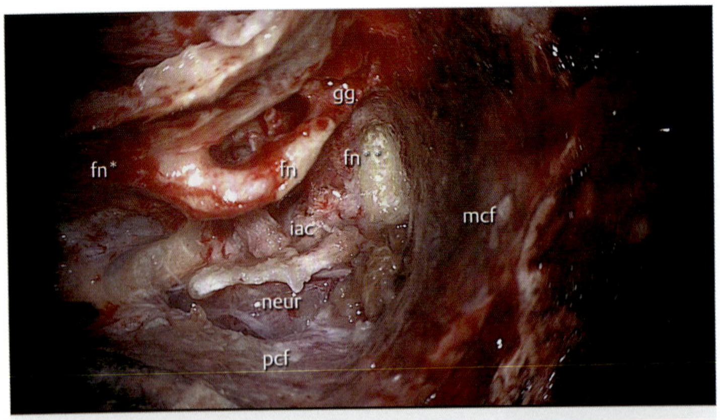

Fig. 2.47 Clinical Case 1, Left side: The dura of posterior fossa is opened using microscissors close to the porus. The tumor in the cerebellopontine angle (CPA) is isolated. *c: chorda tympani; fn: tympanic segment of facial nerve; fn*: mastoid segment of facial nerve; fn**: labyrinthine portion of facial nerve; gg: geniculate ganglion; iac: internal auditory canal; mcf: middle cranial fossa; neur: acoustic neuroma; pcf: posterior cranial fossa.*

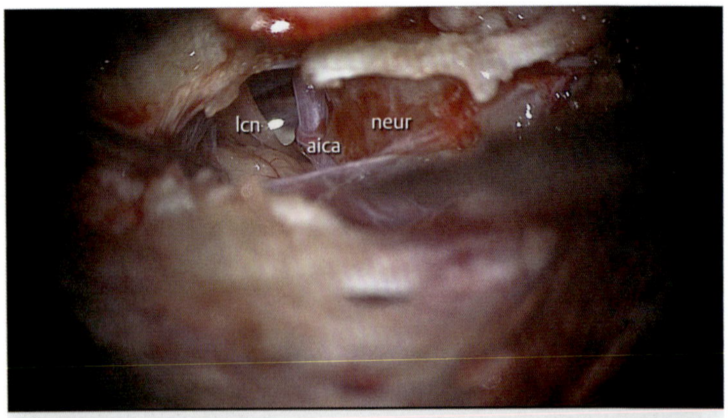

Fig. 2.48 Clinical Case 1, Left side: The lower cranial nerve is visible in the inferior area of the cerebellopontine angle (CPA). The dissection of the tumor starts from the brainstem surface. *lcn: lower cranial nerve; neur: acoustic neuroma.*

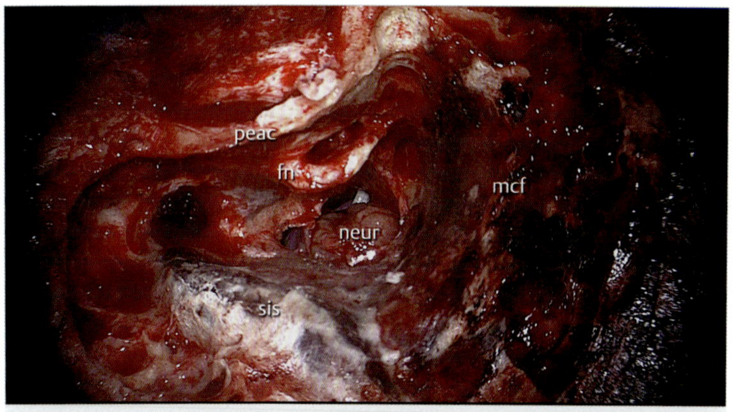

Fig. 2.49 Clinical Case 1, Left side: The tumor is isolated from the internal auditory canal (IAC) to the brainstem preserving the facial nerve. *fn: facial nerve; mcf: middle cranial fossa; neur: acoustic neuroma; pcf: posterior cranial fossa; peac: posterior auditory canal; sis: sigmoid sinus.*

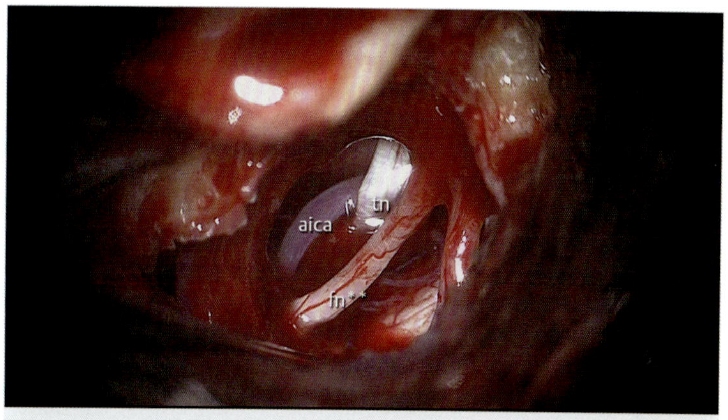

Fig. 2.50 Clinical Case 1, Left side: Microscopic magnification of the facial nerve in the cerebellopontine angle (CPA) after tumor removal. Notice the anatomical relationship between the facial nerve, the trigeminal nerve, and the anterior inferior cerebellar artery (AICA). *fn**: facial nerve at the entry zone; tn: trigeminal nerve.*

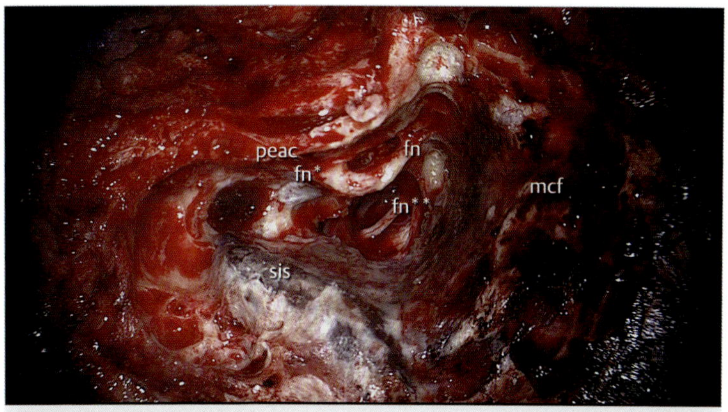

Fig. 2.51 Clinical Case 1, Left side: Final cavity after acoustic tumor removal. The facial nerve can be seen from the stylomastoid foramen to the entry zone of the brainstem. *fn: facial nerve; fn*: mastoid segment of facial nerve; fn**: facial nerve at the cerebellopontine angle (CPA); mcf: middle cranial fossa; peac: posterior auditory canal; sis: sigmoid sinus.*

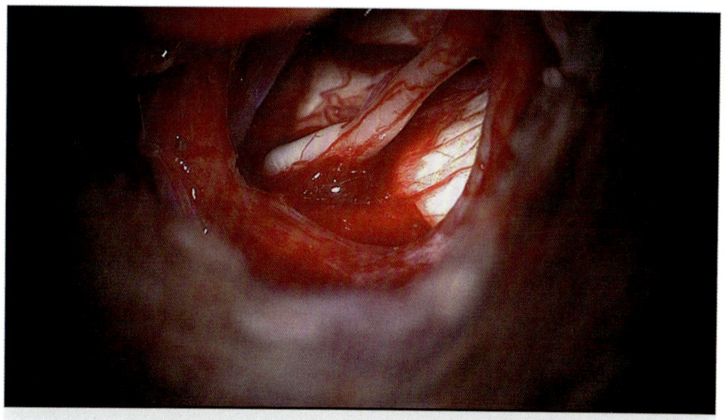

Fig. 2.52 Clinical Case 1, Left side: Microscopic view of the facial nerve entering the entry zone on the brainstem surface.

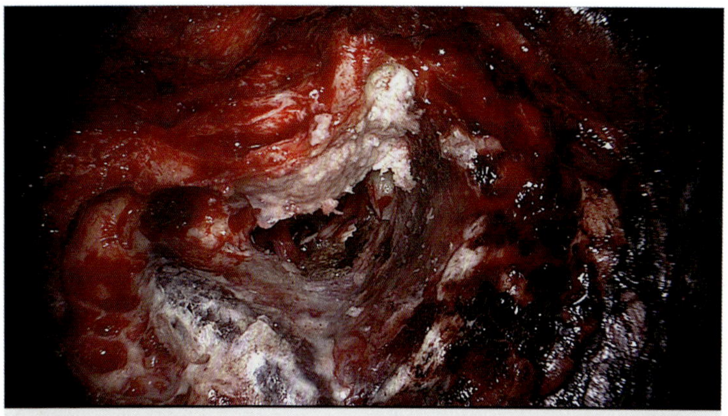

Fig. 2.53 Clinical Case 1, Left side: The antrum and the connection between the tympanic cavity and the mastoid is separated using a fragment of muscle in the aditus, and reinforced with bone paté and fibrin glue.

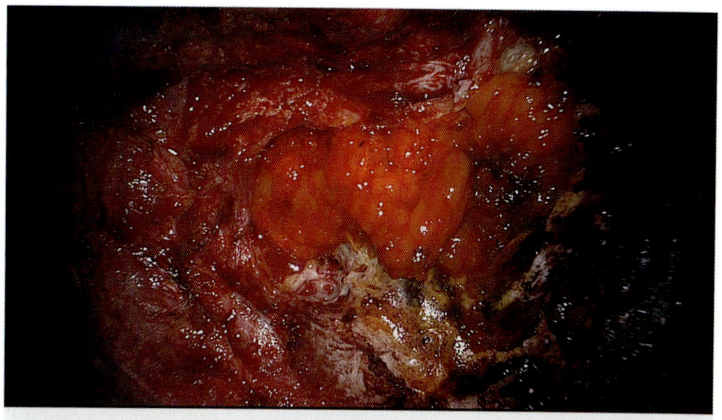

Fig. 2.54 Clinical Case 1, Left side: Abdominal fat is used to obliterate the surgical cavity. The musculoperiosteal flap is replaced to cover the cavity. The subcutaneous tissue and the skin are carefully closed.

portion of the facial nerve in this area could be exposed (see Clinical Case 2 ▶ Fig. 2.61 and ▶ Fig. 2.62). Once the IAC is exposed, the dura of the posterior fossa is opened close to the porus. One needs to be careful as a vascular structure may be present just behind the dural layer. A small incision is suggested (see Clinical Case 2 ▶ Fig. 2.63), and cottonoids should be placed in between the dural layer and the CPA in order to protect the vascular structures, allowing a safe incision of the dura of the posterior fossa along the axis of the temporal bone. Before starting the tumor dissection, the opening of lateral cisterna is suggested. This step leads to a cerebrospinal fluid (CSF) leakage and the brainstem becomes relaxed. The tumor is then progressively dissected from the facial nerve and removed from the CPA (see Clinical Case 2 ▶ Fig. 2.64 and ▶ Fig. 2.65).

- In case of high jugular bulb, a careful dissection of the vein must be carried out. The surgeon should be able to maintain a thin

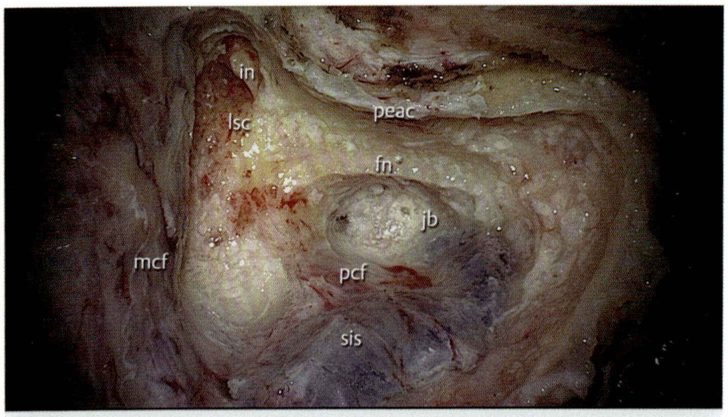

Fig. 2.55 Clinical Case 2, Right side: Before starting the labyrinthectomy, the mastoid segment of the facial nerve until the second genu located just anteriorly to the lateral canal is detected. *fn*: mastoid segment of facial nerve; in: incus; jb: jugular bulb; lsc: lateral semicircular canal; mcf: middle cranial fossa; pcf: posterior cranial fossa; peac: posterior auditory canal; sis: sigmoid sinus.*

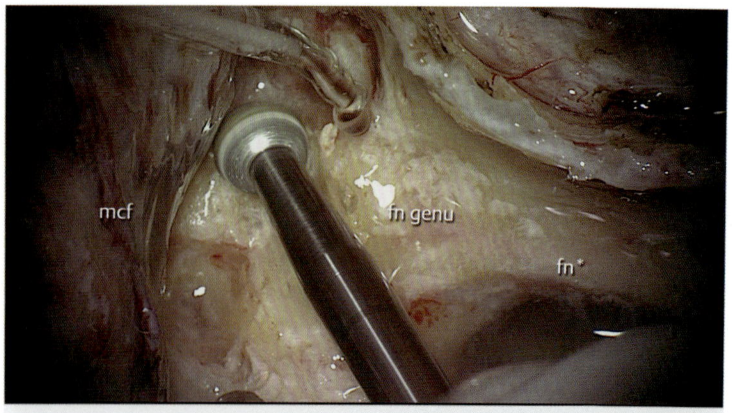

Fig. 2.56 Clinical Case 2, Right side: The labyrinthectomy is started. During this step, a large diamond bur is used and the surgical field carefully irrigated to avoid damage to the facial nerve. *fn*: mastoid segment of facial nerve; fn genu: second genu of facial nerve; mcf: middle cranial fossa.*

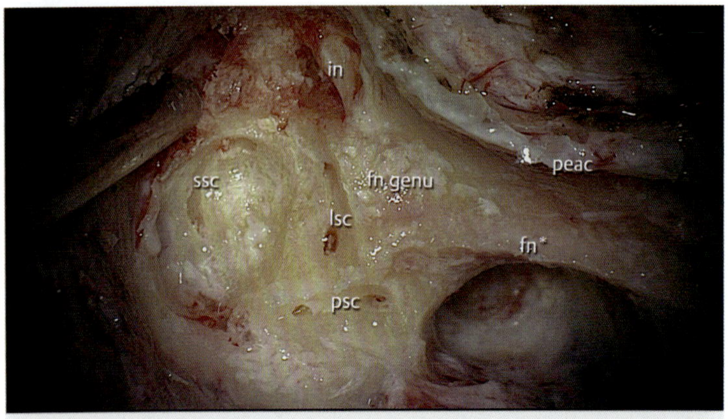

Fig. 2.57 Clinical Case 2, Right side: The lateral, superior, and posterior semicircular canals are opened. The close anatomical relationship between the lateral semicircular canal and the second genu of the facial nerve can be noticed. *fn*: mastoid segment of facial nerve; fn genu: second genu of facial nerve; in: incus; lsc: lateral semicircular canal; peac: posterior wall of external auditory canal; psc: posterior semicircular canal; ssc: superior semicircular canal.*

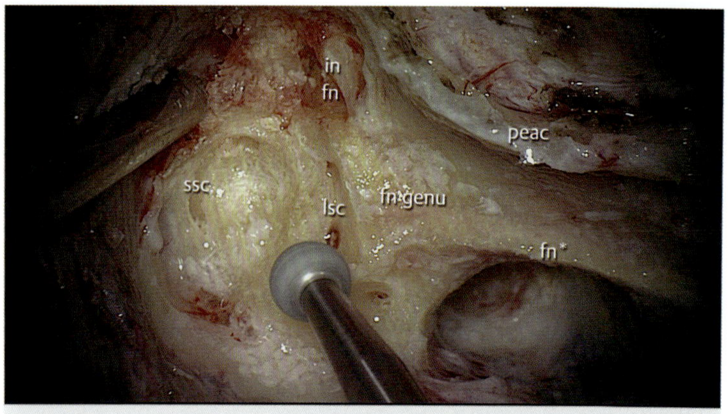

Fig. 2.58 Clinical Case 2, Right side: During the drilling of the semicircular canals, the most anterior portion of the lateral semicircular canal should be kept in place to protect the facial nerve, preventing its damage in close proximity to the second genu. *fn: tympanic segment of facial nerve; fn*: mastoid segment of facial nerve; fn genu: second genu of facial nerve; in: incus; lsc: lateral semicircular canal; peac: posterior wall of external auditory canal; ssc: superior semicircular canal.*

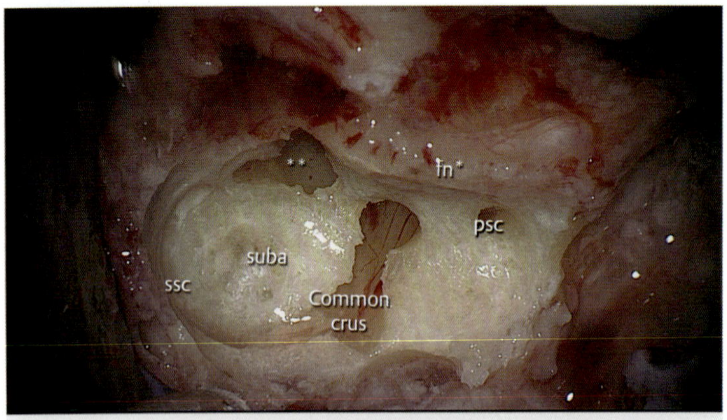

Fig. 2.59 Clinical Case 2, Right side: The superior semicircular canal is opened until the ampullae and the common crus are identified. ***: the joint lateral and superior ampullae; fn*: mastoid segment of facial nerve; psc: posterior semicircular canal; suba: subarquate artery.*

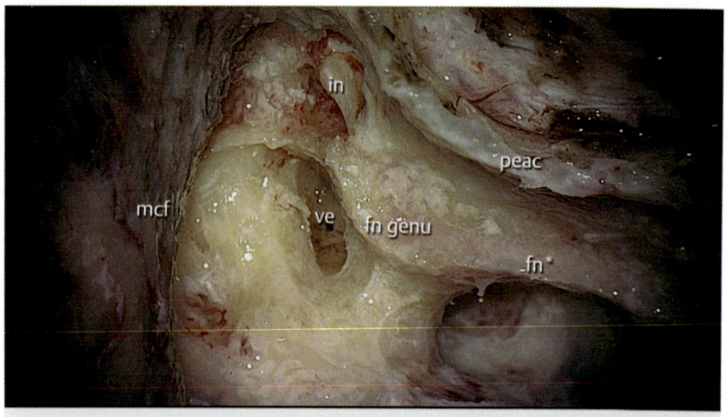

Fig. 2.60 Clinical Case 2, Right side: The vestibule is opened. The labyrinthine portion of the facial nerve runs immediately medially to the most posterior and superior portions of the vestibule, entering the fundus of the internal auditory canal (IAC). *fn*: mastoid segment of facial nerve; fn genu: second genu of facial nerve; in: incus; mcf: middle cranial fossa; peac: posterior wall of external auditory canal; ve: vestibule.*

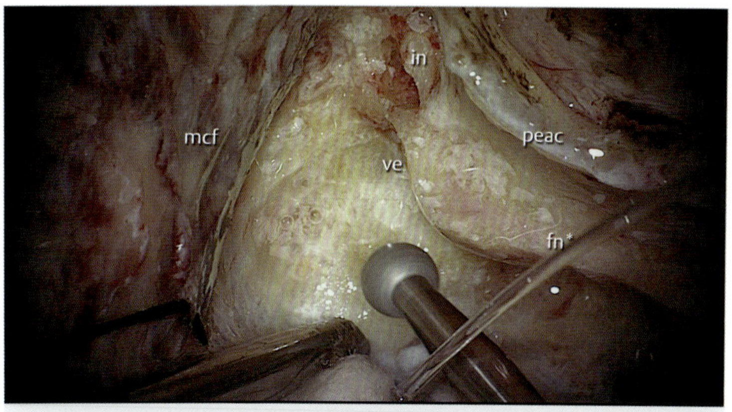

Fig. 2.61 Clinical Case 2, Right side: The surgical field is irrigated and a diamond bur is used to identify the internal auditory canal (IAC). The surgeon must be careful during the detection of the most anterior and superior portions of the IAC close to the fundus, to avoid damage to the labyrinthine portion of the facial nerve in its entrance into the IAC. *fn*: mastoid segment of facial nerve; in: incus; mcf: middle cranial fossa; peac: posterior wall of external auditory canal; ve: vestibule.*

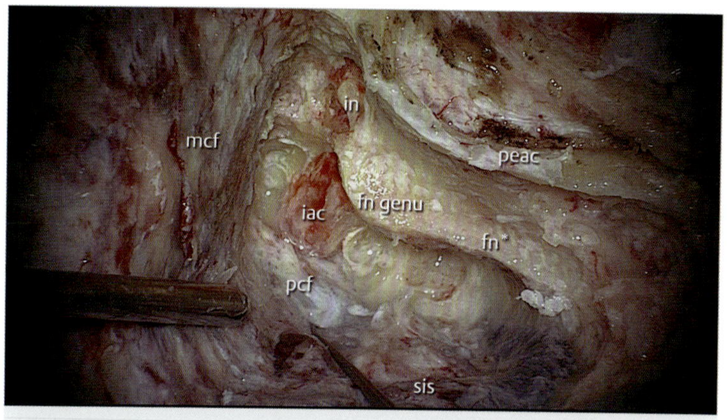

Fig. 2.62 Clinical Case 2, Right side: The internal auditory canal (IAC) is exposed from the fundus until the porus. *fn*: mastoid segment of facial nerve; fn genu: second genu of facial nerve; iac: internal auditory canal; in: incus; mcf: middle cranial fossa; pcf: posterior cranial fossa; peac: posterior wall of external auditory canal; sis: sigmoid sinus.*

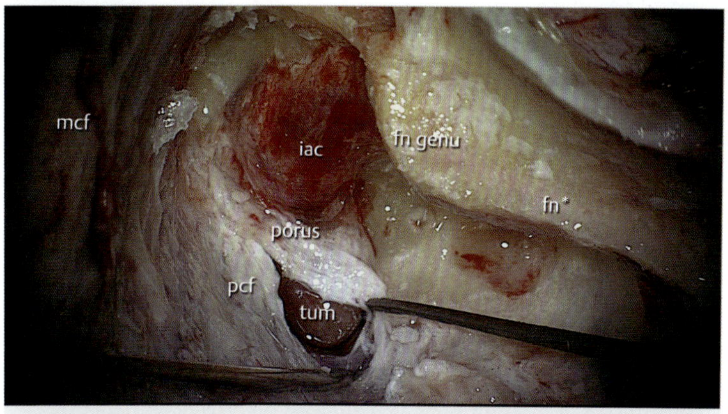

Fig. 2.63 Clinical Case 2, Right side: Before opening the dura of the posterior fossa, a bipolar instrument is used to coagulate the line of incision. Microscissors are used to cut the dura in proximity to the porus, along the surface of the temporal bone to avoid damage to the cerebellum entering the cerebellopontine angle (CPA). *fn*: mastoid segment of facial nerve; fn genu: second genu of facial nerve; iac: internal auditory canal; mcf: middle cranial fossa; pcf: posterior cranial fossa; tum: acoustic tumor.*

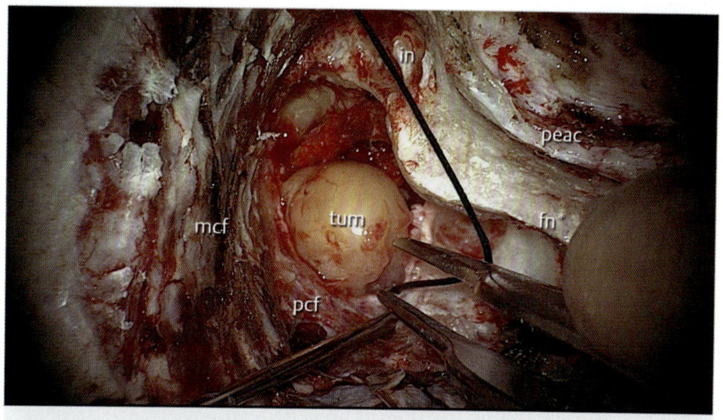

Fig. 2.64 Clinical Case 2, Right side: Before tumor removal, the lateral cisterna is opened allowing cerebrospinal fluid (CSF) leakage. After this step, the cerebellum and the brainstem are relaxed, and tumor removal is easier. *fn*: mastoid segment of facial nerve; in: incus; mcf: middle cranial fossa; pcf: posterior cranial fossa; peac: posterior wall of external auditory canal; tum: acoustic tumor.*

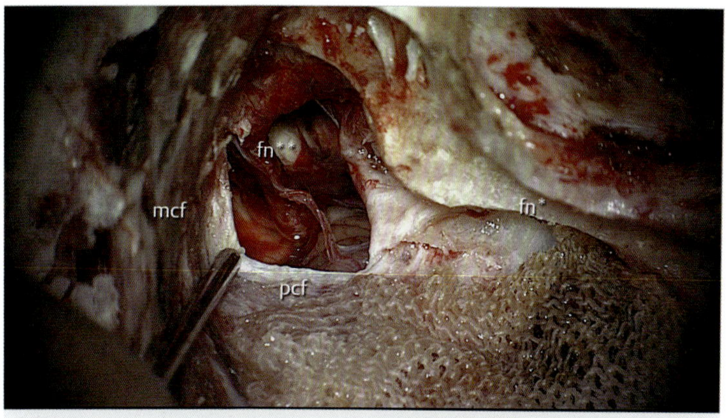

Fig. 2.65 Clinical Case 2, Right side: Final view of the brainstem after tumor removal. *fn*: mastoid segment of facial nerve; fn**: facial nerve into the cerebellopontine angle (CPA); mcf: middle cranial fossa; pcf: posterior cranial fossa.*

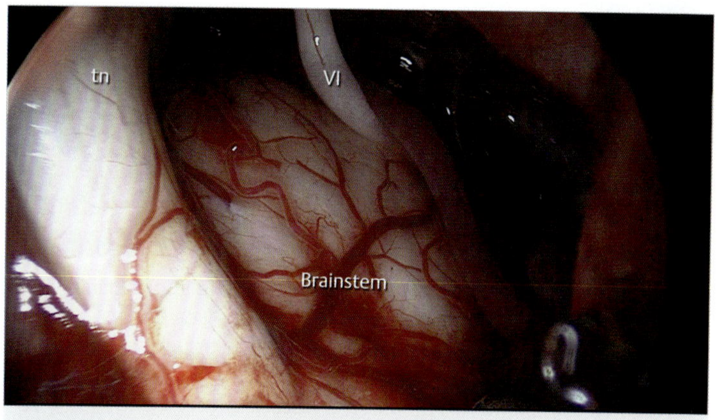

Fig. 2.66 Clinical Case 2, Right side: Endoscopic magnification with 0-degree endoscope of the cerebellopontine angle (CPA) through the translabyrinthine cavity. *tn: trigeminal nerve.*

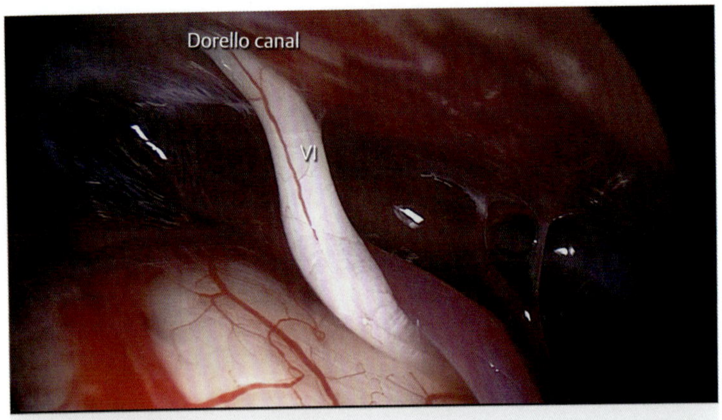

Fig. 2.67 Clinical Case 2, Right side: Endoscopic magnification of the VI cranial nerve inside the cerebellopontine angle (CPA).

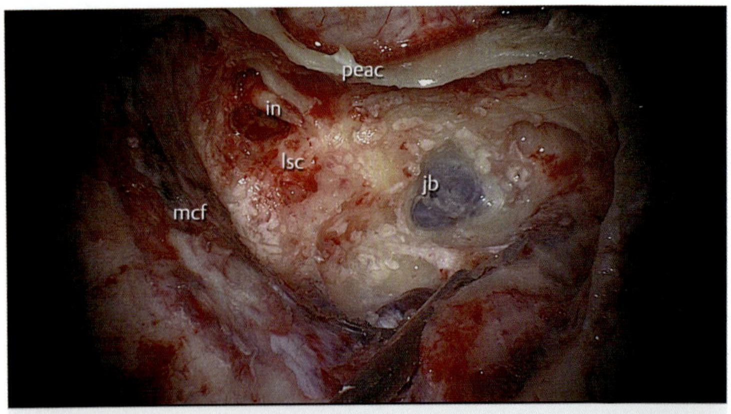

Fig. 2.68 Clinical Case 3, Right side: A high jugular bulb is visible in this patient. The jugular bulb must be skeletonized to define the most superior limit of the vein related to the labyrinthine block. *in: incus; jb: jugular bulb; lsc: lateral semicircular canal; mcf: middle cranial fossa; peac: posterior wall of external auditory canal.*

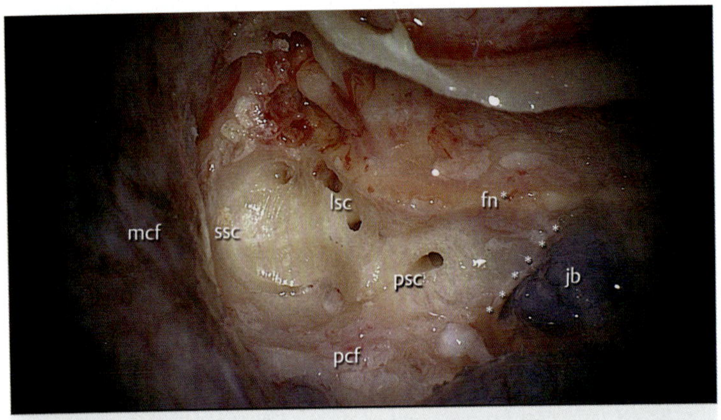

Fig. 2.69 Clinical Case 3, Right side: The labyrinthectomy is started paying attention to the relationship between the jugular bulb and the posterior semicircular canal. During the labyrinthectomy, Surgicel is used over the jugular bulb to protect the vein and suction is used to depress the bulb during the drilling time. *fn*: mastoid segment of facial nerve; jb: jugular bulb; lsc: lateral semicircular canal; mcf: middle cranial fossa; pcf: posterior cranial fossa; psc: posterior semicircular canal; ssc: superior semicircular canal.*

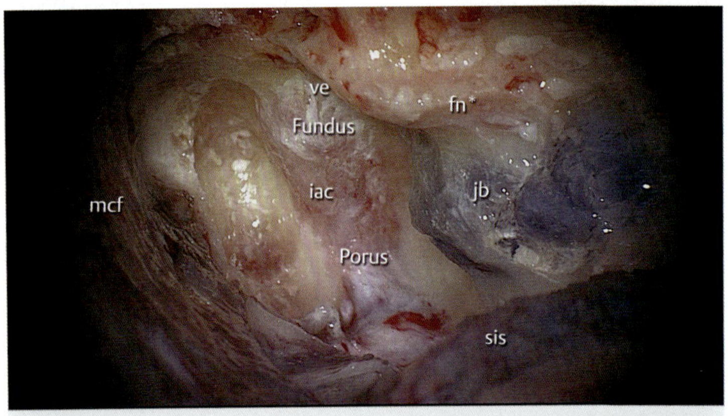

Fig. 2.70 Clinical Case 3, Right side: The internal auditory canal (IAC) is skeletonized. A piece of bone wax may be used to press down the jugular bulb. *fn*: mastoid segment of facial nerve; iac: internal auditory canal; jb: jugular bulb; mcf: middle cranial fossa; sis: sigmoid sinus; ve: vestibule.*

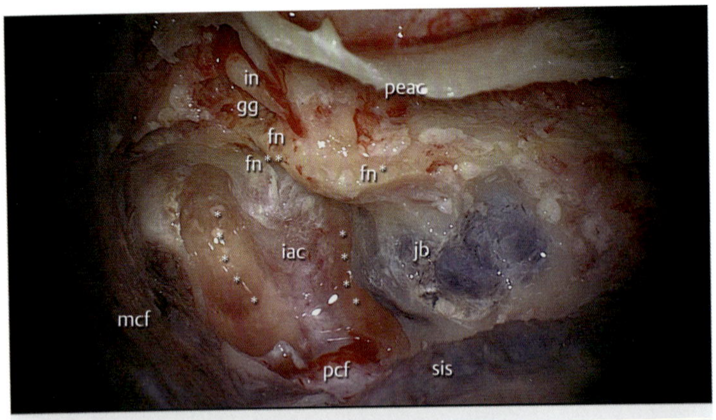

Fig. 2.71 Clinical Case 3, Right side: The internal auditory canal (IAC) is drilled creating two troughs, inferior and superior (see the **** line). During this step one must be careful to create the troughs between the jugular bulb and the inferior portion of the IAC. The jugular bulb should be covered by bone wax to protect the vascular structure and should be pressed down during the drilling. *fn: tympanic segment of facial nerve; fn*: mastoid segment of facial nerve; fn**: labyrinthine portion of facial nerve; gg: geniculate ganglion; iac: internal auditory canal; in: incus; jb: jugular bulb; mcf: middle cranial fossa; pcf: posterior cranial fossa; peac: posterior wall of external auditory canal; sis: sigmoid sinus.*

bony layer over the jugular bulb when the vascular structure is just under the labyrinthine block in order to protect the vein during the tumor dissection into the IAC (see Clinical Case 3). If the vein is uncovered, a piece of Surgicel is placed on the vascular structure in order to protect the jugular bulb during the labyrinthectomy. This enables the surgeon to uncover the most superior aspect of the bulb during the opening of the labyrinthine. After this maneuver, a piece of bony wax may be used to cover and press down the jugular bulb during the drilling to detect the IAC. Control of the jugular bulb should be kept during the whole dissection of the IAC from the fundus to the porus (see Clinical Case 3 ▶ Fig. 2.70 and ▶ Fig. 2.71). The dura of the IAC is opened, exposing the tumor. Cottonoids are used to cover the jugular bulb during tumor removal (see Clinical Case 3 ▶ Fig. 2.72 and ▶ Fig. 2.73).

- In case of a large acoustic neuroma, or neuroma with an anterior extension treatment, a transapical drilling should be performed around the IAC (see Clinical Case 4). In these cases, the IAC is uncovered, removing the bone inferiorly and superiorly to the petrous apex 360 degrees around the canal, circumferentially exposing the IAC (see Clinical Case 5).

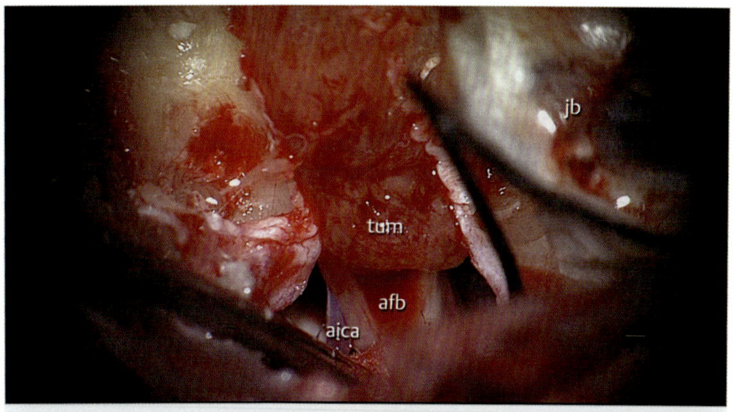

Fig. 2.72 Clinical Case 3, Right side: After opening the dura of the posterior fossa the tumor is visible, spreading into the internal auditory canal (IAC) until the porus. *afb: acousticfacial bundle; jb: jugular bulb; tum: acoustic tumor.*

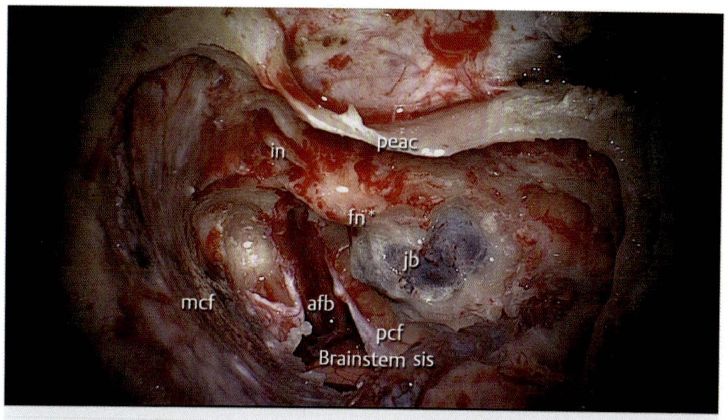

Fig. 2.73 Clinical Case 3, Right side: Final cavity after tumor removal. *afb: acoustic-facial bundle; fn*: mastoid segment of facial nerve; in: incus; jb: jugular bulb; mcf: middle cranial fossa; pcf: posterior cranial fossa; peac: posterior wall of external auditory canal; sis: sigmoid sinus.*

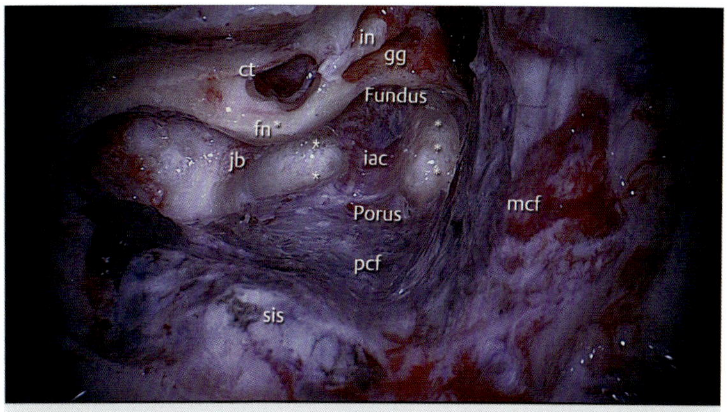

Fig. 2.74 Clinical Case 4, Left side: The bone surrounding the internal auditory canal (IAC) is removed (see the *** line). A transapical extension is performed. *ct: chorda tympani; fn*: mastoid segment of facial nerve; gg: geniculate ganglion; in: incus; jb: jugular bulb; mcf: middle cranial fossa; pcf: posterior cranial fossa; peac: posterior wall of external auditory canal; sis: sigmoid sinus.*

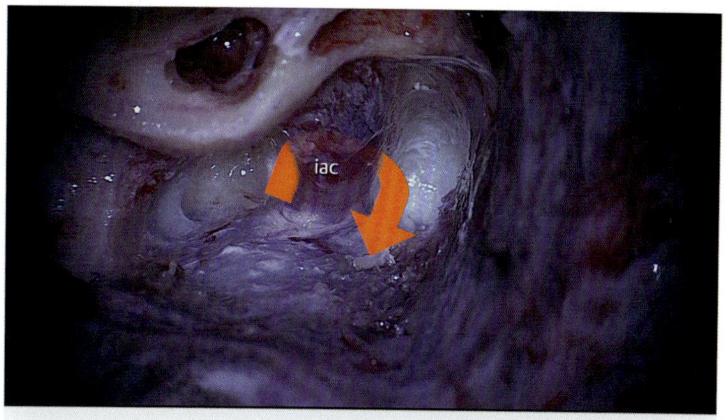

Fig. 2.75 Clinical Case 4, Left side: In an enlarged translabyrinthine approach with transapical extension the bone around the internal auditory canal (IAC) should be removed to drill the internal canal for a 360° circumference (see the *orange arrow*). *iac: internal auditory canal.*

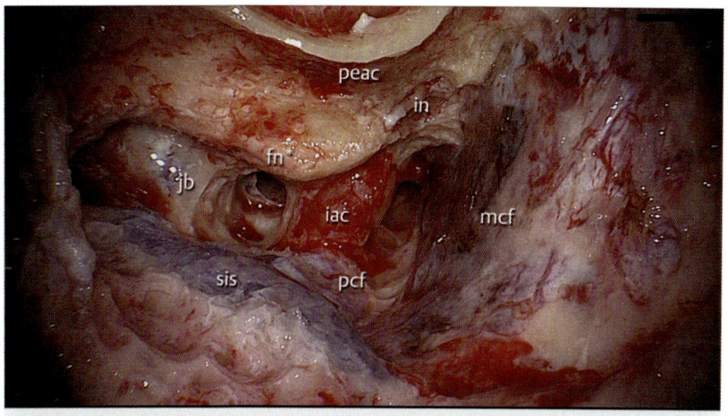

Fig. 2.76 Clinical Case 5, Left side: An enlarged translabyrinthine approach with transapical extension is performed. The petrous apex cells around the internal auditory canal (IAC) are opened. *fn*: mastoid segment of facial nerve; iac: internal auditory canal; in: incus; jb: jugular bulb; mcf: middle cranial fossa; pcf: posterior cranial fossa; peac: posterior wall of external auditory canal; sis: sigmoid sinus.*

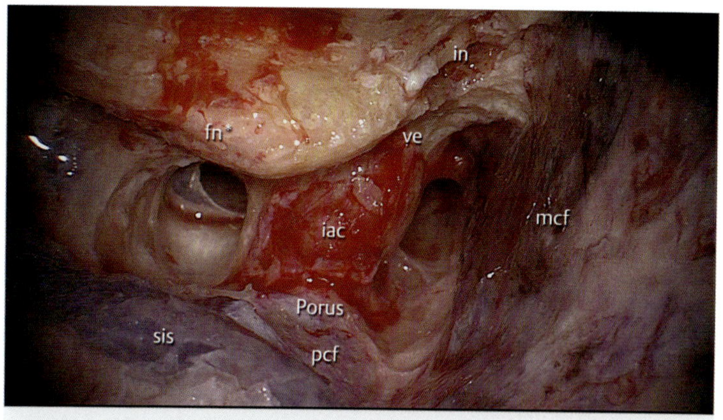

Fig. 2.77 Clinical Case 5, Left side: A microscopic magnification of the internal auditory canal (IAC) after an enlarged translabyrinthine approach with transapical extension. *fn*: mastoid segment of facial nerve; iac: internal auditory canal; in: incus; mcf: middle cranial fossa; pcf: posterior cranial fossa; sis: sigmoid sinus; ve: vestibule.*

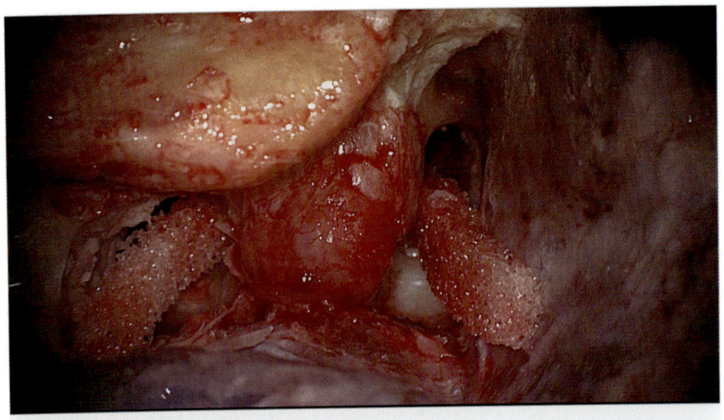

Fig. 2.78 Clinical Case 5, Left side: An enlarged translabyrinthine approach with transapical extension is performed. After drilling all the bone surrounding the internal auditory canal (IAC) (360 degrees) a Gelfoam strip is inserted along the medial portion of the IAC.

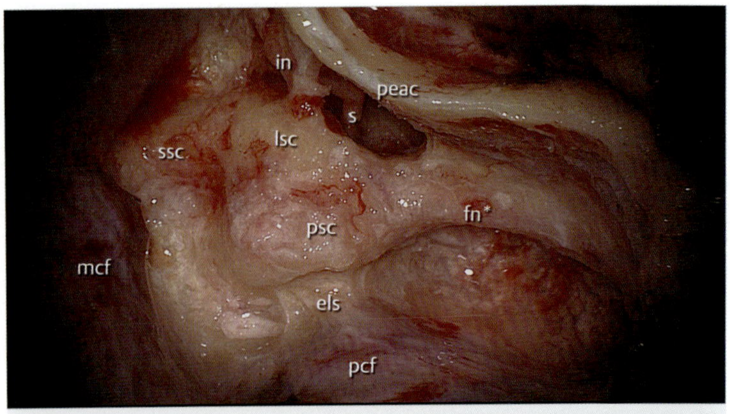

Fig. 2.79 Clinical Case 6, Right side: The labyrinthine block is isolated, the facial nerve is detected, and a posterior tympanotomy is performed to expose the round window niche and the incudostapedial joint. *els: endolymphatic sac; fn*: mastoid segment of facial nerve; in: incus; lsc: lateral semicircular canal; mcf: middle cranial fossa; pcf: posterior cranial fossa; peac: posterior wall of external auditory canal; psc: posterior semicircular canal; s: stapes; ssc: superior semicircular canal.*

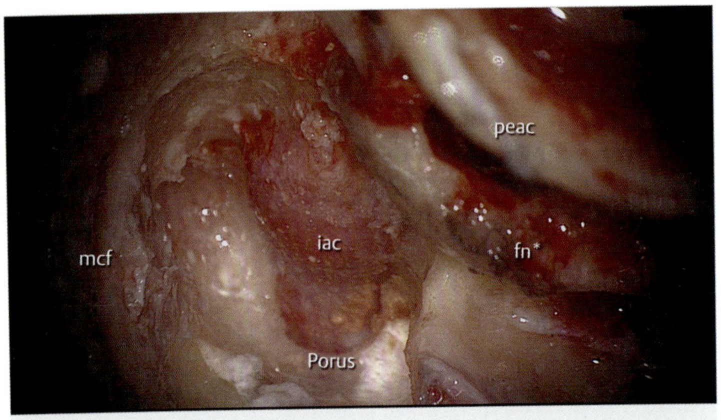

Fig. 2.80 Clinical Case 6, Right side: After the labyrinthectomy the internal auditory canal (IAC) is skeletonized from the fundus to the porus. *iac: internal auditory canal; mcf: middle cranial fossa; peac: posterior auditory canal.*

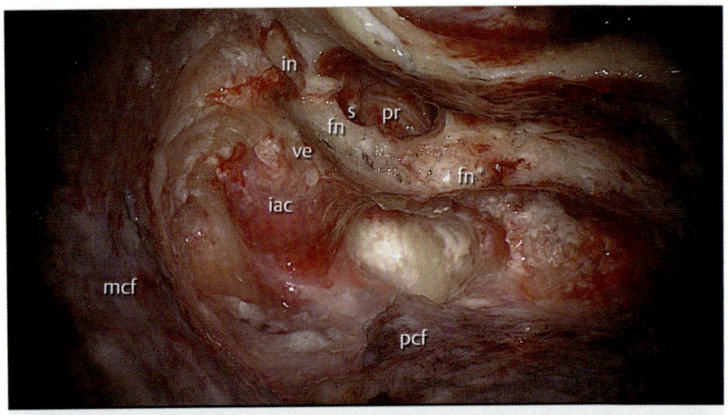

Fig. 2.81 Clinical Case 6, Right side: After internal auditory canal (IAC) exposure, the cochleostomy is started through the tympanotomy. *fn*: mastoid segment of facial nerve; fn: tympanic segment of facial nerve; iac: internal auditory canal; in: incus; mcf: middle cranial fossa; pr: promontory; s: stapes; ve: vestibule.*

2.3 Translabyrinthine Approach and Cochlear Implant

In certain conditions, a simultaneous cochlear implant during translabyrinthine procedure should be considered. To do so, a cochlear nerve intraoperative monitoring is mandatory during surgery, and a soft dissection of the tumor, preserving the acoustic nerve and the cochlea, is necessary.

Despite the feasibility of this procedure, the results in literature are controversial, especially if we have to consider the long-term results in terms of hearing function. At present, we have no guideline regarding the indication.

2.3.1 Indications

The authors recommend the placement of a cochlear implant during translabyrinthine approach in the following situations:

- When a surgical route in the site of the acoustic neuroma for hearing preservation is not recommendable due to unstable conditions, such as chronic otitis media with or without cholesteatoma, in the contralateral ear.
- Receptive hearing loss in the contralateral ear.
- Type 2 neurofibromatosis (NF2) patients with bilateral acoustic neuroma, when a cochlear nerve preservation is possible due to the small dimension of the tumor.

2.3.2 Surgical Steps

The translabyrinthine approach is performed as previously described. A posterior tympanotomy is performed to expose the promontory and the round window niche (see Clinical Case 6). The labyrinthectomy is performed and the IAC is isolated from the fundus to the porus. Once the dura of the posterior fossa and the IAC are uncovered, before opening the dura, the cochleostomy is performed through the posterior tympanotomy using a small diamond bur (see Clinical Case 7). The tegmen, and posterior and anterior pillars of the round window niche are drilled until the round window membrane is identified. The round window is opened, entering the scala tympani (see Clinical Case 6 ▶ Fig. 2.82). Once the scala tympani is detected, a piece of Gelfoam is placed on the cochleostomy, and the IAC dura is opened, isolating the tumor (see Clinical Case 6 ▶ Fig. 2.83 and ▶ Fig. 2.84). The inferior and superior vestibular nerves are cut and the cochlear and facial nerves are isolated. Cottonoids soaked with water are placed in between the tumor and the nerves protecting the nervous structures. During this step, intraoperative monitoring may help the surgeon find the right plane of dissection, separating and preserving the cochlear nerve and the facial

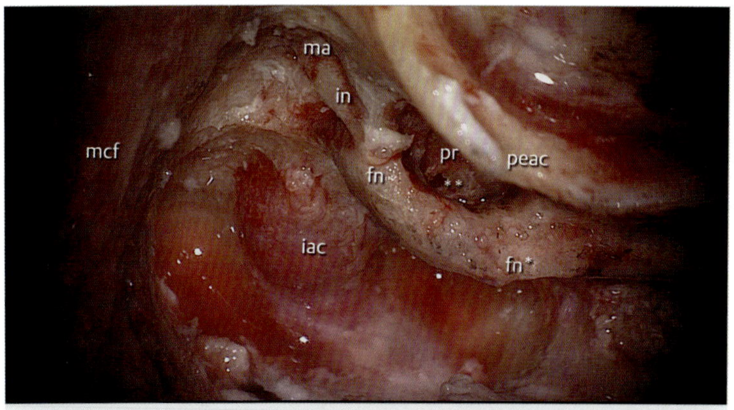

Fig. 2.82 Clinical Case 6, Right side: Using a small diamond bur the round window niche is drilled until the round window membrane is detected. After this step, the round window is opened entering the scala tympani. *fn: tympanic segment of facial nerve; fn*: mastoid segment of facial nerve; iac: internal auditory canal; in: incus; ma: malleus; mcf: middle cranial fossa; pr: promontory; **: round window cochleostomy.*

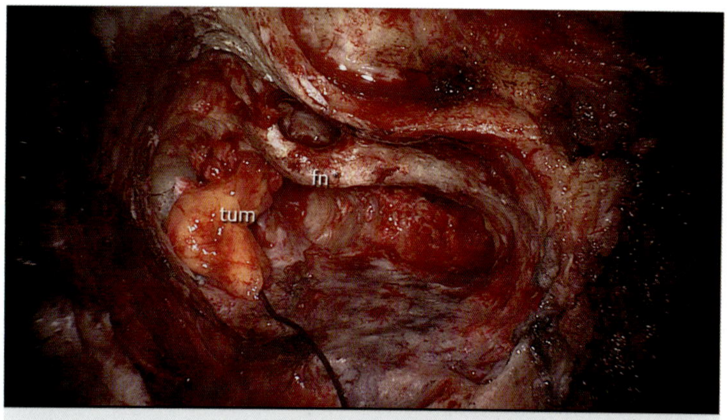

Fig. 2.83 Clinical Case 6, Right side: The tumor is removed from the internal auditory canal (IAC). The surgeon must be careful to preserve the facial nerve and the cochlear nerve. The cochlear nerve lies medially to the inferior vestibular nerve, entering inferiorly to the transverse crest. *fn*: mastoid segment of facial nerve; tum: acoustic tumor.*

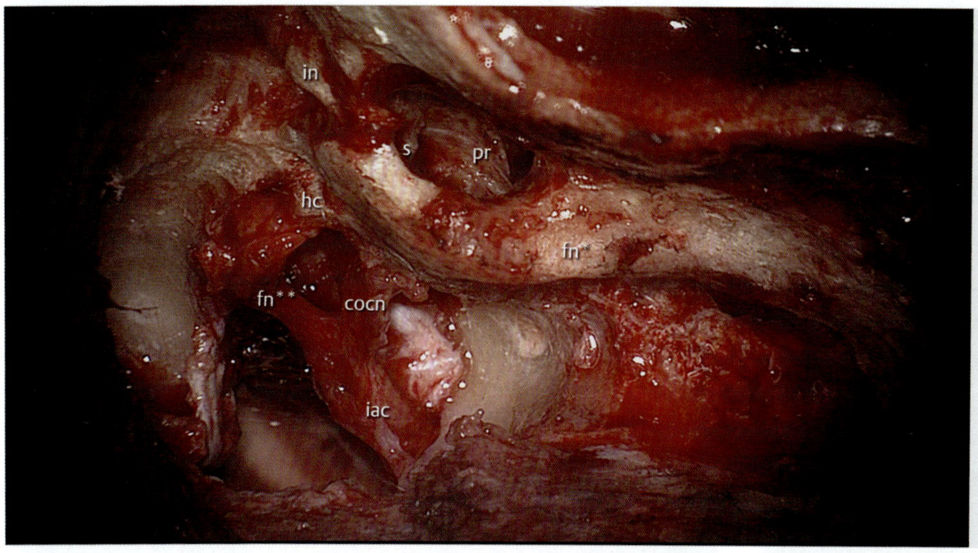

Fig. 2.84 Clinical Case 6, Right side: The cochlear nerve and the facial nerve are preserved and visible in the internal auditory canal (IAC). *cocn: cochlear nerve; fn*: mastoid segment of facial nerve; fn**: facial nerve into the IAC; hc: horizontal (transverse) crest; iac: internal auditory canal; in: incus; pr: promontory; s: stapes.*

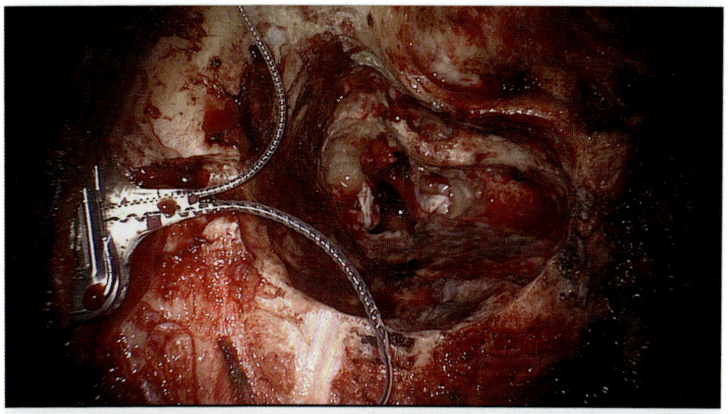

Fig. 2.85 Clinical Case 6, Right side: The receiver-stimulator complex of the implant is fixed in its bed.

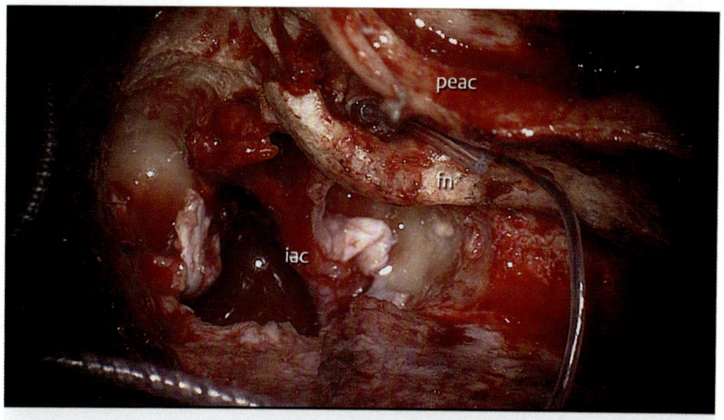

Fig. 2.86 Clinical Case 6, Right side: The array is placed into the cochleostomy, and pulled in a gentle way into the scala tympani until the final marker. *fn*: mastoid segment of facial nerve; iac: internal auditory canal; peac: posterior wall of external auditory canal.*

nerve with a soft dissection (see Clinical Case 7 ► Fig. 2.91 and ► Fig. 2.92), and know the status of the cochlear nerve. After tumor removal, the receiver-stimulator complex of the implant is placed and fixed under the temporalis muscle after drilling the placement, and the array is gently inserted into the cochleostomy (see Clinical Case 6 ► Fig. 2.85 and ► Fig. 2.86). A piece of muscle may help to fix the array to the cochleostomy and a fat pad is used to close the connection of the CPA and the surgical cavity.

The eustachian tube and the posterior tympanotomy are filled with pieces of muscle harvested from the temporalis muscle. Bony dust is placed over the muscle separating the tympanic cavity from

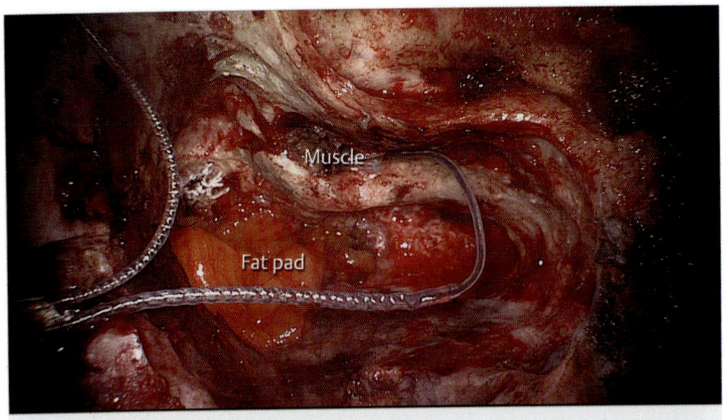

Fig. 2.87 Clinical Case 6, Right side: A fragment of muscle is placed into the posterior tympanotomy to fix the array and to exclude the tympanic cavity from the mastoid cavity. Abdominal fat is used to obliterate the connection between the cerebellopontine angle (CPA) and the mastoid.

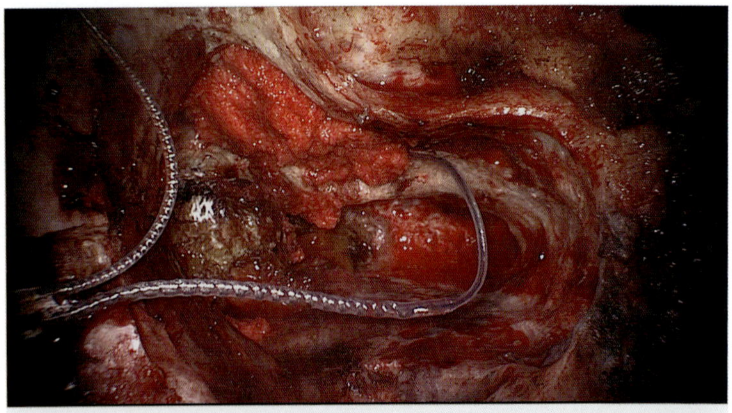

Fig. 2.88 Clinical Case 6, Right side: Bone dust is used to obliterate the posterior tympanotomy and the aditus.

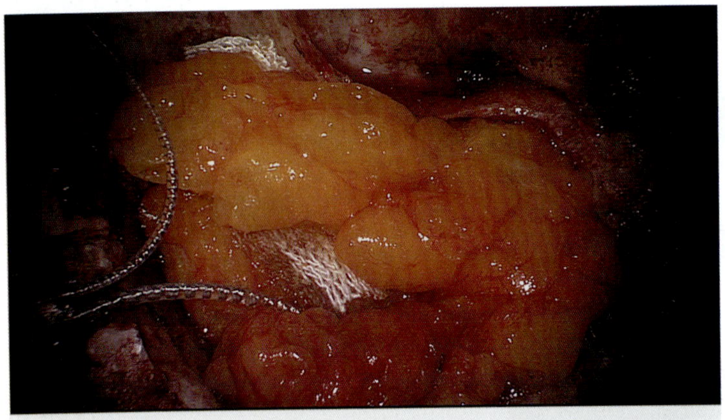

Fig. 2.89 Clinical Case 7, Right side: Abdominal fat is used to fill and obliterate the surgical cavity.

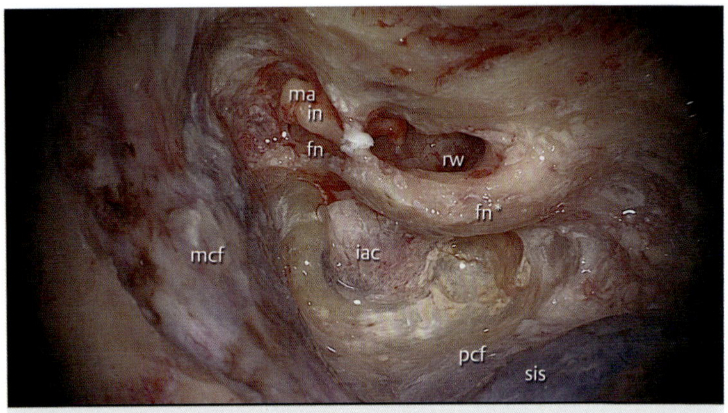

Fig. 2.90 Clinical Case 7, Right side: The posterior tympanotomy is performed and after labyrinthectomy the internal auditory canal (IAC) is exposed. *fn: tympanic segment of facial nerve; fn*: mastoid segment of facial nerve; iac: internal auditory canal; in: incus; ma: malleus; mcf: middle cranial fossa; pcf: posterior cranial fossa; rw: round window; sis: sigmoid sinus.*

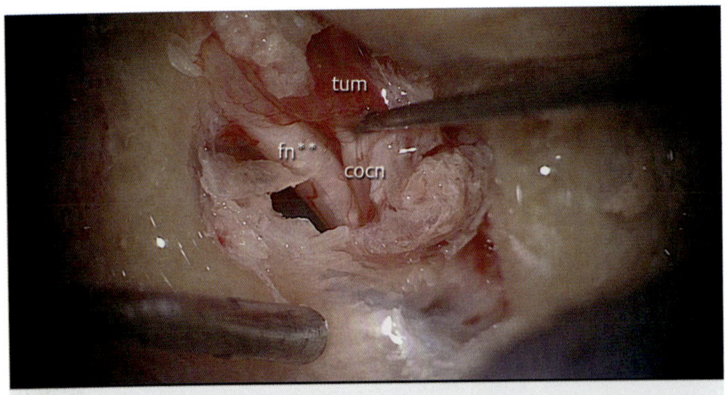

Fig. 2.91 Clinical Case 7, Right side: The acoustic tumor is removed from the internal auditory canal (IAC) and the cochlear nerve is carefully preserved. *cocn: cochlear nerve; fn**: facial nerve into the IAC; tum: acoustic tumor.*

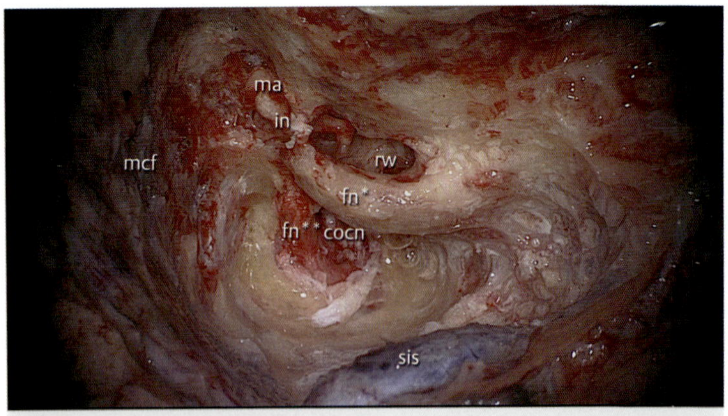

Fig. 2.92 Clinical Case 7, Right side: Final view of the surgical cavity after tumor removal; the round window is exposed through the posterior tympanotomy. *cocn: cochlear nerve; fn*: mastoid segment of facial nerve; fn**: facial nerve into the IAC; in: incus; ma: malleus; mcf: middle cranial fossa; rw: round window; sis: sigmoid sinus.*

the surgical cavity (see Clinical Case 6 ▶ Fig. 2.88). A fibrin glue is used to reinforce the obliteration. Abdominal fat is used to fill the whole surgical cavity (see Clinical Case 6 ▶ Fig. 2.89).

2.4 Translabyrinthine Approach and Brainstem Implant

The translabyrinthine route may also be used for brainstem implant surgery, especially when surgery for patients affected by bilateral acoustic neuroma (NF2) is planned. In that case, depending on the audiological status after tumor removal, a simultaneous brainstem implant should be considered.

2.5 Indications

Indications for brainstem implant are:

- Bilateral acoustic neuroma in NF2 patients according to their audiological status.

- Bilateral cochlear nerve aplasia.
- Bilateral transverse fracture of temporal bone with a bilateral interruption of the cochlear nerve.
- Necessary acoustic neuroma resection in the only hearing ear when it is not possible to preserve the cochlear nerve.

It is necessary to bear in mind that in case of bilateral acoustic nerve hypoplasia, cochlear and inner ear malformations, or cochlear ossification, a cochlear implant should be attempted before considering a brainstem implant, and in such cases, the brainstem implant will be planned in the event of a bad outcome or a failure of the cochlear implant.

2.5.1 Surgical Steps (See Also Chapter 7)

Anatomically, the extremity of the lateral recess forms the foramen of Luschka, which is found at the edge of the bulbopontine sulcus. Just above the foramen, the root of nerves VII and VIII can be seen and below it that of nerves IX and X. The choroid plexus is attached to the inner surface of the choroid tela and protrudes from the foramen of Luschka below the entrance of nerves VII and VIII and it slides to overlap the posterior part of nerves IX and X. The floccule is a cerebellar lobe which protrudes from the margin of the lateral recess and adheres to the rostral margin of the lateral recess and to the foramen of Luschka. The tenia passes across the roof of the lateral recess and outlines the area of the ventral cochlear nucleus.

From a surgical point of view, after a translabyrinthine approach and tumor removal, performed as previously described (see ▶ Fig. 2.68), the receiver-stimulator complex of the brainstem implant is placed and fixed under the temporalis muscle after drilling its placement. The lateral recess should be microscopically detected inside the CPA and the choroid plexus must be identified. This anatomical structure protrudes laterally to the brainstem, and by following it toward the posterior surface, the entrance to the lateral recess can easily be detected. The origin of IX cranial nerve from the brainstem, the stump of the VIII cranial nerve, and the facial nerve and the tinea choroidea should be detected as well, since all these anatomical structures converge on the mouth of the lateral recess. The entrance of the lateral recess is located just above the origin of the glossopharyngeal nerve at the level of the brainstem. This anatomical landmark is important especially after tumor removal since it is consistent, while the surface of the brainstem may be distorted. Once the lateral recess is detected, a careful opening of the recess exposing the foramen of Luschka should be carried out. The electrode plate should be placed carefully with a soft movement over the brainstem, inserting it into the foramen deeply (see Clinical Case 8 ▶ Fig. 2.95 and ▶ Fig. 2.96).

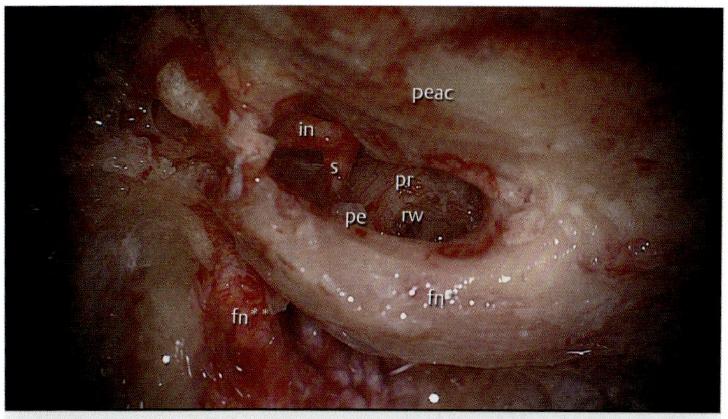

Fig. 2.93 Clinical Case 7, Right side: Microscopic magnification of the round window region through the posterior tympanotomy.
cocn: cochlear nerve; fn: mastoid segment of facial nerve; fn**: facial nerve into the internal auditory canal (IAC); in: incus; pe: pyramidal eminence; peac: posterior wall of external auditory canal; pr: promontory; rw: round window; s: stapes.*

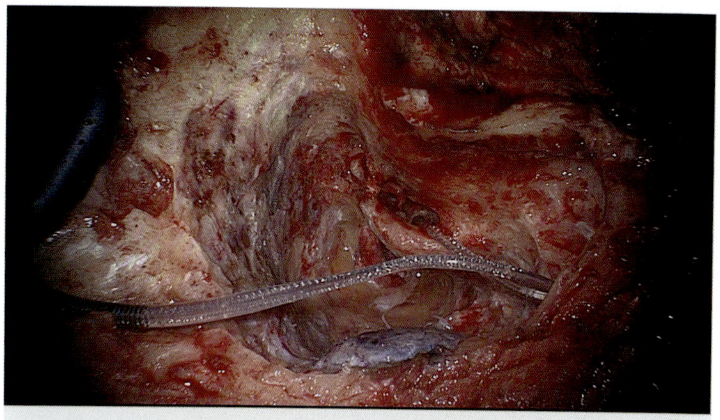

Fig. 2.94 Clinical Case 7, Right side: The cochlear implant is placed under the temporalis muscle and the array is inserted into the cochleostomy.

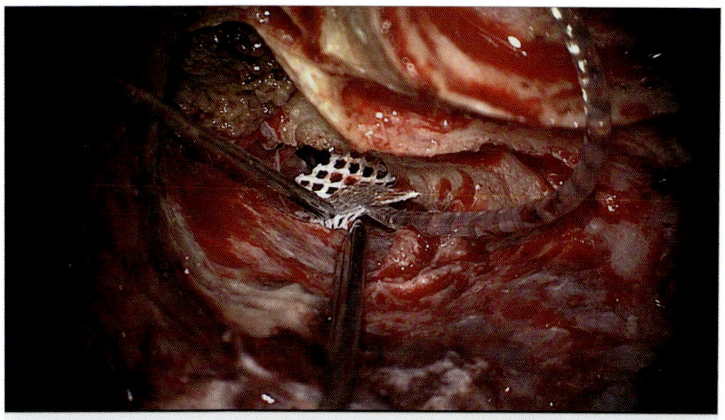

Fig. 2.95 Clinical Case 8, Right side:: Once the lateral recess is detected in between the stump of VIII nerve and IX nerve through the translabyrinthine approach, the receiver-stimulator is placed under the temporalis muscle, and the electrode plate is gently pushed into the cerebellopontine angle (CPA).

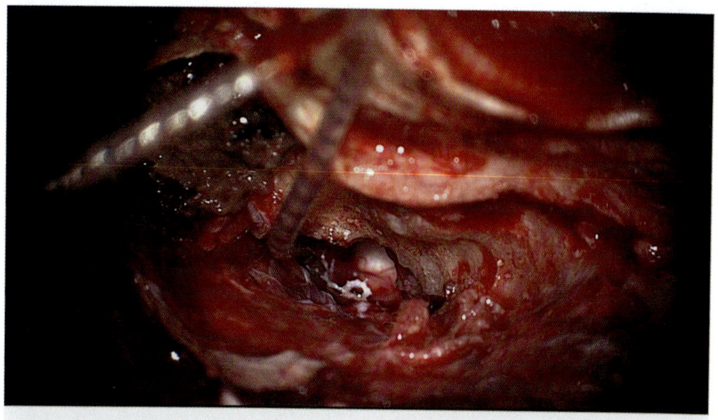

Fig. 2.96 Clinical Case 8, Right side: The electrode plate is gently inserted into the foramen of Luschka through the lateral recess. After this surgical maneuver, the intraoperative electrophysiological test may help to find the best position for the implant.

After placing the electrode plate into the foramen of Luschka, the electrophysiology may help in the right orientation of the implant, looking for the best audiological response and stimulation results of the cochlear nuclei. After the final placement, a piece of muscle is placed between the glossopharyngeal nerve and the electrode plate in order to separate the implant from the nerves to avoid extra-auditive effects. Fibrin glue is used to fix the electrode plate into the foramen. A long strip of abdominal fat is used to obliterate the surgical cavity around the implant in the CPA.

2.5.2 Postoperative Care

Patients need to stay in the intensive care unit for monitoring for 24 hours after surgery.

A computed tomography (CT) scan is performed 6 hours after surgery (see ▶ Fig. 2.97). The patient should maintain a supine position for 2 days, and early progressive deambulation is required in order to reduce the risk of pulmonary embolus or deep vein thrombosis. The compressive bandage is removed 4 days after surgery. Traditionally, the patient is discharged around 7 days after surgery; the suture is removed after 10 days. Magnetic resonance imaging (MRI) is planned 1 year after surgery to check the result.

2.5.3 Complications

Although the translabyrinthine approach is a safe procedure, it is still a neurosurgical procedure and some complications should be considered especially during large tumor removal:

- Postoperative CSF leak
- Cranial nerve deficit (facial nerve and lower cranial nerves)
- Meningitis/Infections
- Postoperative bleeding, CPA hematoma formation
- Infarction or stroke with cerebral ischemia

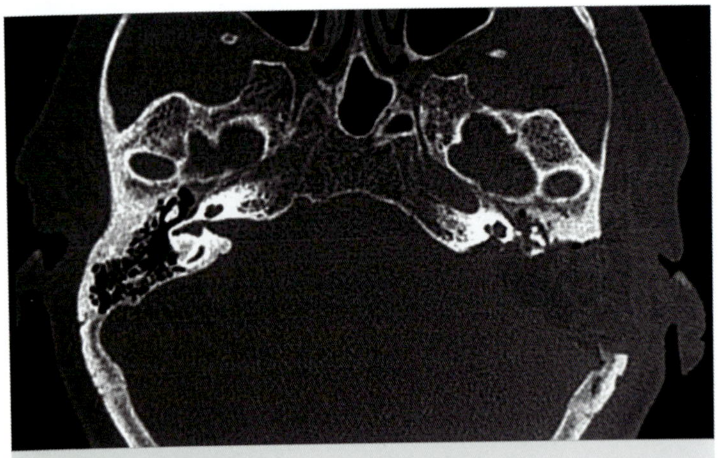

Fig. 2.97 Postoperative computed tomography (CT) scan after a translabyrinthine approach.

2.6 Retrolabyrinthine Approach

2.6.1 Rationale

The retrolabyrinthine approach is a modification of the traditional translabyrinthine approach, passing just behind the labyrinthine block. With this surgical route, the preservation of hearing becomes possible, and the preservation of the cochlear nerve during the tumor removal is mandatory. This approach provides access to the CPA and the most posterior portion of the IAC close to the porus without sacrificing the labyrinthine block; but since the surgical window is limited, an appropriate selection of the patients is crucial to obtain a good result in terms of hearing function.

2.6.2 Indications

The indications for a retrolabyrinthine approach are limited to the following(see ▶ Fig. 2.98):

- Small and medium size tumor located in the CPA or in the porus, without involvement of the most lateral portion of the IAC in patients with a preoperative good hearing function.
- Posterior fossa meningioma with adhesion of the posterior portion of the temporal bone in the proximity of the porus with a preoperative good hearing function (see Clinical Case 10).
- Neurovascular conflict in the entry zone of the acoustic-facial nerve bundle.
- Vestibular nerve section in Meniere's disease.

2.6.3 Advantages

- Direct approach to CPA and the most medial section of the IAC especially the porus with preservation of the hearing function by passing behind the otic capsule.

2.6.4 Limitations

- Inability to expose the fundus and the most lateral portion of the IAC.
- Unsuitable for tumors with IAC involvement.

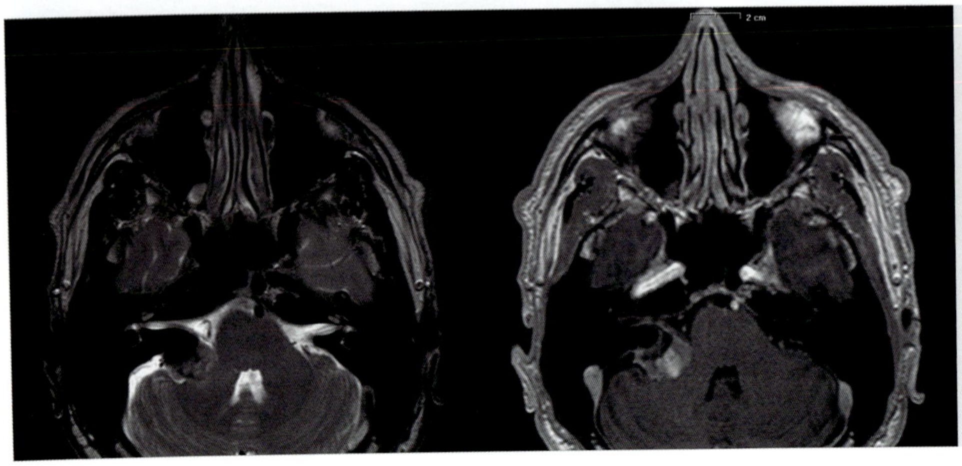

Fig. 2.98 Magnetic resonance imaging (MRI) scan in axial view showing a meningioma of the right posterior fossa.

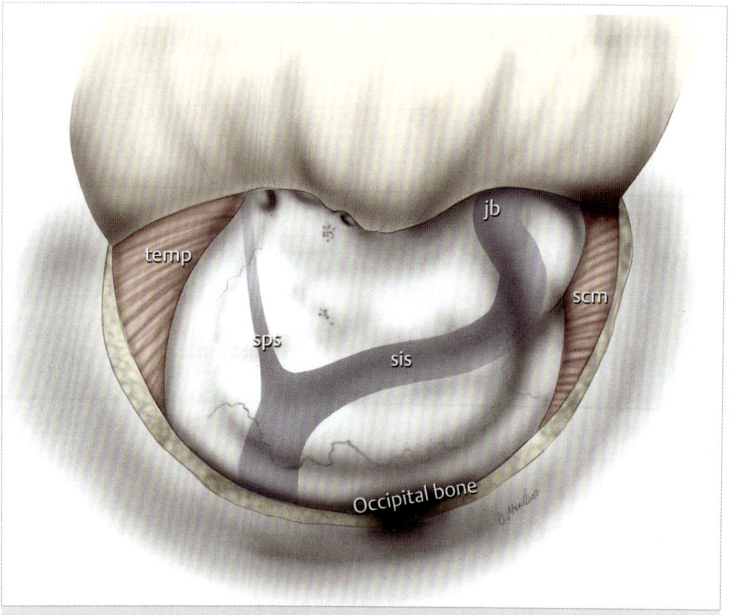

Fig. 2.99 Right side: The flap has been elevated and the mastoid bone uncovered. On the surface on the mastoid bone the route of the sigmoid sinus is noticeable. *jb: jugular bulb; scm: sternocleidomastoid muscle; sis: sigmoid sinus; sps: superior petrosal sinus; temp: temporalis muscle.*

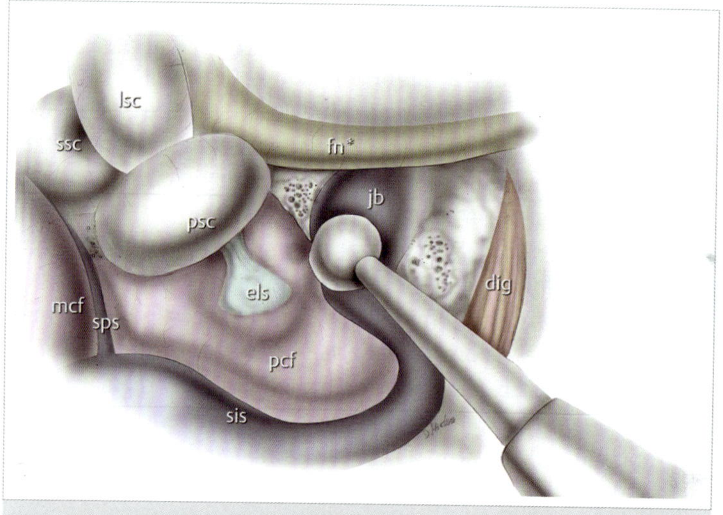

Fig. 2.100 Right side: The mastoid bone is removed to reveal the dura of the posterior fossa. The endolymphatic sac is visible just behind the posterior semicircular canal. *dig: digastric muscle; els: endolymphatic sac; fn*: mastoid segment of facial nerve; jb: jugular bulb; lsc: lateral semicircular canal; mcf: medial cranial fossa; pcf: posterior cranial fossa; psc: posterior semicircular canal; scm: sternocleidomastoid muscle; sis: sigmoid sinus; sps: superior petrosal sinus; ssc: superior semicircular canal; temp: temporalis muscle.*

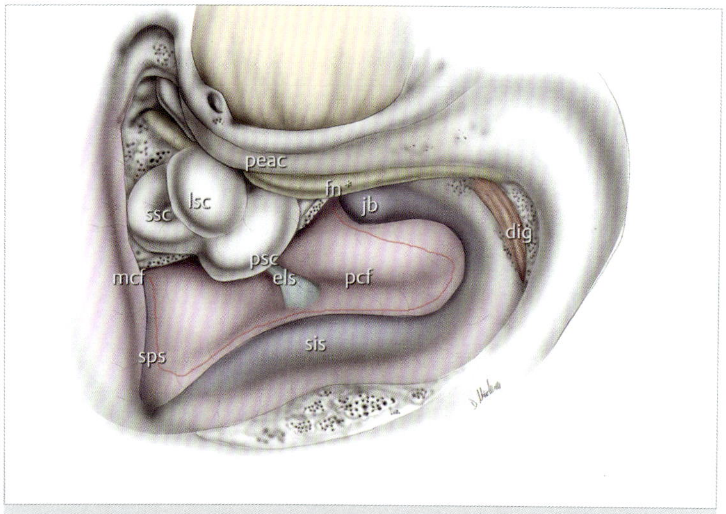

Fig. 2.101 Right side: The red line represents the incision pattern of the dura of the posterior fossa to access the cerebellopontine angle (CPA). It should be parallel to the sigmoid sinus, preserving the endolymphatic sac. *dig: digastric muscle; els: endolymphatic sac; fn*: mastoid segment of facial nerve; jb: jugular bulb; lsc: lateral semicircular canal; mcf: medial cranial fossa; pcf: posterior cranial fossa; peac: posterior wall of external auditory canal; psc: posterior semicircular canal; sis: sigmoid sinus; sps: superior petrosal sinus; ssc: superior semicircular canal; temp: temporalis muscle.*

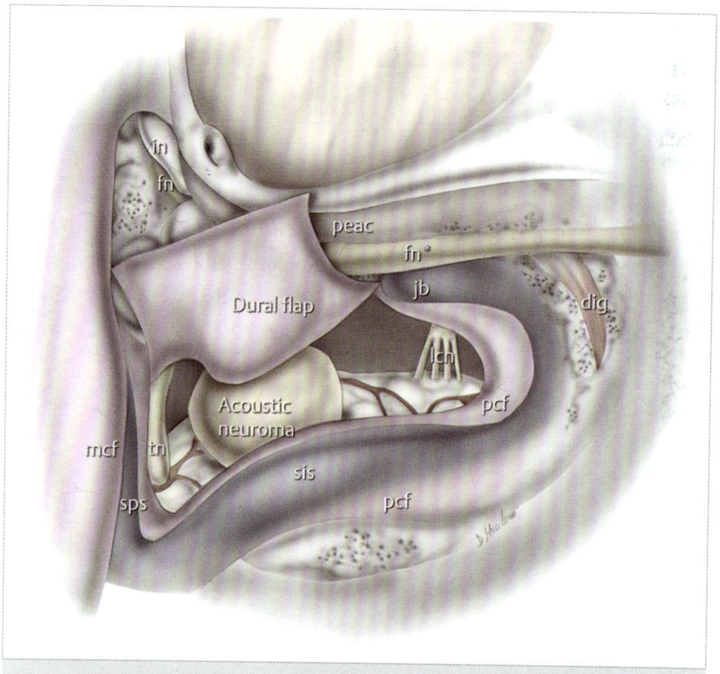

Fig. 2.102 Right side: The dural flap is anteriorly elevated with the endolymphatic sac, exposing the cerebellopontine angle (CPA) with the acoustic neuroma involving the entry zone, the lower cranial nerves inferiorly, and the trigeminal nerve superiorly. *dig: digastric muscle; els: endolymphatic sac; fn: facial nerve; fn*: mastoid segment of facial nerve; in: incus; jb: jugular bulb; lcn: lower cranial nerves; mcf: medial cranial fossa; pcf: posterior cranial fossa; peac: posterior wall of external auditory canal; sis: sigmoid sinus; sps: superior petrosal sinus.*

- Inadequate approach for large tumors due to the limited size of the surgical window.
- In case of high jugular bulb, this surgical route may be difficult because of the very limited surgical field.

2.6.5 Use of the Endoscope

In this technique, endoscopic-assisted surgery should be considered especially to get an adequate exposure of the portion of tumor involving the porus of the IAC. Due to anatomical conformation, the presence of the labyrinthine block in the surgical field may make the microscopical exposure of this anatomical area difficult, forcing the surgeon to perform a blind dissection of the tumor (see Clinical Case 9).

2.6.6 Surgical Technique

The patient is placed in a supine position with the head turned to the contralateral side; facial nerve and cochlear nerve monitoring are used.

A C-shaped incision is made approximately 4 cm behind the retroauricular sulcus in a similar manner to the translabyrinthine approach (see ▶ Fig. 2.2); a fibroperiosteal layer is created and elevated to uncover the occipitomastoid bone (▶ Fig. 2.99); then an enlarged mastoidectomy is performed. The superior trough extends from the zygomatic root to the asterion, just inferior to the linea temporalis. The anterior trough is perpendicular to the superior one and extends from the postero superior rim of the external auditory meatus down to the mastoid tip. The dura of the middle cranial fossa superiorly and the sigmoid sinus posteroinferiorly are widely skeletonized (▶ Fig. 2.100). Approximately 1 cm of posterior fossa dura is exposed behind the sigmoid sinus. This additional bone removal behind the sigmoid sinus allows retraction of the sinus posteriorly, providing an improved exposure medial to the bony labyrinth.

The antrum and the fossa incudis are exposed. The sigmoid sinus and the sinodural angle are widely skeletonized. The sigmoid sinus is then followed inferiorly and anteriorly until the jugular bulb. The digastric ridge is uncovered. This anatomical structure is used as an anatomical landmark for the detection of the most inferior portion of the mastoid segment of the facial nerve close to the stylomastoid foramen. The mastoid segment of the facial nerve is then detected. The mastoid cells between the dura of the middle fossa, the sigmoid sinus, and the labyrinthine block are removed until the dura of the posterior fossa is exposed. During this step, a careful drilling of the infralabyrinthine cells around the labyrinthine block should be performed in order to preserve the otic capsule. The dura of the posterior fossa is progressively skeletonized between the middle fossa superiorly, the sigmoid sinus posteriorly, and labyrinthine block anteriorly. The endolymphatic sac is exposed just behind the posterior semicircular canal; a gentle retraction of the sigmoid sinus can help this procedure. Once the dura of the posterior fossa is completely exposed around the labyrinthine block, the most medial portion of the IAC is skeletonized, close to the porus. When the dura of the posterior fossa is completely exposed between the lateral sinus and the posterior semicircular canal, an incision of the posterior fossa dura is performed just anteriorly and parallel to lateral sinus. The incision must be lateral to the endolymphatic sac in order to preserve it (see ▶ Fig. 2.101). The dural flap is anteriorly elevated with the endolymphatic sac exposing the CPA and leading to CSF leakage. Thus, the tumor is exposed inside the CPA (see ▶ Fig. 2.102). In most patients the porus of the IAC is impossible to expose through this approach because the sigmoid sinus limits a more obtuse viewing angle in relation to the posterior petrous ridge. In these cases an endoscopic assisted procedure is mandatory to remove a tumor located in the porus (see Endoscopic-Assisted Surgery). The ninth and tenth cranial nerves are visible inferiorly, as anterior to the level of the jugular bulb. The fifth cranial nerve and basilar artery can also be examined through this exposure. Cottonoids are used to protect the brainstem around the tumor. Tumors located in the CPA are dissected under a microscopic view in the same manner as with the translabyrinthine approach. A soft dissection of the tumor around the acoustic-facial bundle should be performed in order to preserve the cochlear nerve. The use of a bipolar instrument is useful just around the tumor mass but coagulation of the internal auditory artery must be avoided in order to preserve the hearing function by avoiding damage to the internal acoustic artery (see ▶ Fig. 2.103 and ▶ Fig. 2.104). A Gelfoam may be used over the facial-acoustic bundle in case of bleeding in order to protect the nerves during the dissection of the tumor.

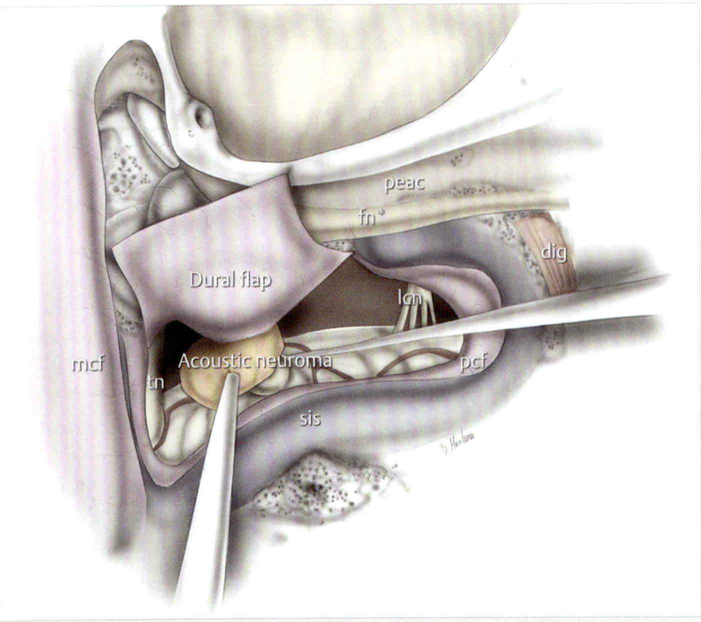

Fig. 2.103 Right side: The tumor is dissected from the acoustic-facial bundle preserving the cochlear nerve. *dig: digastric muscle; els: endolymphatic sac; fn*: mastoid segment of facial nerve; jb: jugular bulb; lcn: lower cranial nerves; mcf: medial cranial fossa; pcf: posterior cranial fossa; peac: posterior wall of external auditory canal; sis: sigmoid sinus; tn: trigeminal nerve.*

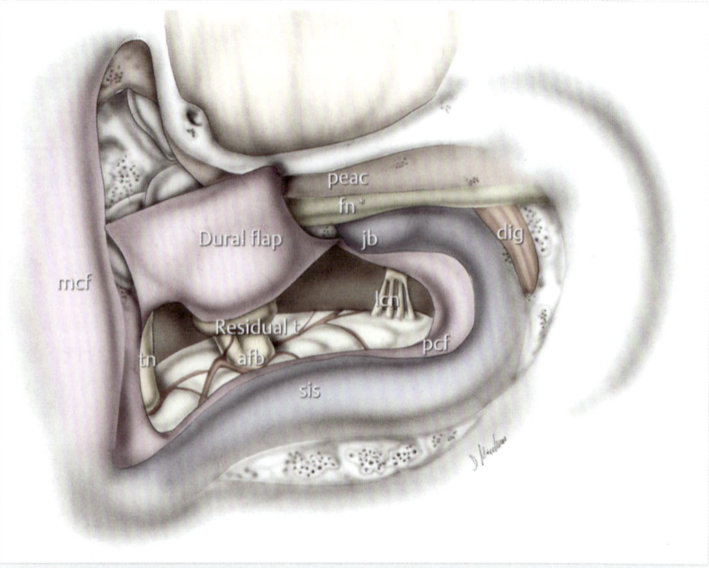

Fig. 2.104 Right side: Any residual tumor in the area of the porus is not visible under microscopic view. The orientation of the internal auditory canal (IAC) prevents a clear exposure of the area. *afb: acoustic-facial bundle; dig: digastric muscle; els: endolymphatic sac; fn*: mastoid segment of facial nerve; jb: jugular bulb; lcn: lower cranial nerves; mcf: medial cranial fossa; pcf: posterior cranial fossa; peac: posterior wall of external auditory canal; sis: sigmoid sinus; tn: trigeminal nerve.*

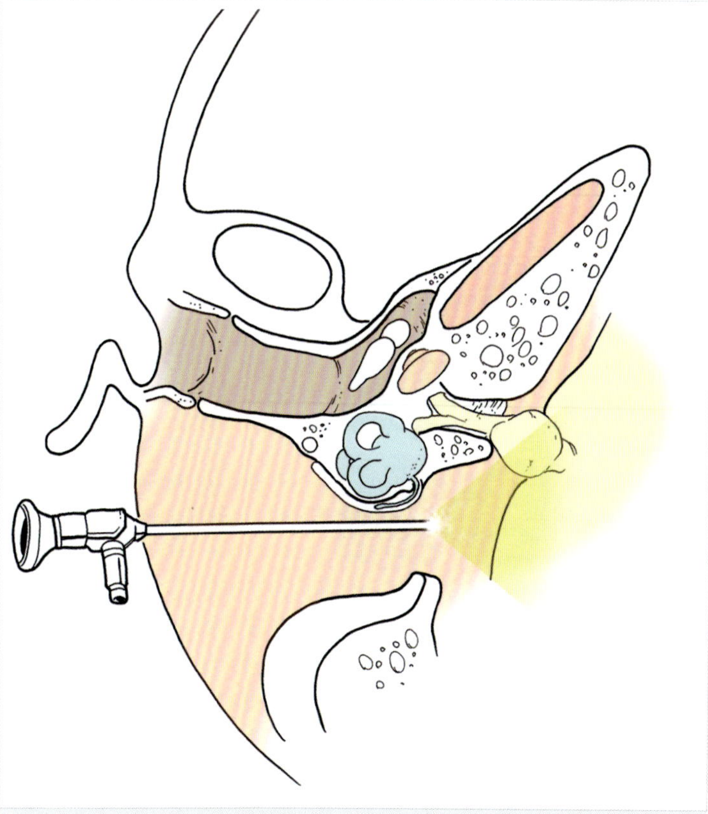

Fig. 2.105 Schematic drawing showing the exposure of cerebellopontine angle (CPA) with the endoscope.

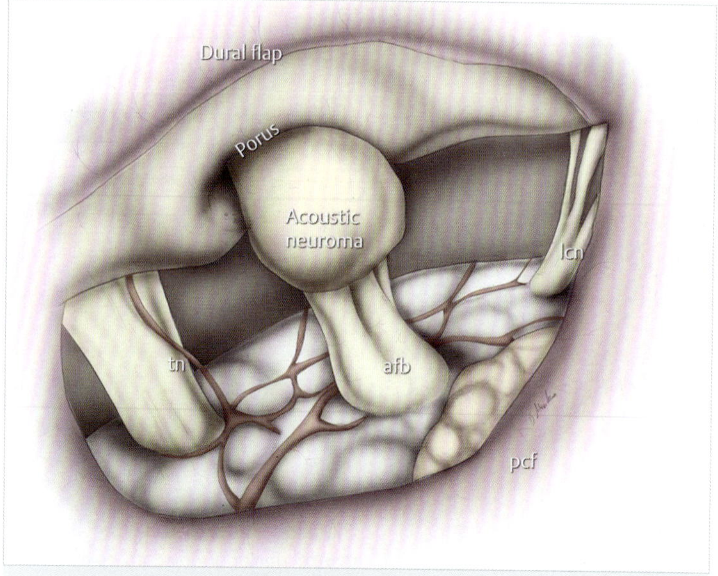

Fig. 2.106 Right side: Endoscopic view of the cerebellopontine angle (CPA). The area of the porus is clearly visible, to remove any residual tumor and ensure radicality. *afb: acoustic-facial bundle; lcn: lower cranial nerves; pcf: posterior cranial fossa; tn: trigeminal nerve.*

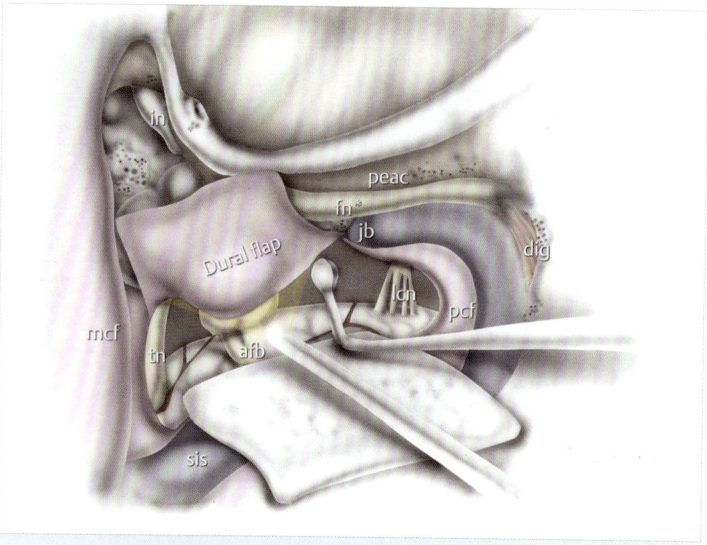

Fig. 2.107 Right side: 45-degree and 70-degree endoscopes along with curved dissectors may be useful to remove the residual tumor and inspect the internal auditory canal (IAC). *afb: acoustic-facial bundle; fn*: mastoid segment of facial nerve; in: incus; jb: jugular bulb; lcn: lower cranial nerves; mcf: medial cranial fossa; peac: posterior wall of external auditory canal; sis: sigmoid sinus; tn: trigeminal nerve.*

Intraoperative neuromonitoring of the cochlear nerve is mandatory in this step in order to avoid damage of the cochlear nerve by informing the surgeon on the status of this nerve during the surgical maneuver.

2.6.7 Endoscopic-Assisted Surgery (see Clinical Case 9)

In case of tumor with porus and medial IAC involvement after the microscopic step endoscopic-assisted surgery should be considered to avoid leaving any residual tumor in the IAC. A 0-degree, 4-mm-diameter, 15-cm-length endoscope is used at first in order to check the surgical cavity after microscopic tumor removal (see ▶ Fig. 2.105). The endoscope allows to magnify the porus and the medial aspect of the IAC behind the labyrinthine block when looking for any residual tumor (see ▶ Fig. 2.106).

A residual tumor may be present under the acoustic-facial bundle and inside the medial IAC. To detect the residual tumor in the IAC, 45-degree and 70-degree endoscopes should be also used. Once a residual tumor is found, a curved dissector (see Chapter 4) is introduced into the surgical cavity, under endoscopic control (see ▶ Fig. 2.107). The surgical maneuver should be soft, from a lateral to a medial direction in order to detach the tumor from the IAC and the nerves, avoiding to stretch the nerves. During the endoscopic maneuver, cottonoids are placed on cerebellum and brainstem to protect these important structures by avoiding direct contact between the instrument and the parenchyma (see ▶ Fig. 2.107 and ▶ Fig. 2.108). In order to remove the residual tumor, the use of suction instruments is not recommended in the IAC and close to nervous structures due to the possibility of damaging the nerves with the suction. In case of difficult view because the IAC is covered with blood, a gentle irrigation of the IAC should be considered in order to clean the surgical field. In case of residual tumor under the nerves, the dissection maneuver must be carried out along the major axis of the nerves (see Clinical Case 9). In case of bleeding from the nerves, a Gelfoam should be placed on the nerve to stop the bleeding. Once the tumor is removed under endoscopic view, a final check of the IAC is performed with a 70-degree endoscope (see ▶ Fig. 2.109).

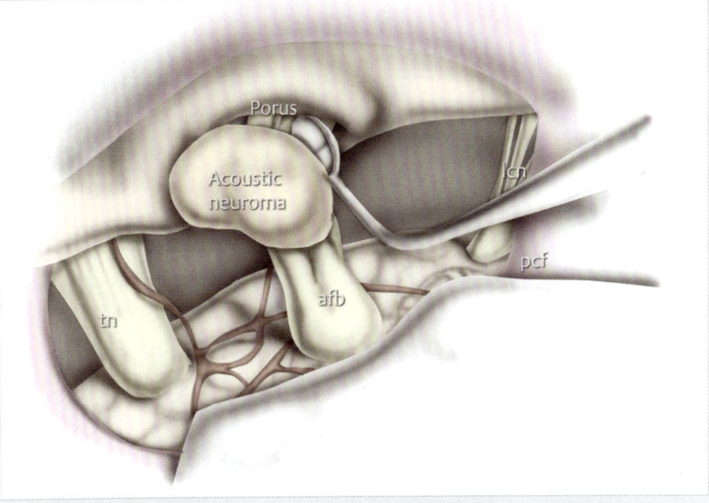

Fig. 2.108 Right side: Removal of the acoustic neuroma from the internal auditory canal (IAC). *afb: acoustic-facial bundle; lcn: lower cranial nerves; pcf: posterior cranial fossa; tn: trigeminal nerve.*

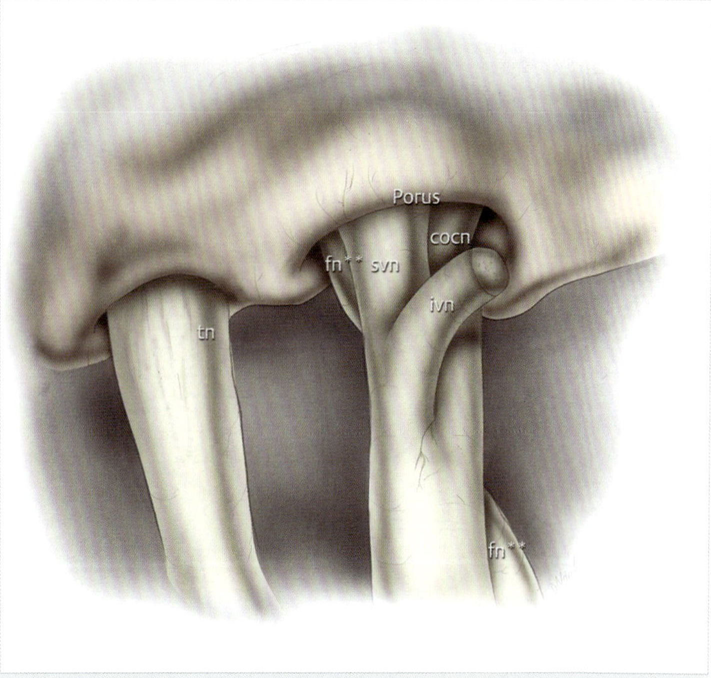

Fig. 2.109 Right side: Final check of the internal auditory canal (IAC) with a 70-degree endoscope. *cocn: cochlear nerve; fn**: facial nerve into the IAC; ivn: inferior vestibular nerve; svn: superior vestibular nerve; tn: trigeminal nerve.*

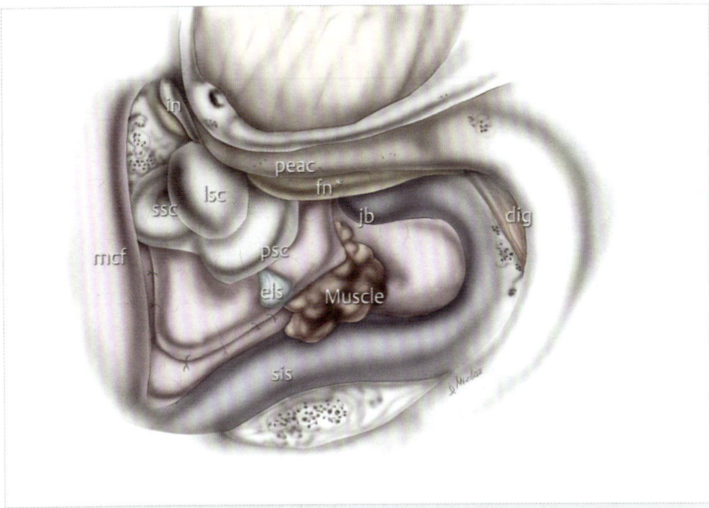

Fig. 2.110 The dural layer is replaced and sutured. In case of dural defect, a muscle fragment is used to obliterate the defect. *dig: digastric muscle; els: endolymphatic sac; fn*: mastoid segment of facial nerve; in: incus; jb: jugular bulb; lsc: lateral semicircular canal; mcf: medial cranial fossa; peac: posterior wall of external auditory canal; psc: posterior semicircular canal; sis: sigmoid sinus; ssc: superior semicircular canal.*

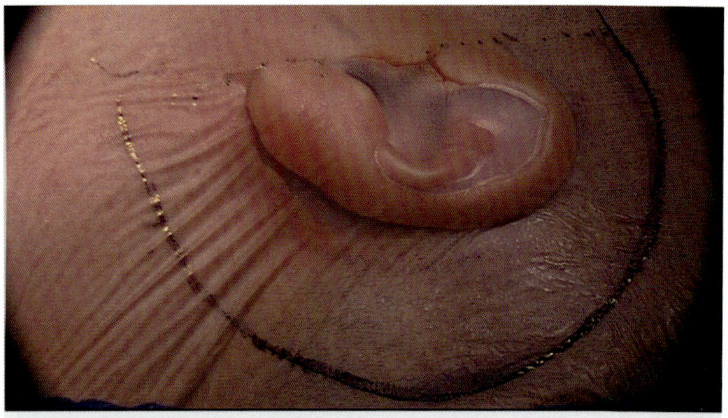

Fig. 2.111 Clinical Case 9, Left side: A C-shaped postauricular incision is made 4 cm behind the retroauricular sulcus. The anterosuperior portion of the incision must be placed over the ear attachment; the anteroinferior part of the incision must be placed just inferiorly on the tip of the mastoid.

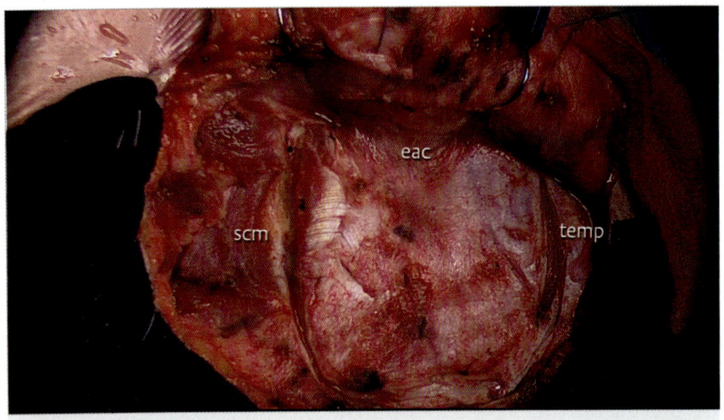

Fig. 2.112 Clinical Case 9, Left side: The skin flap is elevated and the temporalis muscle is incised to create a musculoperiosteal flap. *eac: external auditory canal; scm: sternocleidomastoid muscle; temp: temporalis muscle.*

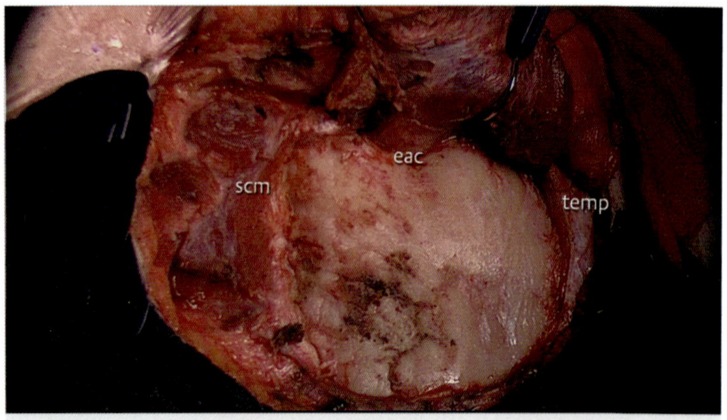

Fig. 2.113 Clinical Case 9, Left side: The mastoid bone is exposed after the elevation of the musculoperiosteal layer. The posterior aspect of external auditory canal (EAC) is detected. *eac: external auditory canal; scm: sternocleidomastoid muscle; temp: temporalis muscle.*

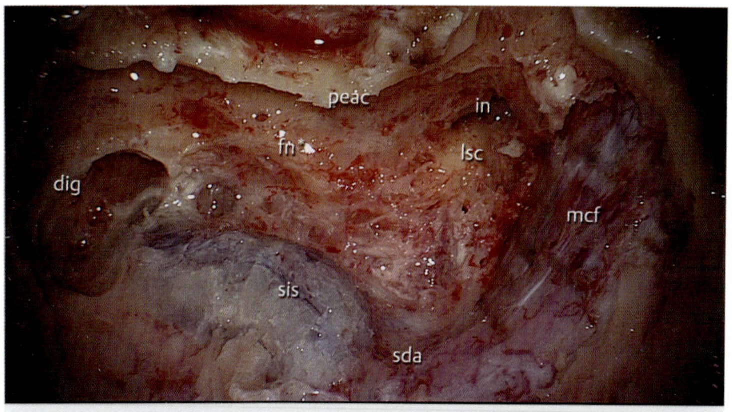

Fig. 2.114 Clinical Case 9, Left side: A mastoidectomy is performed exposing the sigmoid sinus and the sinodural angle posteriorly while the middle fossa dura is in a superior position. The sinodural angle and the middle cranial fossa dura are skeletonized. *dig: digastric ridge; fn*: mastoid segment of facial nerve; in: incus; lsc: lateral semicircular canal; mcf: middle cranial fossa; peac: posterior wall of external auditory canal; sda: sinodural angle; sis: sigmoid sinus.*

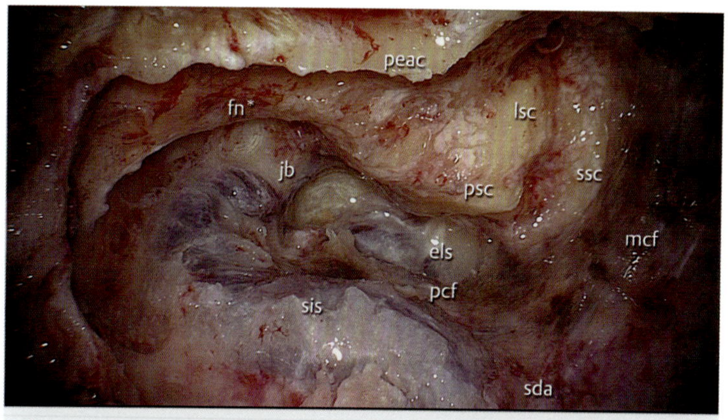

Fig. 2.115 Clinical Case 9, Left side: The dura of the posterior fossa is uncovered revealing the endolymphatic sac which is visible just behind the posterior semicircular canal. *els: endolymphatic sac; fn*: mastoid segment of facial nerve; jb: jugular bulb; lsc: lateral semicircular canal; mcf: middle cranial fossa; pcf: posterior cranial fossa; peac: posterior wall of external auditory canal; psc: posterior semicircular canal; sda: sinodural angle; sis: sigmoid sinus; ssc: superior semicircular canal.*

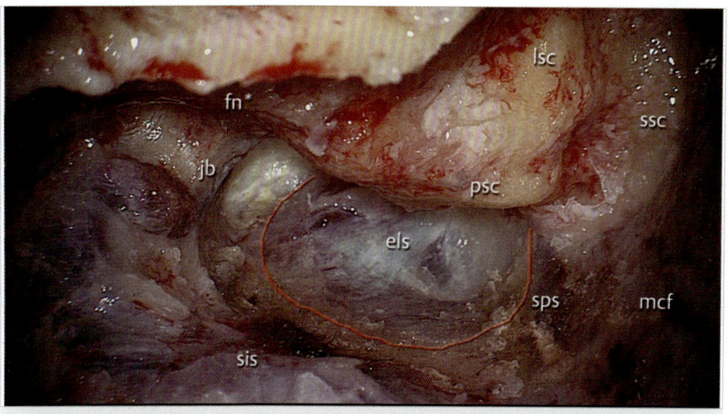

Fig. 2.116 Clinical Case 9, Left side: The *red line* represents the incision pattern of the dura of the posterior fossa to access the cerebello-pontine angle (CPA). It should be parallel to the sigmoid sinus, preserving the endolymphatic sac. *els: endolymphatic sac; fn*: mastoid segment of facial nerve; jb: jugular bulb; lsc: lateral semicircular canal; mcf: middle cranial fossa; psc: posterior semicircular canal; sis: sigmoid sinus; sps: superior petrosal sinus; ssc: superior semicircular canal.*

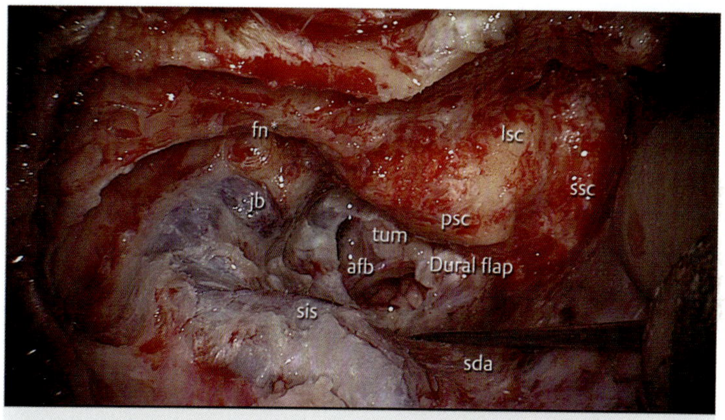

Fig. 2.117 Clinical Case 9, Left side: The dural flap is elevated uncovering the cerebellopontine angle (CPA). The acoustic neuroma is visible involving the acoustic-facial bundle up to the entry zone. *afb: acoustic-facial bundle; fn*: mastoid segment of facial nerve; jb: jugular bulb; lsc: lateral semicircular canal; psc: posterior semicircular canal; sda: sinodural angle; sis: sigmoid sinus; ssc: superior semicircular canal; tum: acoustic tumor.*

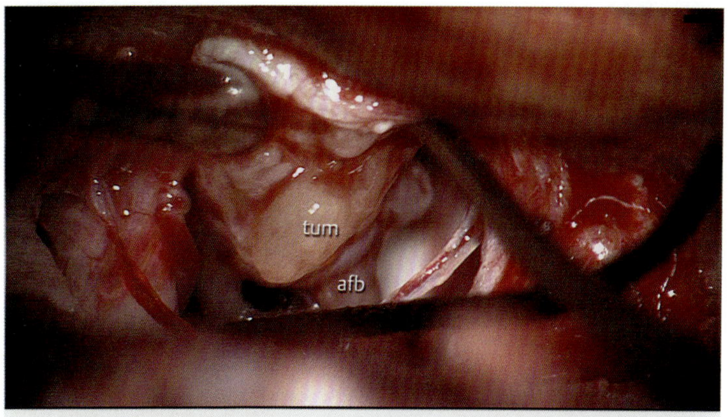

Fig. 2.118 Clinical Case 9, Left side: Removal of the acoustic neuroma. The acoustic-facial bundle is clearly visible in its entrance into the brainstem. *afb: acoustic-facial bundle; tum: acoustic tumor.*

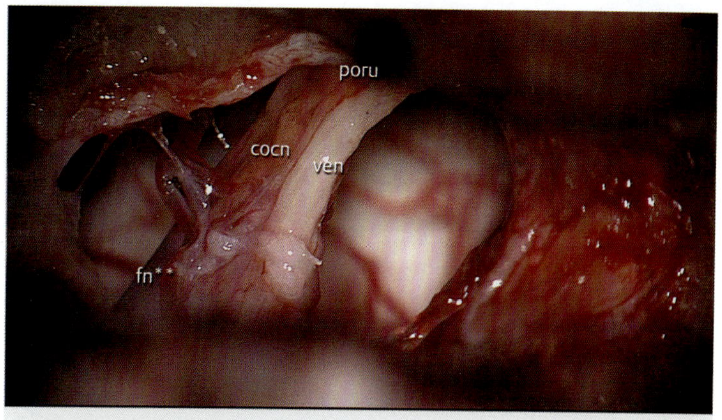

Fig. 2.119 Clinical Case 9, Left side: Acoustic-facial bundle after the removal of the tumor. The cochlear nerve was carefully preserved. *cocn: cochlear nerve; fn**: facial nerve inside the cerebellopontine angle (CPA); ven: vestibular nerve.*

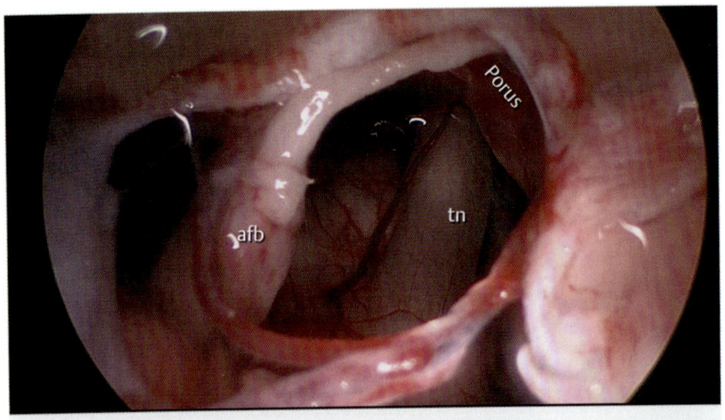

Fig. 2.120 Clinical Case 9, Left side: Endoscopic view of the cerebellopontine angle (CPA). The trigeminal nerve, anteriorly, and the acoustic-facial bundle entering the internal auditory canal (IAC) are visible. *afb: acoustic-facial bundle; tn: trigeminal nerve.*

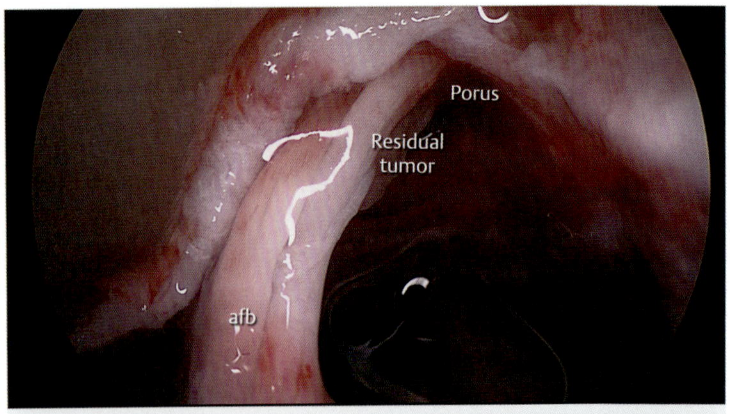

Fig. 2.121 Clinical Case 9, Left side: Under an endoscopic view the residual tumor is evidenced as lying medially to the acoustic-facial bundle, in the porus area. *afb: acoustic-facial bundle.*

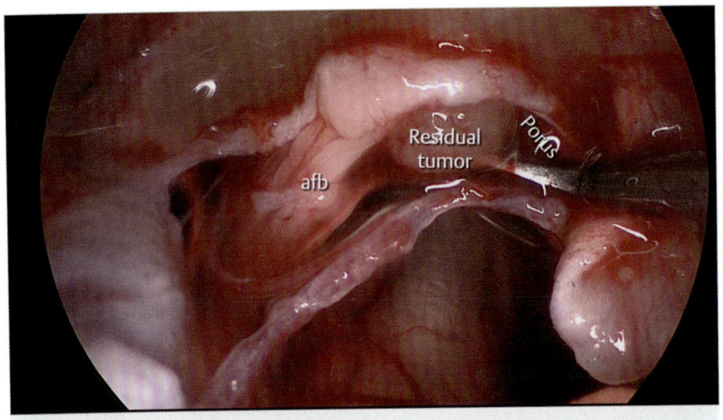

Fig. 2.122 Clinical Case 9, Left side: Curved dissectors may be useful under an endoscopic view to remove the residual tumor. *afb: acoustic-facial bundle.*

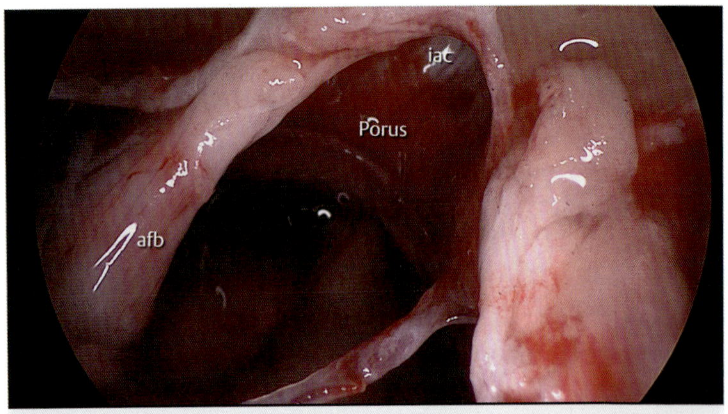

Fig. 2.123 Clinical Case 9, Left side: Final endoscopic inspection of the surgical cavity after tumor removal. *iac: internal auditory artery.*

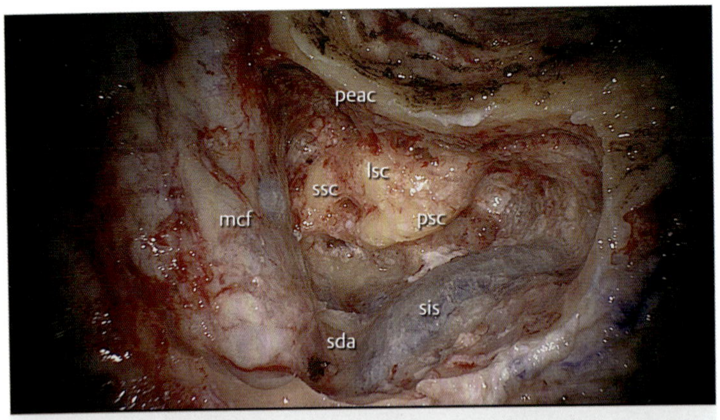

Fig. 2.124 Clinical Case 10, Right side: A wide mastoidectomy is performed to expose the labyrinth anteriorly, the sigmoid sinus posteriorly, and the dura of the middle cranial fossa superiorly. *lsc: lateral semicircular canal; mcf: middle cranial fossa; peac: posterior wall of external auditory canal; psc: posterior semicircular canal; sda: sinodural angle; sis: sigmoid sinus; ssc: superior semicircular canal.*

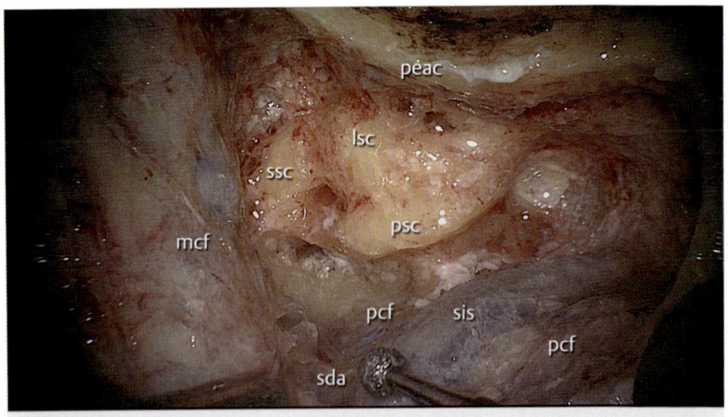

Fig. 2.125 Clinical Case 10, Right side: The dura of the posterior fossa is skeletonized. *lsc: lateral semicircular canal; mcf: middle cranial fossa; pcf: posterior cranial fossa; peac: posterior wall of external auditory canal; psc: posterior semicircular canal; sda: sinodural angle; sis: sigmoid sinus; ssc: superior semicircular canal.*

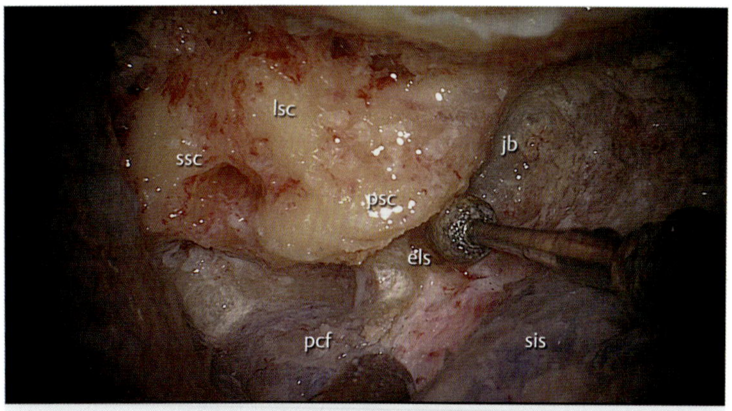

Fig. 2.126 Clinical Case 10, Right side: The endolymphatic sac is exposed just behind the posterior semicircular canal. *els: endolymphatic sac; jb: jugular bulb; lsc: lateral semicircular canal; pcf: posterior cranial fossa; psc: posterior semicircular canal; sis: sigmoid sinus; ssc: superior semicircular canal.*

2.6.8 Final Steps

Once the tumor is removed, a piece of temporalis muscle and bone dust are used to cover the antrum separating the middle ear from the mastoid cavity. The dural layer of the posterior fossa is replaced and sutured wherever possible. In case of dural defect, a muscle is used to obliterate and abdominal fat is used to fill the surgical field (see ▶ Fig. 2.110). The periosteal flap is replaced and sutured, and a watertight suture of the skin is made. A compressive bandage is used to cover the site of the surgery.

2.6.9 Vestibular Nerve Resection (see Clinical Case 11)

The indication is limited, and suitable only in case of intractable vertigo associated with unilateral vestibular disorder (Meniere's disease is the most frequent indication), which does not respond to medical treatment, in patients with a good hearing function.

The surgical procedure is contraindicated in case of bilateral vestibular disorders or in case of vertigo arising from the only hearing ear.

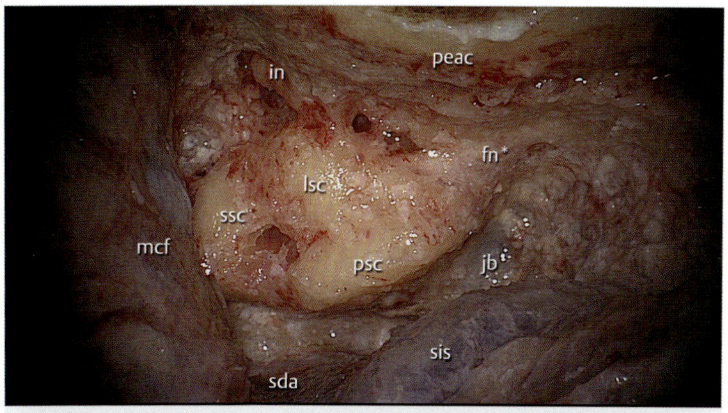

Fig. 2.127 Clinical Case 10, Right side: Anteriorly the incus is visible. The short process of the incus can be used as a landmark for the facial nerve. *fn*: mastoid segment of facial nerve; in: incus; jb: jugular bulb; lsc: lateral semicircular canal; mcf: middle cranial fossa; pcf: posterior cranial fossa; peac: posterior wall of external auditory canal; psc: posterior semicircular canal; sda: sinodural angle; sis: sigmoid sinus; ssc: superior semicircular canal.*

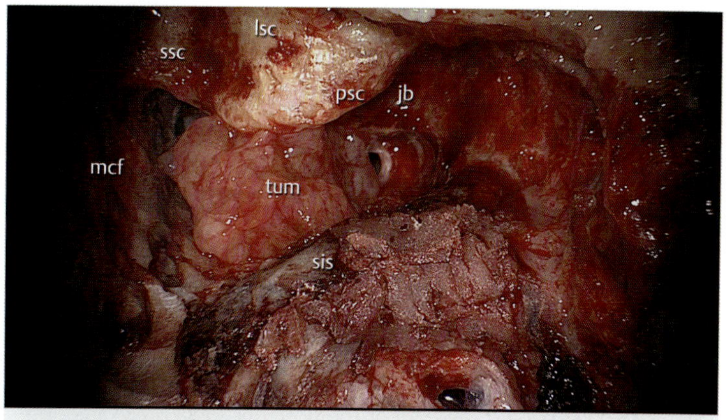

Fig. 2.128 Clinical Case 10, Right side: The dura of the posterior fossa is incised and the meningioma is exposed in the cerebellopontine angle (CPA). *jb: jugular bulb; lsc: lateral semicircular canal; mcf: middle cranial fossa; psc: posterior semicircular canal; sis: sigmoid sinus; ssc: superior semicircular canal; tum: meningioma of the posterior cranial fossa.*

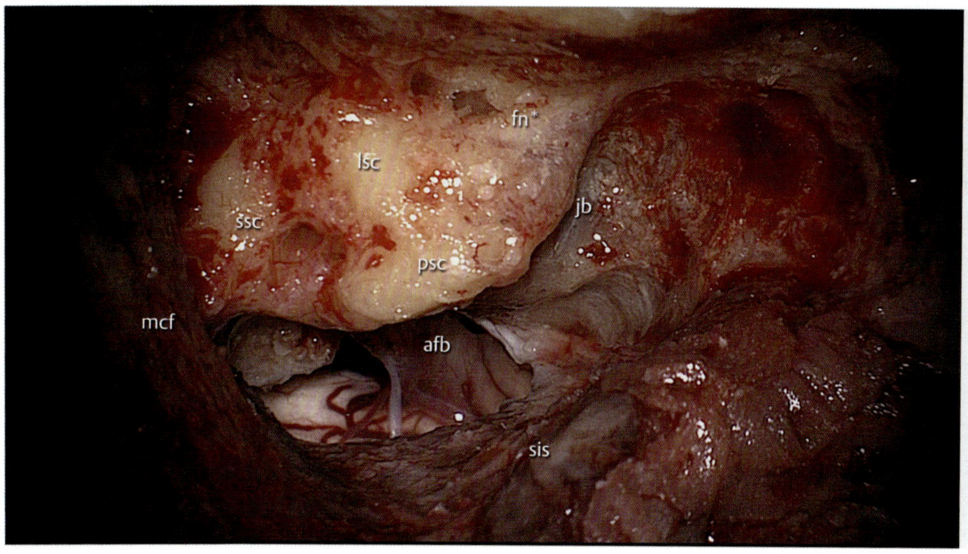

Fig. 2.129 Clinical Case 10, Right side: Final check of the surgical cavity after tumor removal. *afb: acoustic-facial bundle; fn*: mastoid segment of facial nerve; jb: jugular bulb; lsc: lateral semicircular canal; mcf: middle cranial fossa; psc: posterior semicircular canal; sis: sigmoid sinus; ssc: superior semicircular canal.*

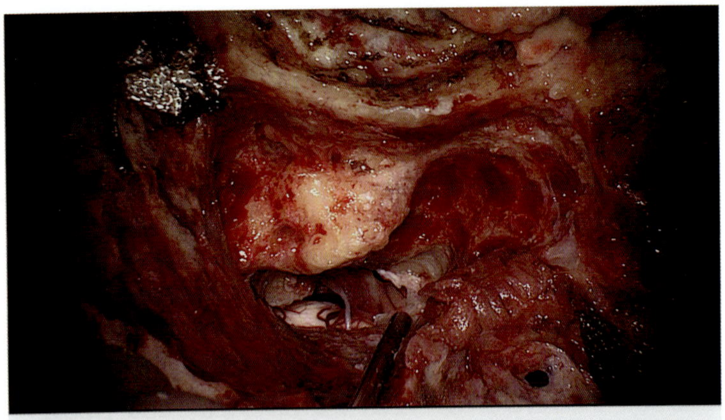

Fig. 2.130 Clinical Case 10, Right side: Global view of the surgical field, the acoustic-facial bundle is visible at the entry zone.

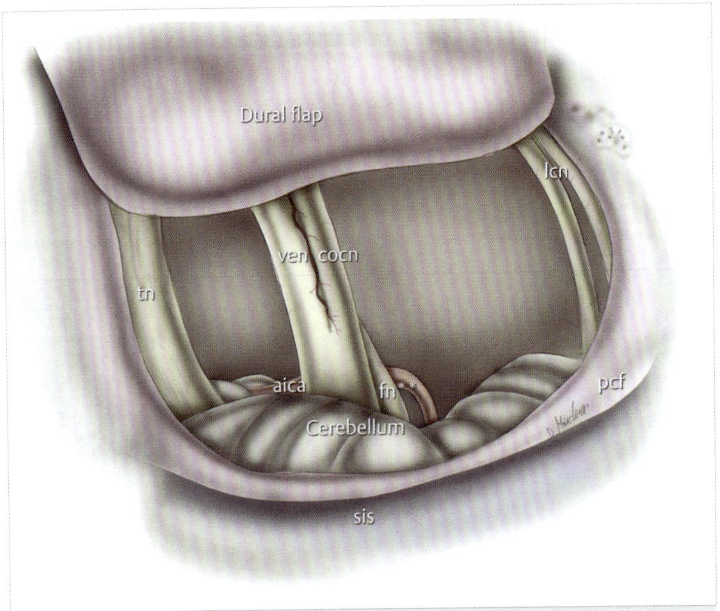

Fig. 2.132 Right side: The dura of the posterior fossa is elevated; the cerebellopontine angle (CPA) is exposed and the acoustic-facial bundle is detected. *aica: anterior inferior cerebellar artery; cocn: cochlear nerve; fn**: facial nerve inside the CPA; lcn: lower cranial nerves; pcf: posterior cranial fossa; sis: sigmoid sinus; tn: trigeminal nerve; ven: vestibular nerve.*

In case of hearing loss on the same side as the vestibular disorder, a transcanal endoscopic selective vestibular nerve resection should be considered.

An anatomical knowledge of the position of the acoustic nerve from the entry zone to the IAC is mandatory in case of retrolabyrinthine approach (see ▶ Fig. 2.131). The surgical approach is the same as previously described. Monitoring of the facial nerve is always performed during the surgical procedure. Intraoperative monitoring of auditory-evoked responses is useful to enhance the surgeon's ability to preserve hearing in a safe way.

After dural flap elevation and dural suspension, the CPA is microscopically exposed and the acoustic-facial bundle is detected (see ▶ Fig. 2.132). The next step is finding the right cleavage plane between the acoustic and vestibular nerves in the CPA. Several landmarks are helpful in finding the cleavage plane: the vestibular nerve often appears grayer, and the cochlear nerve whiter; the cochlear fibers are more numerous than the vestibular nerve fibers; furthermore a fine blood vessel frequently runs on the surface between the cochlear and vestibular fibers (see ▶ Fig. 2.133). A 0-degree, 4 mm diameter, 15 cm length

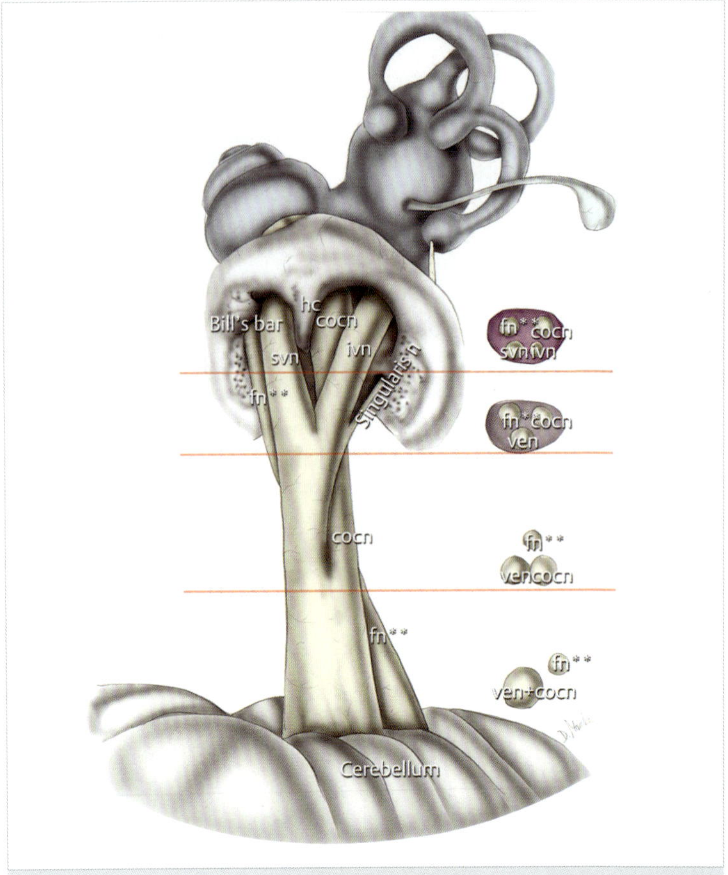

Fig. 2.131 Right side: Schematic drawing of the acoustic-facial bundle from the entry zone and inside the internal auditory canal (IAC). The red lines represent the sectional organization of the nerves in the cerebellopontine angle (CPA) and inside the IAC. *cocn: cochlear nerve; fn**: facial nerve into the IAC and the CPA; hc: horizontal crest; ivn: inferior vestibular nerve; svn: superior vestibular nerve.*

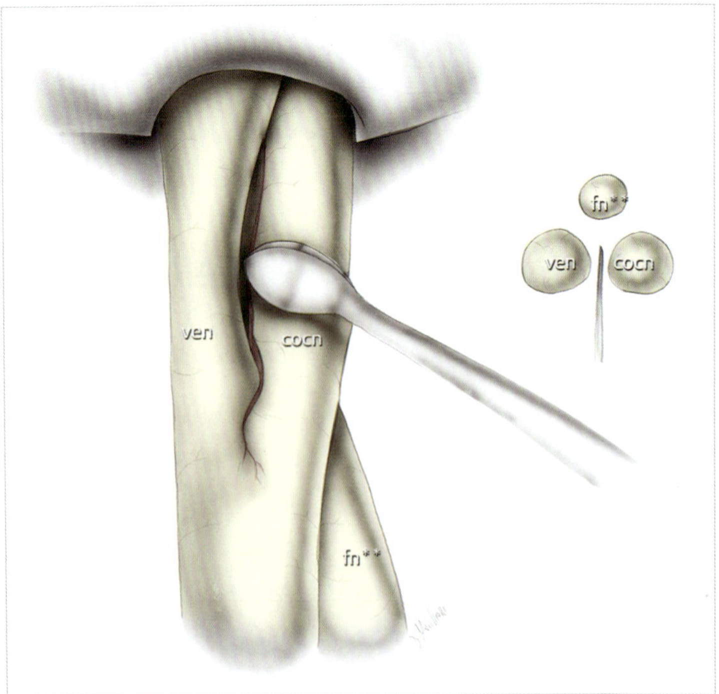

Fig. 2.133 Right side: The right cleavage plane is often pointed out by a fine blood vessel which frequently runs on the surface between the cochlear and vestibular fibers. Furthermore, the vestibular nerve often appears grayer, and the cochlear nerve whiter. *cocn: cochlear nerve; fn**: labyrinthine segment of facial nerve; ven: vestibular nerve.*

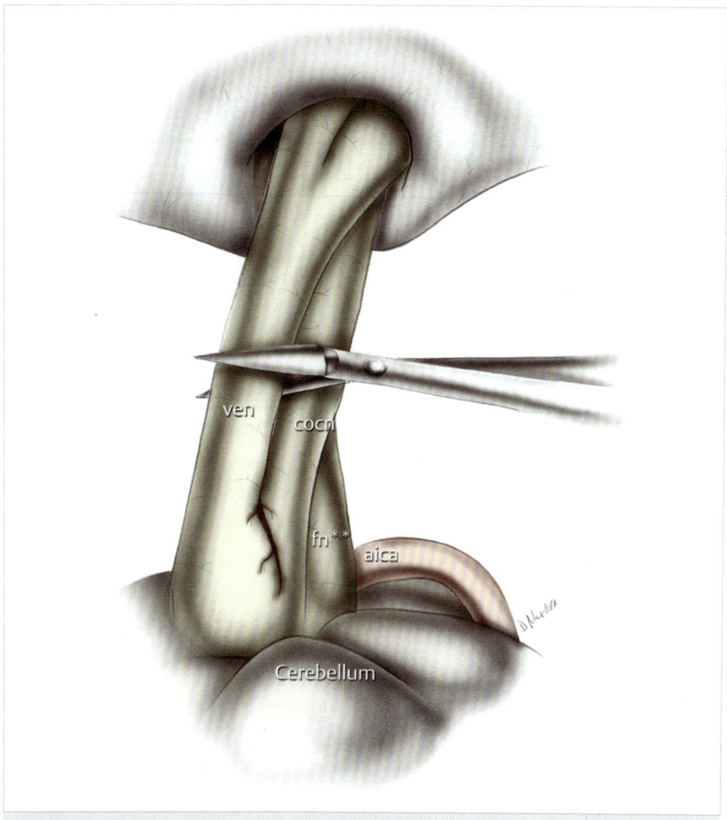

Fig. 2.134 Right side: Microscissors are used to cut the vestibular nerve. *aica: anterior inferior cerebellar artery; cocn: cochlear nerve; fn**: facial nerve inside the cerebellopontine angle (CPA); ven: vestibular nerve.*

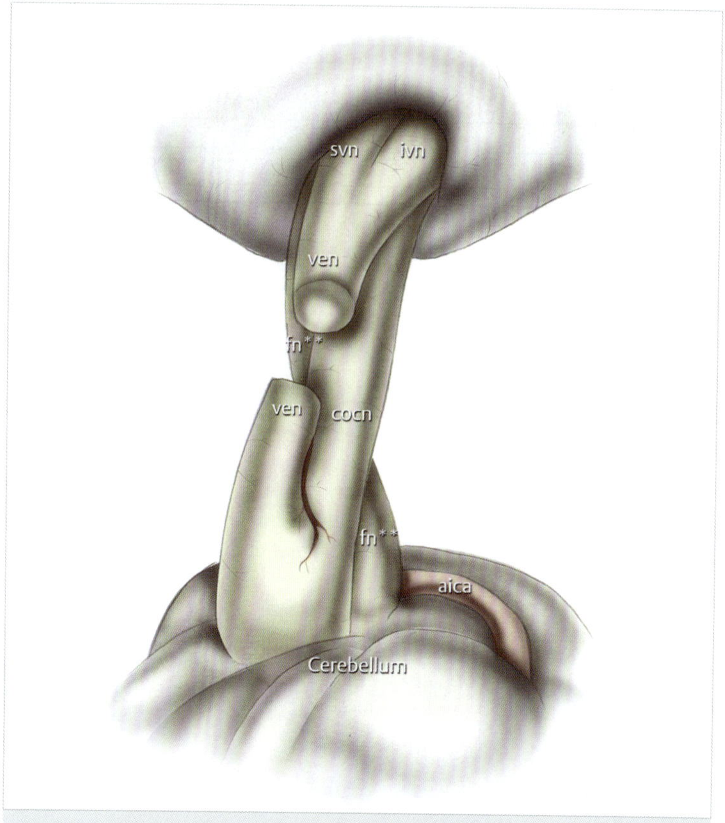

Fig. 2.135 Right side: Schematic drawing of the acoustic-facial bundle after the resection of the vestibular nerve. *aica: anterior inferior cerebellar artery; cocn: cochlear nerve; fn**: facial nerve inside the cerebellopontine angle (CPA); ivn: inferior vestibular nerve; svn: superior vestibular nerve; ven: vestibular nerve.*

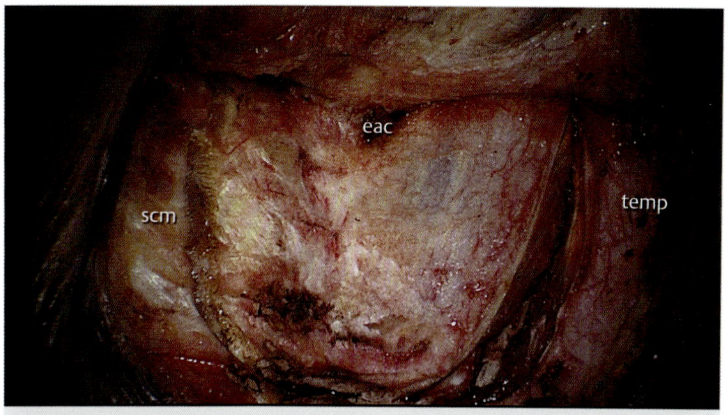

Fig. 2.136 Clinical Case 11, Left side: A C-shaped postauricular incision is made 4 cm behind the retroauricular sulcus; the skin flap is then elevated and the temporalis muscle is incised to create a musculoperiosteal flap. *eac: external auditory canal; scm: sternocleidomastoid muscle; temp: temporalis muscle.*

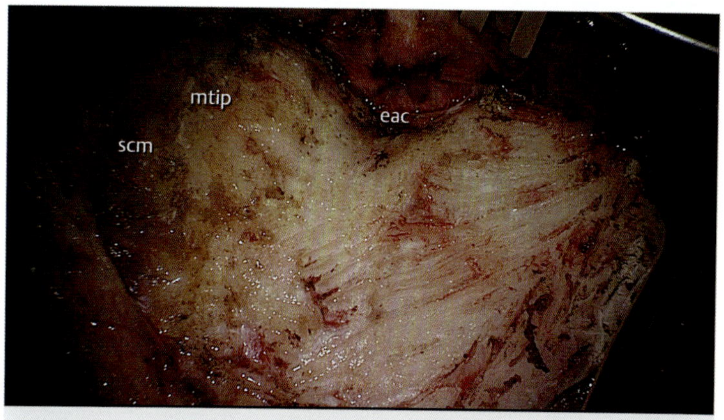

Fig. 2.137 Clinical Case 11, Left side: The mastoid bone is exposed after the elevation of the musculoperiosteal flap. *eac: external auditory canal; mtip: mastoid tip; scm: sternocleidomastoid muscle.*

endoscope can be used through the surgical cavity to view the anterior surface of the eighth nerve, since the cleavage plane is sometimes more visible from this surface. An endoscopic magnification may help the surgeon to have a right orientation regarding the cleavage plane and to detect the different fibers in between the two nerves (see Clinical Case 11). Once the cleavage plane is detected, a dissector is used to gently separate the two nerves; microscissors are used to cut the vestibular nerve (see ▶ Fig. 2.134 and ▶ Fig. 2.135).

The dura flap is replaced and sutured. A fat tissue is placed in the surgical cavity.

2.6.10 Hints and Pitfalls

- During the exposure of the labyrinthine block, the semicircular canals must be carefully skeletonized using a diamond bur alongside the main axis of these canals, avoiding to open the labyrinthine.
- The lateral sinus and the dura of the middle cranial fossa should be widely skeletonized. These structures must be retracted during the surgery, enabling the surgeon to gain more space space in the CPA behind the labyrinthine block.
- A bipolar instrument may be used over the dura of the middle and posterior fossae, under constant irrigation, in order to have a retraction of the dura to gain more surgical space.

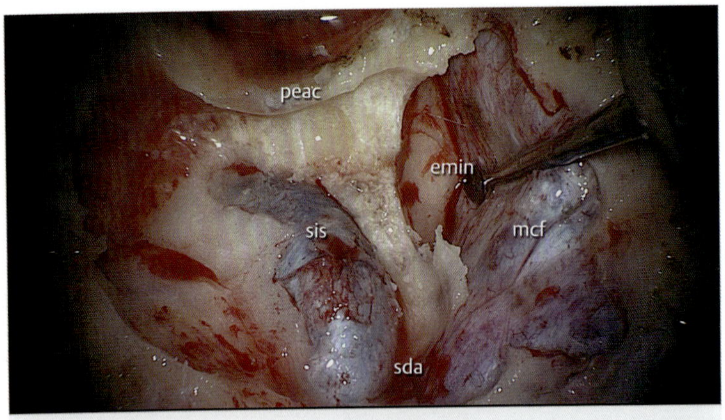

Fig. 2.138 Clinical Case 11, Left side: The middle fossa and the lateral sinus are widely skeletonized. On the superior surface of the petrous bone the arcuate eminence is a landmark for the superior semicircular canal. *emin: arcuate eminence; mcf: middle cranial fossa; peac: posterior wall of external auditory canal; sda: sinodural angle; sis: sigmoid sinus.*

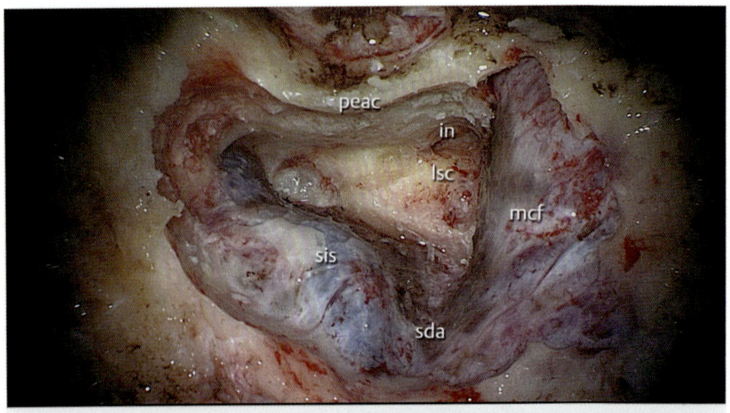

Fig. 2.139 Clinical Case 11, Left side: The antrum and the incudo-malleolar joint are detected; the posterior fossa dura is exposed just anteriorly to the sigmoid sinus. *in: incus; lsc: lateral semicircular canal; mcf: middle cranial fossa; peac: posterior wall of external auditory canal; sda: sinodural angle; sis: sigmoid sinus.*

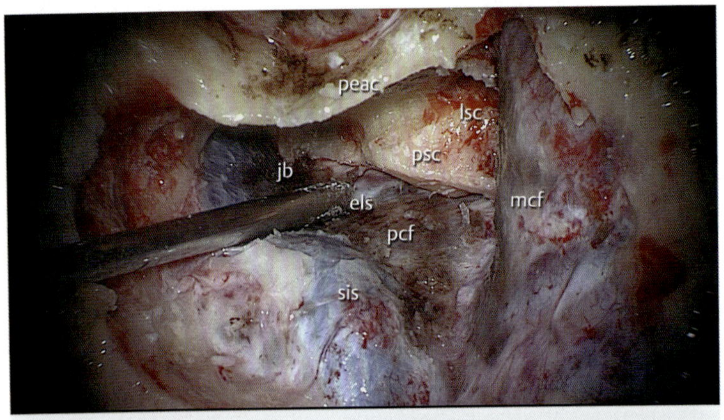

Fig. 2.140 Clinical Case 11, Left side: The dura of the posterior cranial fossa is gently detached from the mastoid bone. A diamond burr is used to remove the mastoid bone, uncovering the dura of the posterior fossa and exposing the endolymphatic sac. *els: endolymphatic sac; lsc: lateral semicircular canal; mcf: middle cranial fossa; pcf: posterior cranial fossa; peac: posterior wall of external auditory canal; psc: posterior semicircular canal; sda: sinodural angle; sis: sigmoid sinus.*

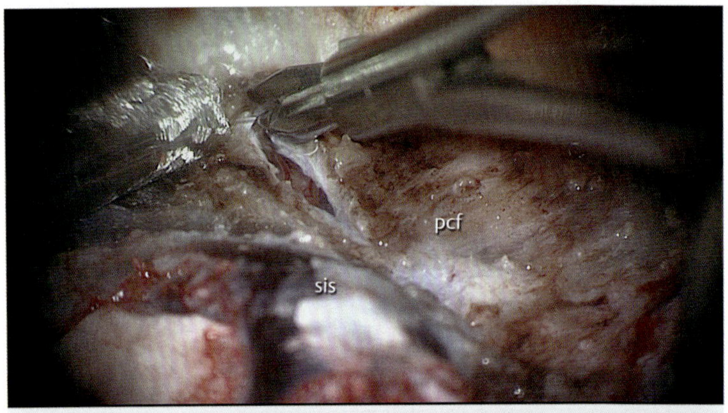

Fig. 2.141 Clinical Case 11, Left side: The dura of the posterior cranial fossa is incised parallel to the sigmoid sinus. *pcf: posterior cranial fossa; sis: sigmoid sinus.*

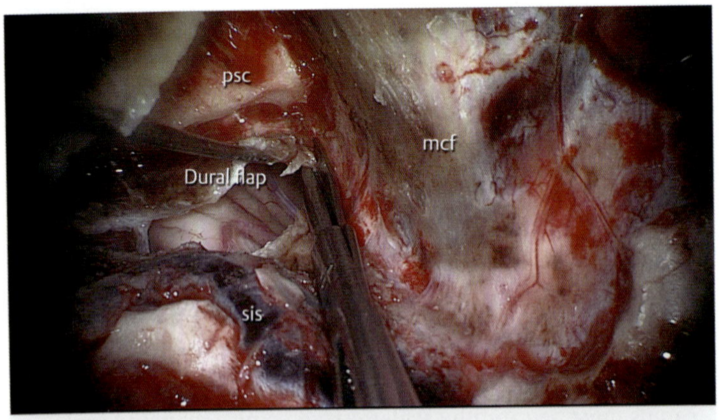

Fig. 2.142 Clinical Case 11, Left side: The dural flap is shaped to expose the cerebellopontine angle (CPA) cutting along the sigmoid sinus and to the middle cranial fossa. *mcf: middle cranial fossa; pcf: posterior cranial fossa; sis: sigmoid sinus.*

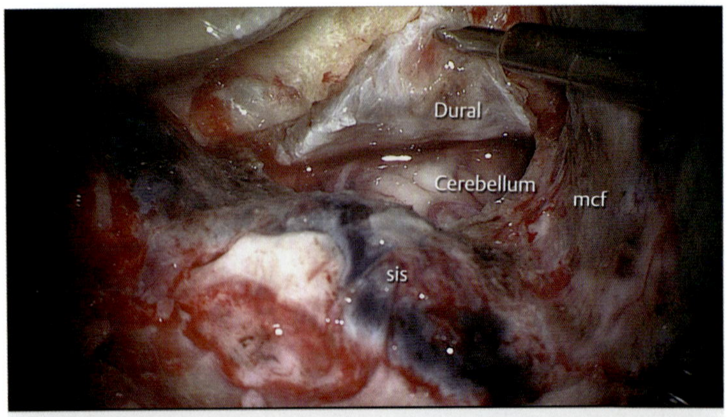

Fig. 2.143 Clinical Case 11, Left side: The dural flap is elevated anteriorly to expose the cerebellopontine angle (CPA). *mcf: middle cranial fossa; sis: sigmoid sinus.*

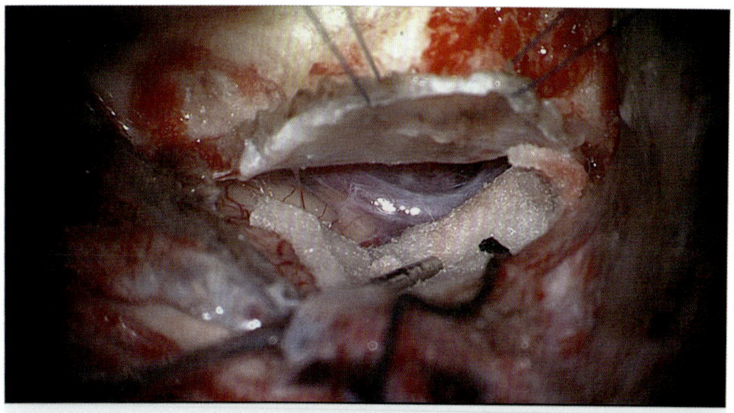

Fig. 2.144 Clinical Case 11, Left side: Stitches can be used to hold the dural flap in position.

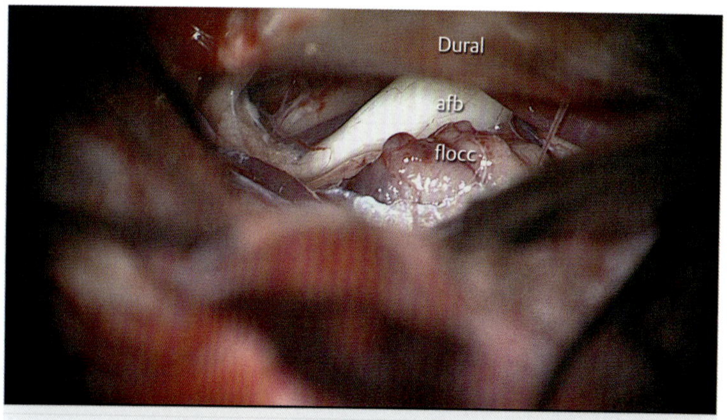

Fig. 2.145 Clinical Case 11, Left side: Microscopic view of the entry zone of the acoustic-facial bundle; the flocculus is visible posteriorly. *afb: acoustic-facial bundle; flocc: flocculus.*

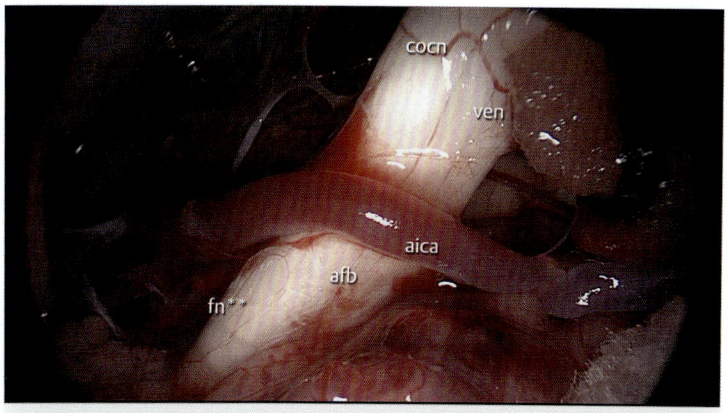

Fig. 2.146 Clinical Case 11, Left side: Endoscopic view of the entry zone of the acoustic-facial bundle. *afb: acoustic-facial bundle; aica: anterior inferior cerebellar artery; cocn: cochlear nerve; fn**: facial nerve inside the cerebellopontine angle (CPA); ven: vestibular nerve.*

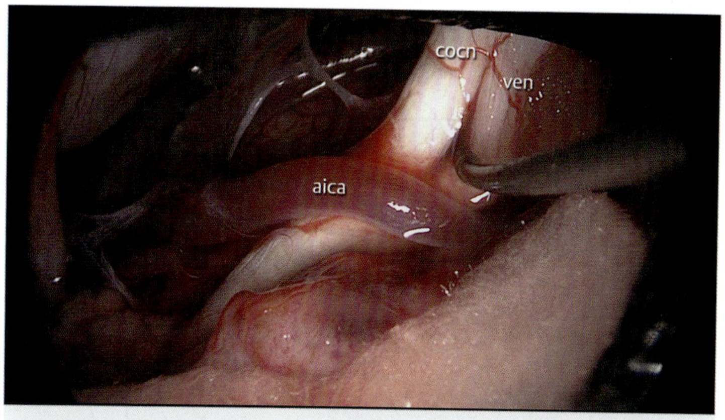

Fig. 2.147 Clinical Case 11, Left side: The right cleavage plane is identified using a sharp instrument. *aica: anterior inferior cerebellar artery; cocn: cochlear nerve; ven: vestibular nerve.*

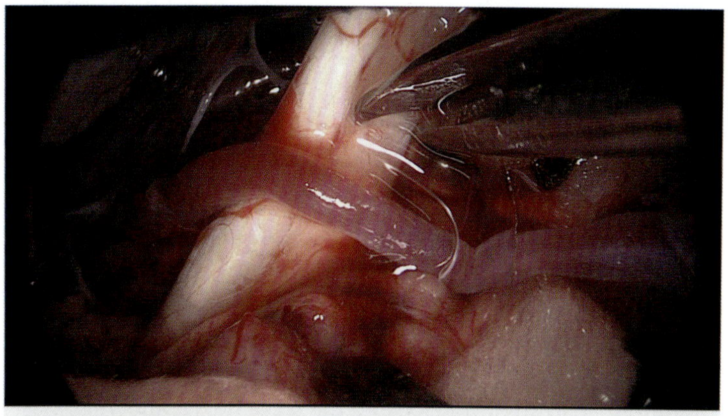

Fig. 2.148 Clinical Case 11, Left side: The vestibular nerve is transected using microscissors.

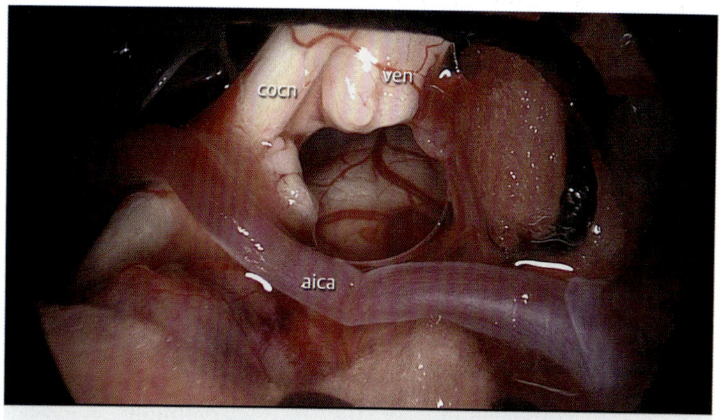

Fig. 2.149 Clinical Case 11, Left side: The nerve has been transected while the cochlear nerve is preserved. The function of the cochlear nerve is intraoperatively monitored. *aica: anterior inferior cerebellar artery; cocn: cochlear nerve; ven: vestibular nerve.*

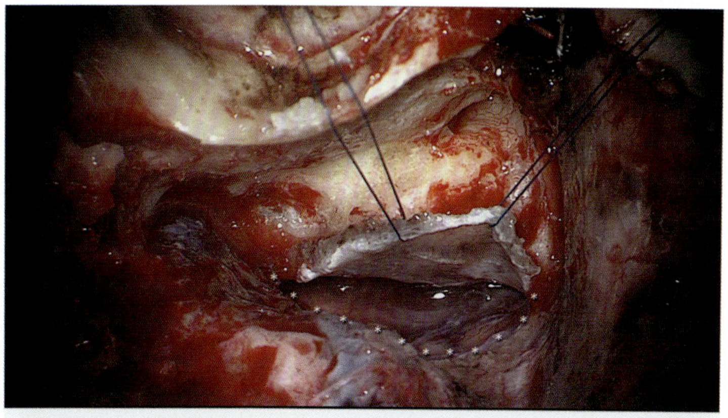

Fig. 2.150 Clinical Case 11: The dural flap is placed back in its original position and the dura is sutured.

- Once the dura is opened, Merocel is placed between the dura and the brainstem in order to avoid damage to the vascular structures running along the medial surface of the dura; the opening is safely performed using microscissors.
- In case of bleeding from the acoustic-facial bundle, Gelfoam is used to pack the nerves in order to stop the bleeding.
- In case of a well-pneumatized mastoid and perilabyrinthine cells, bone dust may be useful to close and obliterate these cells after tumor removal in order to avoid CSF leakage.

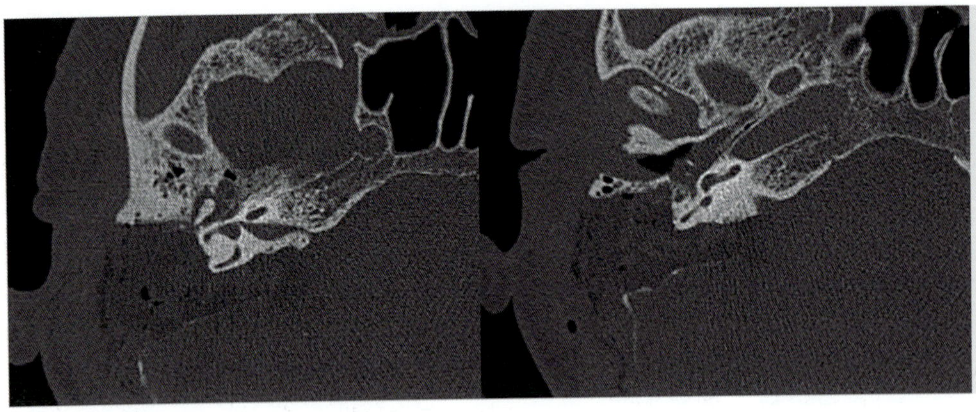

Fig. 2.151 Left side: Postoperative computed tomography (CT) scan, axial view. The labyrinth is preserved and clearly visible.

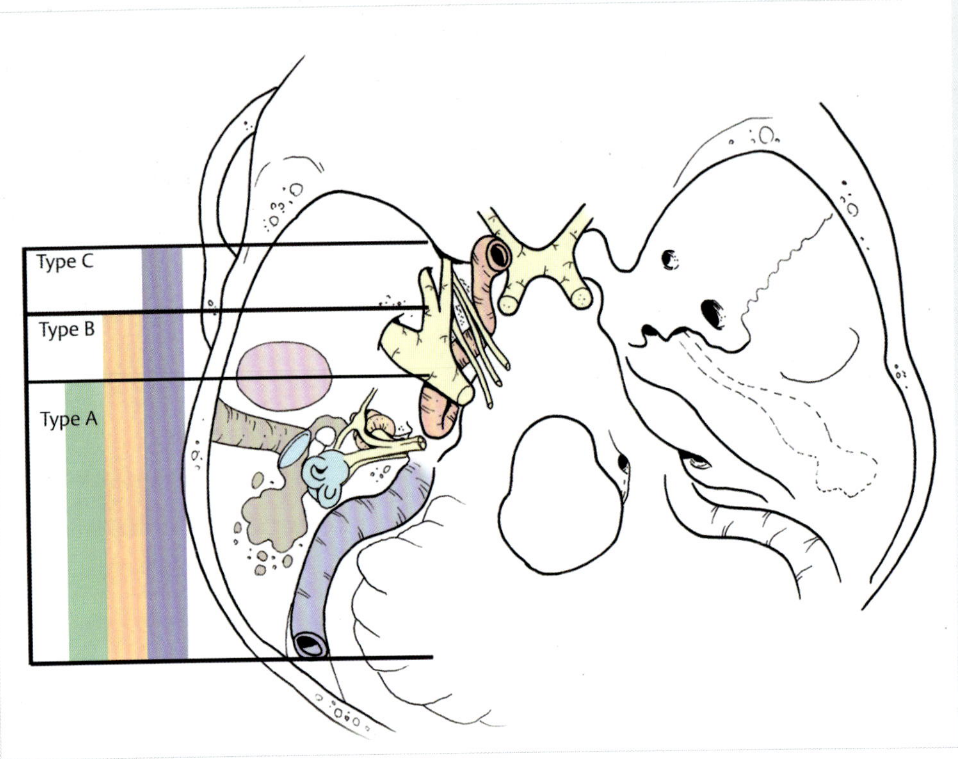

Fig. 2.152 Schematic drawing showing the exposure of different infratemporal fossa approaches (Types A–C).

2.6.11 Postoperative Care and Complications

The postoperative care and the complications that may arise from technique are the same as those found in translabyrinthine approach (see the complication paragraph of the translabyrinthine approach, Section 2.5.3). CT scan is performed in the immediate postoperative time (see ▶ Fig. 2.151).

Potential complications of the retrolabyrinthine approach include bleeding from dural sinus, cerebellar edema, cochlear nerve injury, facial nerve injury, intracranial vascular injury, CSF leakage, postoperative headache, and conductive hearing loss in case abdominal fat graft herniates into the epitympanum.

2.7 Different Infratempoaral Fossa Approaches

The surgical procedures to remove lesions located in the infratemporal fossa were codified by Ugo Fisch.

Fisch divided these techniques into three basic approaches (see ▶ Fig. 2.152):

- ***Type A approach***: In this surgical procedure, a cervical dissection of the vascular structures at the base of skull with subtotal petrosectomy, a jugular vein legation, and an anterior transposition of facial nerve a required in order to have access to the jugular bulb, the vertical petrous carotid, and the posterior infratemporal fossa.
- ***Type B approach***: In this surgical procedure, a subtotal petrosectomy along with V3 and middle meningeal artery sacrifice, and temporalis muscle and zygomatic arch mobilization are required, instead of transposing the facial nerve, allowing access to the petrous apex, clivus, transtemporal horizontal portion of carotid artery, and posterior fossa.
- ***Type C approach***: This surgical procedure is an anterior extension of Type B approach. A V2, V3 transection with pterygoid plate removal is required in order to have the exposure of the infratemporal fossa, pterygopalatine fossa, parasellar region, and rhinopharynx.

2.7.1 Infratemporal Fossa Type A

Indications

- A typical indication is benign tumors located in the jugular foramen with temporal bone and infratemporal fossa extension (glomus jugular tumors of Types C–D, schwannoma of lower cranial nerves) (see ▶ Fig. 2.153).

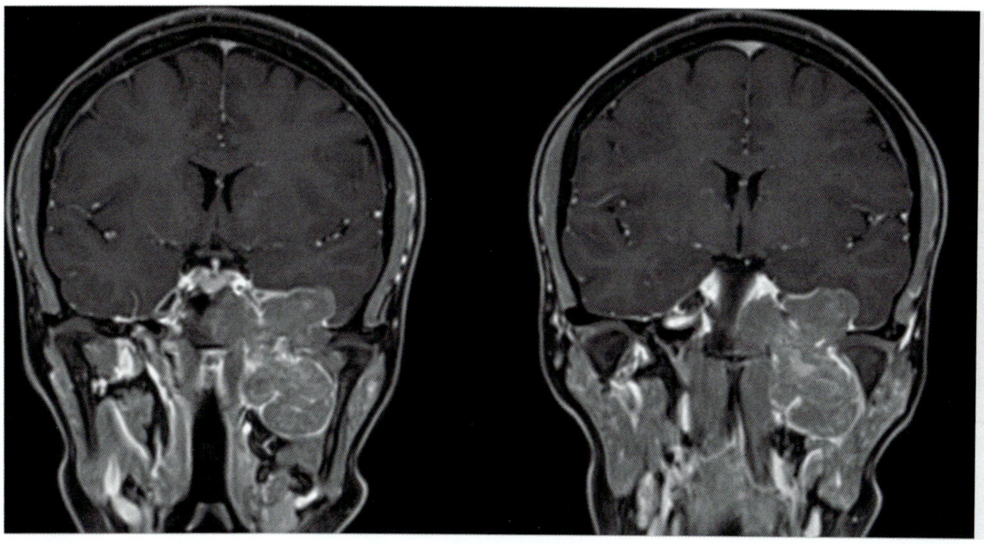

Fig. 2.153 Magnetic resonance imaging (MRI) in coronal view. A Class C4 paragangliomas of the temporal bone is seen.

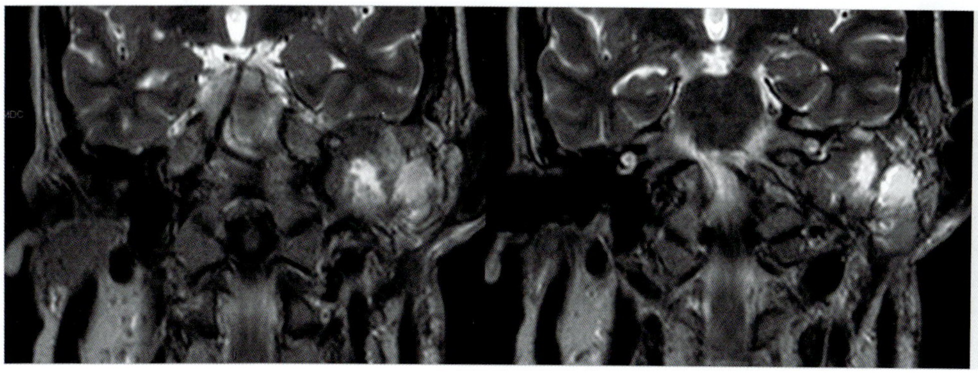

Fig. 2.154 Magnetic resonance imaging (MRI) in coronal view. A malignant tumor of the temporal bone with jugular foramen involvement can be seen.

- Apical or supralabyrinthine cholesteatoma with jugular foramen and petrous apex extension.
- Malignant tumors of the deep lobe of parotid gland (like adenoid cystic carcinoma) with jugular foramen extension or jugular foramen chondrosarcoma (in these cases the facial nerve resection is also considered) (see ▶ Fig. 2.154 and ▶ Fig. 2.202).

Limitations

- Contraindicated in case of contralateral vagus lesion.
- Extensive carotid involvement with poor collateral cerebral circulation or intolerable balloon occlusion test in the preoperative assessment.
- Because of the transposition of the facial nerve, a grade III or IV postoperative facial palsy is to be expected.
- Conductive hearing loss is expected due to the external auditory canal (EAC) closure.
- High risk of lower cranial neve palsy, especially in large tumors.
- Unsuitable for tumors involving the anterior foramen lacerum and the cavernous sinus (Types B–C approaches are combined in such cases).

Use of the Endoscope

- Endoscope use is recommended in these procedures, since bone removal is not always necessary, especially if a C1 tumor is treated.
- In case of a Type A infratemporal fossa bridge technique (described later), a 45-degree endoscope is used to check the presence of remnant disease around the facial nerve (see ▶ Fig. 2.176).
- In C2–C4 or class D glomus jugular tumor, at the end of the microscopic procedure, an endoscopic check with 0-degree and 45-degree endoscopes is suggested especially to check for remnant disease on the medial surface of the vertical carotid artery and along the horizontal portion of the carotid artery until the anterior foramen lacerum.

Preoperative Considerations

Preoperative assessment is crucial to properly evaluate the patient and to select a safe surgical approach:

- In the preoperative examinations a CT scan and a MR with angiography are planned (see ▶ Fig. 2.155). The venous drainage from the brain through the sigmoid sinus must be considered since the jugular vein and the sigmoid sinus are resected during the surgical procedure. In case of dominant sigmoid, due to the transverse sinus venous drainage on the same side of the tumor, this procedure is contraindicated.
- In case of intrapetrous internal carotid artery involvement, a balloon occlusion test is planned, and a closure or a stenting of the internal carotid artery is then considered.
- A grade III/IV (H-B Scale) facial palsy is to be expected in the postoperative period because of the anterior transposition of the facial nerve.
- A lower cranial nerve deficit is to be expected, especially during the treatment of large tumors with the involvement of jugular foramen.
- When a vascular tumor resection is planned (glomus jugular tumors of Types C–D), an angiography with embolization of the vascular branches arising from the external carotid artery must be performed 24–48 hours before surgery.

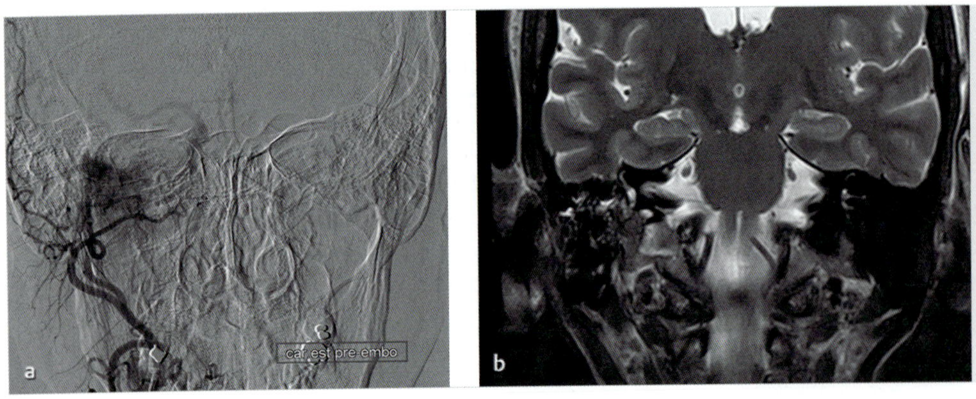

Fig. 2.155 Class C2 paragangliomas of the temporal bone. **(a)** The preoperative angiography study is performed. **(b)** Magnetic resonance imaging (MRI) of the same patient in coronal view.

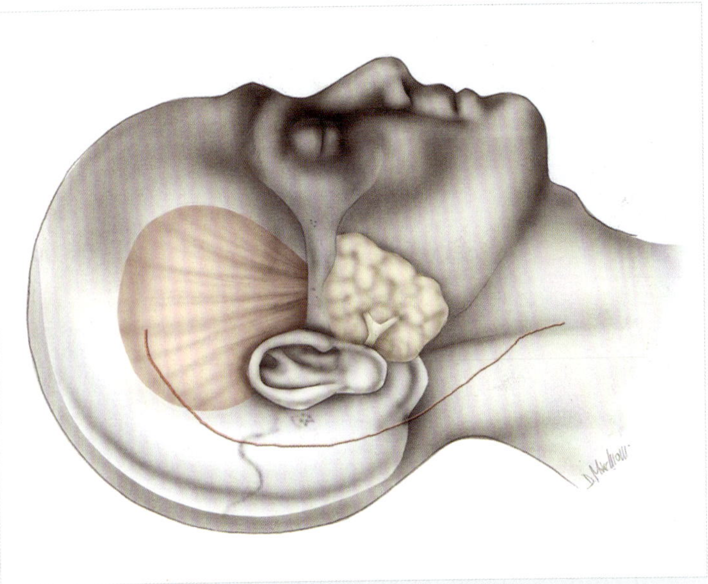

Fig. 2.156 Right side: A C-shaped incision is made starting from the temporalis area, passing 3 to 4 cm behind the retroauricular sulcus, the tip of the mastoid, and ending along the neck.

Surgical Technique (see Clinical Case 12)

The patient is placed in supine position with his head turned around. A facial nerve monitoring device is placed in the orbicularis muscles of the orbit and mouth; lower cranial nerve monitoring is also necessary.

A C-shaped generous incision is performed starting from the temporalis area, passing 3 to 4 cm behind the retroauricular sulcus, the tip of the mastoid, and ending along the neck (see ▶ Fig. 2.156).

A postauricular flap is elevated at the level of the temporalis muscle, the fascia and the periosteum. The flap is anteriorly dissected, and the EAC is circumferentially resected at the bony-cartilaginous junction. The medial skin of the EAC is detached from the cartilage and a suture is made to evert the skin through the meatus, allowing for a blind-sac closure of the EAC. A periosteum flap is created widely uncovering the mastoid bone. This second layer of periosteum may be used to close down the canal (see ▶ Fig. 2.157 and ▶ Fig. 2.158).

The skin of the EAC is circumferentially elevated down to the annulus and removed en bloc with the eardrum (see ▶ Fig. 2.159). Once the tympanic cavity is so exposed, the incudostapedial joint is separated, the incus is removed, and tensor tympani tendon is cut in order to remove the malleus. The stapedial crura are cut with microscissors and the suprastructure of the stapes is removed.

Neck Dissection

At the level of the neck, the anterior border of sternocleidomastoid muscle (SCM) is detected and the great auricular nerve is identified and preserved until the cranial bifurcation in order to use as a graft to reconstruct the facial nerve if necessary at the end of tumor excision.

Neck dissection is then performed. The anterior borders of the SCM and the digastric muscle are dissected at the base of the skull until the major vessels of the neck are identified and initially preserved (see ▶ Fig. 2.160). The internal jugular vein and the common carotid artery with the internal and external branches are gently dissected and exposed in the neck until the base of the skull. The lower cranial nerves are identified at the base of the skull; especially the vagus and the sympathetic trunk are isolated lateroinferiorly to the common carotid artery. The hypoglossal nerve is isolated between the main trunk of the internal jugular vein posteriorly and the common trunk anteriorly. This nerve is isolated and preserved from the neck to the skull base.

A dissection of the lateral process of C-1 and the superior and inferior oblique muscles is performed. At the end of the neck dissection, the internal carotid artery is isolated until the base of the skull and the external carotid artery is ligated just over the bifurcation.

The posterior belly of the digastric muscle is isolated until the mastoid insertion. The tympanomastoid suture is also identified and both anatomical structures are used as landmarks to isolate the main trunk of the facial nerve at the stylomastoid foramen. The insertion of SCM is cut at the level of the mastoid uncovering the occipitomastoid bone (▶ Fig. 2.160). Depending on the extension of the lesion, a partial superficial parotidectomy is performed. The facial nerve is isolated and preserved until the nerve bifurcation at the level of stylomastoid foramen.

Temporal Bone Dissection

A subtotal petrosectomy is then performed, removing the posterior and anterior walls of the EAC until the jugular bulb and

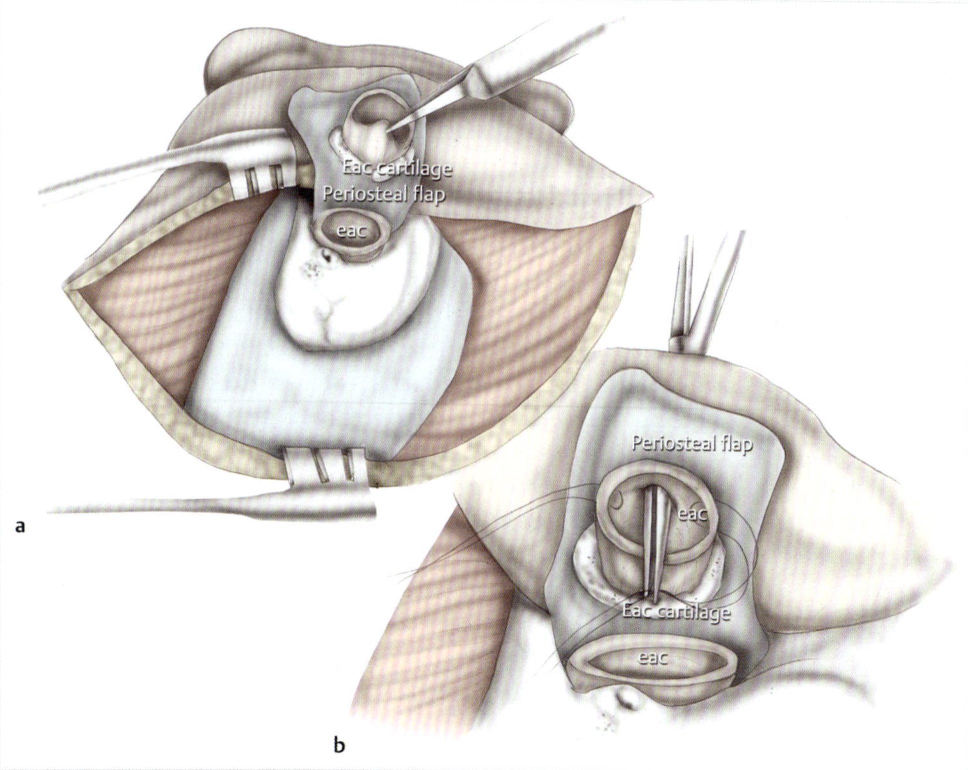

Fig. 2.157 Right side. **(a)** The external auditory canal (EAC) is transected, and a periosteal flap elevated at the same time; the EAC cartilage is detached from the skin of the canal. **(b)** Two sutures are made in the meatus with a curved clamp passing through the external auditory canal. *eac: external auditory canal.*

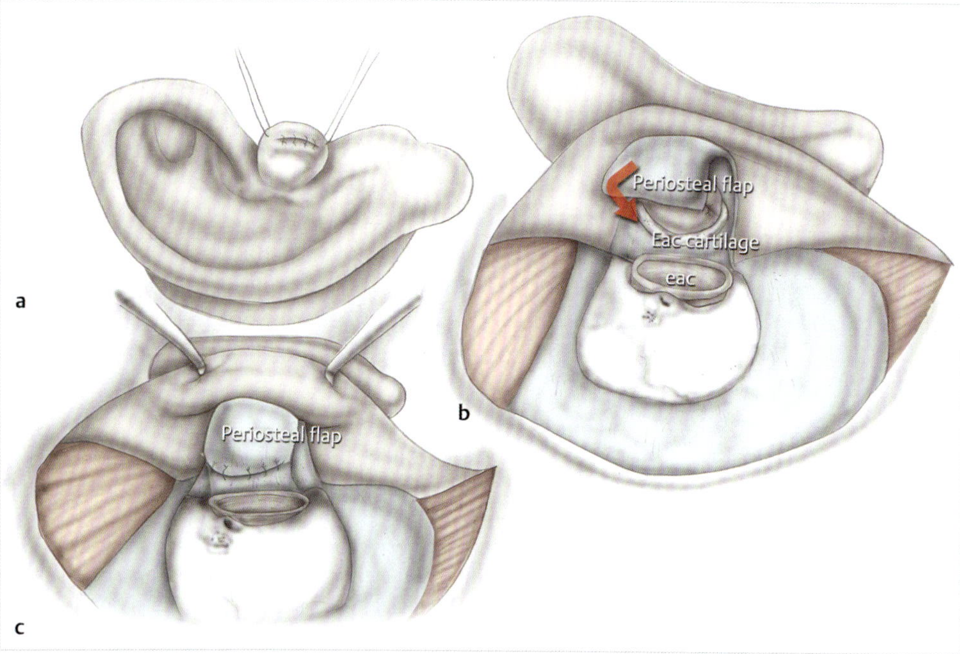

Fig. 2.158 Right side. **(a)** The skin of the external auditory canal (EAC) is everted and closed with 4–0 Vicryl sutures. **(b, c)** The periosteal flap is folded over the medial surface of the meatus, and sutured to the EAC cartilage. *eac: external auditory canal.*

internal carotid artery are visible. The removal of EAC anterior wall uncovers the temporal-mandibular joint in the most posterior portion. A wide mastoidectomy with perilabyrinthine cells removal is performed, and the middle and posterior portions of the fossa dura are widely skeletonized. The sinodural angle is also skeletonized and the sigmoid sinus is detected; following it until the jugular bulb, the facial nerve is skeletonized from the stylomastoid foramen till the geniculate ganglion (see ▶ Fig. 2.161 and ▶ Fig. 2.162). The labyrinthine block is carefully preserved, and the intratemporal vertical internal carotid artery is isolated inside the tympanic cavity just under the eustachian tube orifice.

The fallopian canal is gently removed using a diamond bur, under constant irrigation; the mastoid tip is amputated (see ▶ Fig. 2.163), and with a dissector the bone around the facial nerve is gently removed, uncovering the nerve from the stylomastoid foramen till the geniculate ganglion. A new fallopian canal is created, drilling in the root of the zygoma, above the eustachian tube (see ▶ Fig. 2.164). The bone over the facial nerve is removed for 180 degrees in the tympanic segment and for 270 degrees in the mastoid portion. The facial nerve is freed using scissors at level of the stylomastoid foramen due to the adhesion of the nerve to the surrounding fibrous layer at this level (▶ Fig. 2.165). Then the mastoid segment of the facial nerve is completely uncovered, and the fibrous attachment between the nerve and the fallopian canal is cut using a beaver knife (▶ Fig. 2.166). The facial nerve is gently and progressively elevated from the canal until the geniculate ganglion. The mastoid and tympanic segments of the facial nerve are anteriorly transposed. A tunnel is created on the parotid gland in order to protect the transposed nerve. The tympanic segment of the facial nerve in close proximity to the geniculate ganglion is placed on the previously created canal at the root of zygoma (▶ Fig. 2.167 and ▶ Fig. 2.168). Traditionally the sigmoid sinus is closed inferiorly to the superior petrosal sinus by double ligation through a dural incision close to the sinus using a Vicryl (▶ Fig. 2.169). This procedure has a high risk of CSF leakage. Alternatively, it is possible to close the sinus by extraluminally pressing the vein, packing the vascular lumen with Surgicel (absorbable hemostat), and by pressing the vein to the mastoid bone. The internal jugular vein is double-ligated at the level of the neck and cut. The jugular foramen is exposed and the intraluminal portion of the tumor is isolated. If the tumor presents extradural extension , it must be dissected. Before tumor dissection, an infratemporal fossa retractor may be used with a long blade behind the ascending ramus of the mandible and a short blade placed on the posterior skin margin (▶ Fig. 2.170). This retractor may help to anteriorly displace the mandible, allowing a better view of the entire vertical portion of the carotid artery and the anterior extension of the tumor toward the petrous apex and clivus.

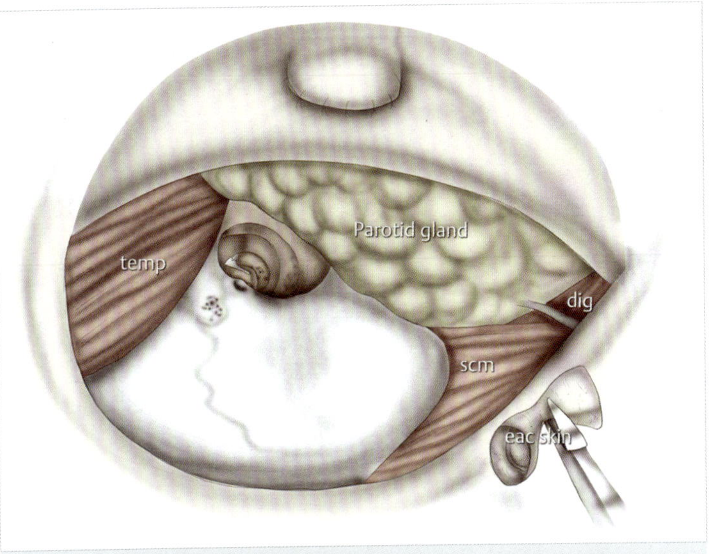

Fig. 2.159 Right side: The skin of the external auditory canal (EAC) and the ear drum is removed. *dig: digastric muscle; scm: sternocleidomastoid muscle; temp: temporalis muscle.*

Tumor Dissection

The lesion is dissected from the jugular foramen, while trying to preserve the previously isolated lower cranial nerves (▶ Fig. 2.171). The lateral wall of the jugular bulb is opened. In this step, bleeding from the openings of the inferior petrosal sinus and the condylar emissary vein is expected. Packing the lumen of the vein with Surgicel may be sufficient to control the bleeding. The medial wall of the jugular bulb and jugular vein at the skull base entrance are preserved in order to protect the lower cranial nerves, since these nerves run from the lacerum foramen to the neck just medially to this vein (▶ Fig. 2.172). The tumor is then removed with the jugular vein and jugular bulb. The infralabyrinthine cells are drilled with a diamond bur in order to remove remnant disease.

When an anterior extension of the tumor over the internal carotid artery is found, a gentle and careful dissection must be performed under microscopic view in order to remove the tumor from the major vascular structures. A diamond bur is used to remove the bone around the vertical portion of the internal carotid artery until the eustachian tube opening. A bipolar instrument is used to coagulate the caroticotympanic artery and to reduce the mass of the tumor around the internal carotid artery. The remnant tumor along the bend of the carotid is eventually removed, because of the risk of damaging the wall of the vascular structure (▶ Fig. 2.173 and ▶ Fig. 2.174).

In case of intradural extension of the tumor, a transjugular craniotomy is performed through the sigmoid–jugular system. After the ligation of the sigmoid sinus, the dura of the posterior fossa is exposed and cut, entering the posterior fossa. With this

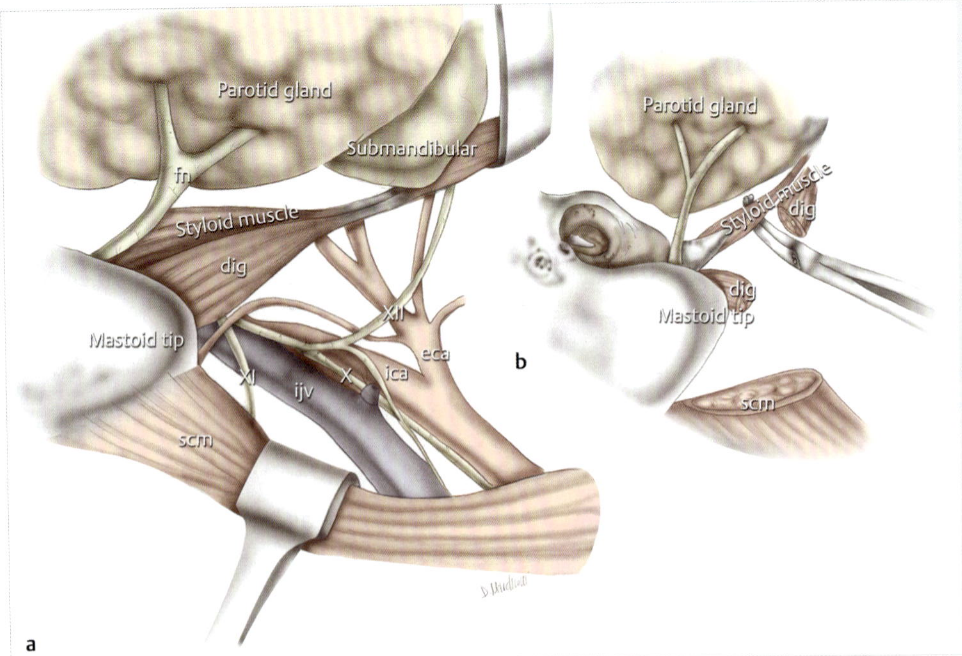

Fig. 2.160 Right side. **(a)** The neck is dissected; the internal jugular vein and the internal and external carotid arteries are isolated; the lower cranial nerve and the hypoglossal nerve are also detected at the base of the skull; the main trunk of the facial nerve is isolated at the stylomastoid foramen level. **(b)** The sternocleidomastoid muscle is cut at its insertion in the mastoid; the digastric and styloid muscles are also cut. *dig: digastric muscle; dig: digastric muscle; eca: external carotid artery; fn: facial nerve; ica: internal carotid artery; ijv: internal jugular vein; scm: sternocleidomastoid muscle.*

approach, the intracranial aspect of the jugular foramen, the lower cranial nerves, the pons, and the upper medulla are well exposed and the tumor is gently removed from the CPA (▶ Fig. 2.175). The dura is repaired using a temporal fascia graft and using abdominal fat.

Fallopian Bridge Technique (see Clinical Case 13)

The bridge technique is a variation of the Type A infratemporal fossa approach: the facial nerve is dissected and the bone over the nerve is partially removed. The facial nerve is left in situ. Avoiding the anterior transposition of the facial nerve, the tumor removal is performed around the facial nerve.

This technique is especially suitable for a schwannoma of the jugular foramen or for Type C 1 glomus tympanicus.

Due to the limitation of the surgical exposure of the jugular bulb and vertical carotid artery because of the presence of the facial nerve, in this technique an endoscopic support is necessary at the end of the microscopic procedure. A 45-degree endoscope is used to check the presence of any residual tumor around the facial nerve and the carotid artery. An angulate dissector is used to remove any residual disease under the mastoid segment of the facial nerve and medial to the carotid artery (see ▶ Fig. 2.176).

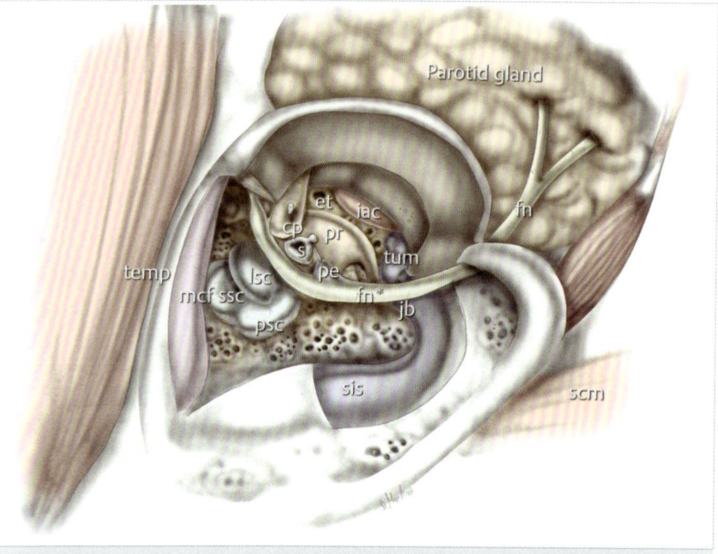

Fig. 2.161 Right side: A subtotal petrosectomy is performed. The facial nerve is skeletonized from the stylomastoid foramen till the geniculate ganglion. *cp: cochleariform process; et: eustachian tube; fn*: mastoid segment of facial nerve; fn: facial nerve; jb: jugular bulb; lsc: lateral semicircular canal; mcf: middle cranial fossa; pe: pyramidal eminence; pr: promontory; psc: posterior semicircular canal; s: stapes; scm: sternocleidomastoid muscle; sis: sigmoid sinus; ssc: superior semicircular canal; temp: temporalis muscle; tum: tumor involving the jugular foramen.*

Closure

A piece of temporalis muscle is used to close the eustachian tube. Abdominal fat is harvested from the abdomen. The cavity is progressively obliterated with this fat. The posterior belly of the digastric muscle is then replaced and sutured. The musculoperiosteal flap is replaced and sutured on the temporalis muscle (▶ Fig. 2.177). A suture of the skin is performed and a compressive bandage is placed.

Hints and Pitfalls

- In case of Class C glomus tumor removal, a single-stage surgery should be considered, since a dissection of the tumor in the second stage of surgery from the vascular structures such as the internal carotid artery and the facial nerve may be difficult due to the scar tissues around these anatomical structures.
- In case of Di glomus tumors (see Chapter 5), a two-stage surgical removal should be considered in order to reduce surgical morbidity as much as possible. In such cases, during the first stage of the operation only the extradural portion of the tumor should be removed and the intradural portion of the tumor must be left in place. A second stage operation will be planned after 6 months from the first procedure.

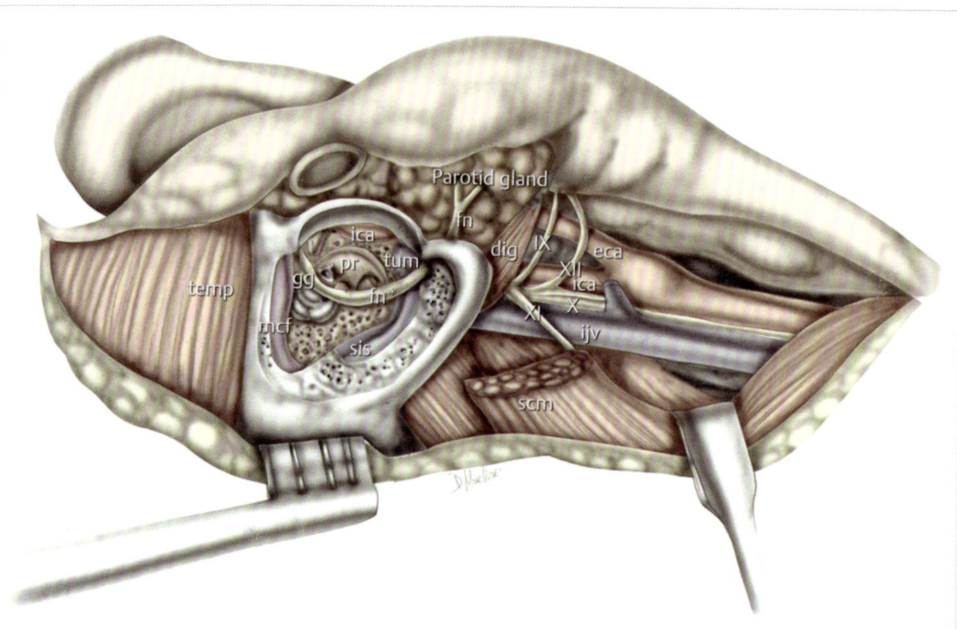

Fig. 2.162 Right side: Global view of the surgical field after temporal bone and neck dissection. *dig: digastric muscle; eac: external carotid artery; fn: facial nerve; fn*: mastoid segment of facial nerve; gg: geniculate ganglion; iac: internal carotid artery; ijv: internal jugular vein; mcf: middle cranial fossa; pr: promontory; scm: sternocleidomastoid muscle; sis: sigmoid sinus; temp: temporalis muscle; temp: temporalis muscle; tum: tumor involving the jugular foramen.*

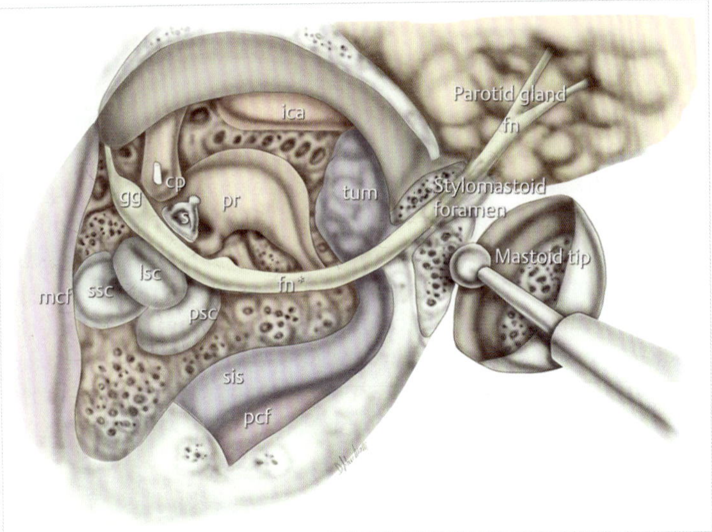

Fig. 2.163 Right side: The tip of the mastoid is removed and the facial nerve at the stylomastoid foramen level is isolated. *cp: cochleariform process; fn*: mastoid segment of facial nerve; fn: facial nerve; ica: internal carotid artery; lsc: lateral semicircular canal; mcf: middle cranial fossa; pcf: posterior cranial fossa; pr: promontory; psc: posterior semicircular canal; s: stapes; sis: sigmoid sinus; ssc: superior semicircular canal; tum: tumor involving the jugular foramen.*

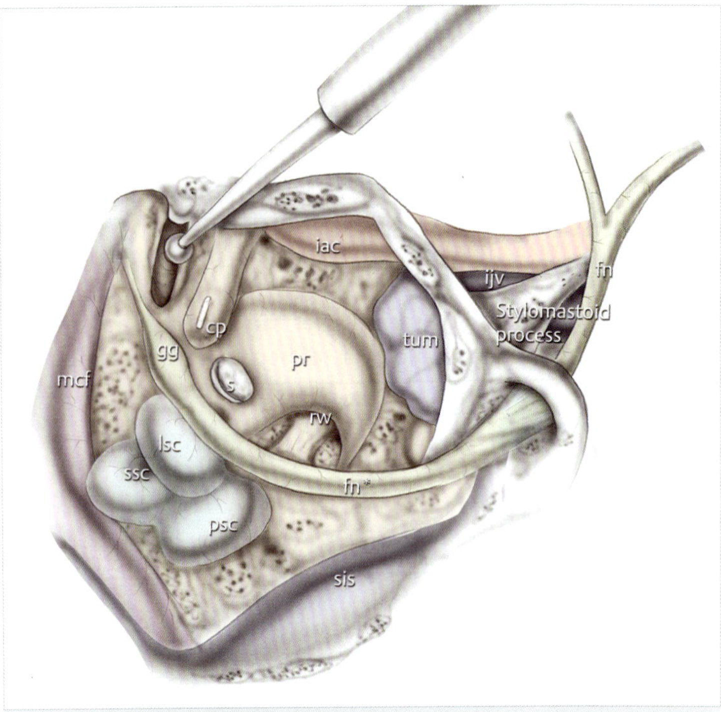

Fig. 2.164 Right side: A new fallopian canal is created, drilling the root of the zygoma, superiorly to the eustachian tube. *cp: cochleariform process; fn: facial nerve; fn*: mastoid segment of facial nerve; ica: internal carotid artery; ijv: internal jugular vein; lsc: lateral semicircular canal; mcf: middle cranial fossa; pr: promontory; psc: posterior semicircular canal; rw: round window; s: stapes; sis: sigmoid sinus; ssc: superior semicircular canal; tum: tumor involving the jugular foramen.*

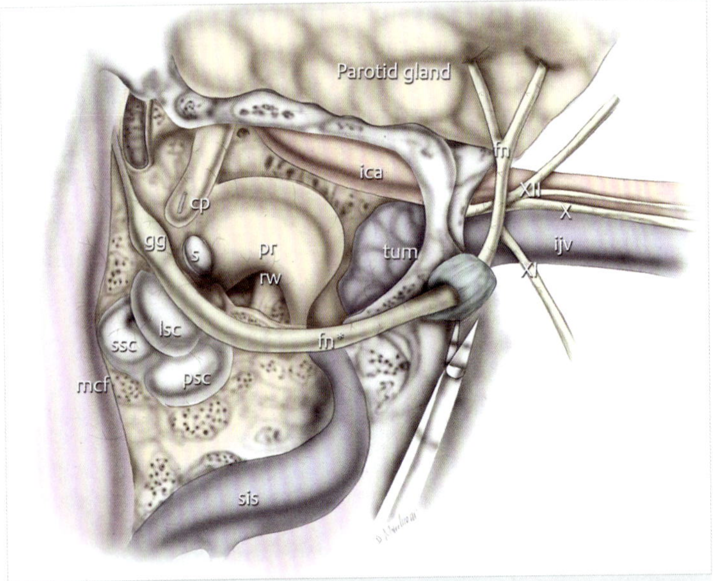

Fig. 2.165 Right side: The facial nerve is freed with scissors at the level of the stylomastoid foramen due to the adhesion of the nerve to the surrounding fibrous layer at this level. *cp: cochleariform process; fn*: mastoid segment of facial nerve; fn: facial nerve; ica: internal carotid artery; ijv: internal jugular vein; lsc: lateral semicircular canal; mcf: middle cranial fossa; pr: promontory; psc: posterior semicircular canal; rw: round window; s: stapes; sis: sigmoid sinus; ssc: superior semicircular canal; tum: tumor involving the jugular foramen.*

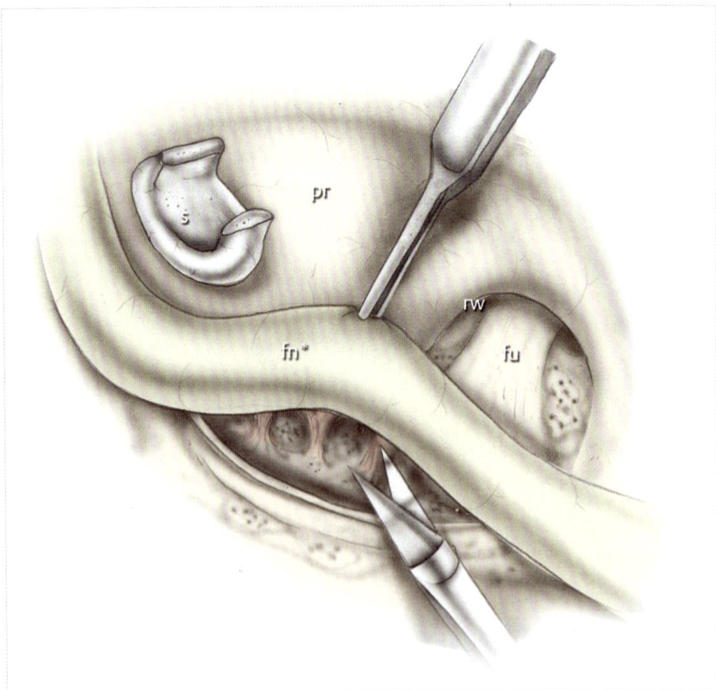

Fig. 2.166 Right side: The facial nerve is displaced from the fallopian canal; the anterior transposition of the facial nerve is started. *fn*: mastoid segment of facial nerve; fu: fustis; pr: promontory; rw: round window; s: stapes.*

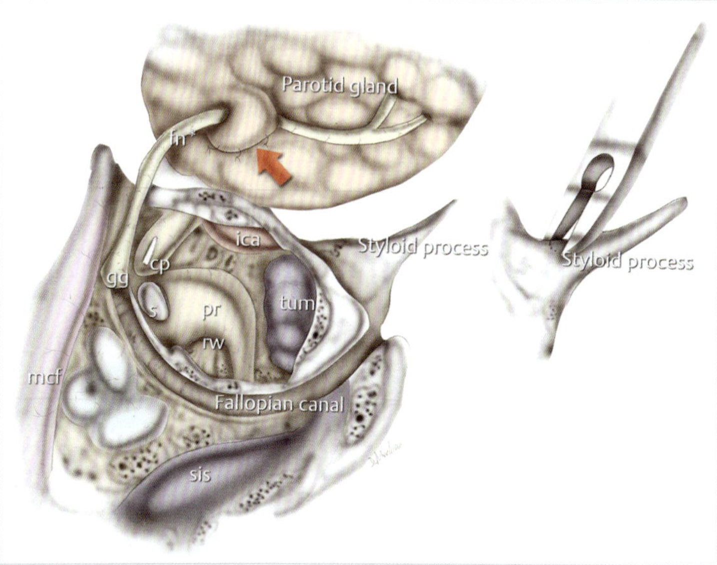

Fig. 2.167 Right side. **(a)** The facial nerve is anteriorly transposed; a groove in the parotid gland is used to place and protect the nerve. **(b)** The styloid process is removed. *cp: cochleariform process; fn*: mastoid segment of facial nerve; ica: internal carotid artery; mcf: middle cranial fossa; pr: promontory; rw: round window; s: stapes; sis: sigmoid sinus; tum: tumor involving the jugular foramen.*

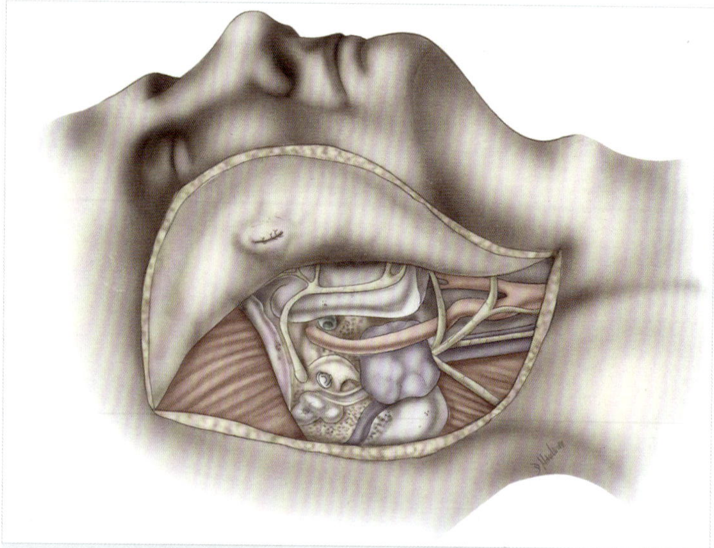

Fig. 2.168 Right side: Global view of the surgical field after the anterior transposition of the facial nerve; the jugular foramen is now approachable.

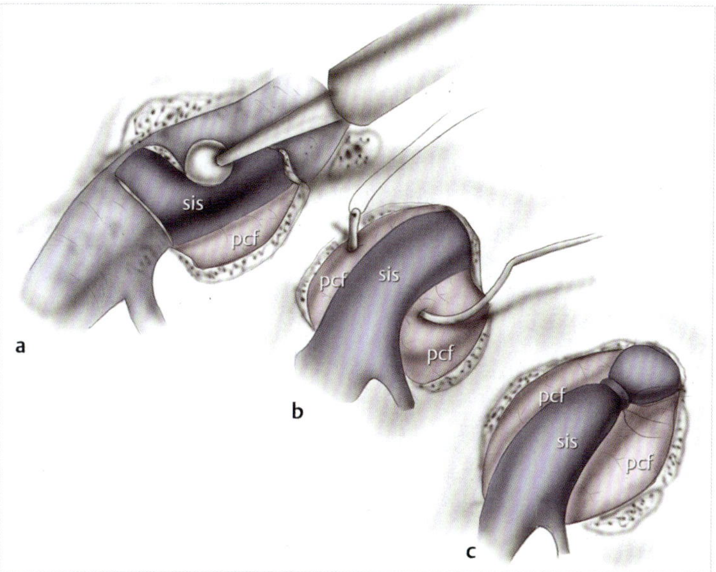

Fig. 2.169 Right side. **(a)** The sigmoid sinus is skeletonized uncovering the dura of the posterior fossa around the vascular structure. **(b)** A blunt tipped aneurysm needle is passed through the dura layer, under the vein; a Vicryl suture is passed through the eye of needle. **(c)** The vein is doubly ligated. *pcf: posterior cranial fossa; sis: sigmoid sinus.*

2.7.2 Infratemporal Fossa Types B and C (see Clinical Case 14)

These approaches are an anterior extension of the Type A infratemporal fossa approach but in Types B–C, the anterior transposition of the facial nerve is not required (see ▶ Fig. 2.203).

Indications for Type B

- Benign lesions involving petrous apex and clivus (see ▶ Fig. 2.204)
- Petrous bone cholesteatoma with involvement of the carotid area (infralabyrinthine, apical)
- Epidermoid or dermoid cysts of the petrous apex/clivus
- Clival chordoma
- Clival chondrosarcoma

Indication for Type C

- Benign lesions spreading into the pterygopalatine fossa, the sellar and parasellar areas, and the rhinopharynx
- Large juvenile nasopharyngeal angiofibroma invading the infratemporal fossa and the intracranial cavity
- Residual malignant nasopharyngeal carcinoma
- Trigeminal neurinoma
- Adenoid cystic carcinoma

Limitations

- This surgical technique requires the sacrifice of the mandibular trigeminal nerve (V3) and a conductive hearing loss is expected.

Endoscopic Support

In Type B and C infratemporal fossa approaches, endoscopic support is strongly recommended especially to remove remnant disease lying in the clivus medial to the vertical and horizontal portions of the internal carotid artery (see ▶ Fig. 2.215 and ▶ Fig. 2.216).

Surgical Technique

The patient is placed in a supine position. Facial nerve monitoring must be used electrodes are placed on the oris and oculi orbicularis muscles.

A wide C-shaped incision behind the postauricular sulcus is made. The incision is extended superiorly on the temporalis area ending above and posterior to the lateral orbital margin, and inferiorly along the neck (▶ Fig. 2.205).

The skin flap is elevated, the anterior border of the SCM is identified, and the greater auricular nerve preserved. Similar to a

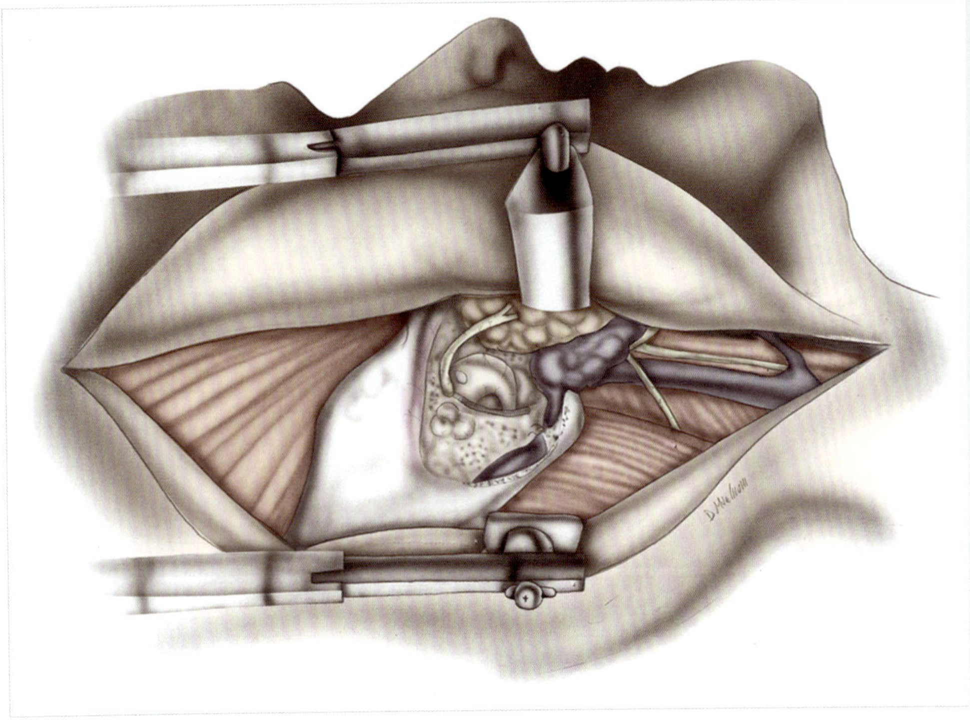

Fig. 2.170 Right side: A temporal fossa retractor is introduced from the top of the head, anteriorly pushing the ascending ramus of the mandible.

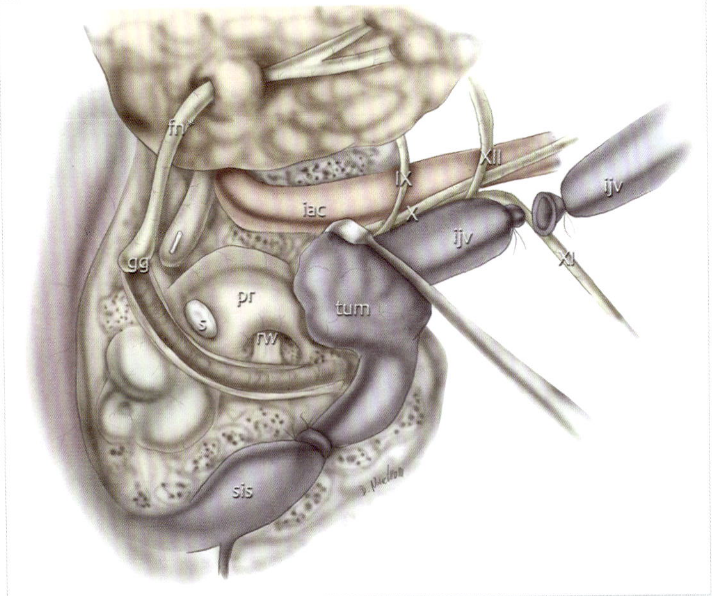

Fig. 2.171 Right side: The internal jugular vein is ligated in the neck at the base of skull. The dissection of the tumor from the jugular foramen and from the intrapetrous vertical portion of internal carotid artery is started. *fn*: mastoid segment of facial nerve; gg: geniculate ganglion; ica: internal carotid artery; ijv: internal jugular vein; pr: promontory; rw: round window; s: stapes; sis: sigmoid sinus; tum: tumor involving the jugular foramen.*

Type A approach, the EAC is transected at the level of the bony-cartilaginous junction and a blind-sac closure of the EAC is performed. The elevation of the flap in the temporalis area must be performed considering the anatomical conformation of the temporalis fascia layers. Anatomically in the temporal area, we have to consider three kinds of fascial layers: the temporoparietal fascia, the superficial layer of the deep temporalis fascia, and the deep layer of the deep temporalis fascia. The temporoparietal fascia (superficial temporalis fascia) is a superficial fascia in continuity with the galea. This fascia envelops the frontal branch of the facial nerve with the superficial temporal artery. The deep temporalis fascia lies on a deeper level than the temporoparietal fascia. The deep temporalis fascia is divided in two layers at the level of the temporalis line: the superficial and the deep layers, both enveloping the zygomatic arch, and a fat pad is present in between the superficial and deep layer of the deep temporalis fascia, just superiorly to the zygomatic arch. For this anatomical reason, the skin flap elevation in the temporalis area should be started on a superficial plane of dissection, superiorly following the temporalis fascia. When the dissection is close to the zygomatic process, the plane of the superficial layer of the deep temporalis fascia should be identified and cut in order to reach the superficial fat pad lying between the superficial and deep layers of deep temporalis fascia. Maintaining this deeper plane of dissection, we are finally able to elevate the skin flap, preserving the frontal branch of the facial nerve and exposing the zygomatic arch (see ▶ Fig. 2.206).

The parotid gland is exposed, and the main trunk of the facial nerve is identified at the stylomastoid foramen at the level of the tragal pointer. The facial nerve is then followed into the parotid gland, exposing the bifurcation of the nerve. The frontal branches are carefully isolated and preserved.

The periosteum of the zygomatic arch is incised along the major axis of the zygoma and elevated, protecting the frontal branches of the facial nerve (▶ Fig. 2.206). A pre-plating is performed on the zygomatic arch, preparing for the osteotomies. The osteotomies are then performed. The zygomatic arch is detached and inferiorly transposed, maintaining the muscular adhesion between the bone and the temporalis muscle (▶ Fig. 2.207). Once the osteotomies are done, the whole temporalis muscle is dissected from the temporal squama and inferiorly transposed with the zygomatic bone, kept attached to the coronoid process, then a retractor is placed over the muscle, allowing

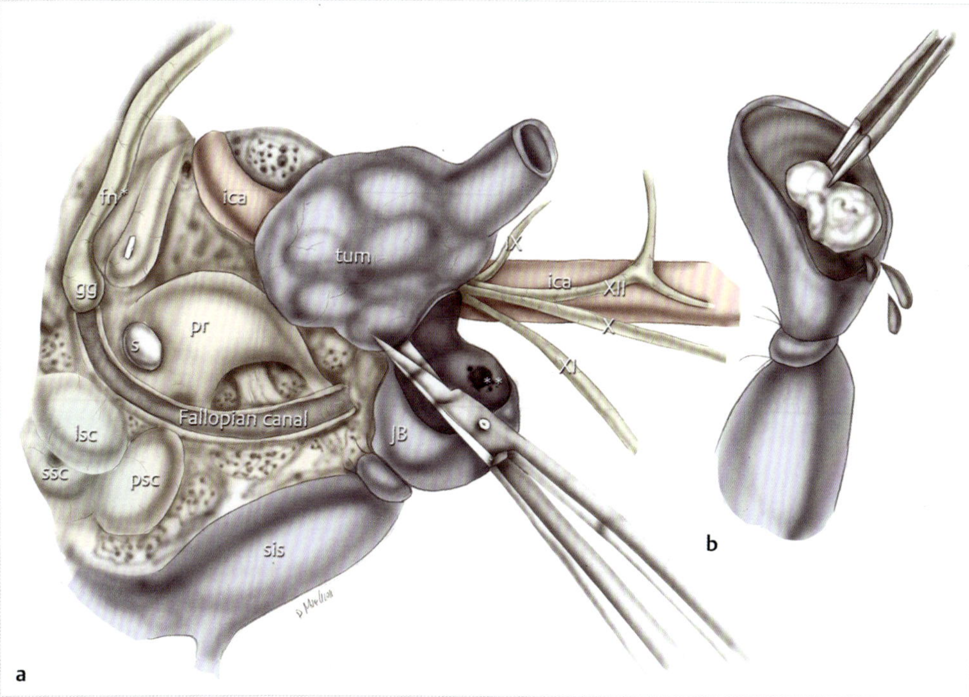

Fig. 2.172 Right side. **(a)** The lateral aspect of the jugular bulb is excised to remove the tumor with the vein; during this maneuver, bleeding is expected due to the opening of the inferior petrosal sinus and the condylar emissary vein in this area. **(b)** A Surgicel is used to pack the jugular lumen. *fn*: mastoid segment of facial nerve; gg: geniculate ganglion; ica: internal carotid artery; jb: jugular bulb; lsc: lateral semicircular canal; pr: promontory; psc: posterior semicircular canal; s: stapes; sis: sigmoid sinus; ssc: superior semicircular canal; tum: tumor involving the jugular foramen; **: the openings of inferior petrosal sinus and condylar emissary vein.*

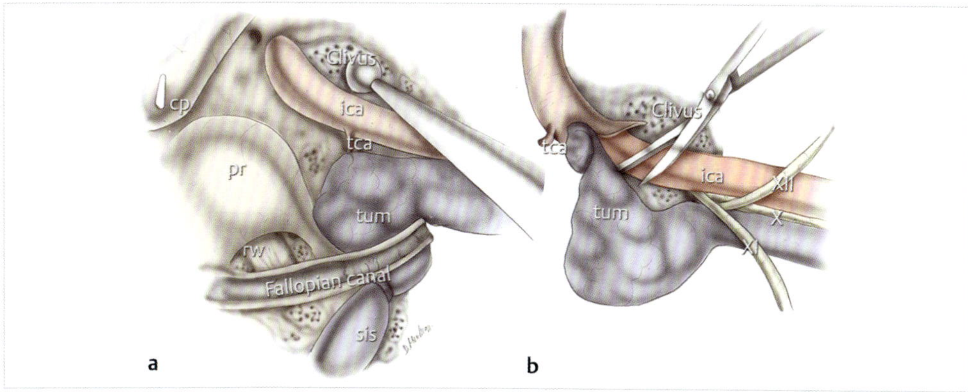

Fig. 2.173 Right side. **(a)** When the intrapetrous carotid artery is involved by the tumor, a diamond bur is used to skeletonize the artery; the caroticotympanic artery is coagulated, and the tumor dissection from the internal carotid artery is performed maintaining the integrity of the arterial wall **(b)**. *ica: internal carotid artery; pr: promontory; rw: round window; sis: sigmoid sinus; tca: caroticotympanic artery; tum: tumor involving the jugular foramen.*

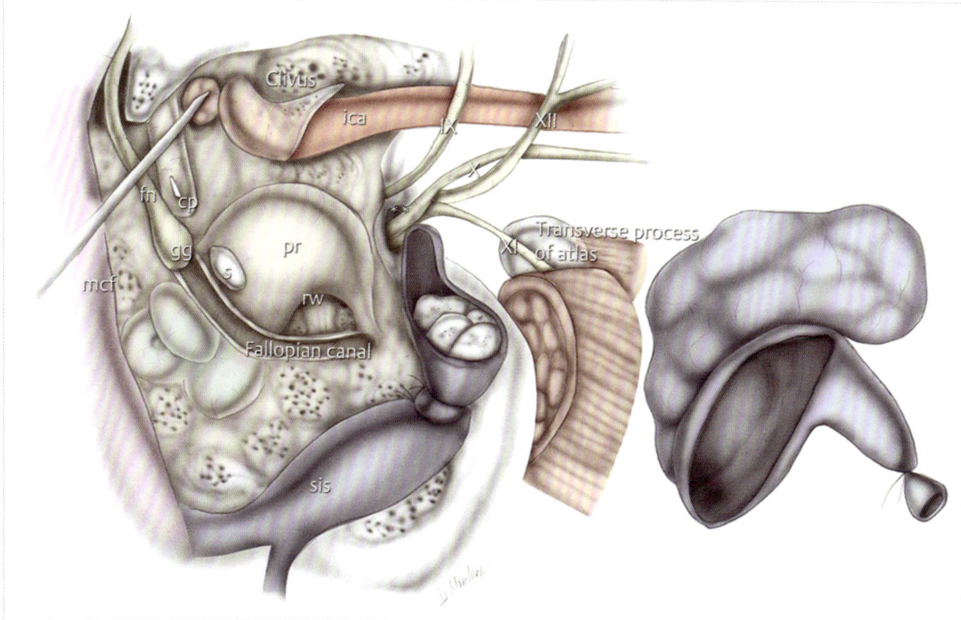

Fig. 2.174 Right side: The tumor is removed with the jugular vein; a piece of muscle harvested from the temporalis muscle is used to obliterate the eustachian tube opening. *cp: cochleariform process; fn: facial nerve; gg: geniculate ganglion; ica: internal carotid artery; mcf: middle cranial fossa; pr: promontory; rw: round window; s: stapes; sis: sigmoid sinus; tum: tumor involving the jugular foramen; **: the openings of inferior petrosal sinus.*

for the inferior transposition of the condyle of the mandible (▶ Fig. 2.208). During this surgical maneuver, damage or stretching of the main trunk of the facial nerve should be avoided. The skin and the eardrum are removed from the EAC as it happens in a Type A infratemporal fossa approach. The ossicular chain is removed, maintaining just the footplate of the stapes. A canal wall down mastoidectomy is performed. The facial nerve is identified and preserved from the geniculate ganglion till the stylomastoid foramen. Using a diamond bur, the tympanic cavity cellularity of the protympanum and hypotympanum is removed, exposing the major vascular structures, the jugular bulb and the carotid artery (see ▶ Fig. 2.209b). During this surgical procedure, the promontory region and the cochlea should be preserved, unless the surgical approach requires the sacrifice of the hearing function. The internal carotid artery is further dissected and isolated from the vertical intrapetrosal portion to the horizontal portion. The cochleariform process and the semicanal of the tensor tympani muscle are removed and the eponymous muscle is removed. The bony portion of the eustachian tube is drilled and opened, allowing for a better isolation of the horizontal portion of the carotid artery and anteriorly following this vascular structure.

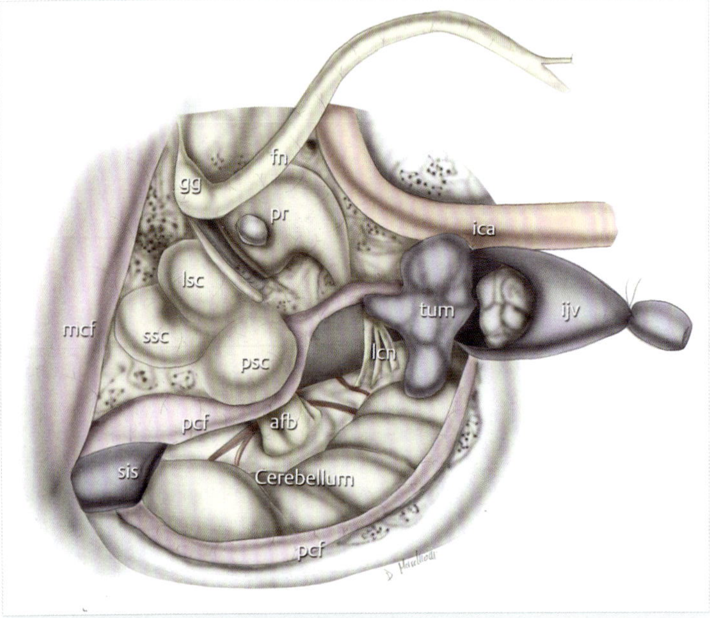

Fig. 2.175 Right side: In case of an intradural extension of the tumor, a transjugular craniotomy is performed through the sigmoid-jugular system. The sigmoid sinus is ligated; the dura of the posterior fossa is excised entering the posterior fossa; the tumor is exposed inside the cerebellopontine angle (CPA) and removed. *afb: acoustic-facial bundle; fn: facial nerve; gg: geniculate ganglion; ica: internal carotid artery; ijv: internal jugular vein; lcn: lower cranial nerves; lsc: lateral semicircular canal; pcf: posterior cranial fossa; pr: promontory; psc: posterior semicircular canal; sis: sigmoid sinus; ssc: superior semicircular canal; tum: tumor involving the jugular foramen and the CPA.*

The floor of the middle cranial fossa is widely exposed using a diamond bur from the sinodural angle till the anterior portion lying close to the zygomatic area. The glenoid fossa is then drilled and removed. The drilling of the floor of the middle cranial fossa allows the surgeon to anteriorly decompress the dura, until the identification of the middle meningeal artery running into the foramen spinosum and the mandibular branch of the trigeminal nerve emerging from the foramen ovale (see ▶ Fig. 2.209a). The middle meningeal artery is coagulated and cut; the V3 is cut allowing access to the infratemporal fossa. A retractor is placed over the temporomandibular joint and over the temporalis muscle in order to anteriorly displace the mandible, exposing the internal carotid artery and the clivus bone (▶ Fig. 2.210). The horizontal portion of the carotid artery is further anteriorly exposed in the petrous apex and clivus with respect to the anterior foramen lacerum, exposing the tumor in the petrous apex (▶ Fig. 2.211; see Clinical Case 15 ▶ Fig. 2.237 and ▶ Fig. 2.238).

Endoscopic Support to Infratemporal Fossa Type B (see also Chapter 6)

Previously in the endoscopic era in case of massive involvement of clivus under the carotid artery, a 360 degrees dissection of the artery should be performed (see ▶ Fig. 2.212) and the carotid had to be carefully and gently transposed and mobilized from the carotid canal to have a good control of the hidden area of the clivus. When necessary, the promontory is drilled and the cochlea is sacrificed in order to drill all the bone around the internal carotid artery, especially if the sacrifice of the hearing function is necessary when the lesion is medial to the cochlea (see ▶ Fig. 2.213). Further bone removal from the wall of the internal

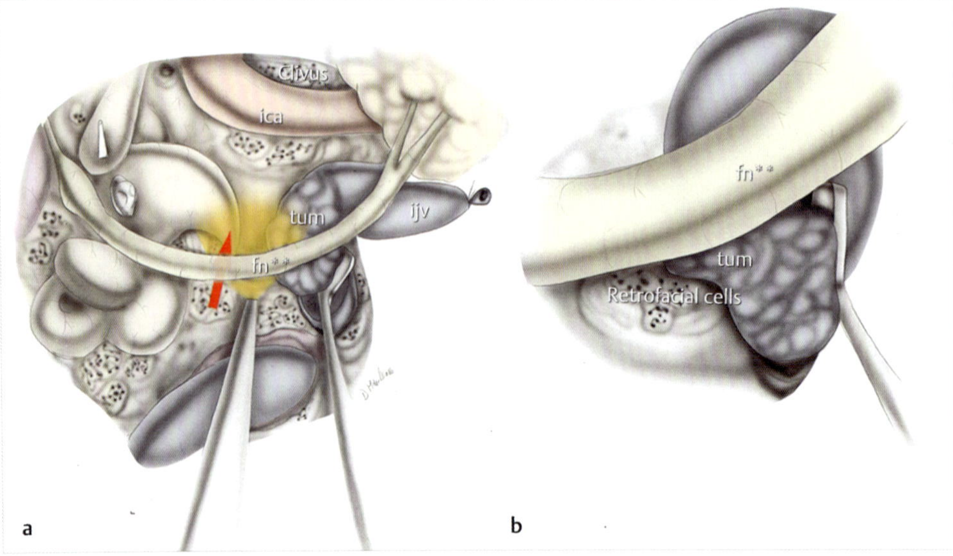

Fig. 2.176 Right side. **(a)** In Class C1 a fallopian bridge technique is performed, maintaining the facial nerve in the fallopian canal; a 0-degree endoscope is used to magnify the jugular foramen and the retrofacial area exposing the tumor. **(b)** A curve dissector may be useful under an endoscopic view to remove the residual tumor lying medial to the fallopian canal. *fn*: mastoid segment of facial nerve; ica: internal carotid artery; ijv: internal jugular vein; tum: tumor involving the jugular foramen.*

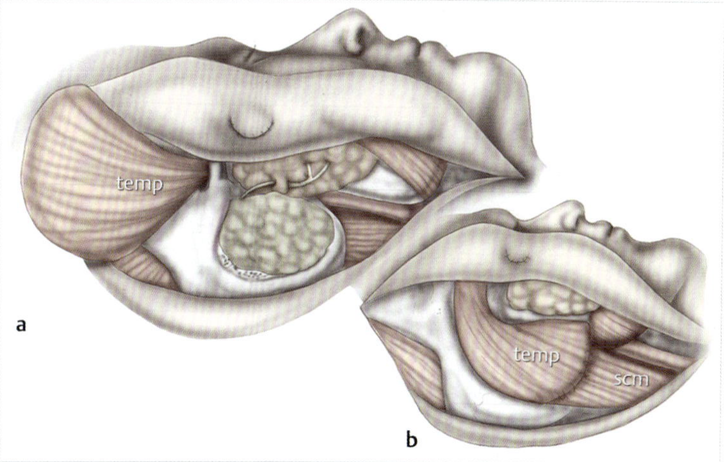

Fig. 2.177 Clinical Case 12, Right side. **(a)** Abdominal fat is used to obliterate the surgical cavity and the temporalis muscle is inferiorly transposed and sutured to the sternocleidomastoid muscle to close the surgical cavity, separating the cavity between the neck and the temporal bone **(b)**. *scm: sternocleidomastoid muscle; temp: temporalis muscle.*

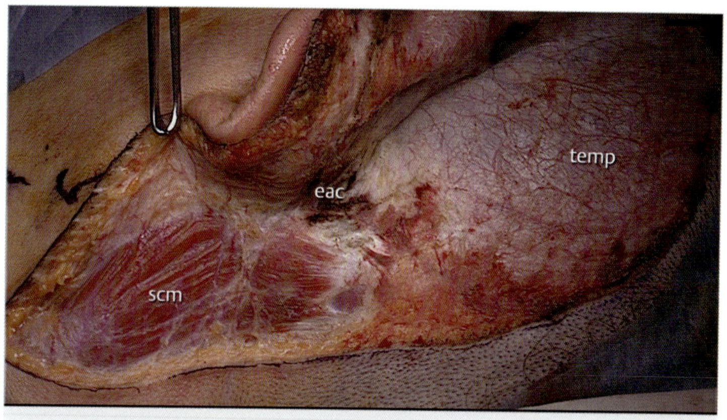

Fig. 2.178 Clinical Case 12, Left side: Class C2 paraganglioma. The skin flap is elevated. *eac: external auditory canal; scm: sternocleido-mastoid muscle; temp: temporalis muscle.*

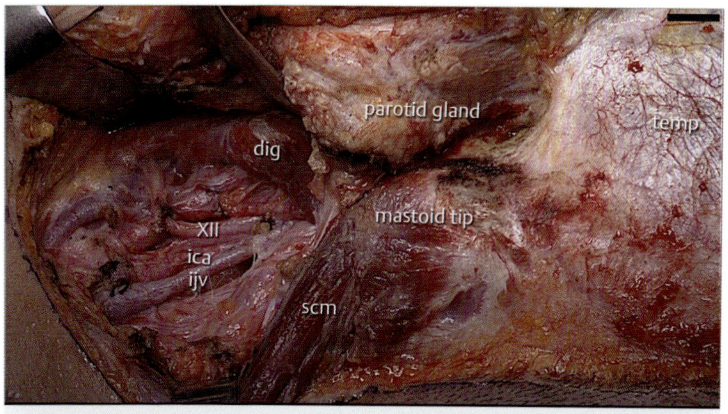

Fig. 2.179 Clinical Case 12, Left side: The external auditory canal (EAC) is transected; the neck is dissected and the major vascular structures with the lower cranial nerves are isolated at the base of skull. *dig: digastric muscle; ica: internal carotid artery; ijv: internal jugular vein; scm: sternocleidomastoid muscle; temp: temporalis muscle.*

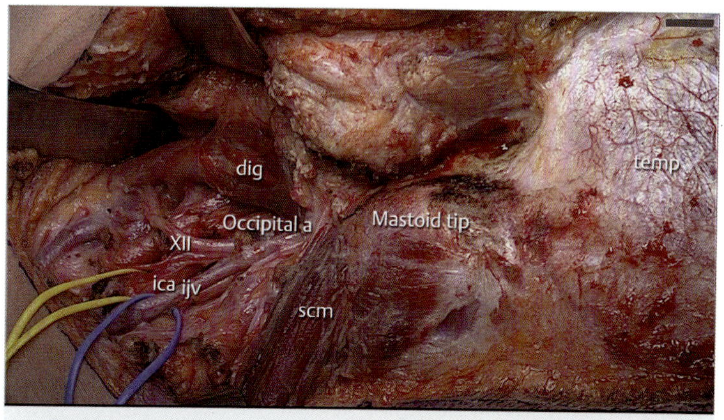

Fig. 2.180 Clinical Case 12, Left side: The internal carotid artery and the internal jugular vein are isolated and marked with different colors in the neck at the base of skull. *dig: digastric muscle; ica: internal carotid artery; ijv: internal jugular vein; occipital a: occipital artery; scm: sternocleidomastoid muscle; temp: temporalis muscle.*

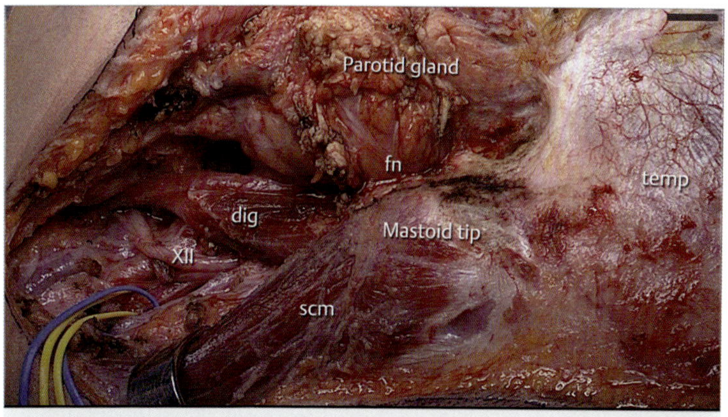

Fig. 2.181 Clinical Case 12, Left side: A superficial parotidectomy is performed and the facial nerve is isolated at the level of stylomastoid foramen. *dig: digastric muscle; fn: facial nerve; scm: sternocleidomastoid muscle; temp: temporalis muscle.*

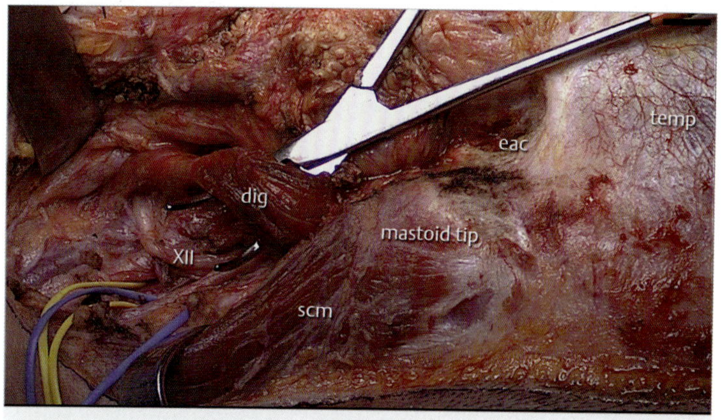

Fig. 2.182 Clinical Case 12, Left side: The digastric and the styloid muscles are cut. *dig: digastric muscle; eac: external auditory canal; scm: sternocleidomastoid muscle; temp: temporalis muscle.*

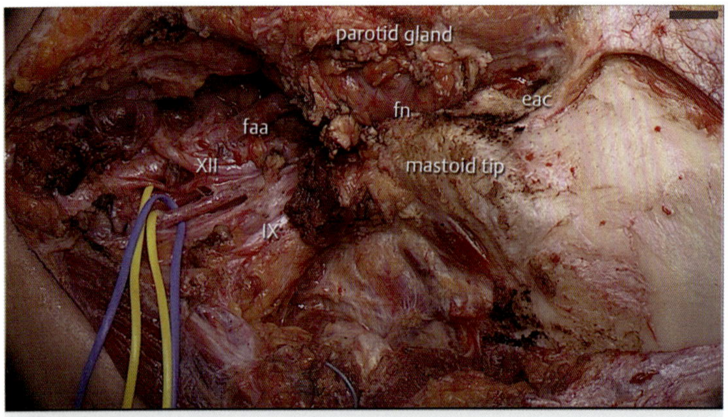

Fig. 2.183 Left side: The sternocleidomastoid muscle is cut at the tip of the mastoid and the periosteal flap is elevated uncovering the occipitomastoid bone. *eac: external auditory canal; faa: facial artery; fn: facial nerve.*

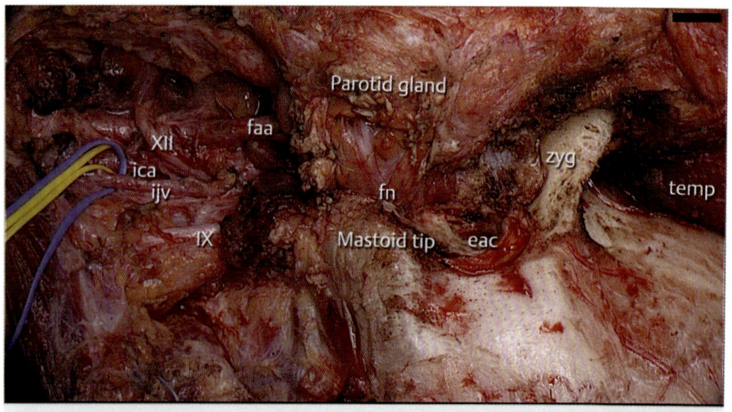

Fig. 2.184 Left side: The zygomatic arch is uncovered and the skin of the external auditory canal (EAC) is removed. *eac: external auditory canal; faa: facial artery; fn: facial nerve; ica: internal carotid artery; ijv: internal jugular vein; temp: temporalis muscle; zyg: zygomatic arch.*

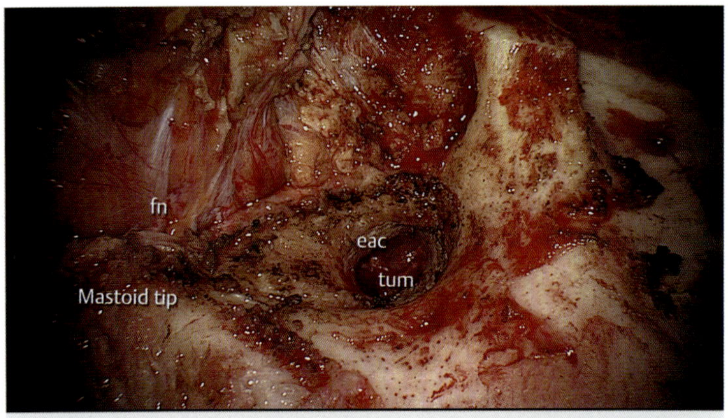

Fig. 2.185 Clinical Case 12, Left side: The skin and the eardrum are removed. The tumor is visible inside the tympanic cavity. *eac: external auditory canal; fn: facial nerve; tum: tumor.*

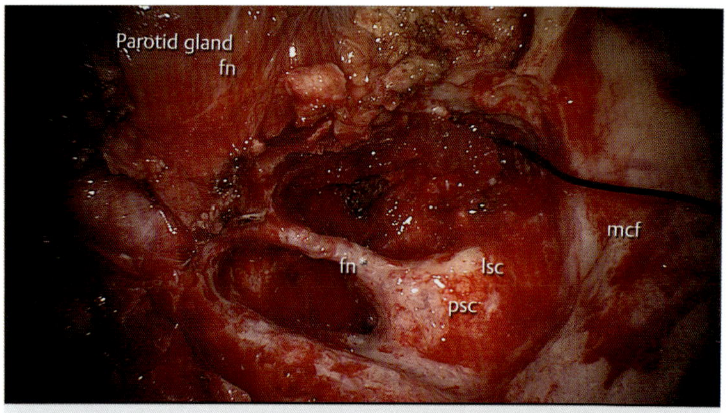

Fig. 2.186 Clinical Case 12, Left side: A subtotal petrosectomy is performed, the ossicular chain is removed, and the tumor is progressively removed from the tympanic cavity; the facial nerve is isolated inside the temporal bone. *fn: facial nerve; fn*: mastoid segment of the facial nerve; lsc: lateral semicircular canal; mcf: middle cranial fossa; psc: posterior semicircular canal.*

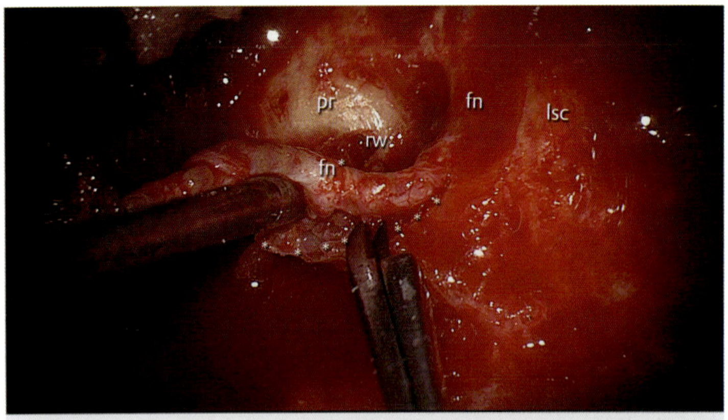

Fig. 2.187 Clinical Case 12, Left side: The anterior transposition of the facial nerve is started; the mastoid segment of the facial nerve is gently transposed; a microscissor is used to remove the adherences between the nerve and the fallopian canal (*****). *fn: facial nerve; fn*: mastoid segment of the facial nerve; lsc: lateral semicircular canal; rw: round window.*

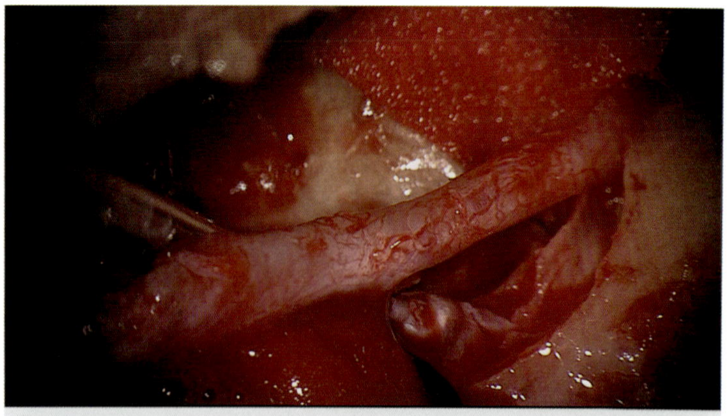

Fig. 2.188 Clinical Case 12, Left side: Gelfoam soaked with corticosteroid is used on the nerve to protect the facial nerve during the anterior transposition.

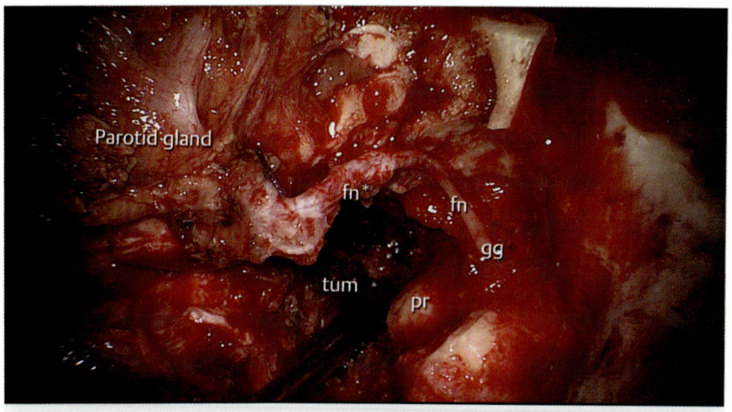

Fig. 2.189 Clinical Case 12, Left side: The anterior transposition is done, exposing the tumor into the jugular foramen. *fn: facial nerve; fn*: mastoid segment of the facial nerve; lsc: lateral semicircular canal; pr: promontory; tum: tumor involving the jugular foramen.*

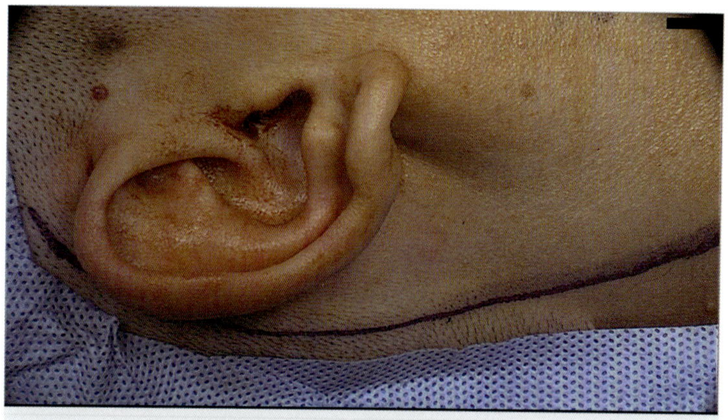

Fig. 2.190 Clinical Case 13, Right side: Class C1 paraganglioma. Fallopian bridge technique. Line of incision.

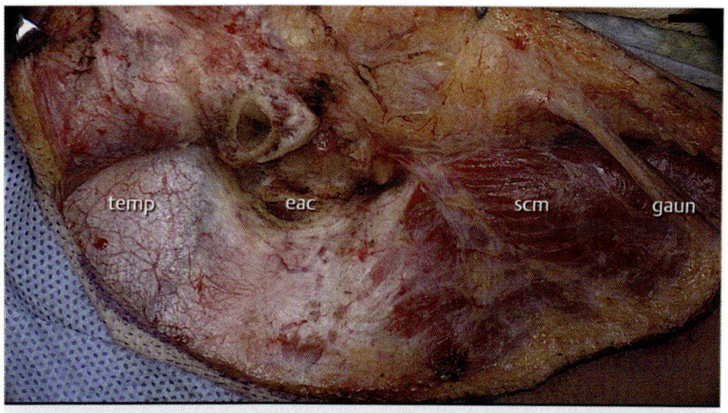

Fig. 2.191 Clinical Case 13, Right side: The skin flap is elevated and the external auditory canal (EAC) is transected. *eac: external auditory canal; gaun: great auricular nerve; scm: sternocleidomastoid muscle; temp: temporalis muscle.*

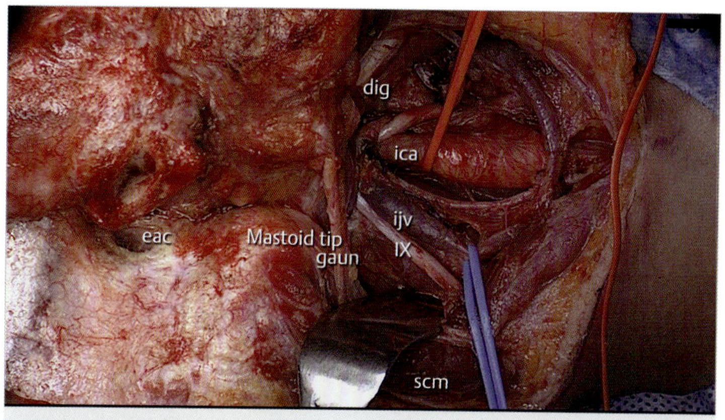

Fig. 2.192 Clinical Case 13, Right side: The major vascular structures and nerves are isolated at the base of the skull. *dig: digastric muscle; eac: external auditory canal; gaun: great auricular nerve; ica: internal carotid artery; ijv: internal jugular vein; scm: sternocleidomastoid muscle.*

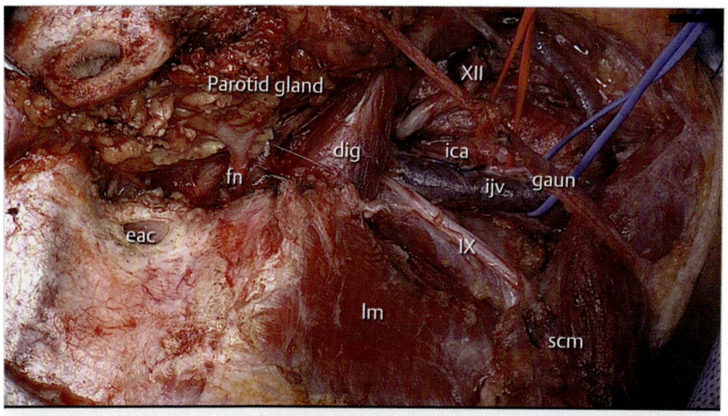

Fig. 2.193 Clinical Case 13, Right side: The internal jugular vein and the internal carotid artery are isolated; the facial nerve is detected at the level of the stylomastoid foramen; the sternocleidomastoid muscle is cut at the tip of the mastoid. *dig: digastric muscle; eac: external auditory canal; gaun: great auricular nerve; ica: internal carotid artery; ijv: internal jugular vein; lm: splenium muscle; scm: sternocleidomastoid muscle.*

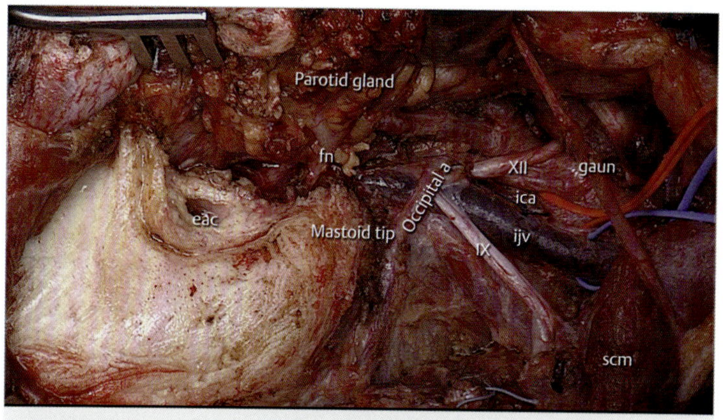

Fig. 2.194 Clinical Case 13, Right side: The digastric and styloid muscles are cut. The periosteal flap is elevated uncovering the occipital-mastoid bone. *dig: digastric muscle; eac: external auditory canal; gaun: great auricular nerve; ica: internal carotid artery; ijv: internal jugular vein; scm: sternocleidomastoid muscle.*

carotid artery allows to move the vascular structure, transposing it anteriorly, uncovering all the clivus lying medial to the carotid (▶ Fig. 2.214).

In case of a lesion with involvement of the areas superior and medial to the carotid artery, the removal of the lesion is extremely difficult, since a small displacement of the horizontal portion of the carotid artery is possible. In these cases, an endoscopic support is mandatory.

Also in cases in which the tumor is located medial to the vertical portion of the internal carotid artery, endoscopic support is strongly suggested since the endoscopic procedure can help the surgeon to remove the lesion in the clivus lying medial to the

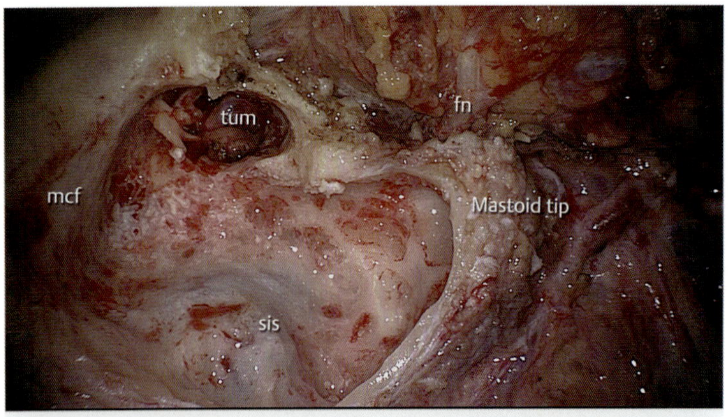

Fig. 2.195 Clinical Case 13, Right side: A subtotal petrosectomy is started; the tumor is seen in the tympanic cavity. *fn: facial nerve; mcf: middle cranial fossa; sis: sigmoid sinus; tum: tumor.*

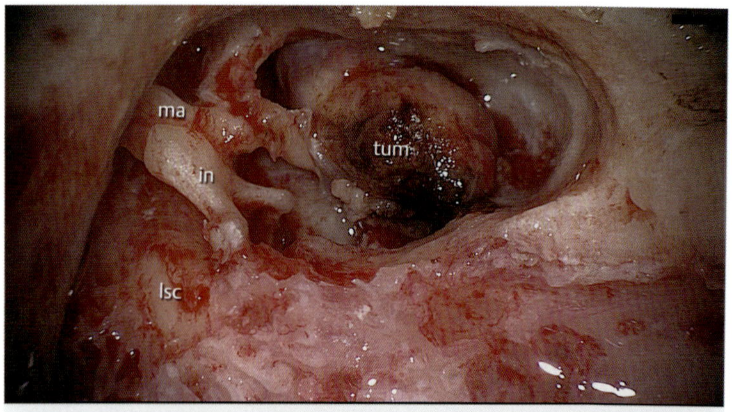

Fig. 2.196 Clinical Case 13, Right side: The tumor is progressively coagulated. *in: incus; lsc: lateral semicircular canal; ma: malleus; tum: tumor.*

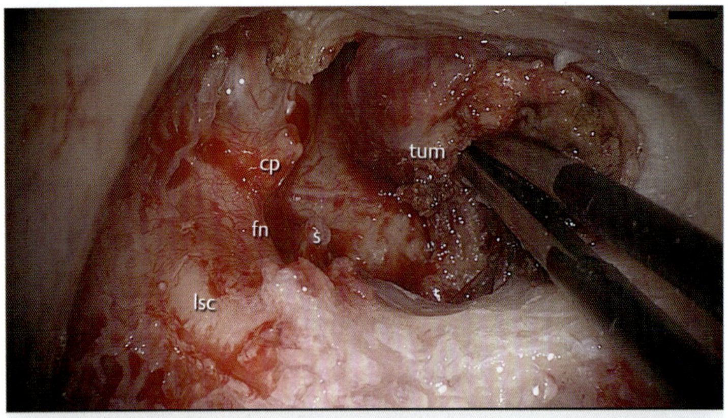

Fig. 2.197 Clinical Case 13, Right side: The ossicular chain is removed; a bipolar instrument is used to coagulate the tumor. *cp: cochleariform process; fn: facial nerve; lsc: lateral semicircular canal; s: stapes; tum: tumor.*

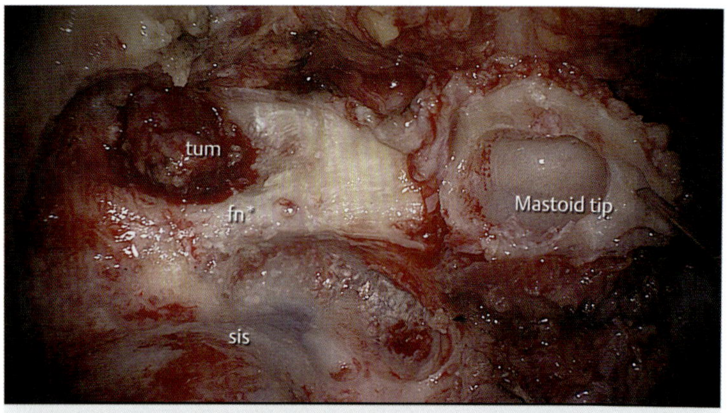

Fig. 2.198 Clinical Case 13, Right side: The tip of the mastoid is removed and the mastoid segment of the facial nerve detected. *fn*: mastoid segment of facial nerve; sis: sigmoid sinus; tum: tumor.*

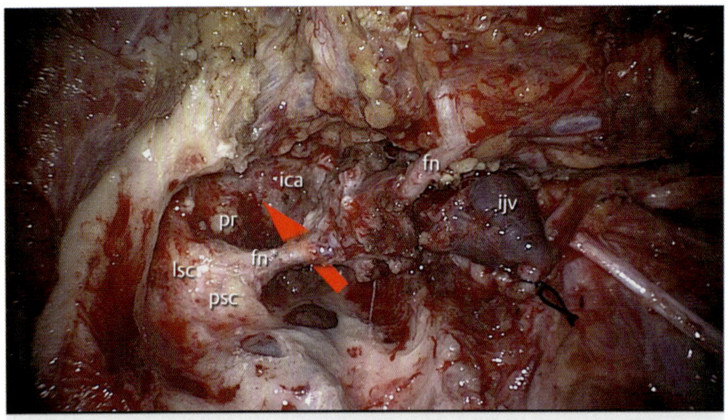

Fig. 2.199 Clinical Case 13, Right side: The facial nerve is isolated from the geniculate ganglion till the parotid portion. The mastoid segment of the facial nerve is kept in place. The retrofacial cells are removed and the tumor is isolated at the level of jugular foramen. The tumor is progressively removed between the neck and the temporal bone working under the facial nerve (see the *red arrow*). The internal jugular vein is ligated at the base of the skull and the jugular bulb is cut with the tumor. *fn*: mastoid segment of facial nerve; ica: internal carotid artery; ijv: internal jugular vein; lsc: lateral semicircular canal; pr: promontory; psc: posterior semicircular canal.*

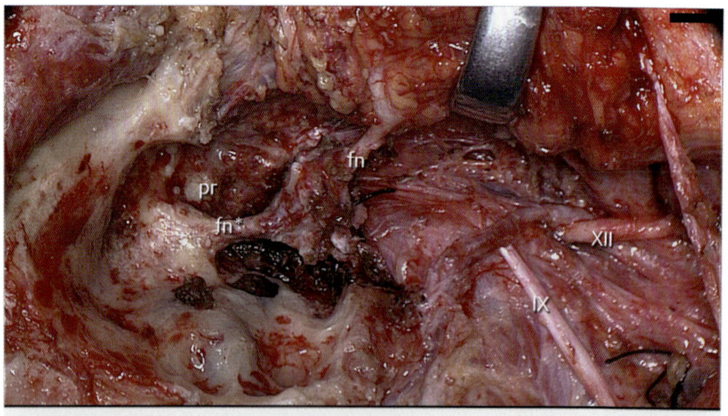

Fig. 2.200 Clinical Case 13, Right side: Final view of the surgical cavity after tumor removal. *fn: facial nerve; fn*: mastoid segment of facial nerve; pr: promontory.*

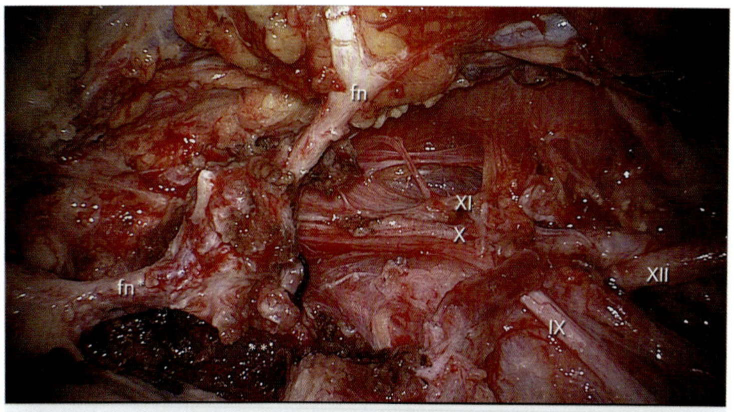

Fig. 2.201 Clinical Case 13, Right side: The lower cranial nerve and the hypoglossal nerve are preserved. The medial portion of the jugular bulb is left in place and packed with Surgicel, closing the opening from the inferior petrosal sinus (**). *fn: facial nerve; fn*: mastoid segment of facial nerve.*

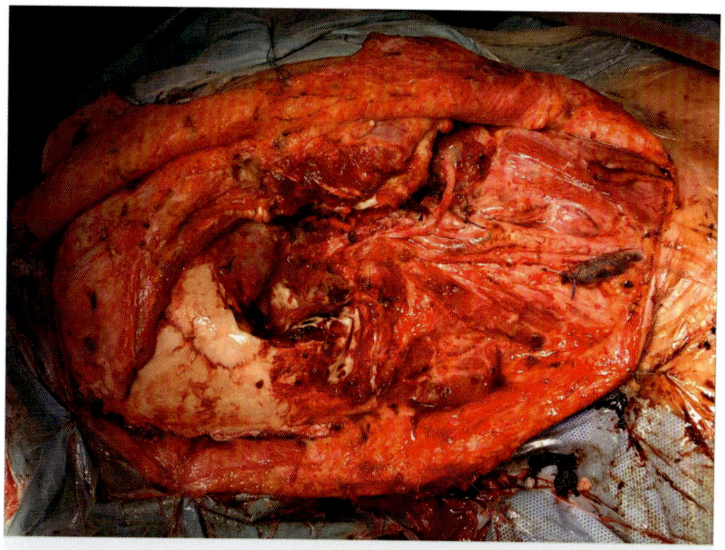

Fig. 2.202 Right side: Clinical Case malignant tumor of the parotid gland with jugular foramen involvement. The final surgical cavity is noted after tumor removal. In this case, an infratemporal fossa Type A is adopted with a sacrifice of facial nerve.

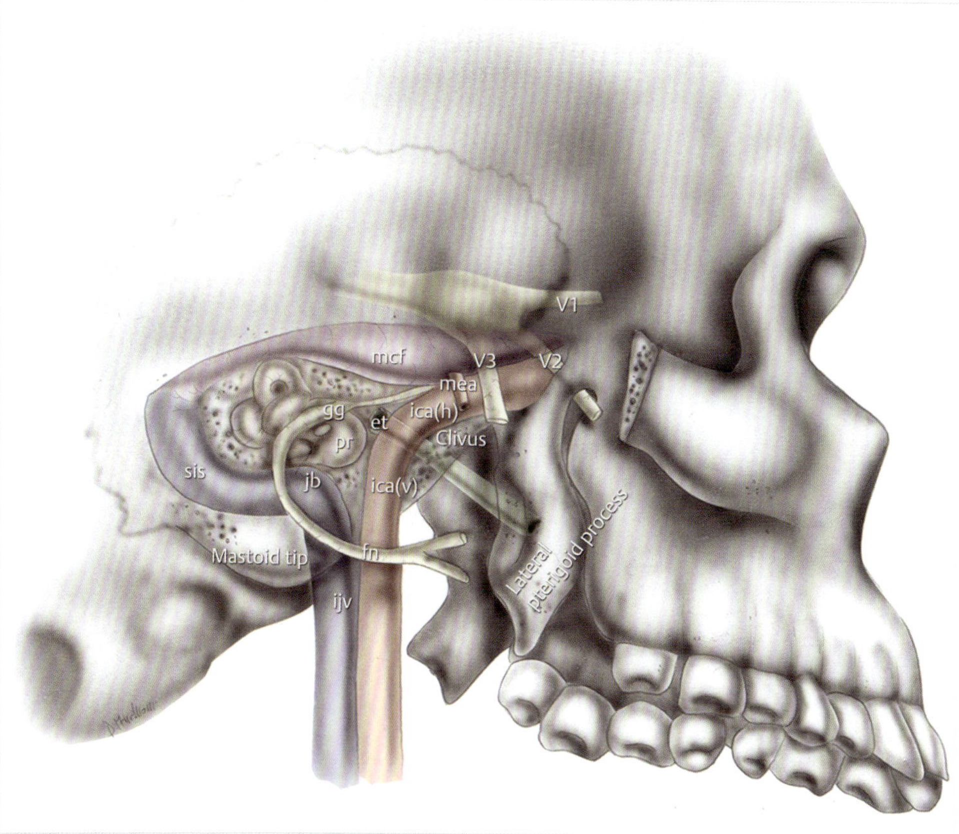

Fig. 2.203 Right side: Schematic drawing showing the anatomical structures involved during the infratemporal fossa approaches, Types B and C. *et: eustachian tube; fn: facial nerve; gg: geniculate ganglion; ica(h): intrapetrous horizontal internal carotid artery; ica(v): intrapetrous vertical internal carotid artery; ijv: internal jugular vein; jb: jugular bulb; mcf: middle cranial fossa; mea: middle meningeal artery; pr: promontory; sis: sigmoid sinus.*

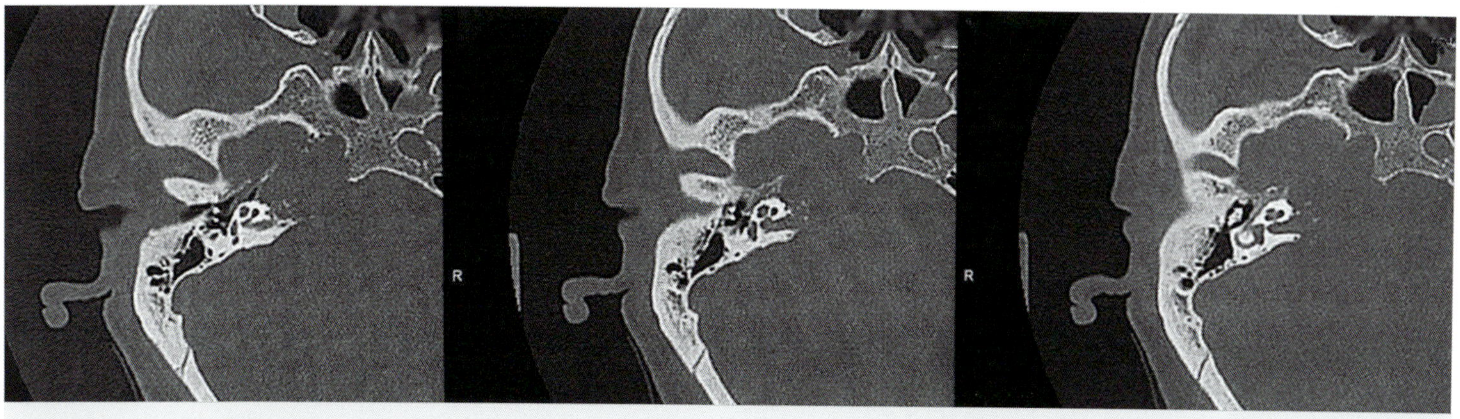

Fig. 2.204 Computed tomography (CT) scan in axial view: A petrous apex lesion extending to the clivus with internal carotid artery involvement can be seen.

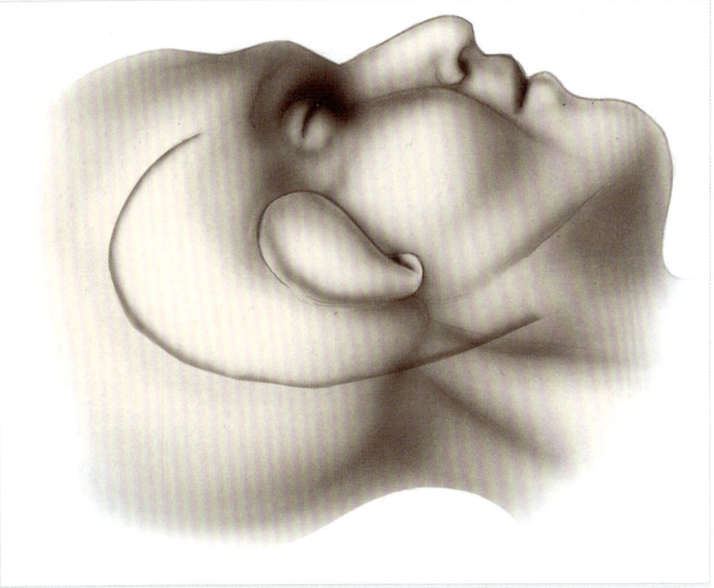

Fig. 2.205 Right side: A C-shaped incision is made from the temporalis area superiorly to the neck inferiorly.

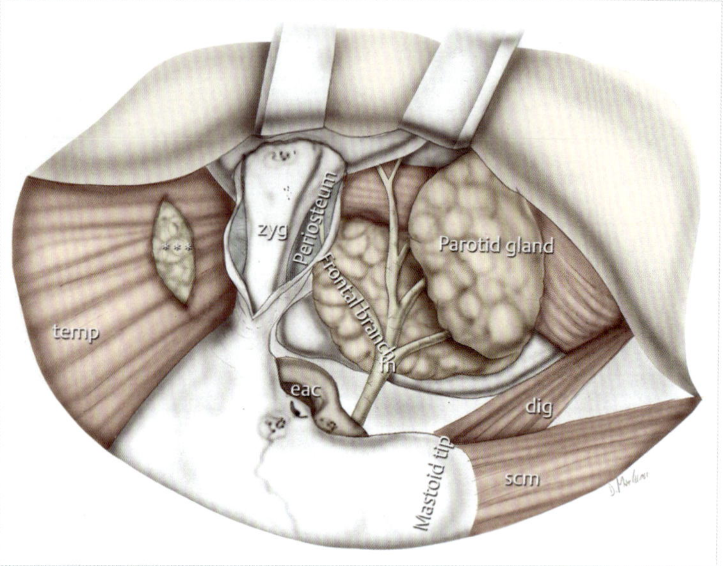

Fig. 2.206 Right side: The external auditory canal (EAC) is transected; the facial nerve is isolated from the stylomastoid foramen till the peripheral branches after superficial parotidectomy; the layers of temporalis fascia are elevated, reaching the superficial fat pad lying between the superficial and deep layers of the deep temporalis fascia and preserving the frontal branch of the facial nerve, exposing the zygomatic arch. *dig: digastric muscle; eac: external auditory canal; fn: facial nerve; scm: sternocleidomastoid muscle; temp: temporalis muscle; zyg: zygomatic arch; ***: superficial fat pad in between the superficial and deep layers of deep temporalis fascia.*

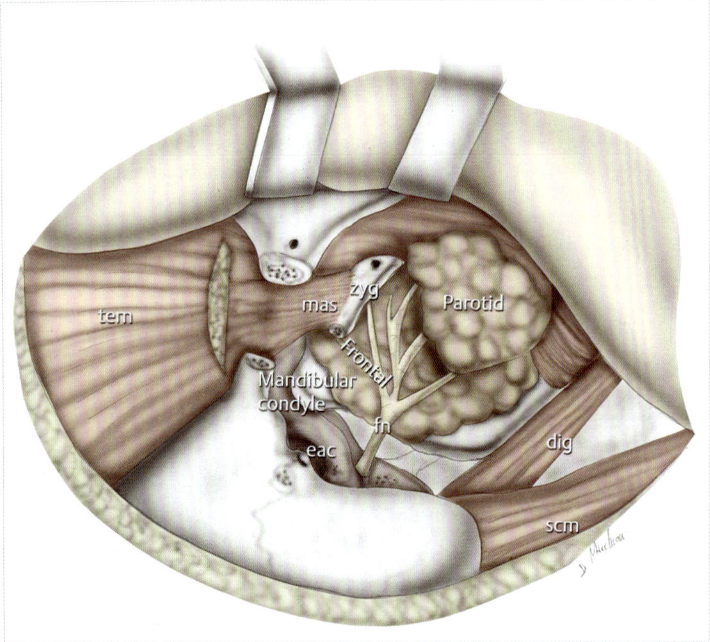

Fig. 2.207 Right side: The zygomatic arch is detached and inferiorly transposed, maintaining the muscular adhesion between the bone and the temporalis muscle. *dig: digastric muscle; eac: external auditory canal; fn: facial nerve; mass: masseter muscle; scm: sternocleidomastoid muscle; temp: temporalis muscle; zyg: zygomatic arch.*

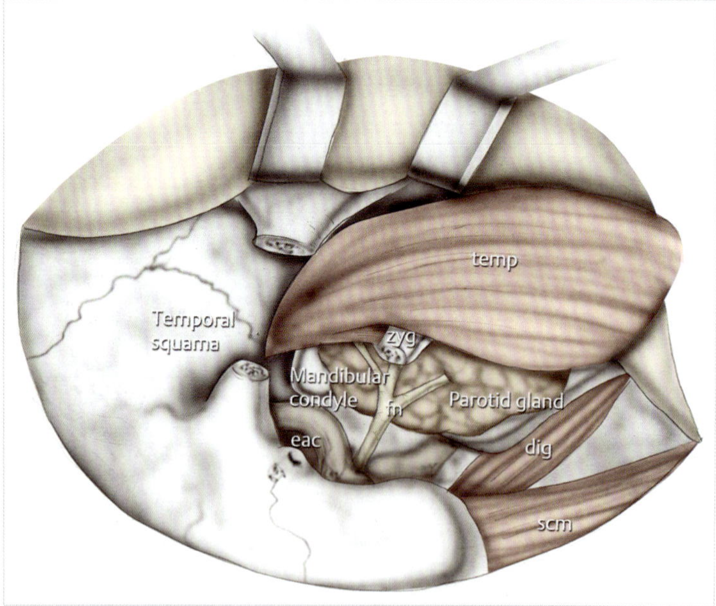

Fig. 2.208 Right side: The temporalis muscle is inferiorly transposed with the zygomatic bone, unremoved from the coronoid process. *dig: digastric muscle; eac: external auditory canal; fn: facial nerve; mass: masseter muscle; scm: sternocleidomastoid muscle; temp: temporalis muscle; zyg: zygomatic arch.*

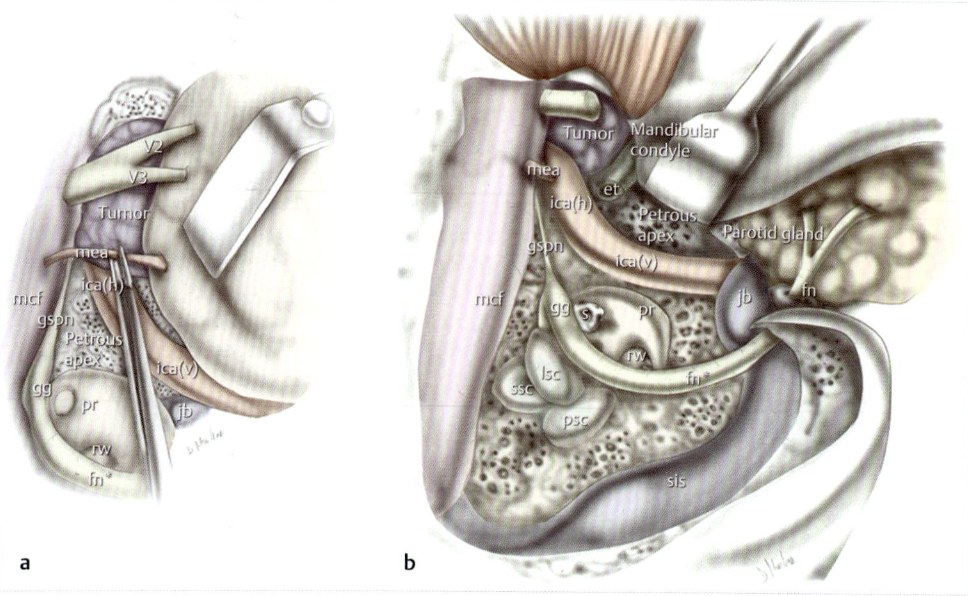

Fig. 2.209 Right side. **(a)** A subtotal petrosectomy is performed; the middle cranial fossa is anteriorly widely exposed anteriorly, uncovering the middle meningeal artery and the trigeminal nerve V3. A bipolar instrument is used to coagulate the meningeal artery. **(b)** The mandibular condyle is exposed and the vertical portion of the internal carotid artery is detected. *et: eustachian tube; fn: facial nerve; fn*: mastoid segment of facial nerve; gg: geniculate ganglion; ica(h): intrapetrous horizontal internal carotid artery; ica(v): intrapetrous vertical internal carotid artery; jb: jugular bulb; lsc: lateral semicircular canal; mcf: middle cranial fossa; mea: middle meningeal artery; pr: promontory; psc: posterior semicircular canal; rw: round window; s: stapes; sis: sigmoid sinus; ssc: superior semicircular canal.*

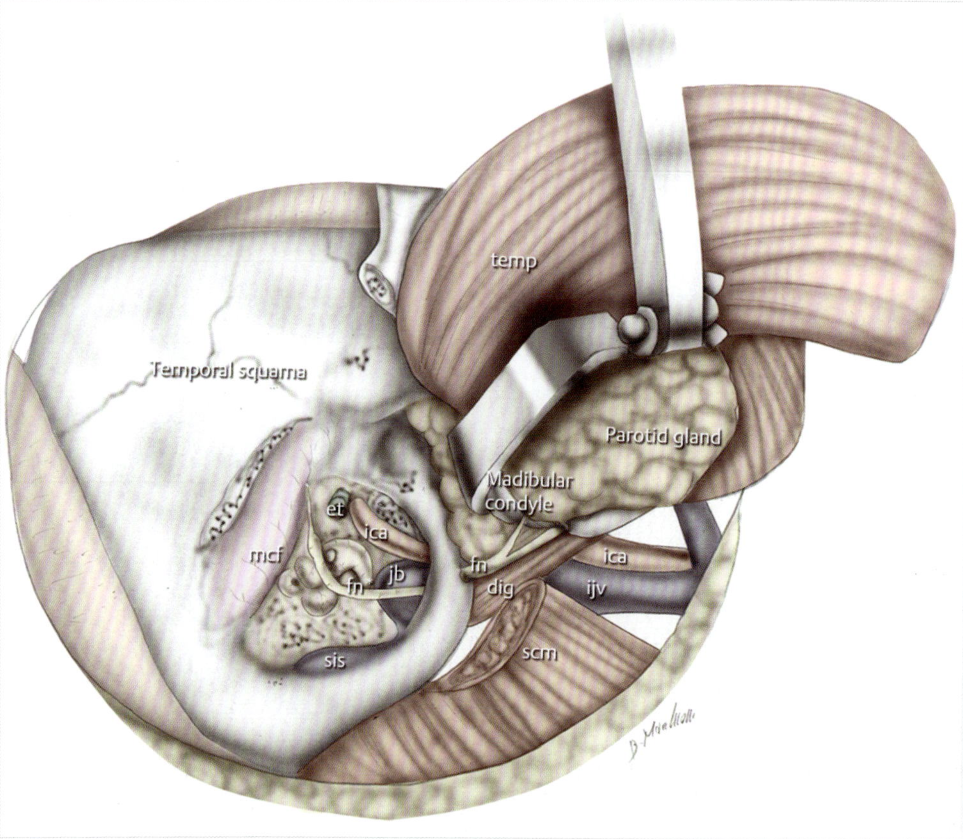

Fig. 2.210 Right side: Once the articular disc of the mandibular condyle is removed, a retractor is placed over the mandibular condyle and over the temporalis muscle to displace anteriorly the mandible, exposing the glenoid fossa and obtaining further access to the infratemporal fossa. *dig: digastric muscle; et: eustachian tube; fn: facial nerve; fn*: mastoid segment of facial nerve; ica: internal carotid artery; ijv: internal jugular vein; jb: jugular bulb; mcf: middle cranial fossa; scm: sternocleidomastoid muscle; sis: sigmoid sinus; temp: temporalis muscle.*

carotid artery, avoiding the mobilization of the artery, by working on the medial portion of the vascular structure.

In case of petrous apex cholesteatoma or epidermoid cyst involving the carotid artery and clivus, a diamond bur is used under a microscopic view to remove the remnant bone around the internal carotid artery. A cottonoid soaked with saline solution should be pulled over the artery in a gentle way to remove the matrix and diseases from the vascular structure (see ▶ Fig. 2.212b). Once the vertical and horizontal segments of the carotid artery are completely exposed and the visible matrix is removed, in order to get control of the hidden area of the clivus, a 45-degree, 15 cm length, 4 mm diameter endoscope is inserted into the surgical field, under the vertical portion of the carotid artery, looking for remnant disease. In case of preservation of the cochlea, the endoscopic procedure should be performed on the opposite side of the affected ear in order to have a view of the most anterior portion of the clivus under the anterior limit of the carotid artery (see ▶ Fig. 2.215). The surgeon must visualize the following anatomical landmarks on the monitor: the position of the vertical and horizontal internal carotid artery, the facial nerve, and the promontory (see ▶ Fig. 2.215 and Chapter 4).

In case of remnant diseases in the clivus, a large cottonoid is placed over the carotid artery to protect the vascular structure and a curve dissector is used under an endoscopic view in order to remove the residual diseases (see ▶ Fig. 2.216). During the dissection of the lesion, an angulated suction and a curve dissector

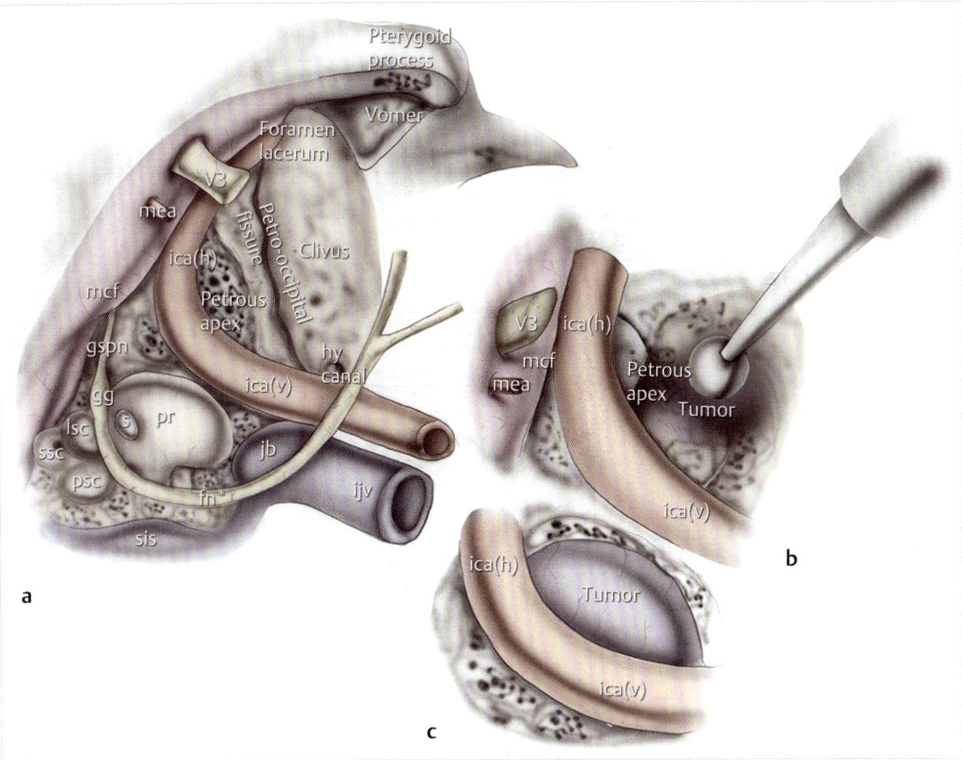

Fig. 2.211 Right side. **(a–c)** The vertical and horizontal portions of the carotid artery are further anteriorly exposed in the petrous apex and clivus with respect to the anterior foramen lacerum, exposing the tumor in the petrous apex. *fn*: mastoid segment of facial nerve; gg: geniculate ganglion; hy: hypoglossal canal; ica(h): intrapetrous horizontal internal carotid artery; ica(v): intrapetrous vertical internal carotid artery; ijv: internal jugular vein; jb: jugular bulb; lsc: lateral semicircular canal; mcf: middle cranial fossa; mea: middle meningeal artery; pr: promontory; psc: posterior semicircular canal; s: stapes; sis: sigmoid sinus; ssc: superior semicircular canal.*

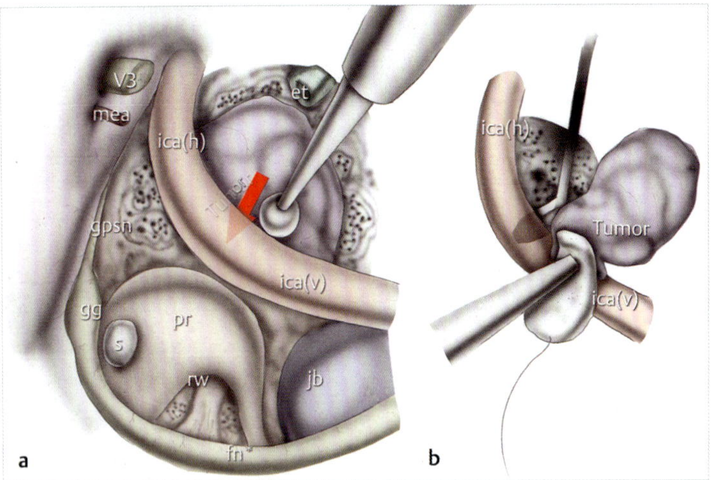

Fig. 2.212 (a, b) Right side: When the tumor is spreading in the petrous apex lying medial to the intrapetrous internal carotid artery (see the *red arrow*), a diamond bur is used around the artery to reach the lesion; a curve dissector is used to dissect the tumor; a microscopic blind dissection should be attempted since the position of the carotid artery is covering the most medial portion of the tumor. *fn*: mastoid segment of facial nerve; gg: geniculate ganglion; gspn: great superficial petrosal nerve; ica(h): intrapetrous horizontal internal carotid artery; ica(v): intrapetrous vertical internal carotid artery; jb: jugular bulb; mea: middle meningeal artery; pr: promontory; rw: round window; s: stapes.*

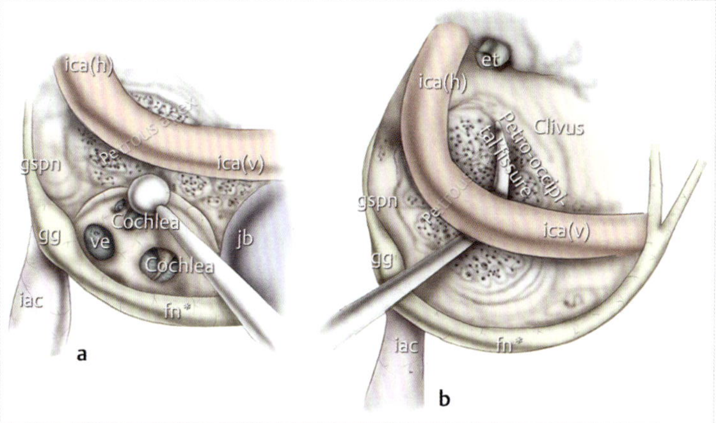

Fig. 2.213 Right side. **(a)** In case of large lesion involving the petrous apex and clivus, labyrinthectomy is performed and vestibule and cochlea are sacrificed passing under the vertical portion of the internal carotid artery reaching the clivus bone **(b)**. *et: eustachian tube; fn*: mastoid segment of facial nerve; gg: geniculate ganglion; gspn: great superficial petrosal nerve; iac: internal auditory canal; ica(h): intrapetrous horizontal internal carotid artery; ica(v): intrapetrous vertical internal carotid artery; jb: jugular bulb; ve: vestibule.*

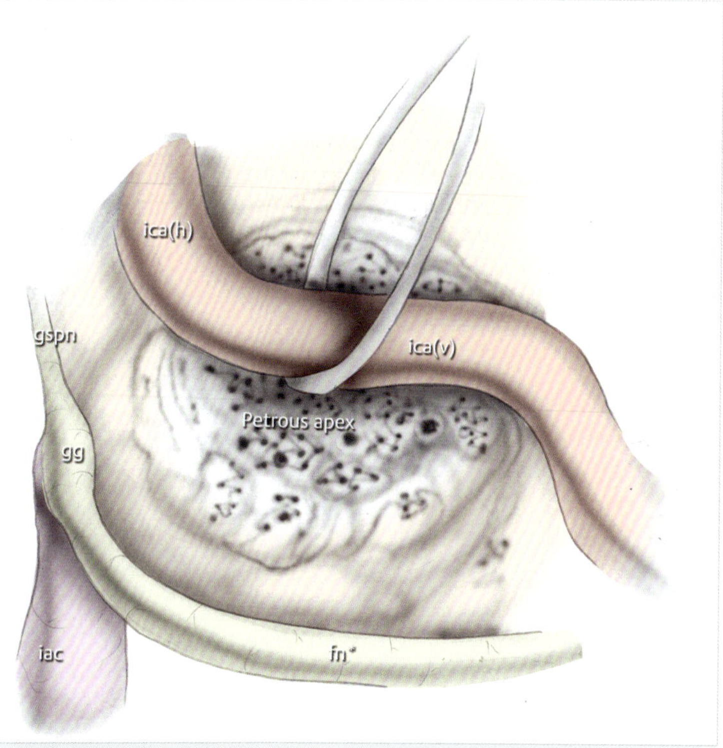

Fig. 2.214 Right side: The internal carotid artery is skeletonized. A gentle anterior displacement of the artery is produced, enabling the surgeon to acquire a microscopic view of the petrous apex. *fn*: mastoid segment of facial nerve; gg: geniculate ganglion; gspn: great superficial petrosal nerve; iac: internal auditory canal; ica(h): intrapetrous horizontal internal carotid artery; ica(v): intrapetrous vertical internal carotid artery.*

could be useful to radically remove the lesion. Once the residual lesion is removed, a diamond bur is used under endoscopic view to radically dissect the clivus bone under the internal carotid artery. A further drilling of the clivus should uncover the dura of the posterior fossa.

In case of lesions such as cholesteatoma or epidermoid cyst with adventitia involvement of the internal carotid artery, a cottonoid is used on the artery in order to microscopically remove the matrix.

Before closing, a final inspection of the cavity is then performed. An endoscopic check is recommended to avoid leaving any remnant disease in the area.

Closure

Some abdominal fat is harvested, and the mastoid cavity is filled and obliterated using the fat pad.

The fatty tissues should be placed around the carotid artery in order to protect the vascular structure. A fibrin glue is used to reinforce the obliteration.

The eustachian tube lumen is sutured and closed with Nylon 4|0 (▶ Fig. 2.217a). A muscular fragment could be used before the suture to obliterate the remnant lumen of the eustachian tube.

The temporalis muscle is inferiorly and posteriorly rotated over the SCM covering the obliterated mastoid cavity (▶ Fig. 2.217b). A meticulous suture is performed between the SCM and the temporalis muscle. The skin is closed in layers and a pressing dressing is made.

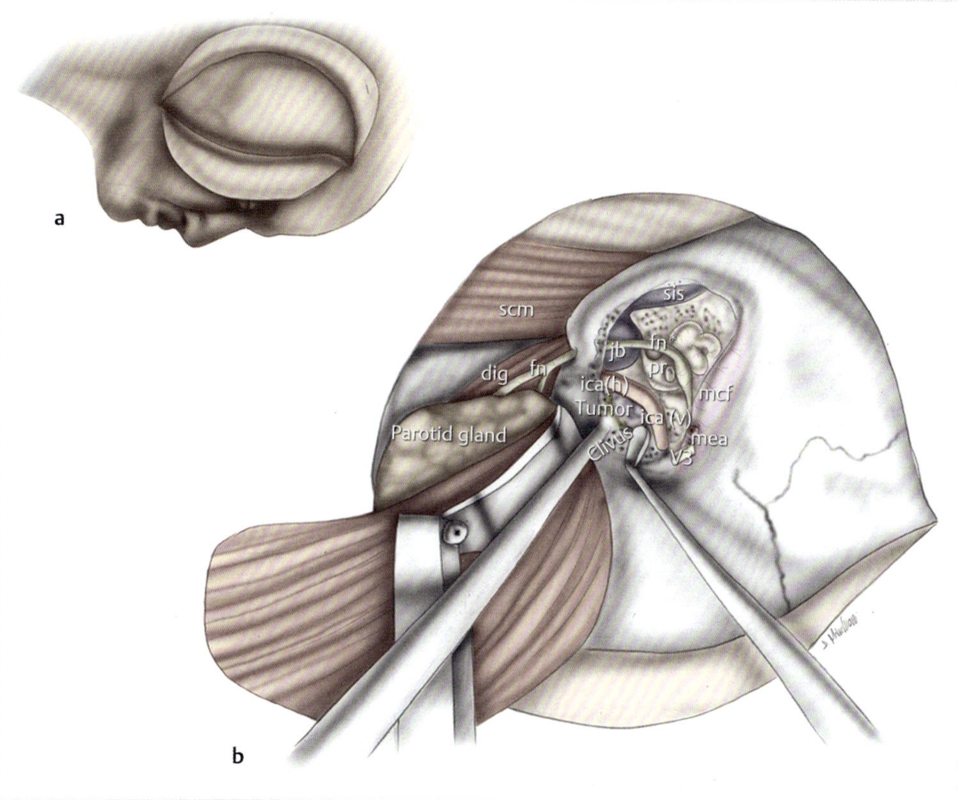

Fig. 2.215 Right side: Endoscopic-assisted surgery for petrous apex lesions. The surgeon must stand on the opposite side of the affected ear (see the surgical view of the head of the patient, **a**). The surgeon should hold an endoscope of 0–45 degrees with the left hand and a curved dissector with the right hand. The endoscope is introduced in the surgical field under the anterior portion of the vertical portion of the internal carotid artery, exposing the medial surface of the petrous apex and clivus to gain access to the whole remaining disease **(b)**. *dig: digastric muscle; fn: facial nerve; fn*: mastoid segment of facial nerve; ica(h): intrapetrous horizontal internal carotid artery; ica(v): intrapetrous vertical internal carotid artery; jb: jugular bulb; mcf: middle cranial fossa; mea: middle meningeal artery; pr: promontory; scm: sternocleidomastoid muscle.*

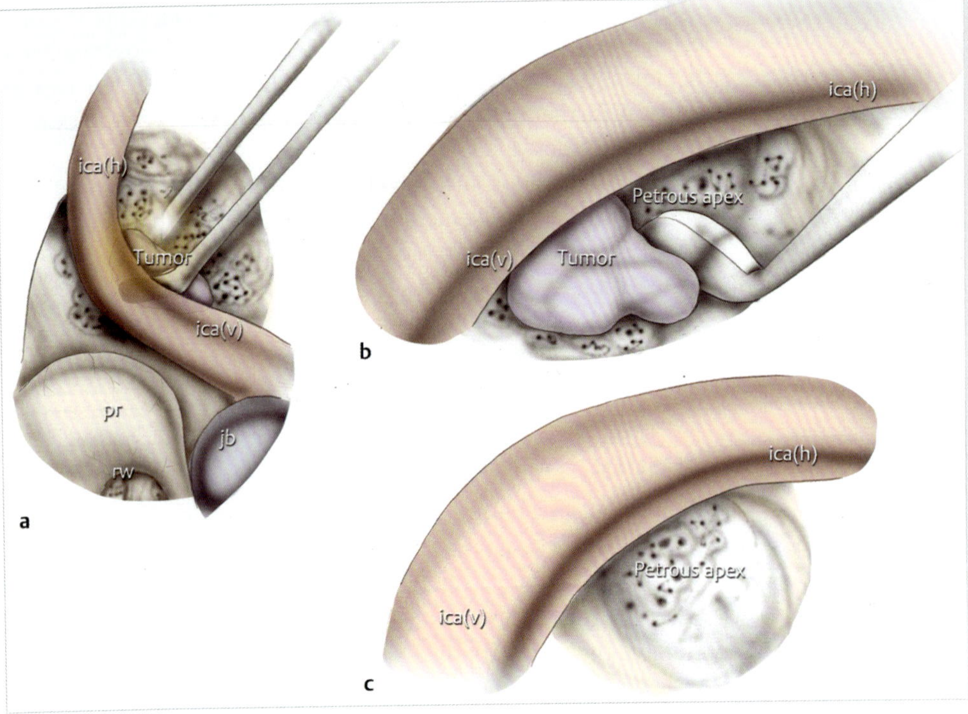

Fig. 2.216 Right side. **(a, b)** The remnant tumor is removed under endoscopic control from the medial portion of the internal carotid artery. **(c)** Clivus bone under the internal carotid artery after tumor removal. *ica(h): intrapetrous horizontal internal carotid artery; ica(v): intrapetrous vertical internal carotid artery; jb: jugular bulb; pr: promontory; rw: round window.*

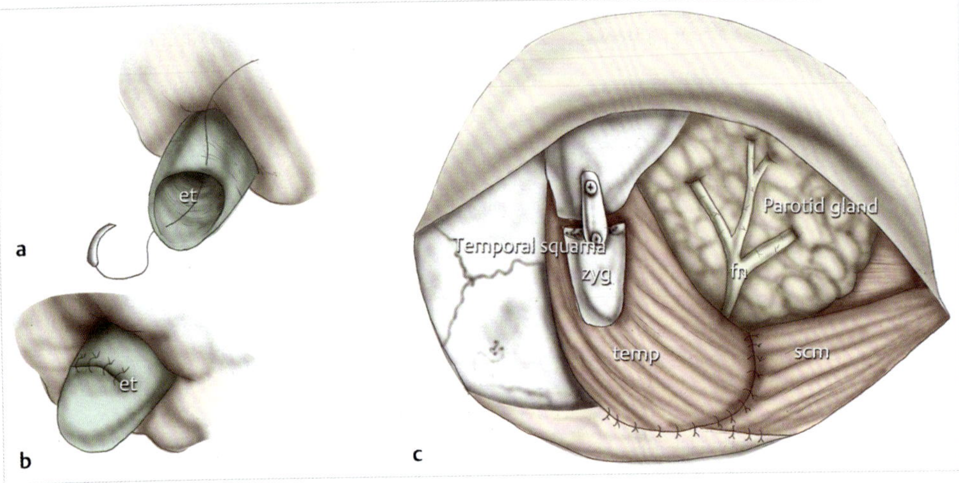

Fig. 2.217 **(a–c)** Right side: The membranous eustachian tube is closed through a Vicryl suture, avoiding contamination of the surgical cavity from rhinopharynx. The cavity is obliterated with abdominal fat. The temporalis muscle is inferiorly rotated, covering the fat, and sutured to the sternocleidomastoid muscle. The zygomatic arch is replaced. *et: eustachian tube; scm: sternocleidomastoid muscle; temp: temporalis muscle; zyg: zygomatic arch.*

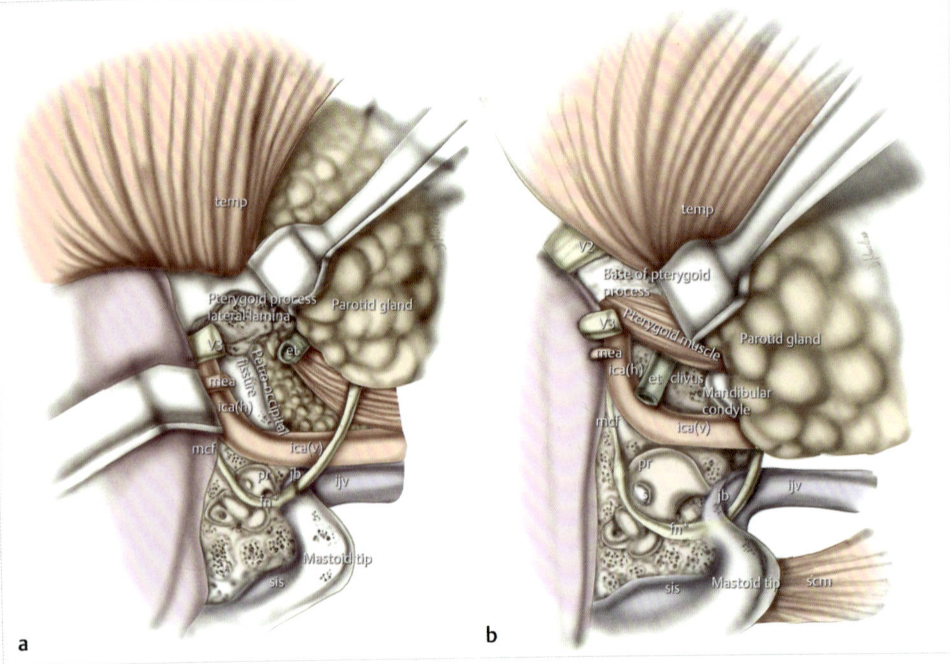

Fig. 2.218 Right side: Type C infratemporal fossa approach. As in the Type B approach, the bone at the base of the middle cranial fossa is removed over the dura. The foramen spinosum with the middle meningeal artery and the foramen ovale with the V3 are exposed. These vascular and nervous structures are cut. The internal carotid artery is exposed until the anterior foramen lacerum. The pterygoid process is exposed and drilled **(a)**, until the exposition of the pterygoid muscles and the lateral wall of the right nasal cavity **(b)**. *et: eustachian tube; fn*: mastoid segment of facial nerve; ica(h): intrapetrous horizontal internal carotid artery; ica(v): intrapetrous vertical internal carotid artery; jb: jugular bulb; mcf: middle cranial fossa; mea: middle meningeal artery; pr: promontory; scm: sternocleidomastoid muscle; sis: sigmoid sinus.*

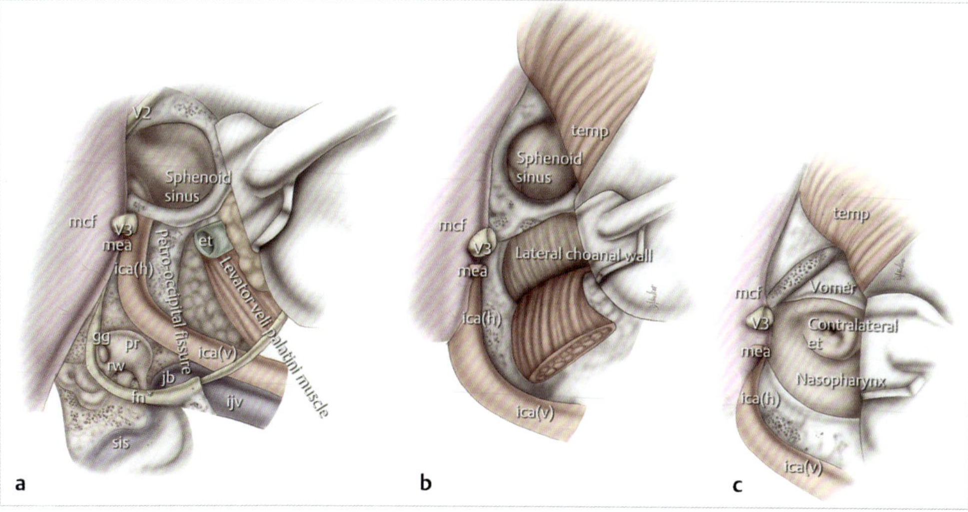

Fig. 2.219 Right side. **(a)** The sphenoid sinus is opened through the infratemporal fossa Type C approach. **(b)** The lateral wall of the right nasal cavity is exposed under the sphenoid sinus. **(c)** The incision is extended along the superior and posterior nasopharyngeal walls. The vomer and the contralateral eustachian tube orifice are identified. *fn*: mastoid segment of facial nerve; gg: geniculate ganglion; ica(h): intrapetrous horizontal internal carotid artery; ica(v): intrapetrous vertical internal carotid artery; jb: jugular bulb; mcf: middle cranial fossa; mea: middle meningeal artery; pr: promontory; rw: round window; sis: sigmoid sinus; temp: temporalis muscle.*

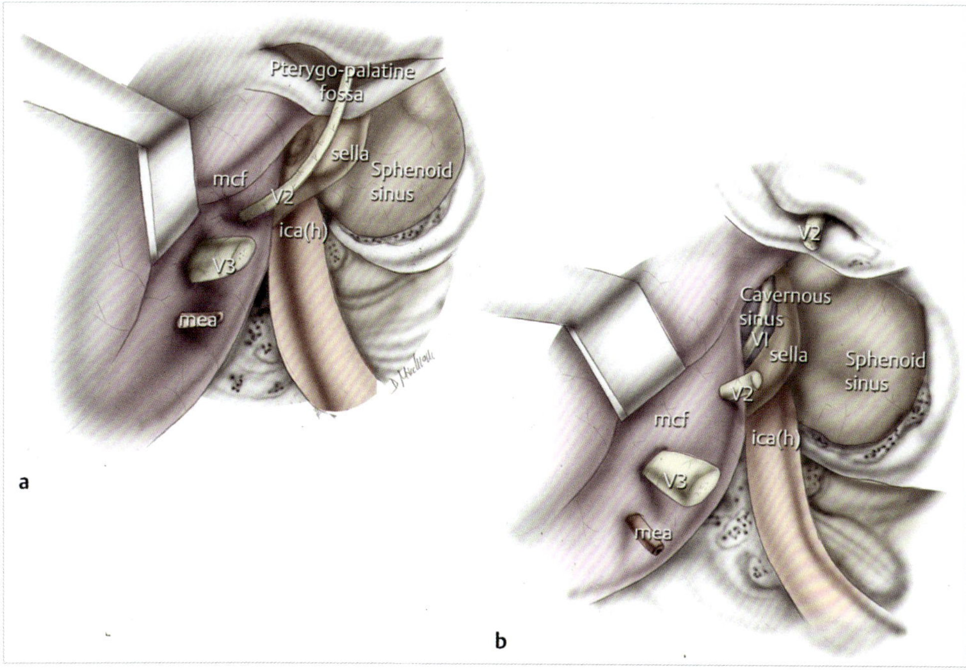

Fig. 2.220 Right side. **(a)** Once the section of middle meningeal artery and V3 is performed, the temporal lobe is elevated to gain access at the level of parasellar and cavernous sinus region; V2 is exposed. **(b)** To expose the cavernous sinus, V2 is cut leading to the exposition of the six cranial nerve running along the lateral wall of the cavernous sinus. *ica(h): intrapetrous horizontal internal carotid artery; mcf: middle cranial fossa; mea: middle meningeal artery.*

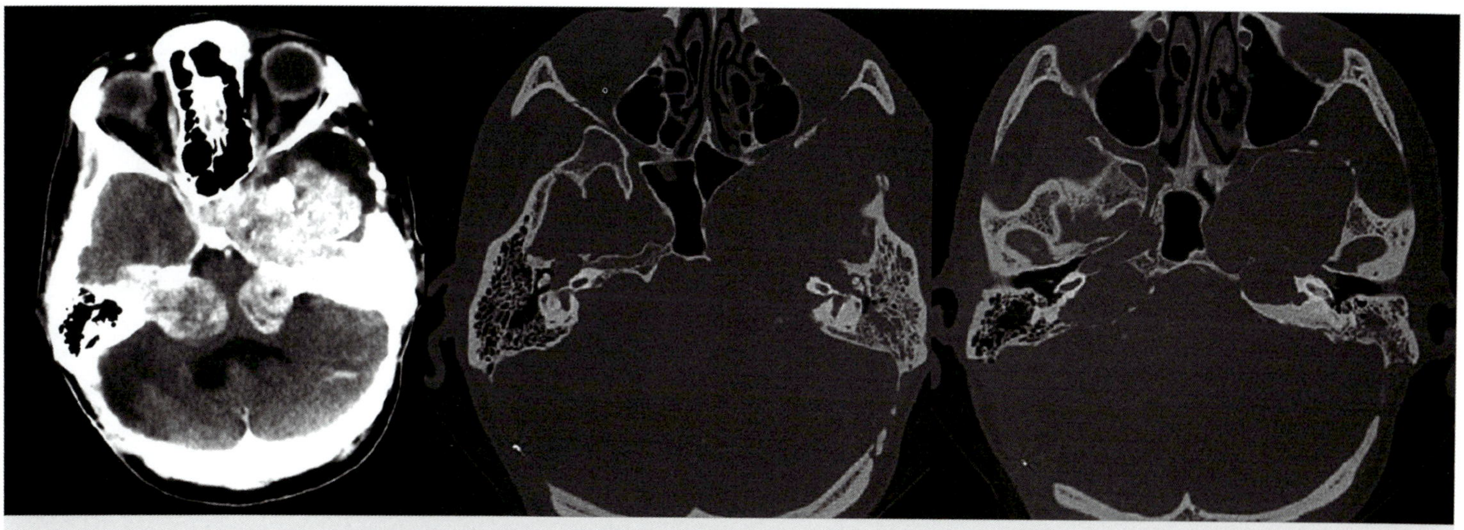

Fig. 2.221 Clinical Case 14: Computed tomography (CT) scan in axial view. Type 2 neurofibromatosis (NF2) disease: Multiple tumors invading the petrous apex, the infratemporal fossa, and the posterior fossa are visible.

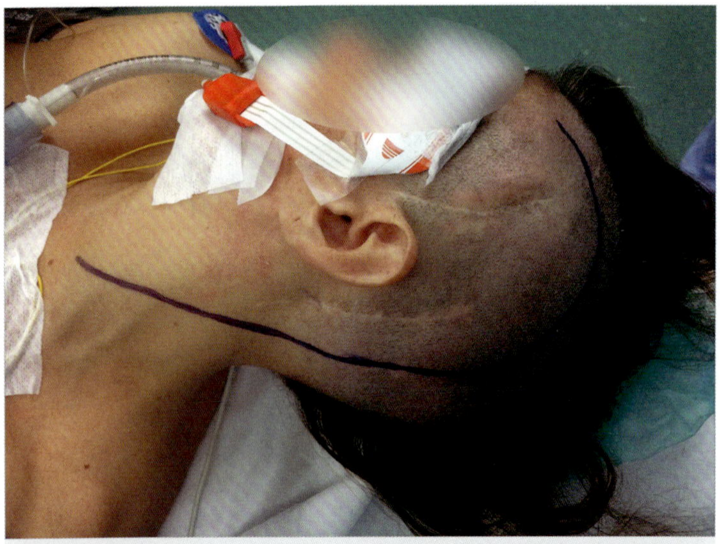

Fig. 2.222 Clinical Case 14, Left side: Infratemporal fossa Type B. The line of incision can seen.

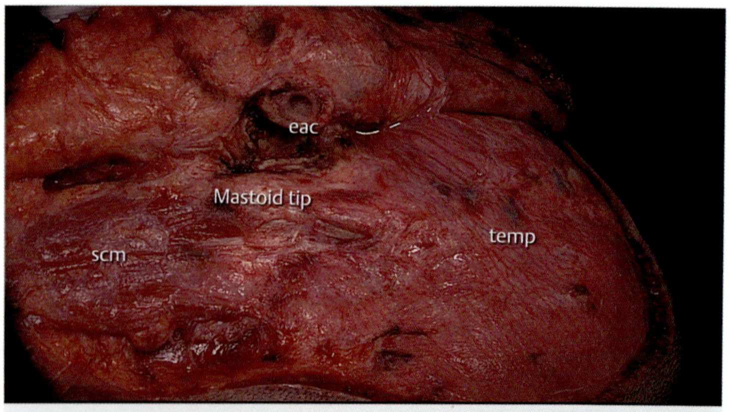

Fig. 2.223 Clinical Case 14, Left side: The skin flap is elevated and the external auditory canal (EAC) transected. *eac: external auditory canal; scm: sternocleidomastoid muscle; temp: temporalis muscle.*

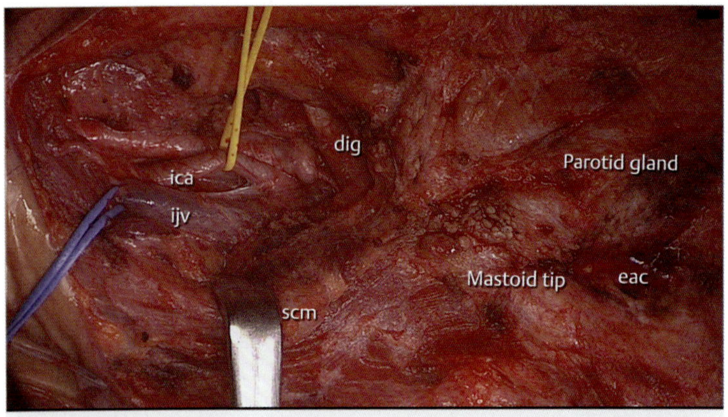

Fig. 2.224 Clinical Case 14, Left side: The major vascular structures are isolated at the base of the skull. *dig: digastric muscle; eac: external auditory canal; ica: internal carotid artery; ijv: internal jugular vein; scm: sternocleidomastoid muscle.*

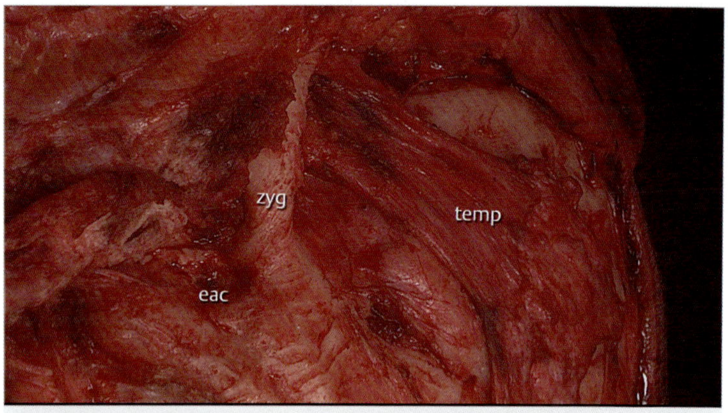

Fig. 2.225 Clinical Case 14, Left side: The zygomatic arch is isolated. *eac: external auditory canal; temp: temporalis muscle; zyg: zygomatic arch.*

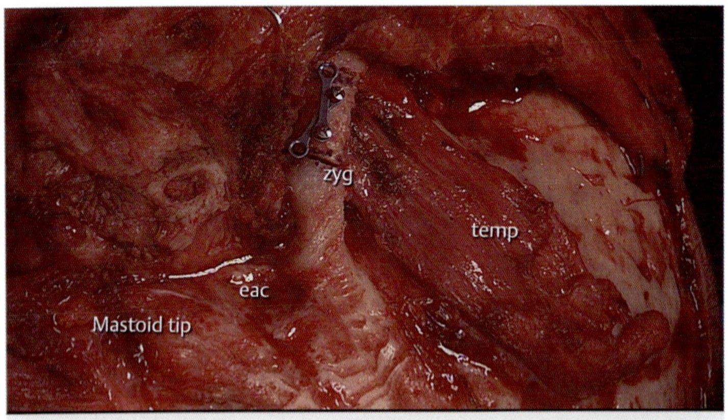

Fig. 2.226 Clinical Case 14, Left side: An osteotomy of the zygomatic arch is performed. *eac: external auditory canal; temp: temporalis muscle; zyg: zygomatic arch.*

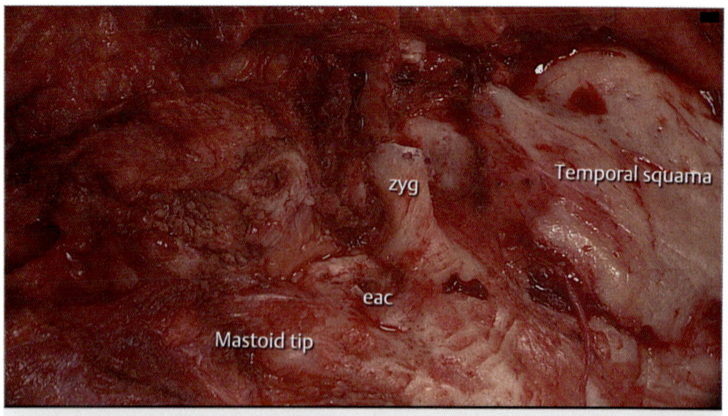

Fig. 2.227 Clinical Case 14, Left side: The temporalis muscle and the zygomatic arch are inferiorly and anteriorly transposed, uncovering the temporalis squama. *eac: external auditory canal; zyg: zygomatic arch.*

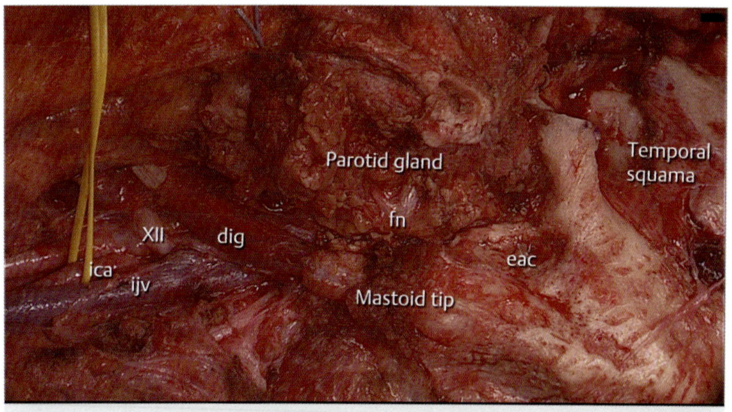

Fig. 2.228 Clinical Case 14, Left side: The facial nerve is detected at the level of the stylomastoid foramen. *dig: digastric muscle; eac: external auditory canal; fn: facial nerve; ica: internal carotid artery; ijv: internal jugular vein.*

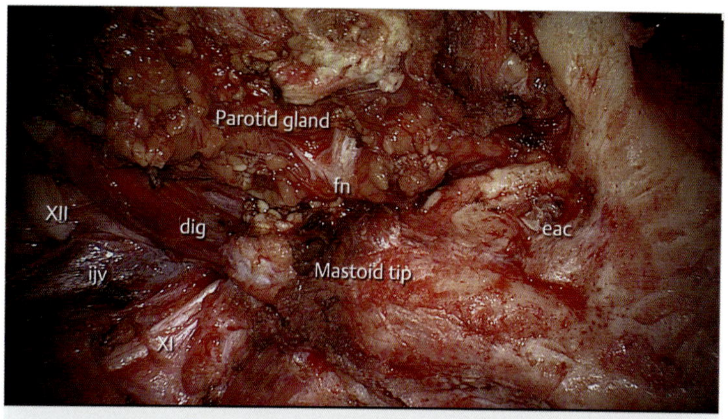

Fig. 2.229 Clinical Case 14, Left side: The external auditory canal (EAC) skin is removed, the occipitomastoid bone is uncovered, and the sternocleidomastoid muscle is detached from the mastoid bone. *dig: digastric muscle; eac: external auditory canal; fn: facial nerve; ijv: internal jugular vein.*

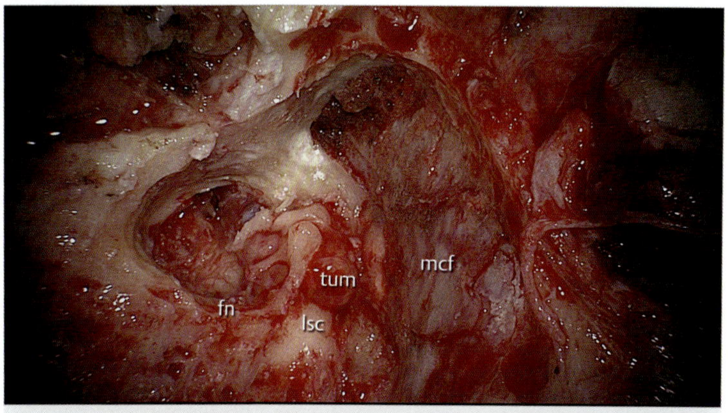

Fig. 2.230 Clinical Case 14, Left side: A subtotal petrosectomy is performed; a facial nerve tumor is seen under the ossicular chain. *fn: facial nerve; lsc: lateral semicircular canal; mcf: middle cranial fossa; tum: tumor.*

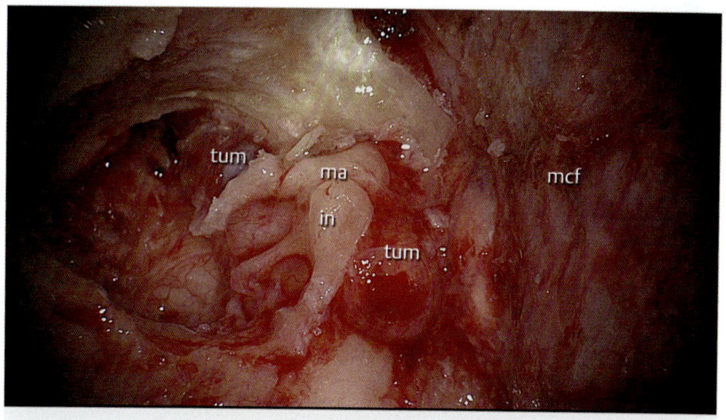

Fig. 2.231 Clinical Case 14, Left side: Microscopic magnification of the facial nerve tumor under the ossicular chain. *in: incus; ma: malleus; mcf: middle cranial fossa; tum: tumor.*

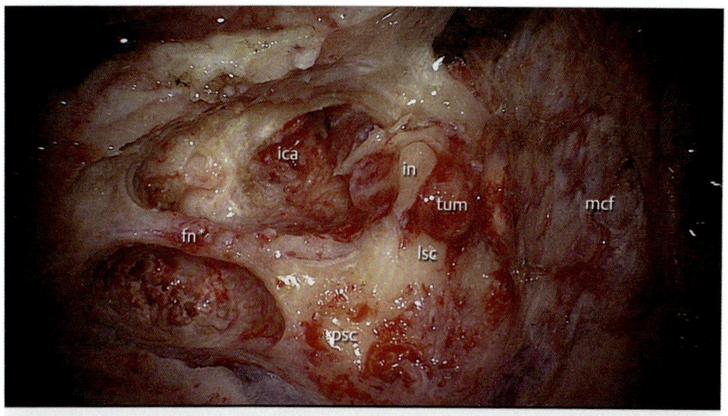

Fig. 2.232 Clinical Case 14, Left side: The mastoid segment of the facial nerve is skeletonized and the vertical portion of the carotid artery is detected. *fn*: mastoid segment of the facial nerve; ica: internal carotid artery; in: incus; lsc: lateral semicircular canal; mcf: middle cranial fossa; psc: posterior semicircular canal.*

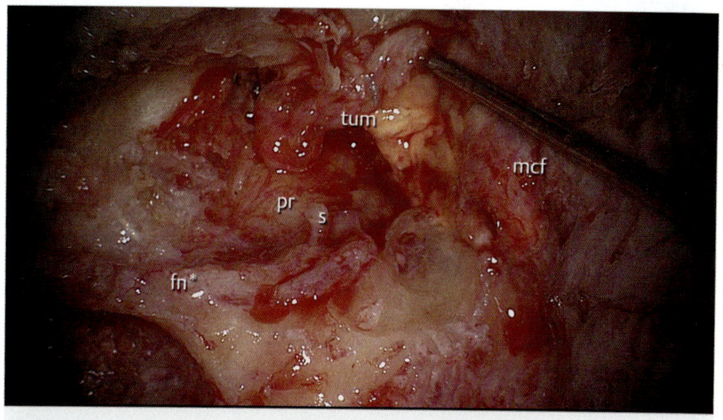

Fig. 2.233 Clinical Case 14, Left side: The facial nerve is cut and the dissection of the tumor is started from the tympanic segment of the facial nerve to the middle cranial fossa. *fn*: mastoid segment of the facial nerve; mcf: middle cranial fossa; pr: promontory; s: stapes; tum: tumor.*

Type C Infratemporal Fossa Approach

This approach is an anterior extension of the Type B approach; the pterygoid plate is exposed, drilled, and removed. The base of the pterygoid and the connected muscles are exposed (see ▶ Fig. 2.218).

The sphenoid sinus is exposed lying superomedial to the base of pterygoid, and the rhinopharynx are exposed through this approach (see ▶ Fig. 2.219).

In case of tumors with cavernous sinus involvement, further anterior drilling of the middle cranial fossa over the sphenoid sinus allows the surgeon to isolate the sella and the V2. The V2 is cut and the cavernous sinus is exposed with the VI cranial nerve (see ▶ Fig. 2.220).

Endoscopic Support

Endoscopic support is also suggested for Type C with the same indications as for Type B approach.

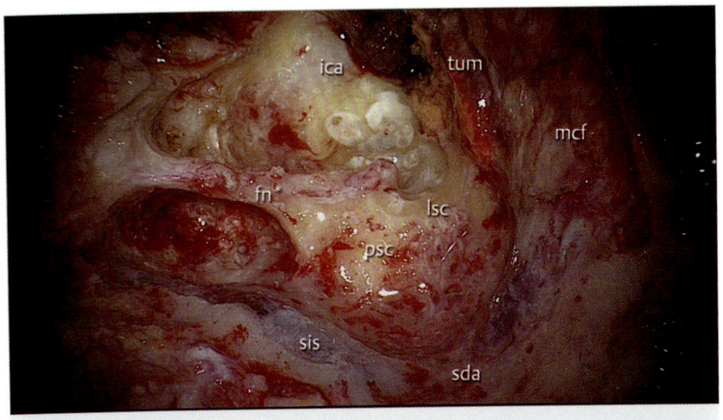

Fig. 2.234 Clinical Case 14, Left side: Microscopic view of the mastoid segment of the facial nerve after the section of this nerve. The middle fossa is progressively exposed uncovering the tumor. *fn*: mastoid segment of the facial nerve; ica: internal carotid artery; lsc: lateral semicircular canal; mcf: middle cranial fossa; psc: posterior semicircular canal; sda: sinodural angle; sis: sigmoid sinus; tum: tumor.*

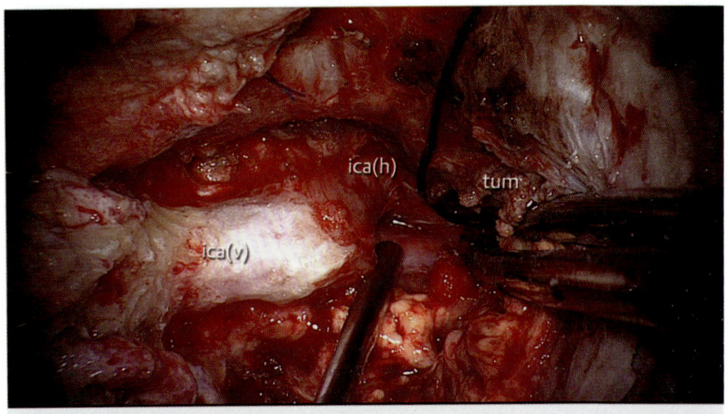

Fig. 2.235 Clinical Case 14, Left side: A Type B infratemporal fossa approach is performed. Once the middle meningeal artery is coagulated and V3 is cut, the tumor is progressively removed from the vertical and horizontal portions of the internal carotid artery. *ica(h): intrapetrous horizontal internal carotid artery; ica(v): intrapetrous vertical internal carotid artery; tum: tumor.*

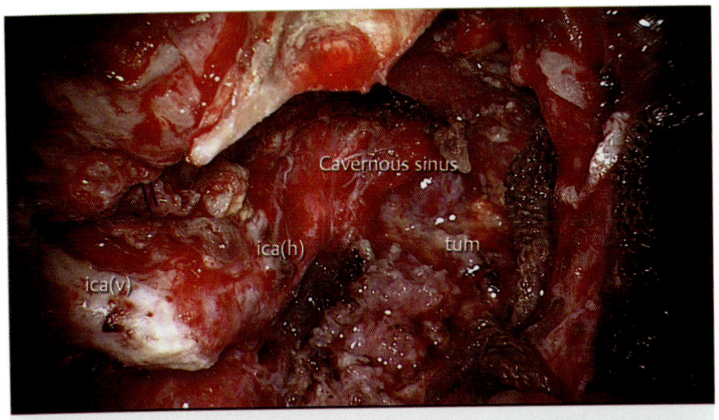

Fig. 2.236 Clinical Case 14, Left side: The carotid artery is exposed till the anterior foramen lacerum; the cavernous sinus is detected and the tumor is progressively removed. *ica(h): intrapetrous horizontal internal carotid artery; ica(v): intrapetrous vertical internal carotid artery; tum: tumor.*

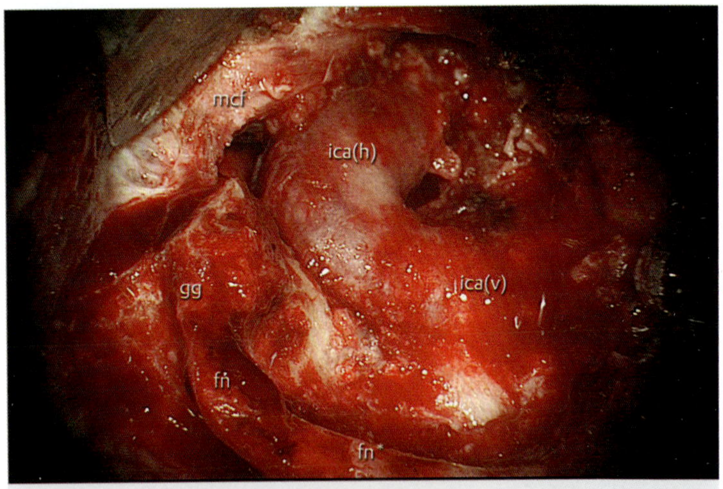

Fig. 2.237 Clinical Case 15, Right side: Clinical case of Type B infratemporal fossa approach. The tumor is removed; the vertical and horizontal portions of the carotid artery can be noticed in the final cavity. *fn: facial nerve; fn*: mastoid portion of facial nerve; gg: geniculate ganglion; ica(h): intrapetrous horizontal internal carotid artery; ica(v): intrapetrous vertical internal carotid artery; mcf: middle cranial fossa.*

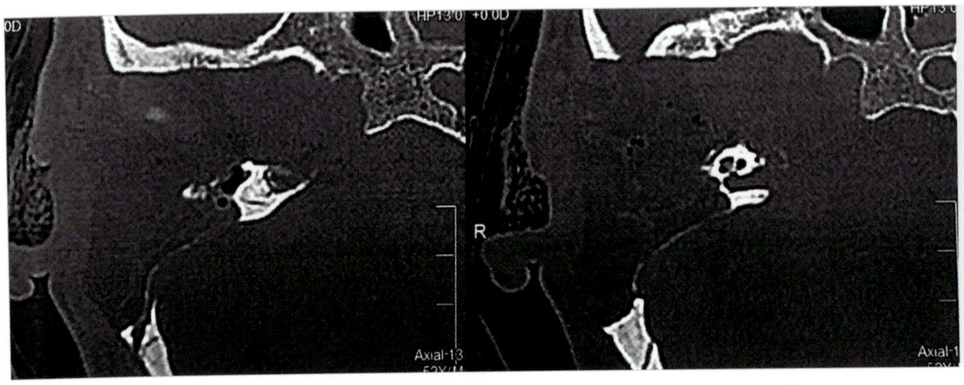

Fig. 2.238 Clinical Case 15: Computed tomography (CT) scan in axial view. Postoperative result after Type B infratemporal fossa approach. The surgical route is noted.

Suggested Readings

Angeli SI, De la Cruz A, Hitselberger W. The transcochlear approach revisited. Otol Neurotol. 2001; 22(5):690–695

Arriaga MA, Lin J. Translabyrinthine approach: indications, techniques, and results. Otolaryngol Clin North Am. 2012; 45(2):399–415, ix

Atlas MD, Moffat DA, Hardy DG. Petrous apex cholesteatoma: diagnostic and treatment dilemmas. Laryngoscope. 1992; 102(12 Pt 1):1363–1368

Browne JD, Fisch U. Transotic approach to the cerebellopontine angle. Otolaryngol Clin North Am. 1992; 25(2):331–346

Chamoun R, MacDonald J, Shelton C, Couldwell WT. Surgical approaches for resection of vestibular schwannomas: translabyrinthine, retrosigmoid, and middle fossa approaches. Neurosurg Focus. 2012; 33(3):E9

Chanda A, Nanda A. Retrosigmoid intradural suprameatal approach: advantages and disadvantages from an anatomical perspective. Neurosurgery. 2006; 59(1) Suppl 1:ONS1–ONS6, discussion ONS1–ONS6

Chen JM, Fisch U. The transotic approach in acoustic neuroma surgery. J Otolaryngol. 1993; 22(5):331–336

Chole RA. Petrous apicitis: surgical anatomy. Ann Otol Rhinol Laryngol. 1985; 94 (3):251–257

Elhammady MS, Telischi FF, Morcos JJ. Retrosigmoid approach: indications, techniques, and results. Otolaryngol Clin North Am. 2012; 45(2):375–397, ix

Fisch U, Fagan P, Valavanis A. The infratemporal fossa approach for the lateral skull base. Otolaryngol Clin North Am. 1984; 17(3):513–552

Fisch U. Infratemporal approach for extensive tumors of the temporal bone and base of skull. In: Siverstein H, Norrel H, eds. Neurological Surgery of the Ear, Vol II. Birmingham: Aesculapius; 1977:34–53

Fisch U, Mattox D. Microsurgery of the Skull Base. Stuttgart: Georg Thieme Verlag; 1988

Fisch U, Pillsbury HC. Infratemporal fossa approach to lesions in the temporal bone and base of the skull. Arch Otolaryngol. 1979; 105(2):99–107

Fisch U. Transtemporal surgery of the internal auditory canal. Report of 92 cases, technique, indications and results. Adv Otorhinolaryngol. 1970; 17:203–240

Gantz BJ, Fisch U. Modified transotic approach to the cerebellopontile angle. Arch Otolaryngol. 1983; 109(4):252–256

Haberkamp TJ. Surgical anatomy of the transtemporal approaches to the petrous apex. Am J Otol. 1997; 18(4):501–506

House WF, Glasscock ME, III. Glomus tympanicum tumors. Arch Otolaryngol. 1968; 87(5):550–554

House WF, Hitselberger WE. The transcochlear approach to the skull base. Arch Otolaryngol. 1976; 102(6):334–342

Isaacson B, Kutz JW, Roland PS. Lesions of the petrous apex: diagnosis and management. Otolaryngol Clin North Am. 2007; 40(3):479–519, viii

Jackson CG. Glomus tympanicum and glomus jugulare tumors. Otolaryngol Clin North Am. 2001; 34(5):941–970, vii

Jacob CE, Rupa V. Infralabyrinthine approach to the petrous apex. Clin Anat. 2005; 18(6):423–427

Jenkins HA, Fisch U. The transotic approach to resection of difficult acoustic tumors of the cerebellopontine angle. Am J Otol. 1980; 2(2):70–76

Lanman TH, Brackmann DE, Hitselberger WE, Subin B. Report of 190 consecutive cases of large acoustic tumors (vestibular schwannoma) removed via the translabyrinthine approach. J Neurosurg. 1999; 90(4):617–623

Mamikoglu B, Wiet RJ, Esquivel CR. Translabyrinthine approach for the management of large and giant vestibular schwannomas. Otol Neurotol. 2002; 23(2):224–227

Martin C, Prades JM. Removal of selected infralabyrinthine lesions without facial nerve mobilization. Skull Base Surg. 1992; 2(4):220–226

Royer MC, Pensak ML. Cholesterol granulomas. Curr Opin Otolaryngol Head Neck Surg. 2007; 15(5):319–322

Sanna M, Bacciu A, Falcioni M, Taibah A. Surgical management of jugular foramen schwannomas with hearing and facial nerve function preservation: a series of 23 cases and review of the literature. Laryngoscope. 2006; 116(12):2191–2204

Sanna M, Zini C, Gamoletti R, et al. Petrous bone cholesteatoma. Skull Base Surg. 1993; 3(4):201–213

Telischi FF, Luntz M, Whiteman ML. Supracochlear approach to the petrous apex: case report and anatomic study. Am J Otol. 1999; 20(4):500–504

Chapter 3

Transcanal Endoscopic Dissection of Lateral Skull Base

3

3 Transcanal Endoscopic Dissection of Lateral Skull Base

Noritaka Komune

Abstract

The aim of this chapter is to showcase the endoscopic anatomy of the temporal bone, along with brief descriptions of the main endoscopic approaches to the lateral skull base, aided by surgical images. First, a general anatomical description of the temporal bone is offered, focusing on the anatomical and spatial relationships of the internal auditory canal. The description is designed in the form of an anatomical dissection, with a progressive removal of the anatomical structures providing guidance through the process. The analysis of the anatomical structure is presented from both the lateral and superior views, in order to mirror the scenarios encountered during lateral skull base surgery. Subsequently, a step-by-step endoscopic dissection of the lateral skull base is presented, with a detailed description of the anatomy of the middle ear and of the spatial relationship of the structures in relation to the facial nerve, the inner ear, the carotid artery, and the jugular vein. Further advancement of the dissection leads to the description of the endoscopic approach to the internal auditory canal and the nervous structures within. Finally, a description of the main endoscopic approaches to the lateral skull base is offered, focusing on the anatomical description and the boundaries of the used corridors.

Keywords: lateral skull base anatomy, internal auditory canal, temporal bone anatomy, tympanic cavity anatomy, petrous apex, endoscopic inner ear anatomy

3.1 Introduction

The endoscope is commonly used in endonasal anterior skull base surgery, and its application of endoscope has recently extended to lateral skull base surgery.[1,2,3,4,5,6,7] Endoscopy has already been applied to middle ear surgery, particularly for the treatment of middle ear cholesteatoma.[8,9] In 2013, Presutti et al stated that the endoscopic approach to the lateral skull base through the external auditory canal was suitable for the treatment of cochlear schwannoma.[10] Studies on the endoscopic approach to the lateral skull base have increasingly been reported and have demonstrated the importance of a transcanal access to the lateral skull base. As the microsurgical anatomy of the temporal bone is complicated, surgeons should be well trained and have a profound anatomical knowledge to successfully perform endoscopic lateral skull base surgery. In this chapter, we will report the findings of our cadaveric study of the microsurgical and endoscopic anatomy of the temporal bone focusing on the transcanal endoscopic approach to the lateral skull base.

3.2 Overview of the Temporal Bone: Microscopic Dissection from Lateral and Above

First, the anatomical structures in the temporal bone from the lateral and superior views to demonstrate the relation between the middle ear and the surrounding skull base structures are respectively shown in ▶ Fig. 3.1 and ▶ Fig. 3.2. The temporal bone is composed of five parts: the squamous, tympanic, mastoid, petrous, and styloid ones. The external auditory canal is composed of three parts of the temporal bone. The roof of the external auditory canal is formed by the squamous part. The tympanic part forms the anterior and inferior parts of the external auditory canal. The mastoid part forms the posterior wall of the external auditory canal. The removal of mastoid air cells reveals the internal structures of the temporal bone and the relation between these structures and the external auditory canal. The facial nerve descends just posteriorly to the posterior wall of the external auditory canal and reaches the neck through the stylomastoid foramen just behind the tympanic bone (▶ Fig. 3.1a). The removal of the vaginal process of the tympanic bone and the lateral wall of the jugular bulb exposes the jugular bulb, the internal jugular vein, and the internal carotid artery (▶ Fig. 3.1b, c). The resection of the posterior half of the external auditory canal and the tympanic membrane reveals the middle ear cavity and the relation between this cavity and the jugular bulb (▶ Fig. 3.1c). The chorda tympani nerve branches off from the mastoid segment of the facial nerve and passes between the malleus and the incus in the middle ear cavity (▶ Fig. 3.1c). The removal of the remaining tympanic bone, the styloid process, the tympanic membrane, the malleus and the incus, and translocating the facial nerve anteriorly reveal the relation among the middle ear, the jugular bulb, and the internal carotid artery (▶ Fig. 3.1d). The sigmoid sinus passes downward in the anteromedial direction to form the jugular bulb just inferior to the posterior semicircular canal and the round window niche. The internal carotid artery ascends from the neck inside the carotid canal and is located anteromedial to the internal jugular vein. In the temporal bone, the internal carotid artery turns anteromedially just medial to the opening of the osseous portion of the eustachian tube (▶ Fig. 3.1d). As shown in this dissection, the middle ear cavity is surrounded by six surfaces. The promontory, the round window, and the oval window form the medial wall. The upper roof is composed by the middle cranial base. The orifice of the bony eustachian tube is a part of the anterior wall of the middle ear cavity. The lateral wall is formed by the tympanic membrane. The inferior wall of the middle ear is the hypotympanum. The posterior wall is composed by the mastoid segment of the facial canal and the semicircular canals.

From the middle cranial fossa, the middle ear is surrounded by the cochlea, the internal acoustic canal, the semicircular canals, and the external auditory canal (▶ Fig. 3.2). The internal acoustic canal is located close to the axial line of the external auditory canal. The cochleariform process is located just lateral and inferior to the geniculate ganglion, which branches off the greater petrosal nerve and the tympanic segment of the facial nerve. The cochlea is positioned in the cochlear angle, between the greater petrosal nerve and labyrinthine part of the facial nerve. The semicircular canals are posteromedial to the middle ear cavity. The tensor tympani muscle partially roofs the eustachian tube. The fundus of the internal acoustic canal is located immediately inferomedial to the tympanic part of the facial nerve.

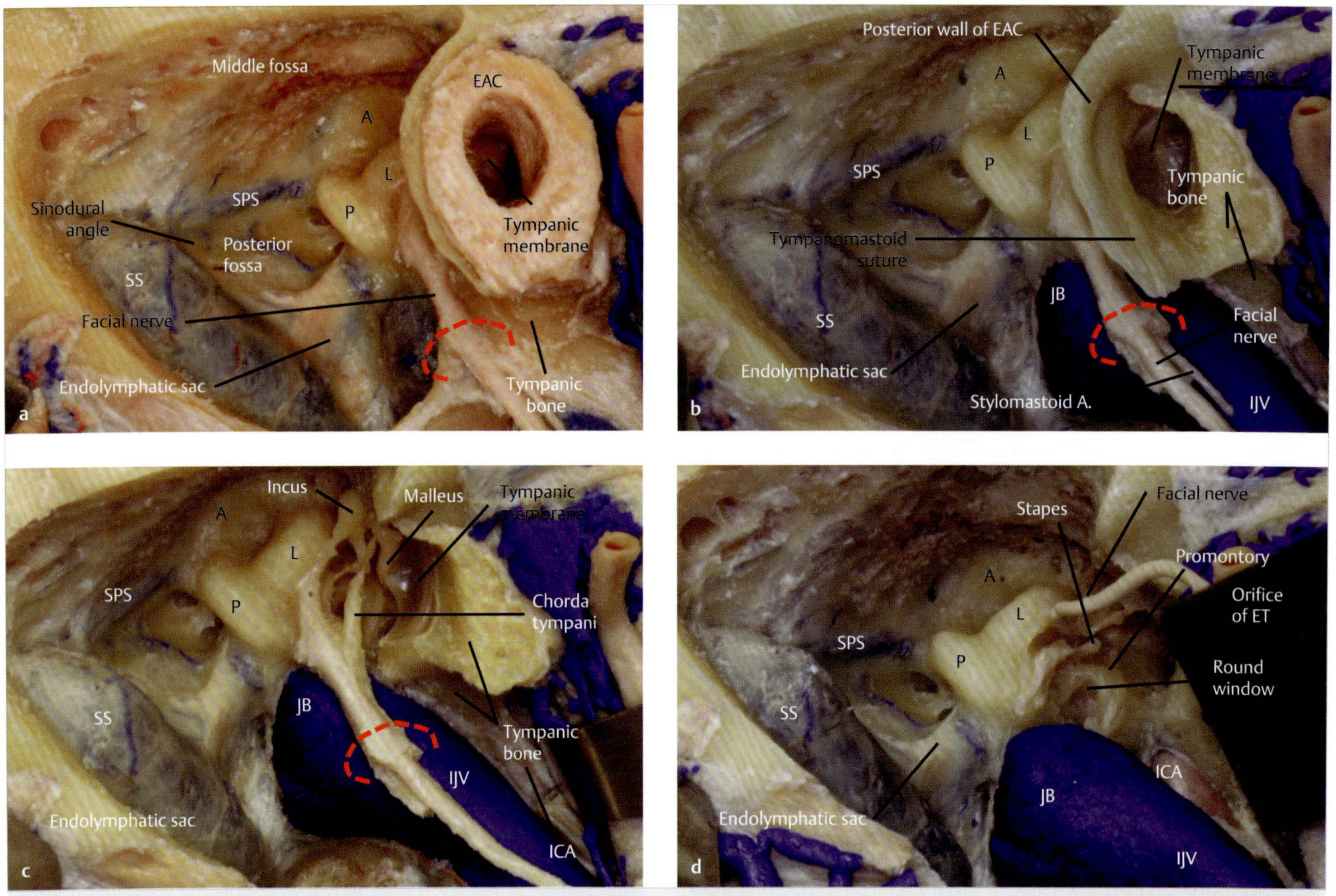

Fig. 3.1 The relation between the middle ear cavity and cranial base can be noticed (*lateral view*). **(a)** A complete mastoidectomy has been performed. The mastoid tip, the digastric muscle, and the lateral part of the vaginal process of the tympanic bone have been removed. **(b)** The lateral wall of the jugular bulb and remaining vaginal process have been removed. **(c)** The posterior wall of the external auditory canal and the posterior half of the tympanic membrane have been removed to reveal the relation of the middle ear cavity with the posterior and inferior structures. **(d)** The anterior wall and the stylomastoid process have been removed. The facial nerve has been anteriorly translocated and the incus and malleus have been removed. *A: anterior semicircular canal; A.: artery; EAC: external auditory canal; IJV: internal jugular vein; JB: jugular bulb; L: lateral semicircular canal; P: posterior semicircular canal; SPS: superior petrosal sinus; SS: sigmoid sinus; Red interrupted line indicates the stylomastoid foramen.*

3.3 Transcanal Endoscopic Dissection to the Lateral Skull Base

Presutti and Marchioni reported a unique technique termed the transcanal exclusive endoscopic technique.[8,10,11] This section describes the step-by-step dissection of a cadaver with an endoscope to access to the fundus of the internal acoustic canal through the external auditory canal and the middle ear cavity. First, the transcanal approach should be started by making a tympanomeatal flap to access the middle ear cavity (▶ Fig. 3.3a, b). The tympanic membrane is also attached to the anterior and inferior malleolar ligaments. The skin of the external auditory canal is firmly attached to the petrotympanic and tympanomastoid fissures. The tympanic part of the temporal bone is respectively articulated with the petrous and mastoid parts at the level of the petrotympanic and tympanomastoid fissures. Through the petrotympanic fissure and tympanomastoid fissure, a branch of the auriculotemporal nerve and Arnold's nerve can be identified (▶ Fig. 3.3b). After the removal of the tympanomeatal flap, the middle ear cavity is exposed. In the middle ear cavity, three small bony structures form the ossicular chain to conduct mechanical vibrations from the tympanic membrane to the inner ear. Before atticotomy, it is not possible to expose the anatomical structures. The chorda tympani passes between the long process of the incus and the handle of the malleus (▶ Fig. 3.3c, d). The removal of the tympanic membrane exposes Prussak's space, which is bounded by the flaccida part of the tympanic membrane laterally, the neck of the malleus medially, the lateral process of the malleus inferiorly, and lateral malleolar ligament superiorly (▶ Fig. 3.3d). The fibers of lateral malleolar ligament arise from the neck of malleus and insert along the rim of the notch of Rivinus. The anterior malleolar ligament delineates the anterior border of Prussak's space. In the protympanum, the opening of the bony eustachian tube is identified. The roof of this opening is composed of the semicanal of the tensor tympani muscle. This muscle posterolaterally runs along this canal to the cochleariform process. The tendon of the tensor tympani leaves the bony wall hooking around the cochleariform process to laterally insert into the medial surface of the manubrium of the malleus (▶ Fig. 3.3e). A bulging bony area can be identified on the medial wall of the opening of the bony eustachian tube. This thin bone is a part of the lateral wall of the carotid canal and it is often defective exposing the petrous carotid artery (▶ Fig. 3.3e).

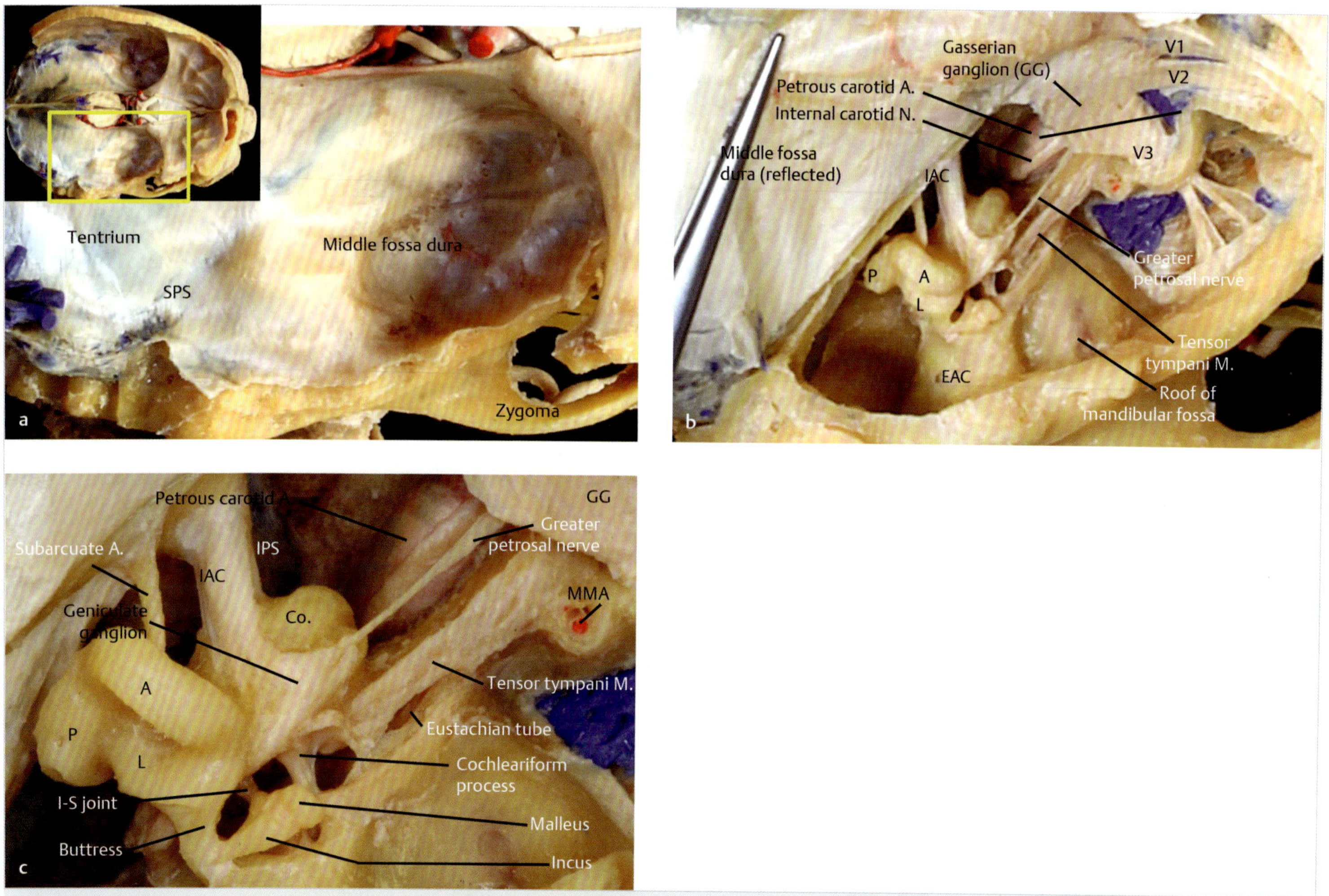

Fig. 3.2 The relation between the middle ear cavity and cranial base (superior view). **(a)** View from the middle cranial base. The yellow rectangle inside in the left on the right upper corner is magnified in **(a)**. **(b)** The middle fossa dura has been folded and the temporal bone has been drilled leaving the important structures. **(c)** The structures surrounding the middle ear have been magnified. *A: anterior semicircular canal; A.: artery; Co.: cochlea; IAC: internal acoustic canal; IPS: inferior petrosal sinus; I-S: incudostapedial; L: lateral semicircular canal; M.: muscle; MMA: middle meningeal artery; P: posterior semicircular canal; SPS: superior petrosal sinus; Yellow rectangle in the insert shows the area of view.*

The removal of the scutum exposes the contents of the attic. This space contains the head of the malleus and the body of the incus, which form an articulation called the incudomalleolar joint which is just inferior to the middle cranial base. Around the malleus, the incus, the stapes and the semicanal for the tensor tympani muscle, several membranous diaphragms can be identified in addition to a ligament attached to the ossicles (▶ Fig. 3.3e, f). After the disconnection of the tensor tympani muscle tendon, the malleus can be removed. The removal of the ossicles reveals the relation between the facial nerve (fallopian canal) and the cochleariform process. This process is inferolateral to the horizontal part of the facial nerve (▶ Fig. 3.3g). The chorda tympani nerve runs just inferior to the cochleariform process towards the petrotympanic fissure (▶ Fig. 3.3g, h). The middle ear cavity can be divided into the protympanum, epitympanum, mesotympanum, hypotympanum, and retrotympanum. On the medial surface of the middle ear cavity, several concavities and convexities can be identified. In the mesotympanum, the prominent convexity is the promontory and the prominent concavity is the round window niche. The overhang of the round window is divided into three parts forming the round window niche: the tegmen, and the anterior and posterior pillars (Fig▶ Fig. 3.3h). In particular, it is important to have a deep knowledge of the medial wall of the retrotympanum for cholesteatoma surgery.[12] The retrotympanum can be divided into the superior and inferior retrotympanum. The finiculus is a bony ridge dividing the inferior retrotympanum from the hypotympanum. The finiculus connects the anterior pillar and the floor of the hypotympanum where the jugular dome is located. The subiculum is also a bony ridge connecting the posterior pillar and the styloid complex, which derives from the superior part of the second branchial arch. The styloid complex is composed of the pyramidal, the styloid, and the chordal eminence. The ponticulus is a bony spicule that runs from the promontory to the pyramidal eminence, which projects from the posterior wall of the middle ear. The ponticulus separates the tympanic sinus from the oval window, which is located immediately inferiorly to the horizontal part of the facial nerve. The tympanic sinus is superoinferiorly inferiorly bordered by the subiculum, laterally by the pyramidal eminence and the facial nerve, and superiorly by the ponticulus. The subtympanic sinus is superoinferiorly bordered by the subiculum, the finiculus anteroinferiorly, and the styloid eminence posterolaterally (▶ Fig. 3.3g, h). On the surface of the promontory, Jacobson's nerve, which forms the tympanic plexus with the branch of the internal carotid nerve (sympathetic fiber), and a branch of the facial nerve can be identified (▶ Fig. 3.3i). This plexus gives off the lesser petrosal nerve, the deep branch to the greater petrosal nerve, and branches to the tympanic cavity.

The genu of the facial nerve passes immediately superior to the oval window, which is covered by the footplate of the stapes bone. Generally, the facial nerve runs along a bony canal called the fallopian canal. However, a bony defect in this canal close to the tympanic segment adjacent to the genu is often observed. The cochleariform process is also located superior to the promontory and just inferolateral to the geniculate ganglion. The removal of the stapes opens the vestibule, which has two distinct depressions: posterosuperiorly the elliptical recess and anteroinferiorly the spherical recess. The utricle is firmly adherent to the elliptical recess and the saccule is adherent to the spherical recess. The vestibular crest is located between the two concavities, which communicate with the vestibular aqueduct. The cochlear recess is located immediately inferior to the two depressions, which the cochlear aqueduct empties into. This recess leads to the scala vestibuli of the cochlea. The scala tympani of the cochlea is adherent to the round window and adjoining the scala vestibule at the level of the helicotrema. The superior vestibular nerve innervates the superior and lateral semicircular canals, and gives off the utricular branch. The inferior vestibular nerve gives off the saccular branch to the spherical recess. The singular nerve, which is the posterior branch of the inferior vestibular nerve, innervates the posterior semicircular canal. The spherical recess is a readily identified landmark of the internal acoustic canal opening.

Through the oval window, the spherical recess of the vestibule can be identified. The spherical recess is located in the cribrose area where the inferior vestibular nerve is attached. To reach the internal acoustic canal while avoiding damage to the facial nerve, the cribrose area of the vestibule and cochleariform process can be used as reliable landmarks. The removal of the bone forming the promontory exposes the basal turn of the cochlea. The internal cavity of the cochlea is divided into three regions: the scala vestibule above, the cochlear duct in the middle, and the scala

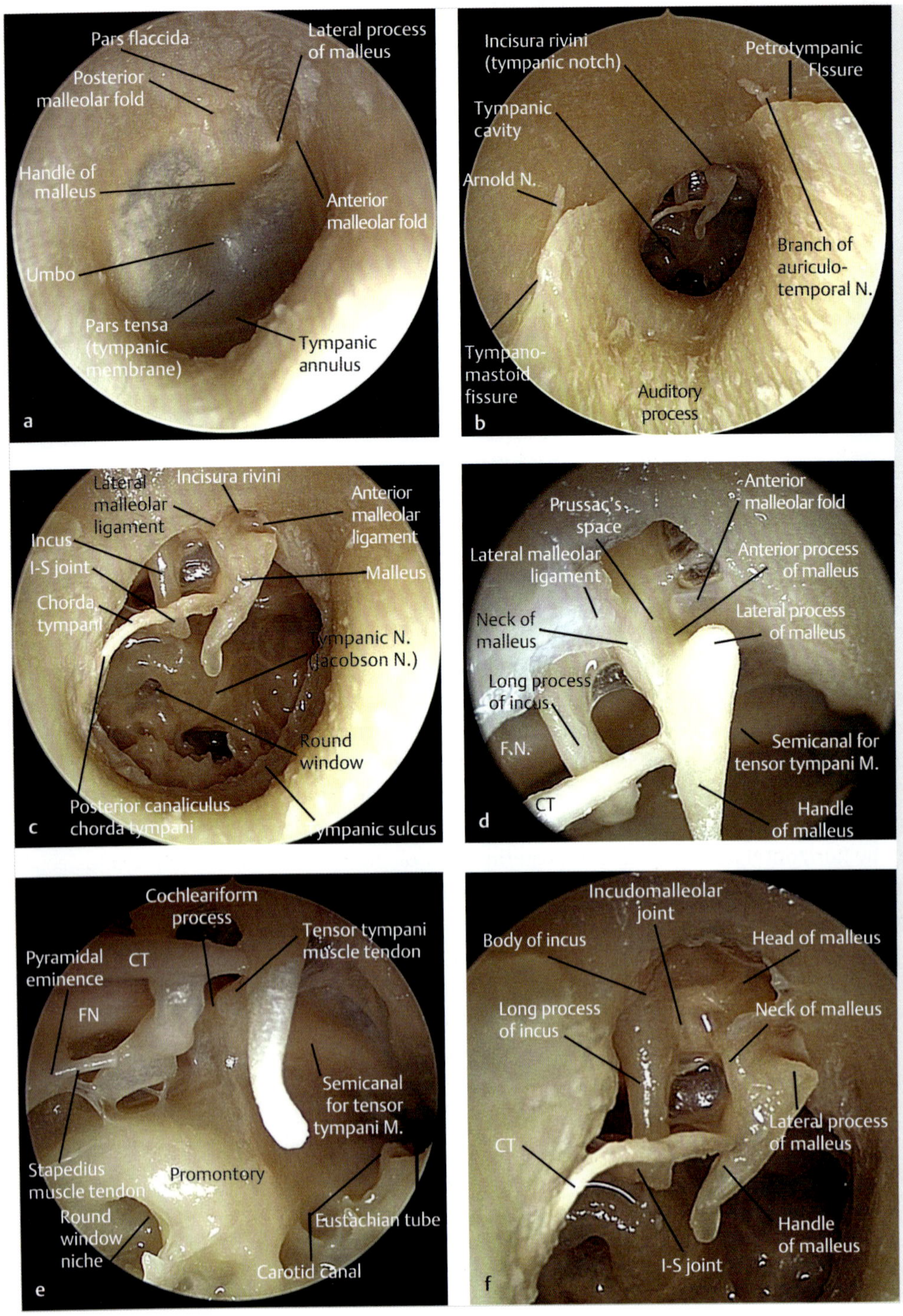

Fig. 3.3 Endoscopic surgical series using the transcanal approach to visualize the internal acoustic canal. **(a)** Normal structures of the tympanic membrane and the external auditory canal. **(b)** After the removal of the tympanomeatal flap, the middle ear cavity is exposed. **(c)** Enlarged view of **(b)**. **(d)** The structures around Prussak's space are shown. **(e)** Enlarged view of the medial wall of the middle ear cavity. **(f)** The removal of the scutum exposes the epitympanum containing the incudomalleolar joint (I-M joint).

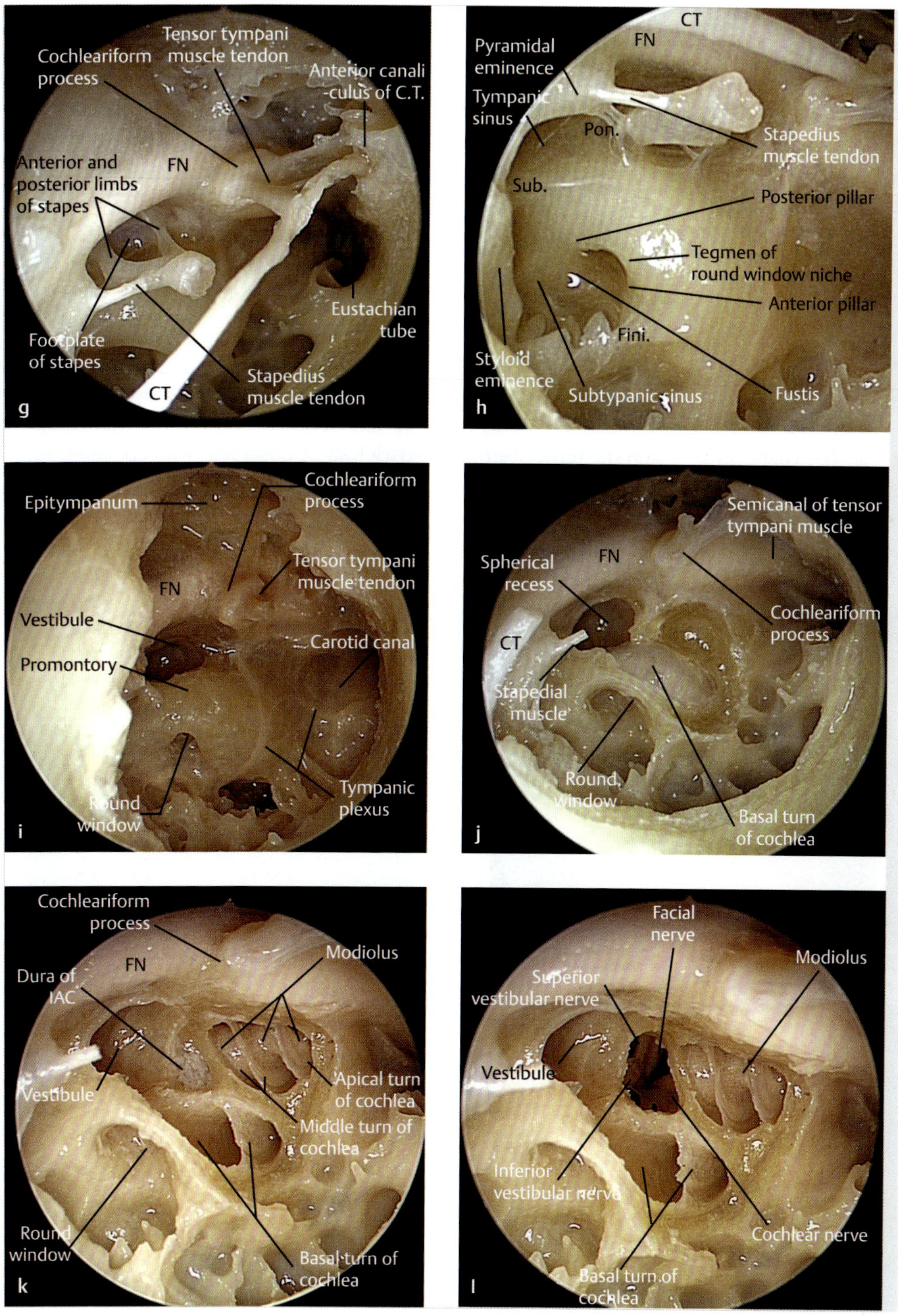

Fig. 3.3 (*Continued*) **(g)** Structures around the oval window niche. **(h)** Structures around the round window niche. **(i)** After the removal of the stapes the vestibule is opened. The triangular landmark composed of the anterior and posterior edges (pillars) and the cochleariform process has been exposed. **(j)** Enlarged view of **(i)**. The spherical recess can be observed through the oval window. The removal of the bone covering the triangular landmark exposes the membranous basal turn of the cochlea. **(k)** Extending bone removal immediately inferior to the cochleariform process allows the opening of the middle and apical turns of the cochlea. Removal of the bone more laterally through the triangular landmark exposes the dura of the internal acoustic canal. **(l)** Opening the dura of the internal acoustic canal clearly exposes cranial nerves (CN) VII and VIII. *C.T.: chorda tympani; F.N.: facial nerve; Fini.: finiculus; I-S: incudostapedial; N.: nerve; M.: muscle; I-M: incudomalleolar joint; Pon.: ponticulus; Sub.: subiculum.*

vestibule below (▶ Fig. 3.3j, k). The scala tympani and vestibule are connected by a small hole, which is called the helicotrema, at the top of the cochlea. Bone drilling immediately inferior to the cochleariform process grants access to the middle and apical turn of the cochlea (▶ Fig. 3.3j). The modiolus of the cochlea is conical and the central axis contains the spiral ganglia which connect to the cochlear nerve (▶ Fig. 3.3k). The modiolus is one of the landmarks of the internal acoustic canal opening. Drilling the bone between the spherical recess of the vestibule and the middle turn of the cochlea exposes the dura of the internal acoustic canal (▶ Fig. 3.3k). Opening the dura exposes the cranial nerves running through the internal acoustic canal: the facial, cochlear, superior and inferior vestibular nerves (▶ Fig. 3.3l).

The triangular area examined in the present study is formed by three points: (1) the cochleariform process; (2) posterior pillar; and (3) anterior pillar, with a mean area of 6.40 ± 2.44 mm^2 (mean ± SD). This shape is almost a complete isosceles triangle.[13] Each side of the triangle is a landmark for the anatomical structures behind the medial wall of the middle ear, with the anterior side corresponding to the cochlea. The internal acoustic canal can be reached by following the modiolus of the cochlea; the posterior side corresponds to the vestibule and genu of the facial nerve, and the top of the triangle, the cochleariform process, is immediately inferolateral to the tympanic segment of the facial nerve. The top of the jugular bulb is inferior to the base of this triangle.

3.4 Endoscopic Approaches to the Lateral Skull Base

The endoscopic assisted approach has become widely accepted. Several microsurgical views using the endoscopic assisted approach during a cadaveric dissection will be shown. The classical microscopic mastoidectomy can expose the middle fossa dura, the posterior fossa dura, the superior petrosal sinus, the sigmoid sinus, the bony labyrinth, the mastoid segment of the facial nerve and the jugular bulb. A lateral tympanotomy can provide access to the middle ear cavity through the mastoid (▶ Fig. 3.4a). However, the bony labyrinth, the cochlea, the jugular bulb, and the facial nerve can prevent access to the deepest areas of the temporal bone. A combined approach with an endoscope often facilitates the access to these areas.

A view of the infralabyrinthine approach (blue shaded area; ▶ Fig. 3.4b) is shown in ▶ Fig. 3.4c, d. After a classical mastoidectomy, the removal of the retrofacial air cells immediately inferior to the posterior semicircular canal and posteromedial to the mastoid segment of the facial nerve with exposure of the jugular bulb is necessary to make room for endoscope insertion. The corridor of this approach is limited by the labyrinth, the cochlea and the internal acoustic canal superiorly, the facial nerve anteriorly, the sigmoid sinus and the posterior fossa dura posteriorly and the jugular bulb inferiorly. When lesions located in the petrosal apex are endoscopically removed, care should be taken to avoid damage to neurovascular structures. With this approach, the petrous carotid artery can be anteriorly and medially identified. The inferior petrosal sinus runs posteroinferiorly toward the jugular bulb, with the internal acoustic meatus, trigeminal nerve, and greater petrosal nerve located superiorly.

A view of the supralabyrinthine suprameatal approach (orange shaded area; ▶ Fig. 3.4b) is shown in ▶ Fig. 3.4e, f. After a classical mastoidectomy, the middle fossa dura is clearly exposed and elevated from the middle cranial base. After the insertion of the endoscope between the bony labyrinth and the middle fossa dura, the geniculate ganglion, the labyrinthine, and tympanic parts of the facial nerve, the middle ear cavity , the greater petrosal nerve, the trigeminal nerve, and the tensor tympani muscle can be observed from above.

A view of the translabyrinthine transcochlear approach (green shaded area; ▶ Fig. 3.4b) is shown in ▶ Fig. 3.4g, h. After a classical mastoidectomy, the labyrinth, the retrofacial air cells, and the

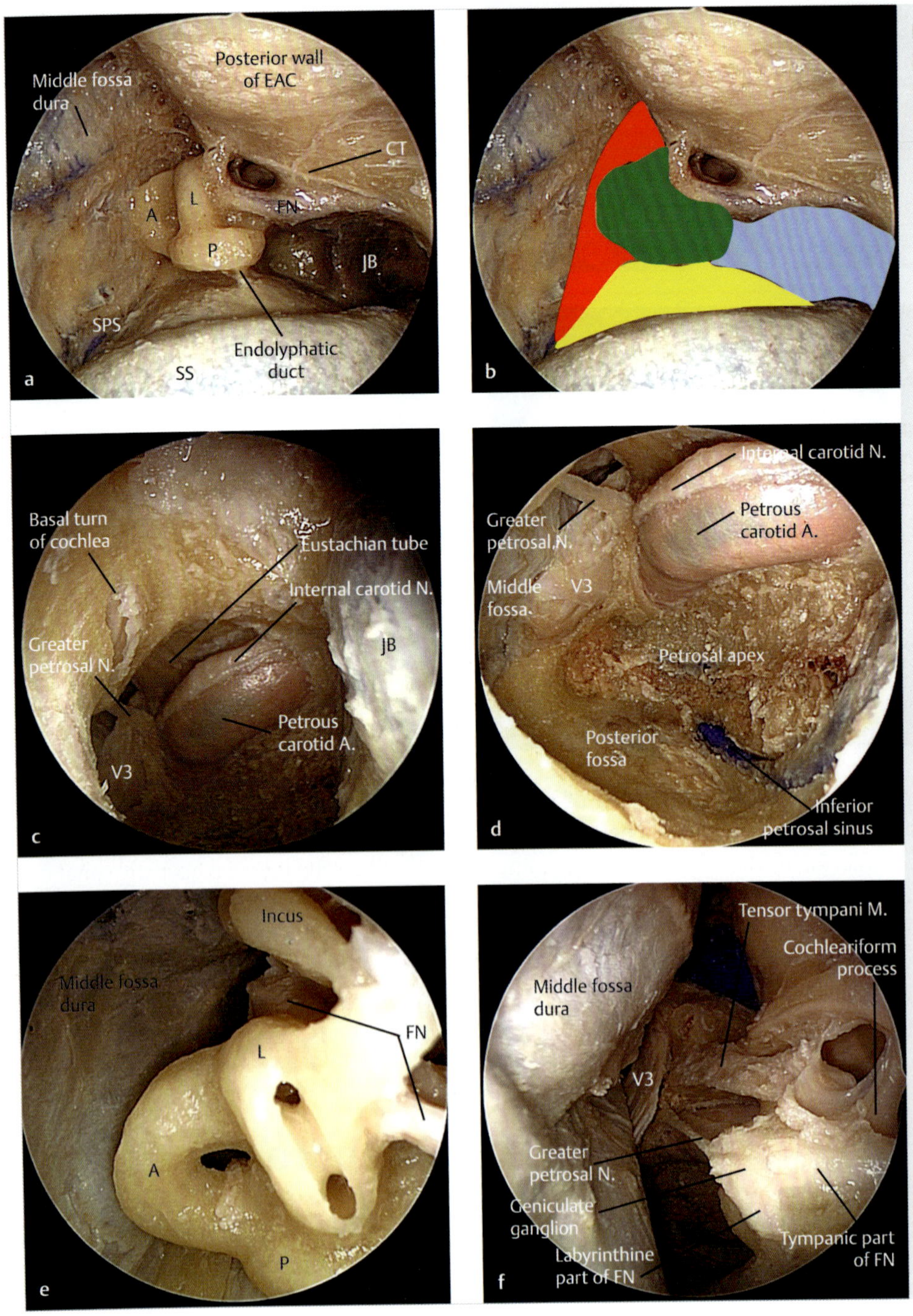

Fig. 3.4 Endoscopic assisted approaches to the lateral skull base. **(a)** A completed conventional mastoidectomy. **(b)** The routes of the previously reported endoscopically assisted approaches are shown. **(c and d)** View of the infralabyrinthine approach. **(e and f)** View of the supralabyrinthine suprameatal approach.

(Continued)

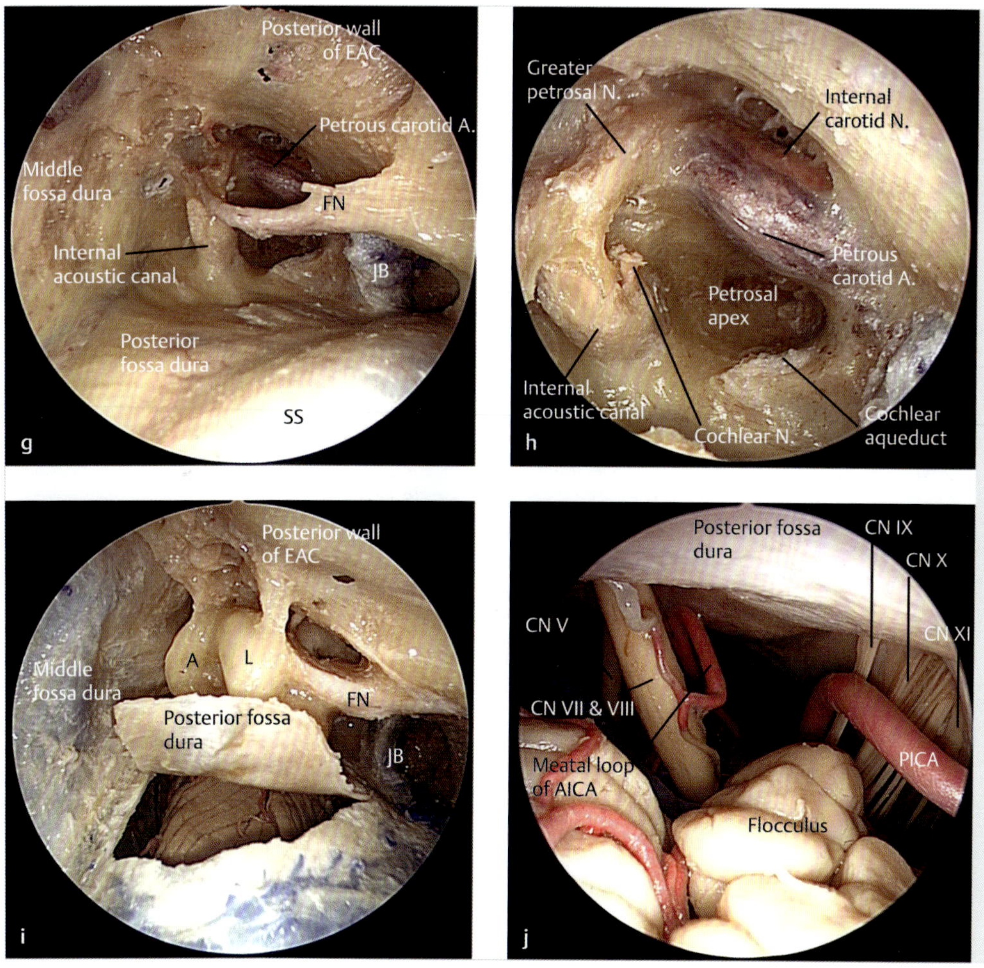

Fig. 3.4 (*Continued*) (**g** and **h**) View of the translabyrinthine transcochlear approach. (**i** and **j**) View of the presigmoid retrolabyrinthine approach. *A: anterior semicircular canal; AICA: anterior inferior cerebellar artery; CN: cranial nerve; EAC: external auditory canal; FN: facial nerve; JB: jugular bulb; L: lateral semicircular canal; N.: nerve; P: posterior semicircular canal; PICA: posterior inferior cerebellar artery; SS: sigmoid sinus.*

cochlea should be drilled preserving the facial nerve from the meatal to the mastoid segment. The genu of the petrous carotid artery is immediately anterior and inferior to the cochlea. Thus, care should be taken to avoid injury to the petrous carotid artery. The greater petrosal nerve branches off and runs under the trigeminal nerve.

A view of the presigmoid retrolabyrinthine approach (yellow shaded area; ▶ Fig. 3.4b) is shown in ▶ Fig. 3.4i, j. After a classical mastoidectomy, sinus skeletonization from the sinodural angle to the jugular bulb is completed. The presigmoid dura is cut along the superior petrosal sinus and the sigmoid sinus. After elevating the dura and the posterior retraction of the sigmoid sinus, the endoscope is inserted. This approach allows access to the internal acoustic canal. Cranial nerves V, VII, and VIII, and the lower cranial nerves (IX–XII) can be observed in detail. Iacoangeli et al reported that the endoscopic assisted presigmoid retrolabyrinthine approach can provide direct access to the CPA along with the labyrinthine complex conservation and a complete visualization of the intracanalicular portion of schwannomas.[14]

Acknowledgments

The author would like to thank the late prof. Albert L. Rhoton, Jr., University of Florida, for giving him the opportunity to study the microsurgical anatomy of the temporal bone.

References

[1] Fortes FS, Carrau RL, Snyderman CH, et al. Transpterygoid transposition of a temporoparietal fascia flap: a new method for skull base reconstruction after endoscopic expanded endonasal approaches. Laryngoscope. 2007; 117 (6):970–976

[2] Hartnick CJ, Myseros JS, Myer CM, III. Endoscopic access to the infratemporal fossa and skull base: a cadaveric study. Arch Otolaryngol Head Neck Surg. 2001; 127(11):1325–1327

[3] Ho B, Jang DW, Van Rompaey J, et al. Landmarks for endoscopic approach to the parapharyngeal internal carotid artery: a radiographic and cadaveric study. Laryngoscope. 2014; 124(9):1995–2001

[4] Hofstetter CP, Singh A, Anand VK, Kacker A, Schwartz TH. The endoscopic, endonasal, transmaxillary transpterygoid approach to the pterygopalatine fossa, infratemporal fossa, petrous apex, and the Meckel cave. J Neurosurg. 2010; 113(5):967–974

[5] Hosseini SM, Razfar A, Carrau RL, et al. Endonasal transpterygoid approach to the infratemporal fossa: correlation of endoscopic and multiplanar CT anatomy. Head Neck. 2012; 34(3):313–320

[6] Kasemsiri P, Solares CA, Carrau RL, et al. Endoscopic endonasal transpterygoid approaches: anatomical landmarks for planning the surgical corridor. Laryngoscope. 2013; 123(4):811–815

[7] Raza SM, Donaldson AM, Mehta A, Tsiouris AJ, Anand VK, Schwartz TH. Surgical management of trigeminal schwannomas: defining the role for endoscopic endonasal approaches. Neurosurg Focus. 2014; 37(4):E17

[8] Tarabichi M, Marchioni D, Presutti L, Nogueira JF, Pothier D. Endoscopic transcanal ear anatomy and dissection. Otolaryngol Clin North Am. 2013; 46(2):131–154

[9] Tarabichi M. Transcanal endoscopic management of cholesteatoma. Otol Neurotol. 2010; 31(4):580–588

[10] Presutti L, Alicandri-Ciufelli M, Cigarini E, Marchioni D. Cochlear schwannoma removed through the external auditory canal by a transcanal exclusive endoscopic technique. Laryngoscope. 2013; 123(11):2862–2867
[11] Marchioni D, Alicandri-Ciufelli M, Rubini A, Presutti L. Endoscopic transcanal corridors to the lateral skull base: initial experiences. Laryngoscope. 2015; 125 Suppl 5:S1–S13
[12] Marchioni D, Alicandri-Ciufelli M, Piccinini A, Genovese E, Presutti L. Inferior retrotympanum revisited: an endoscopic anatomic study. Laryngoscope. 2010; 120(9):1880–1886
[13] Komune N, Matsuo S, Miki K, Rhoton AL, Jr. The endoscopic anatomy of the middle ear approach to the fundus of the internal acoustic canal. J Neurosurg. 2017; 126(6):1974–1983
[14] Iacoangeli M, Salvinelli F, Di Rienzo A, et al. Microsurgical endoscopy-assisted presigmoid retrolabyrinthine approach as a minimally invasive surgical option for the treatment of medium to large vestibular schwannomas. Acta Neurochir (Wien). 2013; 155(4):663–670

Chapter 4

Instruments and Operating Room Setup

4 Instruments and Operating Room Setup

Daniele Marchioni, Alessia Rubini, Stefano De Rossi, Muaaz Tarabichi, and Gabriele Molteni

Abstract

This chapter offers a thorough description of the instrumentation used for endoscopic ear surgery and lateral skull base surgery procedures, as well as illustrations of such instrument and of the setup of the operating room. While lateral skull base surgery is mainly performed under microscopic view, with instruments sets based on traditional microscopic otologic procedures and well known to neurosurgeons and ENT surgeons, in the last few decades new instruments have been developed specifically for endoscopic ear surgery. In addition, the introduction of exoscopes, providing either 2D or 3D images, has enabled the creation of new approaches to the lateral skull base, as well as new tools for teaching anatomy and surgical procedures. First, a complete description of the different operating room settings is offered, with the aid of depictions of devices' and operators' positioning. Second, the main tools used in both microscopic and endoscopic surgery are described, with particular focus on specifications and positioning. Indications on the type of instruments to prefer during the different approaches are provided as well. A section has been dedicated to the description and depiction of dedicated instruments for endoscopic ear surgery. Moreover, tips and tricks for surgery are offered during the description of instruments, to help surgeons at the beginning of their practice (but also more experienced professionals) understand the reasons that brought to the creation, modification, or improvement of the instrument itself.

Keywords: lateral skull base surgery, microscopic surgery, endoscopic surgery, exoscopic approach, dissector instruments, operating room setup

4.1 Introduction

This chapter provides an in-depth description and state-of-the-art illustrations of the devices and instruments used in microscopic and endoscopic lateral skull base surgery. Since lateral skull base surgery is performed mostly under microscopic domain, at present the instrumentation used is based mainly on the traditional otologic and neurotologic surgery sets.

Some special endoscopic equipment and microinstruments specifically designed to fulfill the particular requirements of endoscopic lateral skull base surgery were introduced during the endoscopic ear surgery era. These new specifically designed instruments have widened the indications and refined the surgical skills of the endoscopic approach, which in turn allows a better control of pathology and grants access to previously unreachable or difficult-to-reach anatomical recesses around the facial nerve, internal carotid artery, and internal auditory canal (IAC).

The microscope and the endoscopic tower represent the crucial tools to perform lateral skull base surgery, and the recent introduction of the exoscope enabled the surgeon to have a new approach to lateral skull base; in fact, the exoscopic camera may be used instead of the microscope to perform certain lateral skull base surgery procedures. This new promising tool allows to magnify the surgical field, providing a high-quality view of the anatomical details during the approach. Some exoscopes provide a tridimensional view using 3D glasses, giving also a precise depth perception during the surgical approach.

The operating room setup during lateral skull base surgery must grant all the staff the possibility to follow the surgical approach, and the presence of high-definition (HD) camera with integrated video monitor system is crucial to allow a constant view of the surgical field when performing lateral skull base procedures.

A magnetically operated microscope with built-in HD camera provides continuous video documentation in parallel with the endoscopic surgery performed entirely with the aid of an HD monitor. The availability of continuous video monitoring enables the anesthesiologist, the scrub nurse, and others to observe and follow the operation. Recordings can also be used for teaching purposes.

4.2 Operating Room Setup

Depending on the surgical approach the setting of the operating room may change; we can have three different settings.

4.2.1 Setting for Microscopic and Endoscopic Lateral Skull Base Surgery (see ▶ Fig. 4.1)

The patient is placed supine on the operating room table with the head rotated to the contralateral side with respect to the affected ear.

The microscope is placed in the sterile field ready to be used on the contralateral side with respect to the surgeon, in order to allow the flexible movement of the microscopic tower, and the endoscope is ready to be used too. The endoscopic tower is placed directly facing the surgeon, and the monitor is placed at the same height as the surgeon's eyes. The scrub nurse sits opposite to the surgeon. The other monitor is placed on the contralateral side, to allow the nurse to see the surgical approach.

The anesthesiologist and the anesthesia trolley are located at the foot of the operating table, and this location is adopted for all the various lateral skull base approaches.

4.2.2 Setting for Microscopic and Endoscopic Middle Cranial Fossa Surgery (see ▶ Fig. 4.2)

In case of middle cranial fossa approach the setting is modified as follows: the patient is placed supine on the operating room table with the head rotated to the contralateral side with respect to the affected ear.

The microscope is placed at the head of the operating table, at the level of allow the affected side, in order to flexible movement of the microscopic tower. The endoscopic tower is placed directly facing the surgeon, and the monitor is placed at the same height as the surgeon's eyes contralateral to the affected ear. The scrub nurse sits opposite the endoscopic tower. The anesthesiologist

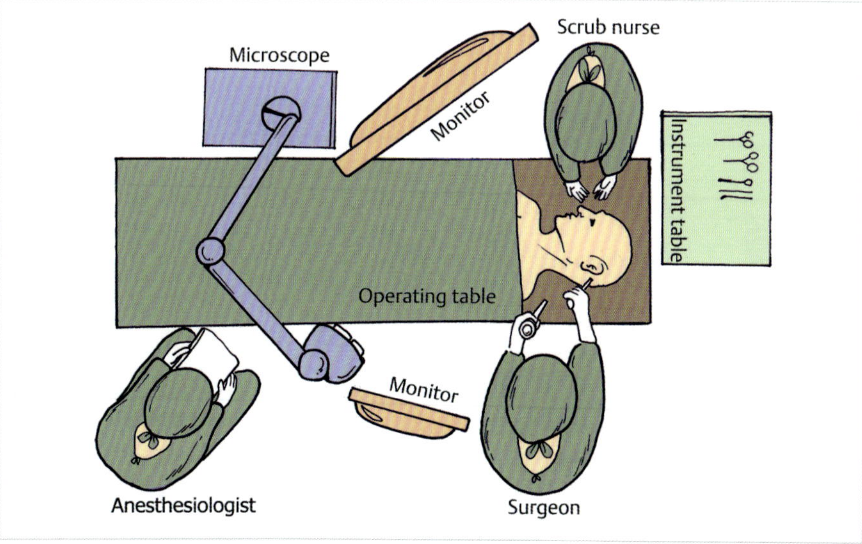

Fig. 4.1 Schematic drawing of the operating room arrangement during most of the microscopic/endoscopic skull base approaches.

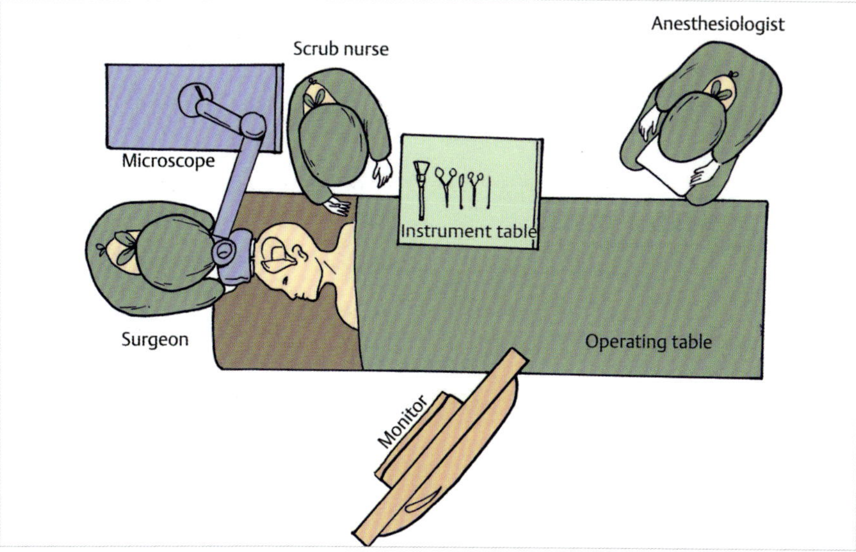

Fig. 4.2 Schematic drawing of the operating room arrangement during middle cranial fossa and anterior petrosectomy approaches.

and the anesthesia trolley are located at the foot of the operating table.

4.2.3 Setting for Exoscopic Lateral Skull Base Surgery (see ▶ Fig. 4.3 and ▶ Fig. 4.4)

In case of exoscopic approach to the lateral skull base the setting should again be modified as follows: the patient is placed supine on the operating room table with the head rotated to the contralateral side with respect to the affected ear.

The 3D exoscope is placed at the head of the operating table, and the camera is placed close to and in front of the surgical field, in order to get an optimal screen vision. The surgeon should use 3D glasses, performing surgery using two hands as it happens for the microscopic technique and watching the monitor like in the endoscopic technique. The assistant surgeon stands opposite the monitor, using 3D glasses and managing a control unit (IMAGE PILOT) to adjust the focus, enlarge or shift the field of view, during surgery. The scrub nurse sits opposite the surgeon, and a second monitor is placed on the opposite side with respect to the nurse, in order to allow the nurse to see the surgical approach. The anesthesiologist and the anesthesia trolley are located at the foot of the operating table.

In the modern operating room, we recognize three different surgical approaches based on the tools used:

- Microscopic approach (using operative microscope)
- Endoscopic approach (using endoscopes with endoscopic tower)
- Exoscopic approach (using the exoscope)

4.3 The Operative Microscope (see ▶ Fig. 4.5 and ▶ Fig. 4.6)

The operating microscope is indispensable for most lateral skull base surgical procedures, since in the majority of cases a large dissection and wide bone drilling are required. The microscope should combine visualization, connectivity, and data management altogether. The microscope must be available, sterile, and ready in the surgical field even when exclusively endoscopic lateral skull base surgery is intended, in order to convert the endoscopic technique to a microscopic one, when required.

The operating microscope should be integrated with an HD camera connected to an HD medical monitor to allow the best visualization. The ergonomic handgrip design and friction-free electromagnetic clutches provide an ideal flexibility in the operating room, allowing an easy alternation between microscope and endoscope throughout the surgical procedure.

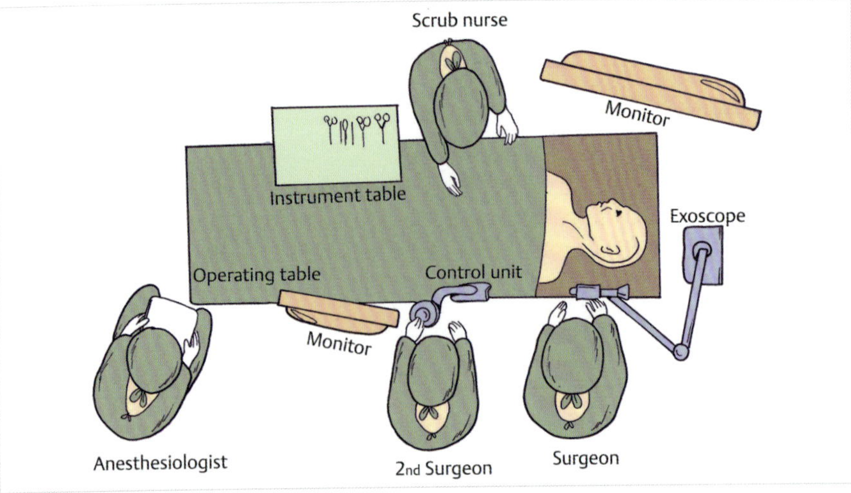

Fig. 4.3 Schematic drawing of the operating room arrangement during exoscopic lateral skull base surgery.

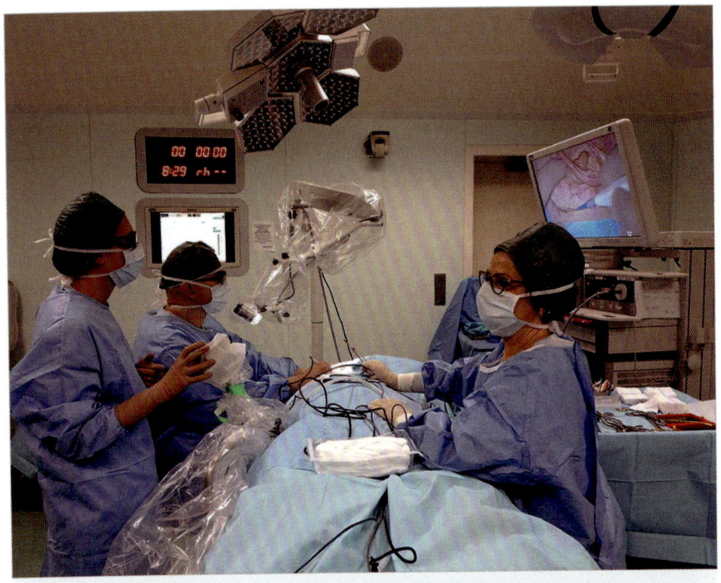

Fig. 4.4 Operating room setup during 3D exoscopic approach to lateral skull base. The surgeon sits opposite the exoscopic tower, facing the monitor, performing surgery with two hands as in microscopic technique, while an assistant surgeon is holding the control unit to adjust the focus and the surgical field. 3D glasses are necessary for 3D vision.

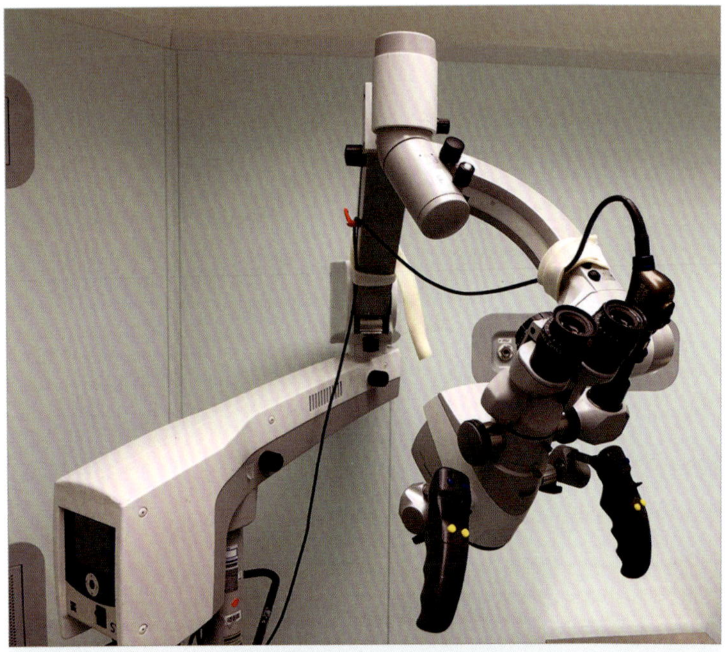

Fig. 4.5 Operative microscope.

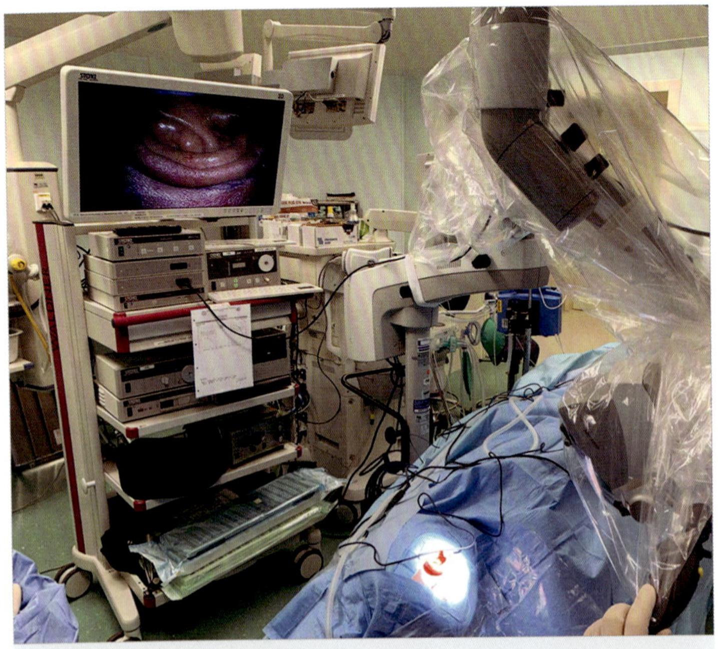

Fig. 4.6 The operating microscope is integrated with a high-definition (HD) camera connected to an HD medical monitor to allow the best visualization for assistant surgeon, nurse, and resident during the surgery.

4.4 The Rigid Endoscopes (see ▶ Fig. 4.7)

The Hopkins rod lens system was developed to provide endoscopes of variable lengths, diameters, and angles of view. The rigid endoscopes commonly used for lateral skull base surgery are either 3 or 4 mm in diameter. All the new endoscopes are now autoclavable. The optimal working lengths for endoscopic lateral skull base surgery are 14 and 15 cm. The larger the diameter, the better the image is displayed and the more light it can transmit to the operative field. For this reason, in open field (like in the cerebellopontine angle [CPA], during transotic/transcochlear approaches), the use of 4 mm diameter scope is suggested; however, in case of fully endoscopic transcanal approaches (such as infracochlear, transpromontorial, or suprageniculate approaches), a 3 mm diameter scope may be used, allowing more comfortable surgical maneuvers.

The 0- and 45-degree angled endoscopes are most commonly used, followed by the 70-degree endoscope. An endoscope with a greater angle, such as 70 degrees, is difficult and disorienting to work with and is only used for inspection and tumor dissection in the fundus of the IAC through the retrosigmoid approach; in this approach, the use of the 70-degree endoscope may be crucial

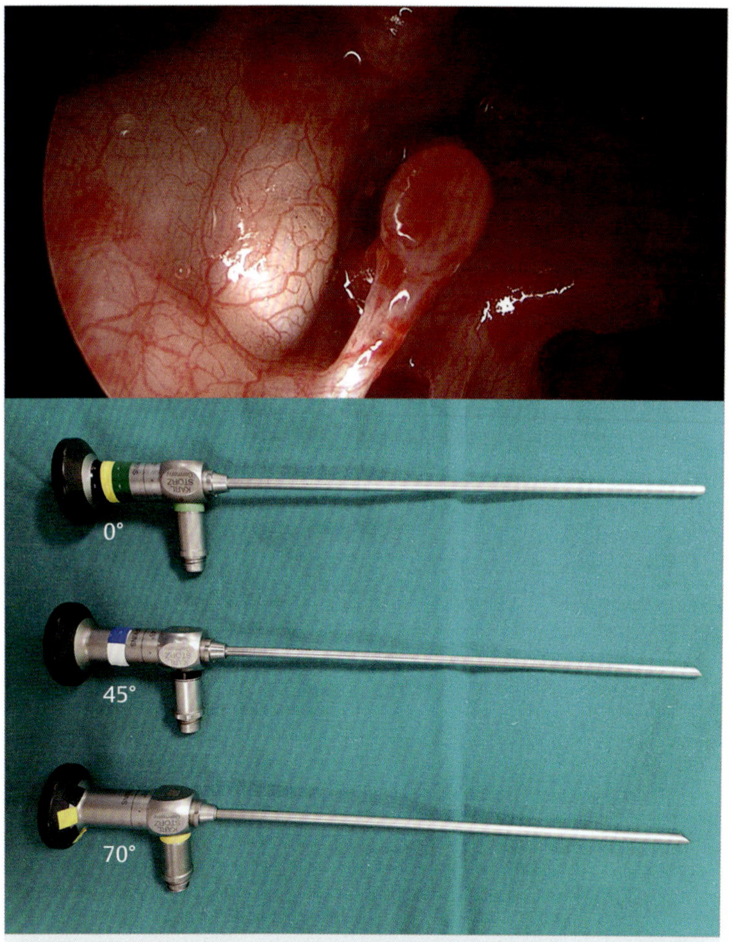

Fig. 4.7 Operative endoscopes with different angles, 4 mm in diameter, 15 cm in length, and the possibility to work close to the field in high definition enables the surgeon to appreciate the anatomical details.

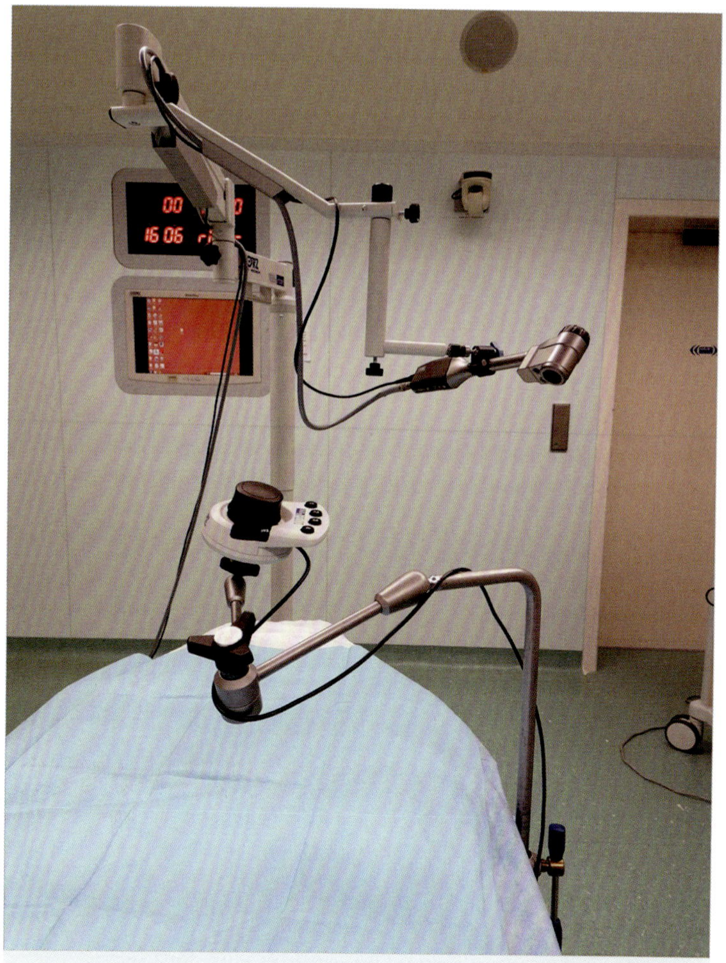

Fig. 4.8 The VITOM 3D exoscope system (Karl Storz GmbH, Tuttlingen, Germany).

in order to have a wide view on the fundus, detecting any residual disease.

During transtemporal approaches, in order to work around the facial nerve and internal carotid artery, 45-degree, 15 cm length, 4 mm diameter endoscope may be used, in search of any residual disease, and at the same time allowing the removal of the disease from hidden areas.

4.5 3D Exoscope (see ▶ Fig. 4.8)

The VITOM 3D exoscope (Karl Storz GmbH, Tuttlingen, Germany) may be used as an exclusive tool instead of the operative microscope in all the skull base procedures requiring open approaches. The system consists of a holding arm for VITOM 3D, placed in front of the surgical field and connected to a camera and fiber optic light cable providing a large field of view which is displayed as a full HD (Nump resolution) image on an N-inch 3D monitor. The screen is placed in front of the surgeon allowing a direct view during surgery. The surgeon should use 3D polarization glasses (or clip-on glasses for those wearing corrective glasses).

The control unit (IMAGE PILOT), used to control the focus, enlarge or shift the field of view, is positioned next to the surgeon and kept in place by another holding arm.

4.6 Xenon Light Sources for Endoscopic Surgery

Illumination is generated by a powerful cold light source and transmitted to the endoscope via a 180 cm long fiberoptic light cable. Different types of light sources (halogen, xenon, LED) offer light of variable brightness. Xenon is currently the chosen source.

4.7 Nerve Integrity Monitor (▶ Fig. 4.9)

A Nerve Integrity Monitor (NIM) is used for facial nerve monitoring during all the lateral skull base procedures. Electrodes are placed in the orbicularis oculi and orbicularis oris muscles to allow a continuous electromyographic monitoring of the facial nerve.

4.8 Instruments

Besides the standard instruments required to set up the surgical approach through the soft tissues (scalpels, forceps, mono/bipolar diathermy, etc.), the neurotological instrument set of special interest includes:

- Self-retaining mastoid retractors of different sizes (▶ Fig. 4.10);
- Instruments for bone drilling: microdrill, micromotor handles (straight and curved);
- Set of different-sized tungsten cutting burs and diamond burs;
- Traditional suction instruments;
- Traditional soft tissue dissectors, large and small scissors, toothed and non-toothed forceps, periosteal raspatory.

In general, a full set of microsurgical instruments is required, and these are very familiar to the practicing otologist: Microforceps (microcup and microalligator); straight and curved delicate

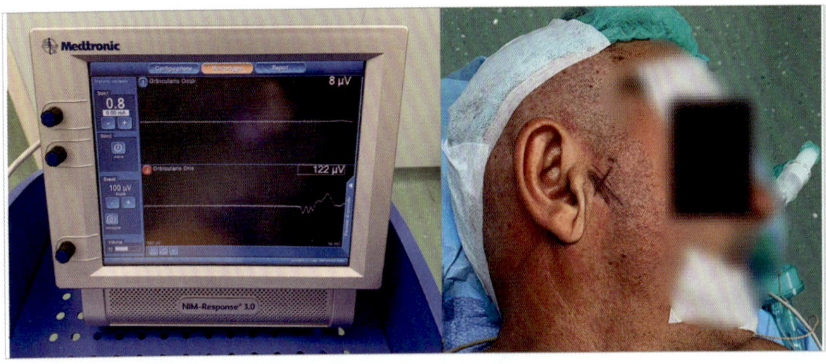

Fig. 4.9 A Nerve Integrity Monitor (NIM) system for facial nerve monitoring during surgery.

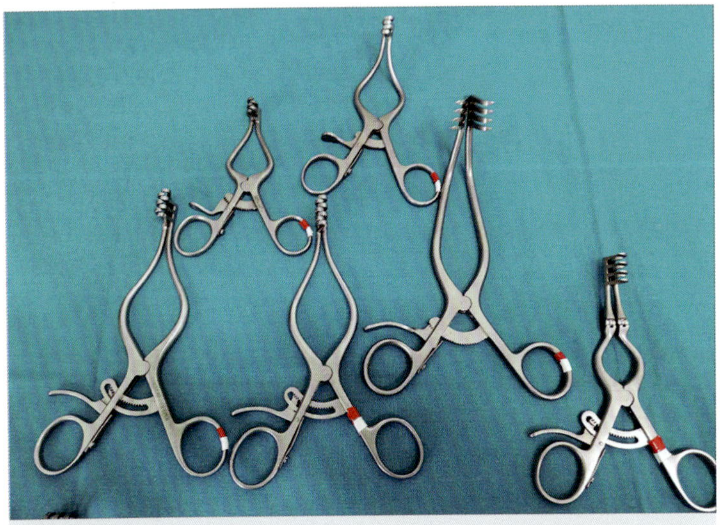

Fig. 4.10 Self-retaining mastoid retractors of different sizes.

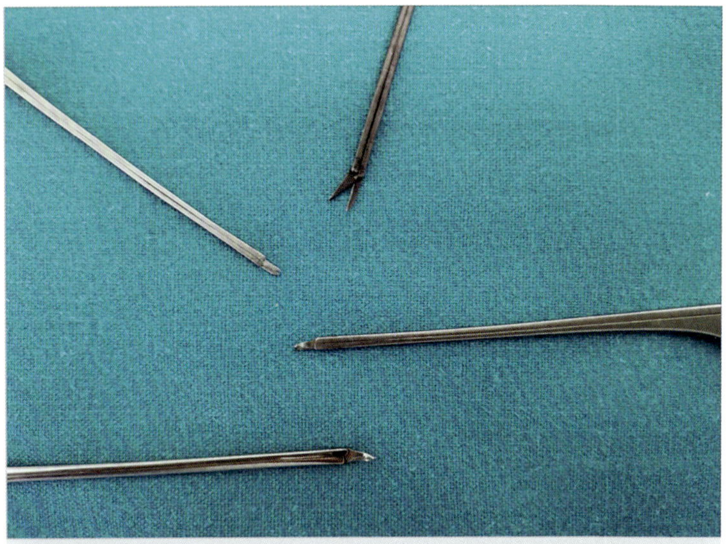

Fig. 4.11 Set of straight and curved microscissors.

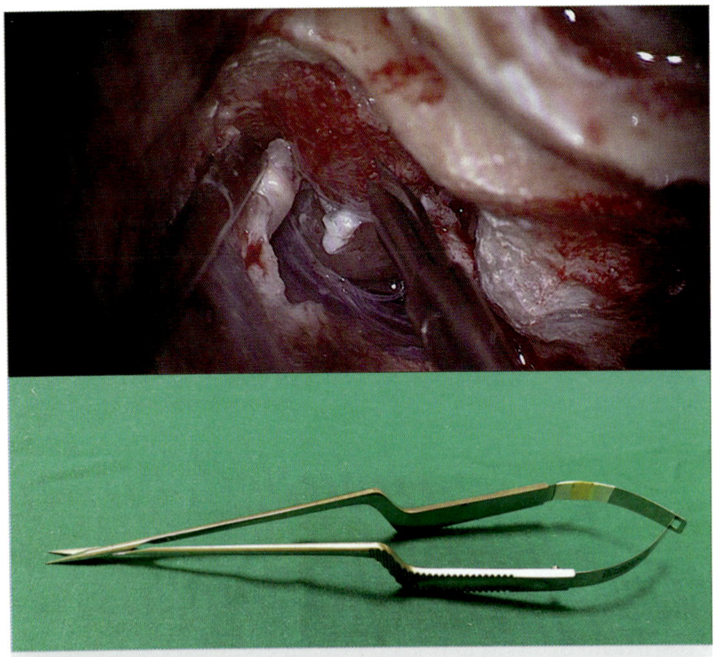

Fig. 4.12 Neurosurgical scissors; this instrument is particularly useful during the dissection of tumor and dural incision.

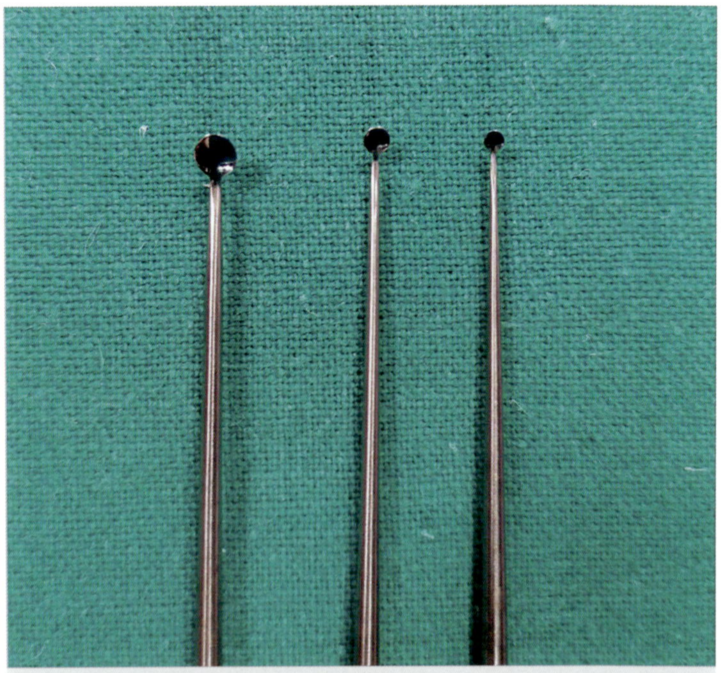

Fig. 4.13 Set of round cutting knives of different sizes.

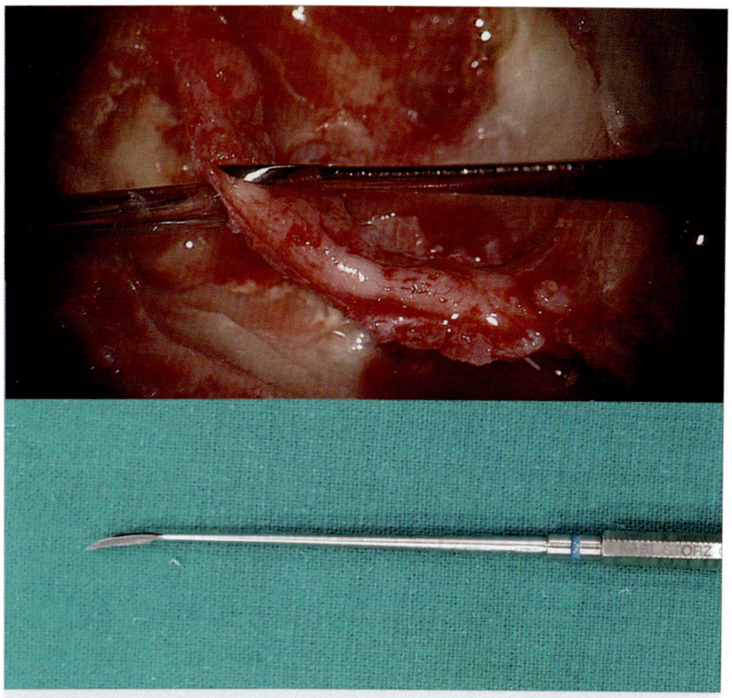

Fig. 4.14 Sickle knives.

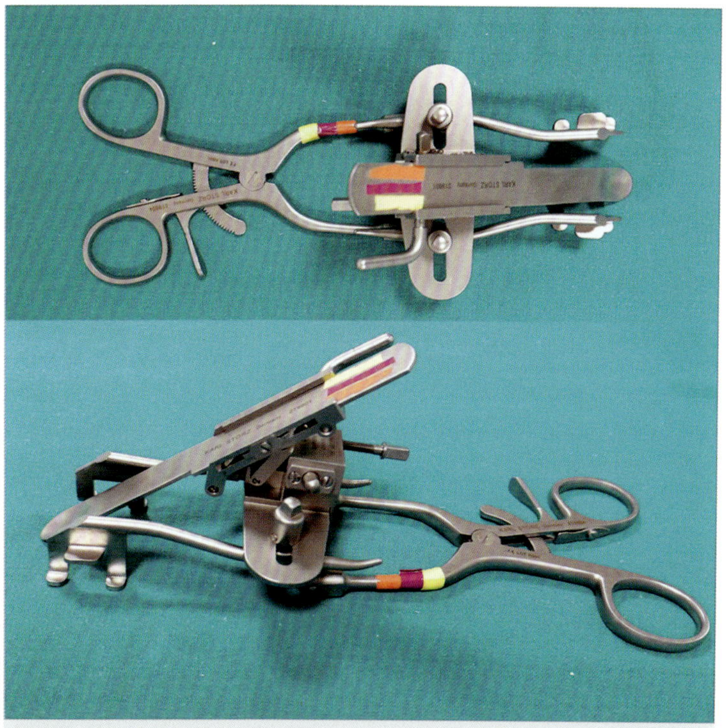

Fig. 4.16 Middle fossa dura Fisch retractor.

microscissors (see ▶ Fig. 4.11); neurosurgical scissors (see ▶ Fig. 4.12); microhooks of different angles and lengths, needles; elevators, knives of different sizes and shapes (e.g., round cutting knife, see ▶ Fig. 4.13), Plester vertical cutting knife, and sickle knives of variable curvatures (see ▶ Fig. 4.14); Rosen elevator; large and small House curette (see ▶ Fig. 4.15); etc.

4.9 Retractor for Lateral Skull Base

Middle fossa dura Fisch retractor is useful during middle cranial fossa or anterior petrosectomy approaches to retract the dura of

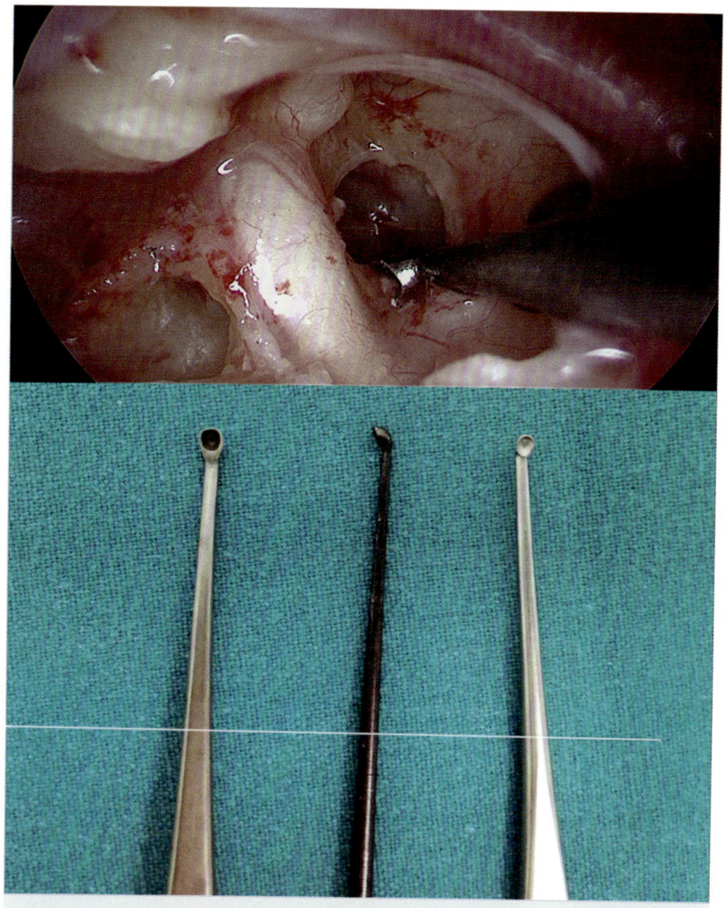

Fig. 4.15 Micro-curettes of different sizes.

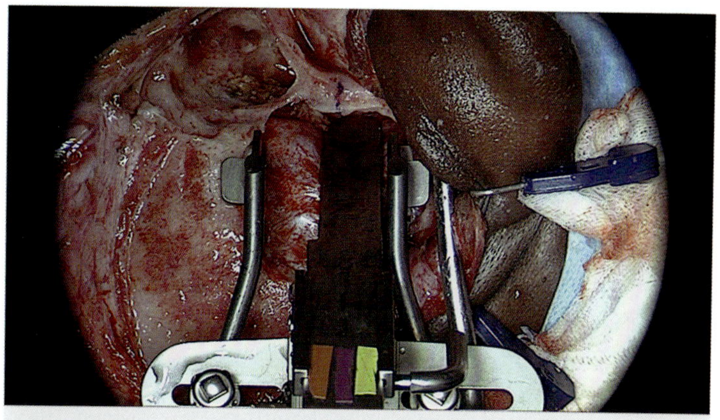

Fig. 4.17 The placement of a middle fossa dura Fisch retractor during middle cranial fossa surgery.

middle fossa allowing surgery in the petrous apex and IAC (see ▶ Fig. 4.16 and ▶ Fig. 4.17).

Leyla retractor of different blade sizes may be useful during the retrosigmoid approach in case a soft cerebellar retraction is necessary to allow for the surgical maneuvers in the CPA, or in case of middle cranial fossa approach to retract the dura of the temporal lobe (see ▶ Fig. 4.18).

4.10 Bone Rongeur

Bone rongeurs of different sizes are useful especially during lateral skull base transtemporal approaches to remove a wide amount of bone after the detachment of the dura from the bony walls (see ▶ Fig. 4.19).

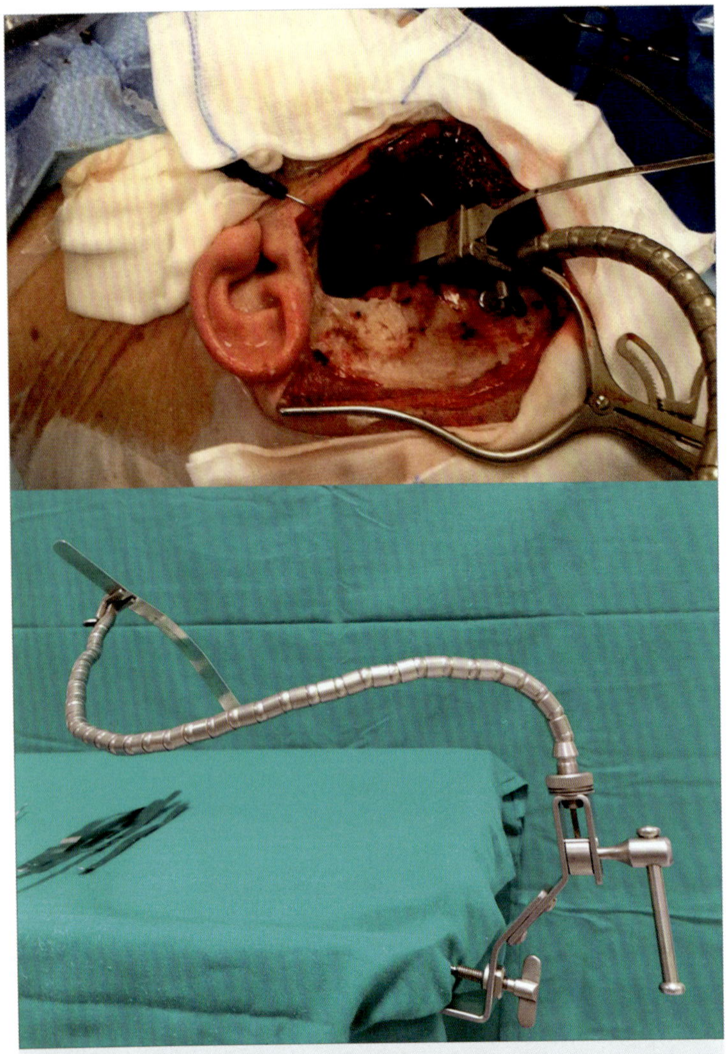

Fig. 4.18 Leya retractor for lateral skull base surgery.

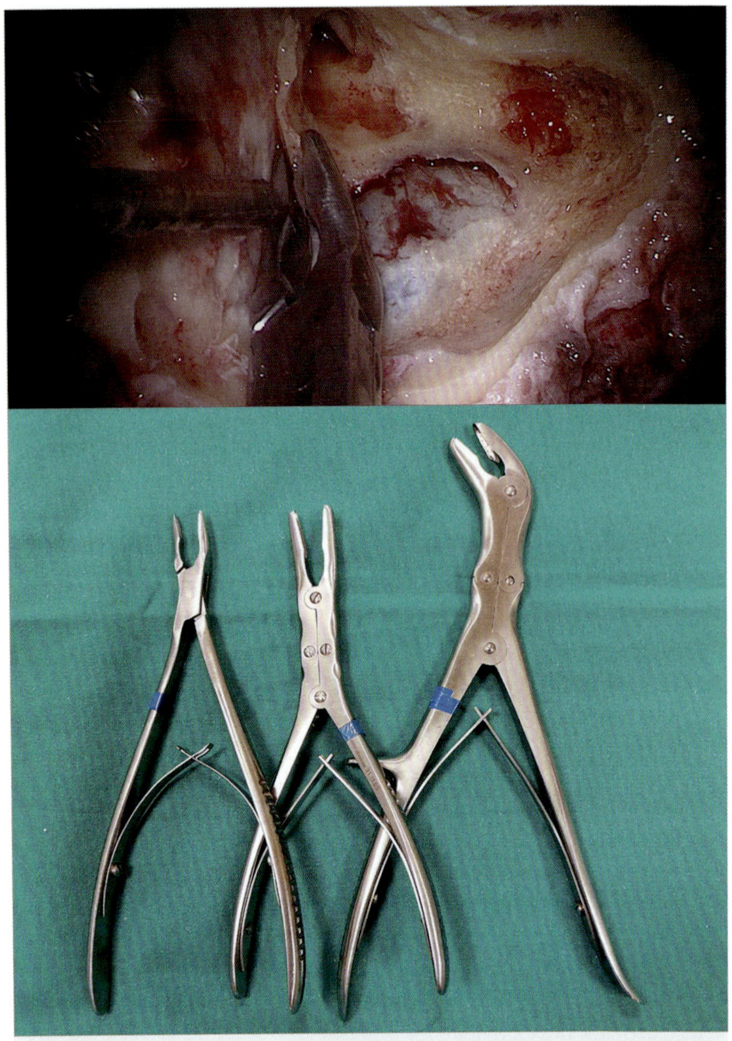

Fig. 4.19 Bone rongeurs of different sizes.

4.11 Special Instruments for Endoscopic/Microscopic Lateral Skull Base Surgery

The endoscope is increasingly used in many neurotological and skull base procedures in combination with the microscope. However, CPA and skull base surgery have their own peculiarities, as the operating field is greatly restricted and usually deeper than that for any standard otological surgery. Standard ear surgery instruments are hence inadequate, mainly with regard to length. Accordingly, a wide range of dedicated microinstruments have been specifically modified and/or designed for use in endoscopic skull base surgery, including microscissors, microdissectors, suction tubes, bipolars, and others. These microinstruments need modification to become longer, thinner, and equipped with angulated microtips. Suction cannulas have also been modified to include longer angulated ones, particularly the Brackmann suction cannulas, to enable the surgeon to work under angled vision inside the IAC or around vital structures.

4.12 Drill and Microdrill

Traditional microdrills are used during most lateral skull base surgery operations. Drills of different sizes and shapes are crucial. A large cutting bur is essential to remove a large amount of bone during transtemporal approaches, while a diamond bur is used on the dura of middle and posterior fossae, as well as in skeletonized lateral sinus and jugular bulb, and to obtain hemostasis on the bony surface (see ▶ Fig. 4.20).

For endoscopic transcanal skull base surgery, pen-style, compact, powerful, lightweight, high-performance microdrills provide the balance and maneuverability that enable the surgeon to work in tight spaces, like for example during suprageniculate transcanal approach or transpromontorial transcanal approach. In particular, the possibility to limit the rotation only to the tip of the drill is crucial to avoid damage on the skin and bone of the external auditory canal while drilling (see ▶ Fig. 4.21).

4.13 Piezosurgery (see ▶ Fig. 4.22)

The Piezosurgery Medical is manufactured by Mectron specifically for bone dissection. Although it does not replace micromotors for bone drilling, piezosurgery offers state of the art technology in bone surgery. The piezoelectric ceramic disks contained in the Piezosurgery Medical handpiece transmit microvibrations to inserts designed specifically for each surgical technique. The system has the advantage of minimizing damage to the soft tissue, maximizing at the same time surgical precision, and offering a blood-free surgical site with ideal intraoperative

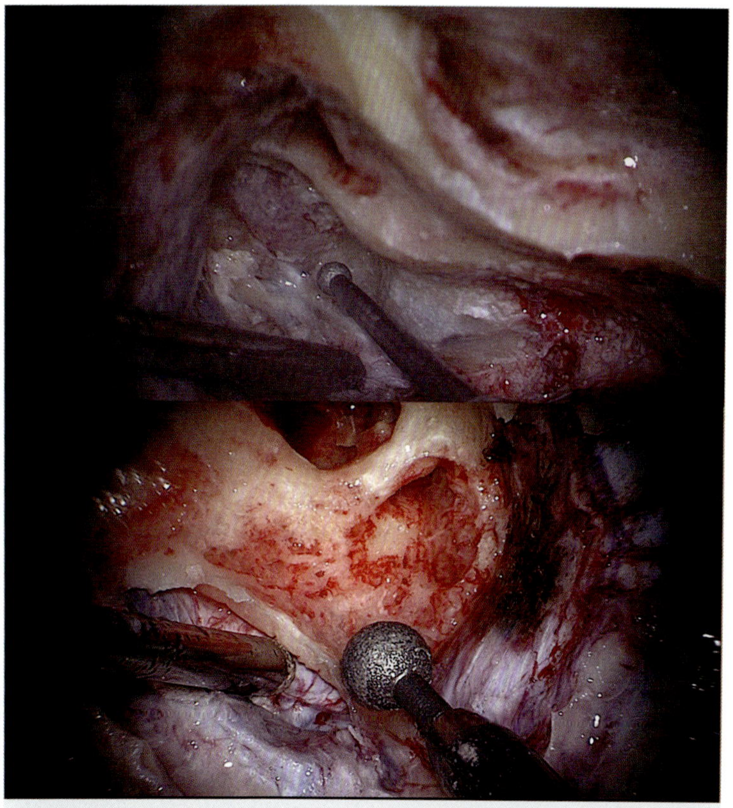

Fig. 4.20 Diamond bur drills of different lengths, are used in particular during the management of the dura of middle and posterior fossae, for instance while skeletonizing of internal auditory canal (IAC).

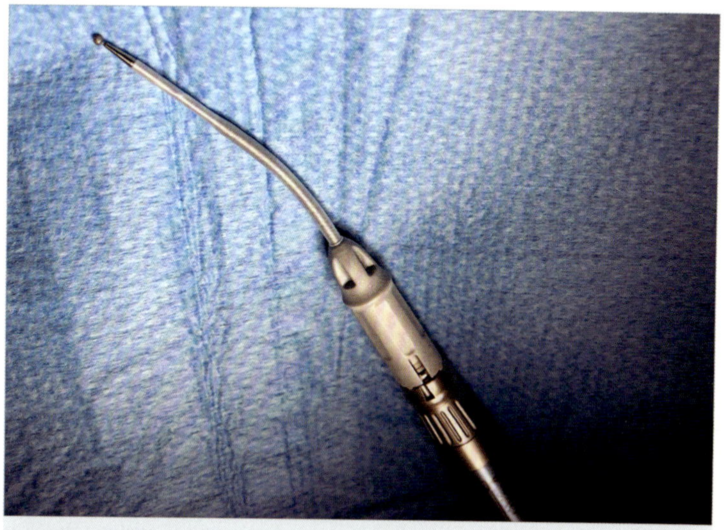

Fig. 4.21 VISAO high-speed otologic microdrill designed for otology and neuro-otology procedures, especially useful for transcanal endoscopic surgery.

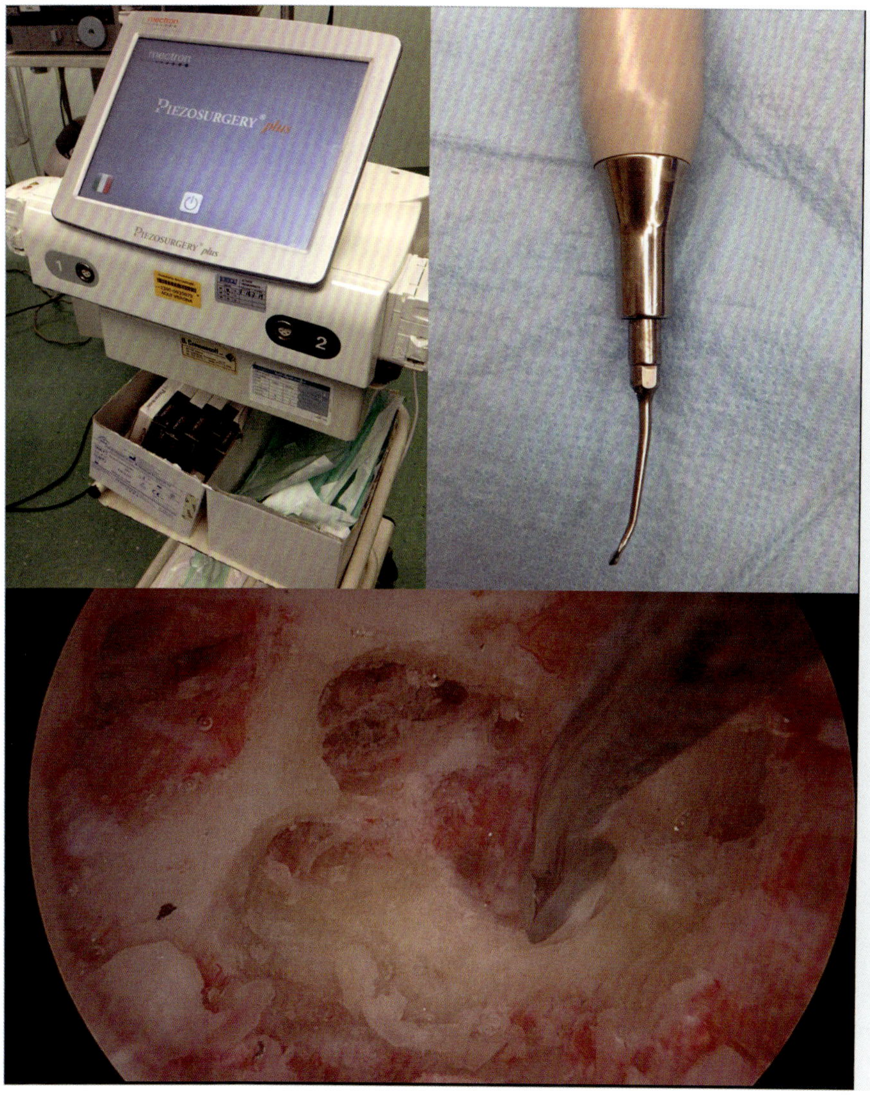

Fig. 4.22 Piezosurgery device with special tip designed for a transcanal endoscopic approach.

visibility. The very fine movement of the cutting inserts (micrometers) allows maximum intraoperative control. It provides a bone cut of only 0.3 to 0.6 mm width, with no bone necrosis. The wide range of surgical inserts makes it easy to use in different fields, including in fully endoscopic lateral skull base surgery. The use of piezosurgery is crucial during transpromontorial and infrapromontorial approaches, as well as during the suprageniculate approach, in order to remove the bone of the fundus of the IAC, avoiding damage and heat dissipation on the nervous structures. The selective removal of bone is performed under water, while constant irrigation allows the surgeon to keep the surgical field clean at all times, thus reducing heat dissipation.

The special tip designed for transcanal endoscopic surgery is a useful tool during precise dissection, such as for decompression of the facial nerve, decompression of the IAC, and transpromontorial bony removal, especially during a transcanal approach. The piezosurgery device is also useful during the bony work on the IAC, as for example during a retrosigmoid approach.

4.14 Bipolar

Bipolar coagulators are crucial during lateral skull base surgery; in particular, different tips and sizes are essential for working on the skull base tumor and on the dura of middle and posterior fossae, as well as intracranially on the CPA. A small size bipolar instrument should be used to coagulate the small vessels around the tumor, and a medium size bipolar tool may be used directly on the tumor in order to debulk the mass, thus controlling the bleeding.

In our practice we make use of Vesalius bipolar, especially during the management of the dura and during intracranial dissection (see ▶ Fig. 4.23). The Vesalius (Telea Electronic Engineering) is a special bipolar/monopolar output device that enables the surgeon to perform surgery in an extremely delicate fashion, preserving both tissues and biological structures. These bipolars can be used to coagulate or to cut tissues, or even a combination of the two.

The tradename Quantum Molecular Resonance (QMR) comes from the particular way the energy is conveyed to the biological tissues in the form of high frequency electrical fields that interact with the tissue itself. The cutting effect does not depend on an increase in the temperature but rather on the rupture of cells due to the induced resonance effect. In the cutting mode, the temperature rises to 45 °C. Coagulation is also obtained using the same resonance for energy transfer. It is important to point out that the cut is not a consequence of the high heat produced in the tissue, as in the case of the standard electro/radiosurgical units, but it is achieved through the breaking of molecular bonds and is therefore accomplished without a temperature rise. In fact, there is a very modest temperature rise to about 63 °C, sufficient to trigger coagulation via the protein denaturation process; cellular necrosis is avoided and consequently the cut and coagulation delivered by the Vesalius are extremely precise and delicate, with minimal thermal damage. The bipolar come in different sizes and lengths, specifically designed for lateral skull base surgery to allow the management of the dura of the middle and posterior fossae and the dissection of tumor inside the CPA, avoiding heat dissipation on the delicate nervous structures.

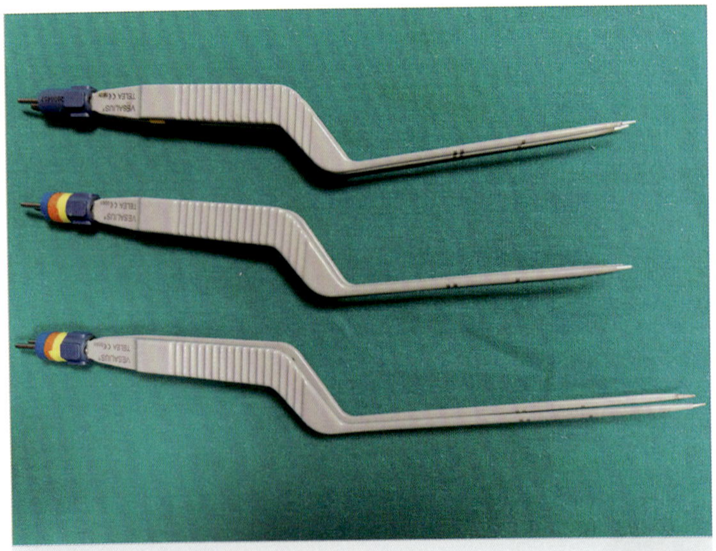

Fig. 4.23 Vesalius bipolar instruments of different lengths and sizes for lateral skull base surgery.

4.15 Dissectors

Dissectors of various sizes, shapes, and lengths are essential during lateral skull base surgery. Rhoton dissectors in particular may be used during the microscopic dissection of the tumor from the facial nerve and other cranial nerves (see ▶ Fig. 4.24), while curved dissectors may be used especially to remove remnant disease along the medial surface of the internal carotid artery or around the facial nerve under endoscopic view (see ▶ Fig. 4.25 and ▶ Fig. 4.26). Long and curved dissectors are crucial during the retrosigmoid approach in order to remove the remnant tumor from the fundus of the IAC under endoscopic control (see ▶ Fig. 4.27).

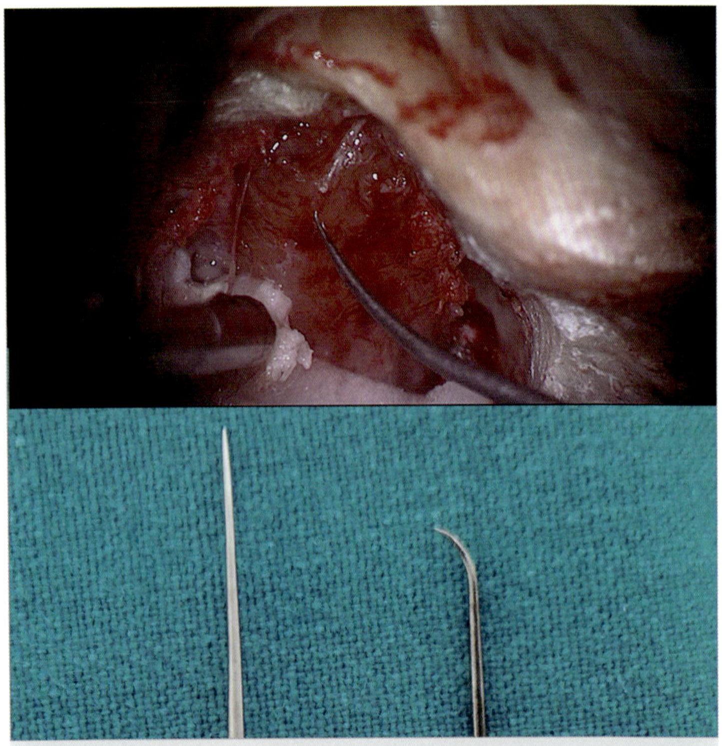

Fig. 4.24 Rhoton microdissectors are especially used for the manipulation and dissection of very fine nerves from tumors of the lateral skull base and cerebellopontine angle (CPA).

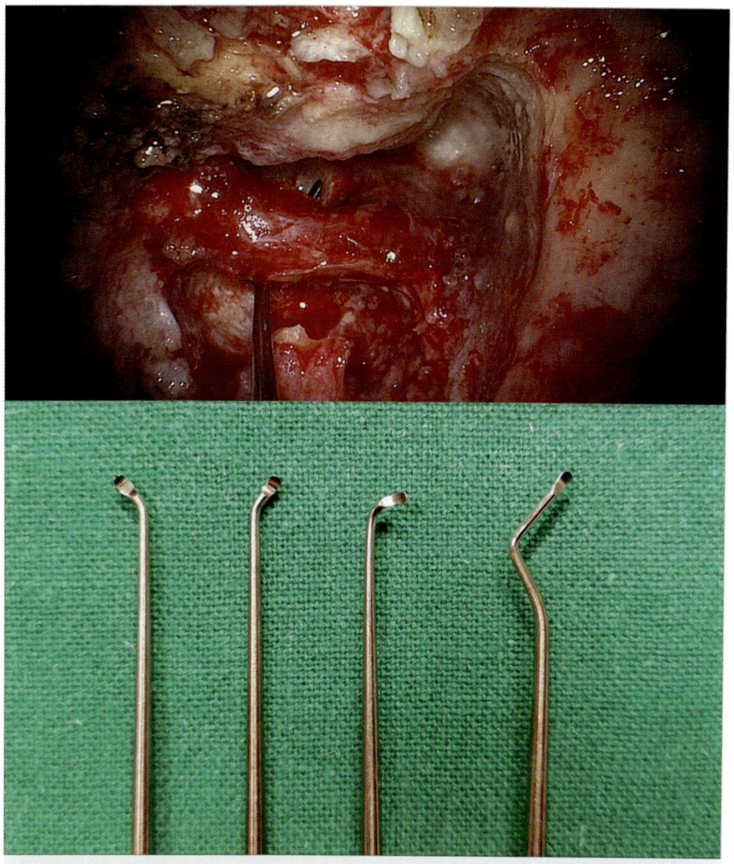

Fig. 4.25 Curved dissectors by Thomassin with different shapes and lengths are useful particularly during transtemporal approaches to control the hidden areas around the internal carotid artery and the facial neve.

4.16 Suction Tubes

Rigid suction instruments of different lengths and shapes are essential particularly during endoscopic surgery. Curved suction instruments are specifically useful during endoscopic assisted surgery in order to remove remnant disease situated around anatomical structures and areas such as the internal carotid artery and the facial nerve, as well as inside the petrous apex and clivus (see ▶ Fig. 4.28).

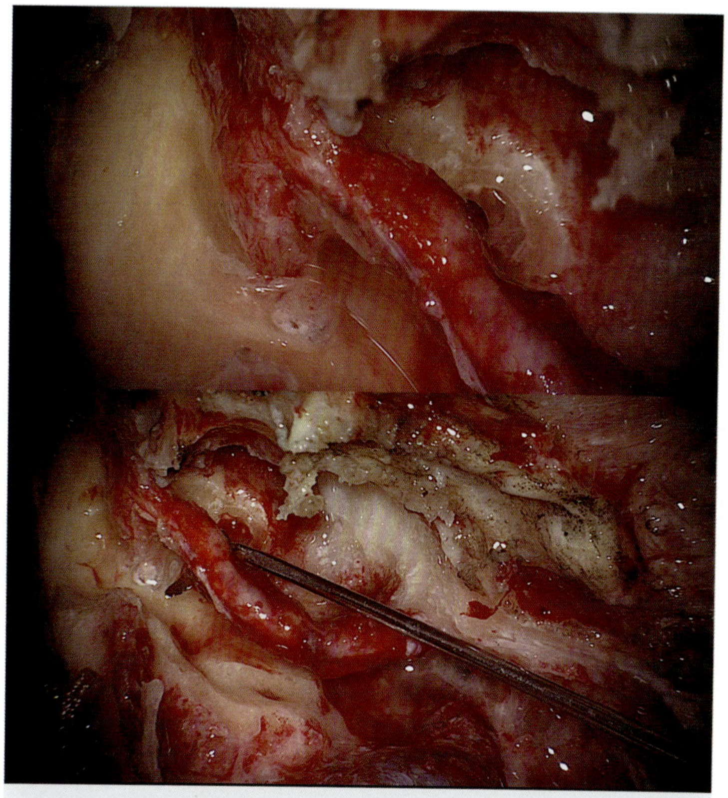

Fig. 4.26 A curved dissector is used to check the presence of residual disease around the facial nerve during a transotic approach.

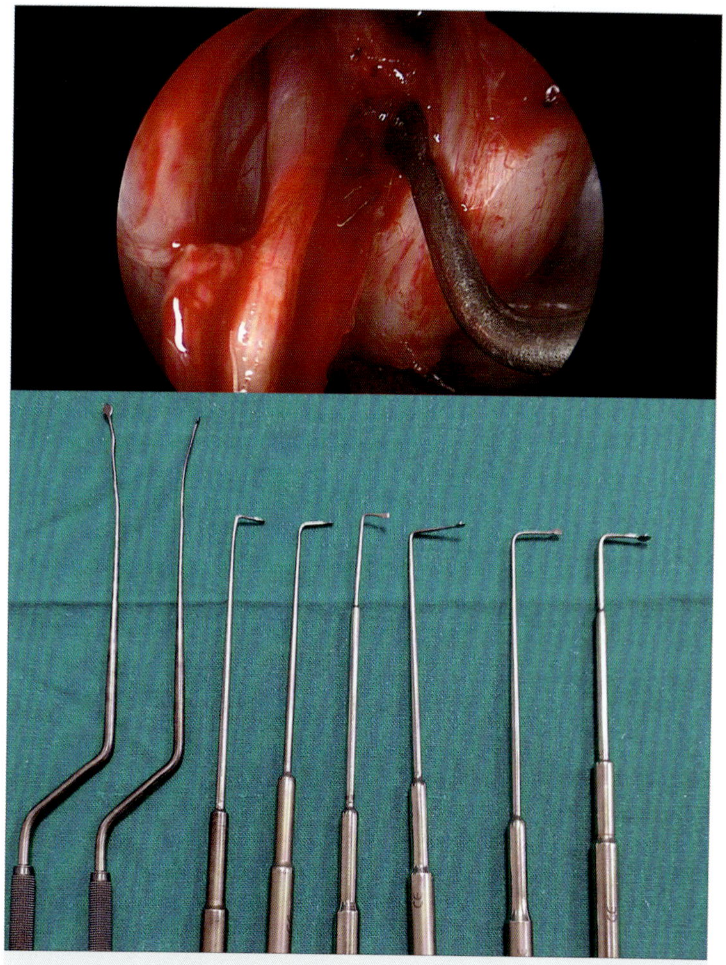

Fig. 4.27 Long and curved dissectors, useful especially to work on the internal auditory canal (IAC) under endoscopic view during a retrosigmoid approach.

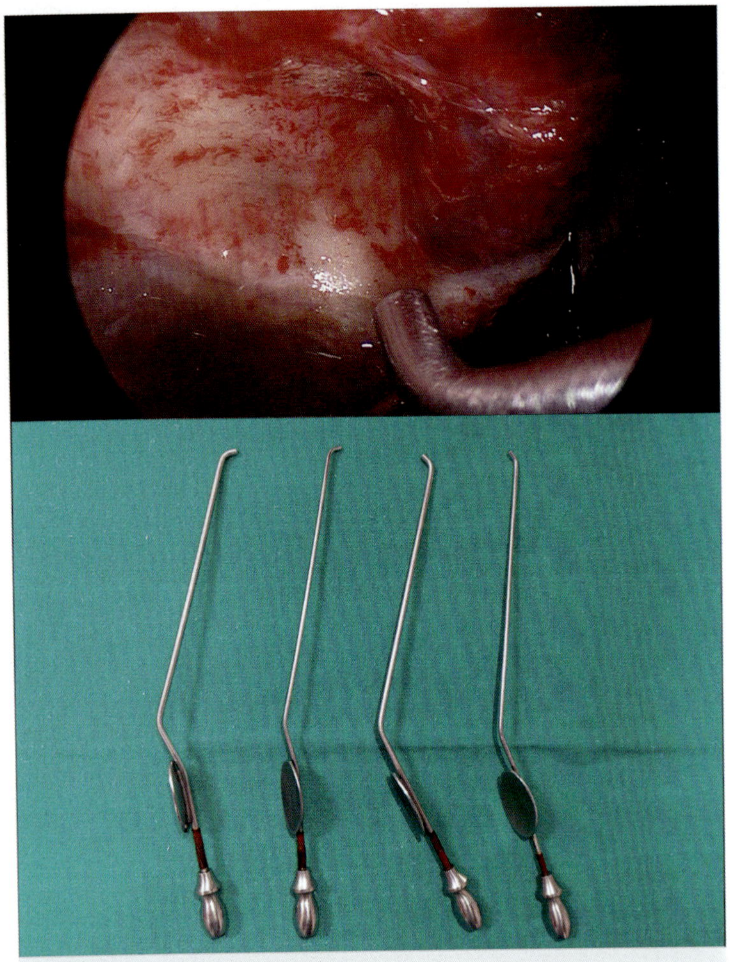

Fig. 4.28 Set of curved suction instruments.

Suggested Readings

Badr-El-Dine M, El-Garem HF, Talaat AM, Magnan J. Endoscopically assisted minimally invasive microvascular decompression of hemifacial spasm. Otol Neurotol. 2002; 23(2):122–128

Badr-El-Dine M, James AL, Panetti G, Marchioni D, Presutti L, Nogueira JF. Instrumentation and technologies in endoscopic ear surgery. Otolaryngol Clin North Am. 2013; 46(2):211–225

Garneau JC, Laitman BM, Cosetti MK, Hadjipanayis C, Wanna G. The use of the exoscope in lateral skull base surgery: advantages and limitations. Otol Neurotol. 2019; 40(2):236–240

Marchioni D, Alicandri-Ciufelli M, Rubini A, Presutti L. Endoscopic transcanal corridors to the lateral skull base: initial experiences. Laryngoscope. 2015; 125 Suppl 5:S1–S13

Marchioni D, Carner M, Rubini A, et al. The fully endoscopic acoustic neuroma surgery. Otolaryngol Clin North Am. 2016; 49(5):1227–1236

Marchioni D, Carner M, Soloperto D, et al. Expanded transcanal transpromontorial approach: a novel surgical technique for cerebellopontine angle vestibular schwannoma removal. Otolaryngol Head Neck Surg. 2018; 158(4):710–715

Marchioni D, De Rossi S, Soloperto D, Presutti L, Sacchetto L, Rubini A. Intralabyrinthine schwannomas: a new surgical treatment. Eur Arch Otorhinolaryngol. 2018; 275(5):1095–1102

Marchioni D, Gazzini L, Boaria F, Pinna G, Masotto B, Rubini A. Is endoscopic inspection necessary to detect residual disease in acoustic neuroma surgery? Eur Arch Otorhinolaryngol. 2019; 276(8):2155–2163

Marchioni D, Rubini A, Nogueira JF, Isaacson B, Presutti L. Transcanal endoscopic approach to lesions of the suprageniculate ganglion fossa. Auris Nasus Larynx. 2018; 45(1):57–65

Marchioni D, Soloperto D, Rubini A, Nogueira JF, Badr-El-Dine M, Presutti L. Endoscopic facial nerve surgery. Otolaryngol Clin North Am. 2016; 49(5):1173–1187

Presutti L, Alicandri-Ciufelli M, Rubini A, Gioacchini FM, Marchioni D. Combined lateral microscopic/endoscopic approaches to petrous apex lesions: pilot clinical experiences. Ann Otol Rhinol Laryngol. 2014; 123(8):550–559

Piezosurgery medical manufactured by Mectron medical technology. Peizosurgery S.R.L., Via Portobello 12, 16039 Sestri Levante (GE), Italy. www.piezosurgery.com

VESALIUS® MC bipolar coagulation/cutting device. By Telea Electronic Engineering. Via Leonardo Da Vinci, 13 – 36066 Sandrigo – Vicenza – Italy. www.vesalius.it; www.teleamedical.com

Chapter 5

Radiologic Assessment in Lateral Skull Base Surgery

5

5 Radiologic Assessment in Lateral Skull Base Surgery

Davide Soloperto, Elisa Ciceri, and Daniele Marchioni

Abstract

The skull base forms the floor of the cranial cavity that separates the brain from the facial structures and the suprahyoid neck. The skull base anatomy is complex and it is not directly accessible for clinical evaluation. Imaging plays a vital role in the diagnosis of certain pathologies, preoperative staging of neoplasms, defining tumor extension and spread, surgical approach planning, detecting tumor recurrences, and follow-up. High-resolution computed tomography (CT) and standard T1- and T2-weighted sequences supplemented with gadolinium in characterizing skull base lesions based on their tissue characteristics and anatomical location are the mainstay in a radiological approach toward skull base lesions. F-fluoro-deoxyglucose positron emission tomography (PET) or PET-CT is often performed to assess the metabolic activity of skull base lesions and to locate the primary tumor or other similar lesions located in areas other than the skull base. Angiography, carotid occlusion test, and carotid stenting are sometimes performed, in combination or in isolation, for the management of head and neck lesions with carotid encasement. Skull base lesions may originate within the skull base or involve it by growth from either the intracranial dura or extracranial structures. A number of challenging tumors and tumor-like non-neoplastic lesions, with different cell types, can thus affect the skull base, so an accurate radiological assessment is mandatory for the correct diagnostic work-up and for the surgical choice.

Keywords: lateral skull base, CT scan, DWI sequences, carotid embolization, radiologic assessment

5.1 Introduction

5.1.1 Anatomy of Lateral Skull Base

The skull base forms the floor of the cranial cavity that separates the brain from the facial structures and suprahyoid neck. The skull base anatomy is complex and it is not directly accessible for clinical evaluation. Imaging plays a vital role in diagnosing certain pathologies, preoperative staging of neoplasms, defining tumor extension and spread, surgical approach planning, detecting tumor recurrences, and during follow-up. The anterior margin of the posterior skull base is formed by the posterior surface of the clivus. The clivus stems from the fusion of the basisphenoid and basioccipital bones. The lateral portion of posterior skull base is formed by the posterior surface of the petrous temporal bone superiorly and the condylar part of the occipital bone inferiorly. The mastoid temporal bone and the squamous occipital bone form the posterior portion of the posterior skull base. The petrous pyramid represents a barrier separating the posterior fossa from the posterolateral extracranial skull base as well as from the petroclival area. The jugular foramen (JF) is seen at the posterior end of petro-occipital suture. Anteriorly the caroticojugular spine separates the JF from the inferior carotid opening. Along the medial portion, an osseous bony bar called the jugular tubercle separates the JF from the hypoglossal canal, which holds the hypoglossal nerve. A fibrous or bony septum divides the JF into anteromedial the pars nervosa and posterolateral pars vascularis. Pars nervosa is smaller and more consistent in size, and holds the IX cranial nerve (glossopharyngeal nerve) with its tympanic branch (Jacobson's nerve) and the inferior petrosal sinus. The pars vascularis is larger and more variable in size, holding the internal jugular vein (IJV), the X cranial nerve (vagus nerve) with its auricular branch (Arnold's nerve), the XI cranial nerve (accessory nerve), and the posterior meningeal artery. The appearance of the JF is anatomically variable, and sometimes both IX and X cranial nerves go through the pars nervosa.

5.2 General Considerations about CT and MRI in Lateral Skull Base

High-resolution computed tomography (HRCT) and standard T1- and T2-weighted sequences supplemented with gadolinium in characterizing skull base lesions based on their tissue characteristics and anatomical location are the mainstay in radiological approach toward skull base lesions. They represent the main choice for evaluation of skull base anatomy and pathology and, due to its complex anatomy and close relationship with osseous structures, skull base lesions are often evaluated with both computed tomography (CT) and magnetic resonance imaging (MRI) for diagnostic and preoperative planning purposes, especially when planning the lesion resection and best surgical approach. Accurate radiologic assessment is mandatory to properly investigate the lesion, understand its nature, make the diagnosis, and plan the best surgical management for the patient. CT is the best choice in defining the bony anatomy of the skull base and depicting the thin cortical margins of skull base neurovascular foramina. In general, it is used to detect bony involvement, such us erosion, reactive bone formation, sclerosis, fibro-osseous skull base lesions, and calcification. Slow-growing lesions that do not infiltrate the bone tend to demonstrate smooth cortical expansion and bone remodeling with preservation of the bony cortex, whereas aggressive tumors or infections typically infiltrate the bone, extensively destroying the adjoining bony cortex. CT scan is also the gold standard technique for the evaluation of base skull fractures and for the detection of cerebrospinal fluid (CSF) leak. With multislice CT scanners, it is possible to acquire 0.5- to 0.6-mm-thin base skull sections and perform a multiplanar reconstruction. The images are reviewed using a bone window and a soft tissue algorithm. Postcontrast evaluation may be performed especially when a vascular mass is suspected. Another use of CT in the skull base is in the identification of bony defects in the evaluation of CSF leaks. Interactive multiplanar evaluation (axial, coronal, sagittal, and oblique planes) is important to identify and correctly describe osseous defects in the evaluation of CSF leaks. In addition to providing important characterization of the bony structures, CT can also provide invaluable information about the relationship of a lesion with the adjacent vascular structures through computed tomography angiography (CTA); in particular for the evaluation of the petrous, cavernous, and supraclinoid internal carotid artery (ICA), it is very important in the preoperative planning for tumors that invade the cavernous sinus. In the postoperative follow-up, HRCT is an excellent tool for evaluating postoperative middle ear and mastoid as it provides a striking contrast between residual or recurrent debris and the air-containing cavity.

Being the modality with better soft tissue resolution, MRI allows precise assessment of the morphology of a lesion and its relation with the surrounding structures. MRI is also superior in the evaluation of vascular invasion, intracranial extension, and for retrocochlear pathologies. MRI is a problem-solving device in many situations where CT and other techniques cannot give the required information. MRI with postcontrast evaluation is usually performed for evaluation of skull base lesions and, for most tumors, for example neuromas, it is the gold standard for the diagnosis. MRI shows intracranial extent (dural, leptomeningeal, and brain parenchyma invasion), perineural and perivascular spread, and bone marrow involvement. Axial and coronal images using fast spin echo T1- and T2-weighted images should be obtained with fat-suppressed, postcontrast images using a smaller field of view with a slice thickness of 3 mm. Additional short-tau inversion recovery (STIR) images are obtained. STIR images have a better fat suppression but take a longer time and are susceptible to pulsatile flow artifacts. Gradient echo T2 images may be useful to demonstrate paramagnetic substances, such as calcifications, blood degradation products, or melanin within a lesion. Diffusion-weighted imaging (DWI) can be used as a noninvasive problem-solving tool in the characterization of skull base lesions, evaluation of pathological grading, and monitoring treatment effects, especially in differentiating malignant tumors from benign ones based on apparent diffusion coefficient (ADC) values. Diffusion imaging has a well-established role in central nervous system (CNS) imaging, and it is the subject of active research for other parts of the body. DWI and ADC have increasingly been used to characterize head and neck tumors and monitor response to treatment. Standard DWI provides single-shot echo-planar imaging (ss-EPI) which is susceptible to artifacts and prone to relatively low resolution at the tissue–air interface such as at the skull base. MRI is also strongly recommended when a postoperative defect is detected in the region of the tegmen or sinus plate. A soft tissue mass protruding through a defect in the tegmen tympani may represent a meningocele or meningoencephalocele. MRI easily identifies the presence or absence of brain tissue within the mass and confirms the contiguity of the mass with adjacent brain. MRI provides crucial information regarding cerebellum and sigmoid sinus in patients with bony defects (see ▶ Fig. 5.1, ▶ Fig. 5.2, ▶ Fig. 5.3).

F-fluoro-deoxyglucose positron emission tomography (PET) or PET-CT is often performed to assess the metabolic activity of skull base lesions and to locate the primary tumor or other similar lesions located in areas other than the skull base. Recurrence and postsurgical fibrosis can easily be differentiated from the primary tumor. However, intense physiological uptake by the brain is a drawback in the evaluation of base skull lesions. Octreotide scintigraphy imaging has been applied for the diagnosis of head and

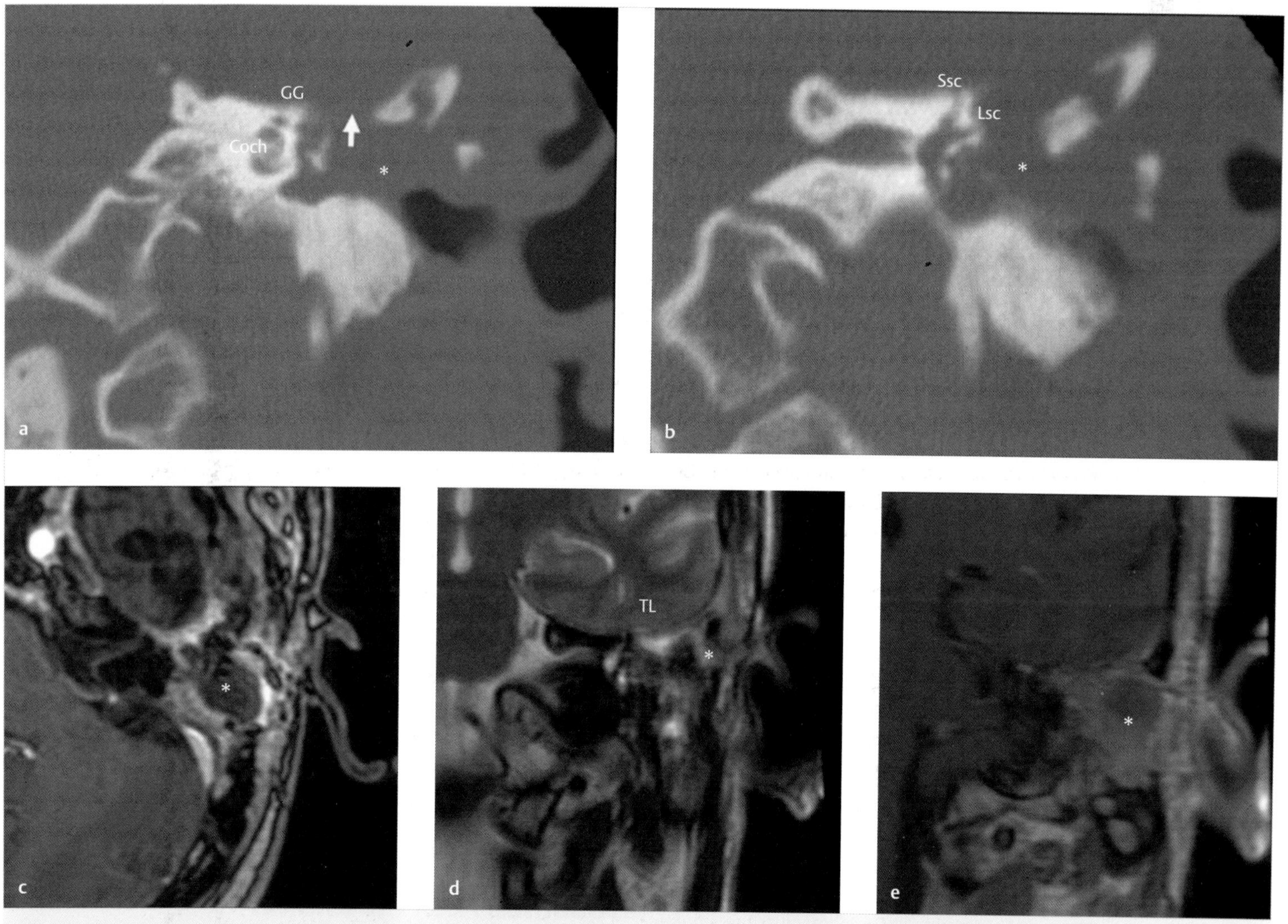

Fig. 5.1 Left extended cholesteatoma, involving the middle ear and the mastoid. **(a)** Erosion of the floor of the middle cranial fossa (*white arrow*). **(b)** Extension into the mastoid, with bone erosion *. **(c–e)** Magnetic resonance imaging (MRI) appearance, with no intradural extension *. *Coch: cochlea; GG: geniculate ganglion; Lsc: lateral semicircular canal; Ssc: superior semicircular canal; TL: temporal lobe.*

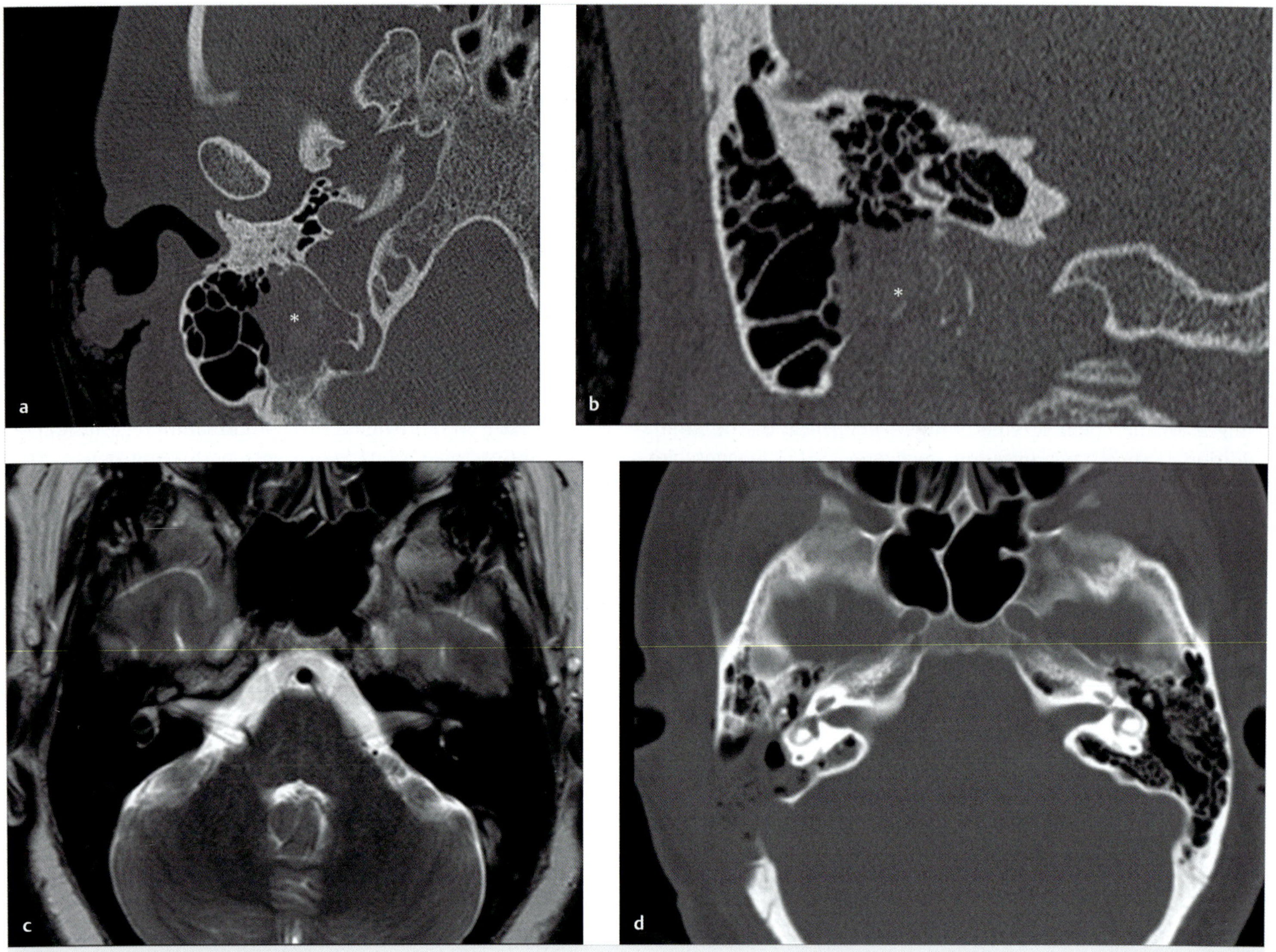

Fig. 5.2 Computed tomography (CT) scan showing right mastoid opacity, located in the retrofacial area. **(a, b)** Mass located near the styloid bone *. **(c)** No evidence on magnetic resonance imaging (MRI) T2 sequence. **(d)** Postoperative CT scan, after a retrolabyrinthine approach.

neck neuroendocrine tumors (NETs) including paragangliomas, Merkel cell carcinomas, medullary thyroid carcinomas, and esthesioneuroblastomas, as well as recurrent paragangliomas. However, a newer generation of radiotracers has been developed, and these more specific molecular markers allow targeted molecular imaging. In addition, the use of positron-emitting radiotracers allows higher resolution images that can easily be matched with CT to create high-quality maps.

Angiography, carotid occlusion test, and carotid stenting are sometimes performed, in combination or individually, for the management of head and neck lesions with carotid encasement (see ▶ Fig. 5.4, ▶ Fig. 5.5). Angiography provides complementary diagnostic information by showing the highly vascular nature of these lesions, usually combined with embolization in the preoperative period. It allows identification of dominant feeding vessels that can then be embolized to reduce blood loss during surgical removal, properly identifying contralateral venous system patency and demonstrating the presence of major venous sinus occlusion on the part of the tumor. Studies have shown decreased operative time and intraoperative blood loss with preoperative embolization of jugular paragangliomas, and preoperative embolization facilitates complete resection of vascular tumors such as jugular paragangliomas or carotid paragangliomas (see ▶ Fig. 5.6).

5.3 Lateral Skull Base Lesions

Skull base lesions may originate within the skull base or involve it after growing from either the intracranial dura or extracranial structures. A number of tumors and tumor-like non-neoplastic lesions, with different cell types, can thus affect the skull base. From a radiological point of view, we can classify lesions spreading into lateral skull base as:

- Lesions involving external auditory canal (EAC), middle ear, and mastoid;
- Lesions involving the internal auditory canal (IAC) and cerebellopontine angle (CPA);
- Lesions involving the JF;
- Lesions involving the petrous apex.

5.3.1 Lesions Involving External Auditory Canal (EAC), Middle Ear, and Mastoid

Squamous Cell Carcinoma

Squamous cell carcinoma (SCC) can spread from the EAC or can originate from the middle ear. It represents the most common

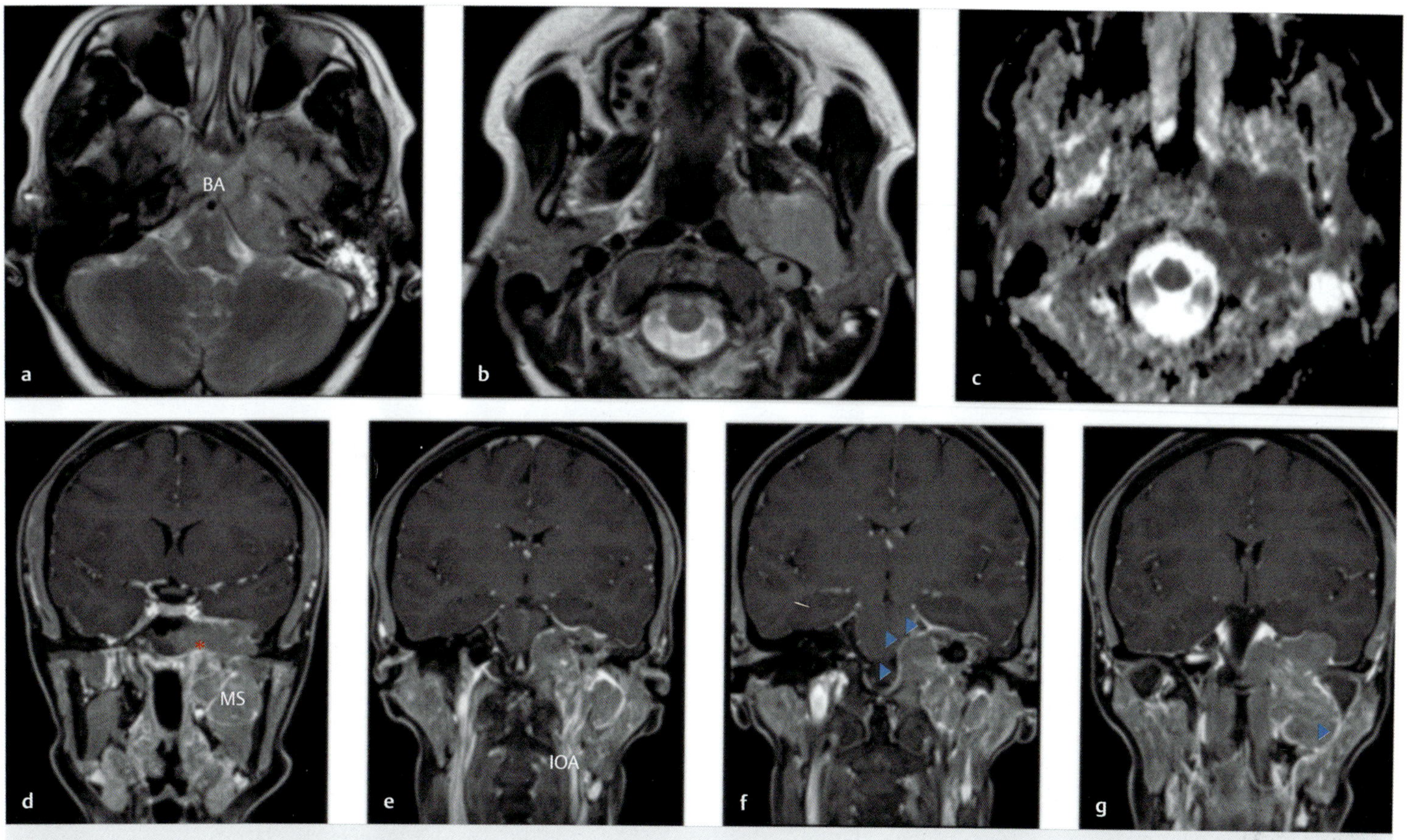

Fig. 5.3 Magnetic resonance imaging (MRI) appearance of neuroesthesioblastoma. **(a, b)** T2 sequences show huge lesion, involving all lateral skull base and neck. **(c)** Diffusion sequence with apparent diffusion coefficient (ADC). **(d–g)** T1 with contrast shows involvement of the cavernous sinus (* in d), compression of the brainstem (*light blue triangles in f*), and masticatory space infiltration (*light blue triangle in g*). *BA: basilar artery; ICA: internal carotid artery; MS: masticatory space.*

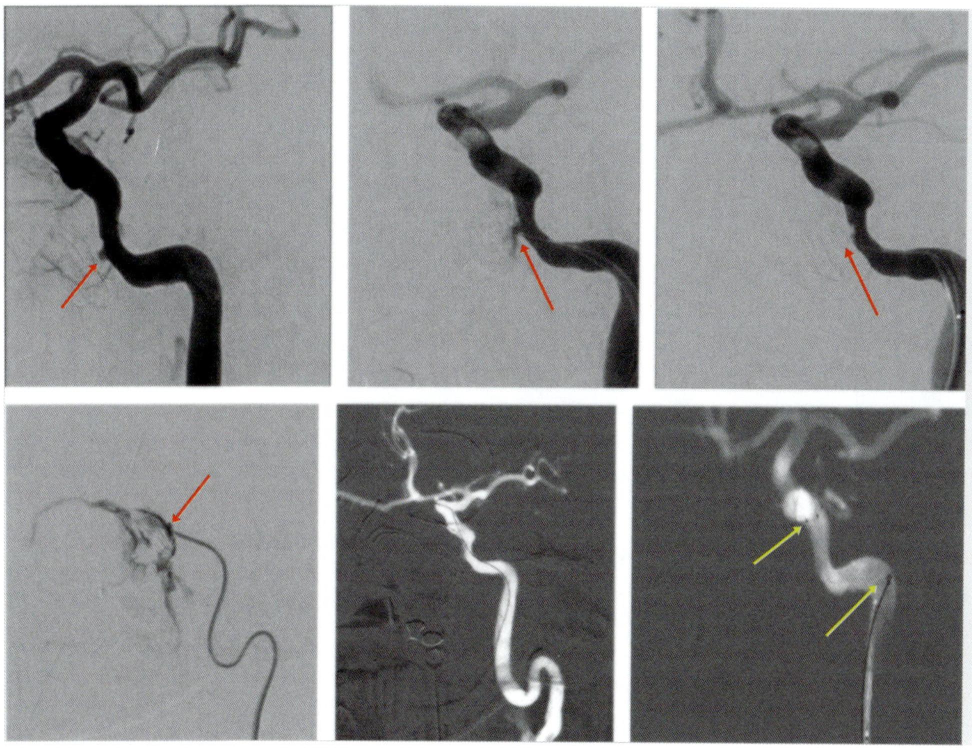

Fig. 5.4 Angiography showing left internal carotid artery (ICA) damage (*red arrow*). Histoacryl glue application and Nitinol stenting to stop the bleeding (*yellow arrows*).

malignant cell type in that location. An association between the middle ear SCC and chronic otitis media and prior radiation are reported as important predisposing factors. Patients are typically older, showing otalgia and otorrhea. SCC is aggressive and locally infiltrative, with the potential to extend intracranially. Tumor spread is multidirectional and may exploit existing anatomic defects, such as the fissures of Santorini, the petrosquamous suture, and the foramen of Huschke (foramen tympanicum), resulting in the extension to the temporomandibular joint (TMJ) and parotid gland without associated bony

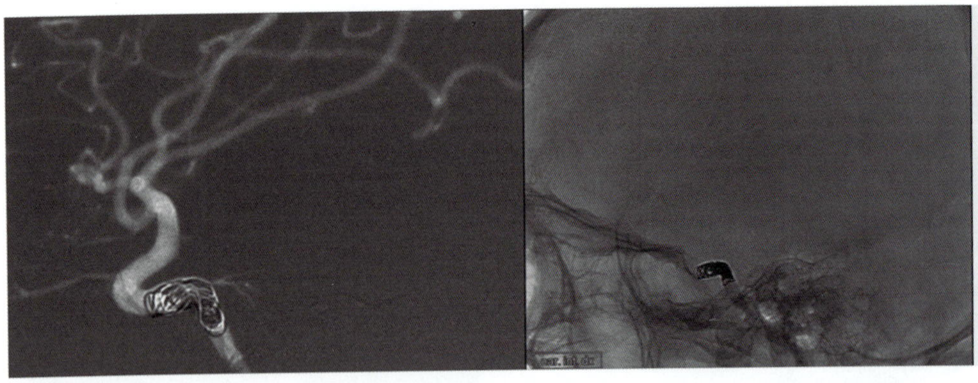

Fig. 5.5 Left internal carotid artery (ICA) closure with coils.

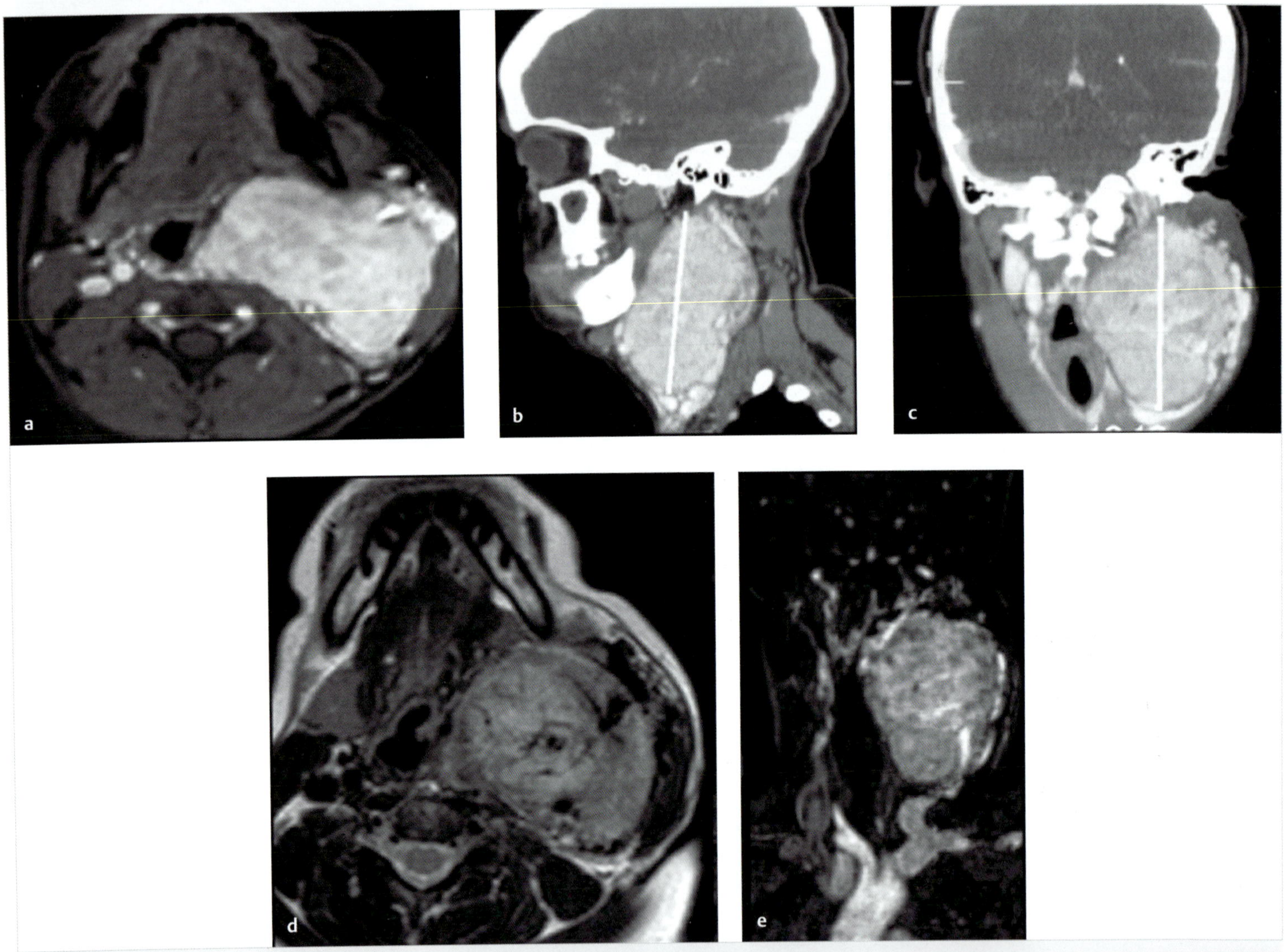

Fig. 5.6 Magnetic resonance imaging (MRI) **(a, d, e)** and computed tomography (CT) **(b, c)** Left carotid paraganglioma. **(d, e)** MRI axial view and coronal view. **(b, c)** Note the extension to the skull base and the compression of the airways.

erosion. A medial extension can lead to middle ear, otic capsule, or eustachian tube involvement. A posterior extension results in mastoid invasion. A craniocaudal extension leads to intracranial, facial nerve, and JF involvement, which is a poor prognostic factor. Nodal metastasis occurs in 10 to 20% of cases, beginning with parotid and periauricular nodes. CT is helpful for delineating the extent of bone destruction, but soft tissue extent is better assessed by MRI, which also allows for a differentiation between tumor tissue and effusion. Nevertheless, imaging is nonspecific, and it may be difficult to differentiate malignant external otitis from carcinoma; tissue biopsy is mandatory for correct diagnosis (see ▶ Fig. 5.7 and ▶ Fig. 5.8).

Middle Ear Cholesteatoma

Cholesteatoma can be a congenital or acquired lesion of the middle ear. Acquired cholesteatoma is subdivided into primary and secondary cholesteatomas:

- Primary, for retraction of pars flaccida or pars tensa;
- Secondary, following eardrum perforation, trauma, or iatrogenic.

These lesions don't usually spread into the lateral skull base, but in advanced stages, they can require a surgical management of the middle and posterior fossa dura, bone repair of the tegmen tympani and antri or the surgical management of the lateral skull

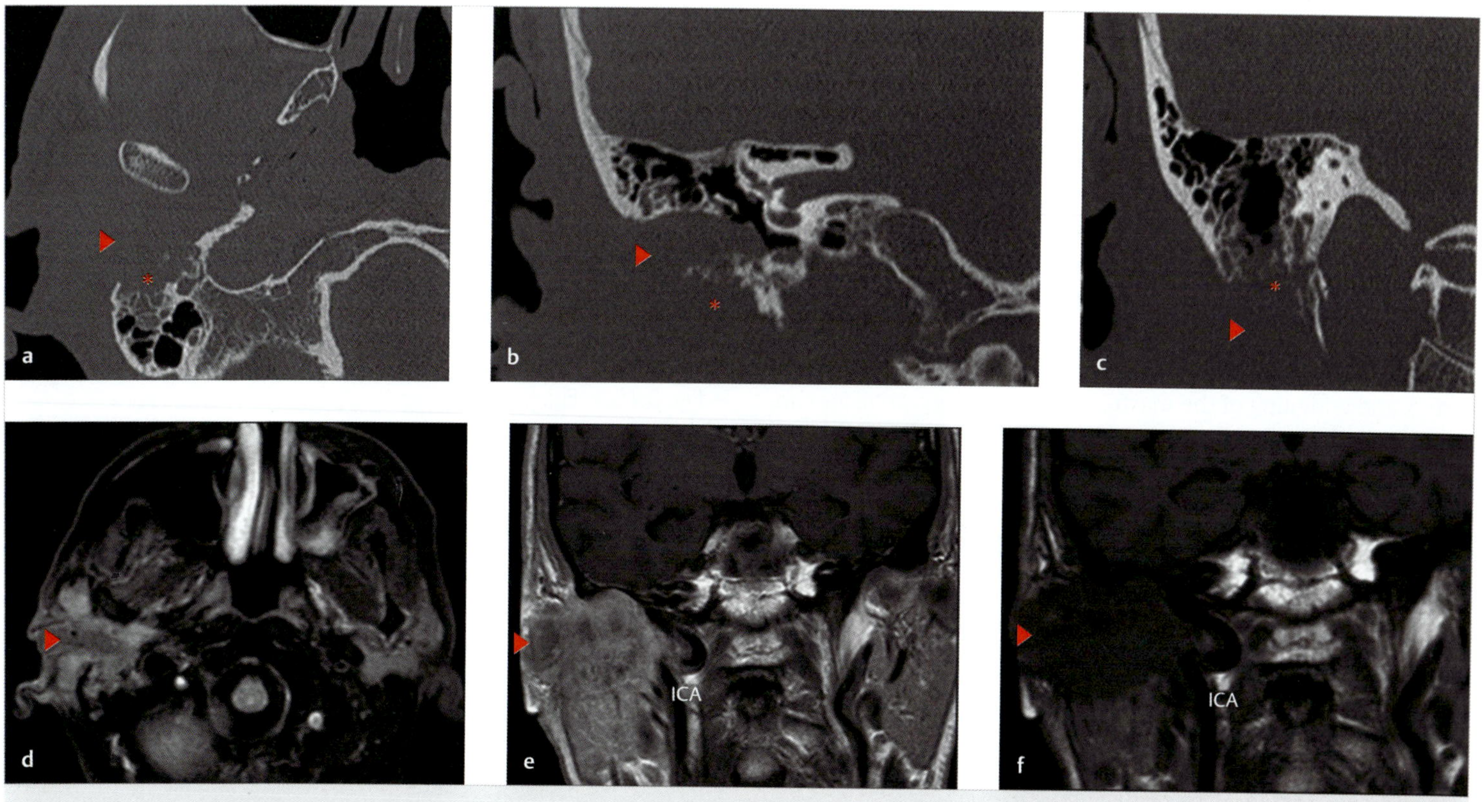

Fig. 5.7 Computed tomography (CT) and magnetic resonance imaging (MRI) showing a right parotid adenocarcinoma (*). **(a–c)** Bone erosion is shown in axial and coronal views (*red triangle*). **(d–f)** MRI better shows the spread of the pathology in different sequences (*red triangle*). ICA: internal carotid artery.

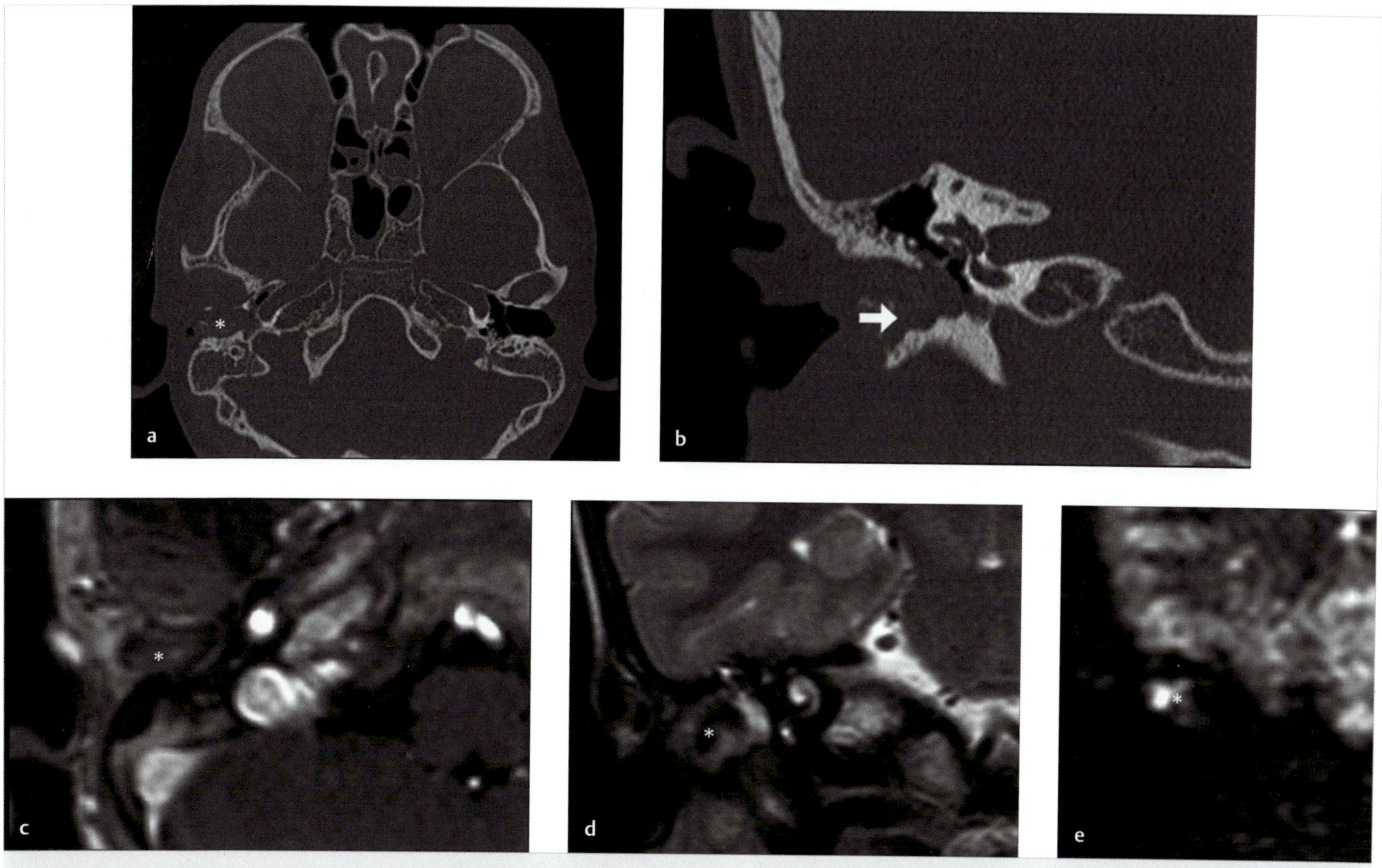

Fig. 5.8 Right pediatric external auditory canal (EAC) cholesteatoma (*). **(a, b)** Computed tomography (CT) scan of axial and coronal views of the cholesteatoma (*). Note the erosion of the inferior canal wall (*white arrow*). **(c–e)** Axial, coronal, and diffusion-weighted sequences.

base when there is an extension of the pathology in the inner ear (see the section Petrous Bone Cholesteatoma). It can cause progressive local destruction with otorrhea, hearing loss, and vertigo if left untreated. Bone erosion being the most important radiological sign of the presence of cholesteatoma, HRCT is usually the main imaging method. Since its introduction in the early 1980s, HRCT of the temporal bone has been the gold standard for imaging cholesteatoma. On CT scan, a nondependent soft tissue, typically with involvement of the epitympanum and Prussak's space, a blunting of the scutum (typically seen in primary acquired attic cholesteatoma), erosion of the ossicles (typically the malleus and incus), and widening of the mastoid aditus are suggestive for cholesteatoma. When ossicular or mastoid bony erosion is seen in association with a soft tissue mass, HRCT can identify a cholesteatoma with specificity between 80 and 90%. Cholesteatoma can also involve other structures, often in asymptomatic patients, eroding the facial nerve canal, the tegmen tympani, the lateral semicircular canal, the sigmoid plate, or the posterosuperior EAC. HRCT is also helpful in order to check the anatomy, revealing specific patterns of pneumatization and aeration or variability in the position of the sigmoid sinus or tegmen, which may help surgical planning by mapping the extent of the disease, in order to plan a transcanal endoscopic or combined approach. Because HRCT doesn't differentiate among soft tissue densities in the temporal bone, sometimes coexisting fluid and inflammation with debris, the addition of MRI, supplemented with nonechoplanar DWI, is valuable in the temporal bone. Generally, MRI is used to better distinguish the recurrence/residual disease in the postoperative follow-up, because recurrent or residual cholesteatoma shows restricted diffusion, while granulation tissue does not, or to investigate intracranial complications, such us temporal abscess or meningocele/meningoencephalocele. On MRI, cholesteatoma appears with intermediate signal on T1-weighted imaging, with high signal on T2-weighted imaging, nonenhancing or a rim-enhancing on delayed contrast enhanced, with high signal on DWI, and with low signal on the ADC map (see ▶ Fig. 5.9, ▶ Fig. 5.10, ▶ Fig. 5.11, ▶ Fig. 5.12, ▶ Fig. 5.13, ▶ Fig. 5.14, ▶ Fig. 5.15, ▶ Fig. 5.16).

Intratemporal Facial Nerve Schwannoma/ Hemangioma

Intratemporal facial nerve schwannoma (FNS) represents less than 1% of temporal bone tumors. According to the tract of the nerve considered, they can be divided into:

- Tympanic and mastoid FNS tract;
- Geniculate ganglion FNS tract;
- Labyrinthic, IAC, and CPA FNS tract.

FNS is the most common schwannoma found in the middle ear, affecting the tympanic segment as a lobulated middle ear mass, resulting in ossicular displacement or erosion leading to

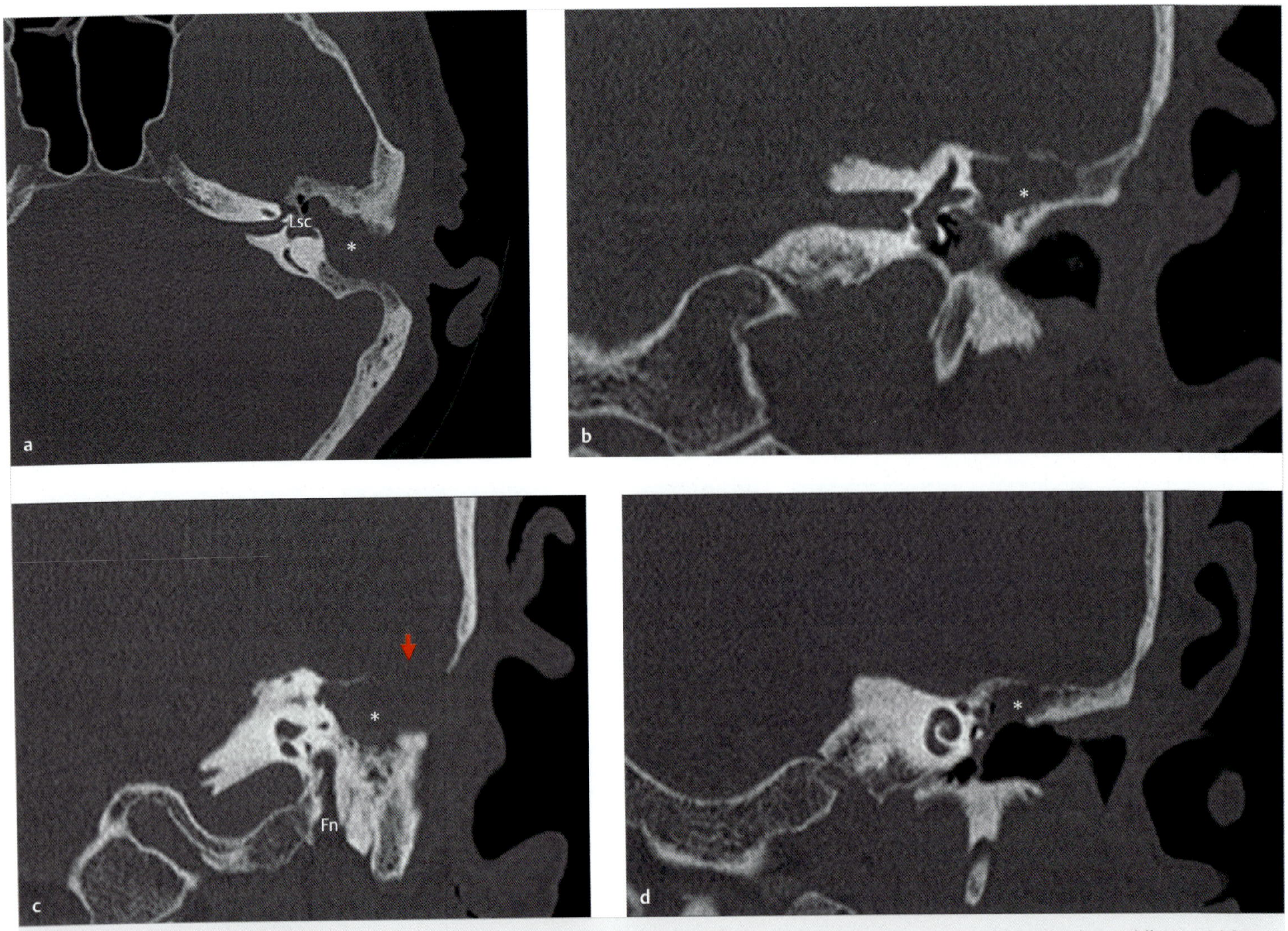

Fig. 5.9 Computed tomography (CT) scan of left cholesteatoma (*). **(a–c)** Mastoid extension (*), with exposure of bone in the middle cranial fossa floor (*red arrow*). **(d)** Cholesteatoma in the geniculate ganglion area (*). Fn: facial nerve mastoid tract; Lsc: lateral semicircular canal.

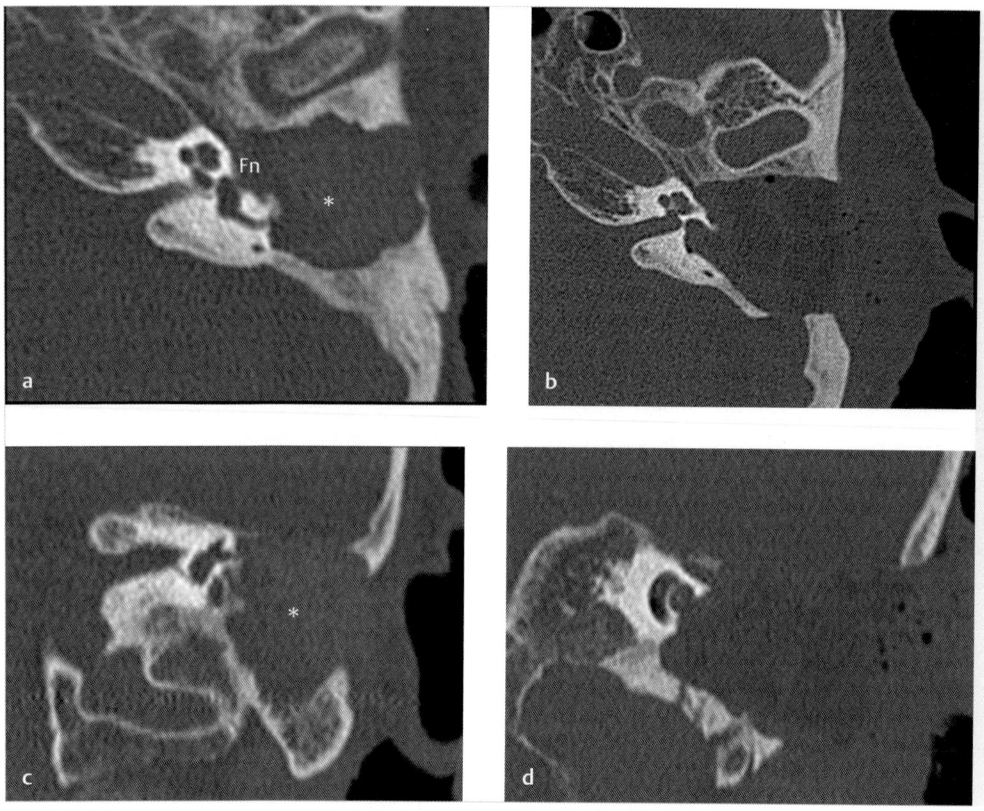

Fig. 5.10 Left cholesteatoma, preoperative and postoperative radiologic aspect after subtotal petrosectomy. **(a, b)** Preoperative and postoperative axial views. **(c, d)** Preoperative and postoperative coronal views. Fn: facial nerve; *: cholesteatoma.

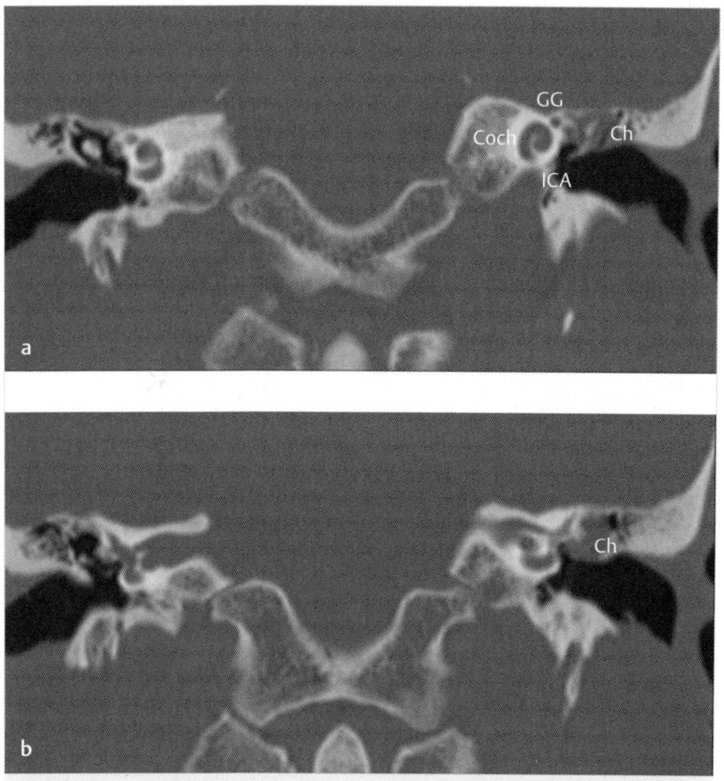

Fig. 5.11 Left epitympanic cholesteatoma. On computed tomography (CT) scan, no tegmen tympani erosion. **(a, b)** Coronal view, showing the left epitympanic cholesteatoma. *Ch: cholesteatoma; Coch: cochlea; GG: geniculate ganglion; ICA: internal carotid artery.*

conductive hearing loss. FNS within the mastoid segment often has irregular bone margins due to the fact that the tumor breaks into mastoid air cells and it may simulate an aggressive lesion. Schwannomas may also arise from the chorda tympani and present as a middle ear mass. Schwannomas cause smooth expansion of the facial canal causing sharply defined bony margins. Geniculate ganglion lesions are better seen on CT than noncontrast MRI. These may show intratumoral bony spicules and irregular margins, best seen on CT. They are isointense to mildly hyperintense on T1-weighted images and markedly hyperintense on T2-weighted images, more than the typical schwannoma. Nonhomogeneous signal intensities corresponding to bony spicules may be seen on MRI. Thin sections and use of contrast-enhanced MRI may improve the MRI results. Facial nerve hemangiomas (FNHs) are rare benign tumors arising from the venous plexus surrounding the facial nerve, most often arising from the region of the geniculate ganglion, due to its rich capillary plexus. This lesion is associated with a more rapid onset of sensorineural hearing loss (SNHL) (for IAC lesions) and facial nerve paresis (for geniculate ganglion lesions) compared to vestibular schwannoma (VS). The bony margins of the lesion are typically irregular and enhancement is considerable but heterogeneous. Intratumoral bone spicules may be identified on CT and MRI (leading to the term "ossifying hemangioma"). Surgical management of these tumors is controversial. Geniculate ganglion FNS grows slowly, but its progression can involve cranial fossae and petrous apex.

"Wait and scan" strategy is suggested as the first choice when normal facial nerve function is shown. However, in case of complete facial palsy, huge dimensions, or fast growth with dural extension, a surgical approach is preferred, with nerve sacrifice and cable graft repair. The goal of surgery is complete tumor removal with restoration of the facial nerve function and preservation of hearing, wherever possible. The most used approches are the translabyrinthine, when hearing loss is present, or/and middle cranial fossa approaches combined with trans-mastoid approach when hearing is normal. A short time ago, an endoscopic transcanal suprageniculate approach to remove geniculate ganglion tumor was described; a great auricular nerve graft was used to reconnect interrupted nerve segments (see Chapter 10; also see ▶ Fig. 5.17 and ▶ Fig. 5.18).

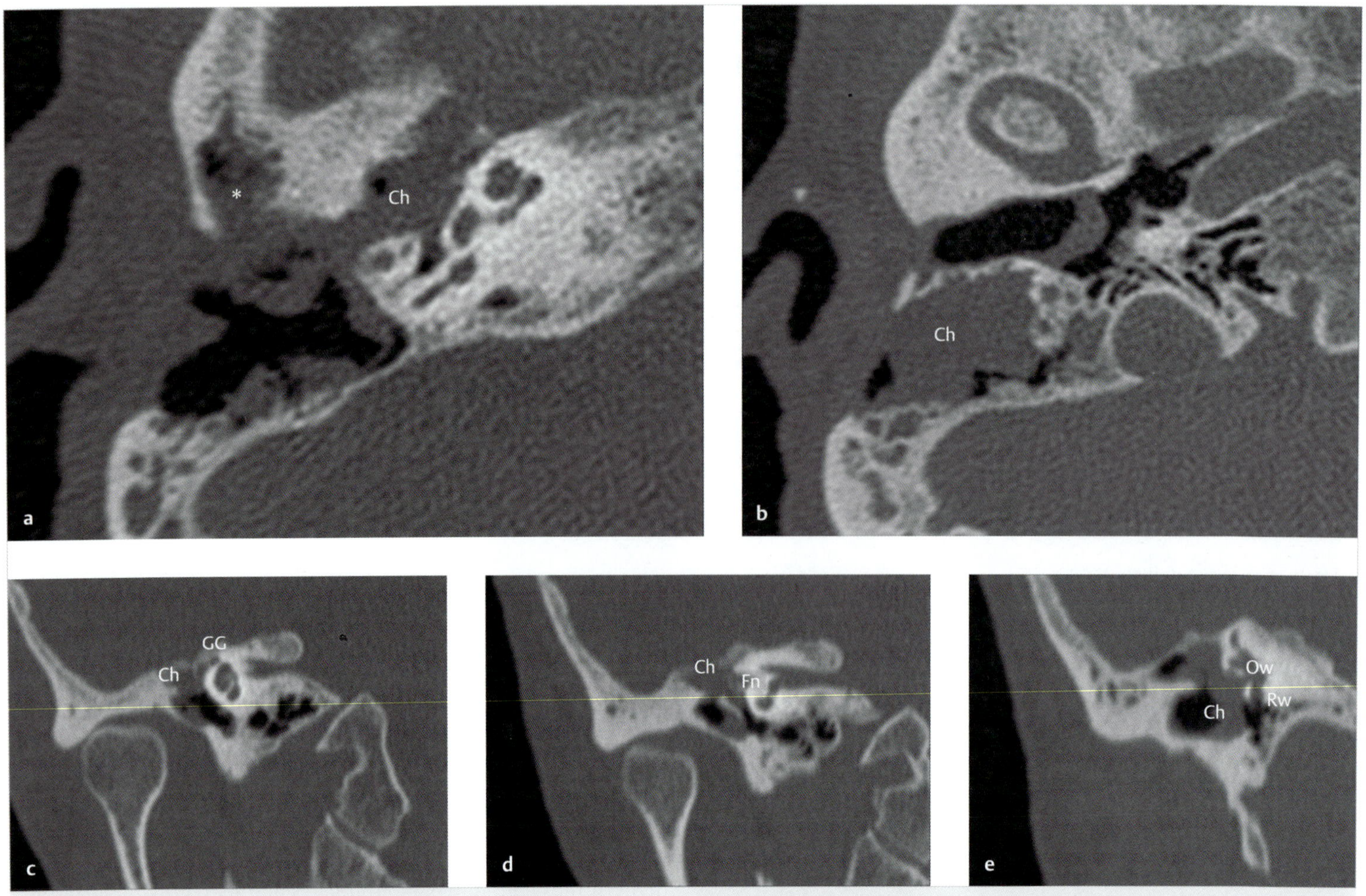

Fig. 5.12 Right cholesteatoma with anterior and mastoid extension. **(a, b)** Computed tomography (CT) scan, axial view (*: anterior extension to zygomatic arch). **(c–e)** CT scan, coronal view. *Ch: cholesteatoma; Fn: facial nerve; GG: geniculate ganglion; Ow: oval window; Rw: round window.*

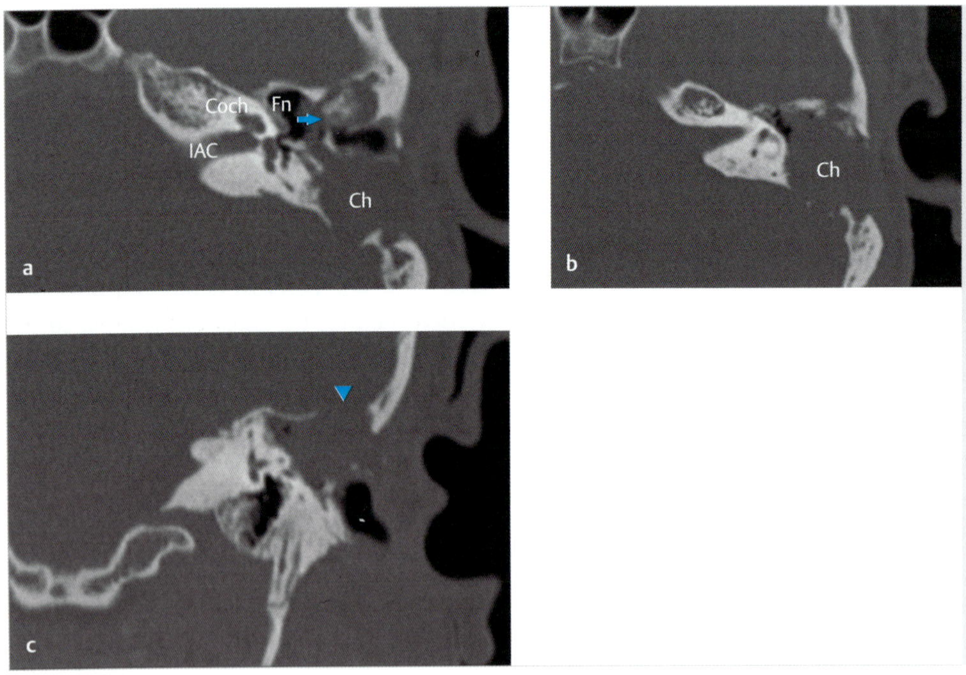

Fig. 5.13 Computed tomography (CT) scan of left cholesteatoma. **(a)** Temporomandibular joint erosion (*light blue arrow*); **(b, c)** Huge mastoid extension, with erosion in the sigmoid sinus and middle fossa area (*light blue triangle*). *Ch: cholesteatoma; Coch: cochlea; Fn: facial nerve; IAC: internal auditory canal.*

Middle Ear and Mastoid Paraganglioma

Head and neck paragangliomas are tumors arising from specialized neural crest cells. Prominent locations are the carotid body along with the vagal, jugular, and tympanic glomus. For petrous bone paragangliomas, Fisch originally classified tympano-jugular paragangliomas into classes A, B, C, and D, according to their location and extension based on HRCT examination (see ▶ Fig. 5.19):

- A: Paragangliomas that arise along the tympanic plexus on the promontory
- B: Paragangliomas with invasion of the hypotympanum; intact cortical bone over jugular bulb

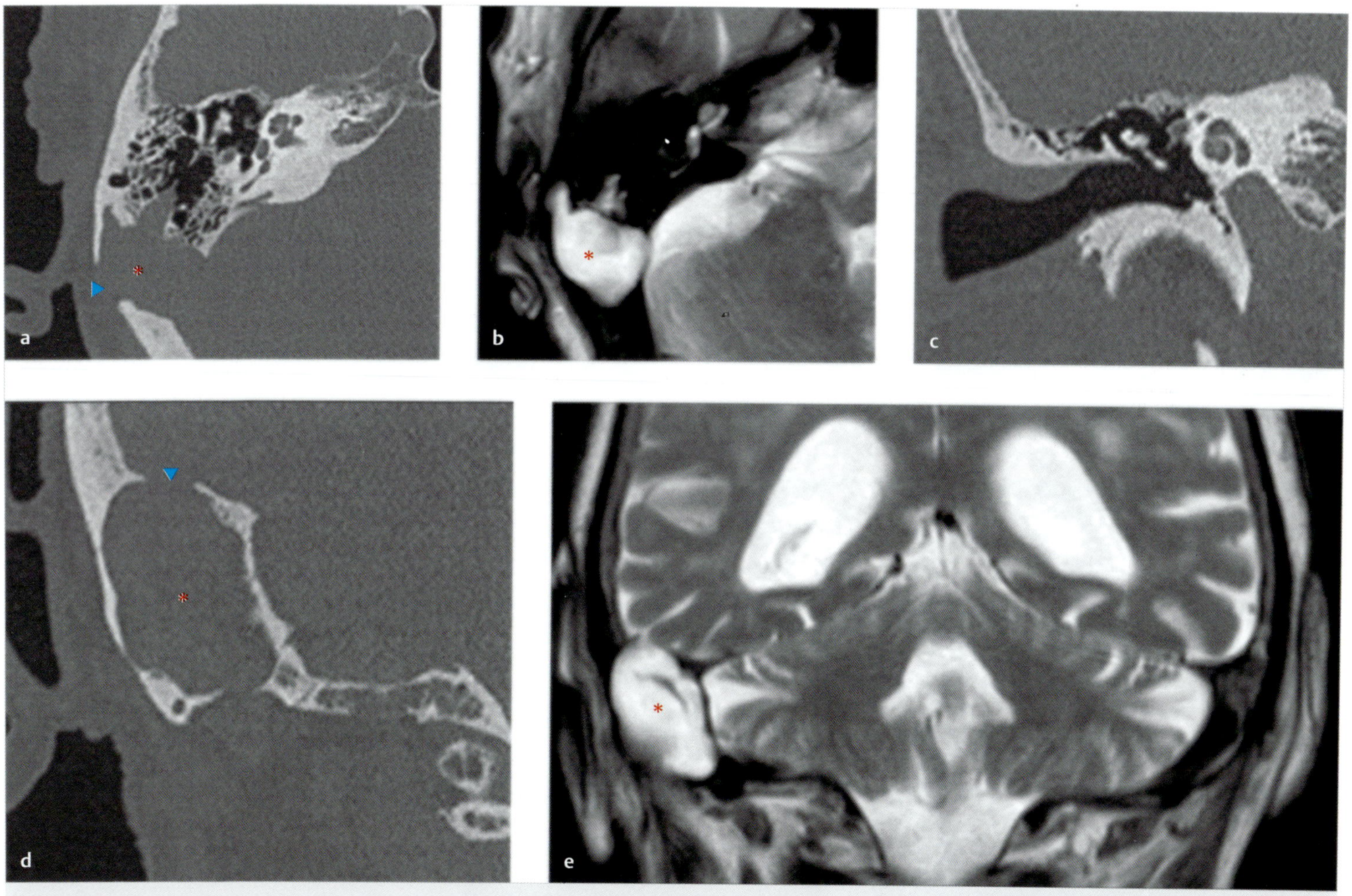

Fig. 5.14 Right retromastoid retrolabyrinthic cholesteatoma. **(a, c, d)** Note the oval-shaped mastoid erosion (*light blue triangle*), with no involvement of the tympanic cavity. **(b, e)** Magnetic resonance imaging (MRI) T2 sequence appearance of the cholesteatoma (*).

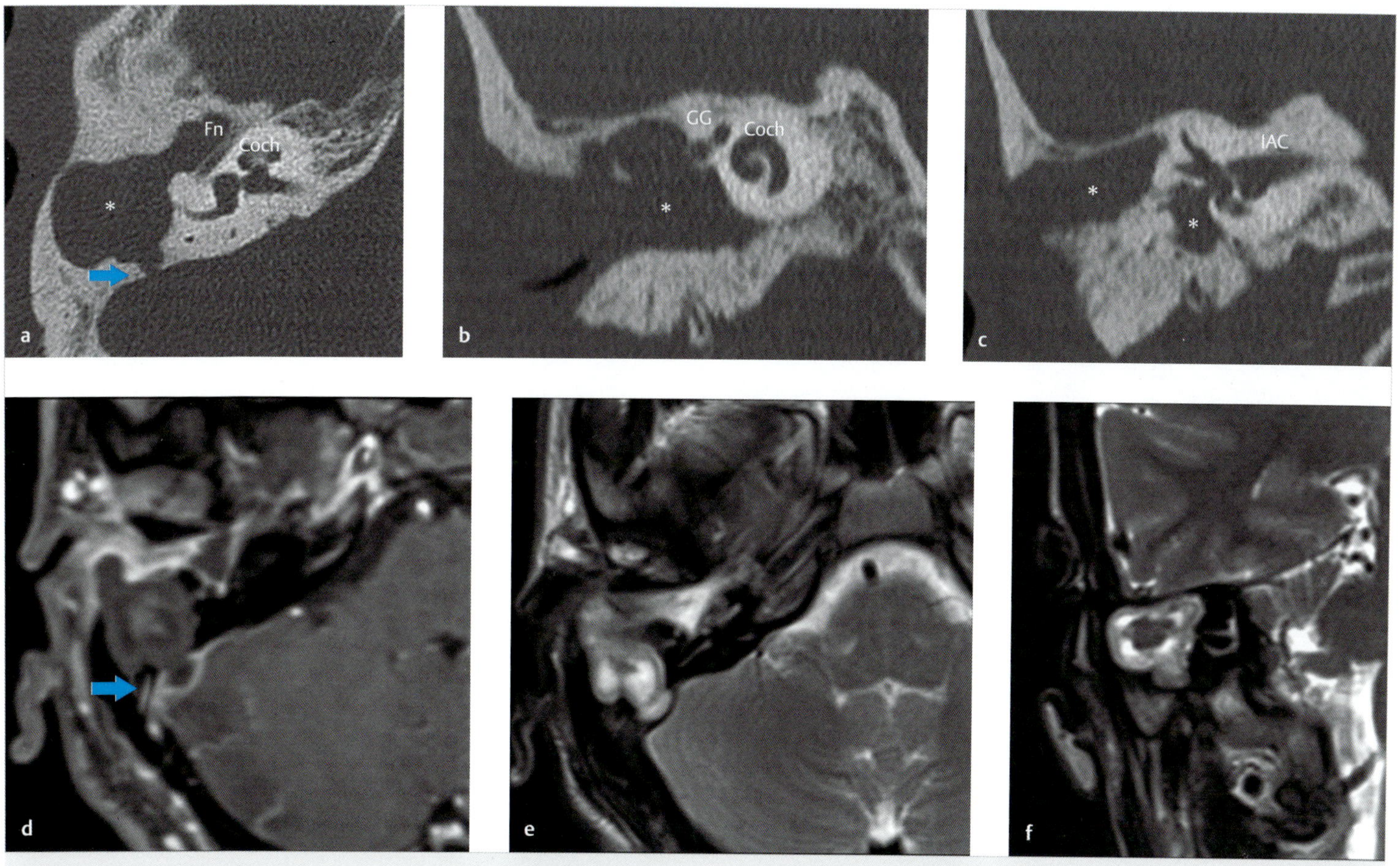

Fig. 5.15 Right extensive cholesteatoma (*). **(a–c)** Axial and coronal computed tomography (CT) scan views. Note the posterior bone erosion in the sigmoid sinus area. **(d–f)** Magnetic resonance imaging (MRI) of the aspect. Note the dural reaction on T1 with contrast and T2 signal (*blue arrow*). *Coch: cochlea; GG: geniculate ganglion; IAC: internal auditory canal; Fn: facial nerve.*

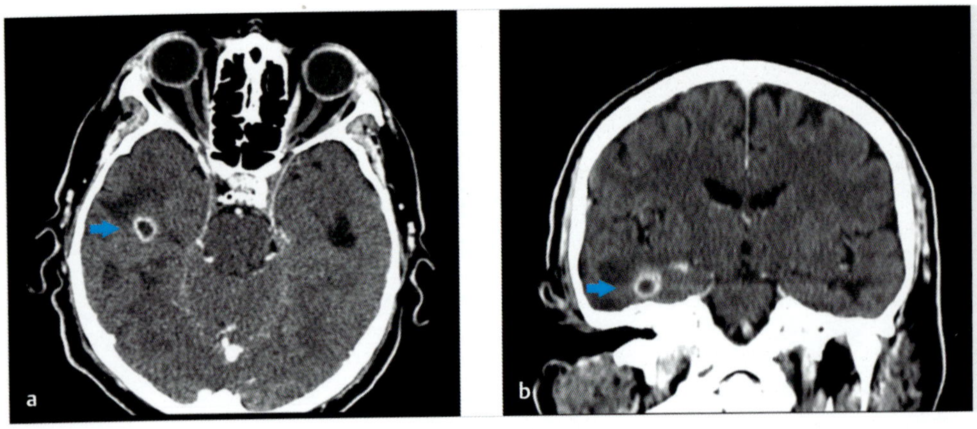

Fig. 5.16 Computed tomography (CT) scan of right temporal lobe abscess in a patient with cholesteatoma (blue arrow). (a) Axial view. (b) Coronal view.

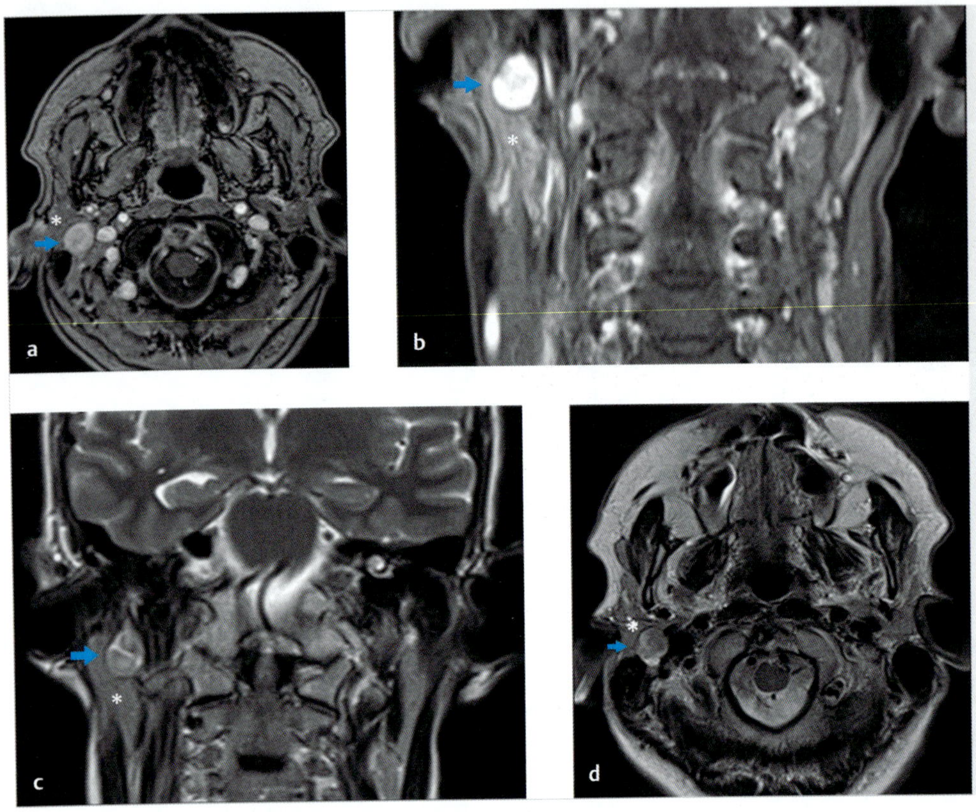

Fig. 5.17 Magnetic resonance imaging (MRI) appearance of a right facial nerve schwannoma. **(a–d)** Axial and coronal views of the tumor (*light blue arrow*) in the parotid tissue (*).

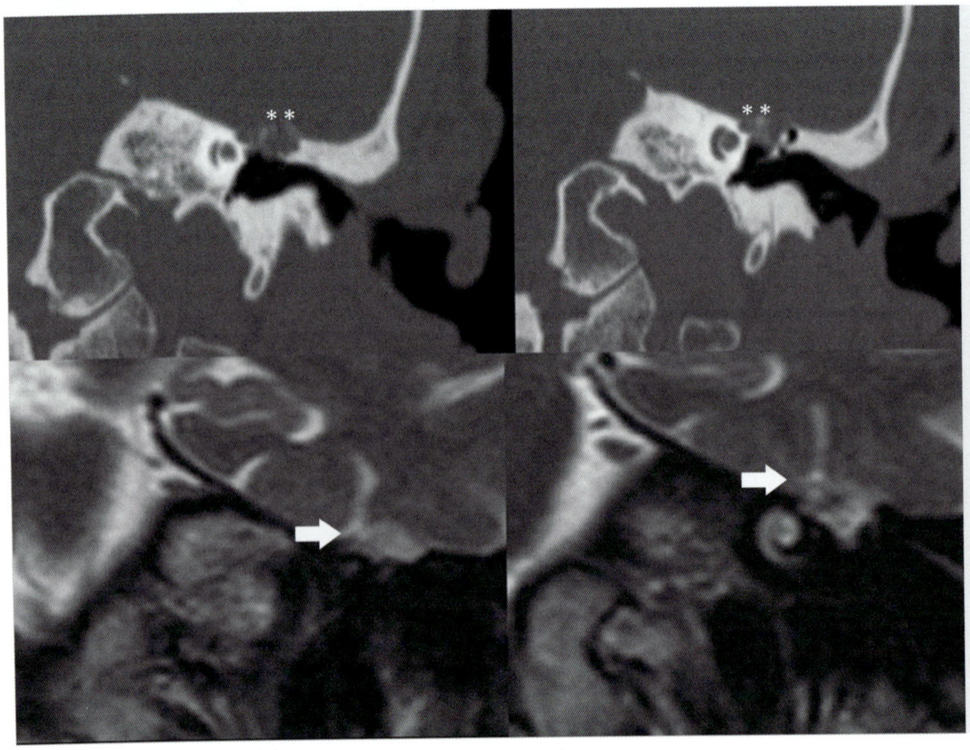

Fig. 5.18 Left facial nerve hemangioma: The computed tomography (CT) scan shows the typical appearance of intratumoral bone spicules (see the **). The magnetic resonance imaging (MRI) shows an infiltrative tumor of the dura of the middle fossa (*white arrow*).

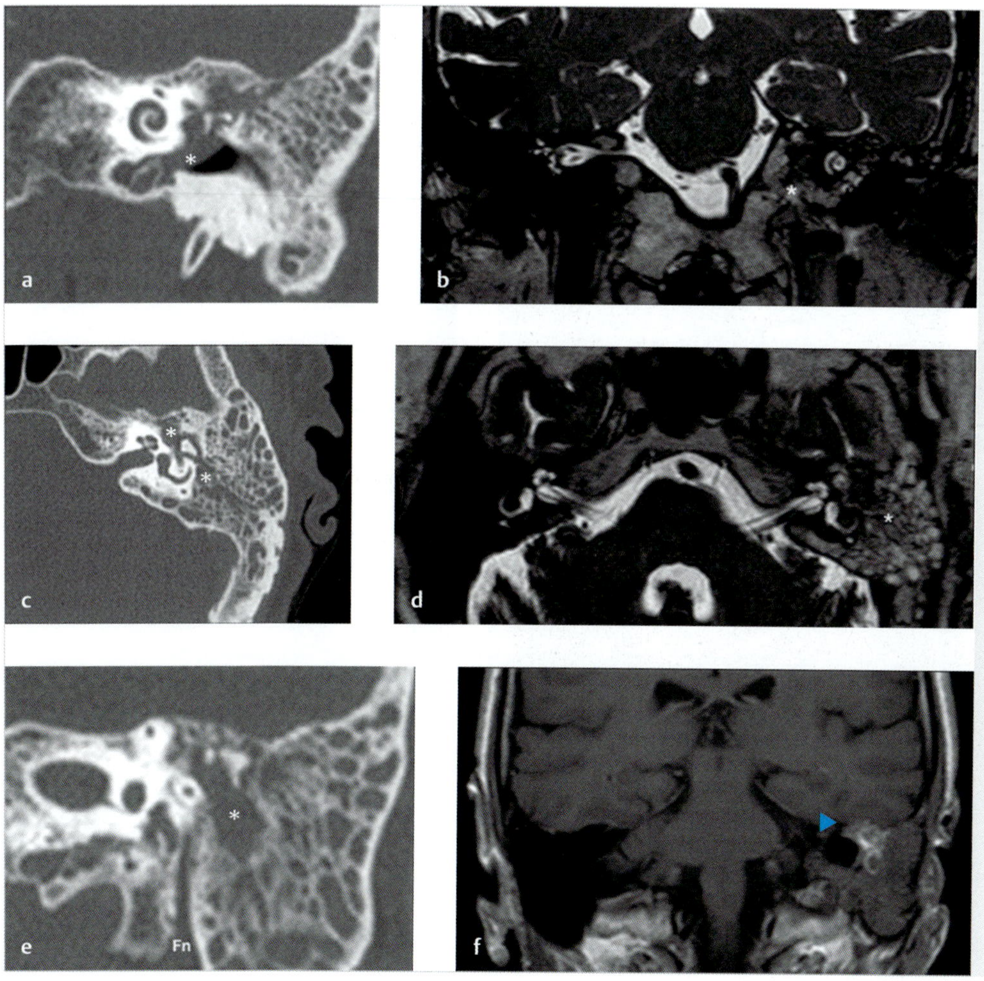

Fig. 5.19 Tympanomastoid paraganglioma. Computed tomography (CT) and magnetic resonance imaging (MRI) scan **(a–f)**. Note the hypotympanum extension and the mastoid involvement (*). *Light blue triangle: dural reaction close to the lesion. Fn: facial nerve.*

- C1: Paragangliomas with erosion of the carotid foramen
- C2: Paragangliomas with destruction of the vertical carotid canal
- C3: Paragangliomas with involvement of the horizontal portion of the carotid canal; intact foramen lacerum
- C4: Paragangliomas with invasion of the foramen lacerum and cavernous sinus
- De 1/2: Paragangliomas with intracranial but extradural extension, according to the displacement of the dura (De 1 < 2 cm, De 2 > 2 cm)
- Di 1/2/3: Paragangliomas with intracranial intradural extension, according to the depth of invasion of the posterior cranial fossa (Di 1 < 2 cm; Di 2 > 2 cm; Di 3 > 4 cm)

Type A paragangliomas represent the most common benign middle ear tumors (glomus tympanicum), which arise from paraganglia located along the tympanic plexus overlying the cochlear promontory. Paragangliomas embryologically stem from the neural crest and represent a proliferation of paraganglion cells within a highly vascularized environment. The clinical presentation is depends on the location of the lesion, with dysfunction of cranial nerves IX–XII in case of jugular lesions and pulsatile tinnitus with conductive hearing loss in case of tympanic lesions.

The presence of a red, pulsatile mass in the middle ear is not an exclusive feature of a paraganglioma and even between the two forms of temporal bone paraganglioma, the clinical presentation can be essentially identical. CT is the ideal modality for imaging assessment, showing a focal mass at the level of the cochlear promontory, which may engulf but not erode the ossicles; mastoid and eustachian tube involvement is also possible. MRI may be used to confirm avid enhancement, distinguishing it from congenital cholesteatoma or chronic otitis media, but the classical "salt-and-pepper" appearance, most evident on T2-weighted sequences and representing prominent intratumoral flow voids, may be difficult to appreciate in small lesions (see ▶ Fig. 5.20, ▶ Fig. 5.21, ▶ Fig. 5.22).

5.3.2 Internal Auditory Canal (IAC) and Cerebellopontine Angle (CPA) Lesions

The CPA cistern is a subarachnoid space containing cranial nerves and vessels bathed in CSF. The CPA is bordered by the pons, the anterior portion of the cerebellum, and the petrous temporal bone covered by dura mater. At its center there is the IAC and it extends caudally from the Vth cranial nerve to the IX–X–XIth cranial nerve complex. VSs account for 70 to 80% of all CPA lesions, meningiomas 10 to 15%, and epidermoid cysts 5%. The few remaining lesions, which represent less than 1% each, are extremely varied and unusual. They include hybrid peripheral nerve sheath tumors, cranial nerve schwannomas, multiforme glioblastomas, metastases, primary adenocarcinomas, arachnoid cysts, lipomas, lipochoristomas, melanomas, and cavernous hemangiomas. MRI is the best assessment tool for the IAC and CPA cistern for a mass lesion. One of the most common indications for imaging is to exclude retrocochlear pathology in patients with asymmetrical SNHL, although only 1 to 7.5% of these patients are ultimately diagnosed with a VS. CT has a limited role in imaging evaluation of IAC pathology, but may be used to assess bone margins (e.g., smooth expansion in VS) and osseous changes such as hyperostosis and sclerosis with a meningioma.

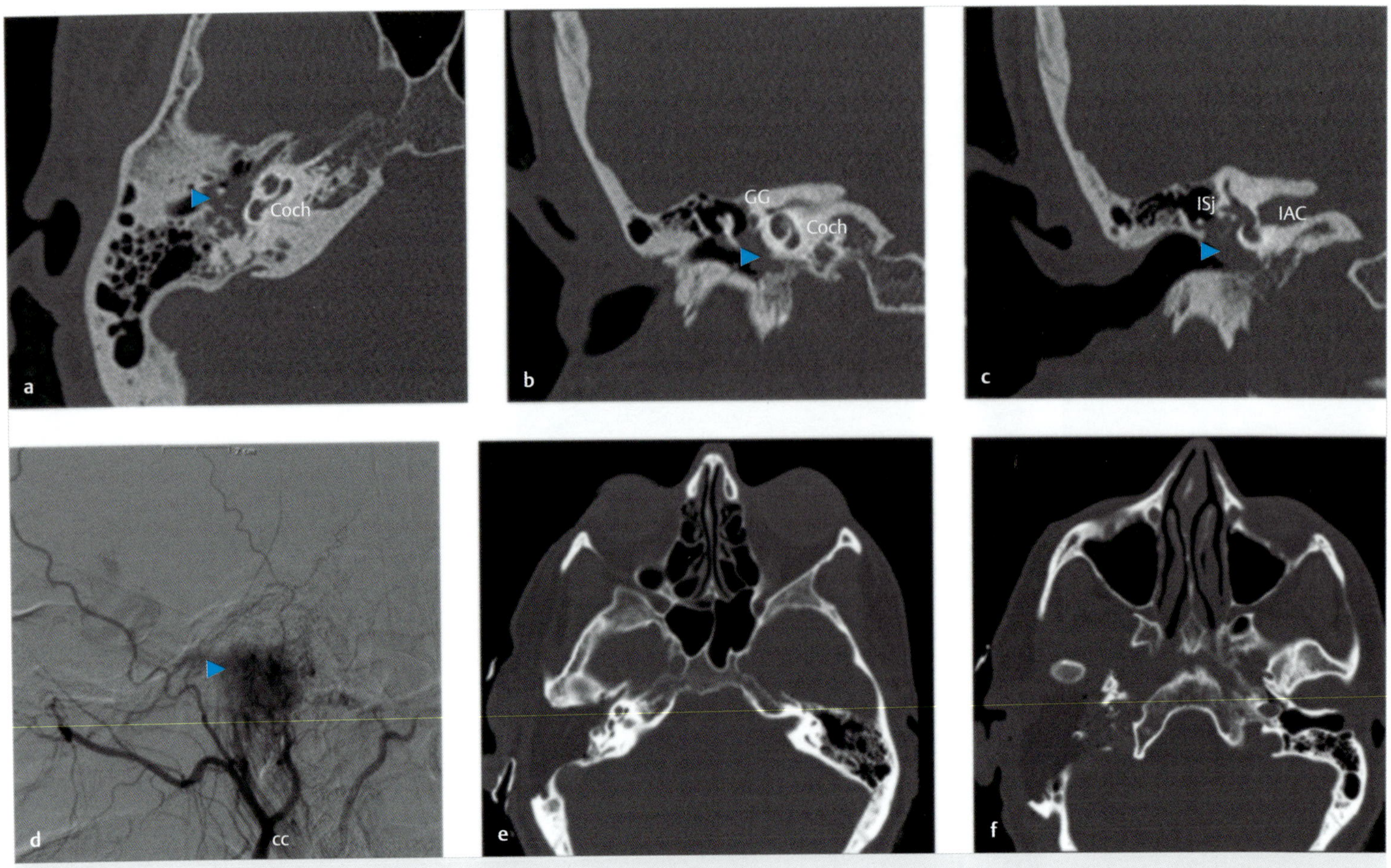

Fig. 5.20 Right tympanomastoid glomus. **(a–c)** Middle ear mass extending to the hypotympanum. **(d)** Angiography and vascularization of the tumor (*light blue triangle*: tympanomastoid glomus). **(e, f)** Postoperative computed tomography (CT) scan. *CC: common carotid trunk; Coch: cochlea; GG: geniculate ganglion; IAC: internal auditory canal; Lsc: lateral semicircular canal.*

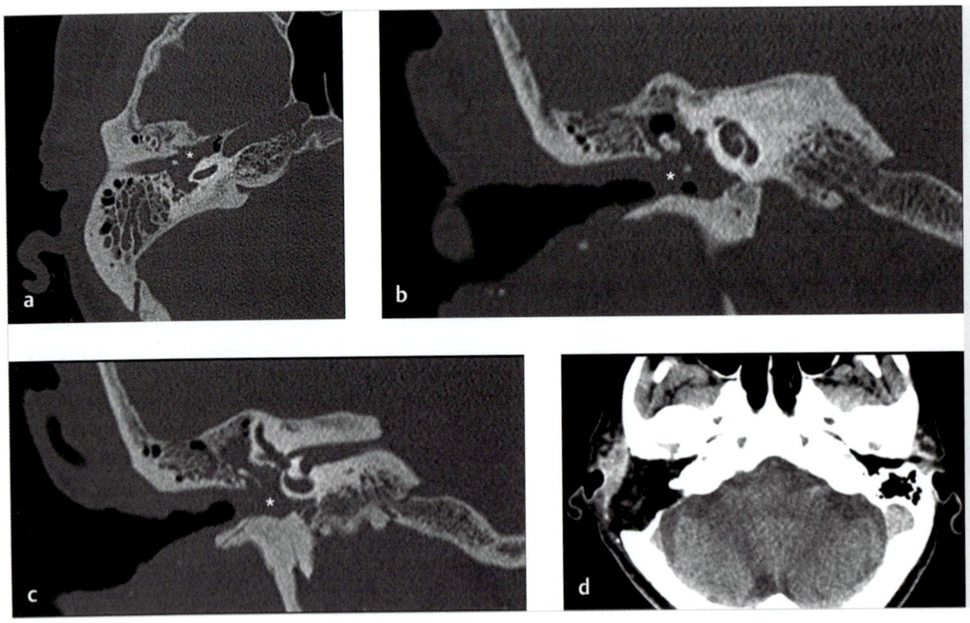

Fig. 5.21 Other examples of right tympanic paragangliomas. **(a–c)** Computed tomography (CT) scan showing the glomus tumor (*). **(d)** Postoperative CT scan.

Vestibular Schwannomas

VS is the most common skull base schwannoma, making up more than 80% of all skull base schwannomas. Different classification systems exist, but the most used is the Koos classification system, introduced in 1998, dividing VS into four grades (see ▶ Fig. 5.23):

- Grade I tumors are completely confined to the IAC;
- Grade II tumors, up to 2 cm, have both intra- and extrameatal components, but do not make contact with the brainstem;
- Grade III tumors make contact with the brainstem but do not compress it, up to 3 cm;
- Grade IV tumors cause brainstem compression, superior to 3 cm.

Most VSs develop from the Schwann sheath of the inferior vestibular nerve in the IAC where they slowly grow. Then, they smoothly erode the posterior edge of the porus acusticus and may give rise to a round or oval component in the CPA cistern,

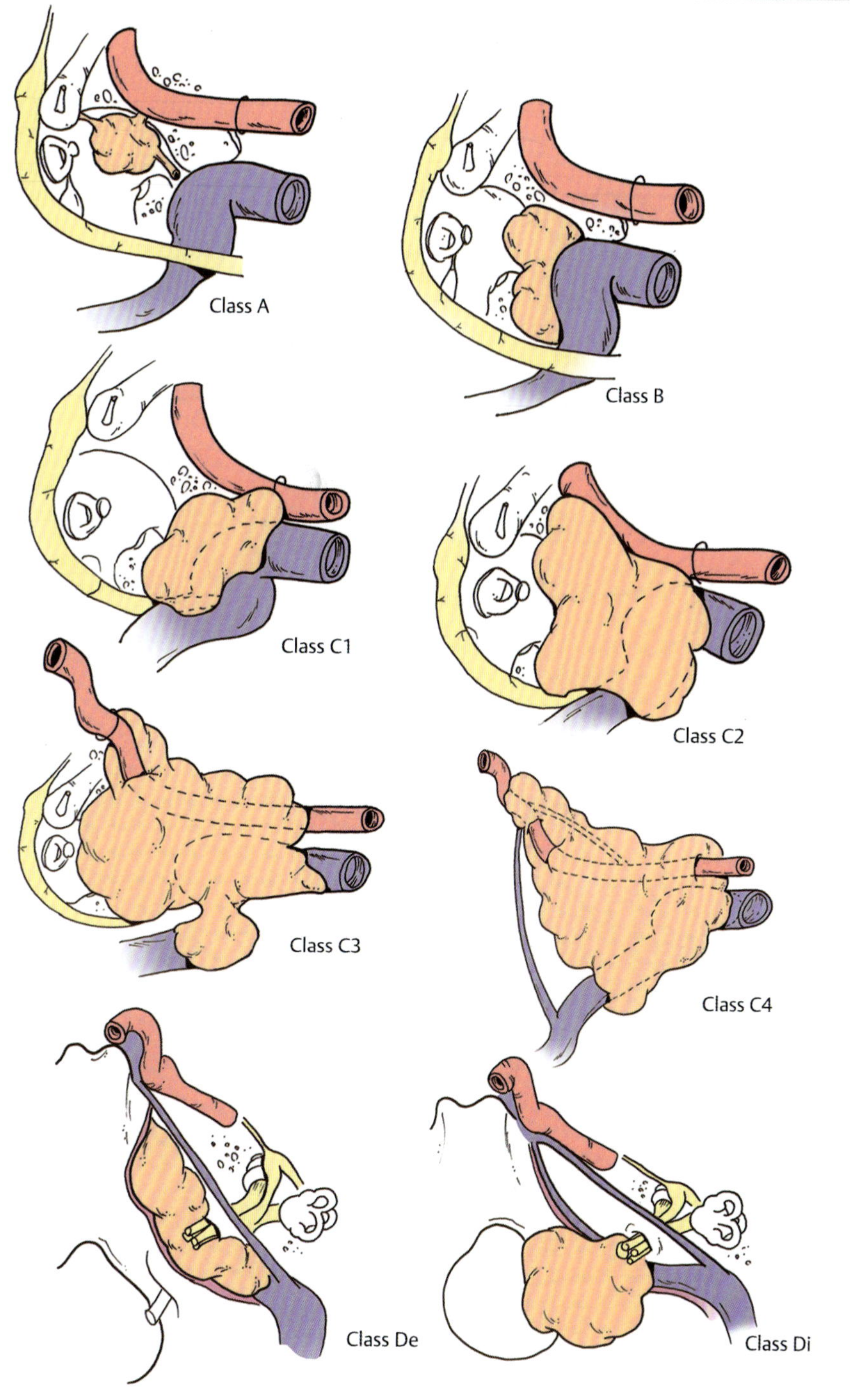

Fig. 5.22 Fisch's classification of temporal bone paragangliomas.

thus giving the typical "ice cream on cone" pattern. The primary differential consideration in imaging for a small intracanicular schwannoma is an infectious/inflammatory lesion, such as the ones seen in Bell's palsy and Ramsay Hunt syndrome. CT scan could show the enlargement of the IAC in case of big lesions and can help in surgical decision-making. On CT, schwannomas are usually isodense and enhance after contrast administration. On MRI, VSs are typically T1-isointense, T2-hyperintense, homogeneously enhancing IAC lesions with variable CPA components. Three different MRI appearances of the tumoral enhancement are described in VSs: homogeneous (50–60%), heterogeneous (30–40%), and cystic (5–15%). Cystic changes occur in up to 48% of cases and are secondary to myxomatous material characteristic of Antoni B areas. High ADC values in VSs are probably related to the presence of increased amounts of extracellular water in the tumor matrix (72). MRI is really important for some considerations about the surgical management of VS.

Besides VSs, rare lesions that have a different management from the more common "acoustic" schwannoma are represented by intralabyrinthine schwannomas (ILS). They are defined as tumors arising primarily from within the membranous labyrinth: cochlea, vestibule, or semicircular canals. They can be classified (*Kennedy classification*) as follows (see ▶ Fig. 5.24):

- Intracochlear—tumor confined to the turns in the cochlea;
- Intravestibular—tumor confined to the vestibule, with or without extension into the semicircular canals;
- Vestibulocochlear—tumors that fill the cochlea and vestibule without extension into the middle ear or IAC;
- Transmodiolar—tumor that extends through the modiolus from the cochlea into the IAC via the cochlear nerve canal;
- Transmacular—tumor that extends through the macula cribrosa from the vestibule into the IAC;
- Transotic—tumor that extends through the labyrinth into the IAC and middle ear.

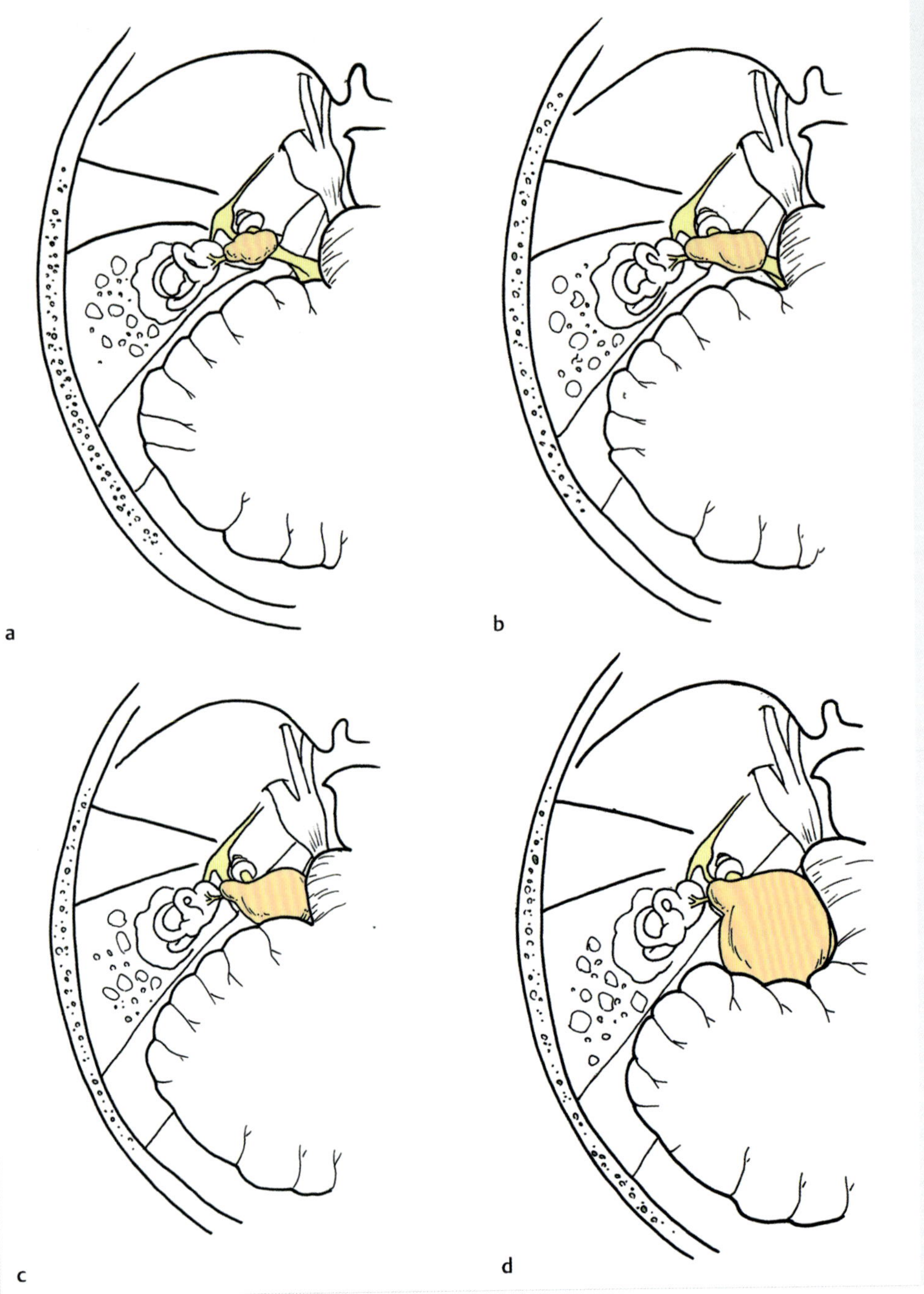

Fig. 5.23 Koos staging system for vestibular schwannomas (VSs). **(a)** Koos I; **(b)** Koos II; **(c)** Koos III; **(d)** Koos IV.

On T2-weighted images, these lesions appear as focal filling defects with replacement of the normal high-signal-intensity fluid. On postgadolinium imaging, they appear as focal homogeneously enhancing masses. The contrast enhancement in the patients who had both T2 and enhanced imaging corresponded to the T2 abnormality. There are other lesions that can mimic ILS on contrast-enhanced MRI, including labyrinthitis (typically viral in etiology), labyrinthitis ossificans, hemorrhage, or lipoma.

Surgical approaches to lesions extending into IAC, such as VSs, are widely known and have been extensively recorded. The retrosigmoid, middle cranial fossa, and translabyrinthine approaches are the most commonly used and well-documented approaches in VS surgery. The choice of the right approach depends on factors such as the surgeon's preferences and habits, the dimension and extension of the pathology, the possibility of hearing preservation, the risk to the facial nerve, and postoperative complications. To access the IAC and CPA, all of these approaches require wide external incisions and a variable degree of temporal bone removal, so an alternative surgical technique was developed for the management of VSs limited to the IAC, minimizing intraoperative and postoperative complications. Starting with the introduction of the endoscope in IAC surgery in combination with the retrosigmoid approach to remove the intracanalicular extension of the tumor under endoscopic control, in 2012, for the first time, an exclusive endoscopic approach to the IAC was described. It was used to remove a VS involving both the IAC and cochlea in a 40 year old patient with hearing loss, tinnitus, and vertigo, who was unresponsive to medical treatment. This approach was called "transcanal transpromontorial approach." Focusing on FN results, overall FN function was perfectly preserved in 95.9% of patients after surgery and results were stable at the last follow-up. These results, if compared with other options ("wait and scan", radiotherapy and traditional microscopic surgeries), are very encouraging and, in the authors' opinion, transcanal surgery, through a total transcanal endoscopic approach (TTEA) and/or an enlarged transcanal approach (ETA) technique, can be added in the "decision-making" algorithm for the management of VS. New studies are changing our perspective on cochlear preservation and cochlear implantation in the future (see

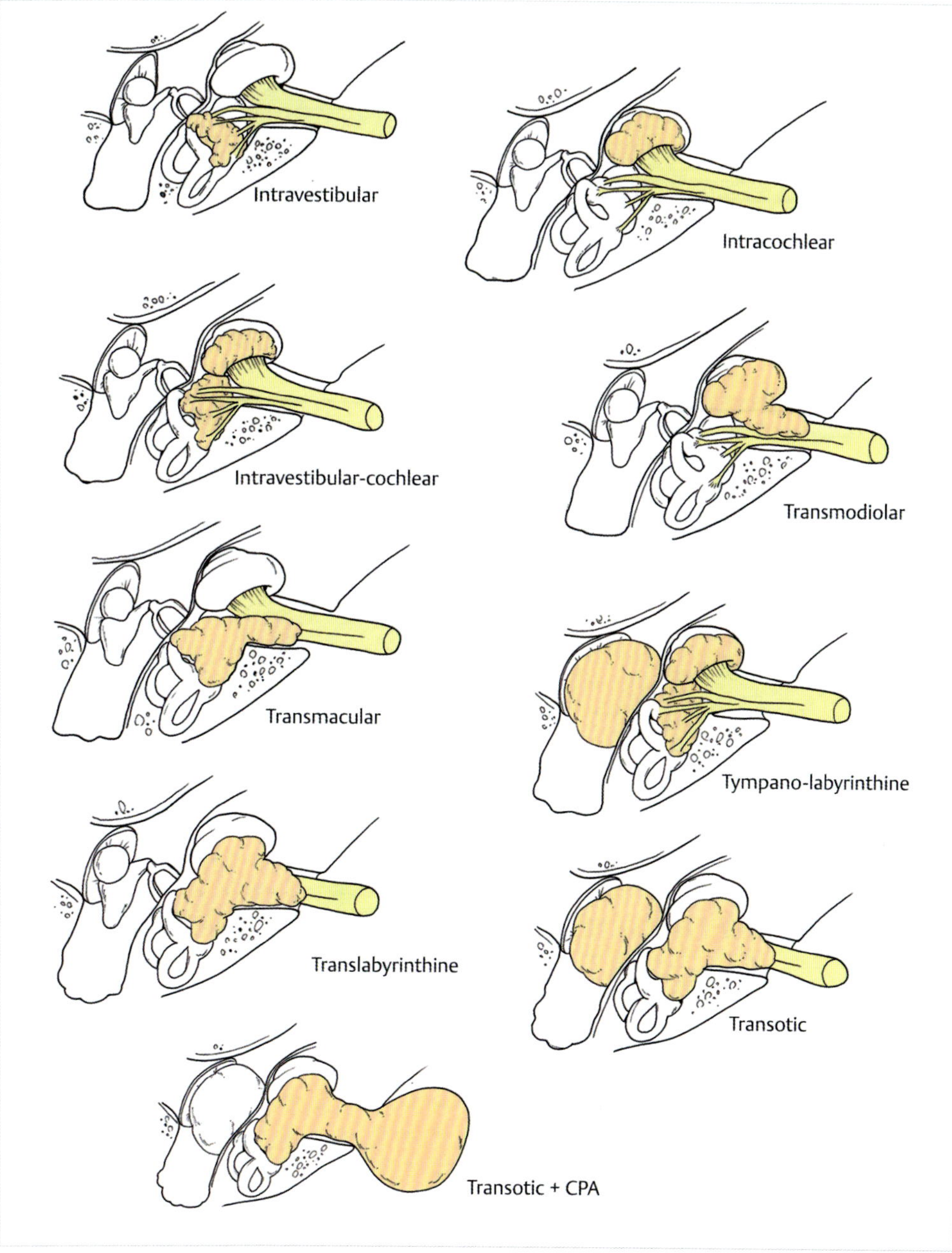

Fig. 5.24 Classification system for intralabyrinthine schwannomas.

▶ Fig. 5.25, ▶ Fig. 5.26, ▶ Fig. 5.27, ▶ Fig. 5.28, ▶ Fig. 5.29, ▶ Fig. 5.30, ▶ Fig. 5.31, ▶ Fig. 5.32, ▶ Fig. 5.33, ▶ Fig. 5.34).

The treatment of ILS depends on the location, symptoms, and the development of the tumor through time. Hearing preservation is actually not possible in the removal of ILS; thus, management is usually observation with serial MRI to avoid excessive morbidity. Surgery is indicated for intractable vertigo or evidence of tumor growth leaving the membranous labyrinth inside the IAC or middle ear. These lesions can be perfectly treated through a transcanal endoscopic approach, which represents in these cases a safe and minimally invasive surgical technique for the surgical management of these tumors.

Some radiological aspects should be kept in mind when an approach is being planned:

- A CT scan is necessary to evaluate:
  - The length and depth of the IAC—short IACs are better for transcanal surgery;
  - The jugular bulb position—a high jugular bulb could make the surgery difficult or impossible;
  - High mastoid pneumatization; obliteration with bone wax is mandatory to avoid postoperative leakage.
- MRI is necessary to evaluate:
  - The dimensions of the neuroma, according to Koos classification, to properly plan the surgery. For Koos I, endoscopic transcanal approach is a possible choice; for Koos grades 2 and 3, an ETA is a possible choice only if the tumor spreads in a straight direction. If the tumor spreads anteriorly to the trigeminal or lower cranial nerves, a translabyrinthine approach is recommended.
  - In case an aberrant course or loops of the anteroinferior cerebellar artery (AICA) into the IAC are found, a two-hand technique is mandatory to manage the vascular structure to avoid intraoperative bleeding.

Meningioma

Meningiomas can be distinguished into petrous bone meningiomas and petroclival meningiomas.

Petrous Bone Meningiomas

They stem from the dura of the temporal bone and are classified as retromeatal, perimeatal, and premeatal, according to the relationship between the main dural attachment and the IAC.

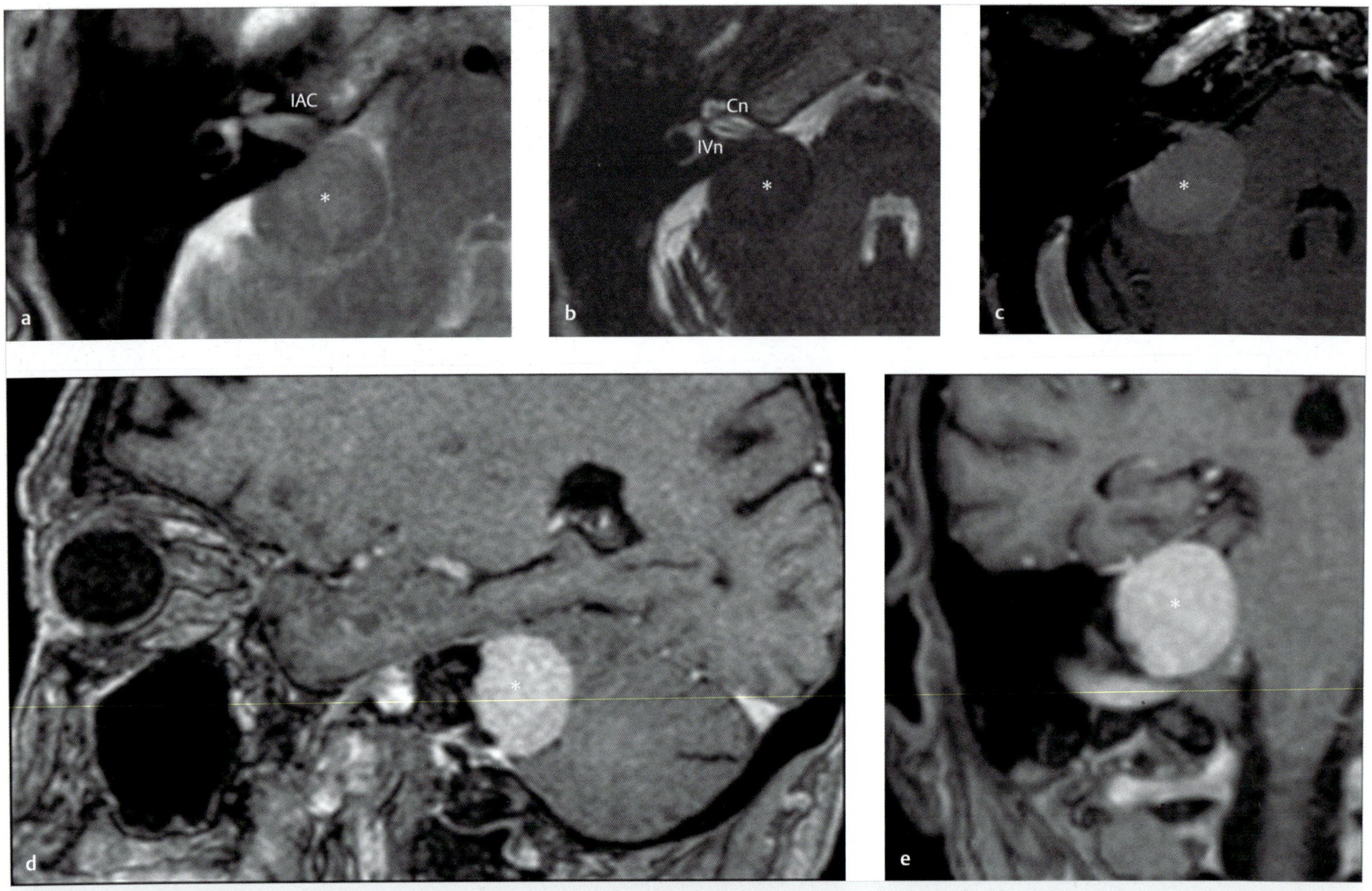

Fig. 5.25 Magnetic resonance imaging (MRI) showing a right vestibular schwannoma (VS, *). **(a–c)** T2 and T1 signal shows a VS of the cerebellopontine angle (CPA), with a minimal intracanalar component. **(d, e)** MRI with contrast shows the lesion with enhancement in sagittal and coronal views. *Cn: cochlear nerve; IAC: internal auditory canal; IVn: inferior vestibular nerve.*

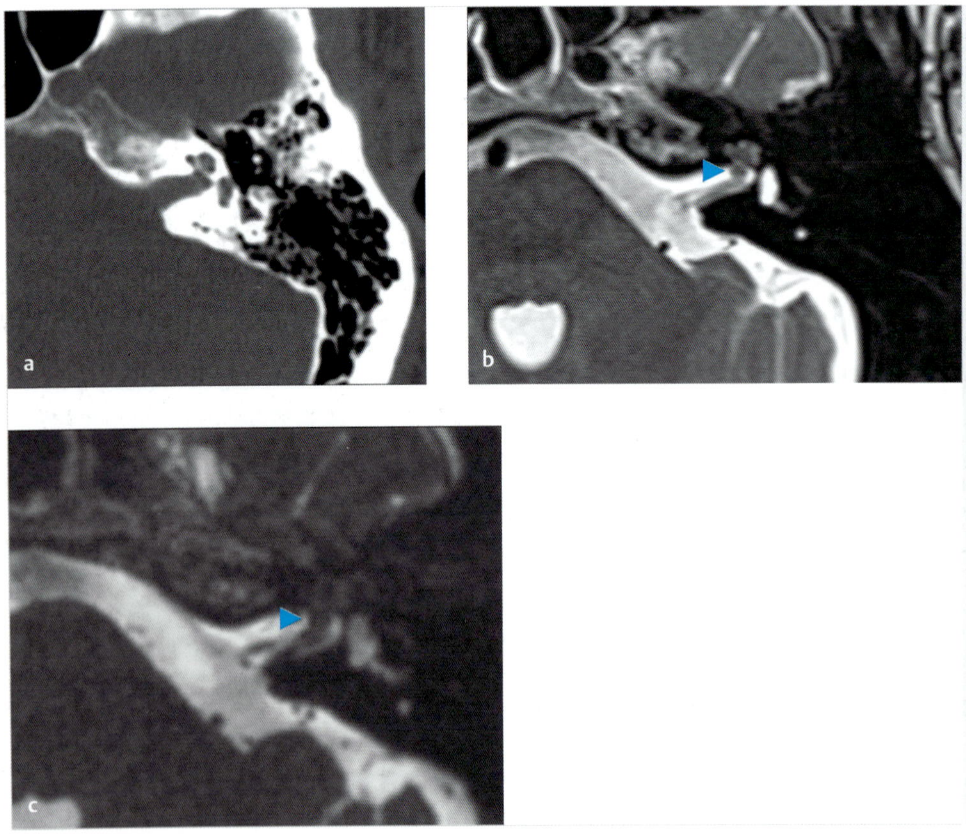

Fig. 5.26 Left intralabyrinthine schwannoma. **(a)** Computed tomography (CT) scan with no enlargement of the internal auditory canal (IAC). **(b, c)** A small cochlear schwannoma is identified close to the cochlea (*light blue triangle*).

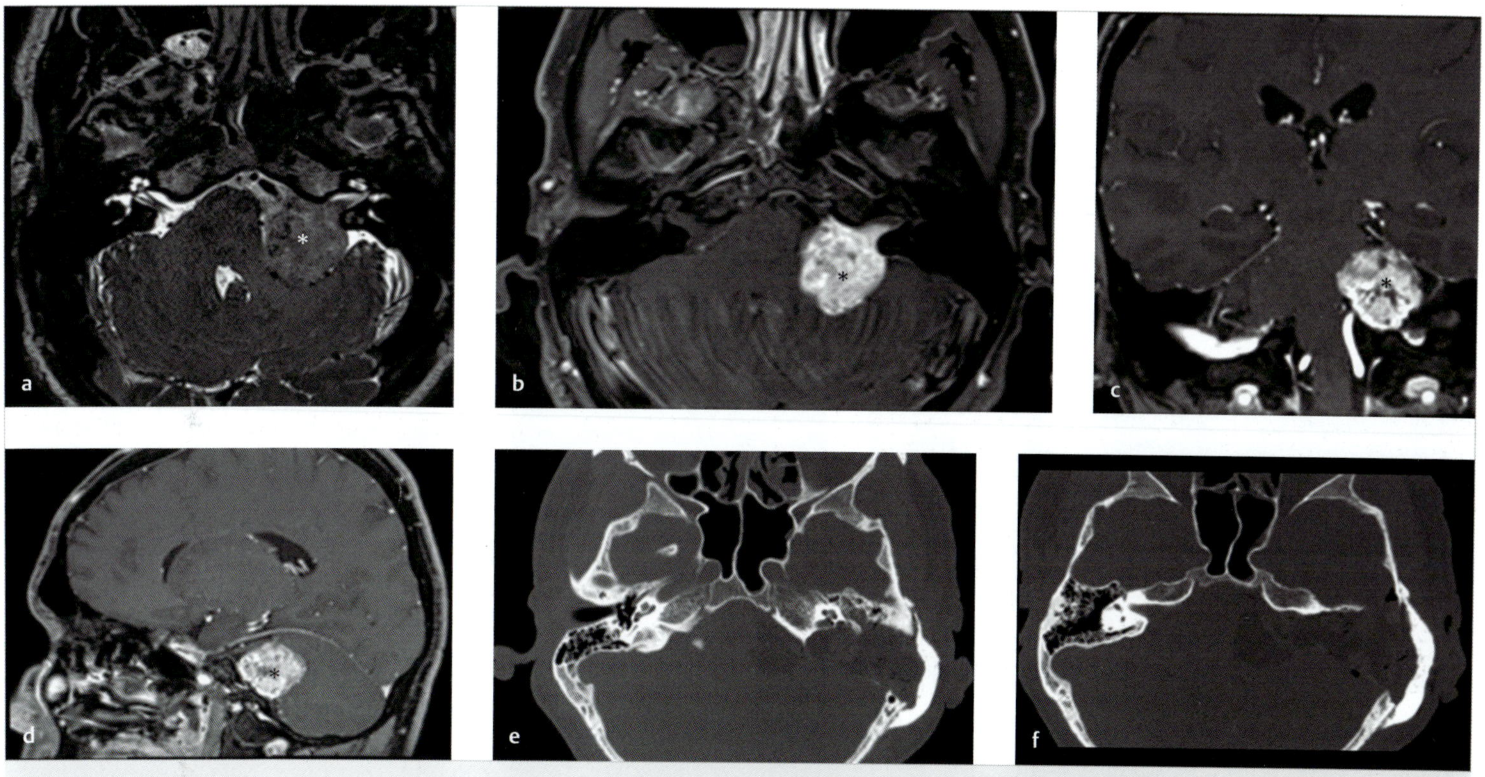

Fig. 5.27 Left vestibular schwannoma (VS, *). **(a–d)** Axial T2, T1 coronal and sagittal T1 with contrast scan showing a huge schwannoma extending from the internal auditory canal (IAC) to the cerebellopontine angle (CPA). **(e, f)** Postoperative computed tomography (CT) scan after a translabyrinthine approach.

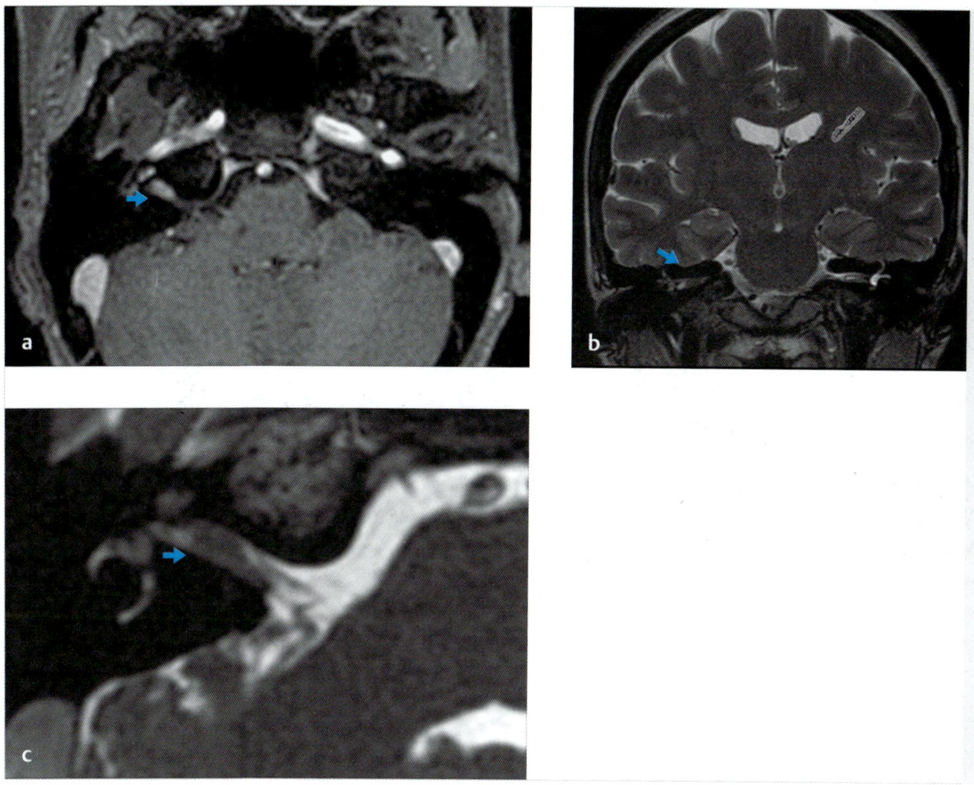

Fig. 5.28 Right vestibular schwannoma (VS). **(a)** T1 with contrast signal. **(b, c)** T2 signal, showing a small internal auditory canal (IAC) VS (*light blue arrow*).

Retromeatal meningiomas (posterior petrous bone [PB] meningiomas) originate from the dura of the posterior PB, between the posterior wall of the IAC and the groove of the sigmoid sinus. They occupy the posterior part of the CPA, usually anterosuperiorly dislocating the acoustic-facial bundle. These lesions can also be removed through a retrolabyrinthine approach. Perimeatal meningiomas arise from the dura in contact with the IAC and the dislocation of the nerves is unpredictable.

Premeatal meningiomas (anterior PB meningiomas) arise from the dura around the porus trigeminalis (petrous apex [PA] meningiomas) or from the dura of the petroclival (PC) junction or directly from the clivus (PC meningiomas). They occupy the anterior part of the CPA and they posteroinferiorly dislocate the acoustic-facial bundle, immediately behind the dura of the posterior PB.

Meningiomas represent the second most common (10–15%) CPA lesions and typically arise in the proximity of the porus acusticus

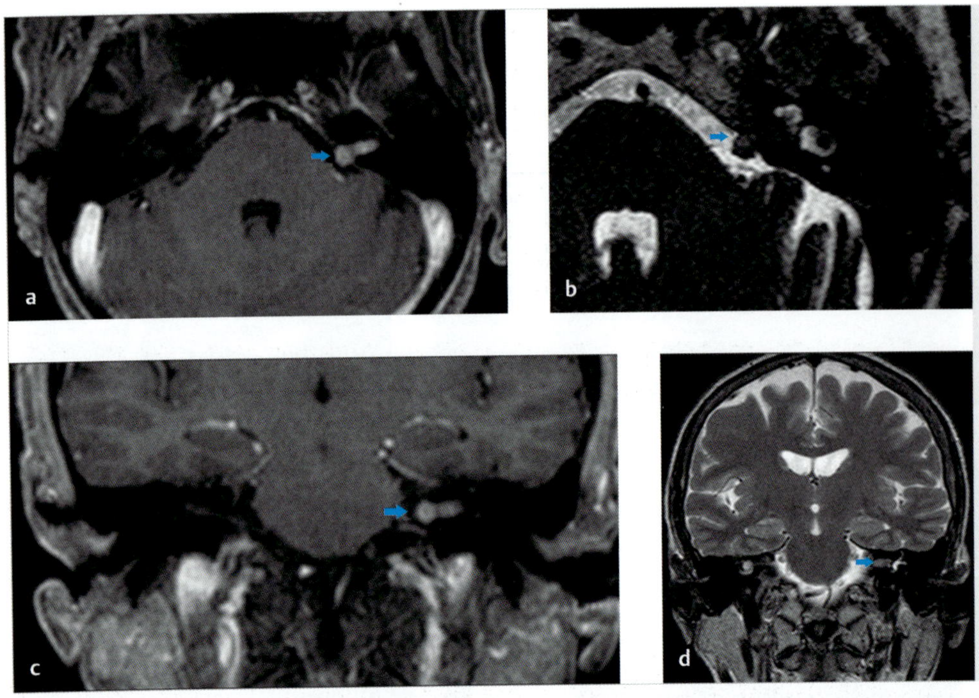

Fig. 5.29 Left vestibular schwannoma (VS). **(a, b)** Axial view showing a lesion extending from the fundus of the internal auditory canal (IAC) to the cerebellopontine angle (CPA). **(c, d)** Coronal view of T1 with contrast and T2 sequences (*light blue triangle:* medial extension to the CPA of VS).

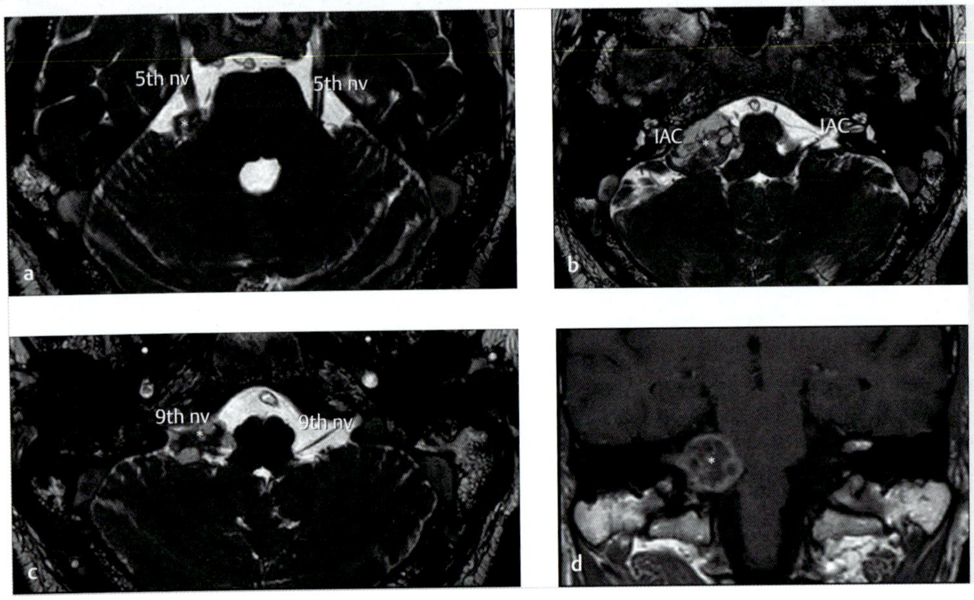

Fig. 5.30 Right vestibular schwannoma (VS) with cystic component. Note the extension from the trigeminal nerve **(a)** to a lower cranial nerve **(b, c)**. **(d)** T1 sequence coronal view. 5th nv: trigeminal nerve; 9th nv: glossopharyngeal nerve; IAC: internal auditory canal.

from where they can extend into the IAC (83%). These slow-growing masses arise from arachnoid meningoepithelial cells and, as it happens with meningiomas elsewhere, they are more frequently seen in individuals above 40 years of age. In the CPA, these tumors tend to arise from the dura of the dorsal aspect of the petrous temporal bone. Unlike VS, hardly ever cause canalicular expansion, may calcify (in ~20% of cases), or can be associated with adjacent hyperostosis; better identified on CT scan, they typically form an obtuse angle with the adjacent bone and may demonstrate transtentorial extension into the middle cranial fossa. On MRI, the masses are isointense to cerebral cortex on T1- and T2-weighted sequences and show avid postcontrast enhancement. Because meningiomas may involve the porus acusticus and extend into the IAC, the detection of a dural tail is key to differentiate meningiomas from VSs (see Figs. ▶ Fig. 5.35, ▶ Fig. 5.36).

Petroclival meningiomas are another group of lesions, developing from the clivus and growing toward the petrous bone, medially to the IAC and upwards, to the upper third of the clivus. They often involve the cavernous sinus and the middle fossa (sphenopetroclival meningiomas).

Most posterior fossa cranial nerves, cerebellar arteries, basilar artery, and its perforating branches, are often involved.

Epidermoid and Arachnoid Cysts

Epidermoid cysts represent around 5% of CPA masses, after meningiomas (6%) and VSs (90%). They also constitute 40% of all intracranial epidermoids, and about two-thirds of the CPA cholesteatomas with trigeminal neuralgia (TN). Few patients can present a mild hemifacial spasm and glossopharyngeal neuralgia (see ▶ Fig. 5.37, ▶ Fig. 5.38, ▶ Fig. 5.39, ▶ Fig. 5.40). They arise during early embryogenesis from inclusion of ectodermal epithelial tissue during neural tube closure. They grow from desquamation and the accumulation of keratin and cholesterol within the cysts. These lobulated malleable masses have a tendency to insinuate between cranial nerves and vessels. Because of this feature, they tend to be diagnosed only when large. Epidermoid tumors have the appearance of nonenhancing cysts on CT and MRI, following the density and intensity of CSF on most sequences. The epidermoid inclusion cyst has a CSF-like appearance on standard MRI sequences, looking isointense on T1-weighted images and hyperintense on T2-weighted images. On these sequences, differentiation with an arachnoid cyst is very difficult, because arachnoid cysts too may have a CSF-like appearance. On heavily T2-

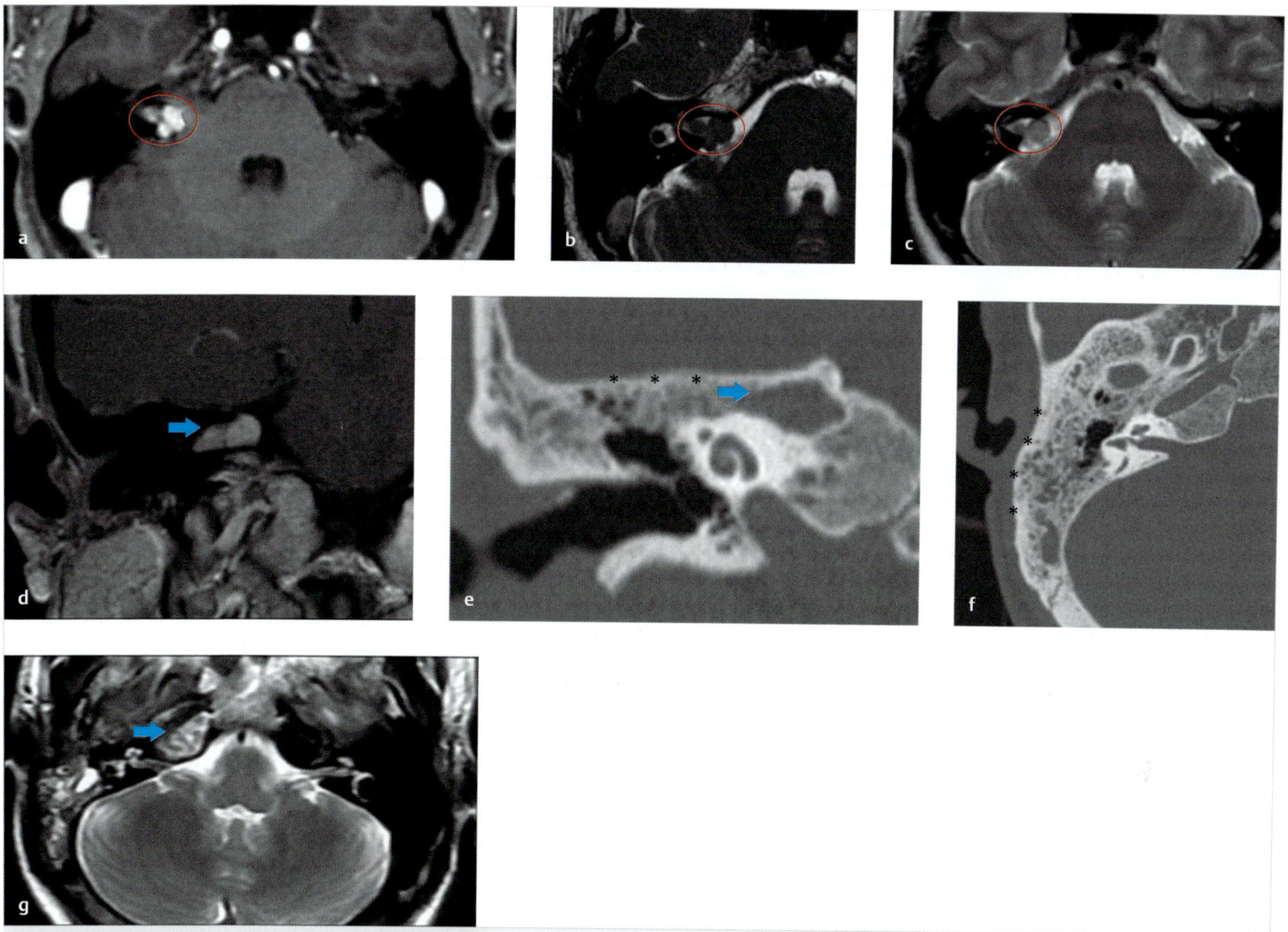

Fig. 5.31 Right vestibular schwannoma (VS) with cystic aspect. **(a–d)** The neuroma is shown in T1 with contrast and T2 axial and coronal views. Note the lobulate appearance inside the internal auditory canal (IAC) (*red circle*). **(e, f)** Right petrous apex opacity (*light blue arrow*), with hard bone in the suprageniculate area (*) in the same patient. **(g)** Magnetic resonance imaging (MRI) of the lesion of the petrous apex (*light blue arrow*), with mastoid fluid signal.

weighted sequences and fluid-attenuated inversion recovery (FLAIR) sequences, arachnoid cysts still have CSF appearance whereas epidermoid inclusion cysts have a mixed hyperintense–hypointense appearance on these heavily T2-weighted sequences and an nonhomogeneous hyperintense appearance on FLAIR sequences. This characteristic of epidermoid tumors helps in the differential diagnosis with arachnoid cysts and is helpful for the detection of any residual tumor in postoperative follow-up. A rare so-called "white epidermoid" demonstrates the opposite signal characteristics on MRI.

Arachnoid cysts are congenital, benign, intra-arachnoid pouch-like lesions filled with normal CSF. Their exact origin is uncertain, but they could result from a splitting of the embryonic meninges. They are usually supratentorial, with about 70% in the temporal fossa, mostly on the left side, anterior to the temporal poles. Only 10% of arachnoid cysts are located in the posterior fossa, where they most commonly develop in the CPA. In neuroimaging, attenuation and signal intensities of uncomplicated arachnoid cysts exactly match those of CSF on all sequences, they do not enhance after contrast, and therefore, may mimic epidermoid cysts on conventional T1- and T2-weighted images. However, arachnoid cysts displace adjacent arteries and cranial nerves rather than encasing them, as epidermoid cysts usually do. They also demonstrate rounded edges, smoothly deforming the adjacent brain or scalloping the bony structures. Additionally, the complete suppression of signal intensity on FLAIR sequence in arachnoid cysts and the lack of diffusion restriction of these lesions on DWI should help exclude epidermoid cysts as a likely differential diagnosis.

Schwannomas of Other Cranial Nerves

Schwannomas in the posterior fossa can arise from any of the cranial nerves from the Vth (trigeminal) to the XIIth (hypoglossal) cranial nerves. These non-VSs share the same CT and MRI features as VSs but they are often different in their presentation symptoms and their precise relation to cranial nerves and skull base foramina. Imaging shows an enhancing tubular mass along the pathway of the parent nerve with a dumbbell shape where it crosses the foramen. On MRI, the T2-weighted sequence can show cystic components within these lesions. CT is the best technique to show associated smooth bone erosion and foraminal widening as the lesion extends through the skull base foramen. Trigeminal schwannoma is the most frequent lesion among non-VSs. It is located cephalad to VS, has an anterior-posterior

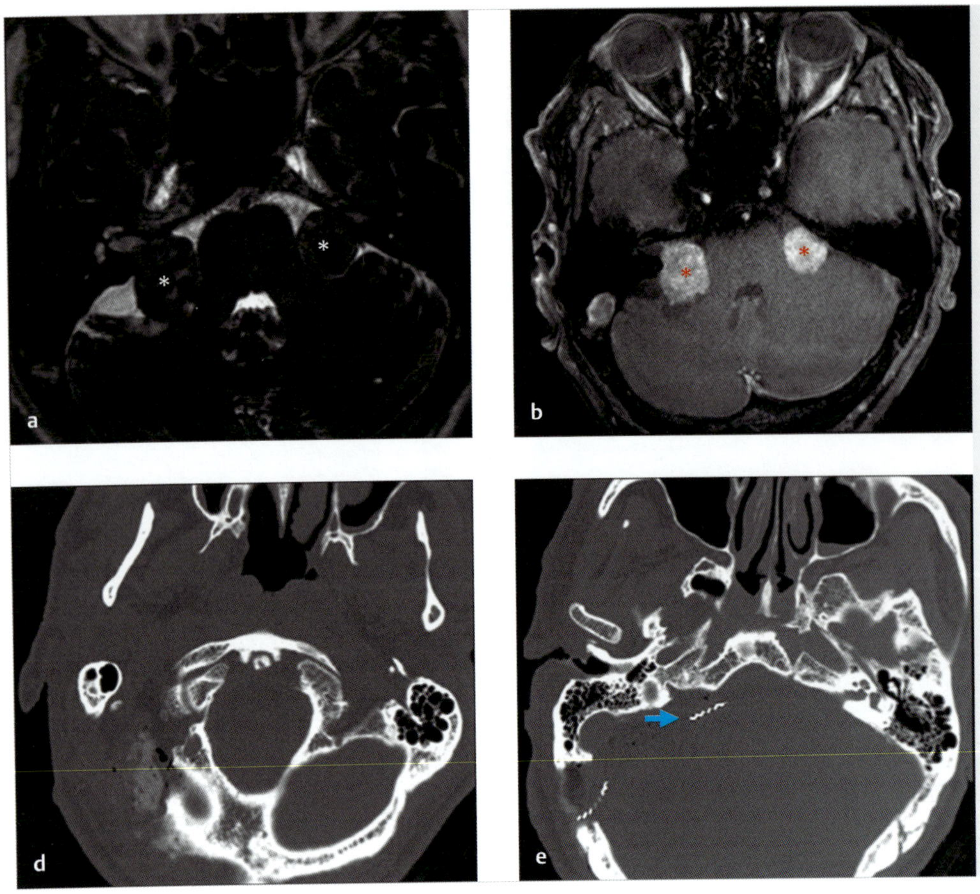

Fig. 5.32 Type 2 neurofibromatosis suffering patient. **(a, b)** Magnetic resonance imaging (MRI) showing the bilateral vestibular schwannoma (VS) (*), with initial compression of the brainstem. **(c, d)** Postoperative computed tomography (CT) scan, with auditory brainstem positioned for hearing rehabilitation (*light blue arrow*).

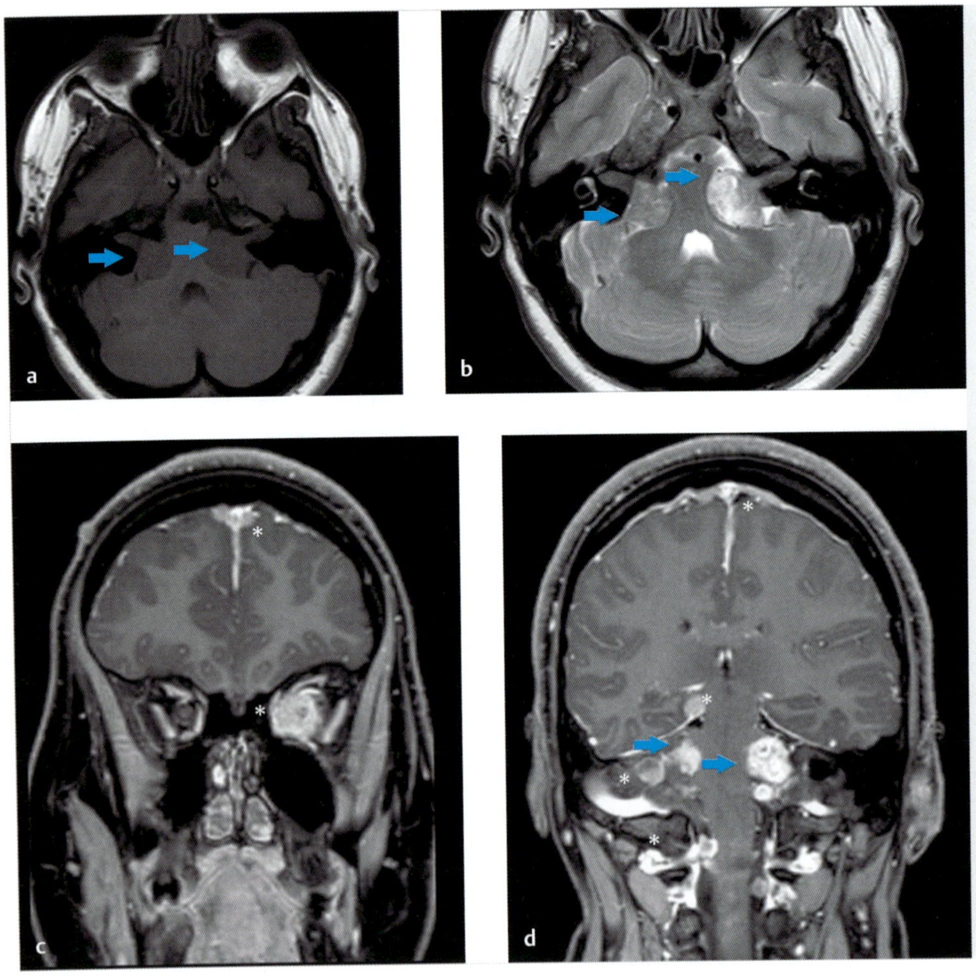

Fig. 5.33 Type 2 neurofibromatosis suffering patient. **(a–d)** Note the bilateral vestibular schwannomas (VSs) (*light blue arrows*), with other meningiomas of the left optic nerve, superior sagittal region, and brainstem (*).

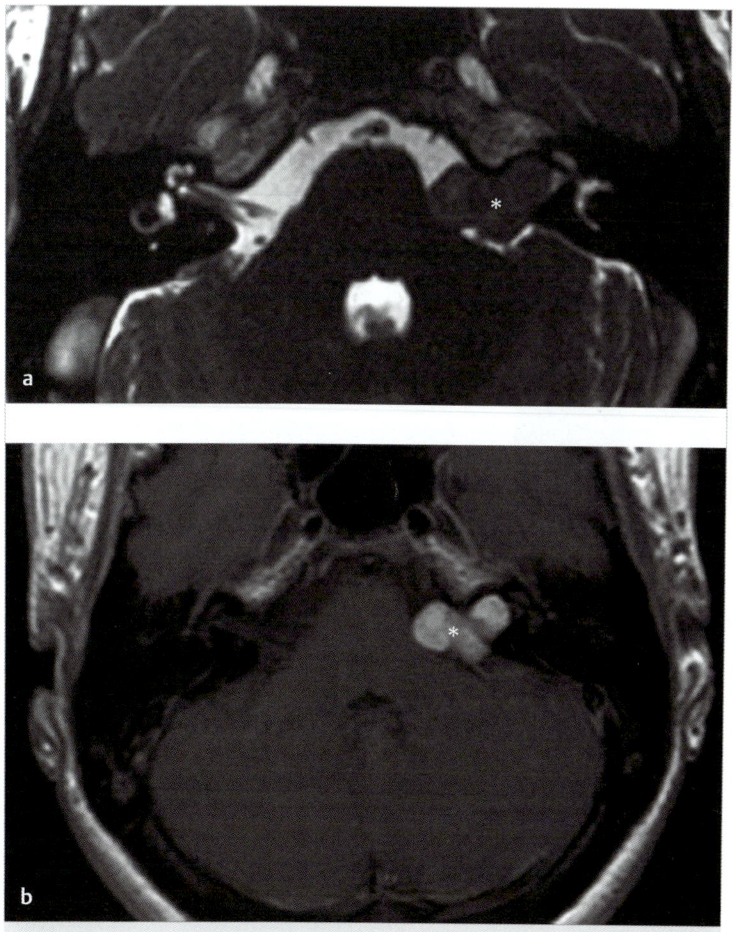

Fig. 5.34 Left vestibular schwannoma (VS). (a, b) note the anterior extension into the cerebellopontine angle (CPA) (*).

direction in the CPA cistern, and may extend into Meckel's cave and along the trigeminal branches. FN schwannomas can sometimes be difficult to distinguish from small VS. On contrast-enhanced MRI, abnormal enhancement can be seen to extend into the labyrinthine segment toward the geniculate ganglion. Trigeminal schwannoma is the most common one and it is classified, according to its location:

- Type I. Predominantly middle fossa tumors;
- Type II. Predominantly posterior fossa tumors with limited middle fossa involvement;
- Type III. Significant middle and posterior fossa components;
- Type IV. Extradural tumors involving the infratemporal fossa and the surrounding structures.

When a facial schwannoma is suspected, CT should be recommended to demonstrate an enlargement of the facial nerve canal. Facial schwannomas in the IAC are more likely to present with SNHL. On MR images, they may present as lobulated masses (when in the CPA cistern, IAC, tympanic segment, and parotid space) or segments of fusiform expansion (when in the labyrinthine and mastoid segments). Finally, glossopharyngeal, vagus, and spinal accessory nerve schwannomas, also called jugular foramen schwannomas, may extend cranially with a large component coming back up in the CPA, especially when cystic, and mimic an intracisternal VS (see the section Schwannomas/Meningiomas). However, a more caudal center and the extension through an enlarged JF are the key features for the diagnosis (see ▶ Fig. 5.41).

Metastasis

Meningeal metastases from lung or breast cancers, melanoma, or more rarely from other cancers, may invade the CPA. CPA metastases should be sought when vertigo or other cranial nerve symptoms appear in a known cancer patient. However, correct preoperative diagnosis is frequently difficult in patients in whom a primary tumor has not been detected at the time of the identification of the lesion in the CPA. The imaging characteristics are nonspecific. These lesions can be detected on CT, MRI, and bone scan. Usually, the presence of multifocal cerebral lesions is highly suggestive of metastases, but CPA metastases may be solitary and mimic benign tumors of the CPA, or be bilateral, mimicking type 2 neurofibromatosis. Metastases from cutaneous melanomas certainly represent the most frequent etiology of melanocytic tumors in the CPA. T1-weighted precontrast imaging is most useful to show replacement of normal fatty marrow and DWI shows restriction caused by the typical increased tumor cellularity. MR spectroscopy shows a predominant peak in lipids in metastasis, another important finding which might be considered suggestive of the diagnosis.

Vascular Anomalies

Vascular masses make up only 3.4% of all CPA lesions, including vascular anomalies, aneurysms, and neoplastic processes. The aneurysms of the posterior inferior cerebellar artery or vertebral artery are the most common lesions. It is not uncommon for a loop of the AICA to enter the porus acusticus, without symptoms. Sometimes, a facial hemispasm and tinnitus can be present.

5.3.3 Lesions Involving Jugular Foramen

The JF is a complex crossroads of neurovascular structures deep in the skull base. It has a complex oblique course running anteriorly, then laterally, and eventually inferiorly through the skull base into the carotid space. It is anteromedially separated from the carotid canal by the caroticojugular spine and inferomedially from the hypoglossal canal by the jugular tubercle. JF lesions may originate from its intrinsic contents, or arise from the surrounding structures and secondarily involve the foramen. Normal variants and imaging artifacts, simulating diseases, are not infrequent in this region. Symptoms include pain, lower cranial nerve palsies, and otological symptoms.

Anatomical Variants (High Jugular Bulb, Dehiscence)

There are a number of important jugular bulb variants and anomalies that should be recognized. Conventionally, a high-riding jugular bulb is defined as a jugular bulb with its roof extending above the inferior tympanic annulus. Some authors have used the inferior margin of the basal turn of cochlea as the criterion of choice. High-riding jugular bulbs are more common on the right side, with an incidence of 4 to 24%. CT scan is really helpful to clearly understand the anatomy of the jugular bulb, particularly for the evaluation of CPA lesions before translabyrinthine or cochlear implant surgery. Sometimes, a high jugular bulb may be associated with focal dehiscence of the jugular (sigmoid) plate, allowing for the superolateral protrusion of the bulb into the posterior hypotympanum. Patients

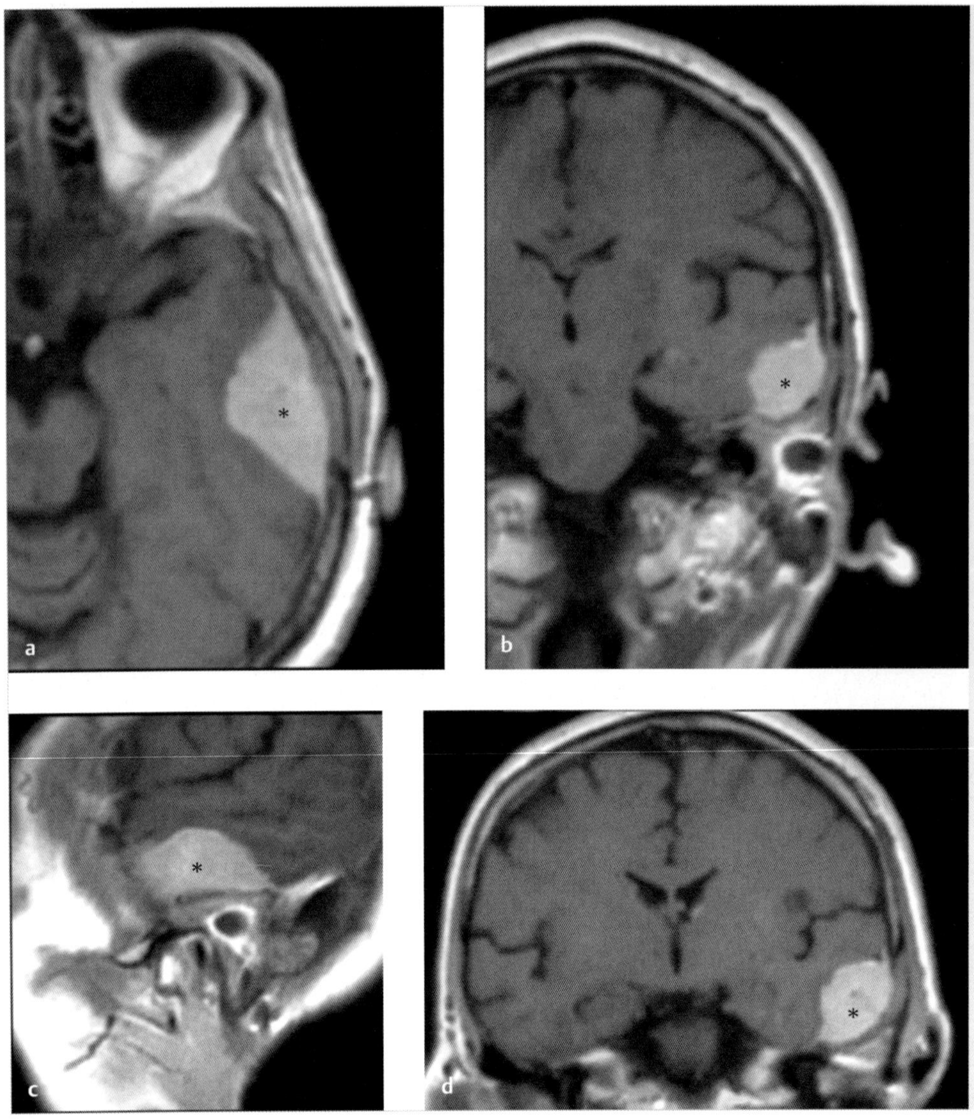

Fig. 5.35 Left temporal lobe meningioma. **(a–d)** Note the presence of a meningioma (*) and the dural reaction with enhancement in the inferior surface.

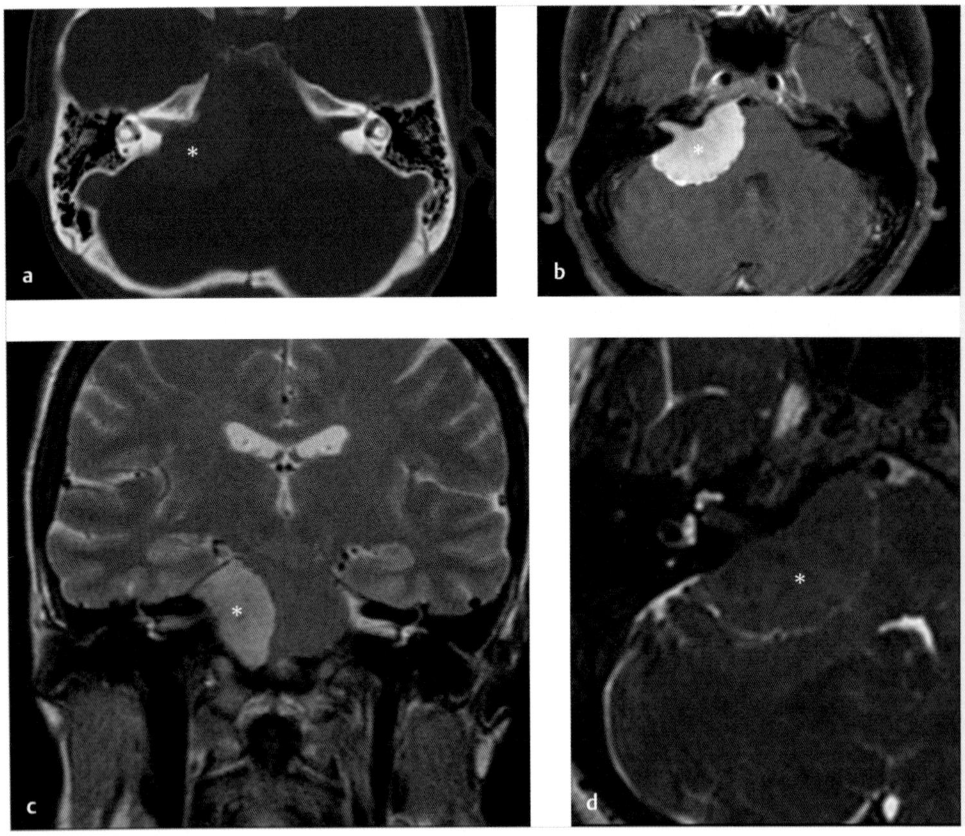

Fig. 5.36 Right cerebellopontine angle (CPA) meningioma. **(a)** Computed tomography (CT) scan; note bone deposition inside the internal auditory canal (IAC). **(b–d)** Magnetic resonance imaging (MRI) aspect. A dural tail is present in the most anterior portion of the lesion. *: meningioma.

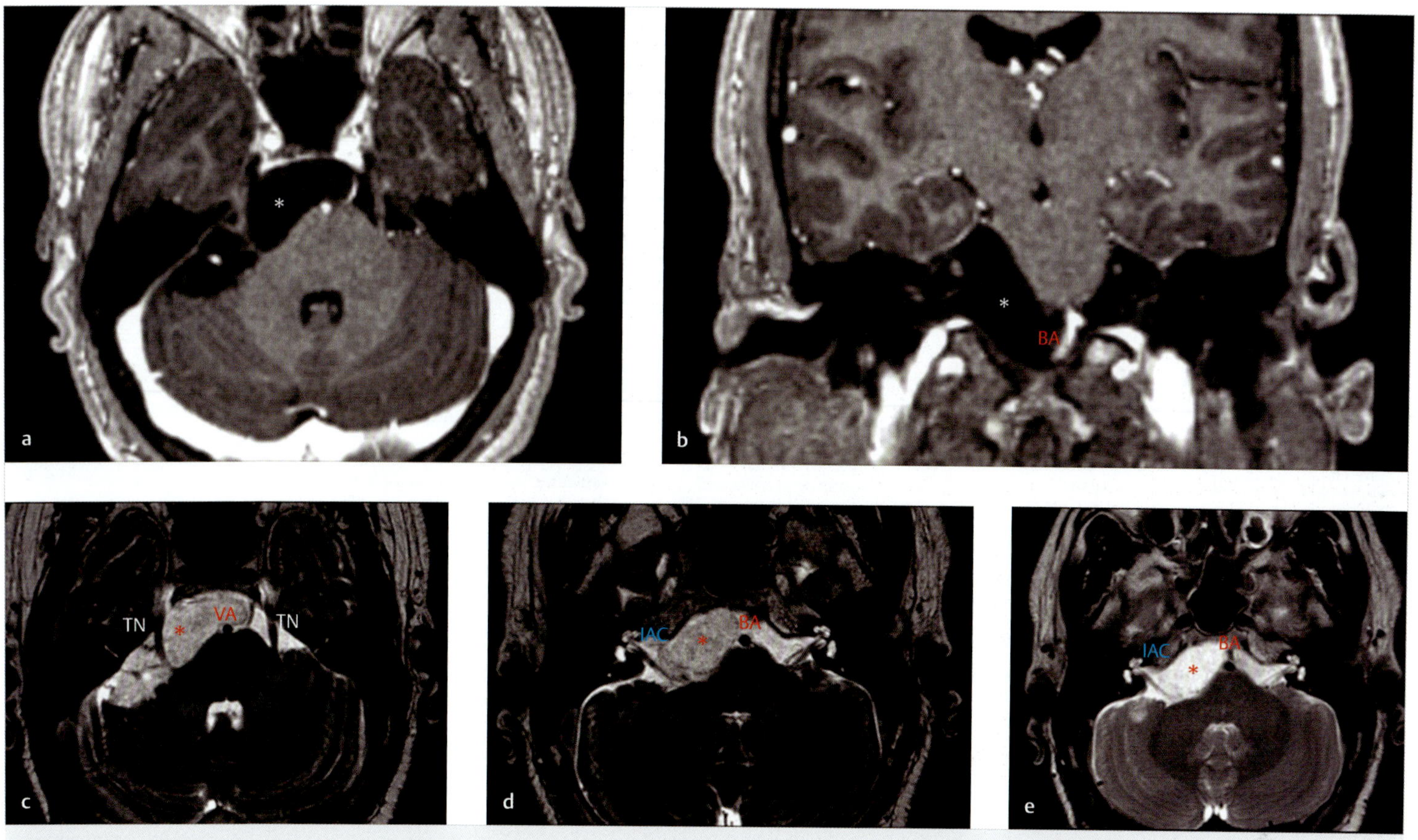

Fig. 5.37 Right epidermoid cyst (*). **(a, b)** Magnetic resonance imaging (MRI) T1 with contrast, showing the medial and contralateral extension of the lesion and the relationship with the basilar artery. **(c–e)** The lesion (*) is seen between the two trigeminal nerves, the basilar artery, and the involvement of right internal auditory canal (IAC). *BA: basilar artery; IAC: internal auditory canal; TN: trigeminal nerve.*

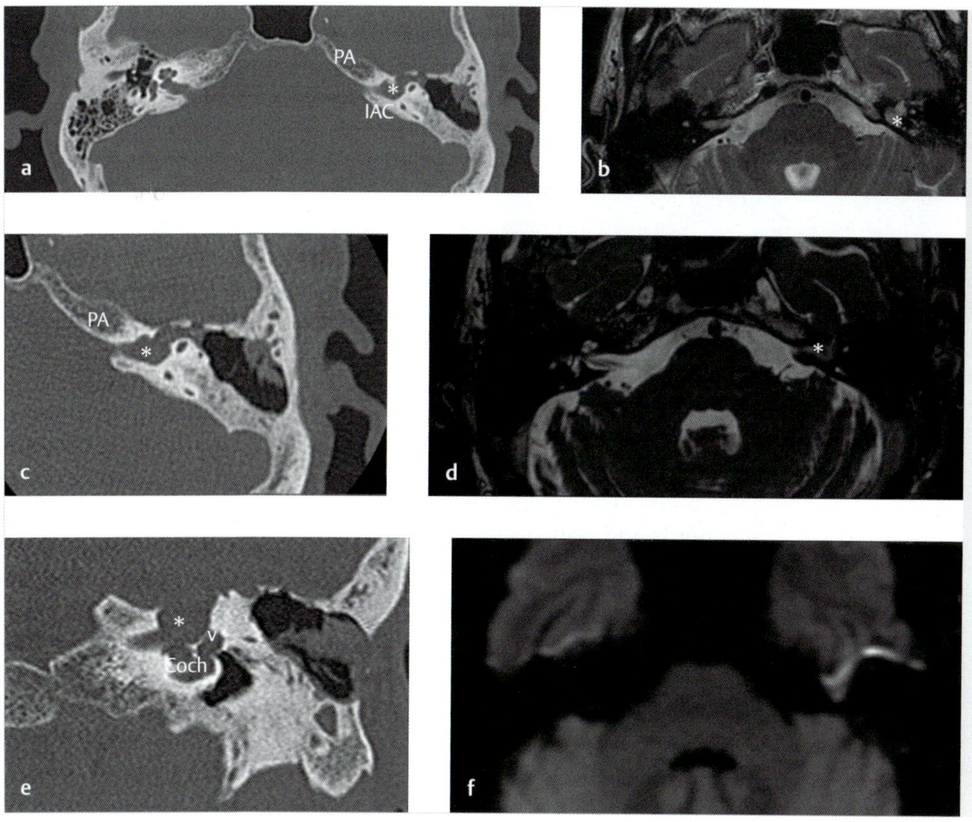

Fig. 5.38 Left petrous bone cholesteatoma (*) in a patient who underwent a mastoidectomy. **(a–d)** Note the computed tomography (CT) scan and magnetic resonance imaging (MRI) showing its extension to the petrous apex and internal auditory canal (IAC). **(e)** Note the superior location of the lesion to the cochlea. **(f)** MRI hyperintensity signal. *Coch: cochlea; IAC: internal auditory canal; PA: petrous apex; V: vestibule.*

can be asymptomatic or show pulsatile tinnitus or conductive hearing loss. It is also important to underline the study of the venous drainage system through the transverse sinus, the jugular bulb, and the IJV, which should be evaluated in all surgical approaches to lateral skull base, and the identification of the predominant site or in rare cases of only one drainage, in order to check if it is possible to close the IJV in a safe way, avoiding cerebral edema in the postoperative period (see ▶ Fig. 5.42).

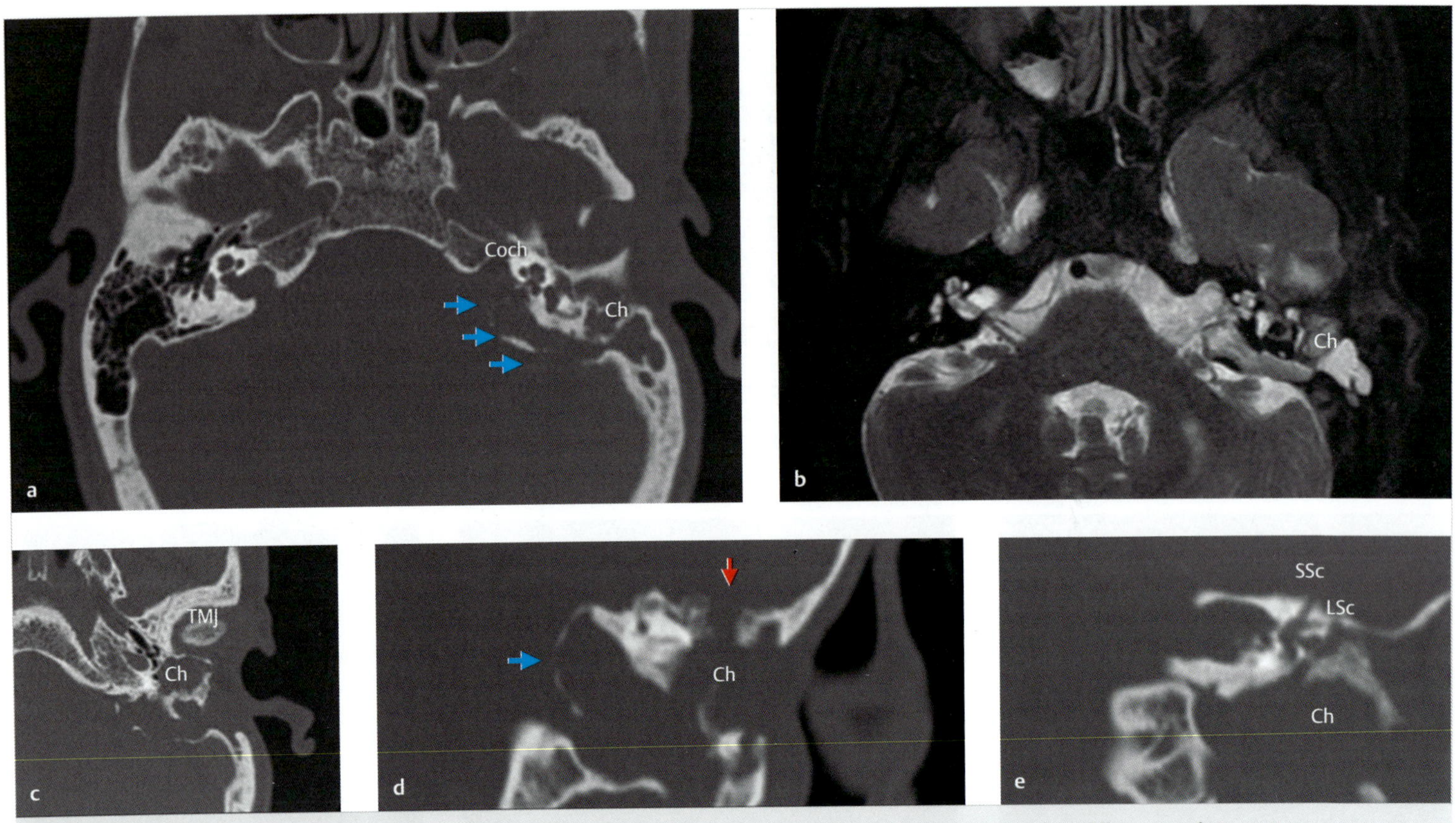

Fig. 5.39 Left petrous bone cholesteatoma (PBC). The patient developed the PBC after radiotherapy for a middle ear embriogenic rhabdomyosarcoma. Bone erosion (**a, c, e**, *light blue arrows*) and middle fossa floor defect (**d**, *red arrow*) are shown. **(b)** T2 magnetic resonance imaging (MRI) of the cholesteatoma. *Ch: cholesteatoma; Coch: cochlea; LSc: lateral semicircular canal; SSc: superior semicircular canal; TMJ: temporomandibular joint.*

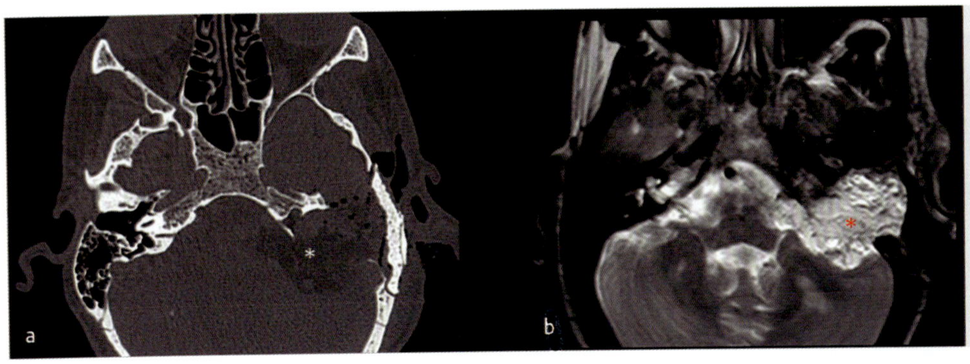

Fig. 5.40 Postoperative imaging after a translabyrinthine...

JF can be involved by:

- Inflammatory conditions;
- Primitive tumors, arising from the JF (paragangliomas, schwannomas, meningiomas);
- Metastasis.

Infection/inflammation

Temporal bone osteomyelitis usually complicates severe external otitis, otitis media, or mastoiditis, with subsequent involvement of the JF. Elderly diabetic patients are particularly susceptible to this problem. CT often shows evidence of bony destruction. MRI shows inflammatory reaction, usually spreading in all temporal bone. Several primary skull base tumors, although uncommon, should also be considered as a differential diagnosis of JF masses. The JF may also be invaded by contiguous spread of temporal bone carcinomas arising from the EAC or the endolymphatic sac. Endolymphatic sac tumors are rare tumors associated with von Hippel-Lindau disease. Posterolateral extension of a nasopharyngeal carcinoma may infiltrate the carotid space and JF, with mixed nerve palsy (see ▶ Fig. 5.43 and ▶ Fig. 5.44).

Primary JF Tumors

Primary JF neoplasms are tumors that arise from the intrinsic structures of the foramen, of which glomus jugulare paraganglioma (GJP) is by far the most common, followed by schwannoma and primary jugular foramen meningioma (PJFM).

Temporal Bone Paragangliomas

Type C and D paragangliomas are the second most common tumors of the temporal bone after VS, and the most common tumors at the JF. They may be multicentric in 5 to 10% of cases, with the incidence rising to 25 to 50% in familial paragangliomas. Associations with type 1 multiple endocrine neoplasia syndrome and type 1 neurofibromatosis are well recognized. GJPs account for up to 80% of primary neoplasms of the JF. They arise from paraganglia in the adventitia of the jugular bulb, the superior ganglion of the Xth nerve, or along Jacobson's and Arnold's nerves. Most GJPs are benign but locally aggressive; malignant degeneration occurs in approximately 3 to 4% of cases. On CT, they show the typical

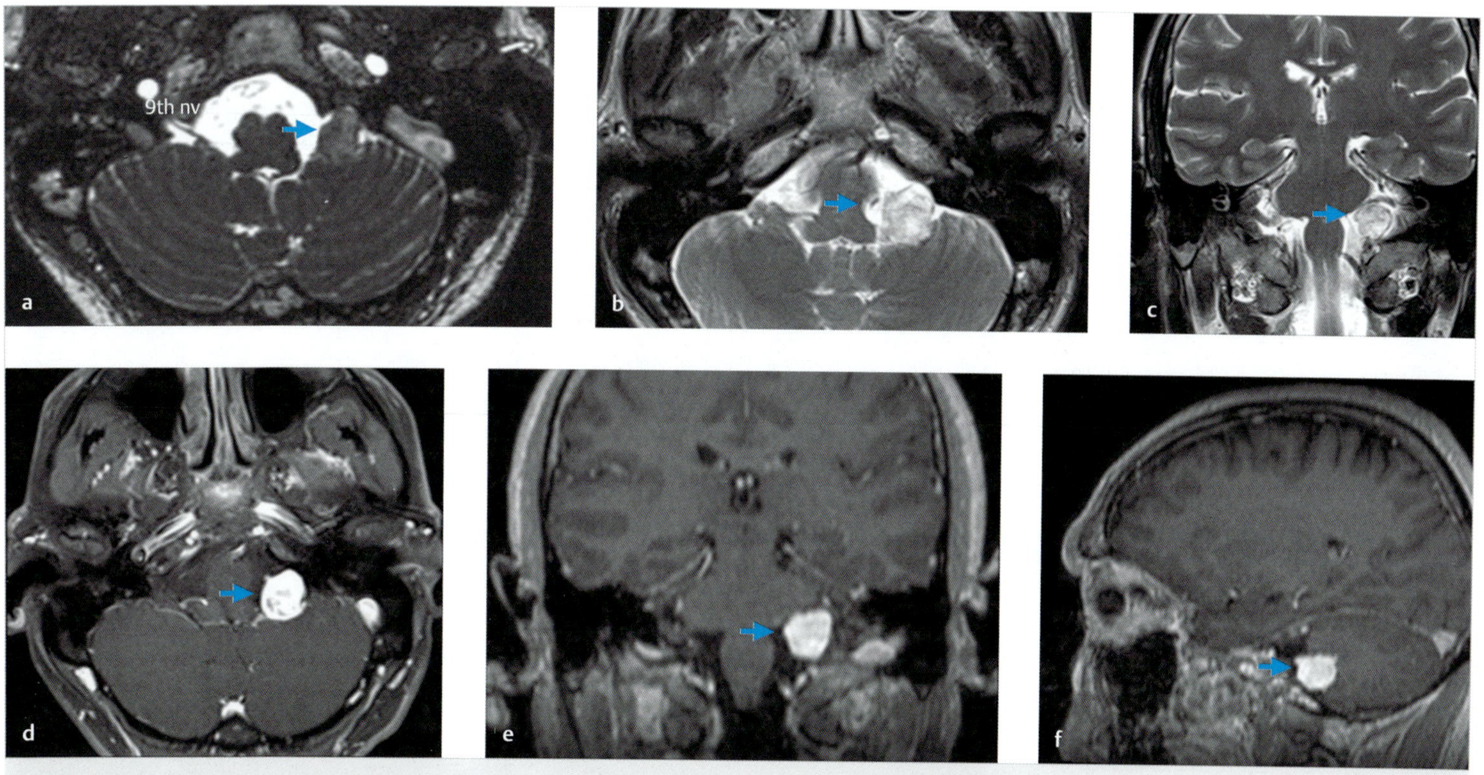

Fig. 5.41 Left mixed nerve schwannoma (*blue arrow*). **(a–c)** T2 magnetic resonance imaging (MRI) signal; note the contralateral glossopharyngeal nerve. **(d–f)** Axial, coronal, and sagittal views in T1 with contrast MRI sequence. 9th nv: glossopharyngeal nerve.

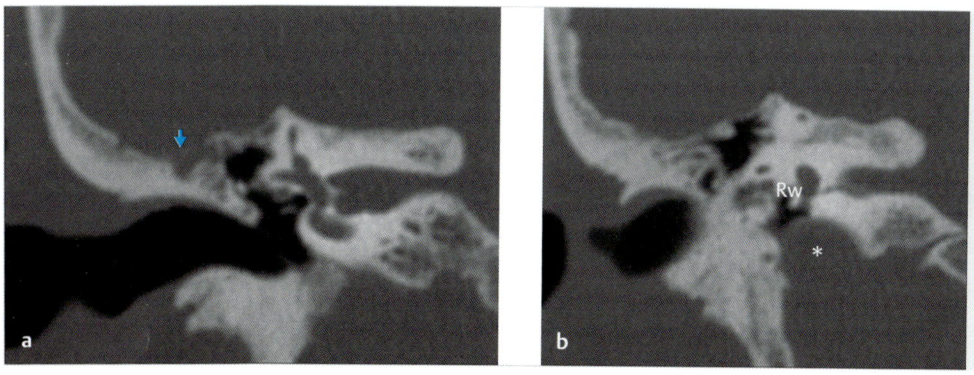

Fig. 5.42 Computed tomography (CT) scan of left temporal bone with meningocele (**a**, *light blue arrow*) and high jugular bulb (**b**, *) in the same patient. The patient underwent an endoscopic assisted cochlear implant with minicraniotomy for the repair of the defect. Rw: round window.

"moth-eaten" permeative-destructive bone changes around the JF, as a result of tumor infiltration through the Haversian canal system. These tumors tend to spread along the "loci minoris resistentiae", particularly through the jugular plate into the middle ear, so they are called "glomus jugulotympanicum paragangliomas." On MRI, larger lesions may demonstrate the characteristic "salt and pepper" appearance on T1-weighted images. The hypointense "pepper" represents high-velocity flow voids of feeding arterial branches within the tumors (which may also be evident on T2-weighted images), whereas the rarely seen hyperintense "salt" is caused by underlying foci of subacute hemorrhage. This feature is not pathognomonic for GJPs, however, because it has been reported in hypervascular metastases and plasmacytomas of the JF. GJPs enhance intensely following intravenous contrast. Conventional angiography provides a vascular road map for surgeons, and preoperative endovascular embolization has been shown to reduce the vascular volume of the tumor mass and decrease intraoperative bleeding.

Type C paraganglioma in its progression can involve the intrapetrous ICA, so according to the Fisch syestem it is classified as (see ▶ Fig. 5.22):

- C1: Tumors destroying the JF and the bulb with limited involvement of the vertical portion of the carotid canal
- C2: Tumors invading the vertical portion of the carotid canal
- C3: Tumors invading the horizontal portion of the carotid canal
- C4: Tumors reaching the anterior foramen lacerum

Class D: Defines only the intracranial tumor extension and should be reported as an addendum to the C stage (De, extradural; Di, intradural):

- De1: Tumors with up to 2 cm dural displacement
- De2: Tumors with more than 2 cm dural displacement
- Di1: Tumors with up to 2 cm intradural extension
- Di2: Tumors with more than 2 cm intradural extension
- Di3: Tumors with inoperable intracranial intradural extension

A preoperative evaluation of these lesions, is mandatory for both the venous drainage system and the arterial supply, because the tumor, which is typically vascularized by the external carotid artery system, can be vascularized also by the ICA system and the vertebral artery system. In Class C tumors the major blood supply comes from the ascending pharyngeal artery. Depending on the involvement of the internal carotid canal, additional blood supply from the ICA can also be present. In Class D tumors the intracranial extradural extensions can be supplied by the meningeal branches

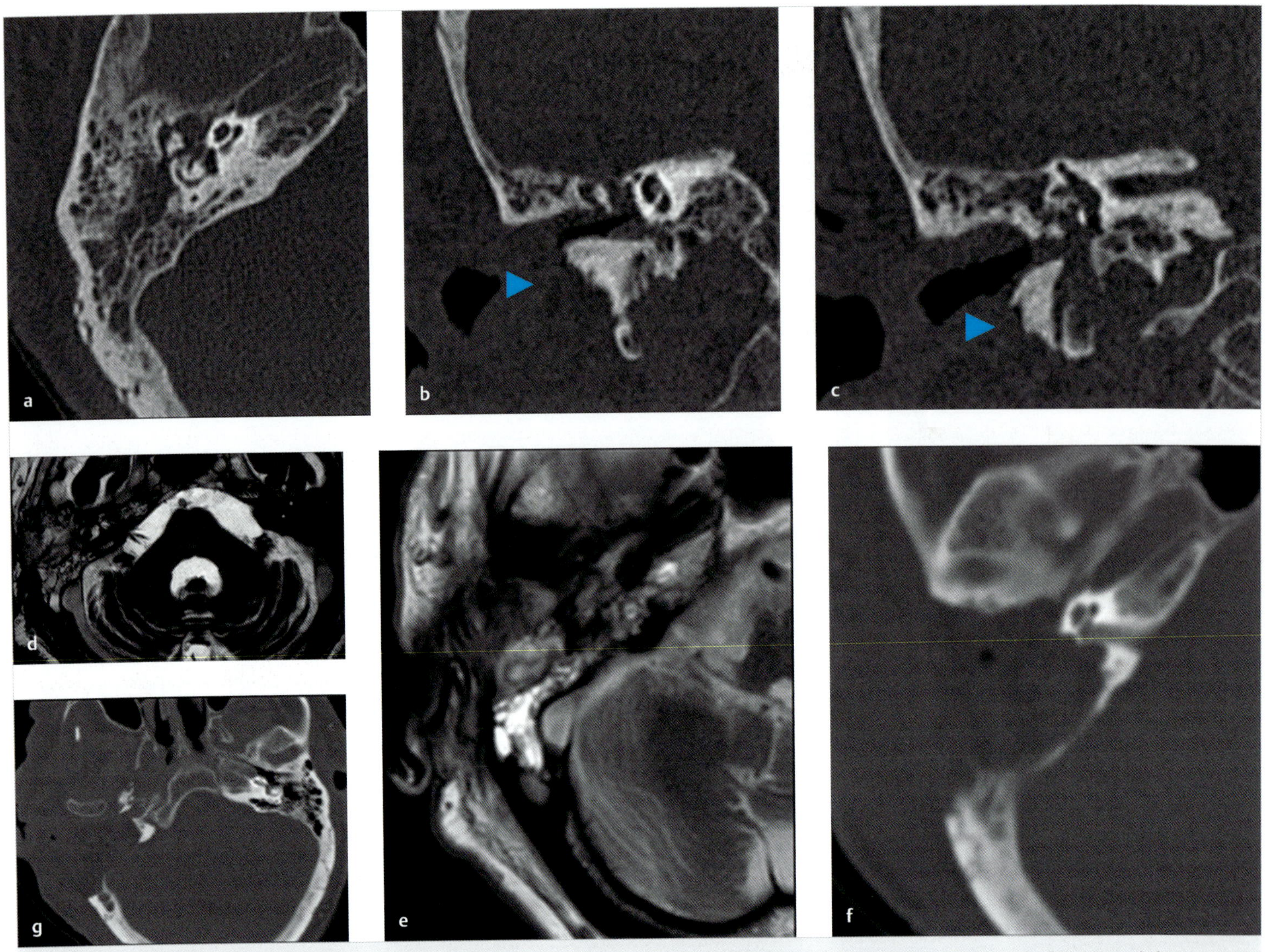

Fig. 5.43 Right temporal bone mycosis. **(a–c)** Computed tomography (CT) scan with erosion of the external auditory canal (EAC) and the mastoid tip (*light blue triangle*). **(d, e)** Magnetic resonance imaging (MRI) shows the real extension of the infection. **(f, g)** Postoperative CT scan after a transotic approach.

of the ascending pharyngeal, occipital, and middle meningeal arteries, by the clival meningeal branches of the ICA, and the meningeal branches of the vertebral artery. Intradural extensions are supplied by the posteroinferior and anteroinferior cerebellar artery.

An accurate angiography should always be carried out to study the arterial supply and to look for any vessel wall abnormalities, especially in the adventitia, suggesting a preoperative treatment of the carotid artery. The vascular preoperative management is done through a direct closure of the damaged tract or through the endovascular positioning of a stent that permits a safe dissection of the tumor from the artery. A lumen stenosis, an involvement of the horizontal intrapetrous tract, or a circumferential carotid encasement can represent other indications for preoperative management of the artery (see ▶ Fig. 5.45).

All these evaluations are performed through an occlusion test, and also when an intraoperative rupture is possible, for example, after radiotherapy. A balloon occlusion test of the ICA is performed before to check for adequate collateral flow. While the balloon remains inflated for 30 minutes during the occlusion test, the patient is awake and is monitored with serial neurological examinations to detect for new deficits and through an angiography to assess the collateral circulation, including the vertebral arteries and contralateral ICA. if the occlusion shows no adverse effects and if the contralateral circulation is satisfactory, the surgeon may be close the ICA during the surgical approach if required (see ▶ Fig. 5.46, ▶ Fig. 5.47, ▶ Fig. 5.48, ▶ Fig. 5.49, ▶ Fig. 5.50).

Schwannomas/Meningiomas

Jugular foramen schwannomas (JFSs) are encapsulated benign tumors arising from Schwann cells wrapping around the IXth to XIth nerves, or less frequently the Jacobson's and Arnold's nerves. They most often originate from the glial Schwann cell junctions, and the Schwann cells around the ganglia of the IXth and Xth nerves within the JF which are particularly susceptible to tumor development. In the absence of type 2 neurofibromatosis, JFSs are rare and constitute only 3% of all intracranial schwannomas. These lesions should be differentiated from VSs, which arise primarily from the internal acoustic canal. CT shows smooth and sharply marginated JF enlargement. Schwannomas may be isodense or hypodense on CT because of their rich lipid content. The low-density appearance on CT is particularly characteristic. They

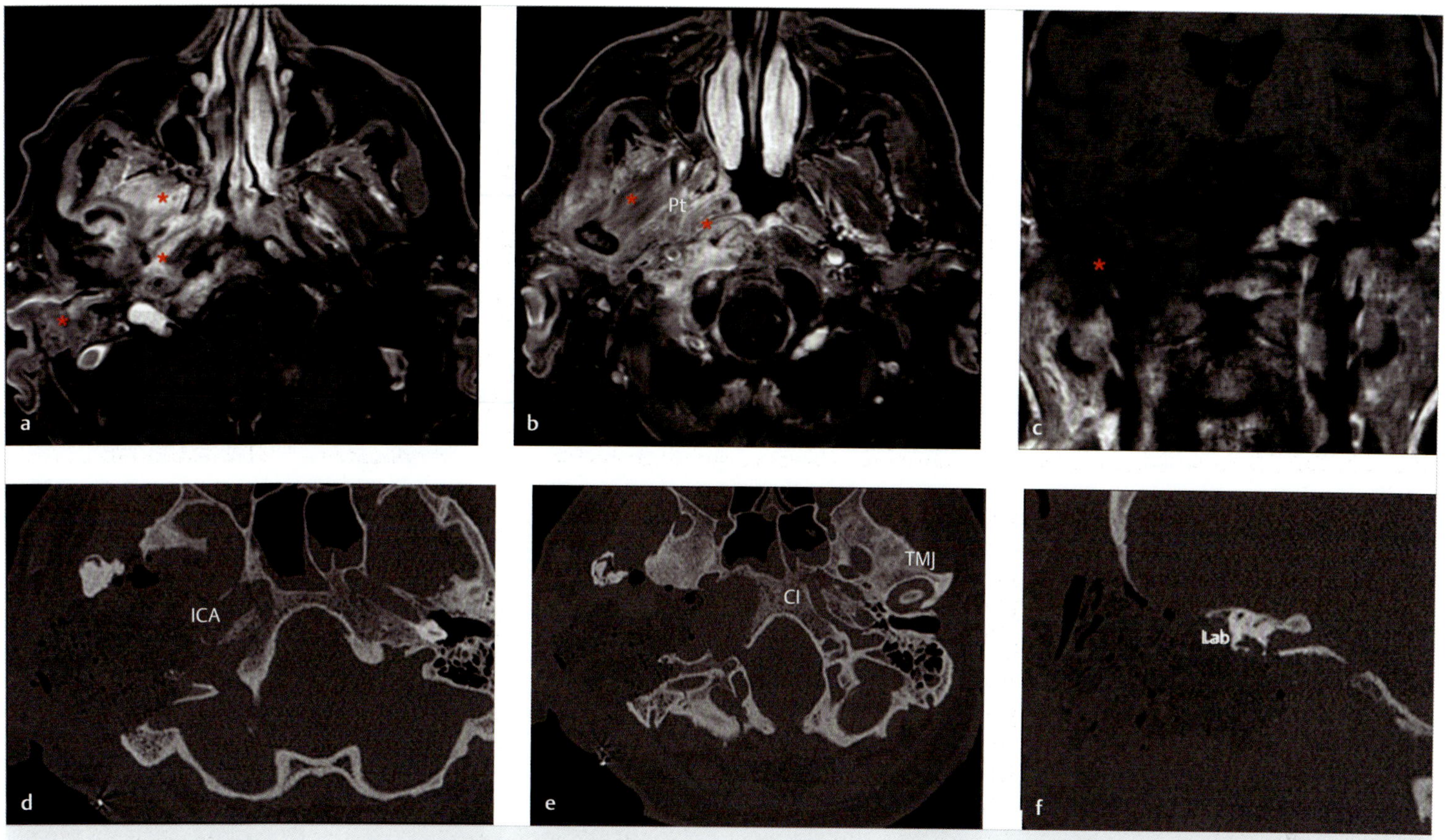

Fig. 5.44 Right mycotic petrositis. **(a–c)** Note the massive involvement of all temporal bone, neck, cerebellopontine angle (CPA), and masticatory space (*). **(d–f)** Postoperative computed tomography (CT) scan after infra temporal fossa type A approach combined with transcochlear approach. *Cl: clivus; ICA: internal carotid artery; Lab: labyrinth; Pt: pterygoid muscles.TMJ: temporomandibular joint.*

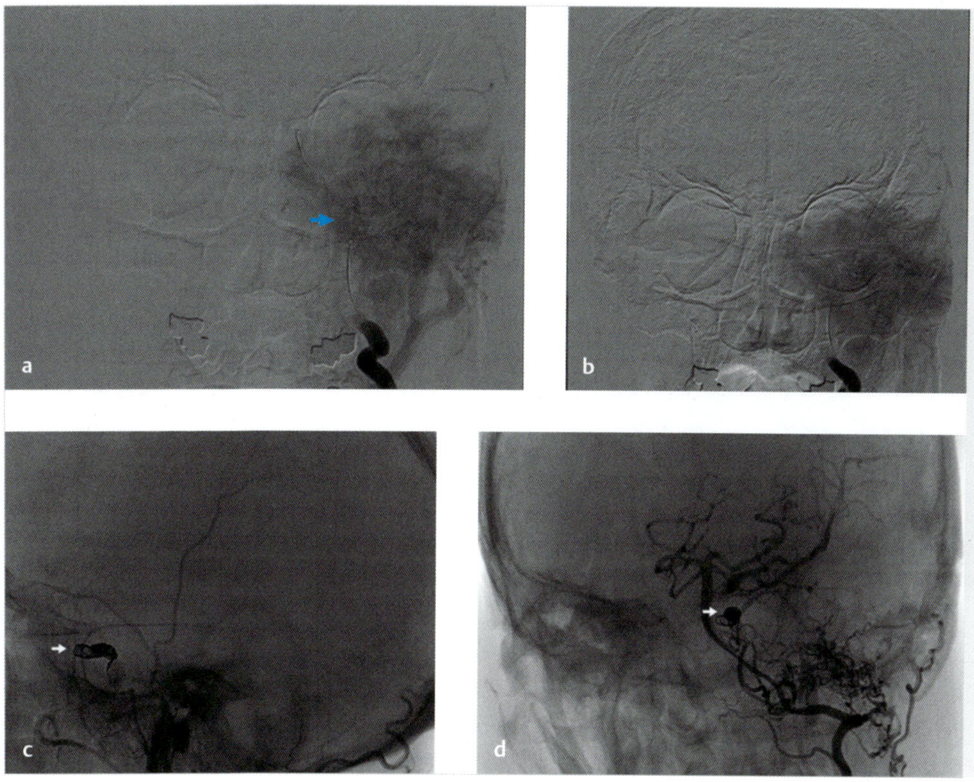

Fig. 5.45 Left huge temporal bone class D paraganglioma. **(a)** Balloon occlusion test (*light blue arrow*). **(b)** Control after 35 days from the closure. **(c, d)** Left internal carotid artery (ICA) closure with coils (*white arrow*).

appear as well-limited masses respectively with low and high signal intensity on T1- and T2-weighted MR images. Avid contrast-enhancement is the norm, with intramural cysts seen in up to 25% of the tumors. Meningiomas have an unusual location in JF, arising from arachnoidal meningothelial cap cells found along the IXth to XIth nerves in the JF. CT shows hyperdense masses, and they are hypointense to isointense on both T1- and T2-weighted MR images. The relative CT hyperattenuation and MRI T2 hypointensity are caused by their underlying dense histology. In addition, the extracranial component of PJFMs shows significantly lower signal intensity than the intracranial component on T1-, T2-, and postcontrast T1-weighted images, possibly because of its

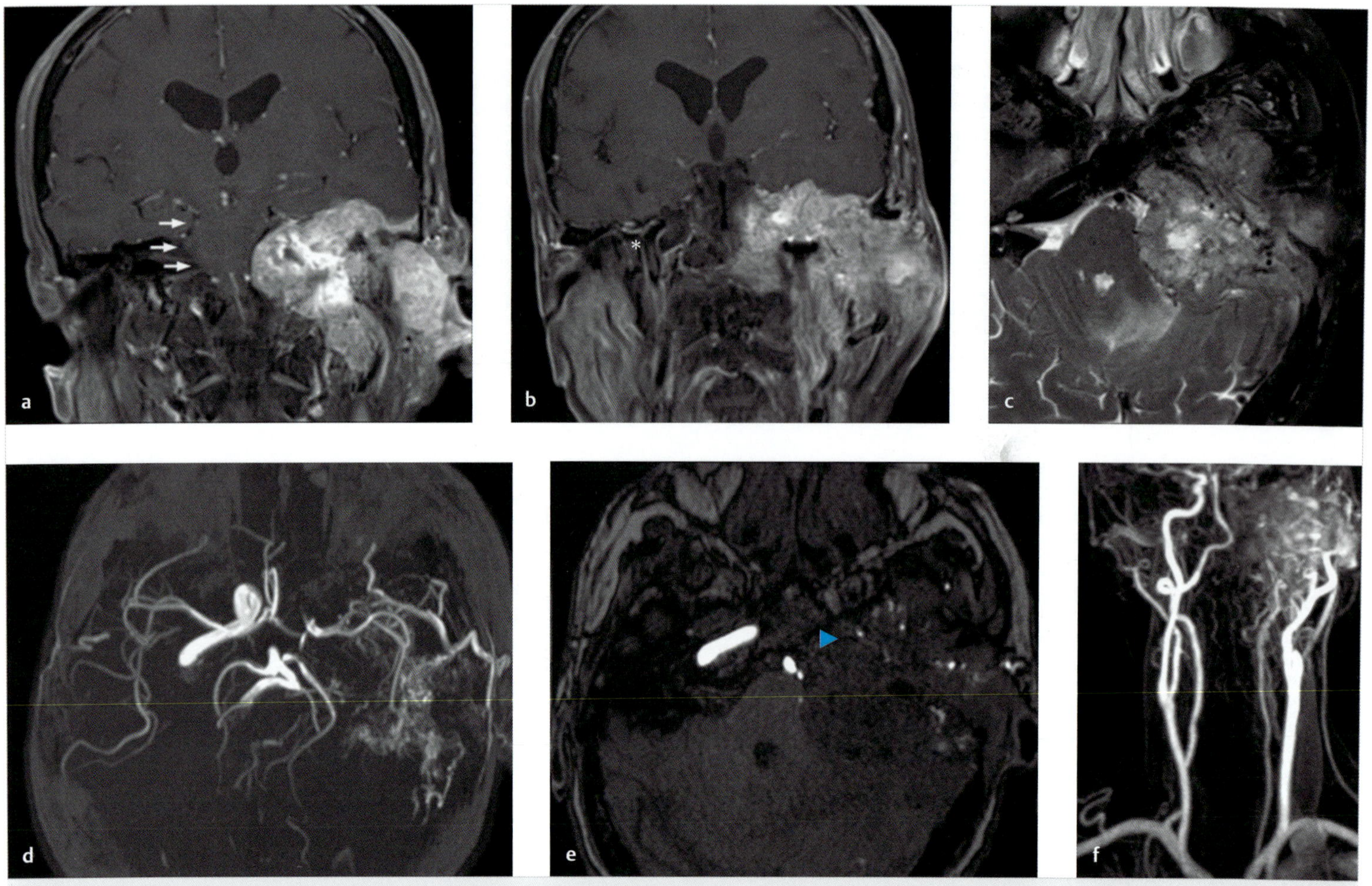

Fig. 5.46 Left huge temporal bone class D paraganglioma. **(a–c)** The magnetic resonance imaging (MRI) shows the extension of the tumor and the compression of the brainstem (*white arrows*). **(d)** Angio MRI demonstrates the vascularization of the tumor. **(e)** Note the absence of signal in the left internal carotid artery (ICA) (*light blue triangle*). **(f)** Coronal view of the tumor.

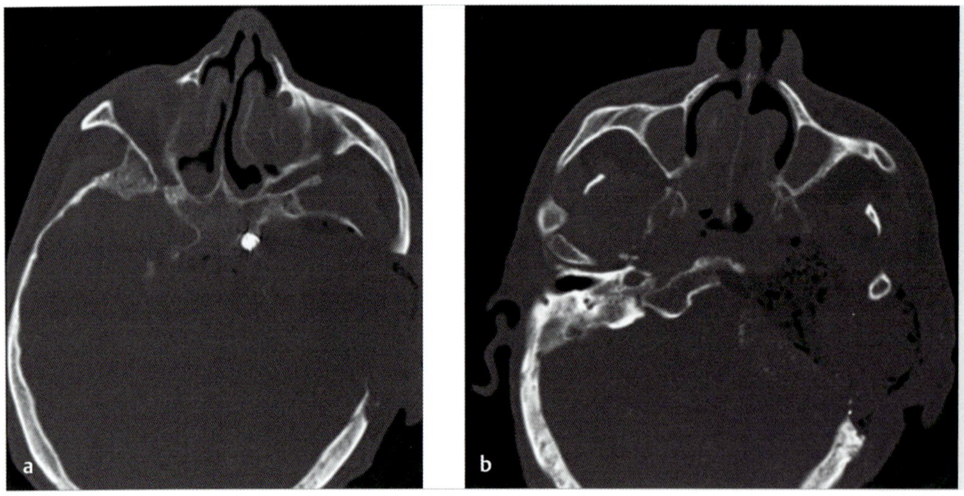

Fig. 5.47 Postoperative computed tomography (CT) scan. **(a)** Internal carotid artery (ICA) closure. **(b)** Regular postoperative appearance after first-time surgery (infratemporal fossa type B + transcochlear approach) for the removal of the extradural component of the tumor; a small intradural residual disease over the cerebellum is left (second-stage surgery should be planned). No compression of the brainstem is now seen.

increased fibrosis and collagen content. "Dural tails," extensive intraosseous infiltration, with hyperostosis, and permeative-sclerotic changes in the surrounding skull base are commonly seen also in these lesions, like in other meningiomas.

Metastasis

Metastatic disease in this area can spread from breast, lung, and prostate cancers. CT usually demonstrates an aggressive lytic lesion invading the skull base around the foramen. Multiple lesions may be present. MRI can display the soft tissue extent of the metastasis, and may detect perineural tumor before bone changes are evident on CT. Vascular metastases from melanoma, renal, and thyroid carcinomas may mimic GJPs on MR images with evidence of intratumoral flow voids or hemorrhage.

Petrous Apex

Because the petrous apex is generally a clinically silent area, diagnostic imaging is often the only means of evaluating potential pathological conditions of the petrous apex. In many cases, petrous apex disease is accidentally discovered while scanning an unrelated problem. Both, HRCT and gadolinium-enhanced MRI are effective in characterizing the various disease processes

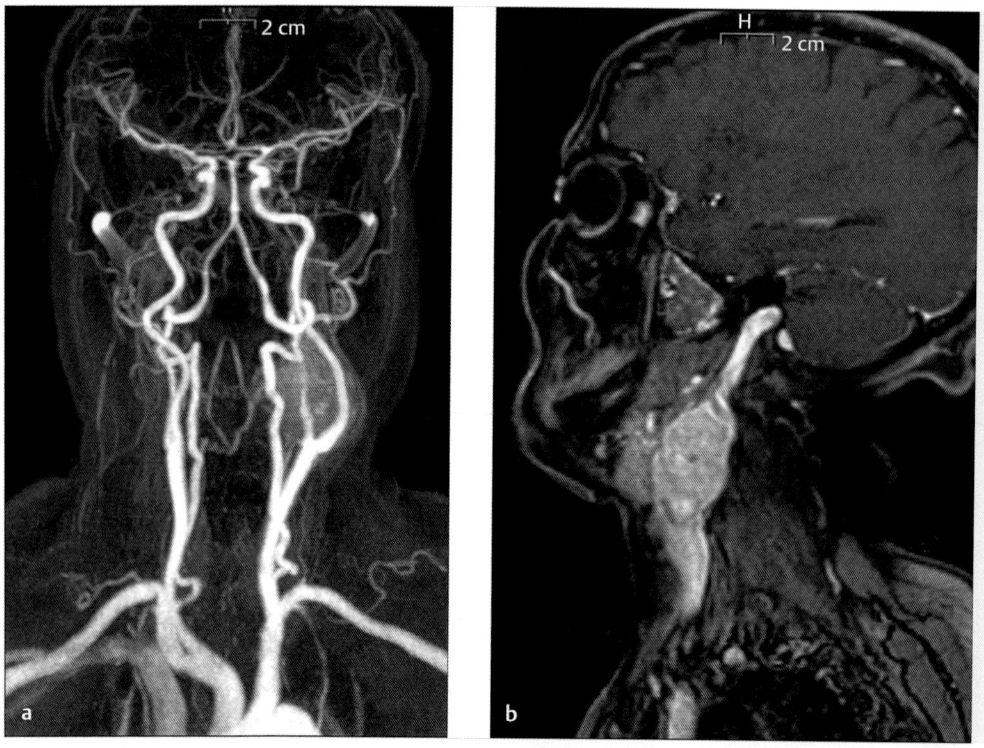

Fig. 5.48 Left carotid paraganglioma. **(a, b)** Angio magnetic resonance imaging (angio MRI), coronal and sagittal views.

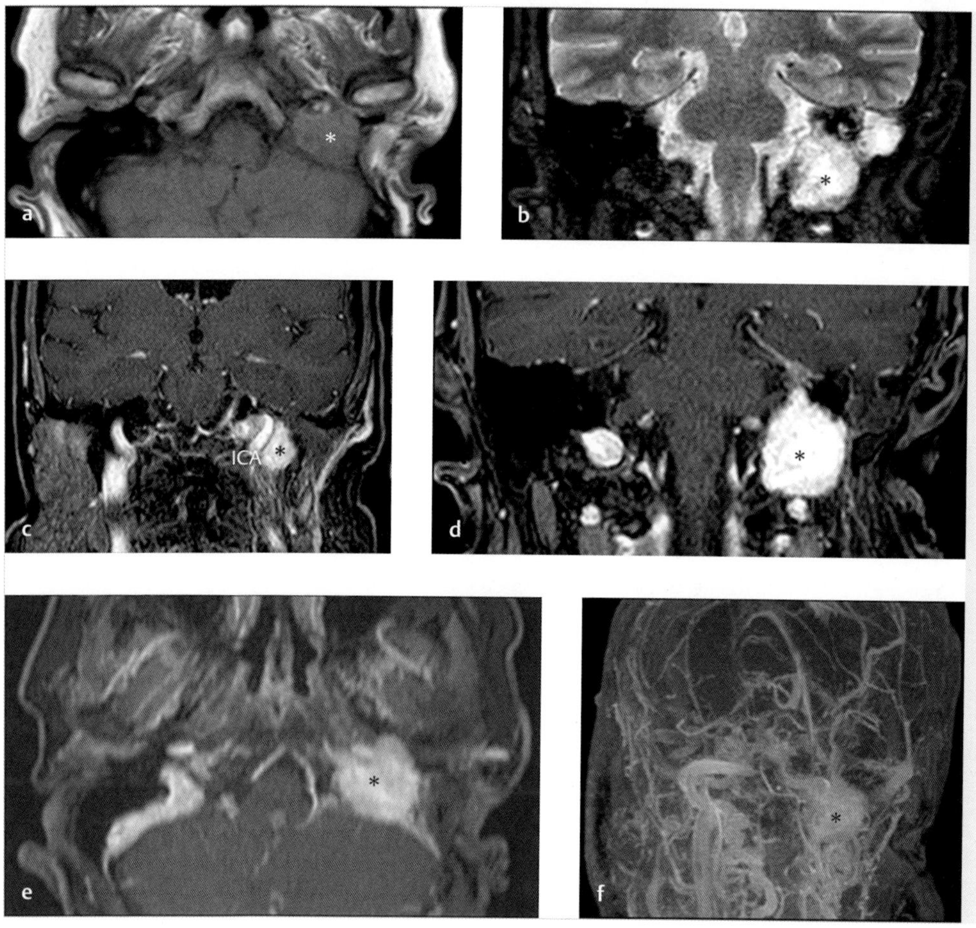

Fig. 5.49 Left jugular foramen (JF) paraganglioma (**a, b**). Note the course of the left ICA **(c)** and the lesion centered on JF (**d–f**, *). **(f)** 3D reconstruction. ICA: internal carotid artery.

involving the petrous apex. MRI typically establishes a diagnosis and identifies the intracranial extension when present. HRCT is useful in characterizing the bone destruction and identifying the relationship between the lesion and the surrounding intratemporal structures, such as the carotid artery, the labyrinth and the IAC. Caution must be used to avoid labeling all imaging asymmetry as pathologic. The most common example is when one petrous apex is made of medullary bone, whereas the opposite side is made of pneumatized bone. The side made of medullary bone shows a bright signal on T1-weighted MRI because of fat content. Pathologic conditions can be excluded when the T2-weighted study reveals a fading signal. A fat-suppression technique also rules out pathologic conditions in such cases. A number of identifiable vascular and neural channels are contained within the petrous apex. The petrous carotid canal and IAC are the largest channels crossing or bordering the petrous apex, but Dorello's canal, the subarcuate canal, the singular canal, and Meckel's cave are smaller channels that are also

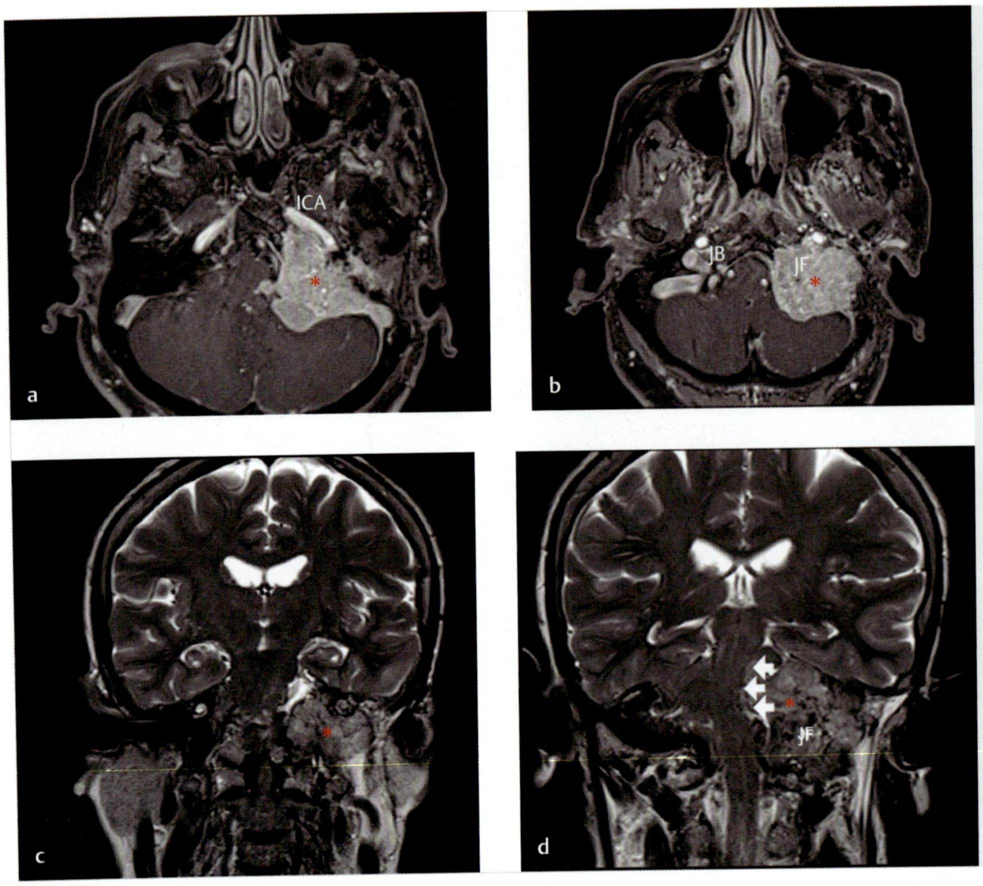

Fig. 5.50 Left jugular foramen (JF) class D paraganglioma. **(a, b)** Magnetic resonance imaging (MRI) with contrast axial view; see the anteromedial component of the tumor in close proximity to the ICA and the JF extension (*). **(c, d)** MRI T2 sequence, coronal view; the compression of the brainstem is well documented (white arrows). *ICA: internal carotid artery; JB: jugular bulb; JF: jugular foramen.*

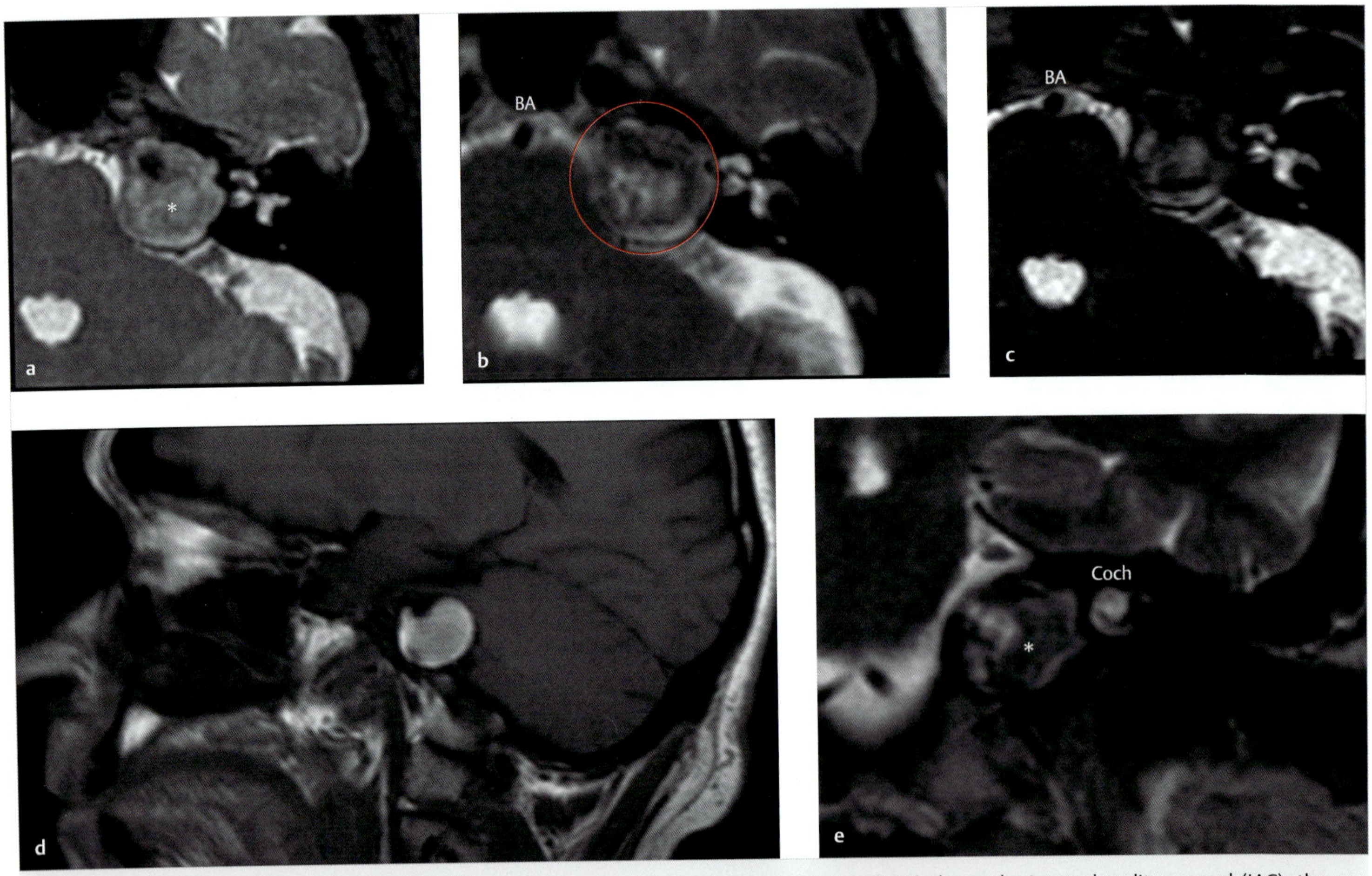

Fig. 5.51 Left vestibular schwannoma (VS) (*, *red circle*). **(a–c)** Magnetic resonance imaging (MRI) shows the internal auditory canal (IAC), the cerebellopontine angle (CPA) and the petrous apex extension of the lesion. **(d, e)** Sagittal view, the relationship of the lesion (*white arrow*) with the cochlea is shown. *BA: basilar artery; Coch: cochlea.*

clearly seen on high-resolution thin-section CT or MR images (see ▶ Fig. 5.51).

Different lesions can spread into the petrous apex:

- Inflammatory processes;
- Mucoceles;
- Cholesterol granulomas;
- Petrous bone cholesteatomas (PBCs);
- Cephaloceles;
- Chordomas;
- Chondrosarcomas;
- Metastases.

Apicitis

Petrous apicitis is probably the most consistently symptomatic petrous apex process. Patients with petrous apicitis usually present with an acute febrile illness and some or all of the symptoms of the classic Gradenigo triad (ear pain, palsy of the VIth cranial nerve, and facial pain). Possible complications of petrous apicitis include meningitis, cerebral abscess formation, and venous sinus thrombosis. Even if the diagnosis can be clinically made, imaging can play a role in identifying abscess formation within the petrous apex or an associated epidural or brain abscess. MRI signal intensifies from the T1- to T2-weighted imaging, and the enhancement with gadolinium is intense. The surrounding dura may also enhance. HRCT demonstrates an opacification and may or may not reveal the destruction of bony septa.

Petrous Apex Trapped Fluid/Mucocele

The petrous apex is pneumatized in nearly one-third of the population via air cell tracts that directly communicate with the middle ear and the mastoid. An asymptomatic sterile fluid collection can also be trapped in the petrous apex air cells, sometimes resulting from remote middle ear cleft infections (petrous apex effusions). Usually fluid signal on T1- and T2-weighted MRI sequences are characteristic of trapped fluid and are not associated with bony erosion on HRCT (see ▶ Fig. 5.52).

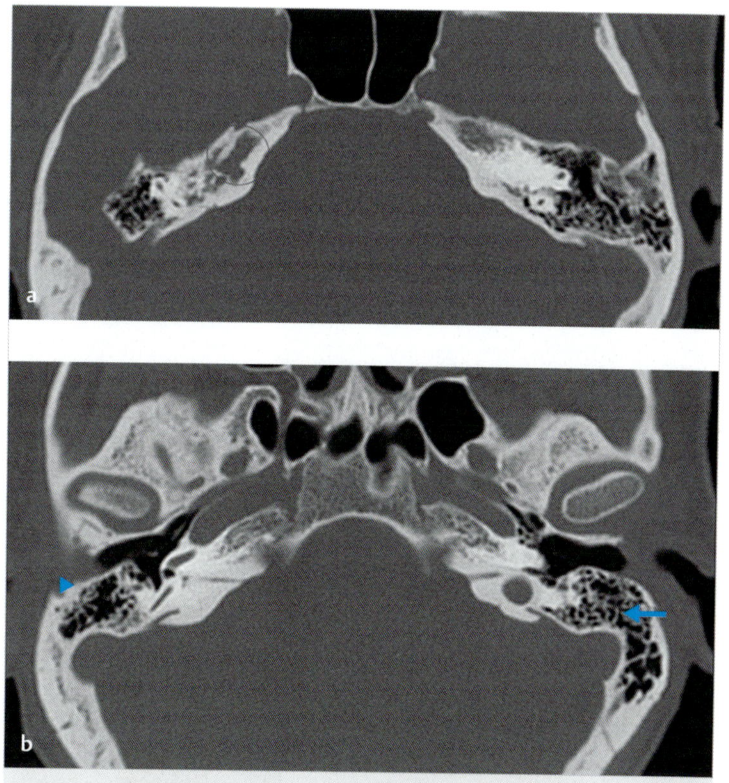

Fig. 5.52 Right petrous apex mucocele. **(a)** See the entrapped fluid located in the petrous apex (*red circle*). **(b)** Normal left temporal bone pneumatization compared with the affected right side.

Cholesterol Granuloma

Cholesterol granulomas are the most common lesions arising in the petrous apex. They usually occur in patients with a pneumatized petrous apex and a long-standing history of otitis media. The cysts are filled with viscous brown fluid, granulation tissue, and cholesterol crystals, which are often contained within a thick fibrous capsule that lacks a true epithelial lining. Cholesterol granulomas can be large at the time of diagnosis. Bone expansion caused by growth of these cysts may lead to "bone gaps" caused by long-standing severe bone remodeling that may be mistaken for bone destruction. A reliable diagnosis of cholesterol granuloma can be made with MRI. Whereas most other petrous apex lesions have low or intermediate signal intensity on T1-weighted images, cholesterol granulomas are usually hyperintense on both T1- and T2-weighted images. Bone marrow in nonpneumatized petrous apices can normally show variations in signal intensity depending on the patient's age. In younger patients, the marrow can show an intermediate signal intensity with conventional sequences because of the high concentration of red marrow. In adults, red marrow is replaced by fatty marrow, which has a higher signal intensity on T1-weighted images. When asymmetric, the high-signal-intensity fatty marrow may be mistaken for a cholesterol granuloma on T1-weighted images. A lack of mass effect and a close observation of the signal intensity with other pulse sequences usually lead to the correct diagnosis. Particularly helpful is the fact that signal from normal fatty bone marrow becomes suppressed on fat-suppressed images. CT demonstrates normal trabeculated bone in the nonpneumatized petrous apex with attenuation similar to that of marrow-containing bone elsewhere in the skull base.

For huge granulomas or growing lesions, a surgical management is required. Surgical options are: middle cranial fossa, transotic, transsphenoidal, and infracochlear approaches, based on the preoperative hearing function and anatomical characteristics of the patient.

The surgical goal is to create a ventilation pathway to the petrous apex, draining entrapped secretions; so a CT scan is very important in order to plan surgery, because it is possible to check:

- The position of the jugular gulf: a high jugular gulf can make it difficult or impossible to perform an endoscopic transcanal infracochlear approach.
- The pneumatization inferior to the cochlea, especially the grade of development of the subcochlear canaliculum. In case of type A subcochlear canaliculus, it is possible to reach the petrous apex with a transcanal infracochlear route.
- The pneumatization of the sphenoid sinus: In case of granulomas located superiorly to the petrous apex, anteriorly to the IAC, it is possible to perform a transnasal transsphenoidal approach.
- Unfavorable anatomical conditions: When facilitating conditions are not present, a transotic approach is recommended, if the preoperative hearing is poor, or a middle cranial fossa approach is recommended, if the preoperative hearing function is to be preserved (see ▶ Fig. 5.53, ▶ Fig. 5.54, ▶ Fig. 5.55, ▶ Fig. 5.56).

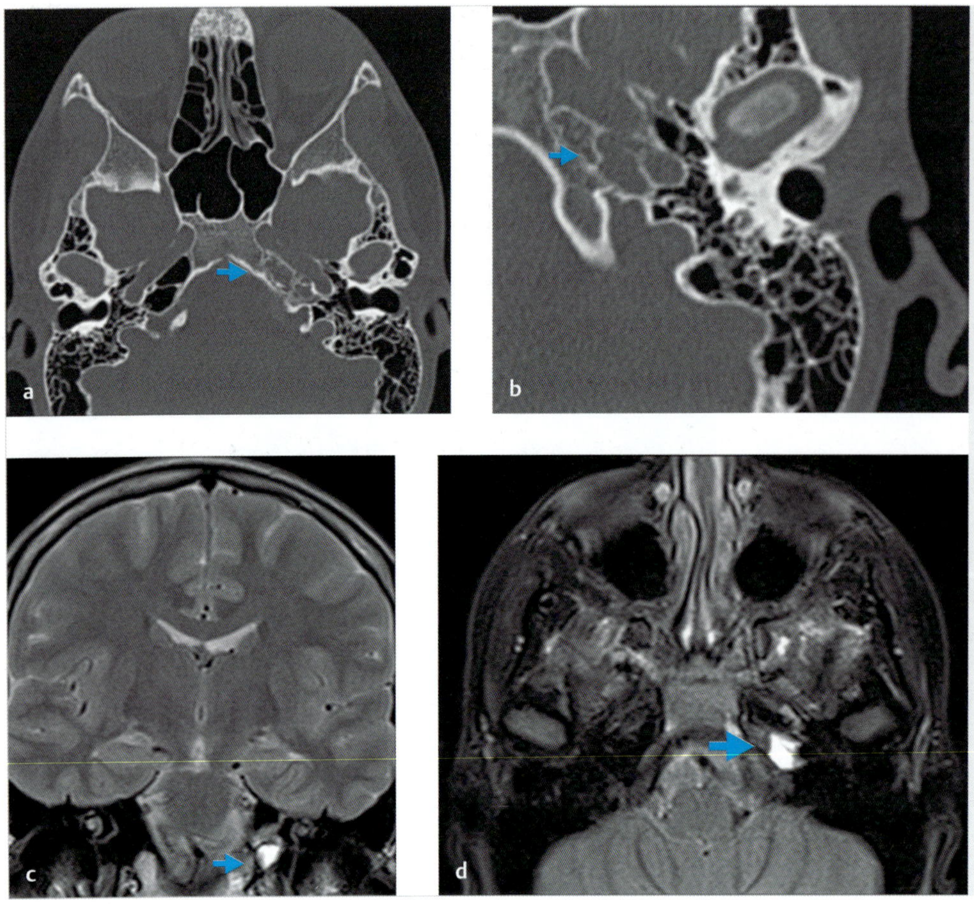

Fig. 5.53 Left cholesterol granuloma of the petrous apex. **(a, b)** Computed tomography (CT) scan; see the lesion compared to the normal pneumatized right side (*light blue arrow*). **(c, d)** Magnetic resonance imaging (MRI) hyperintensity T2 signal of the lesion (*light blue arrow*).

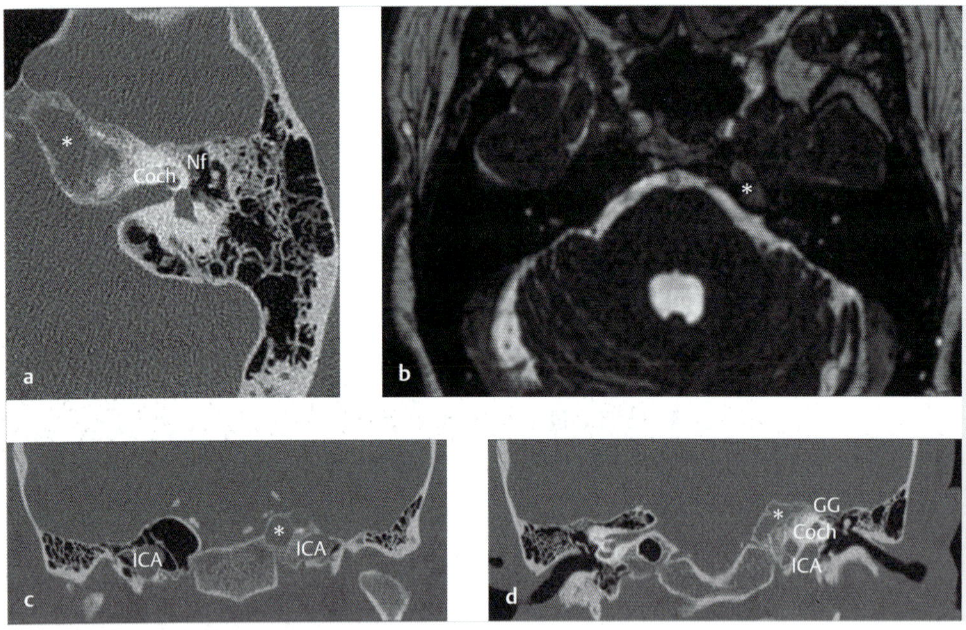

Fig. 5.54 Left petrous apex cholesterol granuloma. **(a–d)** Note the location of the lesion (*) compared to the horizontal and vertical tracts of the ICA and the internal auditory canal (IAC). *Coch: cochlea; Fn: facial nerve tympanic tract; GG: geniculate ganglion; ICA: internal carotid artery.*

Petrous Bone Cholesteatomas

PBCs and epidermoids make up 4 to 9% of all petrous apex lesions. Cholesteatomas may be classified as acquired or congenital, with congenital cholesteatomas of the petrous apex being more common. Congenital cholesteatomas arise from aberrant ectoderm that is trapped during embryogenesis; if histologically analyzed, they consist of cysts lined with stratified squamous epithelium and filled with keratinous debris. A classification of the site and extension of PBCs was initially proposed by Fisch, who separated supra- and infralabyrinthine lesions. In 1993, Sanna et al[120] categorized PBCs into five classes: Class I, supralabyrinthine; Class II, infralabyrinthine; Class III, infralabyrinthine-apical; Class IV, massive; and Class V, apical (see ▶ Fig. 5.57).

Supralabyrinthine

A supralabyrinthine cholesteatoma is characteristically congenital or may result from a deep ingrowth of an acquired tympanic cholesteatoma. It involves the anterior epitympanum and extends medially toward the IAC and anteriorly toward the carotid artery. The cholesteatoma may spread toward the posterior aspect of the bony labyrinth and the retrolabyrinthine mastoid cells.

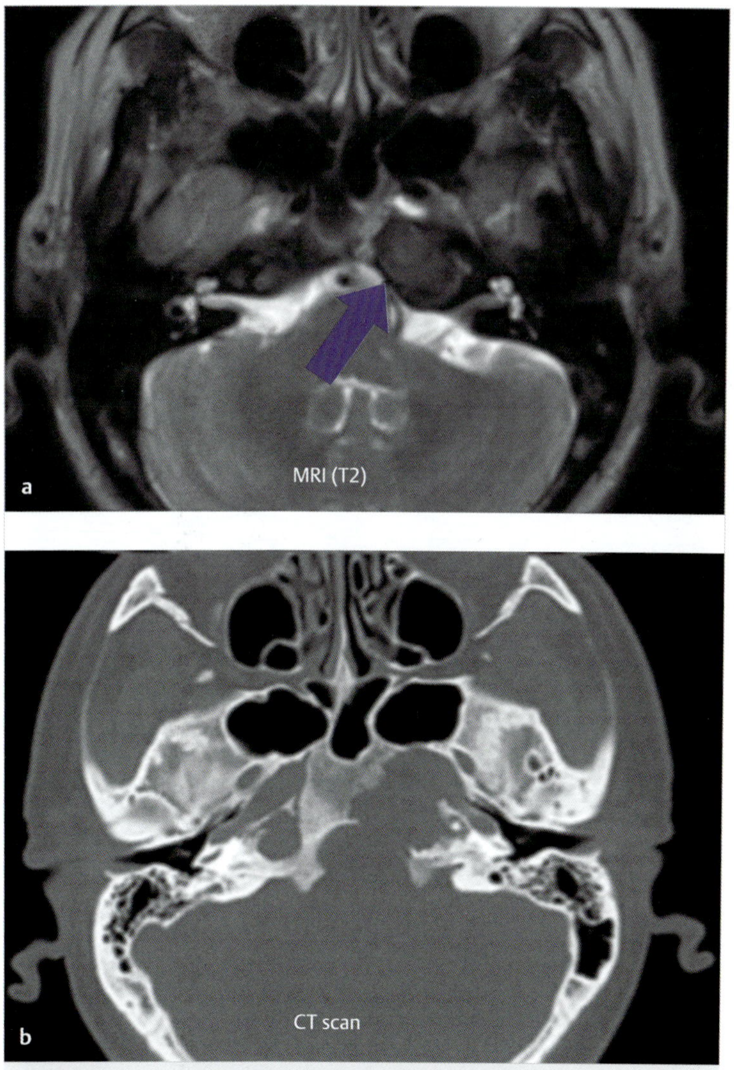

Fig. 5.55 (a) Left cholesterol granuloma surgically treated with transnasal approach (*blue arrow*). (b) Note the conformation of the sphenoid sinus on computed tomography (CT) scan.

Infralabyrinthine

An infralabyrinthine cholesteatoma arises in the hypotympanic and infralabyrinthine regions and extends anteriorly toward the ICA and posteriorly toward the posterior cranial fossa.

Massive labyrinthine

A massive labyrinthine cholesteatoma spreads into the entire posterior and anterior labyrinth. The site of origin results from an extension of supralabyrinthine or infralabyrinthine cholesteatoma. It often develops from a primary acquired cholesteatoma.

Infralabyrinthine-apical

An infralabyrinthine-apical cholesteatoma may arise from the infralabyrinthine or the apical compartments. The former anteriorly extends into the petrous apex and may involve the sphenoid sinus and the horizontal portion of the ICA. The latter arises from the apical compartment and it extends superiorly to the sphenoid sinus and inferoposteriorly to the infralabyrinthine compartment. They are generally congenital in origin.

Apical

It is congenital lesion. It may involve only the apical compartment of the temporal bone. It can cause erosion of the IAC. It may extend toward the posterior cranial fossa or anteriorly to the trigeminal nerve.

In CT scans, cholesteatomas appear as nonenhancing, expansile petrous apex lesions that cause a variable degree of bone destruction. When no or minimal bone destruction is present, they cannot be distinguished from cholesterol granulomas with CT alone. In MRI, cholesteatomas generally have intermediate to low signal intensity on T1-weighted images. On T2-weighted and

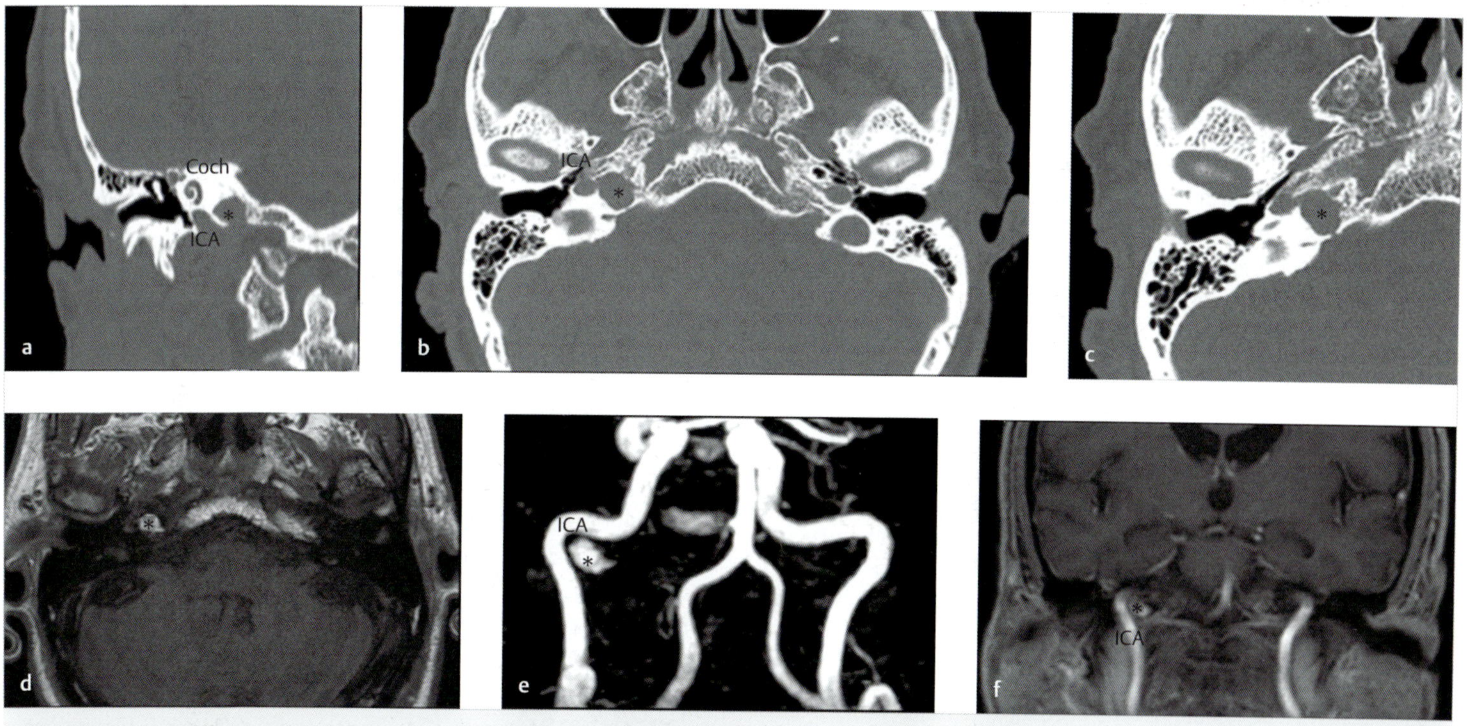

Fig. 5.56 Right petrous apex lesion. (a–c) On computed tomography (CT) scan the lesion is seen medial to the horizontal and vertical tract of internal carotid artery (ICA). (d–f) Magnetic resonance imaging (MRI) confirms the exact location of the pathology. Vascular lesion (*) was suspected on AngioMRI, but the middle fossa approach (MCF), showed the presence of a petrous cholesterol granuloma. *Coch: cochlea.*

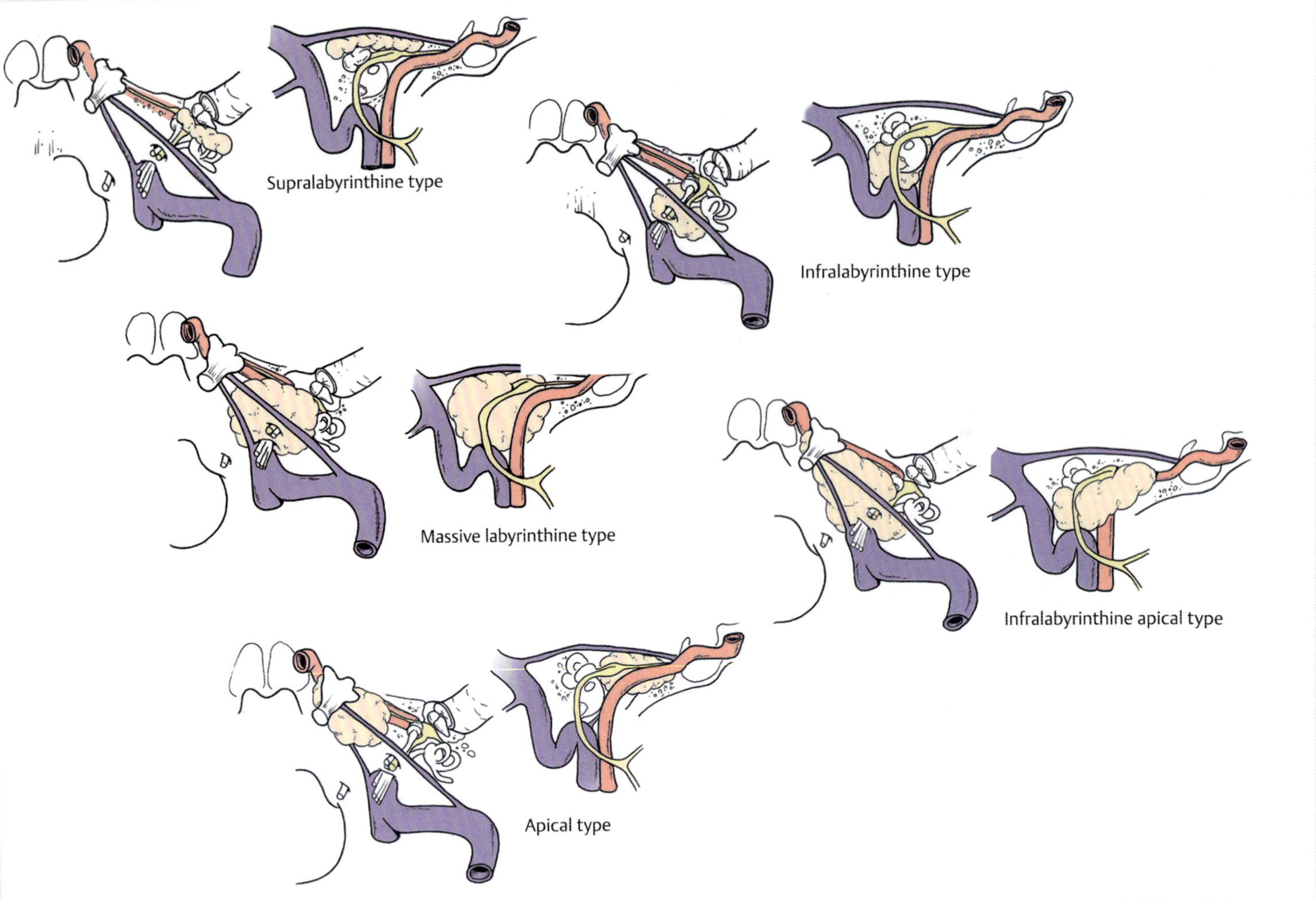

Fig. 5.57 Petrous bone cholesteatoma (PBC) classification.[120]

fluid-attenuated inversion-recovery images, they generally have a high signal intensity. DWI is useful in diagnosis of cholesteatomas, as the lesions often show restricted diffusion, a feature that can be particularly useful for the detection of recurrent cholesteatomas after surgical resection. Radiological evaluation is essential to stage the pathology; especially for what concerns otic capsule, in these cholesteatomas hearing preservation is not possible for a massive involvement of the cochlea and the labyrinth, and a transcochlear or a transotic approach is required. However, in case of small supralabyrinthic cholesteatomas, without posterior extension, it is possible to perform a middle fossa or a transcanal endoscopic suprageniculate approach for hearing preservation. The facial nerve can be infiltrated by the cholesteatoma, so some patients can show a facial nerve palsy before surgery. In these cases, a transcochlear approach, with nerve repair, should be performed, while the endoscopic assisted transotic approach is, in the authors' opinion, a good surgical choice if no palsy is present before surgery. As suggested for paragangliomas, in these cases also, a preoperative evaluation of the vascular system is important.

A carotid encasement should always be excluded and carotid injury avoided with a balloon occlusion test and carotid artery closure or stenting, if necessary.

CT scans and MRI should also be used for the preoperative evaluation of the sigmoid sinus and/or IJV. If a ligation or closure of these structures is required (e.g., type A infratemporal fossa approach), this evaluation is mandatory not to close the only venous drainage system that would cause cerebral edema in the postoperative period.

Finally, dural infiltration should be properly evaluated through MRI, in order to plan dural removal and repair or matrix removal with a bipolar instrument, to preserve the dura too (see ▶ Fig. 5.58 and ▶ Fig. 5.59).

Cephaloceles

Petrous apex cephaloceles are rare lesions representing protrusions of arachnoid or dura mater, usually from Meckel's cave, into the petrous apex. Petrous apex cephaloceles are associated with empty sella and Usher syndrome, they are usually bilateral, and they occur more often in women than in men. The lesions may be incidental findings but they may occasionally erode the otic capsule or the pneumatized petrous apex cells, resulting in headaches, hearing loss, or CSF otorrhea. They are smoothly marginated and have the same signal intensity characteristics as the CSF with all MRI sequences. CT scans may show extensive nonaggressive erosion of the petrous apex with a smooth or scalloped border. Obliteration of the cyst cavity with fat or muscle is recommended for symptomatic lesions, and serial imaging is used for asymptomatic lesions (see ▶ Fig. 5.60, ▶ Fig. 5.61, ▶ Fig. 5.62).

Chordoma

Chordomas are rare tumors that originate from embryologic remnants of the notochord and can occur anywhere from the skull base

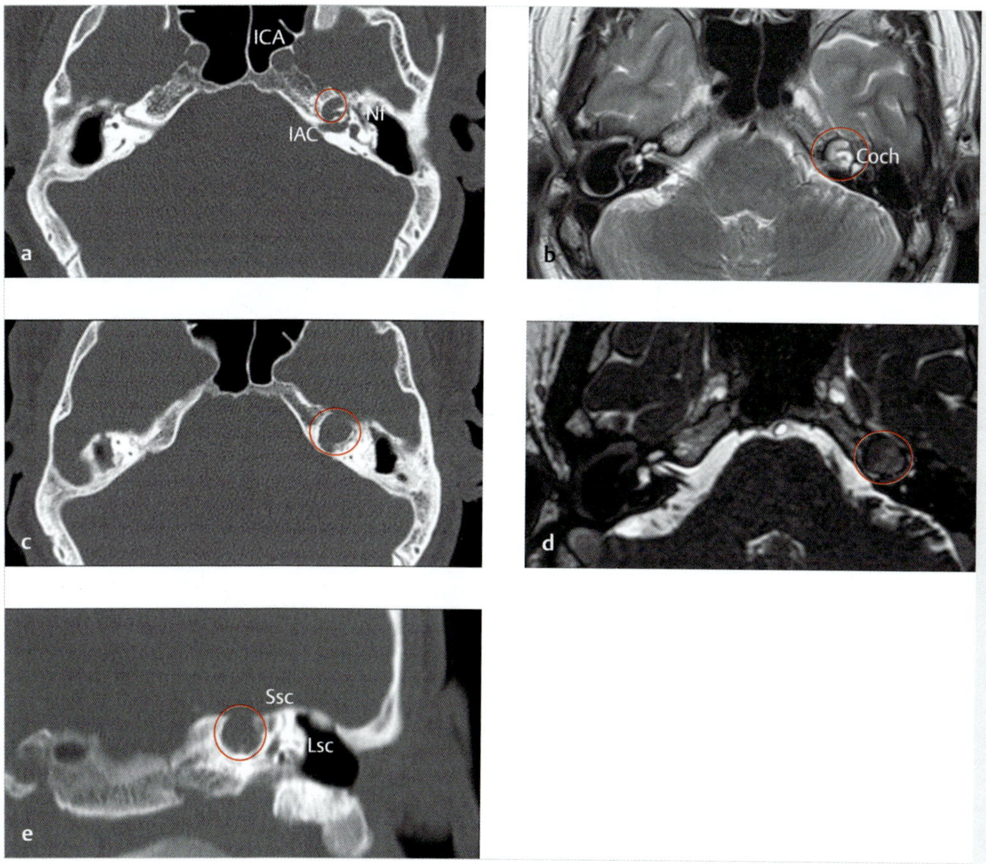

Fig. 5.58 Left petrous bone cholesteatoma (PBC) in a patient who underwent a bilateral open cavity (*red circle*: cholesteatoma). **(a–d)** Computed tomography (CT) and magnetic resonance imaging (MRI) images are compared and show the location of the cholesteatoma in the petrous apex; a canal wall down procedure is seen bilaterally. **(e)** CT scan coronal view; see the lesion medial to the labyrinthine block. Coch: *cochlea; Fn: facial nerve tympanic tract; IAC: internal auditory canal; ICA: internal carotid artery; Lsc: lateral semicircular canal; Ssc: superior semicircular canal.*

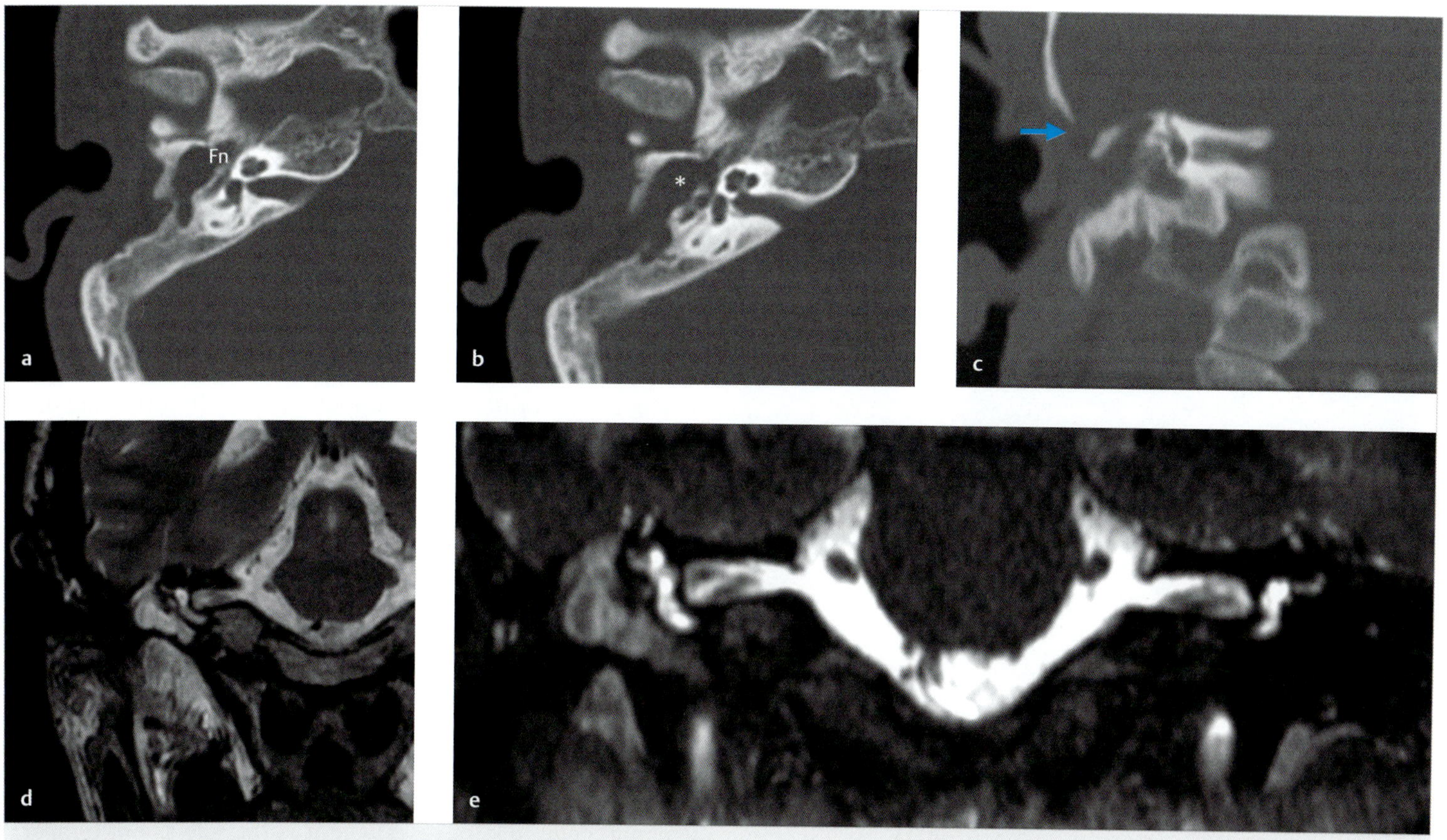

Fig. 5.59 (a–e) Right cholesteatoma. Note the extension into the middle ear (*), the bone erosion of the temporal bone (*light blue arrow*), and its appearance on magnetic resonance imaging (MRI). *Fn: facial nerve.*

to the sacrum. Skull base chordomas are typically midline lesions arising in the clivus but they may laterally extend to involve the petrous apex. In CT scans, skull base chordomas appear as locally destructive soft-tissue masses in the clivus. Calcifications are often evident and represent residual bone trabeculae; true tumor calcifications may occur in the chondroid variant of the chordoma. Low-attenuation areas are occasionally seen and represent portions of the tumor containing gelatinous material. In MRI, chordomas are typically hypointense on T1-weighted images and hyperintense on T2- weighted images. After contrast, they demonstrate variable

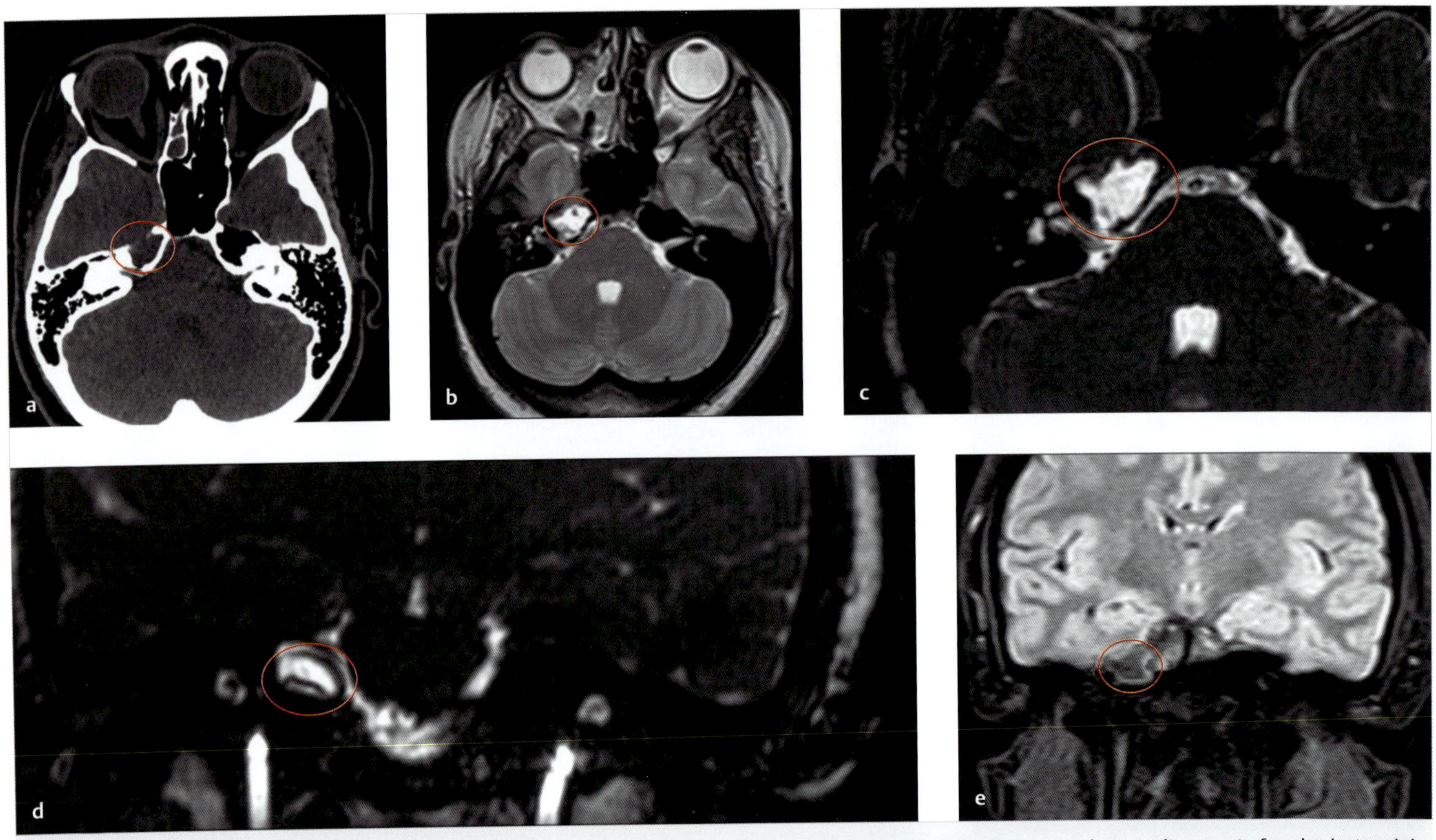

Fig. 5.60 **(a–d)** Right meningoencephalocele of the petrous apex. Magnetic resonance imaging (MRI) T1 coronal view, diagnostic for the lesion **(e)** (*red circle*).

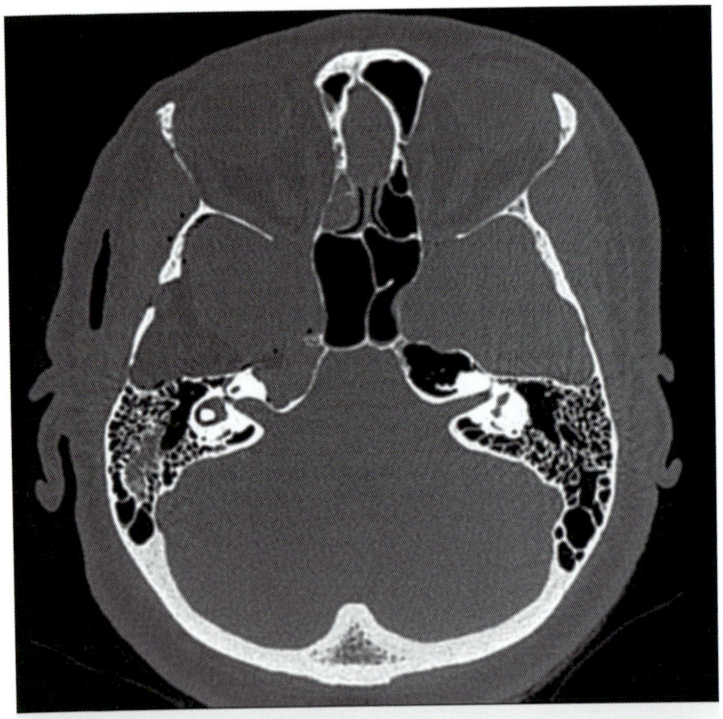

Fig. 5.61 Postoperative computed tomography (CT) scan after right middle cranial fossa approach for meningoencephalocele of the petrous apex.

enhancement and may have a characteristic honeycomb enhancement pattern. Surgery is the best option for these patients, in combination with hadrontherapy. Recently, the endoscopic transnasal technique has been introduced, and it currently represents a good alternative for the surgical management of these lesions, with lower morbidity and postoperative complications when compared to the traditional open approaches, according to the extent and type of pathology (see ▶ Fig. 5.63 and ▶ Fig. 5.64).

Condrosarcomas

Chondrosarcomas are malignant cartilaginous tumors that typically appear in the 2nd and 3rd decades of life. Chondrosarcomas involving the petrous apex typically originate at the level of the petroclival and petrosphenoidal synchondroses. On radiological examination, CT scans show a destructive petrous apex mass containing arcs and rings of calcification, which reflect the chondroid nature of the tumor. In MRI, the lesions have a low to intermediate signal intensity on T1-weighted images and a high signal intensity on T2-weighted images if compared to that of brain tissue. Signal heterogeneity can be seen and may in part be due to the presence of mineralized chondroid matrix. These tumors demonstrate variable degrees of enhancement after contrast material administration. Also, for patients with these lesions, surgery is the best option, in combination with hadrontherapy (see ▶ Fig. 5.65).

Metastasis/Others

The petrous apex is the most common site for metastases in the temporal bone (83% of cases) and it is the sole site of temporal bone involvement in 31% of cases. The most common tumor to metastasize to the petrous apex is breast cancer, followed by lung, prostate, and renal cell carcinomas. The imaging characteristics of petrous apex metastases are nonspecific. Frequently, they demonstrate significant bone destruction and marked enhancement. CT scans usually shows an aggressive lytic lesion destroying the skull base. MRI displays the soft-tissue extent of metastases, which usually have a low to intermediate signal

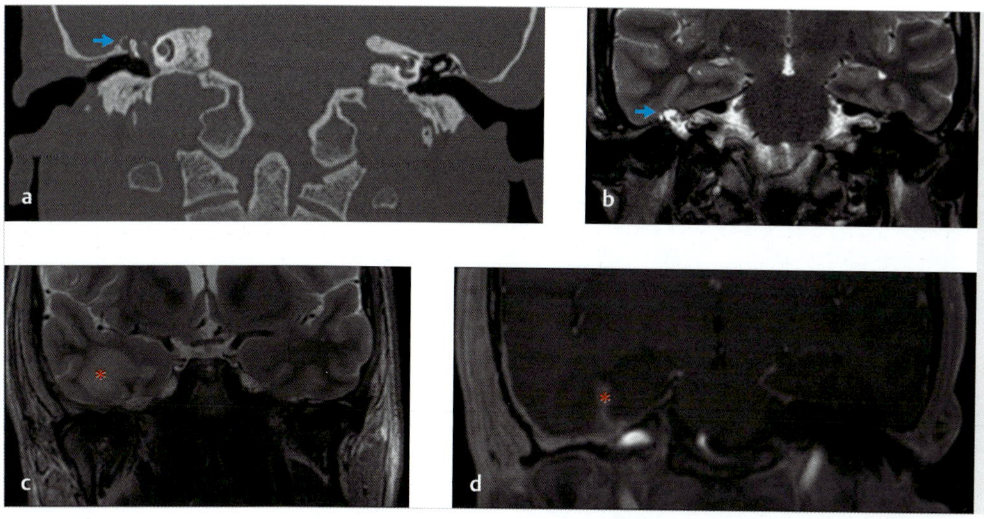

Fig. 5.62 Right epitympanic meningoencephalocele, removed through a middle cranial fossa approach. **(a)** Coronal view of the meningoencephalocele with bone defect of tegmen tympani (*light blue arrow*). **(b)** T2 magnetic resonance imaging (MRI). **(c, d)** Temporal lobe edema after evacuation of abscess, developed 3 weeks after the surgery (*).

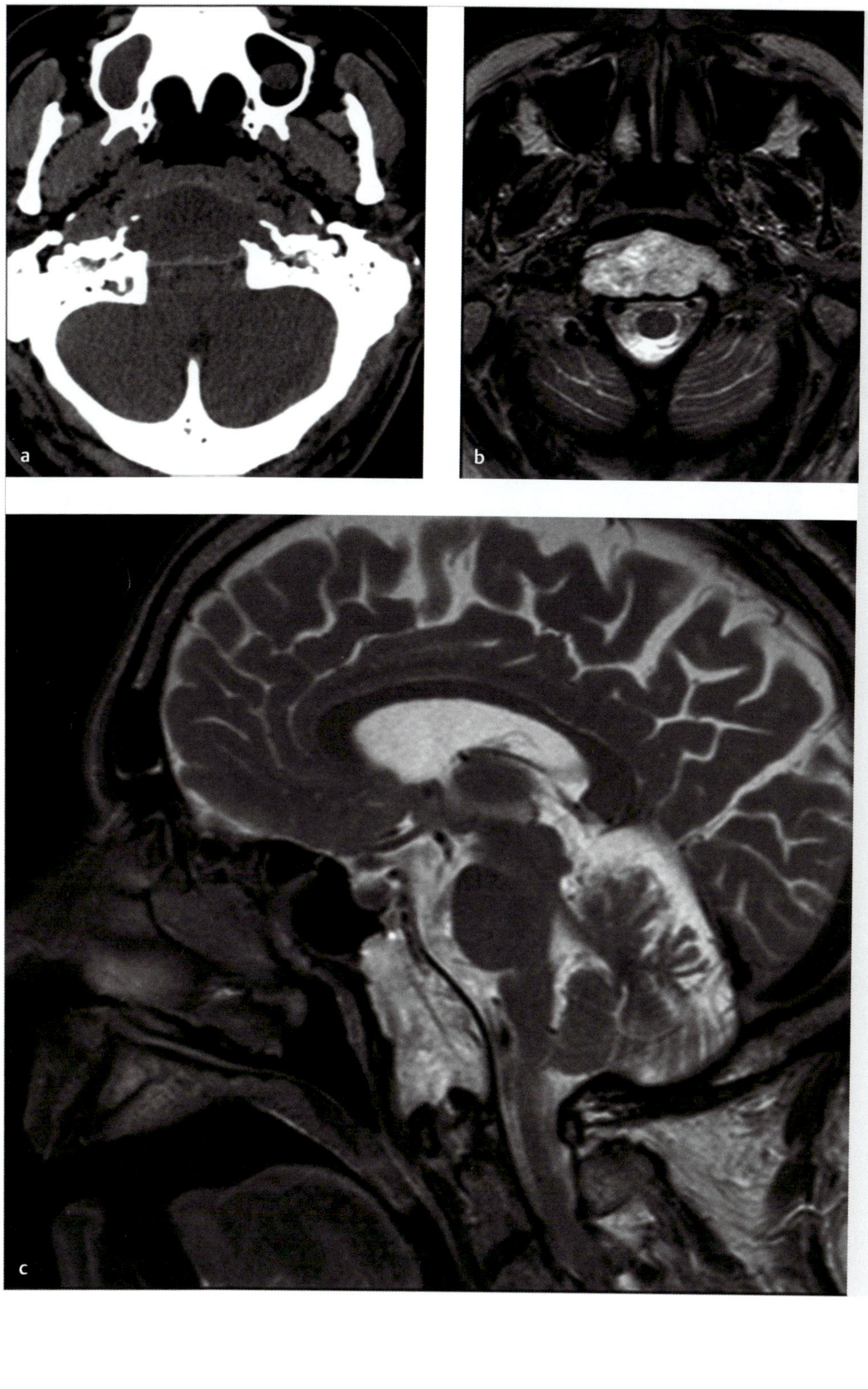

Fig. 5.63 Clivus chordoma. **(a)** Axial computed tomography (CT) scan. **(b, c)** Magnetic resonance imaging (MRI) of the chordoma.

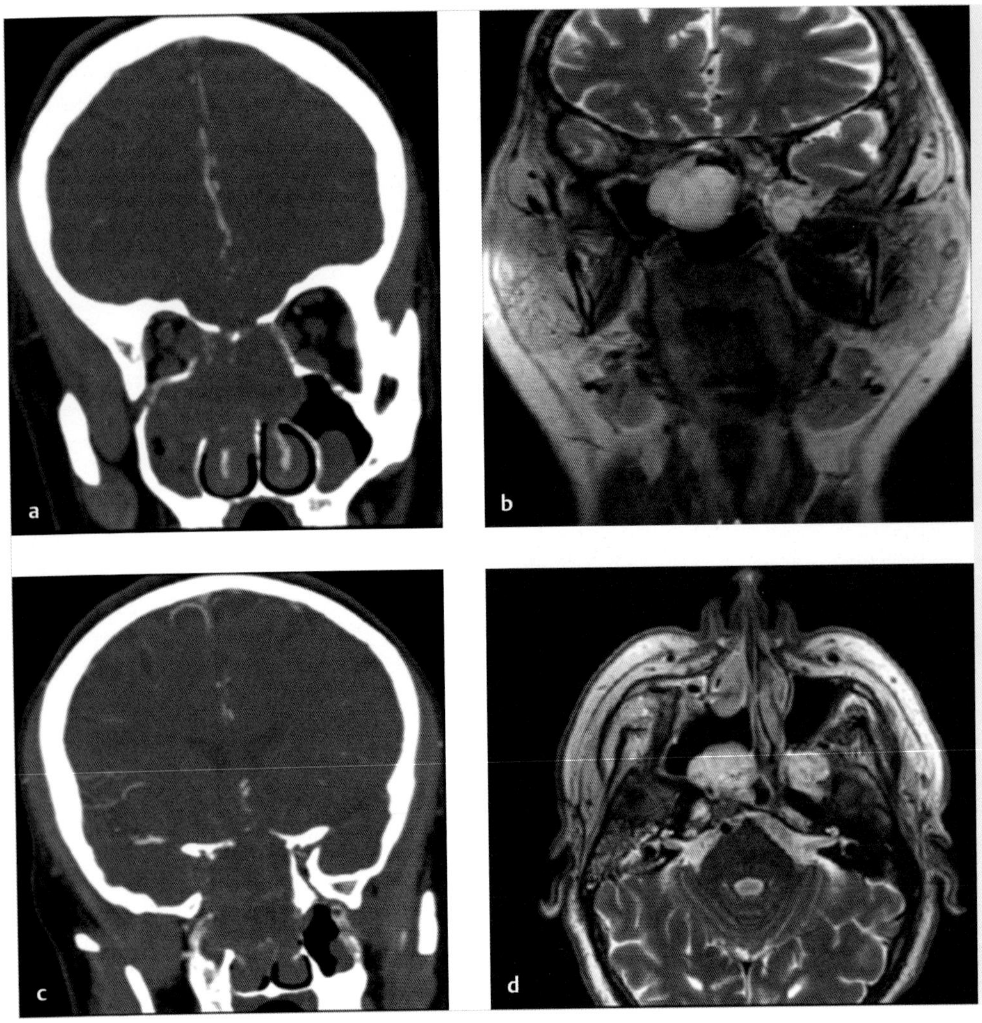

Fig. 5.64 Clivus chordomas. **(a, c)** Computed tomography (CT) scan with contrast of chordoma spreading into the orbit and the right nasal fossa. **(b, d)** Recurrent chordoma spreading into the left infratemporal fossa and the nasal cavity after open and endoscopic transnasal surgery.

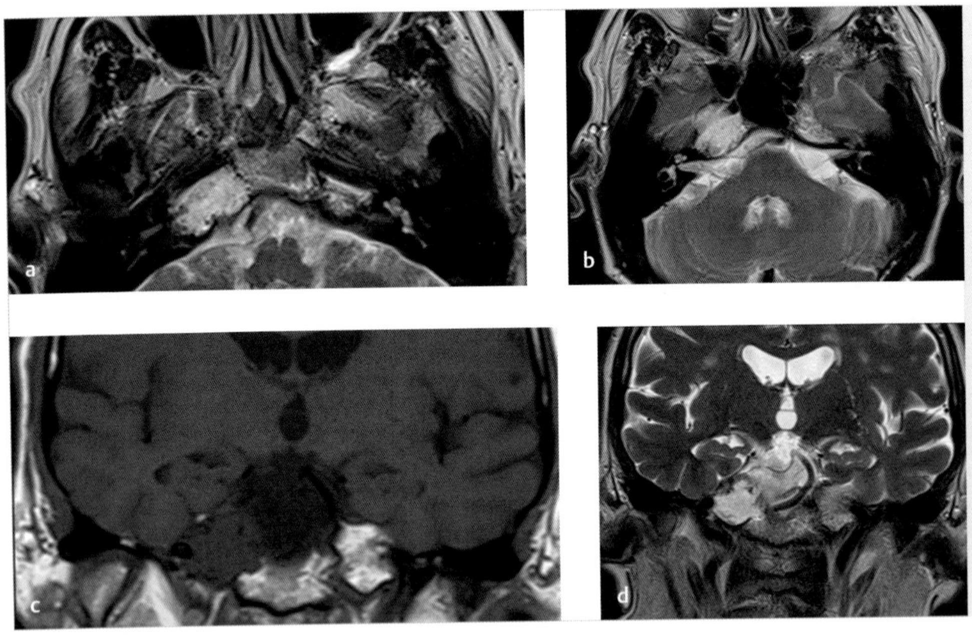

Fig. 5.65 Chondrosarcoma of the right petrous apex. The lesion is laterally located, hypointense in T1 and isointense in T2 **(a–d)**.

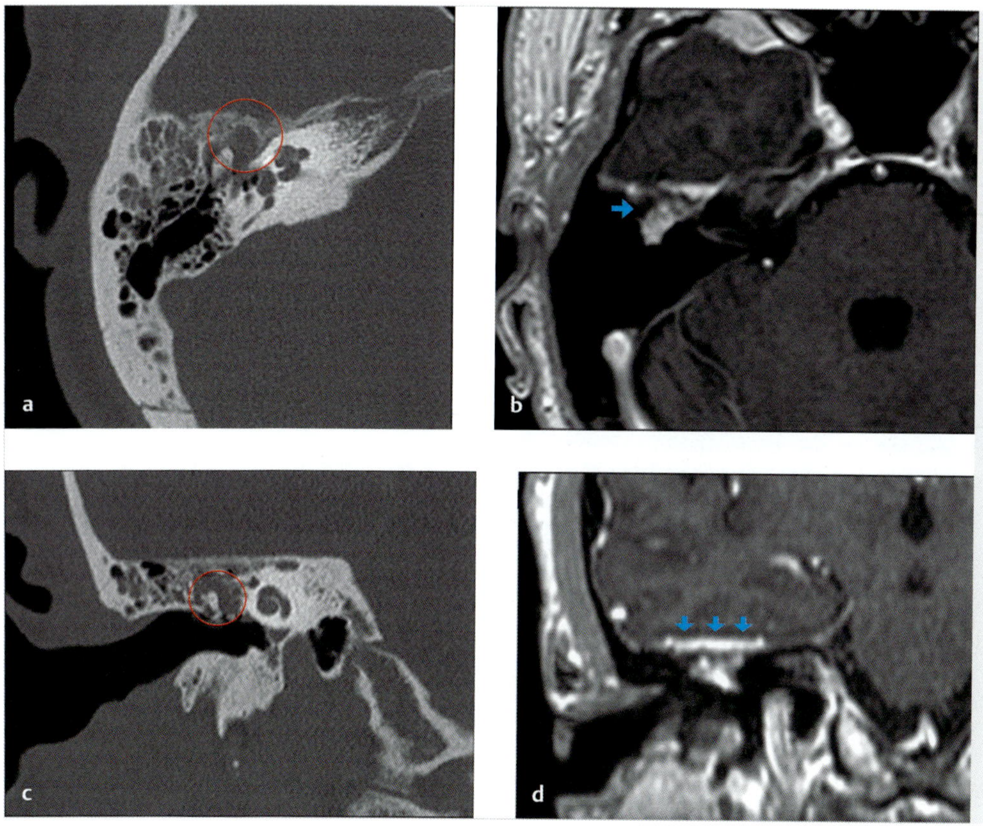

Fig. 5.66 Right meningioma of the middle cranial fossa. **(a, c)** Computed tomography (CT) scan shows an epitympanic mass (*red circle*), medial to the ossicular chain, with no spreading from the geniculate ganglion. **(b, d)** "Dural tail" and enhancement (*light blue arrow*) on T1 magnetic resonance imaging (MRI) sequences.

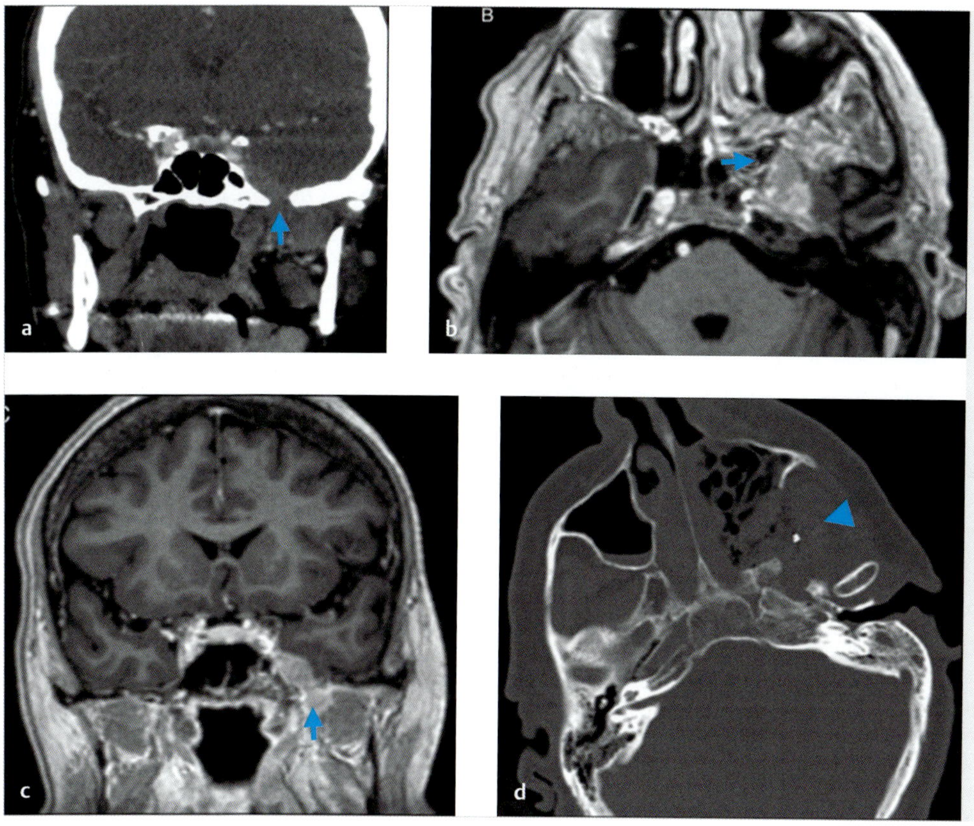

Fig. 5.67 Left infratemporal fossa adenoid cystic adenocarcinoma. **(a–c)** Note the intracranial growth of the tumor through the foramen ovale (*light blue arrow*). **(d)** Computed tomography (CT) scan after transnasal transtemporal approach (*light blue triangle*).

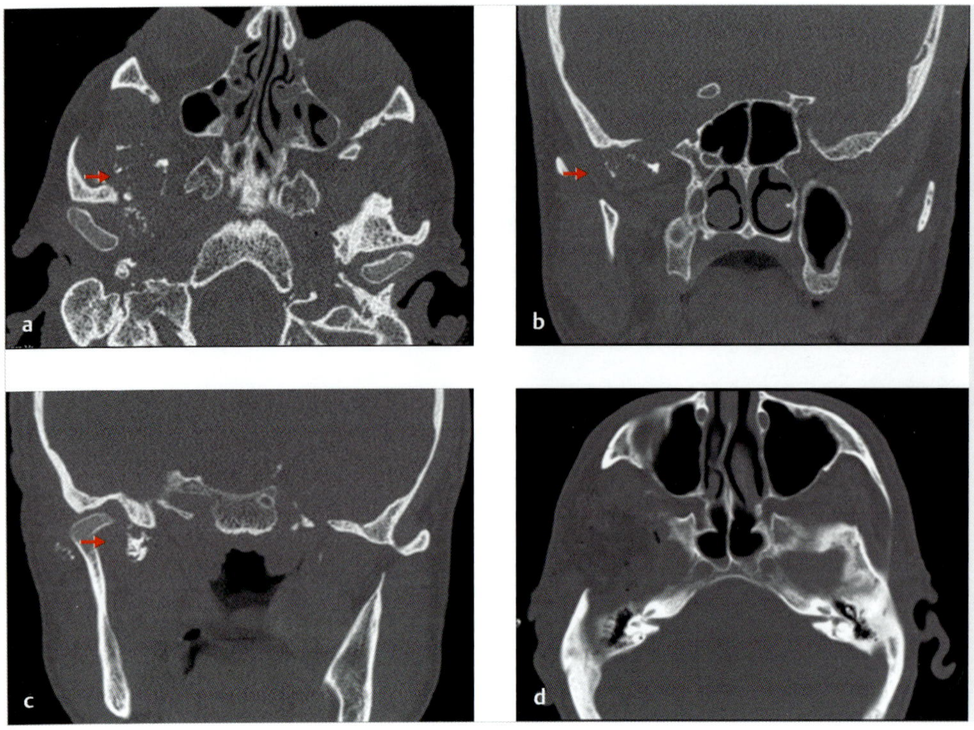

Fig. 5.68 Right infratemporal fossa lesion. **(a–c)** The computed tomography (CT) scan shows in all projections a lesion of the infratemporal fossa with characteristic bone calcifications (*red arrow*). **(d)** CT scan type B infratemporal fossa approach.

intensity on T1-weighted images and a variable signal intensity on T2-weighted images; enhancement is also variable (see ▶ Fig. 5.66, ▶ Fig. 5.67, ▶ Fig. 5.68).

Suggested Readings

Abdel Razek A, Mossad A, Ghonim M. Role of diffusion-weighted MR imaging in assessing malignant versus benign skull-base lesions. Radiol Med (Torino). 2011; 116(1):125–132

Alicandri-Ciufelli M, Marchioni D, Grammatica A, et al. Tympanoplasty: an up-to-date pictorial review. J Neuroradiol. 2012; 39(3):149–157

Alicandri-Ciufelli M, Marchioni D, Kakehata S, Presutti L, Villari D. Endoscopic management of attic cholesteatoma: long-term results. Otolaryngol Clin North Am. 2016; 49(5):1265–1270

Al-Mefty O, Fox JL, Smith RR. Petrosal approach for petroclival meningiomas. Neurosurgery. 1988; 22(3):510–517

Alorainy IA. Petrous apex cephalocele and empty sella: is there any relation? Eur J Radiol. 2007; 62(3):378–384

Atlas MD, Fagan PA, Turner J. Calcification of internal auditory canal tumors. Ann Otol Rhinol Laryngol. 1992; 101(7):620–622

Balkany T, Fradis M, Jafek BW, Rucker NC. Hemangioma of the facial nerve: role of the geniculate capillary plexus. Skull Base Surg. 1991; 1(1):59–63

Bennett M, Haynes DS. Surgical approaches and complications in the removal of vestibular schwannomas. Otolaryngol Clin North Am. 2007; 40(3):589–609, ix–x

Benoit MM, North PE, McKenna MJ, Mihm MC, Johnson MM, Cunningham MJ. Facial nerve hemangiomas: vascular tumors or malformations? Otolaryngol Head Neck Surg. 2010; 142(1):108–114

Bigelow DC, Eisen MD, Smith PG, et al. Lipomas of the internal auditory canal and cerebellopontine angle. Laryngoscope. 1998; 108(10):1459–1469

Bonneville F, Sarrazin JL, Marsot-Dupuch K, et al. Unusual lesions of the cerebellopontine angle: a segmental approach. Radiographics. 2001; 21(2):419–438

Bonneville F, Savatovsky J, Chiras J. Imaging of cerebellopontine angle lesions: an update. Part 1: enhancing extra-axial lesions. Eur Radiol. 2007; 17(10):2472–2482

Bou-Assaly W, Srinivasan A, Mukherji SK. Head and neck high-field imaging: oncology applications. Neuroimaging Clin N Am. 2012; 22(2):285–296, xi

Brown RV, Sage MR, Brophy BPCT. CT and MR findings in patients with chordomas of the petrous apex. AJNR Am J Neuroradiol. 1990; 11(1):121–124

Buis DR, Peerdeman SM, Vandertop WP. Metastatic adenocarcinoma in the cerebellopontine angle, presenting as a meningioma: a case report of rare occurrence. Acta Neurochir (Wien). 2004; 146(12):1369–1372, discussion 1372

Bulakbasi N, Kocaoglu M, Ors F, Tayfun C, Uçöz T. Combination of single-voxel proton MR spectroscopy and apparent diffusion coefficient calculation in the evaluation of common brain tumors. AJNR Am J Neuroradiol. 2003; 24(2):225–233

Bustillo A, Telischi FF. Octreotide scintigraphy in the detection of recurrent paragangliomas. Otolaryngol Head Neck Surg. 2004; 130(4):479–482

Bustillo A, Telischi F, Weed D, et al. Octreotide scintigraphy in the head and neck. Laryngoscope. 2004; 114(3):434–440

Caldemeyer KS, Mathews VP, Azzarelli B, Smith RR. The jugular foramen: a review of anatomy, masses, and imaging characteristics. Radiographics. 1997; 17(5):1123–1139

Calzada AP, Go JL, Tschirhart DL, Brackmann DE, Schwartz MS. Cerebellopontine angle and intracanalicular masses mimicking vestibular schwannomas. Otol Neurotol. 2015; 36(3):491–497

Carvalho GA, Tatagiba M, Samii M. Cystic schwannomas of the jugular foramen: clinical and surgical remarks. Neurosurgery. 2000; 46(3):560–566

Chapman PR, Shah R, Curé JK, Bag AK. Petrous apex lesions: pictorial review. AJR Am J Roentgenol. 2011; 196(3) Suppl:WS26–WS37, Quiz S40–S43

Charabi S, Tos M, Thomsen J, Rygaard J, Fundova P, Charabi B. Cystic vestibular schwannoma—clinical and experimental studies. Acta Otolaryngol Suppl. 2000; 543 S543:11–13

Cheng CJ, Yao NS. Isolated temporal bone metastasis in a patient with non-small cell lung cancer. Eur J Radiol Extra. 2005; 55(3):75–77

Chin RY, Nguyen TBV. Synchronous malignant otitis externa and squamous cell carcinoma of the external auditory canal. Case Rep Otolaryngol. 2013; 2013:837169

Chong VFH, Fan YF. Radiology of the jugular foramen. Clin Radiol. 1998; 53(6):405–416

Chong VF, Khoo JB, Fan YF. Imaging of the nasopharynx and skull base. Neuroimaging Clin N Am. 2004; 14(4):695–719

Connor SE, Leung R, Natas S. Imaging of the petrous apex: a pictorial review. Br J Radiol. 2008; 81(965):427–435

Curtin HD, Jensen JE, Barnes L, Jr, May M. "Ossifying" hemangiomas of the temporal bone: evaluation with CT. Radiology. 1987; 164(3):831–835

Cushing H. Tumors of the Nervus Acousticus and the Syndrome of the Cerebellopontine Angle. Philadelphia, PA: WB Saunders; 1917

De Foer B, Vercruysse JP, Bernaerts A, et al. Middle ear cholesteatoma: non-echo-planar diffusion-weighted MR imaging versus delayed gadolinium-enhanced T1-weighted MR imaging—value in detection. Radiology. 2010; 255(3):866–872

DiMaio S, Mohr G, Dufour JJ, Albrecht S. Distal mycotic aneurysm of the AICA mimicking intracanalicular acoustic neuroma. Can J Neurol Sci. 2003; 30(4):388–392

Fisch UMD. Microsurgery of the Skull Base. Stuttgart: Thieme; 1988

Fleck SK, Baldauf J, Langner S, Vogelgesang S, Siegfried Schroeder HW. Arachnoid cyst confined to the internal auditory canal-endoscope-assisted resection: case report and review of the literature. Neurosurgery. 2011; 68(1):E267–E270

Fortnum H, O'Neill C, Taylor R, et al. The role of magnetic resonance imaging in the identification of suspected acoustic neuroma: a systematic review of clinical and cost effectiveness and natural history. Health Technol Assess. 2009; 13(18):iii–iv, ix–xi, 1–154

Friedman DP, Rao VMMR. MR and CT of squamous cell carcinoma of the middle ear and mastoid complex. AJNR Am J Neuroradiol. 1991; 12(5):872–874

Frisch CD, Jacob JT, Carlson ML, et al. Stereotactic radiosurgery for cystic vestibular schwannomas. Neurosurgery. 2017; 80(1):112–118

Gerganov VM, Hore N, Herold C, et al. Bilateral malignant melanoma metastases to the internal auditory canal/cerebellopontine angle: surgical management and preservation of function. J Neurosurg. 2008; 108(4):803–807

Gillespie MB, Francis HW, Chee N, Eisele DW. Squamous cell carcinoma of the temporal bone: a radiographic-pathologic correlation. Arch Otolaryngol Head Neck Surg. 2001; 127(7):803–807

Ginat DT, Mangla R, Yeaney G, Johnson M, Ekholm S. Diffusion-weighted imaging for differentiating benign from malignant skull lesions and correlation with cell density. AJR Am J Roentgenol. 2012; 198(6):W597–601

Gloria-Cruz TI, Schachern PA, Paparella MM, Adams GL, Fulton SE. Metastases to temporal bones from primary nonsystemic malignant neoplasms. Arch Otolaryngol Head Neck Surg. 2000; 126(2):209–214

Goel A, Muzumdar D, Raman C. Trigeminal neuroma: analysis of surgical experience with 73 cases. Neurosurgery. 2003; 52(4):783–790, discussion 790

Guthikonda B, Theodosopoulos PV, van Loveren H, Tew JM, Jr, Pensak ML. Evolution in the assessment and management of trigeminal schwannoma. Laryngoscope. 2008; 118(2):195–203

Hariharan S, Zhu J, Nadkarni MA, Donahue JE. Metastatic lung cancer in the cerebellopontine angles mimicking bilateral acoustic neuroma. J Clin Neurosci. 2005; 12 (2):184–186

Harnsberger R, Hudgins P, Wiggins R, Davidson C. Diagnostic Imaging: Head and Neck, 1st ed. Salt Lake City, USA: AMIRSYS; 2004

Higgins TS, Antonio SA. The role of facial palsy in staging squamous cell carcinoma of the temporal bone and external auditory canal: a comparative survival analysis. Otol Neurotol. 2010; 31(9):1473–1479

Ikushima I, Korogi Y, Hirai T, et al. MR of epidermoids with a variety of pulse sequences. AJNR Am J Neuroradiol. 1997; 18(7):1359–1363

Isaacson B, Coker NJ, Vrabec JT, Yoshor D, Oghalai JS. Invasive cerebrospinal fluid cysts and cephaloceles of the petrous apex. Otol Neurotol. 2006; 27(8):1131–1141

Isaacson B, Kutz JW, Roland PS. Lesions of the petrous apex: diagnosis and management. Otolaryngol Clin North Am. 2007; 40(3):479–519, viii

Isaacson B, Telian SA, El-Kashlan HK. Facial nerve outcomes in middle cranial fossa vs translabyrinthine approaches. Otolaryngol Head Neck Surg. 2005; 133(6):906–910

Jackler RK, Dillon WP, Schindler RA. Computed tomography in suppurative ear disease: a correlation of surgical and radiographic findings. Laryngoscope. 1984; 94 (6):746–752

Jackson CG. Glomus tympanicum and glomus jugulare tumors. Otolaryngol Clin North Am. 2001; 34(5):941–970, vii

Jackson CG, Welling DB, Chironis P, Glasscock ME, III, Woods CI. Glomus tympanicum tumors: contemporary concepts in conservation surgery. Laryngoscope. 1989; 99(9):875–884

Jain A, Ablett M, Wardrop P. Vanishing tumour of the internal auditory meatus. J Laryngol Otol. 2009; 123(5):563–565

Jazrawy H, Wortzman G, Kassel EE, Noyek AM. Computed tomography of the temporal bone. J Otolaryngol. 1983; 12(1):37–44

Jefferson G. The trigeminal neurinomas with some remarks on malignant invasion of the gasserian ganglion. Clin Neurosurg. 1953; 1:11–54

Kawano H, Tono T, Schachern PA, Paparella MM, Komune S. Petrous high jugular bulb: a histological study. Am J Otolaryngol. 2000; 21(3):161–168

Kaye AH, Hahn JF, Kinney SE, Hardy RW, Jr, Bay JW. Jugular foramen schwannomas. J Neurosurg. 1984; 60(5):1045–1053

Khemani SC, Singh A, Lingam RK, et al. Radiological imaging of cholesteatoma. The Otorhinolaryngologist. 2010; 3(2):69–78

Khemani S, Singh A, Lingam RK, Kalan A. Imaging of postoperative middle ear cholesteatoma. Clin Radiol. 2011; 66(8):760–767

Koos WT, Day JD, Matula C, Levy DI. Neurotopographic considerations in the microsurgical treatment of small acoustic neurinomas. J Neurosurg. 1998; 88(3):506–512

Kumar Y, Khaleel M, Boothe E, Awdeh H, Wadhwa V, Chhabra A. Role of diffusion weighted imaging in musculoskeletal infections: current perspectives. Eur Radiol. 2017; 27(1):414–423

Kumar Y, Wadhwa V, Phillips L, Pezeshk P, Chhabra A. MR imaging of skeletal muscle signal alterations: systematic approach to evaluation. Eur J Radiol. 2016; 85 (5):922–935

La Fata V, McLean N, Wise SK, DelGaudio JM, Hudgins PA. CSF leaks: correlation of high-resolution CT and multiplanar reformations with intraoperative endoscopic findings. AJNR Am J Neuroradiol. 2008; 29(3):536–541

Las Heras F, Martuza R, Caruso P, Rincon S, Stemmer-Rachamimov A. 24-year-old woman with an internal auditory canal mass: hybrid peripheral nerve sheath tumor with schwannoma/perineurioma components. Brain Pathol. 2013; 23 (3):361–362

Lemmerling MM, De Foer B, VandeVyver V, Vercruysse JP, Verstraete KL. Imaging of the opacified middle ear. Eur J Radiol. 2008; 66(3):363–371

Lin ZM, Young YH. Investigating the causes of vertigo in breast cancer survivors. Eur Arch Otorhinolaryngol. 2005; 262(5):432–436

Lo WW, Solti-Bohman LG. High-resolution CT of the jugular foramen: anatomy and vascular variants and anomalies. Radiology. 1984; 150(3):743–747

Mafee MF, Kumar A, Heffner DK. Epidermoid cyst (cholesteatoma) and cholesterol granuloma of the temporal bone and epidermoid cysts affecting the brain. Neuroimaging Clin N Am. 1994; 4(3):561–578

Magnan J, Chays A, Lepetre C, Pencroffi E, Locatelli P. Surgical perspectives of endoscopy of the cerebellopontine angle. Am J Otol. 1994; 15(3):366–370

Majithia A, Lingam RK, Nash R, Khemani S, Kalan A, Singh A. Staging primary middle ear cholesteatoma with non-echoplanar (half-Fourier-acquisition single-shot turbo-spin-echo) diffusion-weighted magnetic resonance imaging helps plan surgery in 22 patients: our experience. Clin Otolaryngol. 2012; 37(4):325–330

Malone A, Bruni M, Wong R, Tabor M, Boyev KP. Pneumatization patterns of the petrous apex and lateral sphenoid recess. J Neurol Surg B Skull Base. 2017; 78 (6):441–446

Marchioni D, Alicandri-Ciufelli M, Rubini A, Masotto B, Pavesi G, Presutti L. Exclusive endoscopic transcanal transpromontorial approach: a new perspective for internal auditory canal vestibular schwannoma treatment. J Neurosurg. 2017; 126 (1):98–105

Marchioni D, Carner M, Soloperto D, et al. Expanded transcanal transpromontorial approach: a novel surgical technique for cerebellopontine angle vestibular schwannoma removal. Otolaryngol Head Neck Surg. 2018; 158(4):710–715

Marchioni D, De Rossi S, Soloperto D, Presutti L, Sacchetto L, Rubini A. Intralabyrinthine schwannomas: a new surgical treatment. Eur Arch Otorhinolaryngol. 2018; 275(5):1095–1102

Marchioni D, Musumeci A, Fabbris C, De Rossi S, Soloperto D. Endoscopic transnasal surgery of clival lesions: our experience. Eur Arch Otorhinolaryngol. 2018; 275 (5):1149–1156

Marchioni D, Soloperto D, Genovese E, Rubini A, Presutti L. Facial nerve hemangioma of the geniculate ganglion: an endoscopic surgical approach. Auris Nasus Larynx. 2014; 41(6):576–581

Marchioni D, Soloperto D, Masotto B, et al. Transcanal transpromontorial acoustic neuroma surgery: results and facial nerve outcomes. Otol Neurotol. 2018; 39 (2):242–249

Marchioni D, Soloperto D, Rubini A, Nogueira JF, Badr-El-Dine M, Presutti L. Endoscopic facial nerve surgery. Otolaryngol Clin North Am. 2016; 49(5):1173–1187

Marchioni D, Soloperto D, Rubini A, et al. Endoscopic exclusive transcanal approach to the tympanic cavity cholesteatoma in pediatric patients: our experience. Int J Pediatr Otorhinolaryngol. 2015; 79(3):316–322

Marchioni D, Veronese S, Carner M, et al. Hearing restoration during vestibular schwannoma surgery with transcanal approach: anatomical and functional preliminary report. Otol Neurotol. 2018; 39(10):1304–1310

Marques E, Brandis A, Samii M, Tatagiba M. Late metastasis of breast adenocarcinoma into internal auditory canal and cerebellopontine angle: case report. Arq Neuropsiquiatr. 2002; 60 3-A:639–642

Martin N, Sterkers O, Murat M, Hahum N. Brain herniation into the middle ear cavity: MR imaging. Neuroradiology. 1989; 31(2):184–186

McKiever ME, Carlson ML, Neff BA. Aberrant petrous carotid artery masquerading as a glomus tympanicum. Otol Neurotol. 2014; 35(8):e228–e230

Megerian CA, McKenna MJ, Nadol JB, Jr. Non-paraganglioma jugular foramen lesions masquerading as glomus jugulare tumors. Am J Otol. 1995; 16(1):94–98

Megerian CA, McKenna MJ, Nuss RC, et al. Endolymphatic sac tumors: histopathologic confirmation, clinical characterization, and implication in von Hippel-Lindau disease. Laryngoscope. 1995; 105(8 Pt 1):801–808

Meng L, Yuguang L, Feng L, Wandong S, Shugan Z, Chengyuan W. Cerebellopontine angle epidermoids presenting with trigeminal neuralgia. J Clin Neurosci. 2005; 12(7):784–786

Moffat D, Chiossone-Kerdel J, Da Cruz M. Squamous cell carcinoma. In: Jackler RK, Driscoll CLW, eds. Tumors of the Ear and Temporal Bone. Philadelphia: Lippincott Williams & Wilkins; 2000:67–77

Moody SA, Hirsch BE, Myers EN. Squamous cell carcinoma of the external auditory canal: an evaluation of a staging system. Am J Otol. 2000; 21(4):582–588

Moore KR, Fischbein NJ, Harnsberger HR, et al. Petrous apex cephaloceles. AJNR Am J Neuroradiol. 2001; 22(10):1867–1871

Mundada P, Purohit BS, Kumar TS, Tan TY. Imaging of facial nerve schwannomas: diagnostic pearls and potential pitfalls. Diagn Interv Radiol. 2016; 22(1):40–46

Murphy TP, Brackmann DE. Effects of preoperative embolization on glomus jugulare tumors. Laryngoscope. 1989; 99(12):1244–1247

Nakamura M, Roser F, Mirzai S, Matthies C, Vorkapic P, Samii M. Meningiomas of the internal auditory canal. Neurosurgery. 2004; 55(1):119–127, discussion 127–128

Neely JG. Reversible compression neuropathy of the eighth cranial nerve from a large jugular foramen schwannoma. Arch Otolaryngol. 1979; 105(9):555–560

Nemec S, Donat M, Hoeftberger R, Matula C, Czerny C. Chondrosarcoma of the petrous apex: a diagnostic and therapeutic challenge. Eur J Radiol Extra. 2005; 54:87–91

Nofsinger YC, Mirza N, Rowan PT, Lanza D, Weinstein G. Head and neck manifestations of plasma cell neoplasms. Laryngoscope. 1997; 107(6):741–746

Noonan PT, Choi IS. Diagnostic imaging, angiography, and interventional techniques for jugular foramen tumors. Oper Tech Neurosurg. 2005; 8:13–18

Oghalai JS, Buxbaum JL, Jackler RK, McDermott MW. Skull base chondrosarcoma originating from the petroclival junction. Otol Neurotol. 2005; 26(5):1052–1060

Ong CK, Fook-Hin Chong V. Imaging of jugular foramen. Neuroimaging Clin N Am. 2009; 19(3):469–482

Ong CK, Pua U, Chong VFH. Imaging of carcinoma of the external auditory canal: a pictorial essay. Cancer Imaging. 2008; 8(1):191–198

Ong CK, Pua U, Chong VF. Imaging of carcinoma of the external auditory canal: a pictorial essay. Cancer Imaging. 2008; 8:191–198

Osborn AG, Preece MT. Intracranial cysts: radiologic-pathologic correlation and imaging approach. Radiology. 2006; 239(3):650–664

Overton SB, Ritter FN. A high placed jugular bulb in the middle ear: a clinical and temporal bone study. Laryngoscope. 1973; 83(12):1986–1991

Parmar H, Gujar S, Shah G, Mukherji SK. Imaging of the anterior skull base. Neuroimaging Clin N Am. 2009; 19(3):427–439

Pisaneschi MJ, Langer B. Congenital cholesteatoma and cholesterol granuloma of the temporal bone: role of magnetic resonance imaging. Top Magn Reson Imaging. 2000; 11(2):87–97

Pont E, Mazón M, Ferrer ÁR. Cerebellopontine angle epidermoid cyst. Acta Otorrinolaringol Esp. 2015; 66(1):63–64

Presutti L, Alicandri-Ciufelli M, Cigarini E, Marchioni D. Cochlear schwannoma removed through the external auditory canal by a transcanal exclusive endoscopic technique. Laryngoscope. 2013; 123(11):2862–2867

Quaranta N, Cassano M, Maselli Del Giudice A, Quaranta A. A rare case of jugular foramen schwannoma arising from Jacobson's nerve. Acta Otolaryngol. 2007; 127 (6):667–672

Rao AB, Koeller KK, Adair CF, Armed Forces Institute of Pathology. From the archives of the AFIP. Paragangliomas of the head and neck: radiologic-pathologic correlation. Radiographics. 1999; 19(6):1605–1632

Raut AA, Naphade PS, Chawla A. Imaging of skull base: pictorial essay. Indian J Radiol Imaging. 2012; 22(4):305–316

Razek AA, Huang BY. Lesions of the petrous apex: classification and findings at CT and MR imaging. Radiographics. 2012; 32(1):151–173

Robertson JH, Gardner G, Cocke EW, Jr. Glomus jugulare tumors. Clin Neurosurg. 1994; 41:39–61

Roditi RE, Kesarwani P, Barker EM, Yeaney GA, Walter KA, Crane BT. Imaging case of the month: bilateral internal auditory canal melanoma. Otol Neurotol. 2012; 33 (9):e77–e78

Rohlfs AK, Burger R, Viebahn C, et al. Uncommon lesions in the internal auditory canal (IAC): review of the literature and case report. J Neurol Surg A Cent Eur Neurosurg. 2012; 73(3):160–166

Roland PS, Meyerhoff WL, Judge LO, Mickey BE. Asymmetric pneumatization of the petrous apex. Otolaryngol Head Neck Surg. 1990; 103(1):80–88

Roser F, Nakamura M, Dormiani M, Matthies C, Vorkapic P, Samii M. Meningiomas of the cerebellopontine angle with extension into the internal auditory canal. J Neurosurg. 2005; 102(1):17–23

Safronova MM, Vaz AR, Resende M, Pereira JR, Honavar M, Casselman JW. Cavernous malformation of the internal auditory canal: a diagnostic challenge. Otol Neurotol. 2009; 30(7):1015–1017

Salzman KL, Childs AM, Davidson HC, Kennedy RJ, Shelton C, Harnsberger HR. Intralabyrinthine schwannomas: imaging diagnosis and classification. AJNR Am J Neuroradiol. 2012; 33(1):104–109

Samii M, Migliori MM, Tatagiba M, Babu R. Surgical treatment of trigeminal schwannomas. J Neurosurg. 1995; 82(5):711–718

Sanna M, Zini C, Gamoletti R, et al. Petrous bone cholesteatoma. Skull Base Surg. 1993; 3(4):201–213

Saunders JE, Kwartler JA, Wolf HK, Brackmann DE, McElveen JT, Jr. Lipomas of the internal auditory canal. Laryngoscope. 1991; 101(10):1031–1037

Schmalfuss IM. Petrous apex. In Skull Base Imaging. Elsevier; 2018:233–246

Schmalfuss IM. Petrous apex. Neuroimaging Clin N Am. 2009; 19(3):367–391

Schweinfurth JM, Johnson JT, Weissman J. Jugular foramen syndrome as a complication of metastatic melanoma. Am J Otolaryngol. 1993; 14(3):168–174

Sener RN. Diffusion magnetic resonance imaging of solid vestibular schwannomas. J Comput Assist Tomogr. 2003; 27(2):249–252

Shimono T, Akai F, Yamamoto A, et al. Different signal intensities between intra- and extracranial components in jugular foramen meningioma: an enigma. AJNR Am J Neuroradiol. 2005; 26(5):1122–1127

Shinogami M, Yamasoba T, Sasaki T. Bilateral isolated metastases of malignant melanoma to the cerebellopontine angle. Otolaryngol Head Neck Surg. 1998; 118 (2):276–279

Smith JD, Harvey RN, Darr OA, et al. Head and neck paragangliomas: a two-decade institutional experience and algorithm for management. Laryngoscope Investig Otolaryngol. 2017; 2(6):380–389

Snow JB, Wackym PA. Ballenger's Otorhinolaryngology Head and Neck Surgery. 17th ed. Shelton (CT); Hamilton (Canada); London: People's Medical Publishing House/BC Decker; 2009

Som PM, Curtin HD. Head and Neck Imaging. 4th ed. St Louis: Mosby 2003;1275–1360

Song MH, Lee HY, Jeon JS, Lee JD, Lee HK, Lee WS. Jugular foramen schwannoma: analysis on its origin and location. Otol Neurotol. 2008; 29(3):387–391

Stark TA, McKinney AM, Palmer CS, Maisel RH, Truwit CL. Dilation of the subarachnoid spaces surrounding the cranial nerves with petrous apex cephaloceles in Usher syndrome. AJNR Am J Neuroradiol. 2009; 30(2):434–436

Sweeney AD, Carlson ML, Wanna GB, Bennett ML. Glomus tympanicum tumors. Otolaryngol Clin North Am. 2015; 48(2):293–304

Tahara A, de Santana PA, Jr, Calfat Maldaun MV, et al. Petroclival meningiomas: surgical management and common complications. J Clin Neurosci. 2009; 16(5):655–659

Tasar M, Yetiser S. Glomus tumors: therapeutic role of selective embolization. J Craniofac Surg. 2004; 15(3):497–505

Tien R, Dillon WP, Jackler RK. Contrast-enhanced MR imaging of the facial nerve in 11 patients with Bell's palsy. AJNR Am J Neuroradiol. 1990; 11(4):735–741

Wanna GB, Sweeney AD, Carlson ML, et al. Subtotal resection for management of large jugular paragangliomas with functional lower cranial nerves. Otolaryngol Head Neck Surg. 2014; 151(6):991–995

Wackym PA, Friedman I. Unusual tumors of the middle ear and mastoid. In: Jackler RK, Driscoll CLW, eds. Tumors of the Ear and Temporal Bone. Philadelphia: Lippincott Williams & Wilkins; 2000:128–143

Weber PC, Patel S. Jugulotympanic paragangliomas. Otolaryngol Clin North Am. 2001; 34(6):1231–1240, x

Weiss RL, Zahtz G, Goldofsky E, Parnes H, Shikowitz MJ. High jugular bulb and conductive hearing loss. Laryngoscope. 1997; 107(3):321–327

Wester K, Svendsen F, Hugdahl K. [Intracranial arachnoidal cysts—localization, gender and sidedness]. Tidsskr Nor Laegeforen. 1999; 119(28):4162–4164

Wharton SM, Davis A. Familial paraganglioma. J Laryngol Otol. 1996; 110(7):688–690

Wiggins RH, III, Harnsberger HR, Salzman KL, Shelton C, Kertesz TR, Glastonbury CM. The many faces of facial nerve schwannoma. AJNR Am J Neuroradiol. 2006; 27(3):694–699

Wilson MA, Hillman TA, Wiggins RH, Shelton C. Jugular foramen schwannomas: diagnosis, management, and outcomes. Laryngoscope. 2005; 115(8):1486–1492

Wu B, Liu W, Zhu H, Feng H, Liu J. Primary glioblastoma of the cerebellopontine angle in adults. J Neurosurg. 2011; 114(5):1288–1293

Yuh WT, Mayr-Yuh NA, Koci TM, et al. Metastatic lesions involving the cerebellopontine angle. AJNR Am J Neuroradiol. 1993; 14(1):99–106

Som PM, Curtin HD. Head and Neck Imaging. USA: Elsevier Health Sciences; 2002

Chapter 6

Transcochlear and Transotic Endoscopic Assisted Approaches

6

6 Transcochlear and Transotic Endoscopic Assisted Approaches

Daniele Marchioni, George Wanna, Mustafa Kapadia, Nicola Bisi, and Luca Bianconi

Abstract

The group of transcochlear/transotic approaches are transtemporal approaches that require the sacrifice of the hearing function passing through the otic capsule. These techniques are meant to deal with extensive petrous bone lesions involving the jugular bulb, the petrous internal carotid artery, and the cerebellopontine angle till the prepontine cistern up to the basilar artery. The transcochlear approach is an anterior extension of the translabyrinthine approach with the additional removal of the external auditory canal, the middle ear contents, and the cochlea. The transotic approach is similar except for the fact that the facial nerve is not mobilized and kept in its fallopian canal like a bridge, in order to preserve the facial nerve function. These surgical techniques allow a direct and wide access to the petrous apex, the internal acoustic canal, the jugular bulb, the petrous internal carotid artery, and the cerebellopontine angle with the possibility to anteriorly extend the dissection and expose the structures up to the basilar artery without cerebellar retraction. In these techniques, an endoscopic assisted procedure is not always necessary, but can be very useful because it allows exploration of hidden areas such as the medial portion of the petrous internal carotid artery without retraction of the medial section of the facial nerve, in the transotic approach, and for the removal of any pathological remnants.

Keywords: lateral skull base surgery, transotic approach, transcochlear approach, acoustic neuroma surgery, cerebellopontine angle surgery, microscopic lateral skull base surgery, endoscopic assisted surgery

6.1 Introduction

The group of transcochlear/transotic approaches passing through the otic capsule requires the sacrifice of the hearing function. The transcochlear approach is an anterior extension of the translabyrinthine approach with the additional removal of the external auditory canal (EAC), the middle ear contents, and the cochlea. This surgical technique enables the surgeon to access the petrous apex before the internal auditory canal (IAC) and around the internal carotid artery (ICA) but a posterior transposition of the facial nerve is mandatory in order to have a surgical exposure of the clivus, the petrous ICA, and the jugular bulb inferiorly. The transcochlear approach described by House and Hitselberger in 1976 was used to access large petrous apex meningiomas and cholesteatomas.

But the mobilization of the facial nerve during the surgery provoked an immediate, dense facial weakness in the postoperative period with a variable recovery.

Gantz and Fisch proposed a variation of this approach. In fact, they codified the transotic approach. This approach required an anterior rerouting of the facial nerve. Because of the poor results in terms of facial nerve function in the postoperative time, this approach was subsequently modified so as to leave the facial nerve within the fallopian canal to preserve the facial nerve integrity, with the complete exenteration of the otic capsule and access to the anterior petrous apex.

6.2 Transcochlear Approach

6.2.1 Indications

- Extensive cerebellopontine angle (CPA) lesions extending into the prepontine cistern, lying ventral to the brainstem (see ▶ Fig. 6.1c);
- Clival chordomas;
- Petroclival meningiomas, meningiomas with temporal bone involvement (see Clinical Case 2);
- Petrous bone cholesteatomas with facial nerve palsy and no serviceable hearing function (see Clinical Case 1).

6.2.2 Advantages

- Direct approach to the ventral brainstem and to the CPA;
- Direct intradural exposure of clivus, basilar artery, brainstem, and cranial nerves (bilateral XI cranial nerves, V, VII, VIII, IX, X and XII) without the need for brain retraction.

6.2.3 Limits

- Due to the posterior transposition of the facial nerve a palsy of this nerve is expected after surgery.
- The sacrifice of the hearing function is mandatory since this approach passes through the otic capsule.

6.2.4 Use of the Endoscope

This technique does not always require endoscopic assisted surgery. Only in case of an epidermoid lesion or a petrous bone cholesteatoma is the use of the endoscope at the end of the microscopic resection of the tumor recommended in order to detect any residual disease in the brainstem and around the ICA.

6.2.5 Surgical Approach

The patient is placed in a supine position with the head turned to the contralateral side; facial nerve monitoring is standard procedure. A "C"-shaped incision is made approximately 5 cm behind the retroauricular sulcus, starting about 1 cm above the auricle in the temporalis muscle area, and ending inferiorly in the neck close to the angle of the mandible (see ▶ Fig. 6.2a). Especially when the involvement of the intrapetrous carotid artery is expected, the skin incision should be prolonged into the neck along the sternocleidomastoid muscle, in order to dissect the neck close to the skull base to isolate the ICA and the internal jugular vein with the lower cranial nerves, to have the control of the major vascular structures (see Clinical Case 1, ▶ Fig. 6.16).

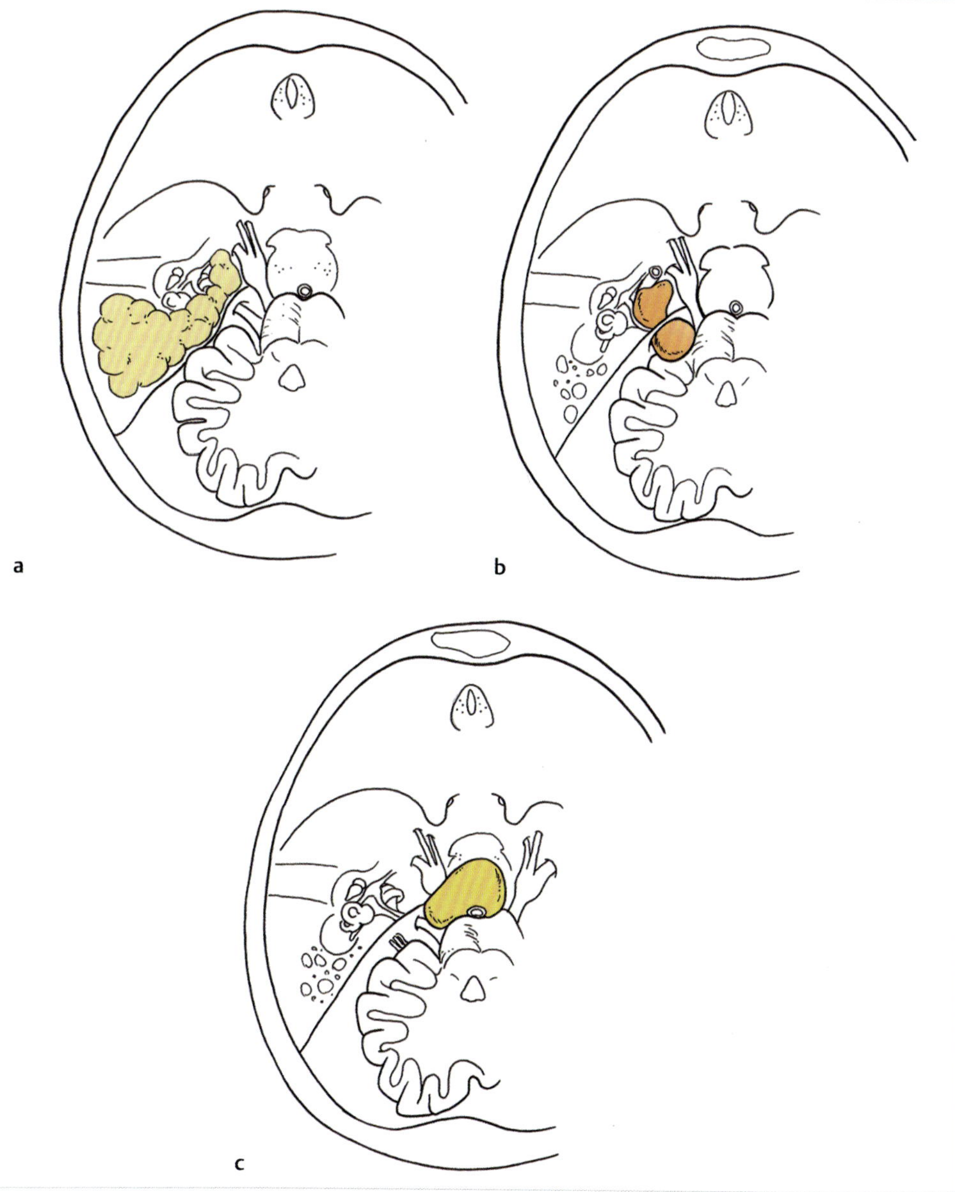

Fig. 6.1 Schematic drawing representing the major surgical indications for a transotic approach. **(a)** A petrous apex supralabyrinthine cholesteatoma is seen. **(b)** Cochlear schwannoma involving the petrous apex. **(c)** A lesion involving the brainstem midline, typical indication for a transcochlear approach.

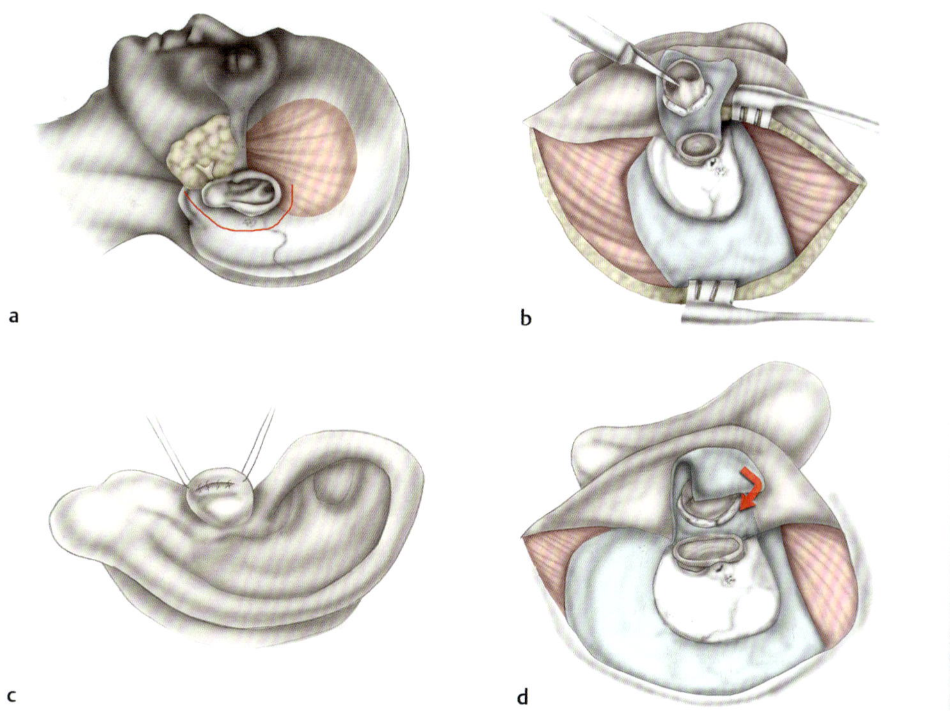

Fig. 6.2 Left ear. **(a)** A C-shaped incision is made approximately 5 cm behind the retroauricular sulcus. **(b)** The skin of the external auditory canal (EAC) is circumferentially cut at level of the osteo-cartilaginous junction. **(c)** The canal skin of the EAC is everted outside and sutured. **(d)** A periosteal layer is reversed on the internal layer of the EAC and sutured to close the canal.

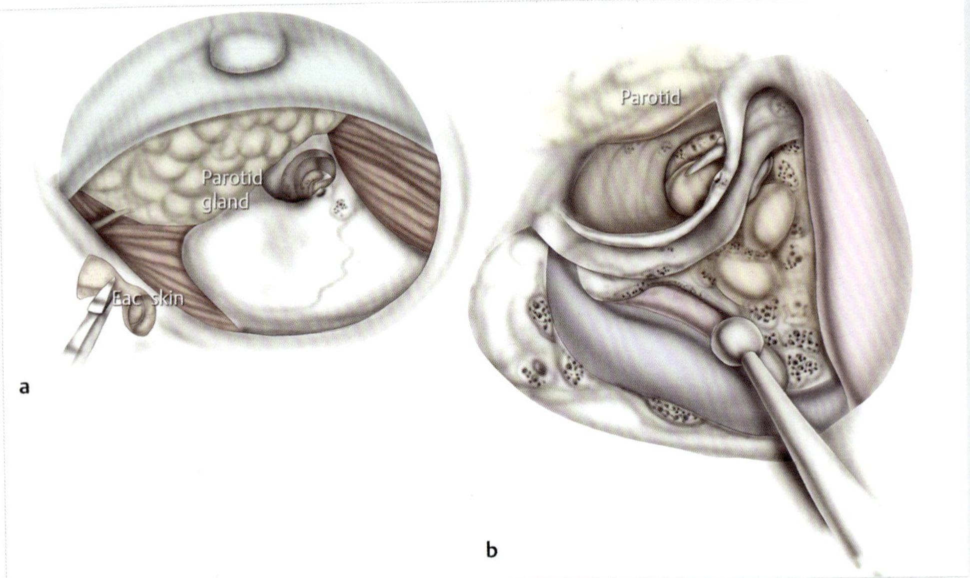

Fig. 6.3 Left ear. **(a)** The mastoid bone is uncovered and the skin of the external auditory canal (EAC) and the eardrum is removed. **(b)** A wide mastoidectomy are performed, uncovering the dura of the middle and posterior fossa, and the sinodural angle with the sigmoid sinus. *eac: external auditory canal; in: incus; lsc: lateral semicircular canal; ma: malleus; mcf: middle cranial fossa; pcf: posterior cranial fossa; psc: posterior semicircular canal; scm: sternocleidomastoid muscle; sis: sigmoid sinus; temp: temporalis muscle; tmj: temporal mandibular joint.*

A skin flap is elevated uncovering the fascia of the temporal muscle. The flap is anteriorly dissected until the detection of the posterior EAC. The skin of the EAC is circumferentially cut at the level of the osteo-cartilaginous junction (see ▶ Fig. 6.2b). The elevation of the flap is anteriorly continued above the superficial fascia of the parotid gland. This maneuver allows circumferential exposure of the EAC skin. The skin of the EAC is transected and the cartilage is separated from the skin. Everting stitches are placed in the superior and inferior portions of the EAC skin. The stitches are pulled out through the ear canal, everting the skin tube. The suture of the skin is made with 3–0 Vicryl (see ▶ Fig. 6.2c–d). A superior based mastoid-periosteal and temporal muscle flap is created and superiorly elevated uncovering the mastoid-occipital bone and the roof of the zygoma.

After a blind sac closure of the EAC, the remaining skin of the EAC and the eardrum is removed en bloc when possible (see ▶ Fig. 6.3a). A wide mastoidectomy is performed uncovering the dura of the middle fossa, the sigmoid sinus, and the sinodural angle (see ▶ Fig. 6.3b). Also, the lateral sinus is skeletonized in its posterior portion, exposing the suboccipital dura. During this step the mastoid emissary vein is detected and coagulated. The mastoidectomy is completed and the antrum with the fossa incudis and the lateral semicircular canal (LSC) are exposed. The perilabyrinthine cells are drilled around the labyrinthine block. The mastoid segment of the facial nerve is detected using the orientation of the LSC as a landmark to find the second genu of the facial nerve superiorly. The digastric ridge is used as a landmark to find the mastoid segment of the facial nerve close to the stylomastoid foramen. After the identification of the mastoid segment of the facial nerve the bone canal of the EAC is removed, exposing the tympanic cavity. During this step, a diamond bur is used to remove the anterior bone wall of the EAC. The temporomandibular joint is detected as the anterior limit of the dissection. The superior, posterior, and inferior portions of the EAC are also drilled until the whole tympanic cavity is under the microscopic view (see ▶ Fig. 6.4). The ossicular chain is removed and the facial nerve is exposed from the geniculate ganglion till the stylomastoid foramen. The dissection proceeds anteriorly to the lateral sinus, drilling the intersinusofacial cells and the retrofacial cells, uncovering the posterior fossa dura, and along the lateral sinus inferiorly exposing the jugular bulb. During this step the cochlear aqueduct is removed. The petrous ridge bone covering the superior petrosal sinus is carefully removed using rongeurs or diamond burs to avoid any bleeding. The endolymphatic duct is transected and the bone overlying the presigmoid dura is removed till the porus acusticus is identified.

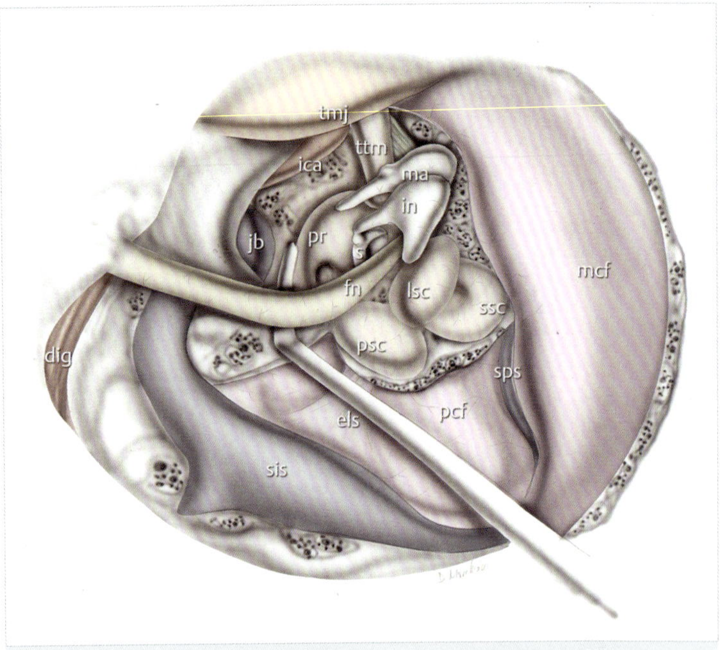

Fig. 6.4 Left ear. The bone wall of the external auditory canal (EAC) is removed; the facial nerve is skeletonized from the stylomastoid foramen to the tympanic segment; the dura of the posterior fossa and the middle fossa is widely exposed, and the sigmoid sinus is decompressed until the jugular bulb; the retrofacial cells are removed (notice the position of the curved dissector). The vertical portion of the carotid artery is detected. The labyrinthine block is isolated. *dig: digastric sulcus; els: endolymphatic sac; fn: facial nerve; ica: internal carotid artery; in: incus; jb: jugular bulb; lsc: lateral semicircular canal; ma: malleus; mcf: middle cranial fossa; pcf: posterior cranial fossa; pr: promontory; psc: posterior semicircular canal; s: stapes; sis: sigmoid sinus; sps; superior petrosal sinus; ssc: superior semicircular canal; tmj: temporal mandibular joint; ttm: tensor tympani muscle canal.*

The labyrinthectomy is then performed in the same fashion as the translabyrinthine approach (see ▶ Fig. 6.5). The lateral, superior, and posterior semicircular canals are exposed and drilled until the vestibule is identified; then it is removed together with the saccule and utricle. The IAC is exposed from the fundus to the porus drilling and exposing the lateral, superior, and inferior portions of the dura of the IAC. The falciform crest (transverse crest) and Bill's bar (vertical crest) are detected in the fundus of the IAC. These anatomical structures are used as landmarks to find the facial nerve in the fundus.

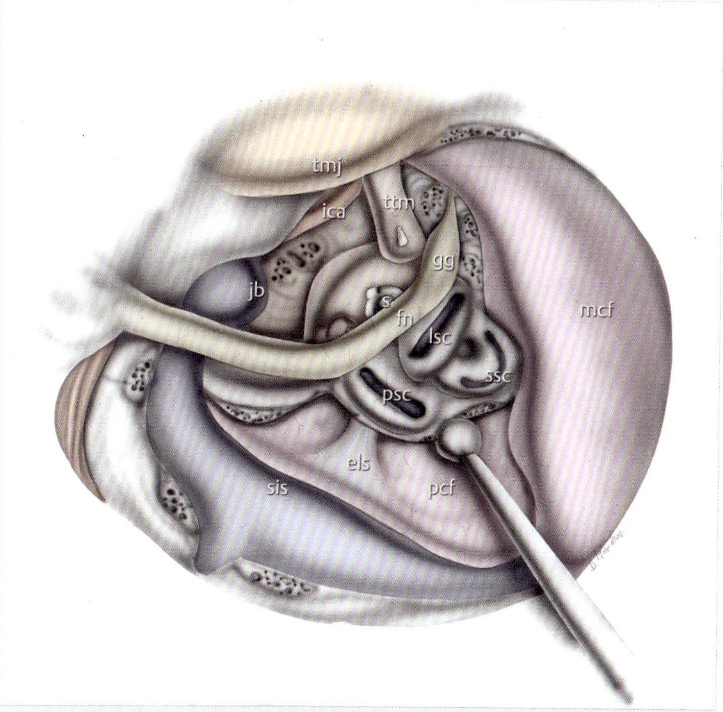

Fig. 6.5 Left ear. The labyrinthectomy is performed. *els: endolymphatic sac; fn: facial nerve; gg: geniculate ganglion; ica: internal carotid artery; jb: jugular bulb; lsc: lateral semicircular canal; mcf: middle cranial fossa; pcf: posterior cranial fossa; psc: posterior semicircular canal; s: stapes; sis: sigmoid sinus; ssc: superior semicircular canal; tmj: temporal mandibular joint; ttm: tensor tympani muscle canal.*

A 270-degree skeletonization of the IAC is performed from the fundus to the porus.

The cochleariform process is carefully removed and the muscle of the malleus is anteriorly pulled, uncovering the geniculate ganglion (see ▶ Fig. 6.6). The next step is the posterior rerouting of the facial nerve; it is exposed by 270 degrees in its vertical segment and 180 degrees in its horizontal part to facilitate its mobilization. The greater superficial petrosal nerve is isolated and detached

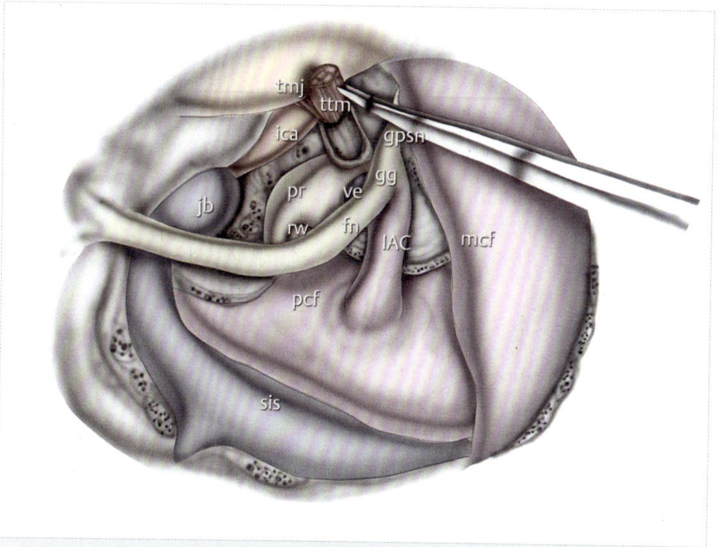

Fig. 6.6 Left ear. Once the labyrinthectomy has been performed, the internal auditory canal (IAC) is skeletonized. The stapes is removed exposing the vestibule. The cochleariform process with the tensor tympani muscle of the malleus are removed exposing the geniculate ganglion with the greater petrosal superficial nerve. *fn: facial nerve; gg: geniculate ganglion; gpsn: greater petrosal superficial nerve; iac: internal auditory canal; ica: internal carotid artery; jb: jugular bulb; mcf: middle cranial fossa; pcf: posterior cranial fossa; sis: sigmoid sinus; tmj: temporal mandibular joint; ttm: tensor tympani muscle canal.*

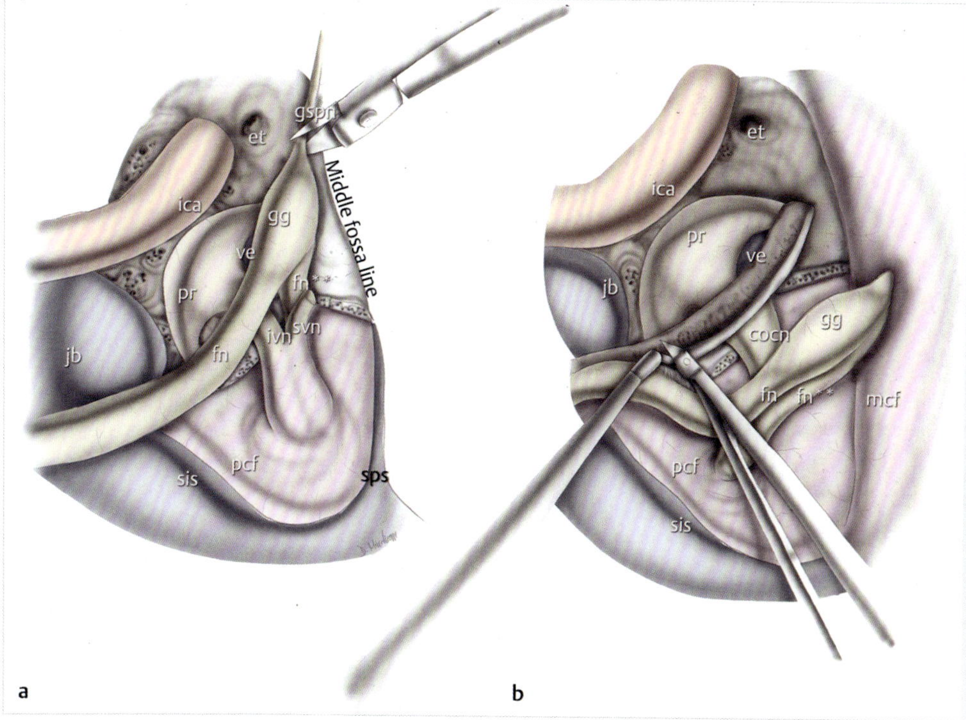

Fig. 6.7 Left ear. **(a)** The facial nerve is completely decompressed from the stylomastoid foramen to the internal auditory canal (IAC) segment. The dura of the IAC is opened and the superior vestibular nerve is cut, exposing the facial nerve inside the IAC. The greater superficial petrosal nerve is isolated and separated from the dura of the middle cranial fossa and cut. **(b)** The facial nerve is posteriorly transposed. A sharp dissection is necessary to mobilize the facial nerve from the fallopian canal. *cocn: cochlear nerve; et: eustachian tube; fn: facial nerve; fn**: facial nerve into the IAC; gg: geniculate ganglion; gspn: greater superficial petrosal nerve; iac: internal auditory canal; ica: internal carotid artery; ivn: inferior vestibular nerve; jb: jugular bulb; mcf: middle cranial fossa; pcf: posterior cranial fossa; pr: promontory; sis: sigmoid sinus; sps: superior petrosal sinus; svn: superior vestibular nerve; ve: vestibule.*

from the dura of the middle cranial fossa. Then this nerve is sharply cut at the level of the anterior end of the geniculate ganglion (see ▶ Fig. 6.7a). This step is performed to prevent unnecessary traction and kinking of the facial nerve during mobilization. A sharp dissection from the stapedius muscle is needed, especially near the mastoid genu, and the entire facial nerve is posteriorly folded and mobilized from the IAC to the stylomastoid foramen. The nerve is kept wet and throughout the operation it is protected from the rotating shaft of the drill (▶ Fig. 6.7b; also see ▶ Fig. 6.41).

Key Points

When required, especially in case of a tumor with jugular bulb involvement, a transcochlear approach with an anterior rerouting of the facial nerve should be considered in order to have a direct access to the inferior surface of temporal bone (see Clinical Case 2).

Once the facial nerve has been transposed, the cochlear nerve is transected at the level of its insertion into the cochlea.

The promontory is now well exposed. Starting with its basal turn the cochlea is completely exenterated (see ▶ Fig. 6.8a). The apical and middle turns of the cochlea are removed and the drilling continues anteriorly to completely skeletonize the intrapetrous carotid artery along its vertical and horizontal segments. Bone removal extends inferiorly to completely expose the jugular bulb and the inferior petrosal sinus. Superiorly bone removal follows the superior petrosal sinus to Meckel's cave and medially into the clivus.

The anterior limit of bone removal, under the vertical portion of the ICA, is the deep limit where the dura–bone interface "straightens" representing the posterior face of the clivus in the midline. Since bleeding from the clivus cells is expected, bone wax and Surgicel may help to control the bleeding in this area during this step (see ▶ Fig. 6.8b).

This extensive bone removal defines a triangular space covered by dura; Meckel's cave forms its apex, the superior petrosal sinus forms its superior border, and the inferior petrosal sinus forms its inferior border. Bone removal extends anteriorly to the petrous carotid artery and medially into the clivus.

In case of extradural extension of the lesion, as it happens with petrous bone cholesteatoma, the integrity of the dural layer of the posterior and middle fossae should be maintained whenever possible. In revision surgery, a variable defect of the posterior dural layer is to be expected, since the epidermization of the dural layer requires a careful surgical management of the dura in order to avoid leaving any residual disease, and at the end of the surgical procedure, the dural layer may be interrupted (see Clinical Cases 1). A bipolar forceps is used over the dural layer to detach the epidermization; microscissors are also used to peel the dural layer, removing the remnants of the cholesteatoma.

In case of intradural extension of the lesion, the dura is opened depending on the type and extension of the pathology. The opening is extended as anteriorly as possible for a safe and complete tumor removal (see ▶ Fig. 6.9a, see Clinical Case 2).

After dural incision, a wide access to the CPA is obtained; especially the midline and the prepontine cistern are exposed (see ▶ Fig. 6.9b). The anterior and lateral faces of the pons, with both sixth cranial nerves and the basilar artery, are visible without brainstem retraction. The tumor with intracranial extension is exposed and progressively removed (see Clinical Case 2). In case of acoustic neuroma with anterior extension in the midline, a central debulking is performed, and a careful detachment of the arachnoidal layers from the surrounding vascular and nervous structures around the tumor is carried out, same as with the translabyrinthine surgical approach.

6.2.6 Endoscopic Assisted Surgery

After the microscopic surgery has been completed and the tumor microscopically removed, an endoscopic check of the cavity is recommended in order to look for residual disease and to make the dissection radical, avoiding remnants.

A 0-degree, 4 mm diameter, 15 cm length endoscope is used as the first step to have the right orientation of the whole surgical cavity. The endoscope is gently inserted into the surgical cavity; the left hand holds the endoscope and the right hand holds the surgical instruments. A whole recognition of the surgical field is made.

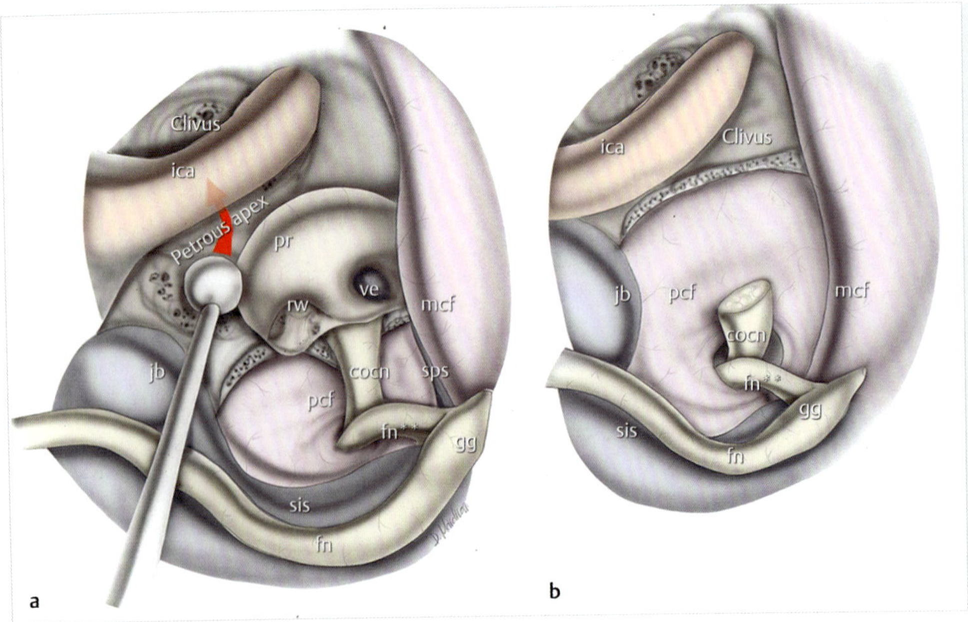

Fig. 6.8 Left ear. **(a)** Once the posterior rerouting of the facial nerve has been performed, the internal carotid artery (ICA) has been skeletonized and a drill is used to remove the promontory with the cochlea, and to reach the petrous apex under the carotid artery (see the *red arrow*). **(b)** The bone around the vertical portion of the carotid artery is removed and the petrous apex is reached until the clivus bone. The cochlear nerve is cut and the posterior fossa dura is widely exposed. *cocn: cochlear nerve; fn: facial nerve; fn**: facial nerve into the internal auditory canal (IAC); gg: geniculate ganglion; ica: internal carotid artery; jb: jugular bulb; mcf: middle cranial fossa; pcf: posterior cranial fossa; pr: promontory; rw: round window; sis: sigmoid sinus; sps: superior petrosal sinus; ve: vestibule.*

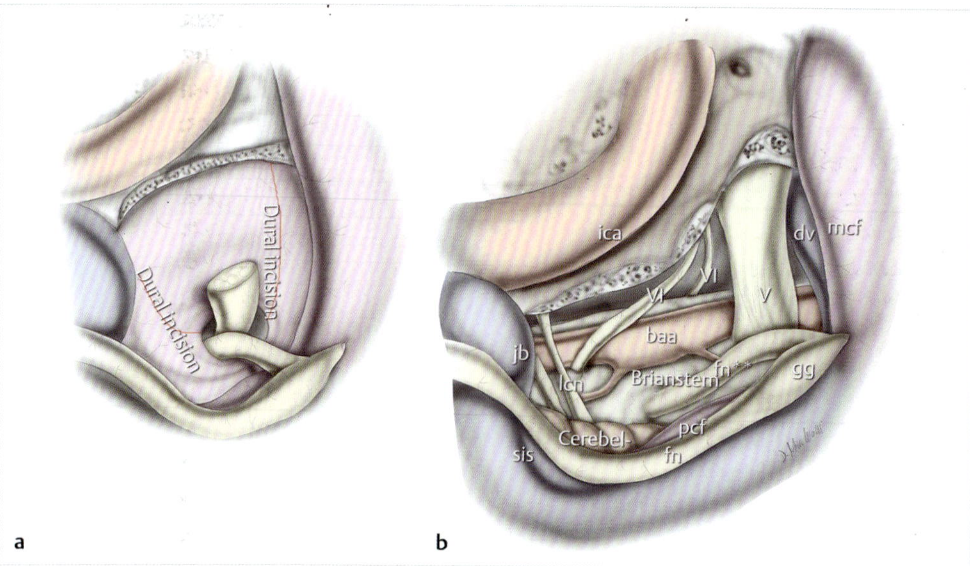

Fig. 6.9 Left ear. **(a)** In case of intradural lesion, the dura of the posterior fossa is cut (see the *red line*), entering the cerebellopontine angle (CPA). **(b)** A panoramic view of the neurovascular structures after dural opening. The exposure of the midline of the brainstem can be noticed. *baa: basilar artery; dv: the vein of Dandy; fn: facial nerve; fn**: internal auditory canal (IAC) component of facial nerve; gg: geniculate ganglion; ica: internal carotid artery; jb: jugular bulb; lcn: lower cranial nerves; mcf: middle cranial fossa; pcf: posterior cranial fossa; sis: sigmoid sinus; sps: superior petrosal sinus.*

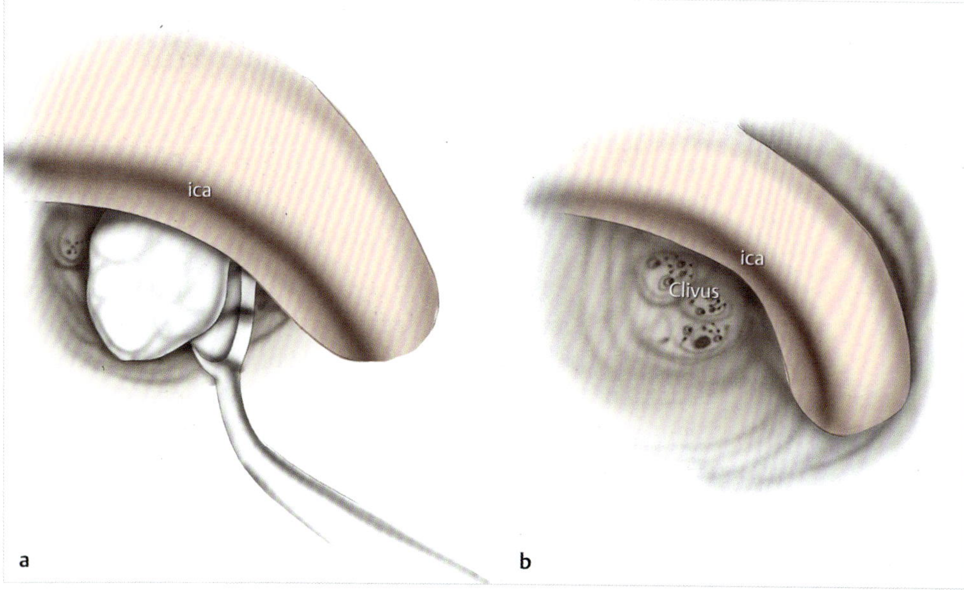

Fig. 6.10 Left ear. **(a)** Endoscopic view with a 45-degree endoscope of the petrous apex and the clivus around the internal carotid artery (ICA); a residual disease can be seen; a curved dissector is used to remove the remnants. **(b)** Endoscopic view of the clivus bone after tumor removal. *ica: internal carotid artery.*

6.2.7 Extradural Lesions

The intrapetrous carotid artery with the deepest portion of the clivus bone lying underneath is the most frequent site where extradural remnants may be present. Especially in case of petrous bone cholesteatoma, residual disease in the medial section of the vertical and horizontal portions of the carotid is to be expected. In these cases, endoscopic support is recommended to avoid the microscopic mobilization of the artery with the consequent important manipulation of the vascular structure.

A 45-degree, 4 mm diameter, 15 cm length endoscope may be useful to detect the residual disease lying along the medial surface of the ICA. A curved suction instrument should be carefully used to detach the remnants from the vascular structure, and wet cottonoids may be used over the artery to protect and clean the vascular structure. Moreover, a soft dissection may be done using curved dissectors (see ▶ Fig. 6.10; see Clinical Case 1).

Key Points

When a two-hand surgical technique is required, the second surgeon can hold the endoscope to detect the remnants so that the first surgeon will be able to use both hands to dissect the residual disease.

This three-hand technique is recommended especially during open surgery in critical areas such as the medial surface of the ICA and in the CPA to remove remnants (especially epidermoid cysts of the CPA) in the midline along the basilar artery.

6.2.8 Intradural Lesions

A final endoscopic check of the CPA is suggested especially in case of epidermoid lesions or acoustic neuromas and petroclival meningiomas.

Epidermoid cysts are generally located off the midline and arise from ectodermal inclusions during neural tube closure in the third to fifth week of embryogenesis. The lesions grow to encase vessels and nerves, and their content consists of layered anucleate squames produced by a well-differentiated squamous epithelium, often with keratohyalin granules.

The endoscope is extremely helpful when removing tumor parts that are hidden behind the dura, for example, in the tentorium, or bony corners along the petrous bone surface inside the cranial nerve foramina as well as behind the neurovascular

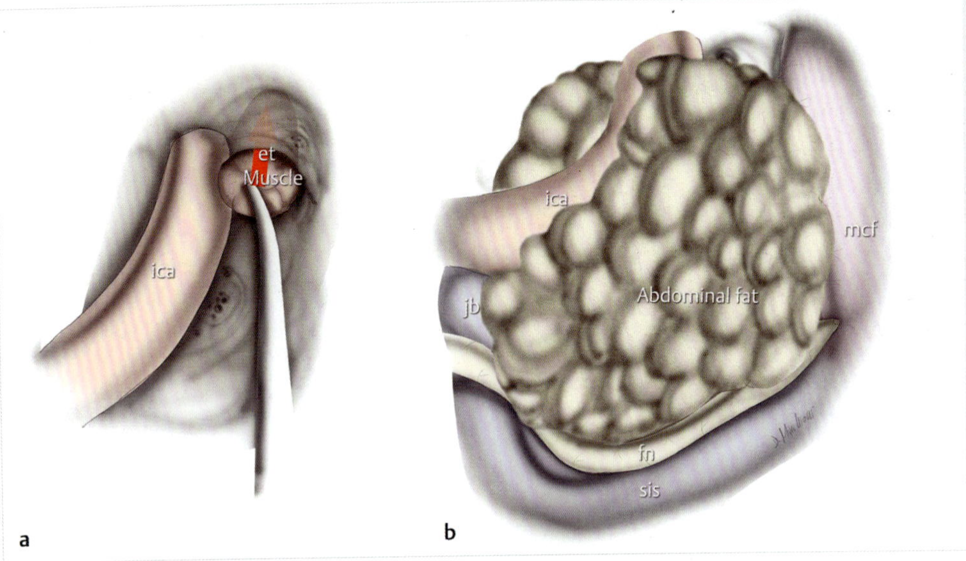

Fig. 6.11 Left ear. **(a)** A piece of muscle is pushed into the eustachian tube orifice to close it. **(b)** Abdominal fat is used to seal the surgical cavity. *et: eustachian tube; fn: facial nerve; ica: internal carotid artery; jb: jugular bulb; mcf: middle cranial fossa; sis: sigmoid sinus.*

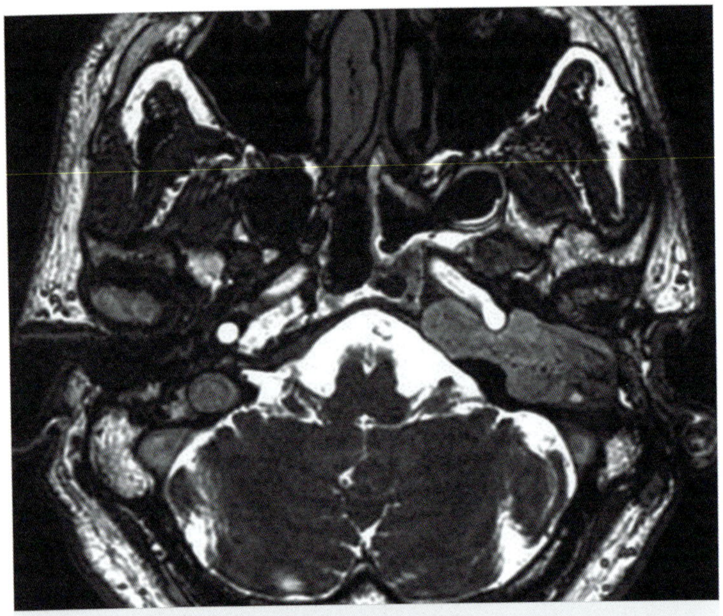

Fig. 6.12 Clinical Case 1: Magnetic resonance imaging (MRI) in axial view. A recurrence of petrous bone cholesteatoma is seen in a patient with facial palsy.

structures. Irrigation is mandatory during the endoscopic procedures to avoid heat dissipation from the tip of the endoscope to the vascular structures. Curved and straight suction instruments are carefully used along the vascular and nervous structures during the dissection of the residual disease.

6.2.9 Final Steps

Once tumor removal is complete, hemostasis is secured with Surgicel and a careful bipolar cautery before closure. If possible, several interrupted sutures are placed to close the dura. The eustachian tube is plugged with muscle, Surgicel, and bone wax (see ▶ Fig. 6.11a). The facial nerve is anteriorly folded. The dural and skull base defect is closed with strips of abdominal fat (see ▶ Fig. 6.11b) and the musculoperiosteal skin flap is closed in a watertight fashion in three layers.

A compressive dressing is placed and the patient is closely observed in the ICU for the first 24 hours after surgery.

The main disadvantage of the transcochlear approach is that the hearing function is completely lost and the rerouting of the facial nerve invariably causes an incomplete postoperative recovery of the facial nerve function. Although it usually improves after surgery, it infrequently exceeds grade III on the House-Brackmann grading scale. This approach is preferable especially when the patient already has grade III or IV facial palsy with a compromised hearing function.

6.3 Transotic Approach

The major drawback of the transcochlear approach is an incomplete postoperative facial nerve recovery due to the posterior rerouting of the facial nerve. The transotic approach described by Fisch and Mattox was similar to that of the transcochlear approach except for the fact that the facial nerve is not mobilized and kept in its fallopian canal (see Clinical Case 3; ▶ Fig. 6.81, ▶ Fig. 6.82, ▶ Fig. 6.83).[5] The transotic approach is mainly used for extensive petrous apex cholesteatomas with anterior extension and large vestibular schwannomas with cochlear involvement. The only disadvantage is that the facial nerve is left in place, and it runs like a bridge in the surgical field limiting the surgical corridor to the anterior CPA, but the use of the endoscope enables the surgeon to work around the facial nerve and the ICA in order to allow radical tumor removal, minimizing the manipulation of the facial nerve and the ICA.

6.3.1 Indications

- Petrous bone cholesteatomas in patients with a normal function of the facial nerve (see ▶ Fig. 6.1a; Clinical Case 4 and Clinical Case 6)
- Petrous apex lesions (such as cholesterol granuloma) in patients with nonserviceable hearing (see Clinical Case 5)
- Acoustic neuromas with anterior temporal bone invasion along the petrous apex or extending into the cochlea and vestibule (see ▶ Fig. 6.1b; see Clinical Case 7 and Clinical Case 8)
- Large CPA lesions with midline involvement or in subjects with a high jugular bulb

6.3.2 Use of the Endoscope

An endoscopic support, in this surgical technique, is always suggested at the end of the microscopic dissection in order to detect

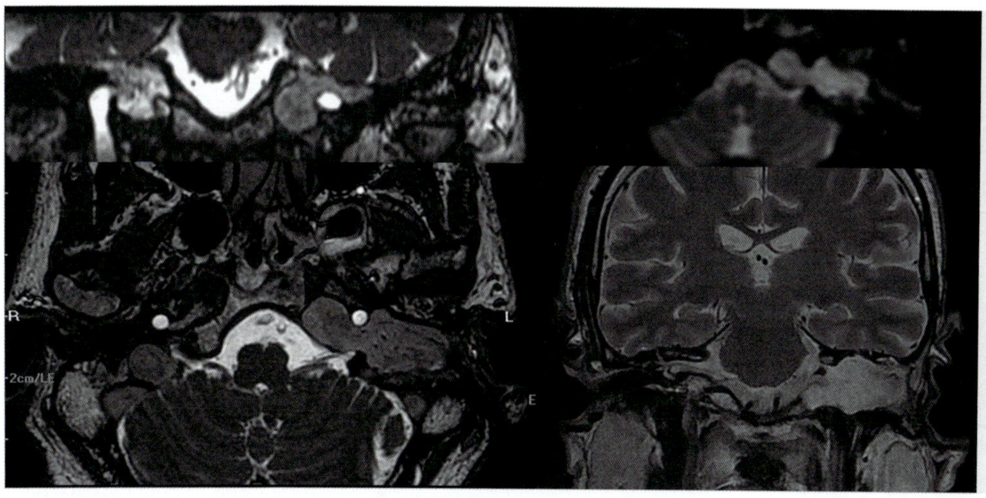

Fig. 6.13 Clinical Case 1: Magnetic resonance imaging (MRI) study. Petrous bone cholesteatoma invading the petrous apex around the vertical and horizontal portions of the internal carotid artery (ICA) reaching the clivus.

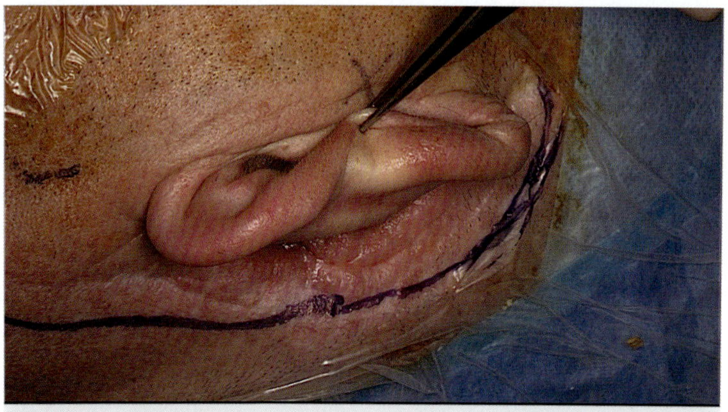

Fig. 6.14 Clinical Case 1, Left ear: An incision is made from the temporal region to the neck passing the retroauricular area. The previous scar is noted.

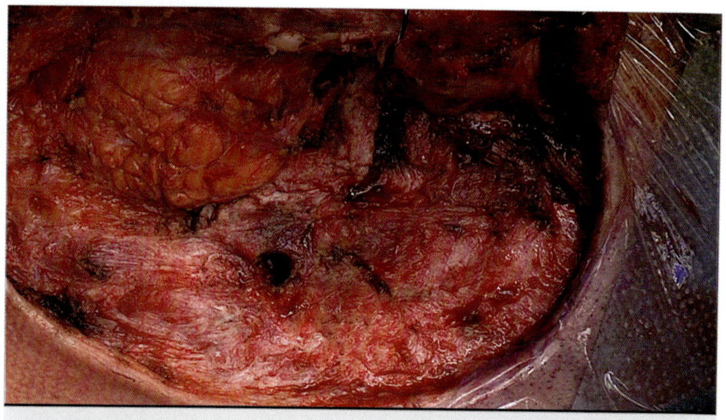

Fig. 6.15 Clinical Case 1, Left ear: The cutaneous flap is elevated, the external auditory canal (EAC) is transected, and the flap is anteriorly dissected progressively exposing the parotid gland. The zygomatic arch is detected.

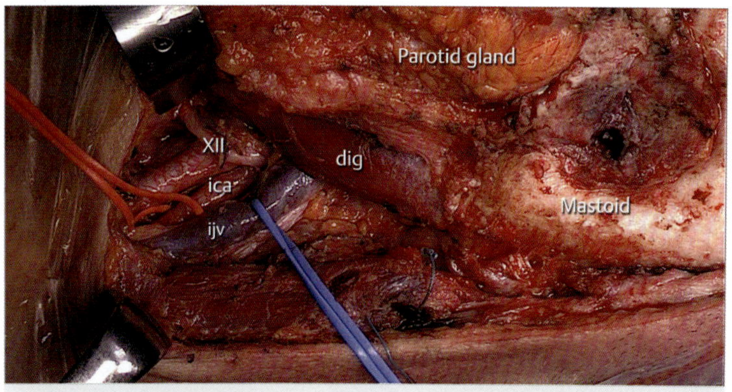

Fig. 6.16 Clinical Case 1, Left ear: The neck around the skull base is dissected; the internal carotid artery (ICA) and the internal jugular vein are marked. *dig: digastric muscle; ica: internal carotid artery; ijv: internal jugular vein.*

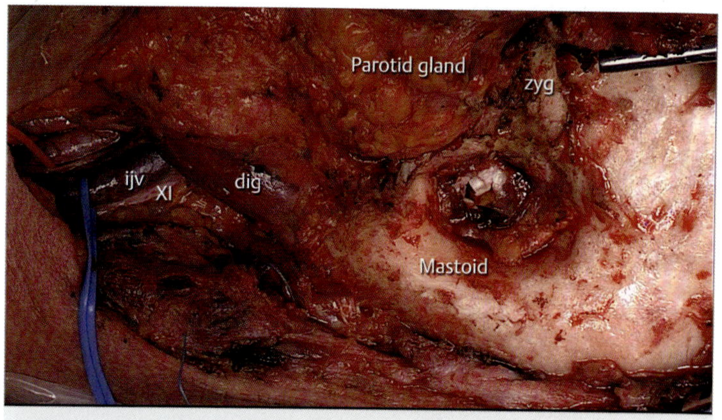

Fig. 6.17 Clinical Case 1, Left ear: The mastoid bone is widely exposed; the cholesteatoma is seen inside the previous surgical cavity. *dig: digastric muscle; ijv: internal jugular vein; zyg: zygomatic arch.*

any residual disease lying in the medial portion of the facial nerve and the ICA.

6.3.3 Surgical Approach

Most of the surgical steps are similar to the ones of the transcochlear approach.

A postauricular incision is made from the temporal region to the mastoid tip inferiorly ending in the neck approximately 4 to 5 cm behind the retroauricular sulcus. When required, the inferior section of the incision may be prolonged along the sternocleidomastoid muscle in the neck, in order to isolate the major vascular and nervous structures (see Fig. 6.2a).

The skin flap is elevated following the same plane as the one of the temporalis muscle fascia. The EAC is transected. The cartilage of the EAC is removed from the skin and the skin is reverted and a blind sac closure is performed in the same fashion as for the transcochlear approach (see ▶ Fig. 6.2b–d). The skin of the bony EAC with the eardrum is removed en bloc using the microscope (see ▶ Fig. 6.3a). The bone walls of EAC are removed. The temporomandibular joint is detected as the anterior limit of the dissection and a subtotal petrosectomy is performed under a

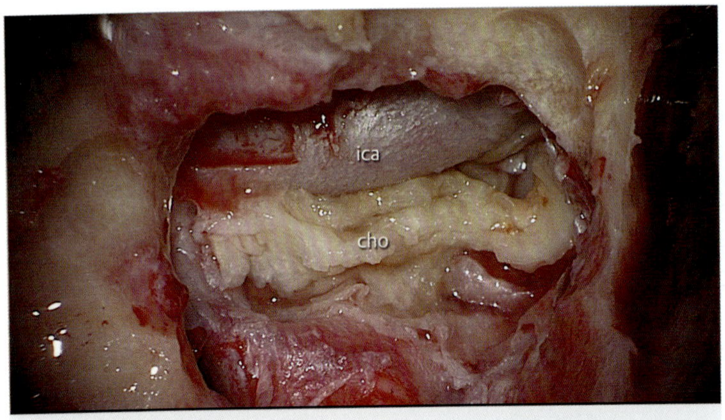

Fig. 6.18 Clinical Case 1, Left ear: A transcochlear approach is performed. An invasive cholesteatoma involving the vertical portion of intrapetrous carotid artery is noted. *cho: cholesteatoma; ica: internal carotid artery.*

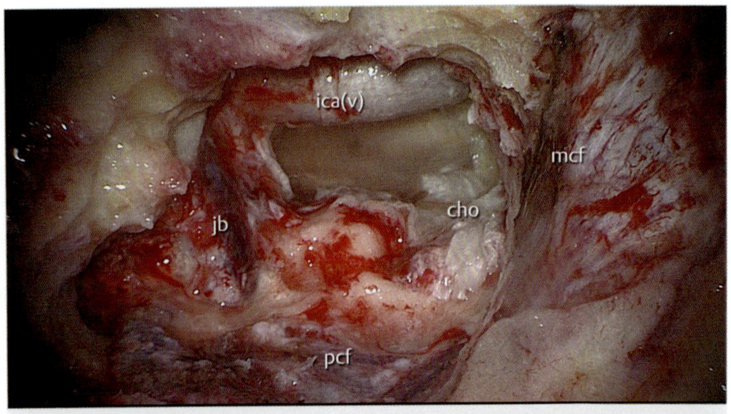

Fig. 6.19 Clinical Case 1, Left ear: The facial nerve which was previously surgically damaged is cut. A wide petrosectomy is performed, exposing the dura of the posterior and middle fossae. *cho: cholesteatoma; ica(v): vertical portion of internal carotid artery; jb: jugular bulb; mcf: middle cranial fossa; pcf: posterior cranial fossa.*

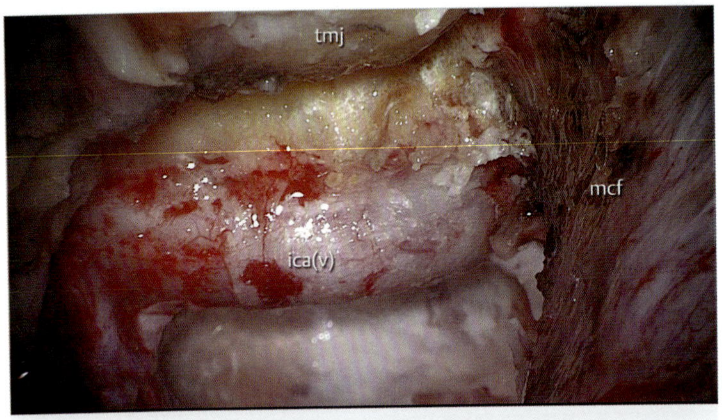

Fig. 6.20 Clinical Case 1, Left ear: The cholesteatoma is progressively removed from the vertical portion of the internal carotid artery (ICA). *ica(v): vertical portion of internal carotid artery; mcf: middle cranial fossa; tmj: temporomandibular joint.*

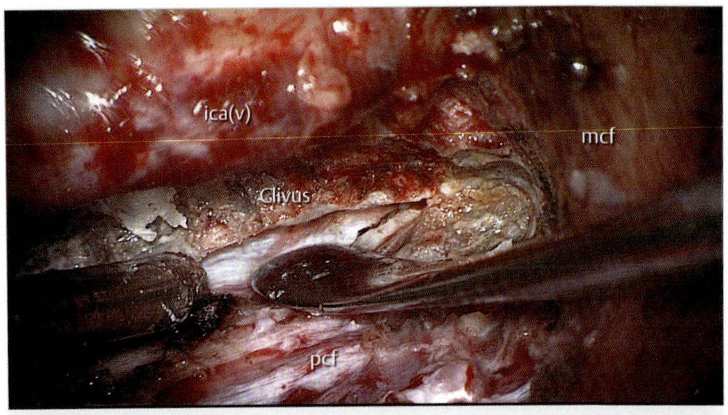

Fig. 6.21 Clinical Case 1, Left ear: The cholesteatoma is progressively removed from the petrous apex and clivus. Using a diamond bur, the bone of the petrous apex is removed reaching the clivus under the internal carotid artery (ICA). *ica(v): vertical portion of internal carotid artery; mcf: middle cranial fossa; pcf: posterior cranial fossa.*

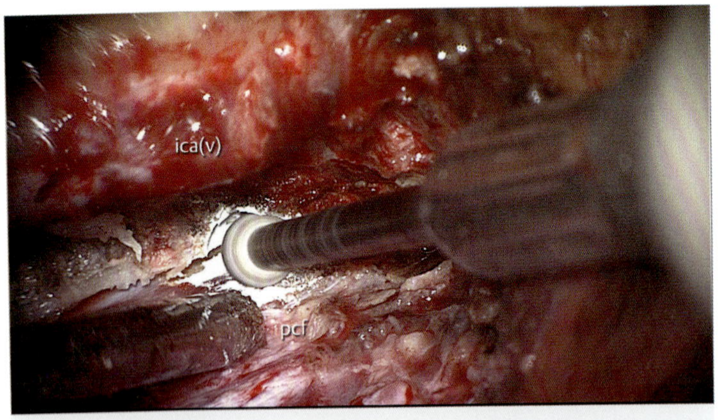

Fig. 6.22 Clinical Case 1, Left ear: The clivus bone is drilled to radicalize the cholesteatoma dissection. *ica(v): vertical portion of internal carotid artery; pcf: posterior cranial fossa.*

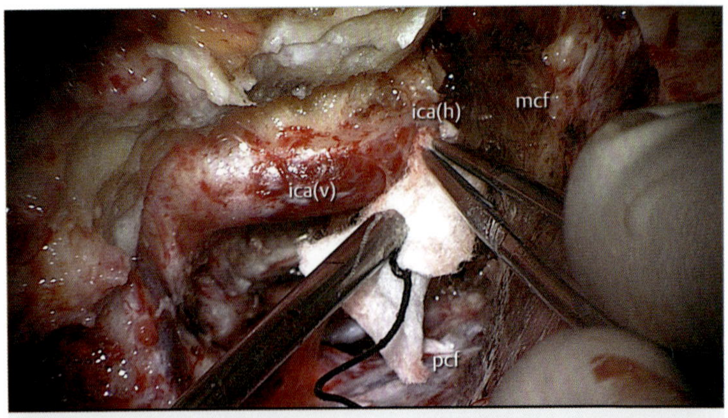

Fig. 6.23 Clinical Case 1, Left ear: A wet cottonoid is gently used over the carotid artery to remove the epidermization around the vascular structure. *ica(h): horizontal portion of internal carotid artery; ica(v): vertical portion of internal carotid artery; mcf: middle cranial fossa; pcf: posterior cranial fossa.*

microscopic view, including a wide mastoidectomy uncovering the dura of the posterior cranial fossa, the dura of the middle fossa, the sinodural angle, and the lateral sinus (see ▶ Fig. 6.3b). The retrolabyrinthine and supralabyrinthine cells are removed. The lateral sinus is inferiorly skeletonized until the jugular bulb. The digastric ridge is identified and anteriorly followed, using it as a landmark to find the facial nerve at the level of the stylomastoid foramen. The facial nerve is skeletonized from the stylomastoid foramen until the geniculate ganglion, maintaining a thin bone wall to cover and protect the nerve (see ▶ Fig. 6.4). Once the jugular bulb is skeletonized, the hypotympanic and protympanic cells are drilled detecting the vertical portion of the

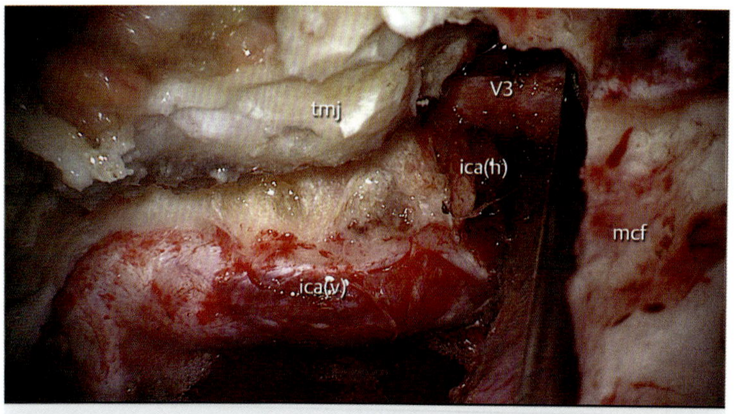

Fig. 6.24 Clinical Case 1, Left ear: The cartilaginous portion of eustachian tube is partially removed exposing the horizontal portion of internal carotid artery (ICA); the zygomatic process is drilled; the middle cranial fossa is widely exposed anteriorly and the middle meningeal artery coagulated. *ica(h): horizontal portion of internal carotid artery; ica(v): vertical portion of internal carotid artery; mcf: middle cranial fossa; tmj: temporal mandibular joint.*

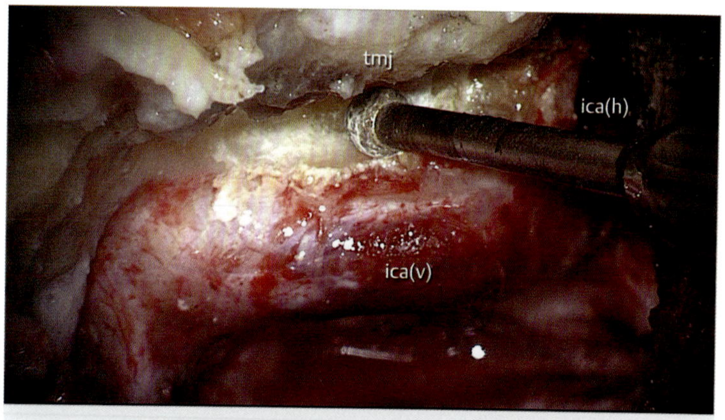

Fig. 6.25 Clinical Case 1, Left ear: The bone in between the temporomandibular joint and the internal carotid artery (ICA) is removed. *ica(h): horizontal portion of internal carotid artery; ica(v): vertical portion of internal carotid artery; tmj: temporal mandibular joint.*

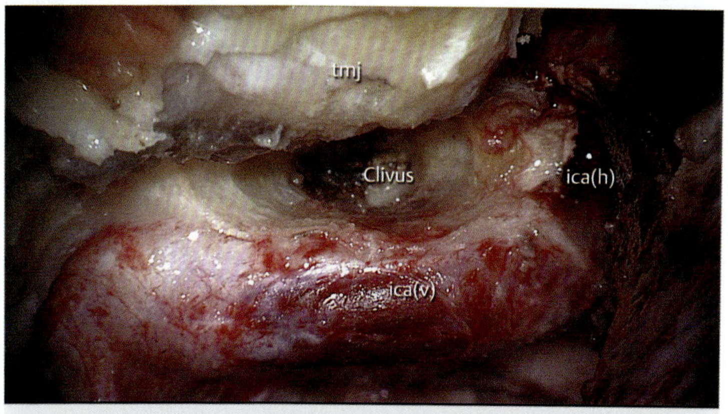

Fig. 6.26 Clinical Case 1, Left ear: The clivus is reached anteriorly to the internal carotid artery (ICA). *ica(h): horizontal portion of internal carotid artery; ica(v): vertical portion of internal carotid artery; tmj: temporal mandibular joint.*

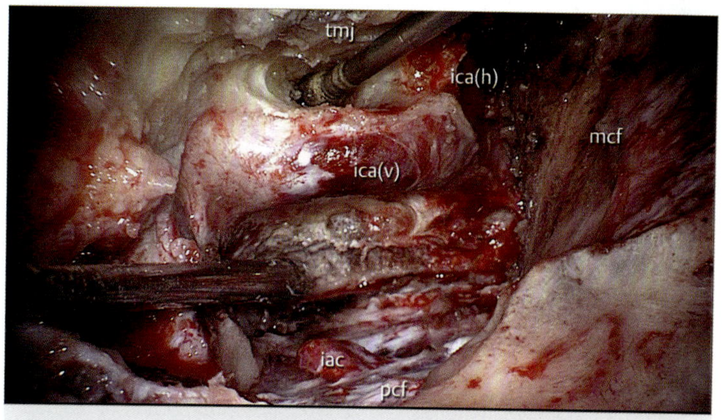

Fig. 6.27 Clinical Case 1, Left ear: A progressive dissection of the intrapetrous internal carotid artery (ICA) is performed. *iac: internal auditory canal; ica(h): horizontal portion of internal carotid artery; ica(v): vertical portion of internal carotid artery; mcf: middle cranial fossa; pcf: posterior cranial fossa; tmj: temporal mandibular joint.*

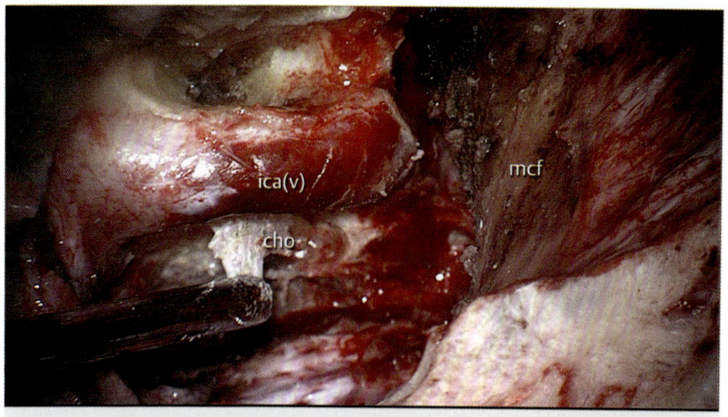

Fig. 6.28 Clinical Case 1, Left ear: A residual cholesteatoma is seen under the vertical portion of the carotid artery. *cho: cholesteatoma; ica (v): vertical portion of internal carotid artery; mcf: middle cranial fossa.*

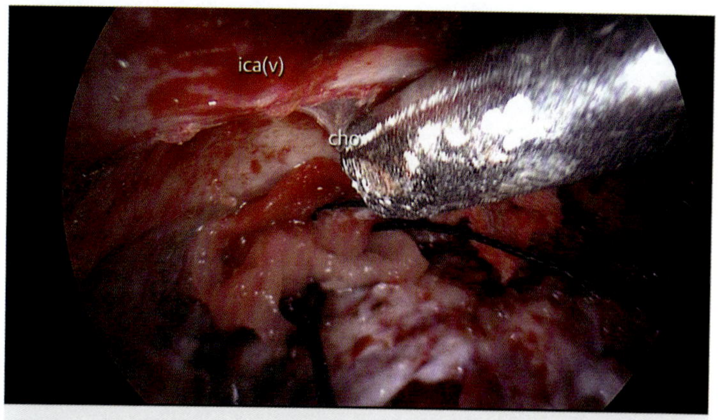

Fig. 6.29 Clinical Case 1, Left ear: A 0-degree endoscope is introduced into the surgical cavity under the carotid artery, detecting the residual cholesteatoma. A curved suction instrument is used gently to remove the residual disease. *cho: cholesteatoma; ica(v): vertical portion of internal carotid artery.*

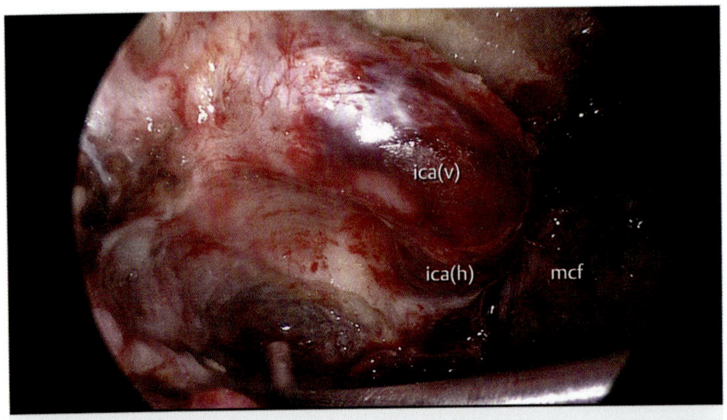

Fig. 6.30 Clinical Case 1, Left ear: A 45-degree endoscopic view of the internal carotid artery (ICA) and clivus after cholesteatoma removal. *ica(h): horizontal portion of internal carotid artery; ica(v): vertical portion of internal carotid artery; mcf: middle cranial fossa.*

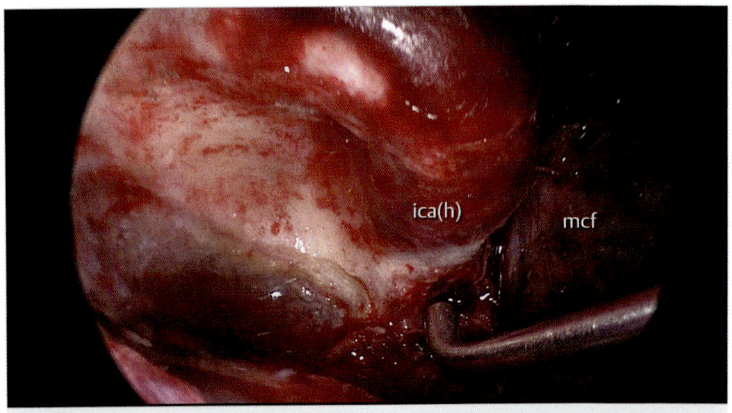

Fig. 6.31 Clinical Case 1, Left ear: Endoscopic magnification of horizontal portion of internal carotid artery (ICA). *ica(h): horizontal portion of internal carotid artery; mcf: middle cranial fossa.*

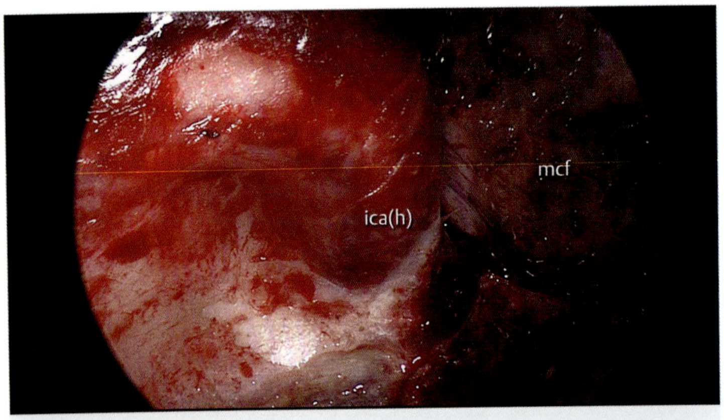

Fig. 6.32 Clinical Case 1, Left ear: Once the cholesteatoma has been removed, a 45-degree endoscope is used to magnify the surgical field looking for any remaining disease. *ica(h): horizontal portion of internal carotid artery; mcf: middle cranial fossa.*

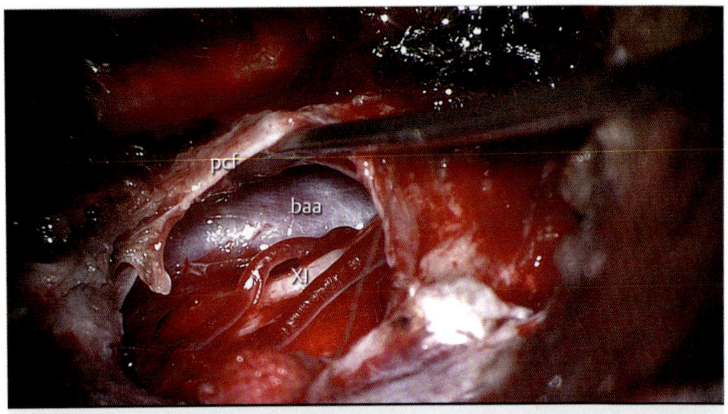

Fig. 6.33 Clinical Case 1, Left ear: A defect of the posterior fossa dura is noted. The brainstem with the basilar artery is seen through the opening. *baa: basilar artery; pcf: posterior cranial fossa dura.*

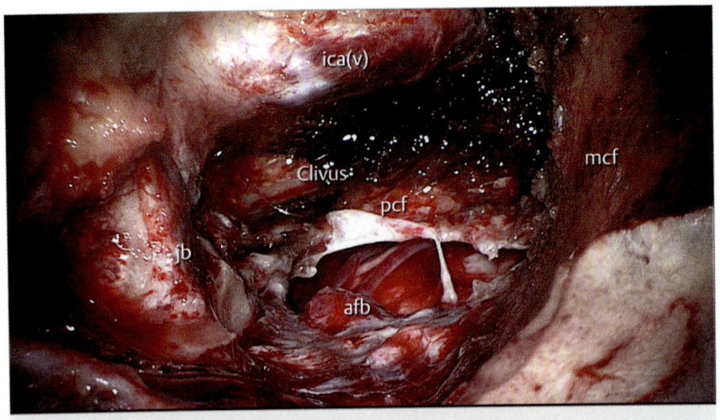

Fig. 6.34 Clinical Case 1, Left ear: Surgicel is used to pack the clivus bone. *afb: acoustic facial bundle; ica(v): vertical portion of internal carotid artery; jb: jugular bulb; mcf: middle cranial fossa; pcf: posterior cranial fossa dura.*

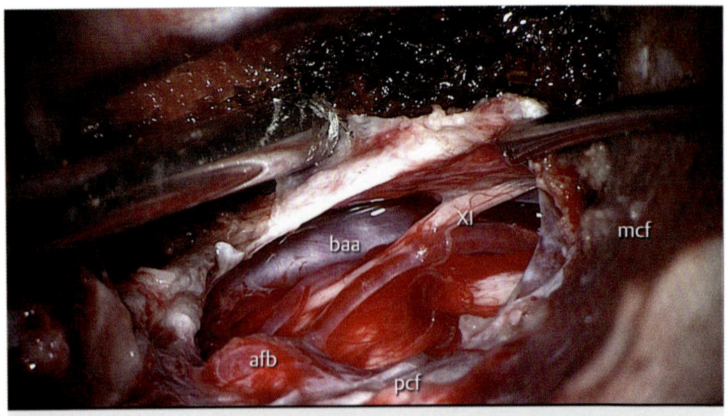

Fig. 6.35 Clinical Case 1, Left ear: The sixth cranial nerve is noted through the dural defect of the posterior fossa. *afb: acoustic facial bundle; baa: basilar artery; mcf: middle cranial fossa; pcf: posterior cranial fossa dura.*

carotid artery. The retrofacial cells are drilled, connecting the mastoid cavity with the hypotympanic cells.

A labyrinthectomy is performed, removing the three semicircular canals together with the vestibule. The IAC is skeletonized from the fundus crest to the porus as it happens in the translabyrinthine approach (see ▶ Fig. 6.5).

Once the dura of the posterior fossa and the IAC has been detected, the bony canal of the tensor tendon muscle is removed with the muscle (see ▶ Fig. 6.6). The promontory is drilled and the cochlea is progressively removed (see ▶ Fig. 6.67). A large diamond bur is used to skeletonize the vertical portion of the ICA until the horizontal portion close to the eustachian tube orifice (see ▶ Fig. 6.68). When required, the petrous apex is exposed under the carotid artery until the clivus bone (see ▶ Fig. 6.69). Once the cochlea and promontory have been removed, the cells in the medial portion of the tympanic, the mastoid segments of

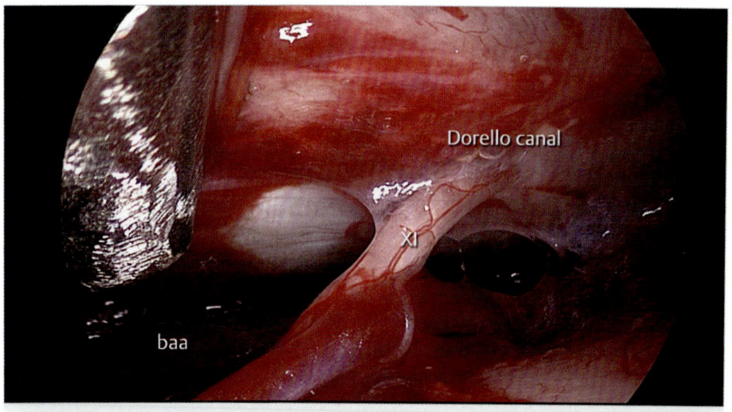

Fig. 6.36 Clinical Case 1, Left ear: Endoscopic view of the sixth cranial neve. *baa: basilar artery.*

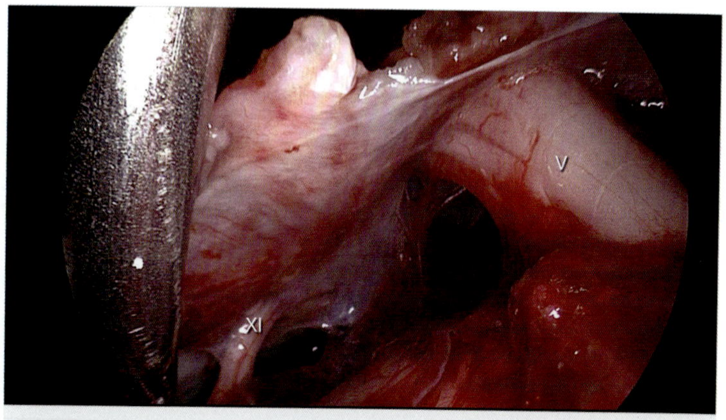

Fig. 6.37 Clinical Case 1, Left ear: The defect of the posterior cranial fossa dura is endoscopically analyzed.

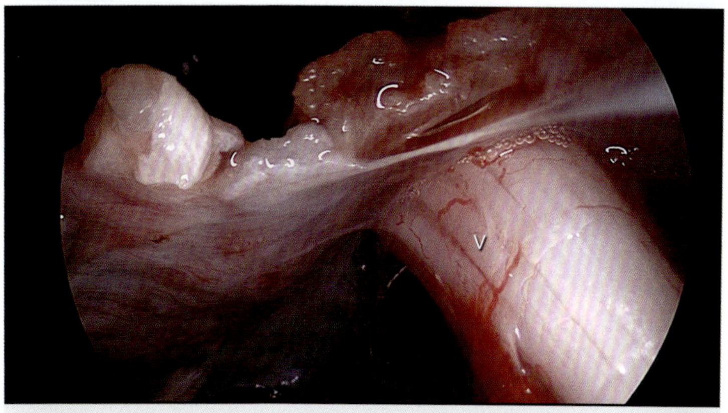

Fig. 6.38 Clinical Case 1, Left ear: Endoscopic view of the trigeminal nerve.

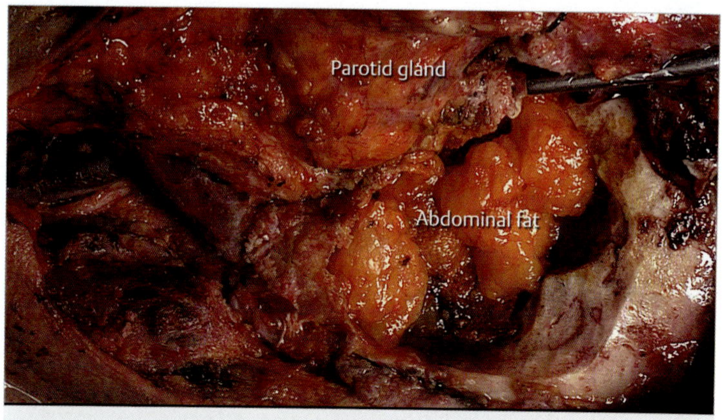

Fig. 6.39 Clinical Case 1, Left ear: Abdominal fat is used to seal the surgical cavity.

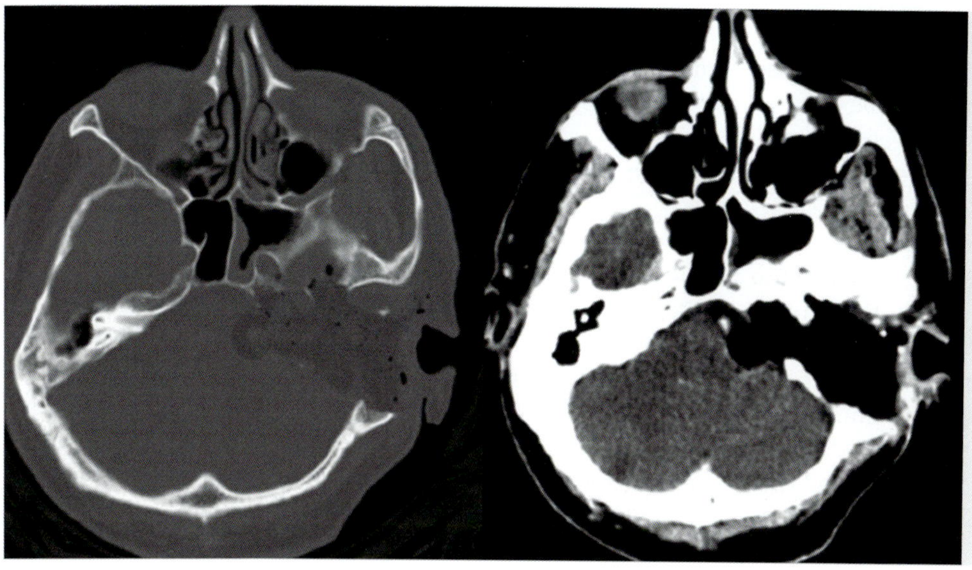

Fig. 6.40 Clinical Case 1, Left ear: Postoperative computed tomography (CT) scan in axial view showing the temporal bone dissection.

the facial nerve, and the IAC are drilled. At the end of this surgical procedure, the facial nerve resembles a bridge in the middle of the field (see Clinical Case 3; ▶ Fig. 6.81, ▶ Fig. 6.82, ▶ Fig. 6.83). The bone under the fallopian canal should be preserved as much as possible to get support for the nerve, to avoid the fracture of the nerve during the dissection of the tumor. When required, the ICA is also skeletonized, carefully removing the bone all around the artery creating a bridge on the vertical portion, exposing the clivus bone (see Clinical Case 5; ▶ Fig. 6.128 and ▶ Fig. 6.129). During this procedure, when the lesion does not infiltrate the vascular structure, it is mandatory to maintain a thin bone layer over the artery in order to protect the ICA during the further surgical maneuvers in the petrous apex, especially if endoscopic use is required to remove any remnants in the medial portion of the carotid artery (petrous bone cholesteatoma, petrous apex epidermoid cyst, cholesterol granuloma).

6.3.4 Endoscopic Assisted Surgery

In case of petrous bone cholesteatomas with a medial involvement of the petrous apex with respect to the facial nerve, the endoscopic support is mandatory in order to maintain the facial nerve in place avoiding the posterior rerouting of the nerve. Once a facial bridge has been created, a microscopic dissection of the

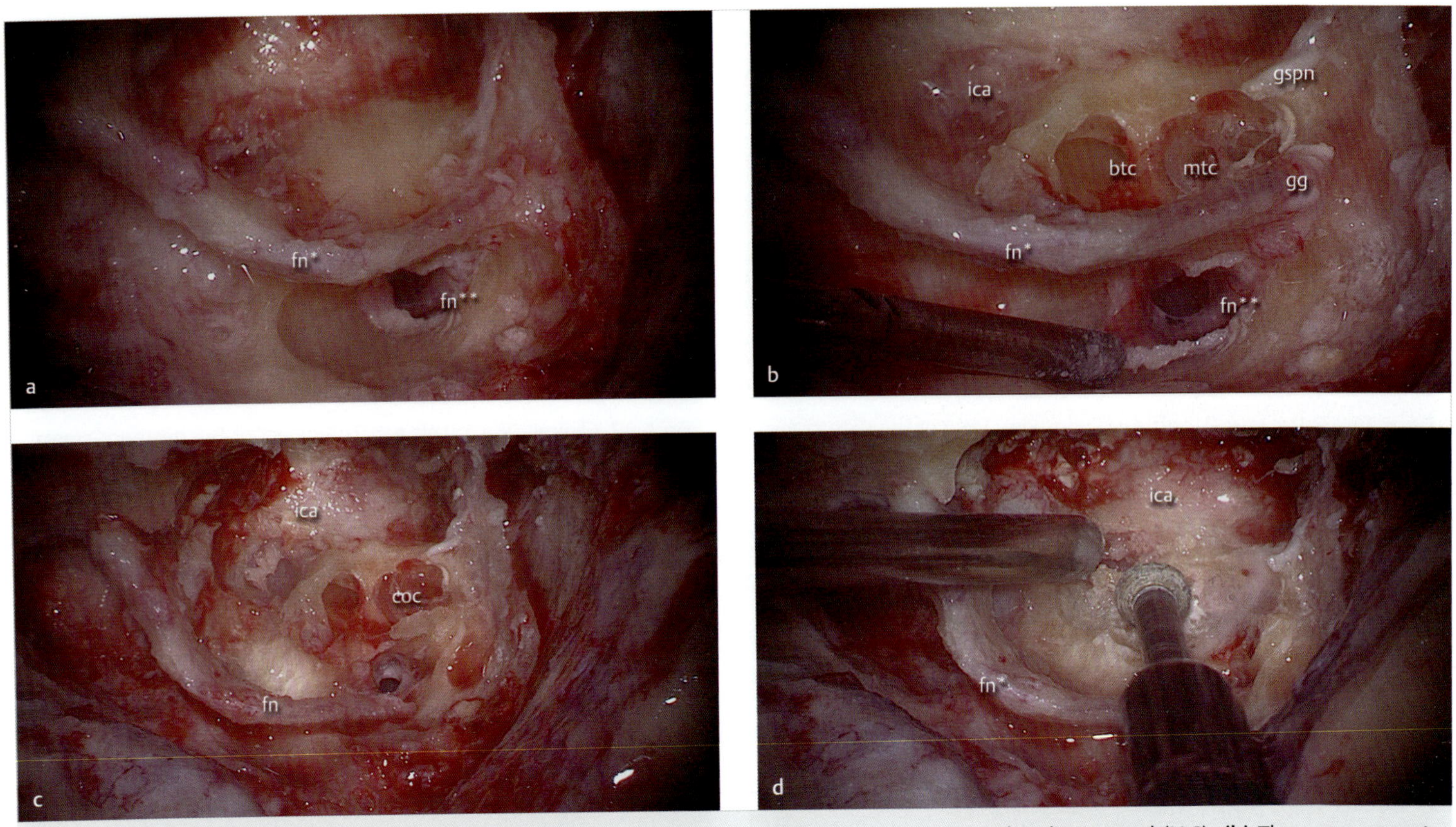

Fig. 6.41 Left ear. **(a)** The facial nerve is decompressed from the stylomastoid foramen to the internal auditory canal (IAC). **(b)** The promontory is drilled and the cochlea is removed. The greater superficial petrosal nerve is cut. **(c)** A posterior rerouting of the facial nerve is made. **(d)** A diamond bur is used to remove the promontory. The vertical portion of internal carotid artery (ICA) is detected, exposing the petrous apex. *btc: basal turn of the cochlea; coc: cochlea; fn*: mastoid portion of facial nerve; fn**: facial nerve into the internal auditory canal; gg: geniculate ganglion; gspn: greater petrosal superficial nerve; ica: internal carotid artery; mtc: middle turn of the cochlea.*

cholesteatoma is performed with an angulated instrument around the nerve, in order to remove the cholesteatoma from the petrous apex (see ▶ Fig. 6.70a,b). A cottonoid may be used to detach the residual disease from the medial surface of the nerve. Once the microscopic step has been performed, an endoscope with different angles (0–45 degree) is introduced into the surgical field to magnify the medial surface of the facial nerve, especially the geniculate ganglion and the labyrinthine portion of the facial nerve (see ▶ Fig. 6.71a). Remnants located in the petrous apex and on the medial surface of the facial nerve are detected under endoscopic view (see ▶ Fig. 6.71b). Curved dissectors and suction instruments may be useful to remove the remnant disease on the medial surface of the facial nerve under endoscopic view. When required, a three-hand technique may be used. The second surgeon can assist the first surgeon by holding the endoscope; the first surgeon can use both hands to remove the remnant disease as in the microscopic technique (see ▶ Fig. 6.72a,b). When a petrous apex involvement under the ICA is found, an endoscopic support is mandatory to remove the remnant disease in the medial section of the vertical and horizontal segments of the vascular structure avoiding the mobilization of the artery, as it happens in the previously described trascochlear approach (see Section 6.2.7, Extradural Lesions, and see ▶ Fig. 6.73 and ▶ Fig. 6.74 and also ▶ Fig. 6.10). The 0-degree and 45-degree endoscopes can magnify the clivus bone under the carotid artery, and the medial surface of the horizontal portion of the artery until the anterior foramen lacerum. In case of acoustic neuroma with cochlea-vestibule extension, once the tumor has been removed, an endoscopic check of the surgical cavity is suggested, especially to detect any remnants of the disease located under the facial nerve bridge, close to the vestibule (see ▶ Fig. 6.75, ▶ Fig. 6.76, ▶ Fig. 6.77, ▶ Fig. 6.78, ▶ Fig. 6.79).

6.3.5 Final Steps

Once the tumor has been removed, the eustachian tube is closed with muscle. In case of dural defect in the posterior fossa, long strips of fat harvested from the abdomen are inserted into the CPA to close the cavity; abdominal fat is also used to fill the extradural surgical cavity (see ▶ Fig. 6.80). Fibrin glue is used to seal off the cavity. Only in cases in which a connection between the skull base and the neck is present in the final cavity, a reconstruction of the lateral and inferior walls linking the base with the neck is mandatory, using synthetic bone materials, to avoid possible CSF leaks in the neck during the postoperative time. The musculoperiosteal layer is carefully closed using an absorbable suture. The subcutaneous tissue and skin are closed and a pressure dressing is applied.

6.4 Postoperative Care

In case of an intradural dissection of a large tumor, the patient needs monitoring in the intensive care unit for 24 hours after surgery.

A computed tomography (CT) scan is performed 6 hours after surgery (see ▶ Fig. 6.97). The patient must keep a supine position for 2 days, and early progressive mobilization is required in order to reduce the risk of pulmonary embolus or deep vein thrombosis. The compressive bandage is removed 4 days after surgery.

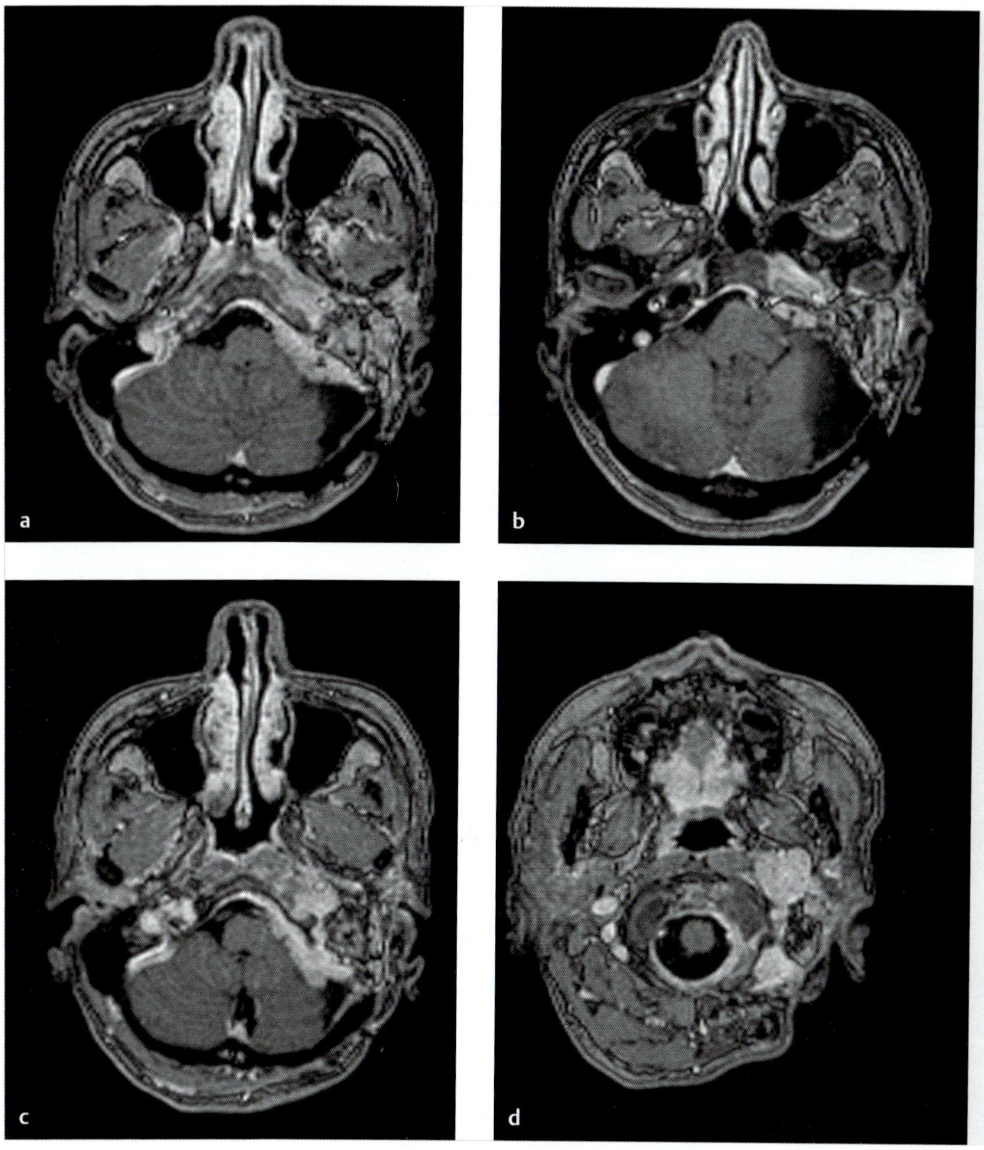

Fig. 6.42 (a–d) Clinical Case 2; Left ear: Magnetic resonance imaging (MRI) in axial view showing an invasive meningioma of the left temporal bone invading the jugular foramen.

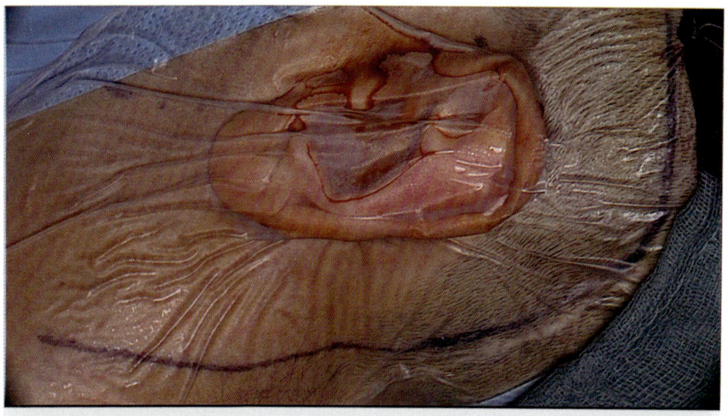

Fig. 6.43 Clinical case 2; Left ear: A retroauricular incision starting from the temporalis area to the neck is performed.

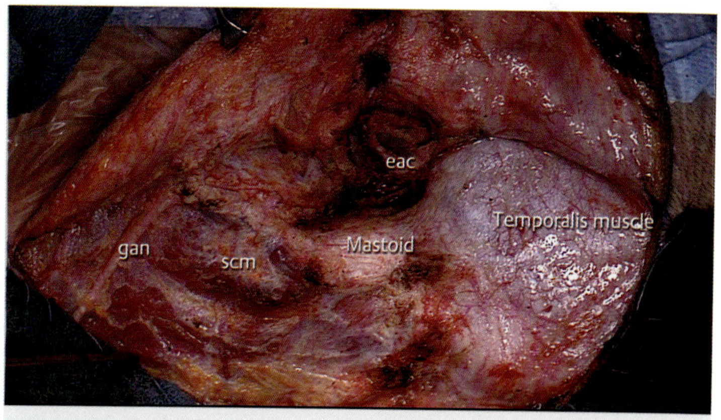

Fig. 6.44 Clinical Case 2; Left ear: The skin flap is elevated uncovering the occipital-mastoid area. The external auditory canal (EAC) is transected. *eac: external auditory canal; gan: greater auricular nerve; scm: sternocleidomastoid muscle.*

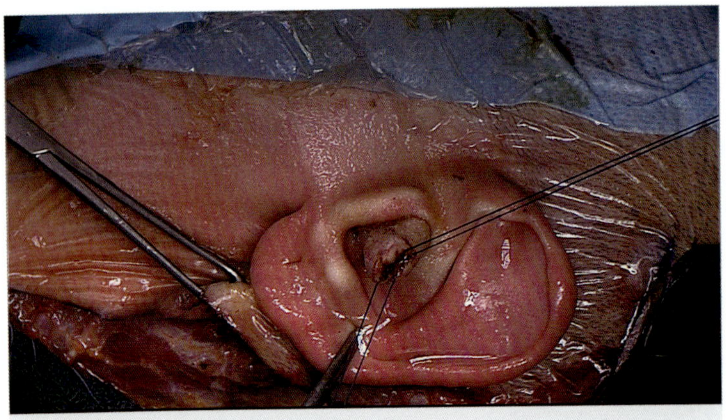

Fig. 6.45 Clinical Case 2, Left ear: The skin of the external auditory canal (EAC) is everted and sutured.

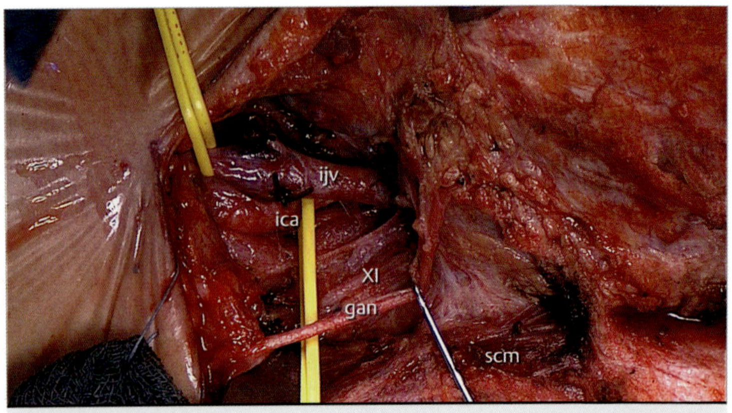

Fig. 6.46 Clinical Case 2; Left ear: The internal carotid artery (ICA) and the internal jugular vein are isolated and marked in the neck at the base of the skull. *gan: greater auricular nerve; ica: internal carotid artery; ijv: internal jugular vein; scm: sternocleidomastoid muscle.*

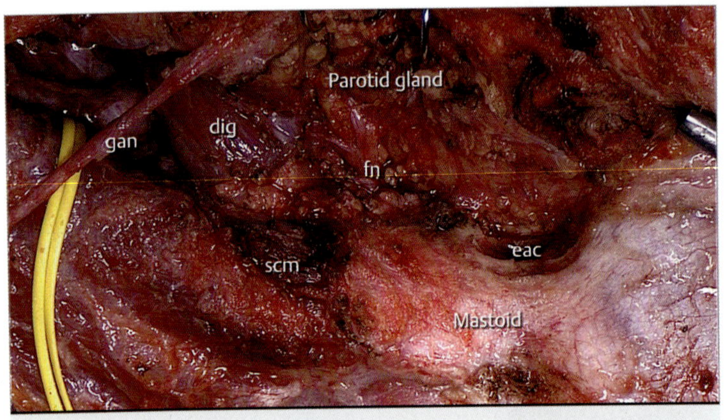

Fig. 6.47 Clinical Case 2; Left ear: The main trunk of the facial nerve is isolated outside the stylomastoid foramen, inside the parotid gland. *dig: digastric muscle; eac: external auditory canal; fn: facial nerve; gan: greater auricular nerve; scm: sternocleidomastoid muscle.*

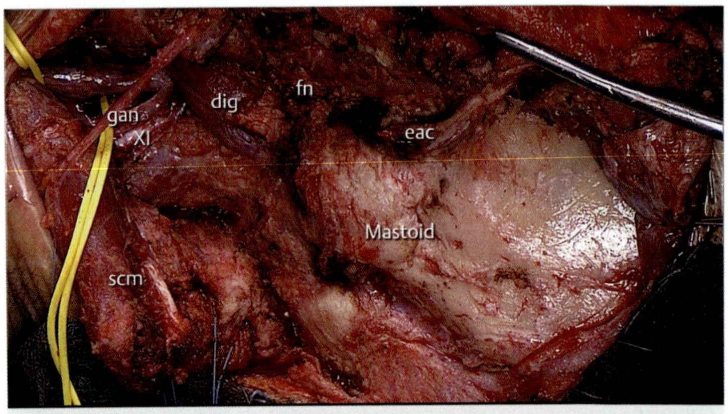

Fig. 6.48 Clinical Case 2; Left ear: The mastoid bone is uncovered and the sternocleidomastoid muscle is cut at the mastoid insertion, exposing the occipital bone. *dig: digastric muscle; eac: external auditory canal; fn: facial nerve; gan: greater auricular nerve; scm: sternocleidomastoid muscle.*

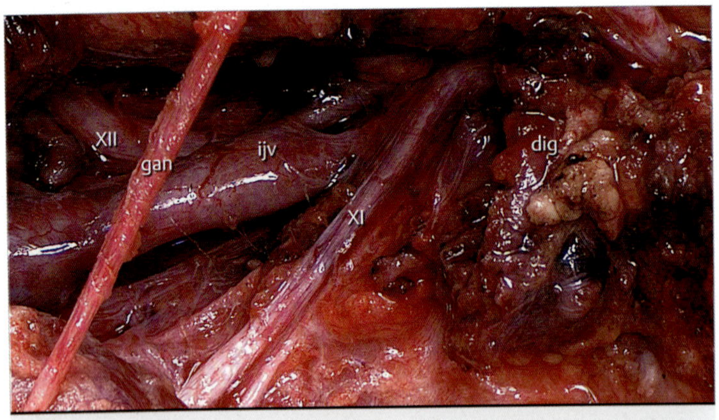

Fig. 6.49 Clinical Case 2; Left ear: The digastric muscle is cut and the lower cranial nerves are isolated at the base of the skull. *dig: digastric muscle; gan: greater auricular nerve; ijv: internal jugular vein.*

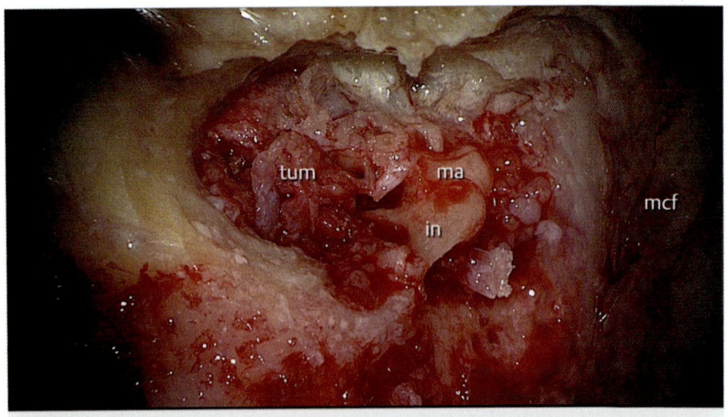

Fig. 6.50 Clinical Case 2; Left ear: A subtotal petrosectomy is performed; the tumor (meningioma) is seen invading the tympanic cavity around the ossicular chain. *in: incus; ma: malleus; mcf: middle cranial fossa; tum: tumor.*

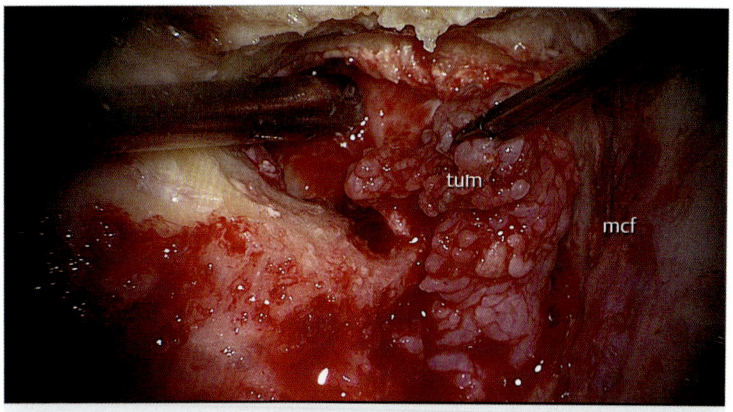

Fig. 6.51 Clinical Case 2; Left ear: The ossicular chain is removed and the tumor is progressively removed from the tympanic cavity. *mcf: middle cranial fossa; tum: tumor.*

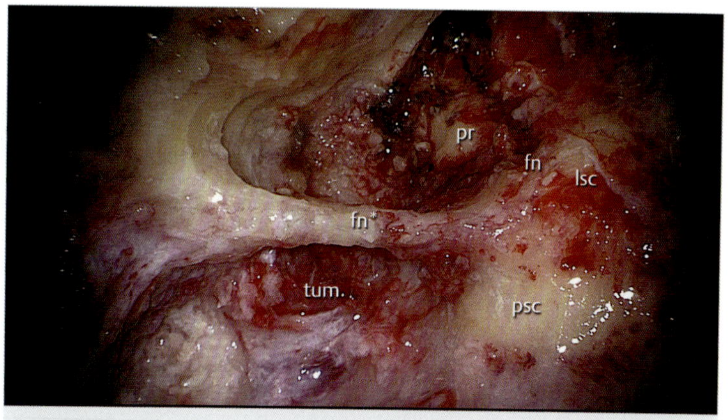

Fig. 6.52 Clinical Case 2; Left ear: Since the tumor involves the jugular foramen, a transcochlear approach with anterior rerouting of the facial nerve is planned. The facial nerve is progressively isolated in the temporal bone. *fn: tympanic segment of facial nerve; fn*: mastoid segment of facial nerve; lsc: lateral semicircular canal; pr: promontory; psc: posterior semicircular canal; tum: tumor.*

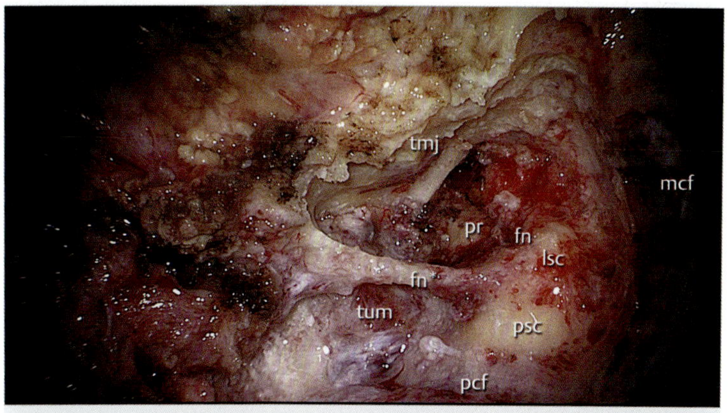

Fig. 6.53 Clinical Case 2; Left ear: The temporomandibular joint is detected, and the mastoid tip removed; the facial nerve at the level of the stylomastoid foramen is isolated. The infiltration of the jugular bulb from the tumor is noted. *fn: tympanic segment of facial nerve; fn*: mastoid segment of facial nerve; lsc: lateral semicircular canal; mcf: middle cranial fossa; pcf: posterior cranial fossa; pr: promontory; psc: posterior semicircular canal; tmj: temporal mandibular joint; tum: tumor.*

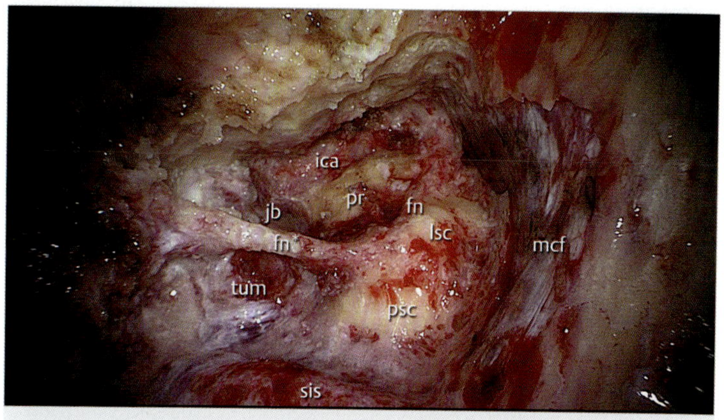

Fig. 6.54 Clinical Case 2; Left ear: The anterior wall of the external auditory canal (EAC) is removed and the vertical portion of the internal carotid artery (ICA) is isolated in the temporal bone. The infiltration of the jugular bulb and the sigmoid sinus from the tumor is noted. *fn: tympanic segment of facial nerve; fn*: mastoid segment of facial nerve; ica: internal carotid artery; lsc: lateral semicircular canal; mcf: middle cranial fossa; pr: promontory; psc: posterior semicircular canal; sis: sigmoid sinus; tum: tumor.*

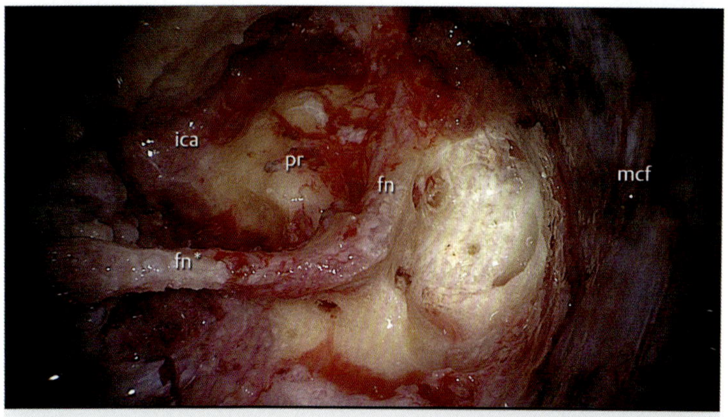

Fig. 6.55 Clinical Case 2; Left ear: The labyrinthectomy is started. *fn: tympanic segment of facial nerve; fn*: mastoid segment of facial nerve; ica: internal carotid artery; mcf: middle cranial fossa; pr: promontory.*

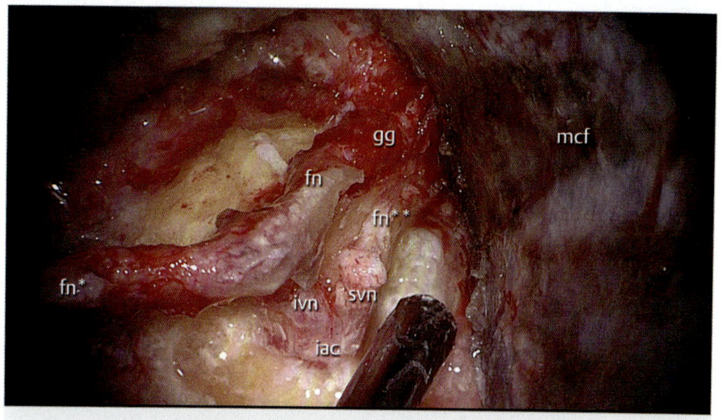

Fig. 6.56 Clinical Case 2; Left ear: The geniculate ganglion and the fundus of the internal auditory canal (IAC) are progressively isolated. *fn: tympanic segment of facial nerve; fn*: mastoid segment of facial nerve; fn**: labyrinthine portion of facial nerve; gg: geniculate ganglion; iac: internal auditory canal; inv: inferior vestibular nerve; svn: superior vestibular nerve.*

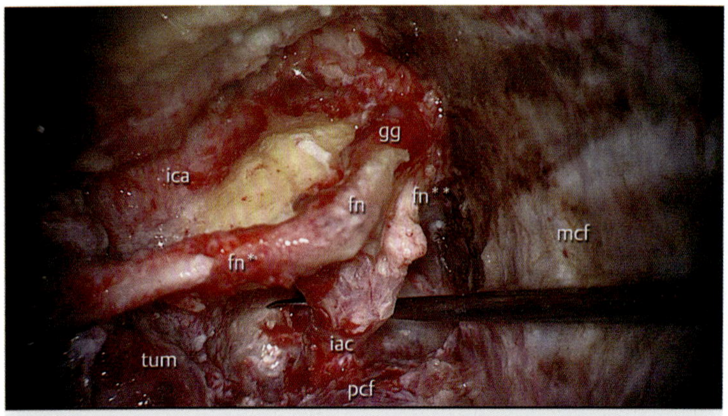

Fig. 6.57 Clinical Case 2; Left ear: The internal auditory canal (IAC) is fully isolated, performing a labyrinthectomy with a transapical extension. *fn: tympanic segment of facial nerve; fn*: mastoid segment of facial nerve; fn**: labyrinthine portion of facial nerve; gg: geniculate ganglion; iac: internal auditory canal; ica: internal carotid artery; mcf: middle cranial fossa; pcf: posterior cranial fossa; tum: tumor.*

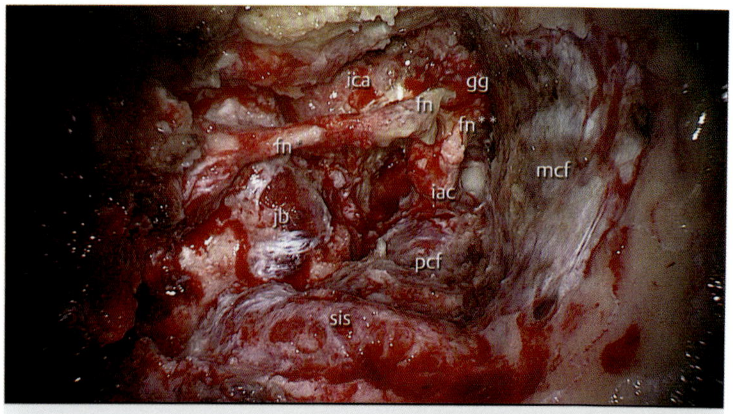

Fig. 6.58 Clinical Case 2; Left ear: The facial neve in the temporal bone is isolated. *fn: tympanic segment of facial nerve; fn*: mastoid segment of facial nerve; fn**: labyrinthine portion of facial nerve; gg: geniculate ganglion; iac: internal auditory canal; ica: internal carotid artery; jb: jugular bulb; mcf: middle cranial fossa; pcf: posterior cranial fossa; sis: sigmoid sinus.*

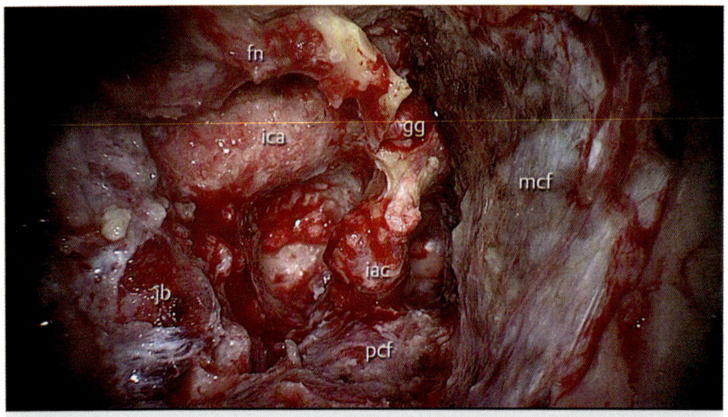

Fig. 6.59 Clinical Case 2; Left ear: An anterior rerouting of the facial nerve is made; the promontory and the cochlea are removed as in the transcochlear approach; the petrous apex is drilled and the vertical portion of the internal carotid artery (ICA) is isolated. *fn: tympanic segment of facial nerve; gg: geniculate ganglion; iac: internal auditory canal; ica: internal carotid artery; jb: jugular bulb; mcf: middle cranial fossa; pcf: posterior cranial fossa; sis: sigmoid sinus.*

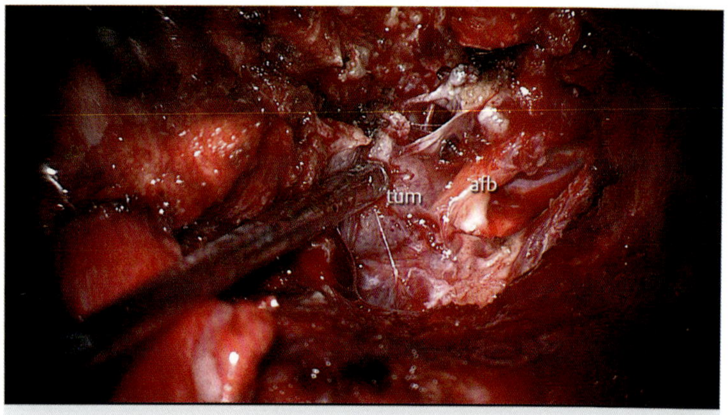

Fig. 6.60 Clinical Case 2; Left ear: The dura of the posterior fossa is cut gaining access to the cerebellopontine angle (CPA). The tumor is seen close to the entry zone of the acoustic-facial bundle. *afb: acoustic-facial bundle; tum: tumor.*

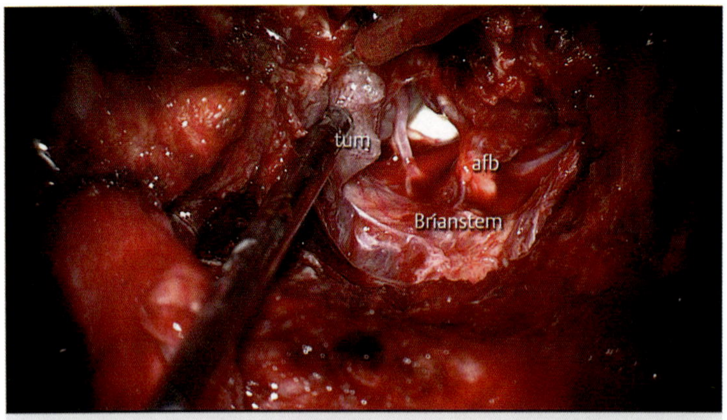

Fig. 6.61 Clinical Case 2; Left ear: The tumor is progressively removed from the brainstem preserving the acoustic-facial bundle. *afb: acoustic-facial bundle; tum: tumor.*

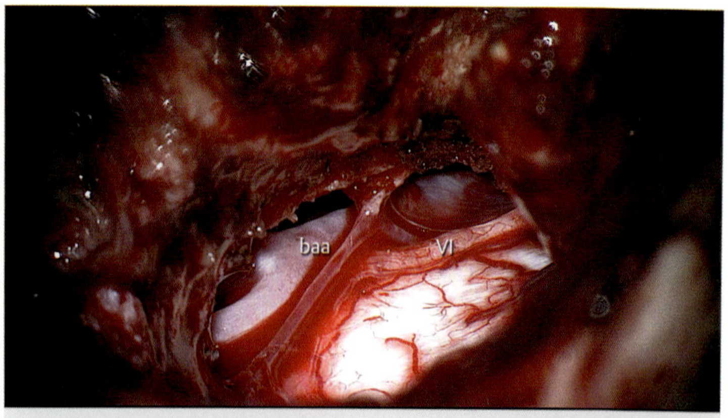

Fig. 6.62 Clinical Case 2; Left ear: Microscopic view of the brainstem midline through the dural defect after tumor removal. *baa: basilar artery.*

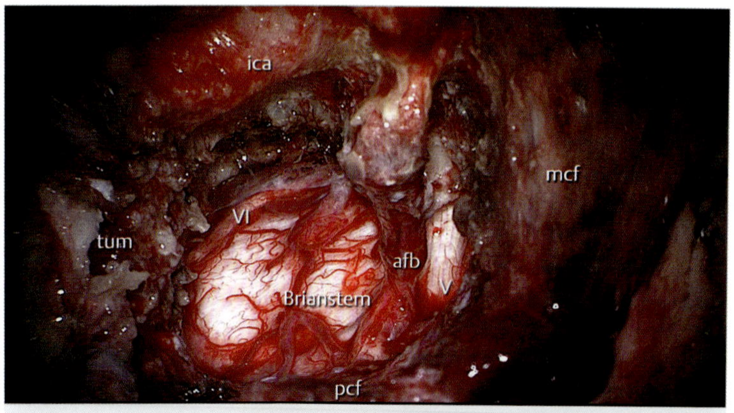

Fig. 6.63 Clinical Case 2; Left ear: The intradural portion of the tumor is removed and the brainstem is decompressed; a progressive dissection of the tumor from the clivus and the jugular bulb is started. *afb: acoustic-facial bundle; ica: internal carotid artery; mcf: middle cranial fossa; pcf: posterior cranial fossa; tum: tumor.*

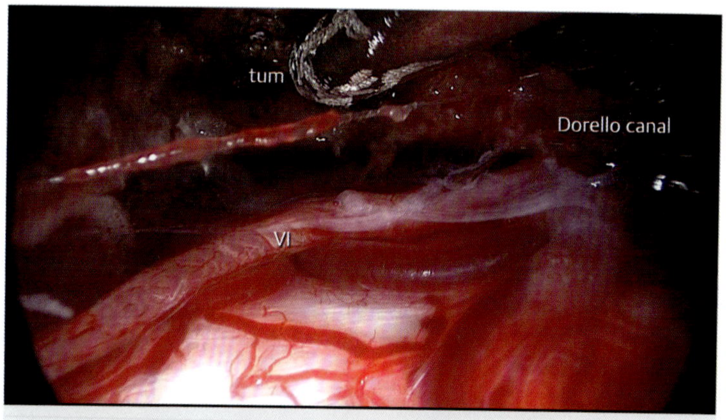

Fig. 6.64 Clinical Case 2; Left ear: Once the internal jugular vein and the jugular bulb have been removed with the tumor as in the infratemporal fossa type A procedure (see Chapter 2), a 45-degree, 4 cm diameter endoscope is used to remove the residual tumor located in the clivus bone under the internal carotid artery (ICA), close to the Dorello canal. *tum: tumor.*

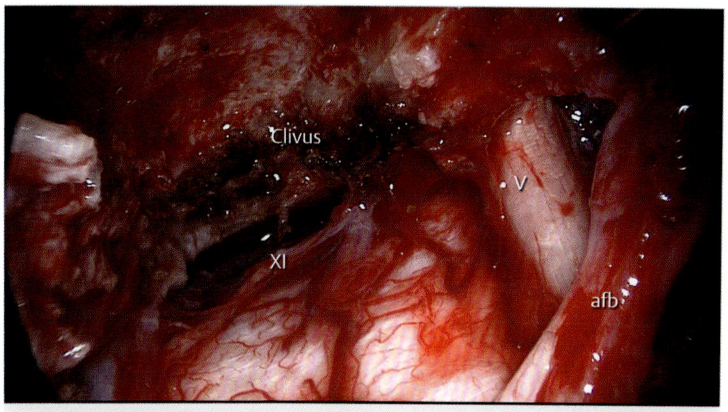

Fig. 6.65 Clinical Case 2; Left ear: Using an endoscopic assisted technique, the residual tumor is progressively removed from the clivus and the petrous apex. *afb: acoustic-facial bundle.*

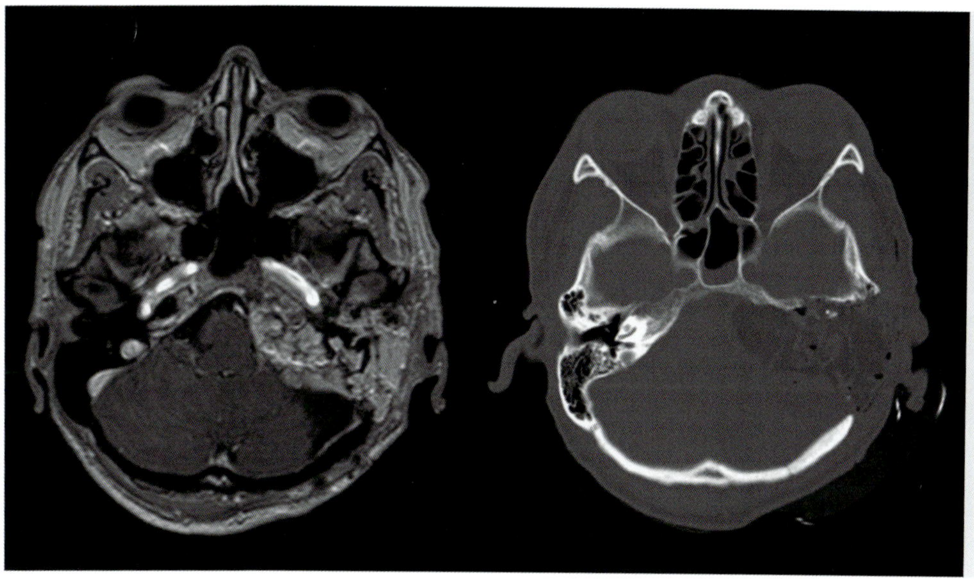

Fig. 6.66 Clinical Case 2; Left ear: Postoperative magnetic resonance imaging (MRI) and computed tomography (CT) scan in axial view showing the temporal bone dissection.

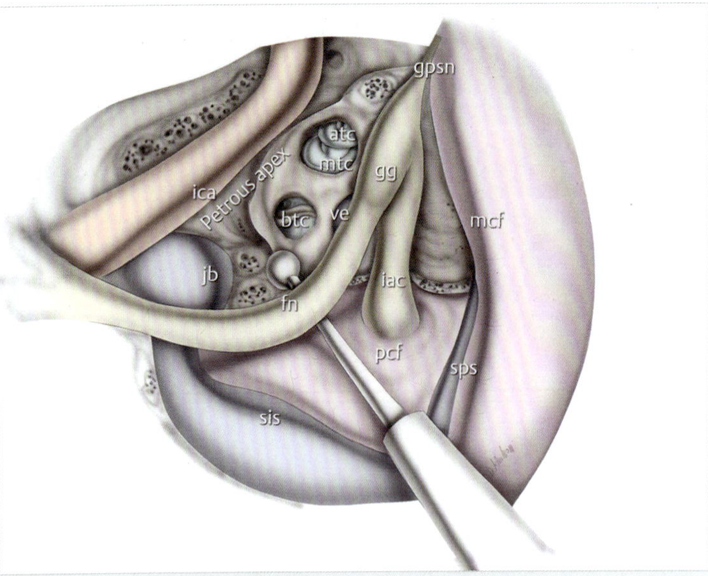

Fig. 6.67 Left ear: The facial nerve is maintained in the fallopian canal; the promontory is removed exposing the cochlea; the jugular bulb is skeletonized and the retrofacial cells are removed under the facial nerve bridge. *atc: apical turn of the cochlea; btc: basal turn of the cochlea; fn: facial nerve; gg: geniculate ganglion; gpsn: greater petrosal superficial nerve; iac: internal auditory canal; ica: internal carotid artery; jb: jugular bulb; mcf: middle cranial fossa; mtc: middle turn of the cochlea; pcf: posterior cranial fossa; sis: sigmoid sinus; sps: superior petrosal sinus; ve: vestibule.*

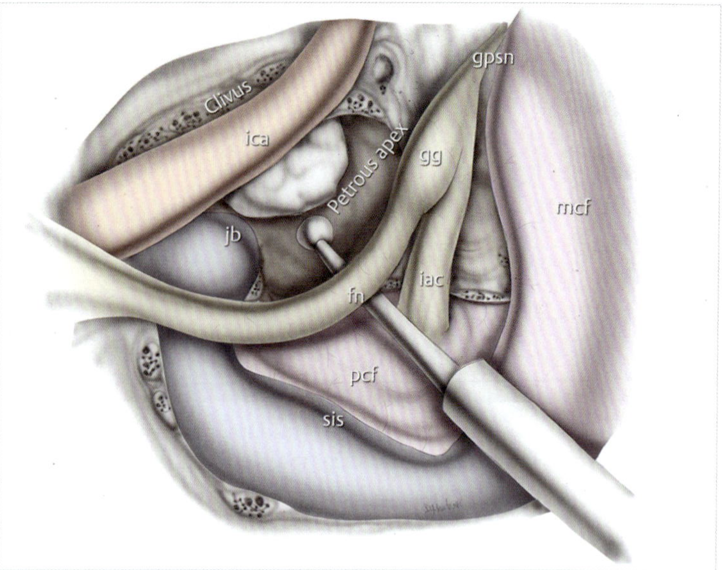

Fig. 6.68 Left ear: The internal carotid artery (ICA) and the jugular bulb are progressively skeletonized. A diamond bur is used to remove the bone under the carotid artery reaching the lesion located in the petrous apex. *fn: facial nerve; gg: geniculate ganglion; gpsn: greater petrosal superficial nerve; iac: internal auditory canal; ica: internal carotid artery; jb: jugular bulb; mcf: middle cranial fossa; pcf: posterior cranial fossa; sis: sigmoid sinus.*

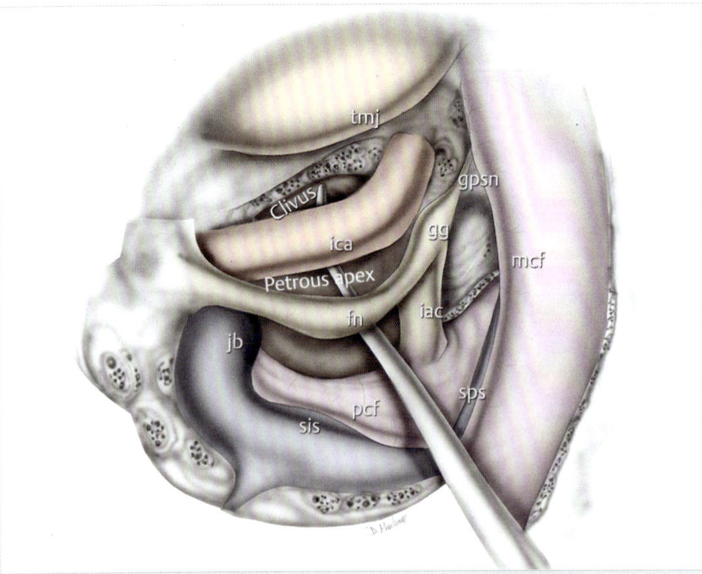

Fig. 6.69 Left ear: When required, the clivus bone under the carotid artery is removed and the vertical portion of internal carotid artery (ICA) is fully skeletonized. *fn: facial nerve; gg: geniculate ganglion; gpsn: greater petrosal superficial nerve; iac: internal auditory canal; ica: internal carotid artery; jb: jugular bulb; mcf: middle cranial fossa; pcf: posterior cranial fossa; sis: sigmoid sinus; tmj: temporal mandibular joint.*

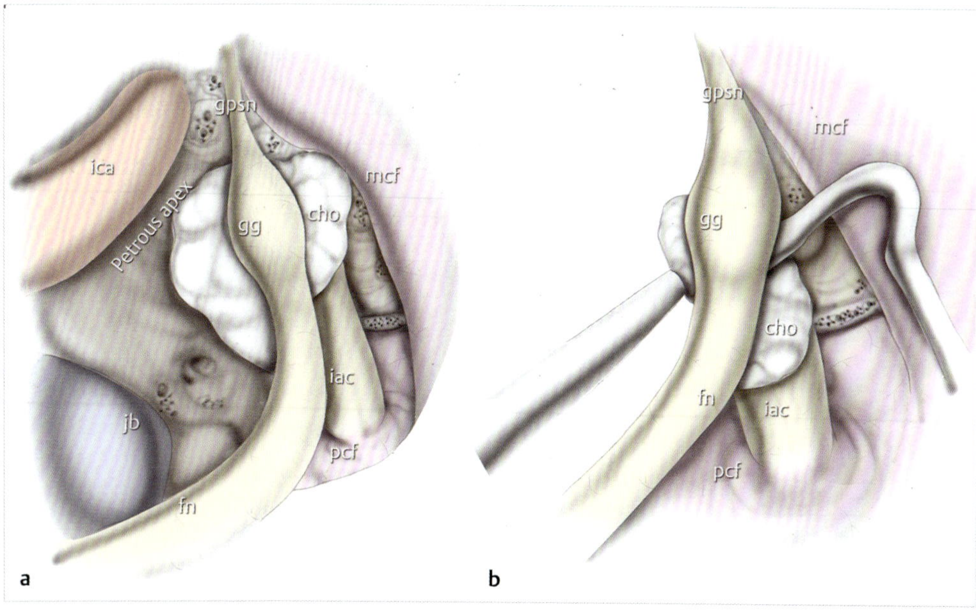

Fig. 6.70 Left ear. **(a)** Microscopic view of a cholesteatoma involving the petrous apex, lying in the medial portion of the geniculate ganglion. **(b)** A curved dissector is used to microscopically remove the cholesteatoma around the facial nerve. *cho: cholesteatoma; fn: facial nerve; gg: geniculate ganglion; gpsn: greater petrosal superficial nerve; iac: internal auditory canal; ica: internal carotid artery; jb: jugular bulb; mcf: middle cranial fossa; pcf: posterior cranial fossa.*

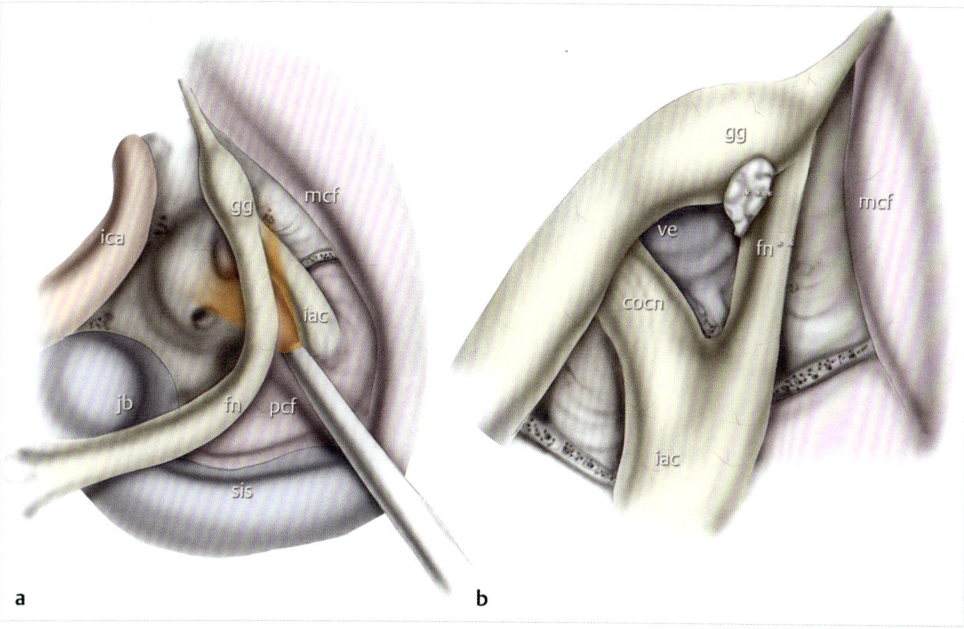

Fig. 6.71 Left ear. **(a)** A 45-degree endoscope is introduced into the surgical field under the facial nerve. **(b)** A residual disease is endoscopically detected on the medial surface of the geniculate ganglion. *cocn: cochlear nerve; fn: facial nerve; fn**: labyrinthine portion of facial nerve; gg: geniculate ganglion; iac: internal auditory canal; ica: internal carotid artery; jb: jugular bulb; mcf: middle cranial fossa; pcf: posterior cranial fossa; sis: sigmoid sinus; ve: vestibule; ***: residual cholesteatoma.*

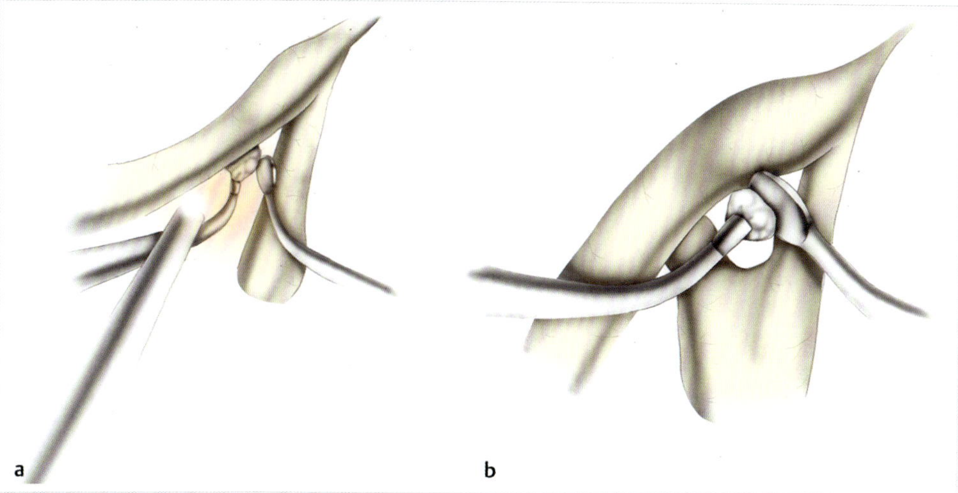

Fig. 6.72 Left ear. **(a, b)** Three-hand technique: The second surgeon holds the endoscope detecting the remnant disease; the first surgeon is using two hands to perform the dissection of the residual disease around the facial nerve.

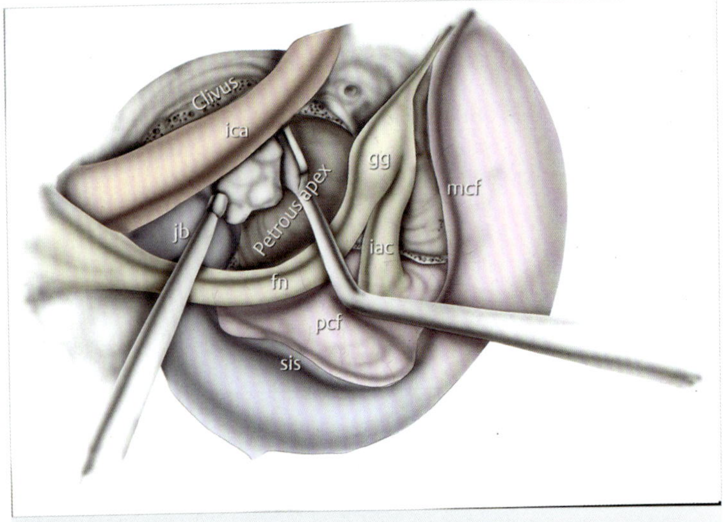

Fig. 6.73 Left ear: The lesion in the petrous apex is microscopically removed. A poor control of the disease located in the petrous apex medial to the internal carotid artery (ICA) is seen. *fn: facial nerve; gg: geniculate ganglion; gspn: greater superficial petrosal nerve; iac: internal auditory canal; ica: internal carotid artery; jb: jugular bulb; mcf: middle cranial fossa; pcf: posterior cranial fossa.*

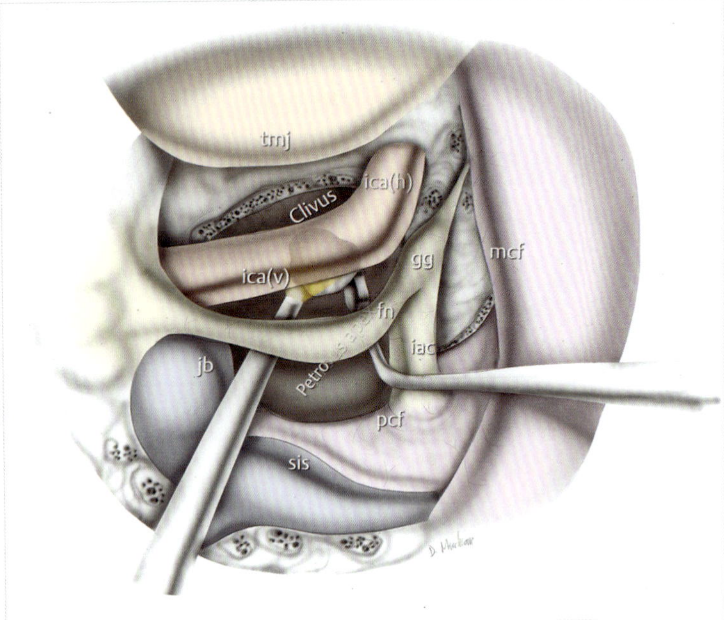

Fig. 6.74 Left ear: The endoscope is introduced into the surgical field to visualize the residual disease located in the petrous apex, medial to the internal carotid artery (ICA); a curved dissector is used to remove the lesion. *fn: facial nerve; gg: geniculate ganglion; iac: internal auditory canal; ica(h): horizontal portion of internal carotid artery; ica(v): vertical portion of internal carotid artery; jb: jugular bulb; mcf: middle cranial fossa; pcf: posterior cranial fossa; sis: sigmoid sinus; tmj: temporal-mandibular joint.*

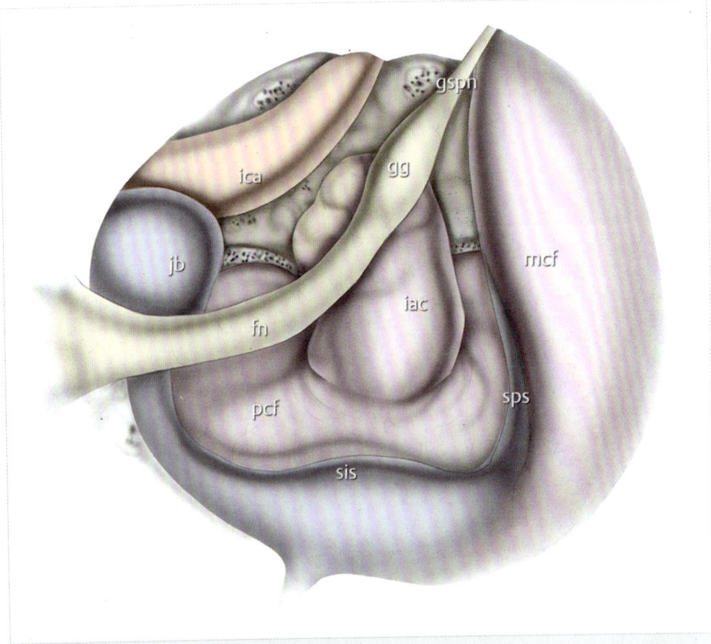

Fig. 6.75 Left ear: A transotic approach for an acoustic neuroma with an anterior extension into the cochlea and involving the cerebello-pontine angle (CPA) is performed. *fn: facial nerve; gg: geniculate ganglion; gspn: greater superficial petrosal nerve; iac: internal auditory canal; ica: internal carotid artery; jb: jugular bulb; mcf: middle cranial fossa; pcf: posterior cranial fossa; sis: sigmoid sinus.*

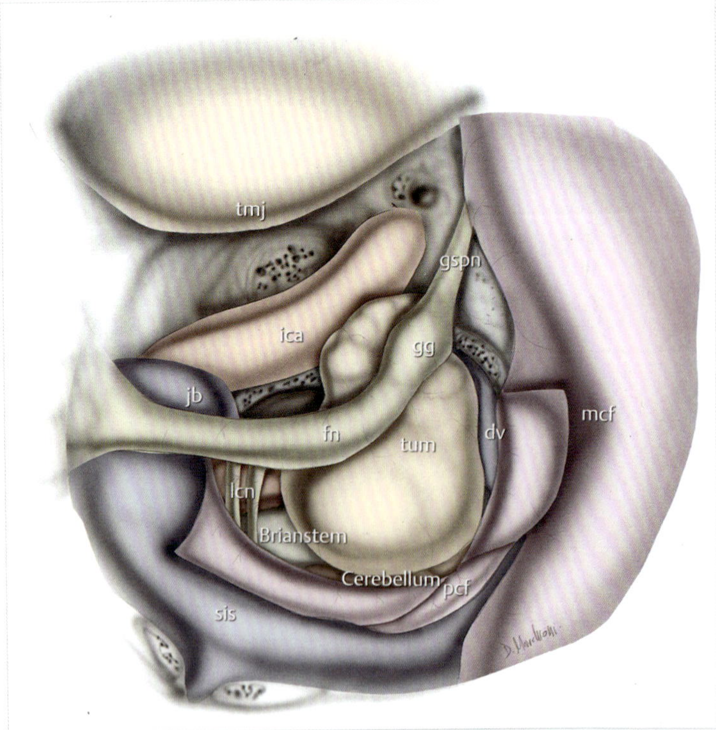

Fig. 6.76 Left ear: The dura of the internal auditory canal (IAC) and of the posterior cranial fossa is opened and the tumor is exposed. *dv: the vein of Dandy; fn: facial nerve; gg: geniculate ganglion; gspn: greater superficial petrosal nerve; ica: internal carotid artery; jb: jugular bulb; lcn: lower cranial nerve; mcf: middle cranial fossa; pcf: posterior cranial fossa; sis: sigmoid sinus; tmj: temporomandibular joint.*

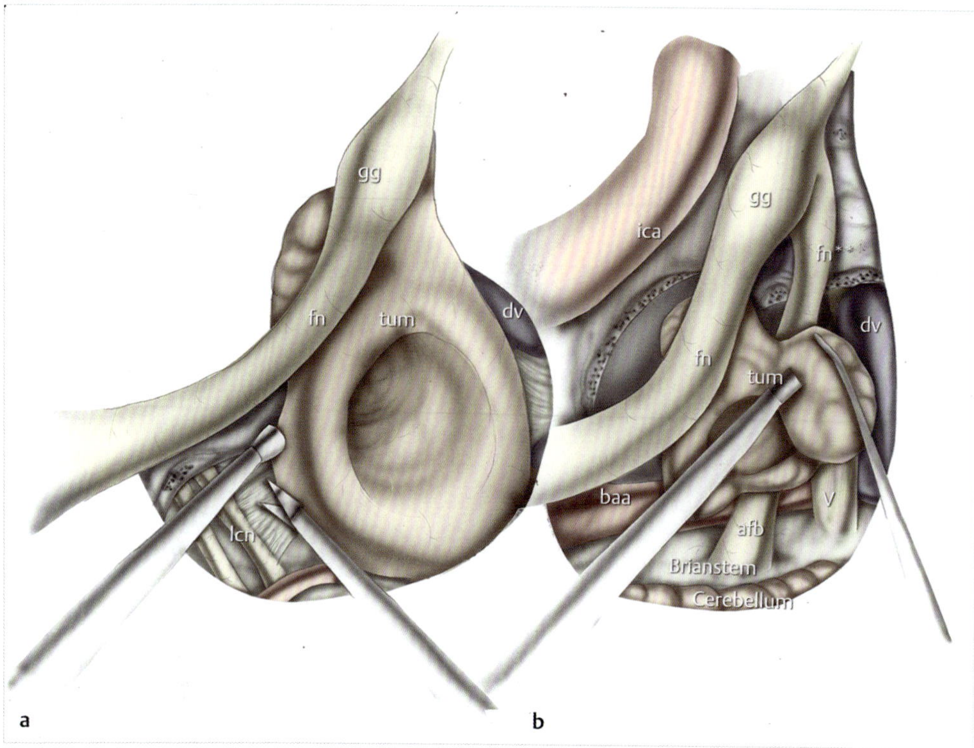

Fig. 6.77 Left ear. **(a)** A central debulking of the tumor is made; the tumor is progressively removed from the cerebellopontine angle (CPA), preserving the facial nerve **(b)**. *afb: acoustic-facial bundle; baa: basilar artery; dv: the vein of Dandy; fn**: labyrinthine portion of facial nerve; fn: facial nerve; gg: geniculate ganglion; ica: internal carotid artery; lcn: lower cranial nerve; tum: tumor.*

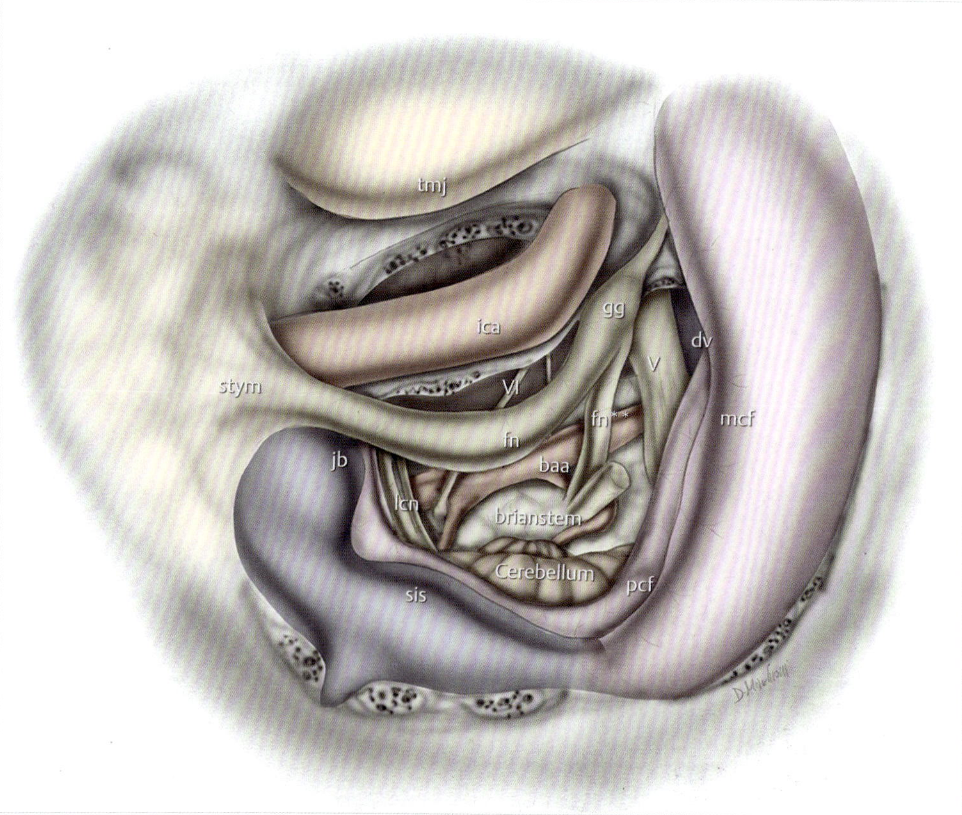

Fig. 6.78 Left ear: Final surgical cavity after tumor removal. *baa: basilar artery; dv: the vein of Dandy; fn: facial nerve; fn**: cerebellopontine angle (CPA) portion of facial nerve; gg: geniculate ganglion; ica: internal carotid artery; lcn: lower cranial nerve; mcf: middle cranial fossa; pcf: posterior cranial fossa; stym: stylomastoid foramen; tmj: tempo-mandibular joint.*

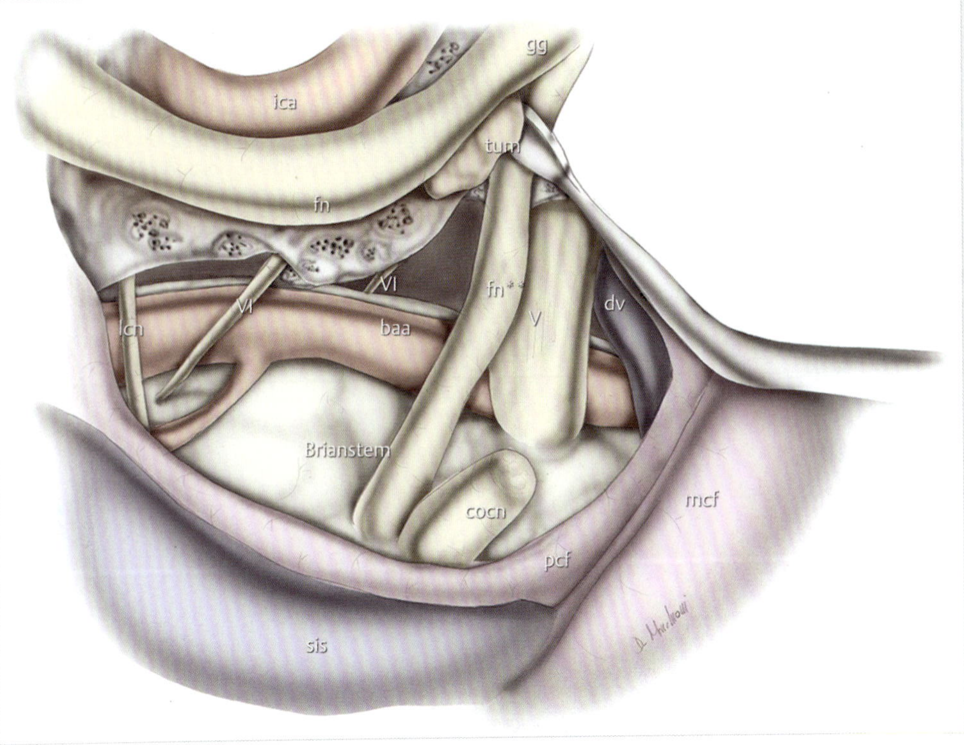

Fig. 6.79 Left ear: Once the tumor has been microscopically removed, an endoscopic check of the surgical cavity is performed. A residual tumor under the facial nerve bridge is seen and removed using an angulated dissector. *baa: basilar artery; cocn: cochlear nerve; dv: the vein of Dandy; fn: facial nerve; fn**: cerebellopontine angle (CPA) portion of facial nerve; gg: geniculate ganglion; ica: internal carotid artery; lcn: lower cranial nerve; mcf: middle cranial fossa; pcf: posterior cranial fossa.*

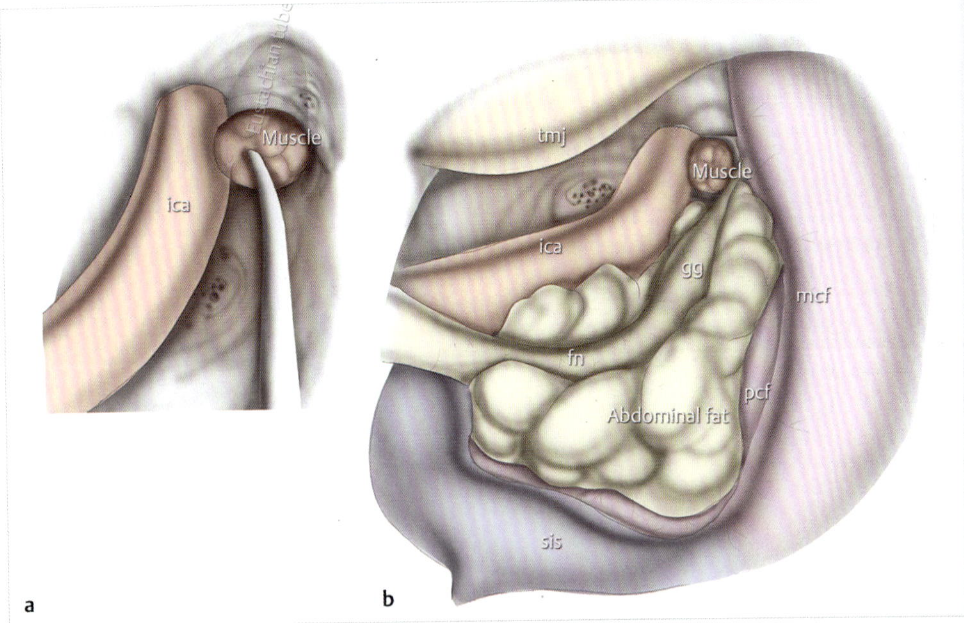

Fig. 6.80 Left ear. **(a)** A piece of muscle is used to obliterate the eustachian tube orifice. **(b)** The surgical cavity is sealed using abdominal fat. *fn: facial nerve; gg: geniculate ganglion; ica: internal carotid artery; mcf: middle cranial fossa; pcf: posterior cranial fossa; tmj: temporomandibular joint.*

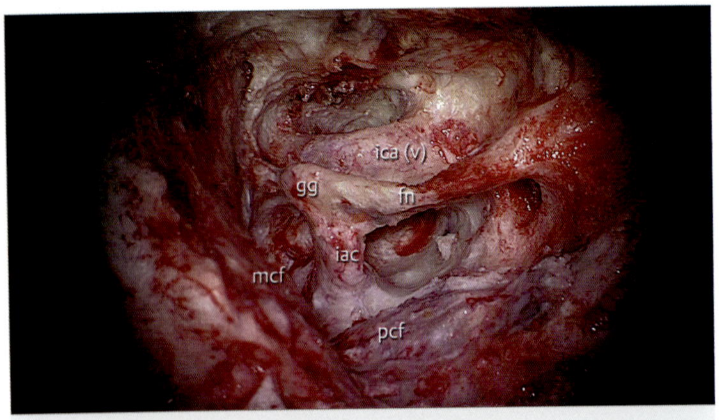

Fig. 6.81 Clinical Case 3, Right ear: Surgical cavity after tumor removal through a transotic approach. The facial nerve bridge in the middle of the surgical field is noted. *fn: facial nerve; gg: geniculate ganglion; iac: internal auditory canal; ica(v): vertical portion of internal carotid artery; mcf: middle cranial fossa; pcf: posterior cranial fossa.*

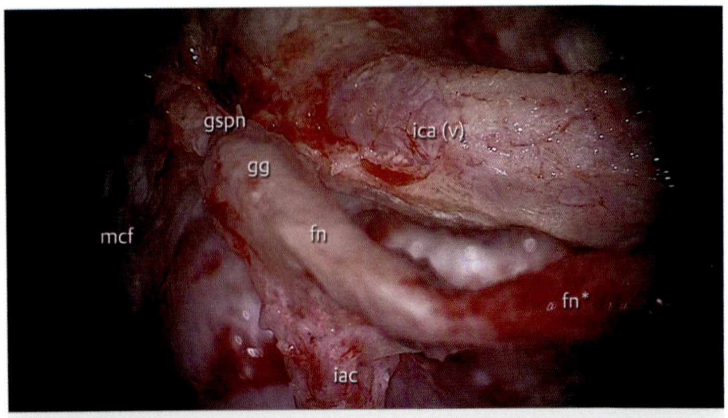

Fig. 6.82 Clinical Case 3, Right ear: Transotic approach: anatomical detail of the vertical portion of the carotid artery. *fn: facial nerve; fn*: mastoid portion of facial nerve; gg: geniculate ganglion; gspn: greater superficial petrosal nerve; iac: internal auditory canal; ica(v): vertical portion of internal carotid artery; mcf: middle cranial fossa.*

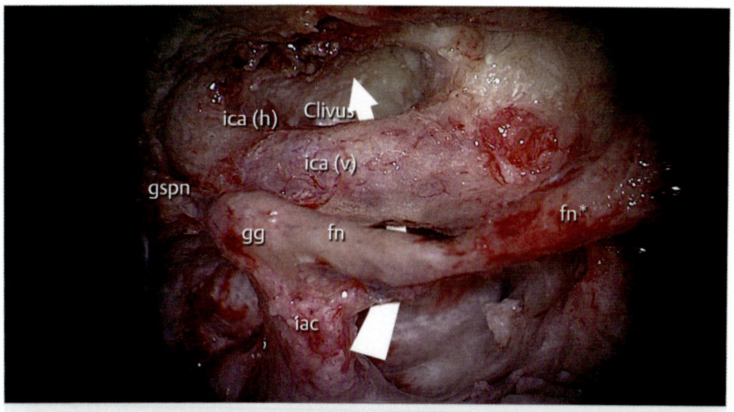

Fig. 6.83 Clinical Case 3, Right ear: The *white arrow* shows the required microscopic bony work under the facial nerve bridge and the internal carotid artery (ICA) which is necessary to expose the petrous apex and the clivus. *fn: facial nerve; fn*: mastoid portion of facial nerve; gg: geniculate ganglion; gspn: greater superficial petrosal nerve; iac: internal auditory canal; ica(h): horizontal portion of internal carotid artery; ica(v): vertical portion of internal carotid artery.*

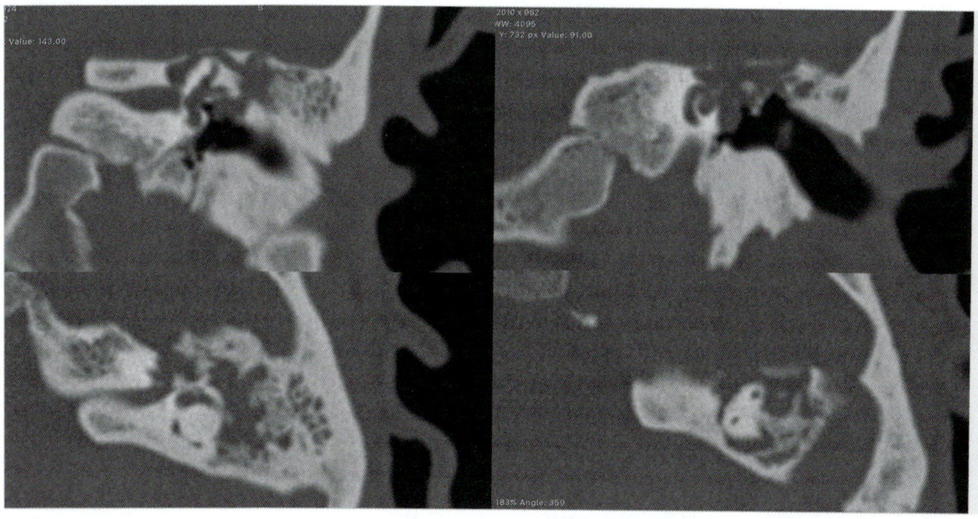

Fig. 6.84 Clinical Case 4, Left ear: Computed tomography (CT) scan in coronal and axial views showing a petrous apex cholesteatoma with a supralabyrinthine extension.

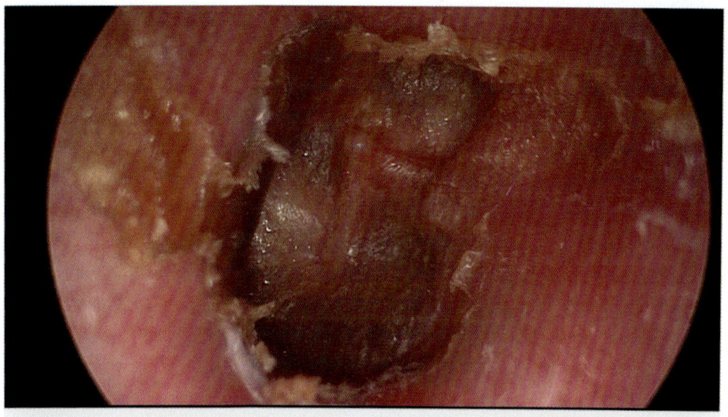

Fig. 6.85 Clinical Case 4, Left ear: Endoscopic view of the eardrum.

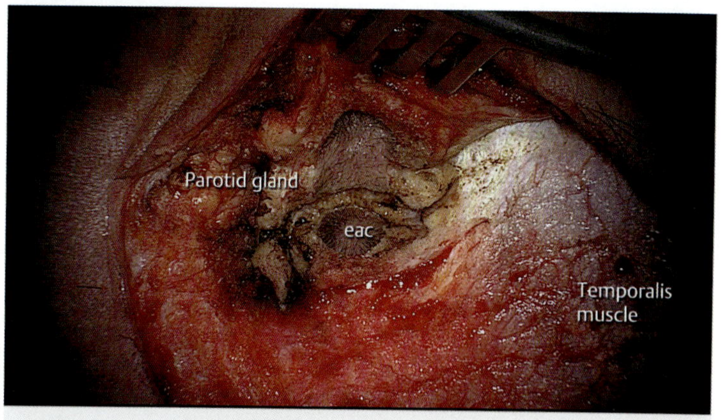

Fig. 6.86 Clinical Case 4, Left ear: The cutaneous flap is elevated and the external auditory canal (EAC) is transected. *eac: external auditory canal.*

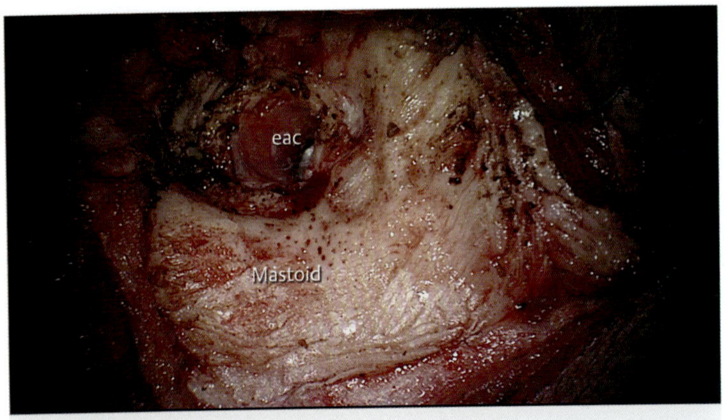

Fig. 6.87 Clinical Case 4, Left ear: The mastoid is uncovered; the external auditory canal (EAC) is seen. *eac: external auditory canal.*

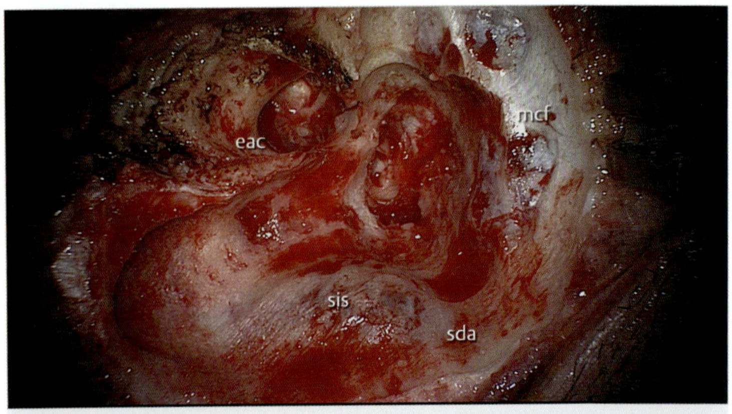

Fig. 6.88 Clinical Case 4, Left ear: A mastoidectomy with a canal wall down procedure is started. *eac: external auditory canal; mcf: middle cranial fossa; sda: sinodural angle; sis: sigmoid sinus.*

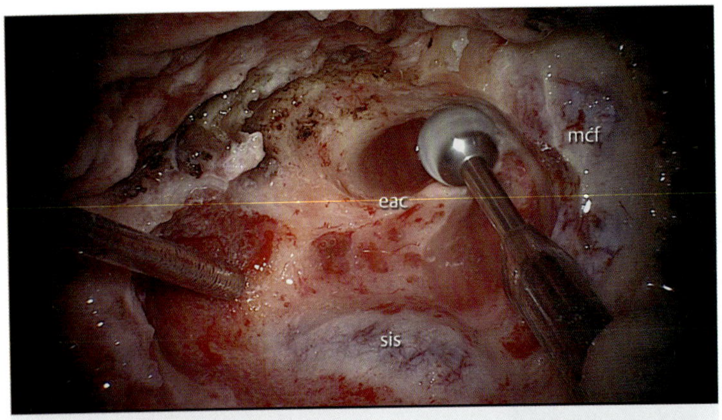

Fig. 6.89 Clinical Case 4, Left ear: The bony wall of the external auditory canal (EAC) is removed. *eac: external auditory canal; mcf: middle cranial fossa; sis: sigmoid sinus.*

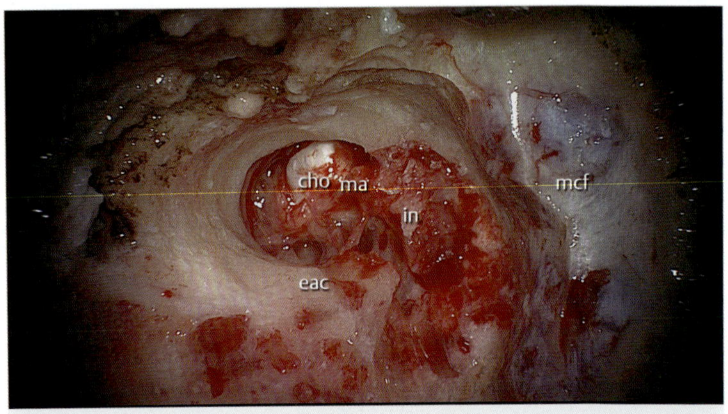

Fig. 6.90 Clinical Case 4, Left ear: The cholesteatoma in the tympanic cavity is noted. *cho: cholesteatoma; eac: external auditory canal; in: incus; ma: malleus; mcf: middle cranial fossa.*

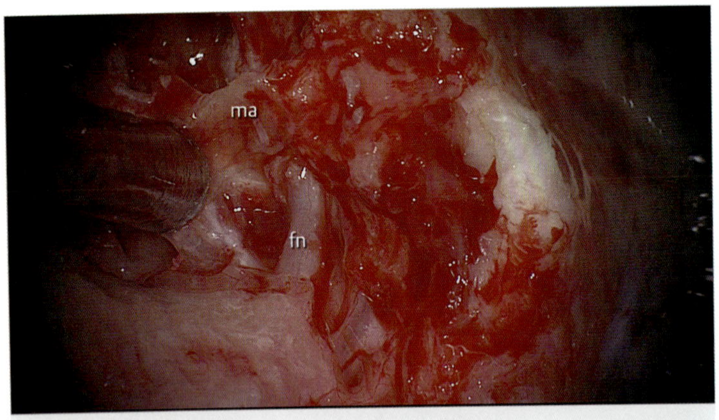

Fig. 6.91 Clinical Case 4, Left ear: The ossicular chain is removed and the tympanic segment of facial nerve is detected. *fn: facial nerve; ma: malleus.*

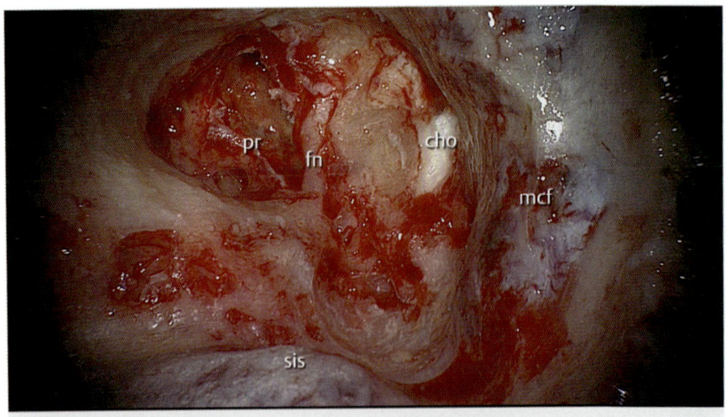

Fig. 6.92 Clinical Case 4, Left ear: The labyrinthectomy is started; a cholesteatoma with a supralabyrinthine extension is seen. *cho: cholesteatoma; fn: facial nerve; mcf: middle cranial fossa; pr: promontory; sis: sigmoid sinus.*

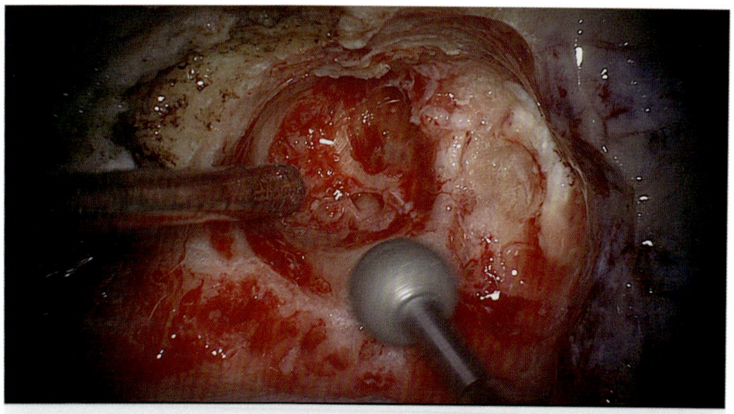

Fig. 6.93 Clinical Case 4, Left ear: The facial nerve is skeletonized.

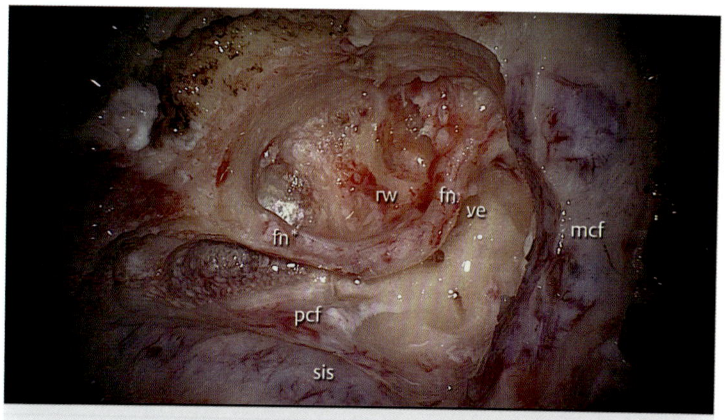

Fig. 6.94 Clinical Case 4, Left ear: A facial nerve bridge is created. Once the labyrinthectomy has been performed the vestibule is detected. *fn: tympanic segment of facial nerve; fn*: mastoid portion of facial nerve; mcf: middle cranial fossa; pcf: posterior cranial fossa; rw: round window; sis: sigmoid sinus; ve: vestibule.*

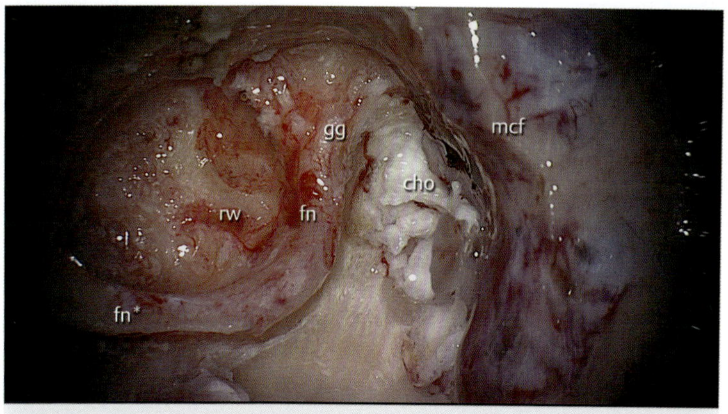

Fig. 6.95 Clinical Case 4, Left ear: A further bone removal between the geniculate ganglion and the dura of the middle cranial fossa (suprageniculate fossa) allows to detect the petrous apex cholesteatoma. *cho: cholesteatoma; fn: tympanic segment of facial nerve; fn*: mastoid portion of facial nerve; gg: geniculate ganglion; mcf: middle cranial fossa; rw: round window.*

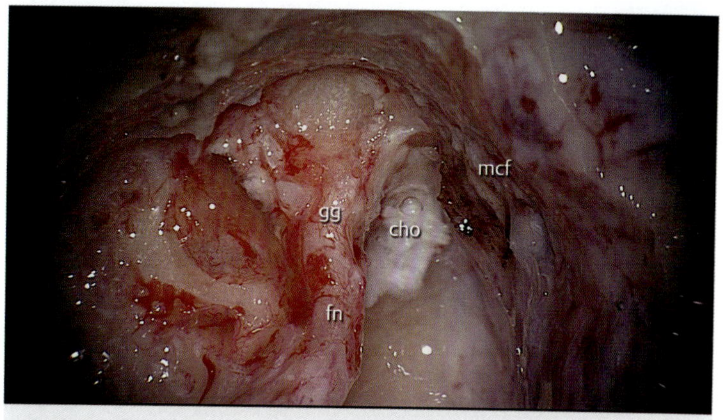

Fig. 6.96 Clinical Case 4, Left ear: Cholesteatoma involving the petrous apex around the geniculate ganglion. *cho: cholesteatoma; fn: tympanic segment of facial nerve; gg: geniculate ganglion; mcf: middle cranial fossa.*

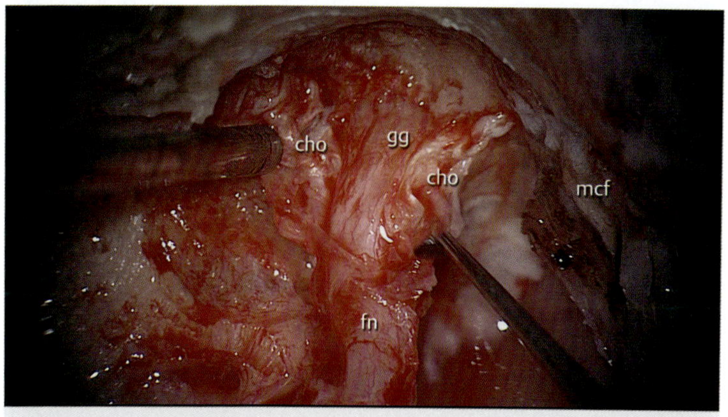

Fig. 6.97 Clinical Case 4, Left ear: The tympanic segments of the facial nerve and geniculate ganglion are decompressed; a curved dissector is used to remove the cholesteatoma in the medial portion of the nerve. *cho: cholesteatoma; fn: tympanic segment of facial nerve; gg: geniculate ganglion; mcf: middle cranial fossa.*

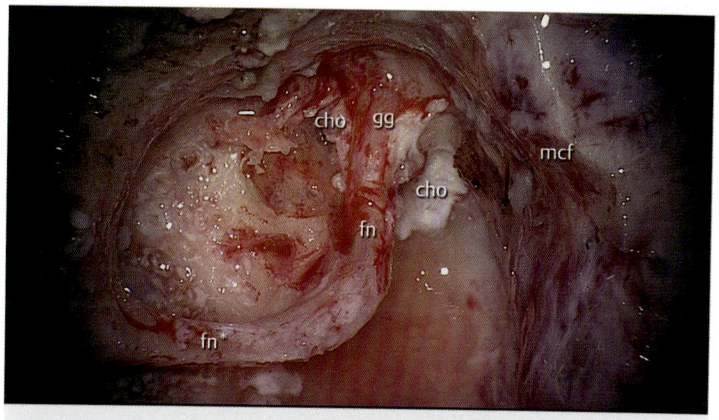

Fig. 6.98 Clinical Case 4, Left ear: The cholesteatoma is progressively removed from the petrous apex. *cho: cholesteatoma; fn: tympanic segment of facial nerve; fn*: mastoid portion of facial nerve; gg: geniculate ganglion; mcf: middle cranial fossa.*

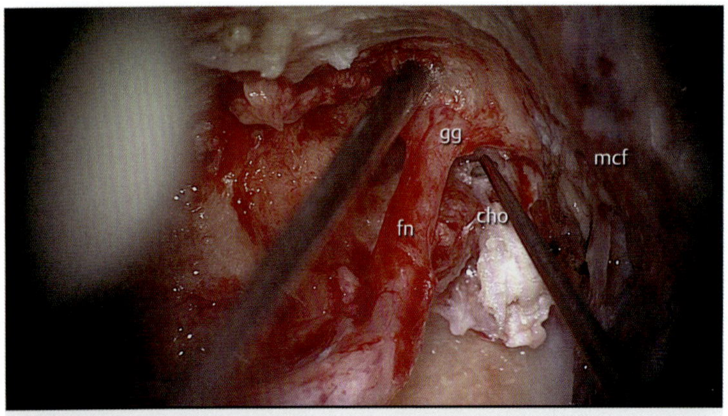

Fig. 6.99 Clinical Case 4, Left ear: The petrous apex extension of the cholesteatoma is seen. *cho: cholesteatoma; fn: tympanic segment of facial nerve; gg: geniculate ganglion; mcf: middle cranial fossa.*

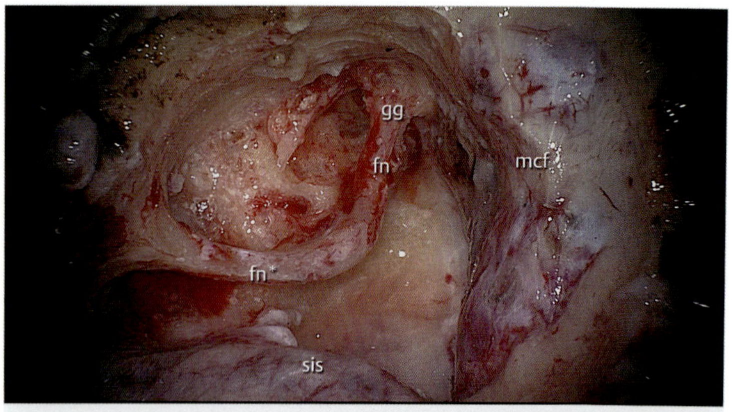

Fig. 6.100 Clinical Case 4, Left ear: Microscopic view after cholesteatoma removal. *fn: tympanic segment of facial nerve; fn*: mastoid segment of facial nerve; gg: geniculate ganglion; mcf: middle cranial fossa; sis: sigmoid sinus.*

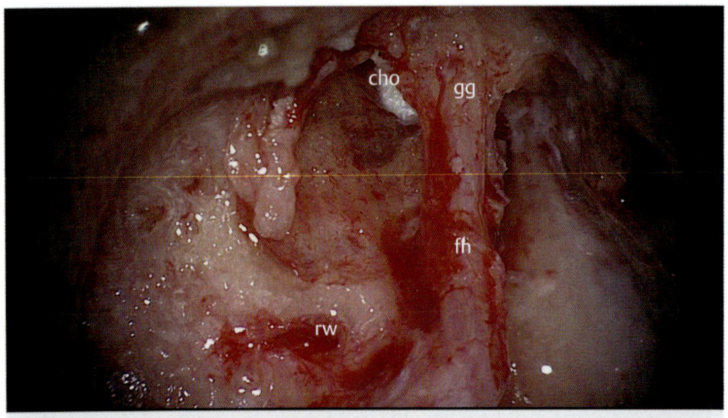

Fig. 6.101 Clinical Case 4, Left ear: A residual cholesteatoma is seen in the petrous apex under the geniculate ganglion. *cho: cholesteatoma; fn: tympanic segment of facial nerve; gg: geniculate ganglion; rw: round window.*

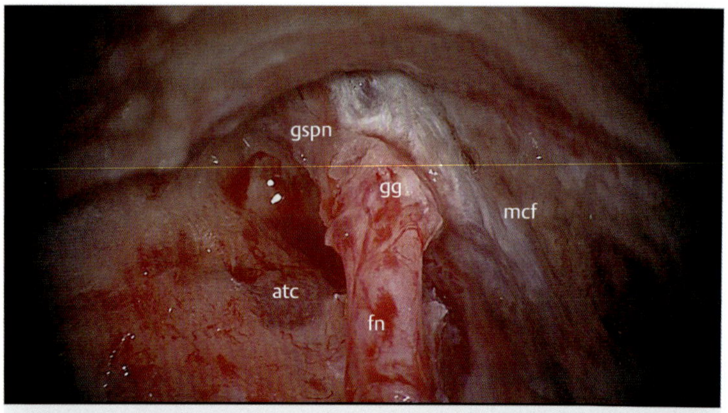

Fig. 6.102 Clinical Case 4, Left ear: Microscopic close view of the geniculate ganglion. The anatomical relationship between the geniculate ganglion and the middle cranial fossa dura is noted. *atc: apical turn of the cochlea; fn: tympanic segment of facial nerve; gg: geniculate ganglion; mcf: middle cranial fossa.*

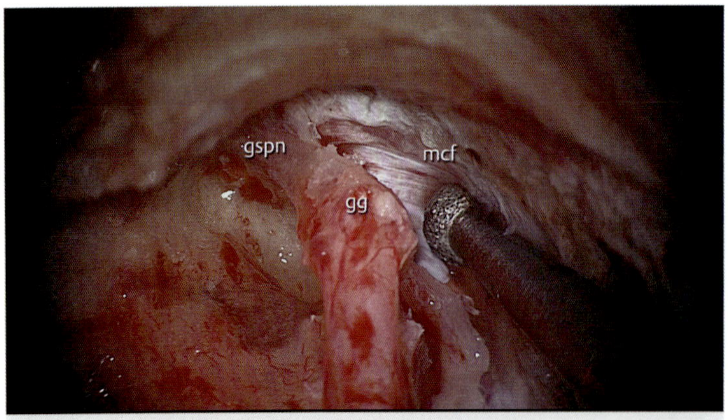

Fig. 6.103 Clinical Case 4, Left ear: The dura of the middle cranial fossa is gently elevated from the geniculate ganglion to check the presence of any residual disease. *gg: geniculate ganglion; gspn: greater superficial petrosal nerve; mcf: middle cranial fossa.*

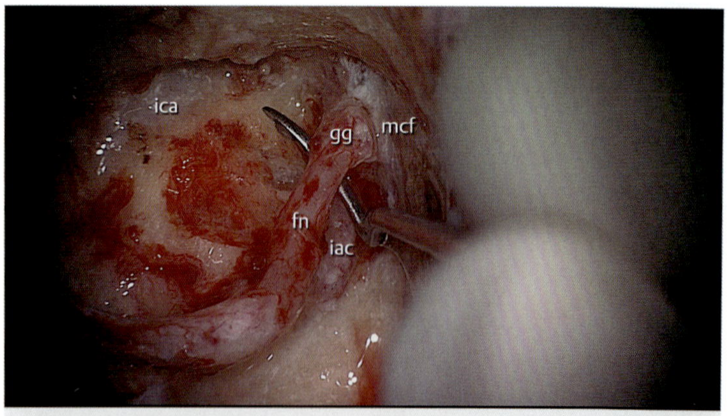

Fig. 6.104 Clinical Case 4, Left ear: A curved dissector is introduced under the facial nerve to detect the presence of any residual disease. *gg: geniculate ganglion; iac: internal auditory canal; ica: internal carotid artery; mcf: middle cranial fossa.*

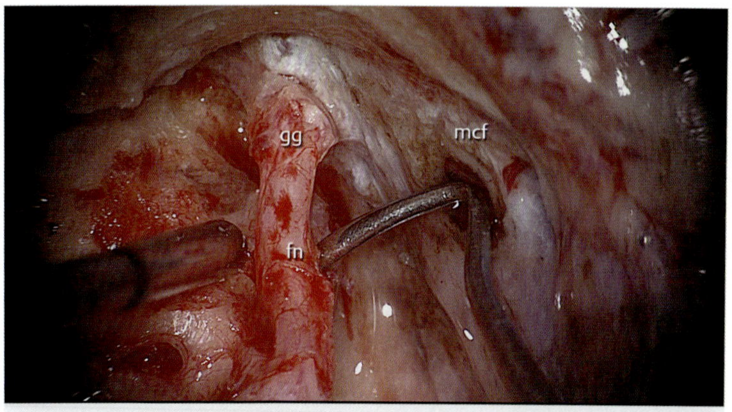

Fig. 6.105 Clinical Case 4, Left ear: The curved dissector is used to remove any residual disease under the facial nerve. *fn: facial nerve; gg: geniculate ganglion; mcf: middle cranial fossa.*

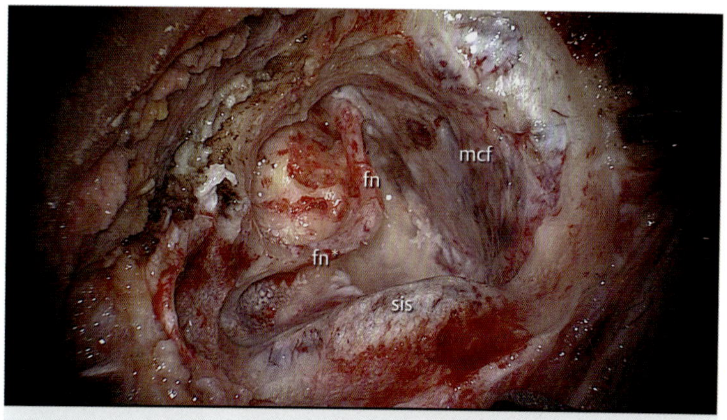

Fig. 6.106 Clinical Case 4, Left ear: Final cavity after microscopic work. *fn: tympanic segment of facial nerve; fn*: mastoid segment of facial nerve; mcf: middle cranial fossa; sis: sigmoid sinus.*

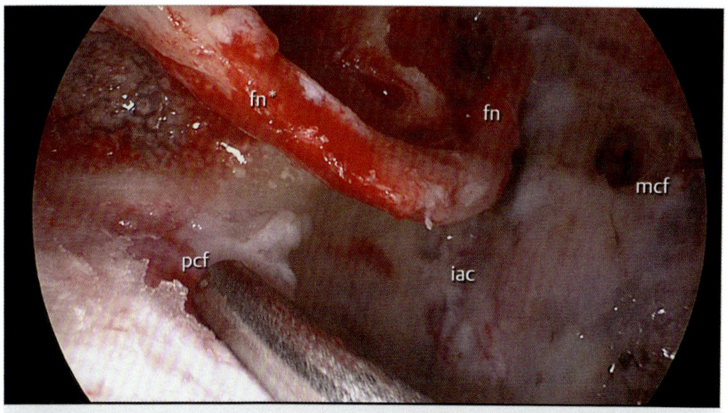

Fig. 6.107 Clinical Case 4, Left ear: After microscopic time, a 45-degree endoscope is used to detect a possible residual cholesteatoma around the facial nerve. *fn: tympanic segment of facial nerve; fn*: mastoid segment of facial nerve; iac: internal auditory canal; mcf: middle cranial fossa; pcf: posterior cranial fossa.*

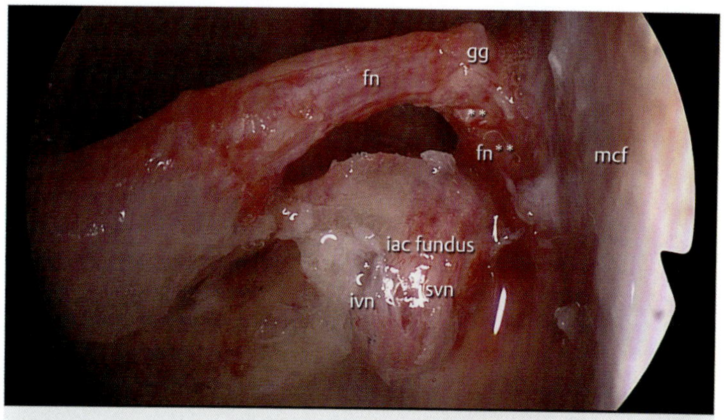

Fig. 6.108 Clinical Case 4, Left ear: Endoscopic check of the geniculate ganglion and the labyrinthine portion of facial nerve. A residual disease on the medial surface of geniculate ganglion is seen. *fn: tympanic segment of facial nerve; fn**: labyrinthine segment of facial nerve; gg: geniculate ganglion; iac: internal auditory canal; ivn: inferior vestibular nerve; mcf: middle cranial fossa; svn: superior vestibular nerve.*

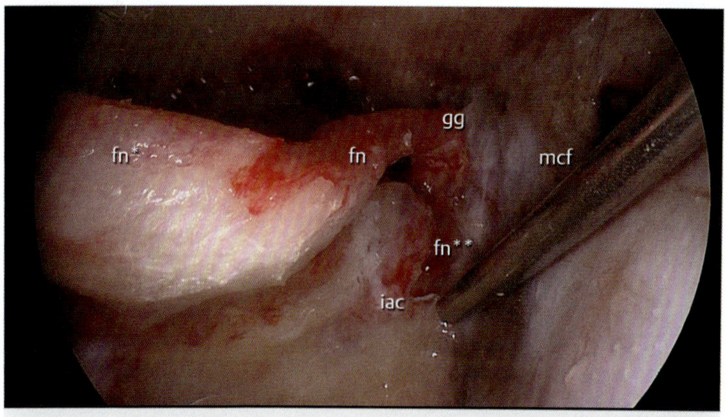

Fig. 6.109 Clinical Case 4, Left ear: A suction instrument is used to remove the residual cholesteatoma. *fn: tympanic segment of facial nerve; fn**: labyrinthine segment of facial nerve; gg: geniculate ganglion; iac: internal auditory canal; mcf: middle cranial fossa.*

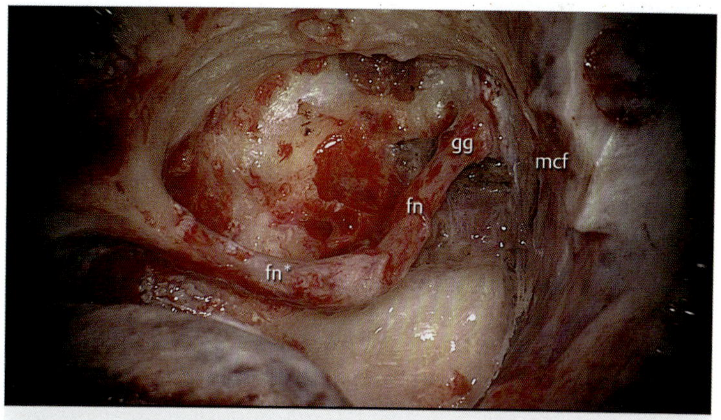

Fig. 6.110 Clinical Case 4, Left ear: Once the cholesteatoma has been radicalized, a piece of muscle is placed in the internal auditory canal around the facial nerve. *fn: tympanic segment of facial nerve; fn*: mastoid segment of facial nerve; gg: geniculate ganglion; mcf: middle cranial fossa.*

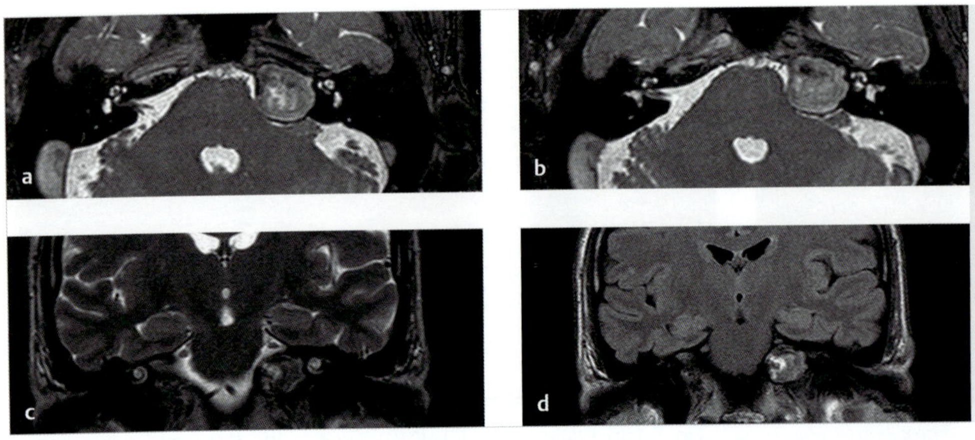

Fig. 6.111 (a–d) Clinical Case 5, Left ear: Magnetic resonance imaging (MRI) in axial and coronal views: a cholesterol granuloma of the petrous apex, developing along the horizontal portion of the internal carotid artery (ICA), involving the internal auditory canal (IAC) is seen. The patient has a profound sensorineural hearing loss.

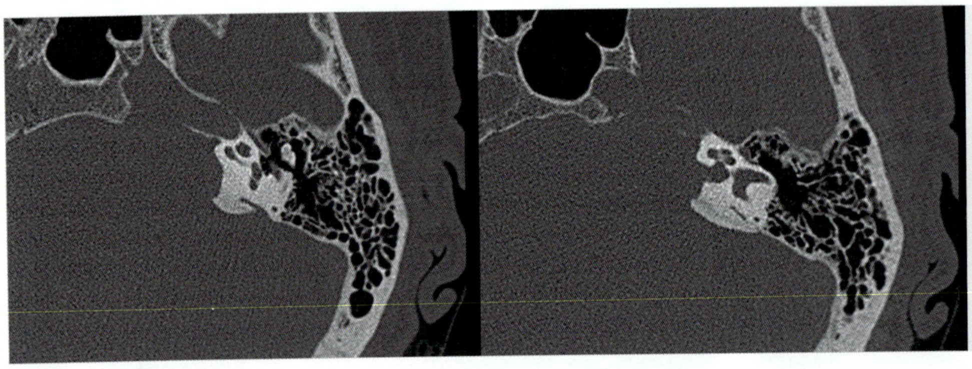

Fig. 6.112 Clinical Case 5, Left ear: Computed tomography (CT) scan in axial view showing the bony defect in the petrous apex till the clivus.

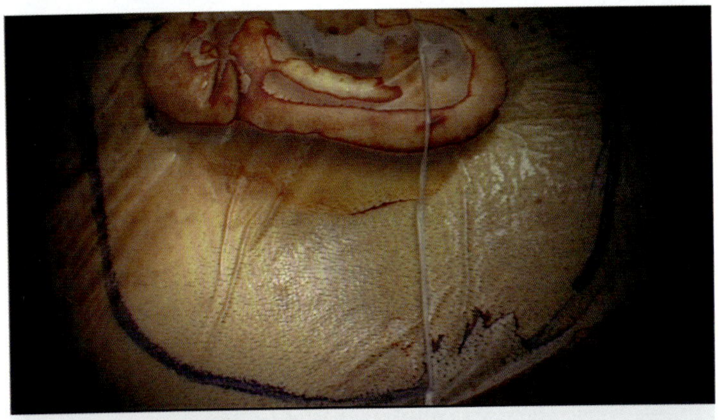

Fig. 6.113 Clinical Case 5, Left ear: A C-shaped incision, about 5 cm from the retroauricular sulcus is performed.

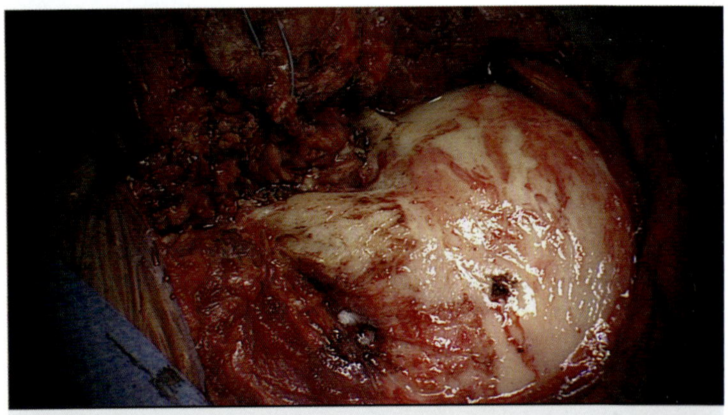

Fig. 6.114 Clinical Case 5, Left ear: The occipital-mastoid bone is uncovered and the external auditory canal (EAC) is transected.

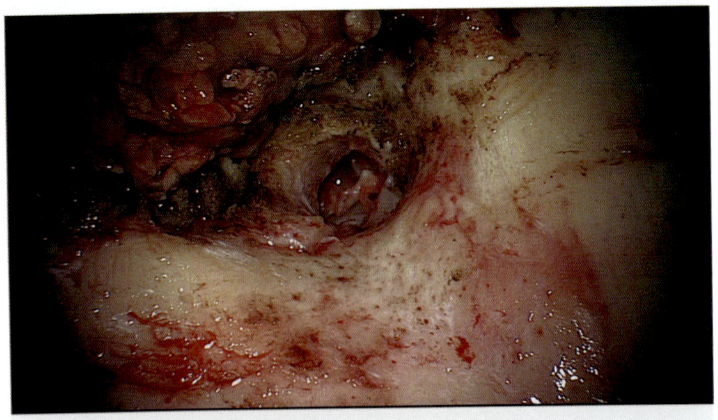

Fig. 6.115 Clinical Case 5, Left ear: The skin of the external auditory canal (EAC) and of the eardrum is removed.

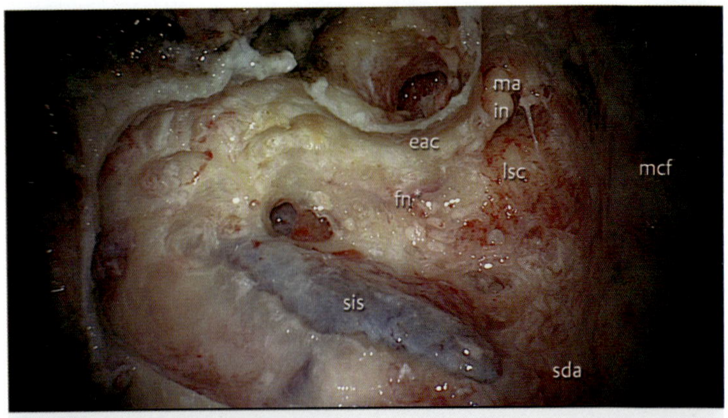

Fig. 6.116 Clinical Case 5, Left ear: A wide mastoidectomy is performed; the mastoid segment of the facial nerve is detected. *eac: external auditory canal; fn*: mastoid segment of facial nerve; in: incus; lsc: lateral semicircular canal; ma: malleus; mcf: middle cranial fossa; sda: sinodural angle; sis: sigmoid sinus.*

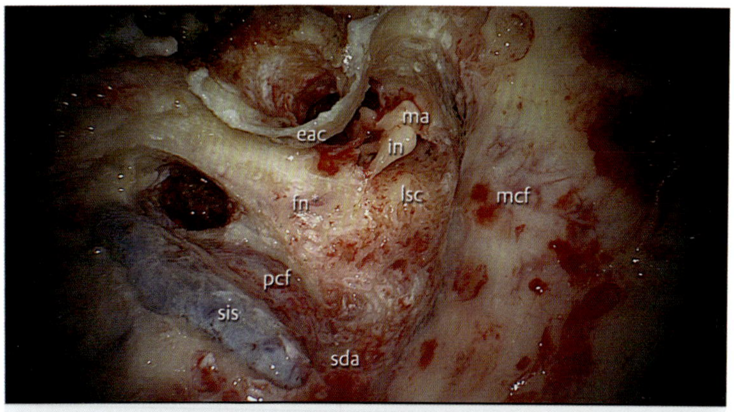

Fig. 6.117 Clinical Case 5, Left ear: The bony walls of the external auditory canal (EAC) are progressively removed. The mastoid portion of the facial nerve is also progressively skeletonized. The anatomical relationship between the bony EAC and the facial nerve is noted. *eac: external auditory canal; fn*: mastoid segment of facial nerve; in: incus; lsc: lateral semicircular canal; ma: malleus; mcf: middle cranial fossa; pcf: posterior cranial fossa; sda: sinodural angle; sis: sigmoid sinus.*

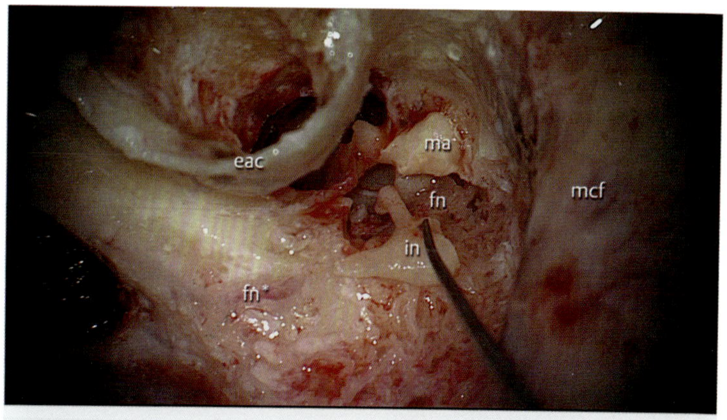

Fig. 6.118 Clinical Case 5, Left ear: The incus is removed. *eac: external auditory canal; fn: tympanic segment of facial nerve; fn*: mastoid segment of facial nerve; in: incus; ma: malleus; mcf: middle cranial fossa.*

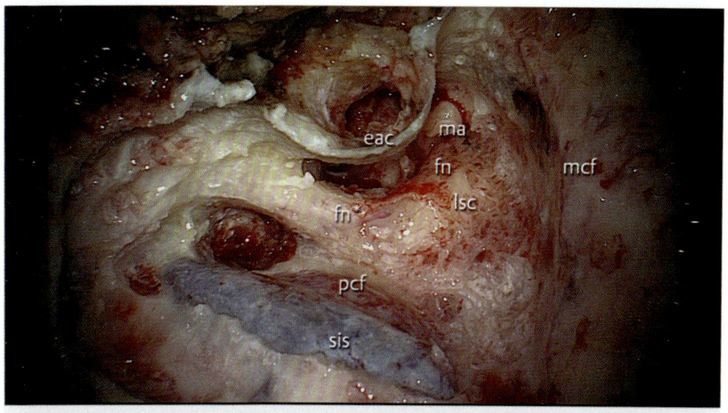

Fig. 6.119 Clinical Case 5, Left ear: The bony walls of the external auditory canal (EAC) are progressively removed. The mastoid portion of the facial nerve is also progressively skeletonized. The anatomical relationship between the bony EAC and the facial nerve is noted. *eac: external auditory canal; fn*: mastoid segment of facial nerve; lsc: lateral semicircular canal; ma: malleus; mcf: middle cranial fossa; pcf: posterior cranial fossa; sis: sigmoid sinus.*

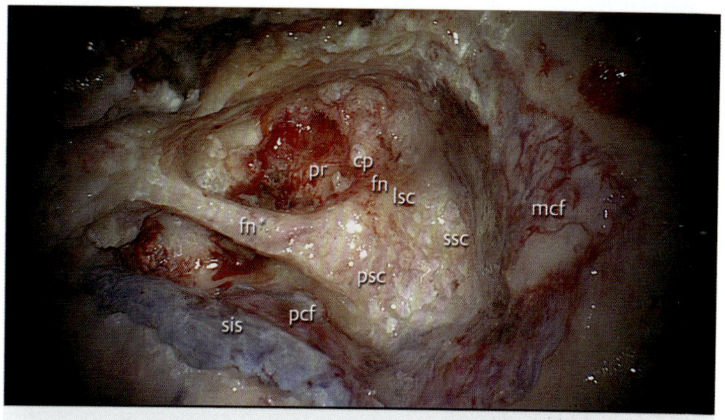

Fig. 6.120 Clinical Case 5, Left ear: Once the external auditory canal (EAC) has been removed, the mastoid and tympanic portions of the facial nerve are visible. *cp: cochleariform process; fn*: mastoid segment of facial nerve; lsc: lateral semicircular canal; mcf: middle cranial fossa; pr: promontory; psc: posterior semicircular canal; sis: sigmoid sinus; ssc: superior semicircular canal.*

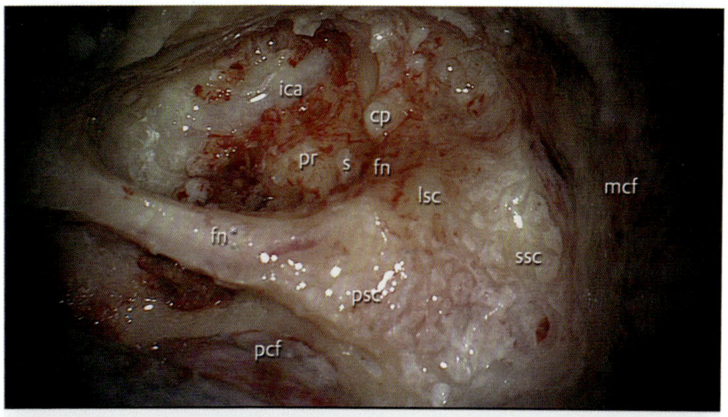

Fig. 6.121 Clinical Case 5, Left ear: The facial nerve is progressively skeletonized; the retrofacial cells are drilled and the vertical portion of internal carotid artery (ICA) is detected. *cp: cochleariform process; fn: tympanic segment of facial nerve; fn*: mastoid segment of facial nerve; ica: internal carotid artery; lsc: lateral semicircular canal; mcf: middle cranial fossa; pr: promontory; psc: posterior semicircular canal; s: stapes; ssc: superior semicircular canal.*

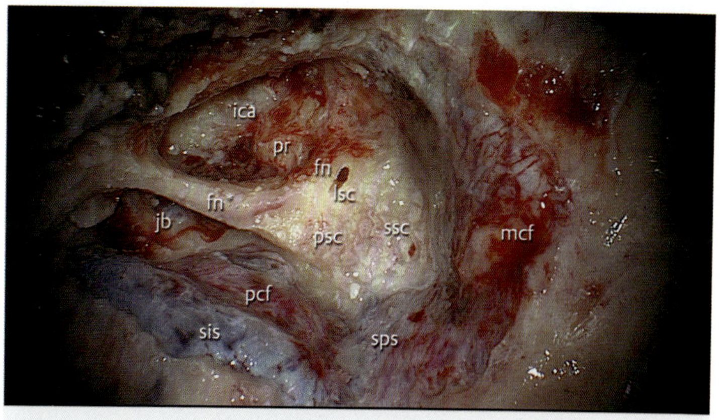

Fig. 6.122 Clinical Case 5, Left ear: The Jugular bulb is detected under the facial neve bridge and the labyrinthectomy is started. The opening of the lateral semicircular canal is seen. *fn: tympanic segment of facial nerve; fn*: mastoid segment of facial nerve; ica: internal carotid artery; jb: jugular bulb; lsc: lateral semicircular canal; mcf: middle cranial fossa; pr: promontory; psc: posterior semicircular canal; sps: superior petrosal sinus; ssc: superior semicircular canal.*

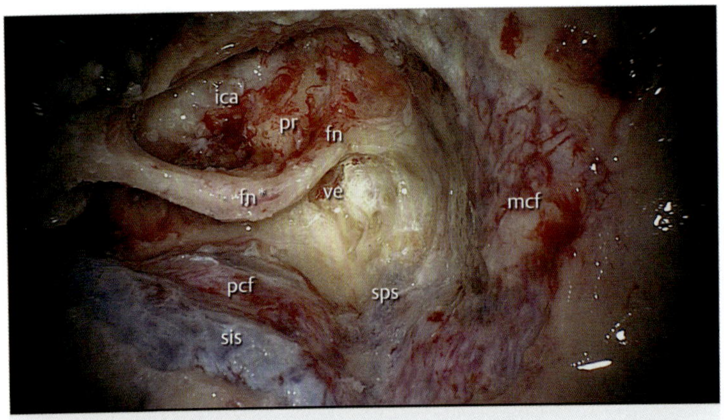

Fig. 6.123 Clinical Case 5, Left ear: Once the labyrinthectomy has been performed the vestibule is exposed. *fn: tympanic segment of facial nerve; fn*: mastoid segment of facial nerve; ica: internal carotid artery; mcf: middle cranial fossa; pcf: posterior cranial fossa; pr: promontory; sps: superior petrosal sinus; ve: vestibule.*

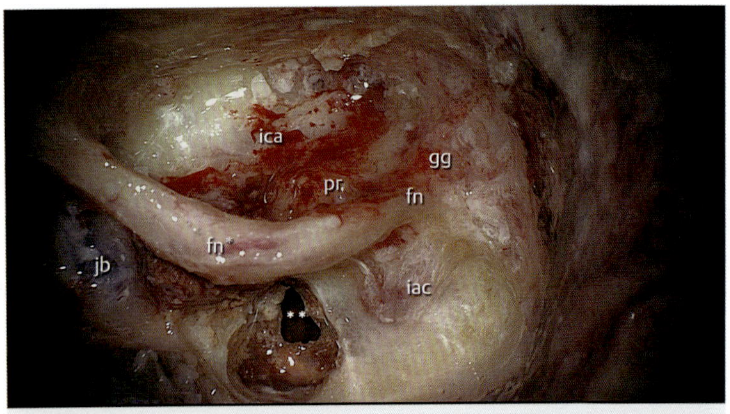

Fig. 6.124 Clinical Case 5, Left ear: The internal auditory canal (IAC) is skeletonized and the lesion lying in the petrous apex is exposed (see the **). *fn: tympanic segment of facial nerve; fn*: mastoid segment of facial nerve; gg: geniculate ganglion; iac: internal auditory canal; ica: internal carotid artery; jb: jugular bulb; pr: promontory.*

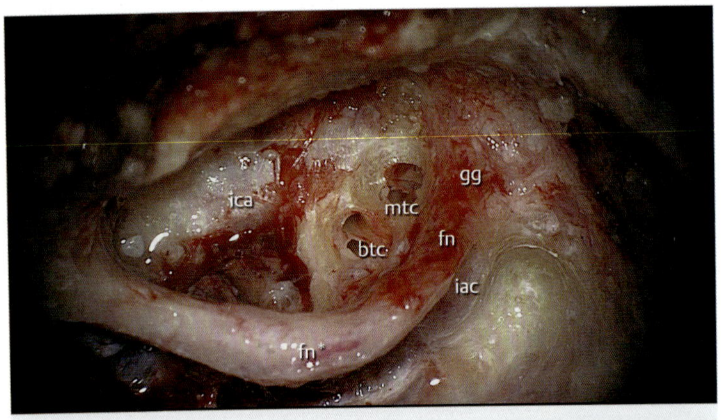

Fig. 6.125 Clinical Case 5, Left ear: The promontory is drilled and the cochlea is opened. *btc: basal turn of cochlea; fn: tympanic segment of facial nerve; fn*: mastoid segment of facial nerve; gg: geniculate ganglion; iac: internal auditory canal; ica: internal carotid artery; mtc: middle turn of cochlea.*

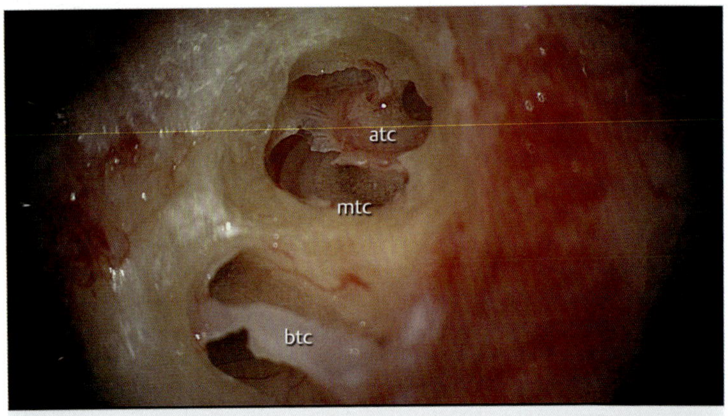

Fig. 6.126 Clinical Case 5, Left ear: Microscopic magnification of the cochlea. *atc: apical turn of cochlea; btc: basal turn of cochlea; mtc: middle turn of cochlea.*

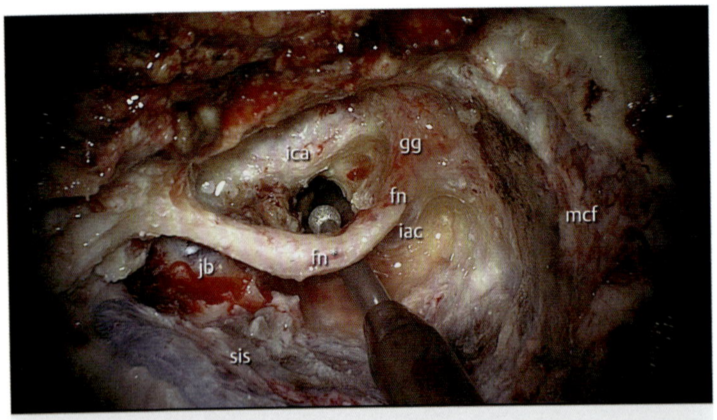

Fig. 6.127 Clinical Case 5, Left ear: The petrous apex with the lesion is exposed under the facial nerve bridge. The vertical portion of internal carotid artery (ICA) is progressively skeletonized. *fn: tympanic segment of facial nerve; fn*: mastoid segment of facial nerve; gg: geniculate ganglion; iac: internal auditory canal; ica: internal carotid artery; jb: jugular bulb; mcf: middle cranial fossa; sis: sigmoid sinus.*

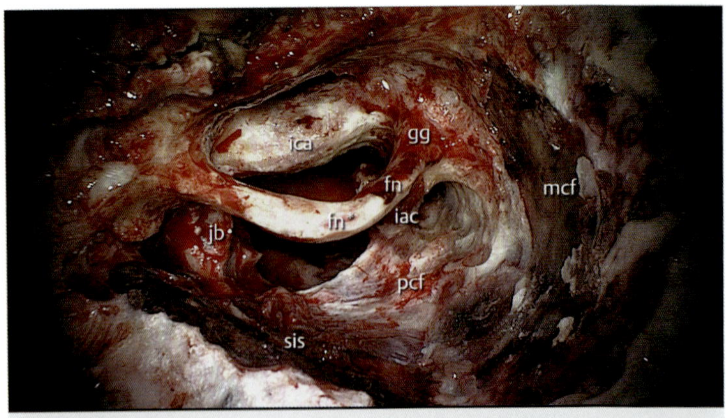

Fig. 6.128 Clinical Case 5, Left ear: The petrous apex is exposed. The lesion is progressively removed maintaining the facial nerve bridge in the middle of the surgical field. The internal carotid artery (ICA) is skeletonized. *fn: tympanic segment of facial nerve; fn*: mastoid segment of facial nerve; gg: geniculate ganglion; iac: internal auditory canal; ica: internal carotid artery; jb: jugular bulb; mcf: middle cranial fossa; pcf: posterior cranial fossa; sis: sigmoid sinus.*

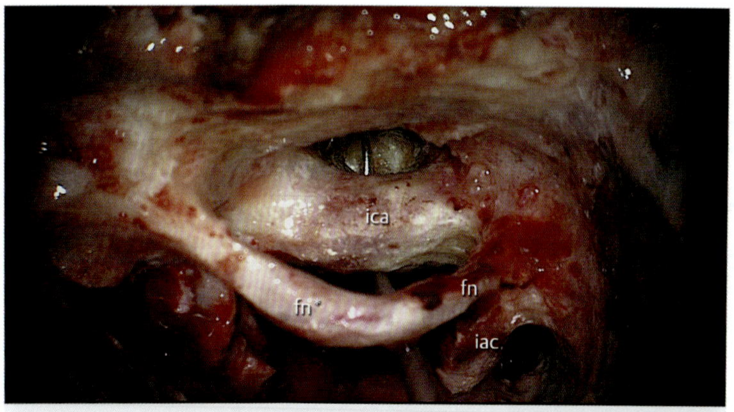

Fig. 6.129 Clinical Case 5, Left ear: The tumor is removed and the petrous apex cells are drilled under the internal carotid artery (ICA) connecting with the clivus bone (see the curve dissector). *fn: tympanic segment of facial nerve; fn*: mastoid segment of facial nerve; iac: internal auditory canal; ica: internal carotid artery.*

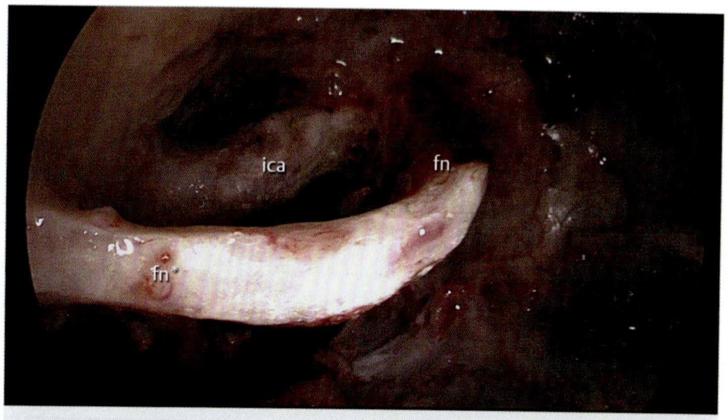

Fig. 6.130 Clinical Case 5, Left ear: Once the microscopic tumor removal is complete, a 45-degree endoscope is introduced into the surgical field under the facial nerve bridge looking for residual disease. *fn: tympanic segment of facial nerve; fn*: mastoid segment of facial nerve; ica: internal carotid artery.*

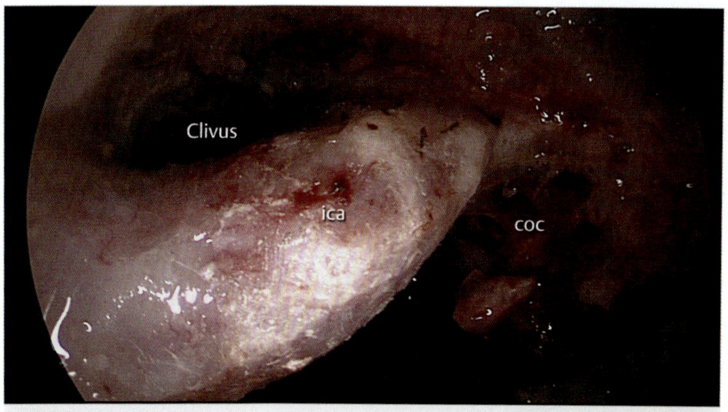

Fig. 6.131 Clinical Case 5, Left ear: Endoscopic magnification of the vertical portion of internal carotid artery (ICA). *coc: cochlea; ica: internal carotid artery.*

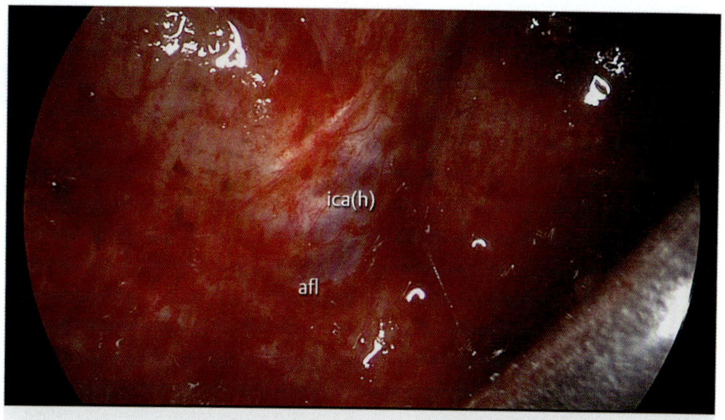

Fig. 6.132 Clinical Case 5, Left ear: The endoscope is introduced under the internal carotid artery (ICA). The horizontal portion of the ICA is endoscopically detected until the anterior foramen lacerum. *afl: anterior foramen lacerum; ica(h): horizontal portion of internal carotid artery.*

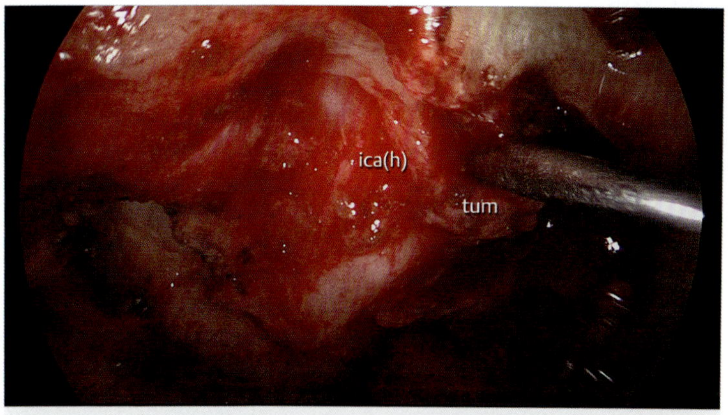

Fig. 6.133 Clinical Case 5, Left ear: A residual disease is detected and removed from the horizontal portion of internal carotid artery (ICA) under endoscopic view. *iac(h): horizontal portion of internal carotid artery; tum: tumor.*

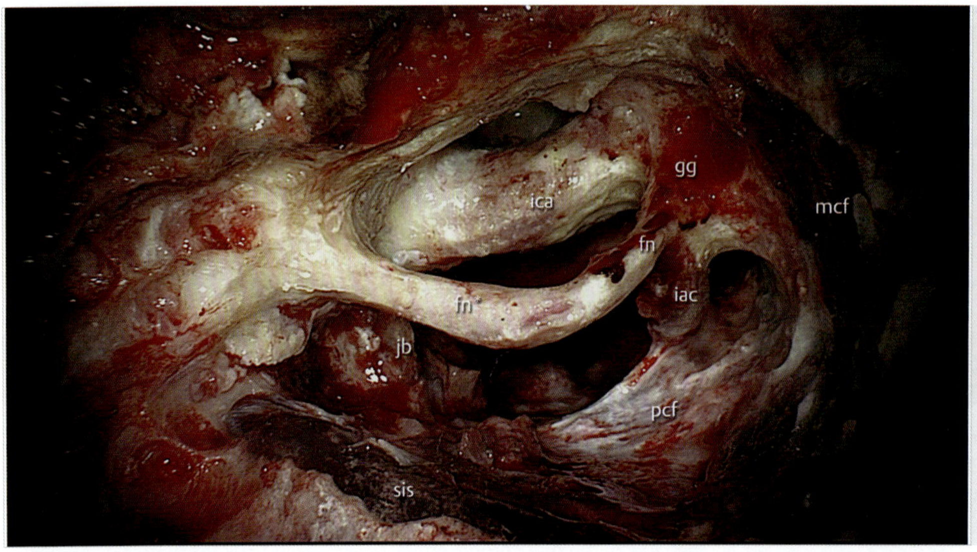

Fig. 6.134 Clinical Case 5, Left ear: Final surgical cavity after tumor radicalization. *fn: tympanic segment of facial nerve; fn*: mastoid segment of facial nerve; gg: geniculate ganglion; iac: internal auditory canal; ica: internal carotid artery; jb: jugular bulb; mcf: middle cranial fossa; pcf: posterior cranial fossa; sis: sigmoid sinus.*

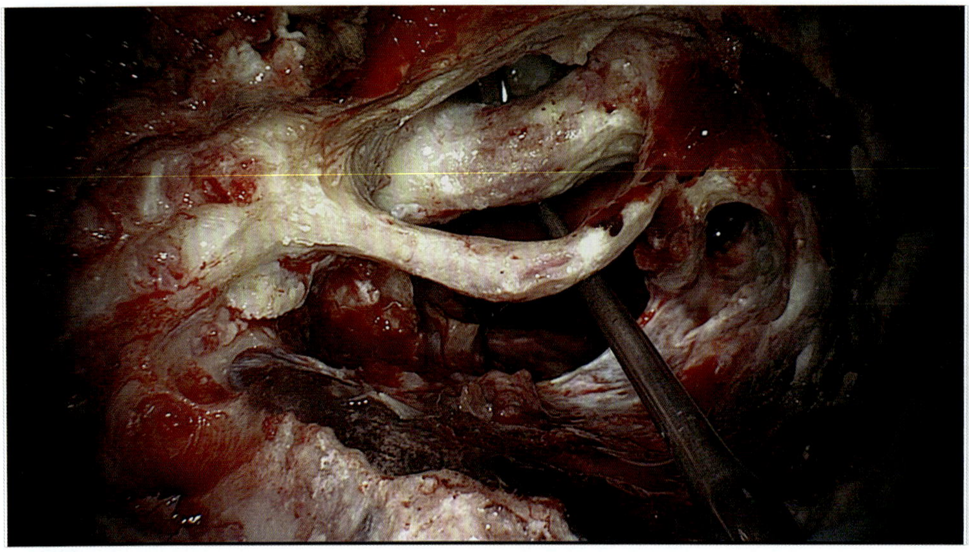

Fig. 6.135 Clinical Case 5, Left ear: A curved dissector shows the transotic surgical corridor to the petrous apex and clivus under the facial nerve bridge and the internal carotid artery (ICA).

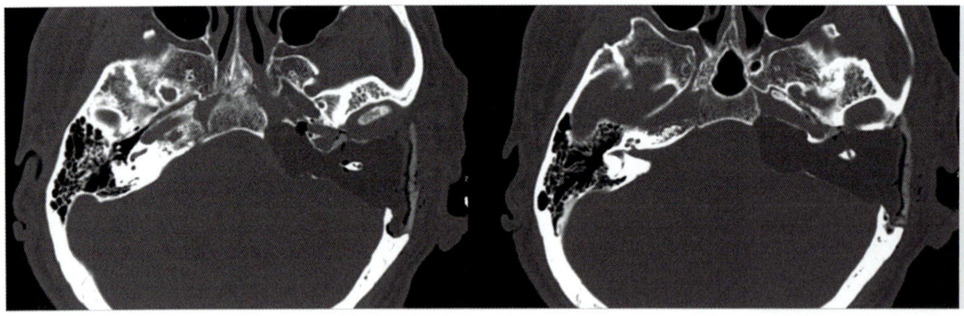

Fig. 6.136 Clinical Case 5, Left ear: Postoperative computed tomography (CT) scan in axial view showing the temporal bone dissection. The facial nerve bridge is seen in the middle of the surgical field.

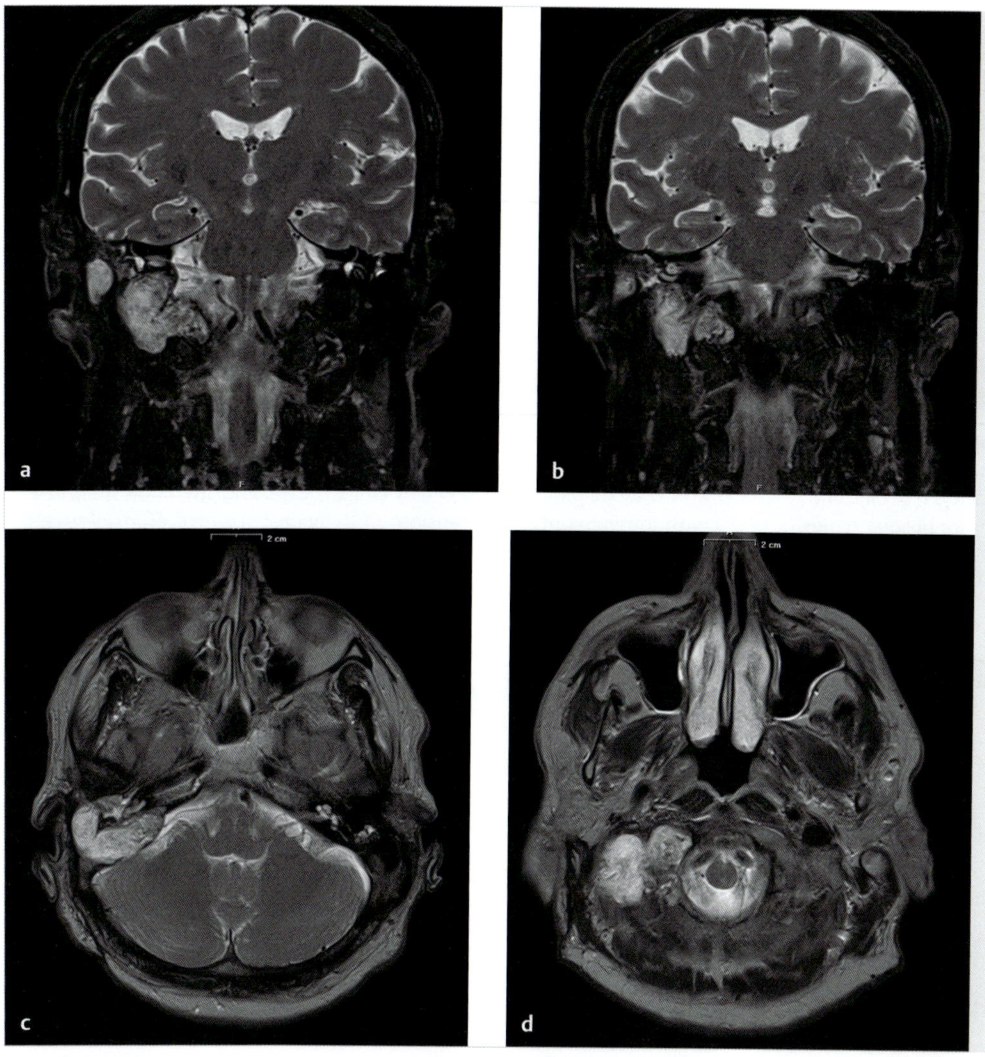

Fig. 6.137 (a–d) Clinical Case 6, Right ear: Magnetic resonance imaging (MRI) in coronal and axial views showing a recurrence of infralabyrinthine-apical petrous bone cholesteatoma in a patient with a normal facial nerve function and a profound hearing loss.

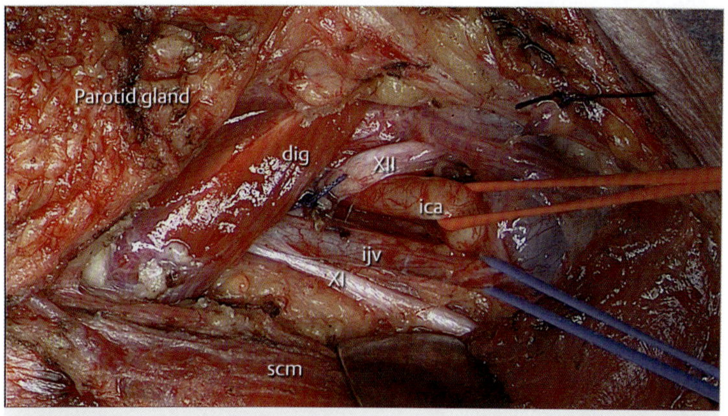

Fig. 6.138 Clinical Case 6, Right ear: After the elevation of the skin flap, the internal carotid artery (ICA) and the internal jugular vein are isolated and marked in the neck at the base of skull. The lower cranial nerves and the hypoglossal nerve are detected. *dig: digastric muscle; ica: internal carotid artery; ijv: internal jugular vein; scm: sternocleidomastoid muscle.*

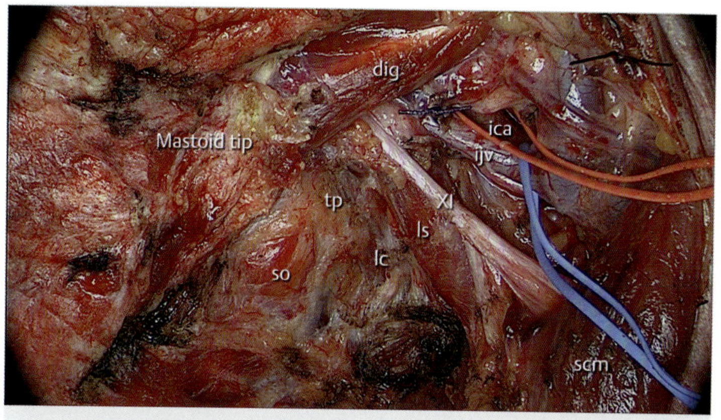

Fig. 6.139 Clinical Case 6, Right ear: The sternocleidomastoid muscle is cut at the level of the mastoid insertion. The mastoid tip and the occipital bone are exposed. *dig: digastric muscle; ica: internal carotid artery; ijv: internal jugular vein; lc: longissimus capitis muscle; ls: levator scapulae muscle; scm: sternocleidomastoid muscle; so: oblique capitis superior; tp: transverse process of atlas.*

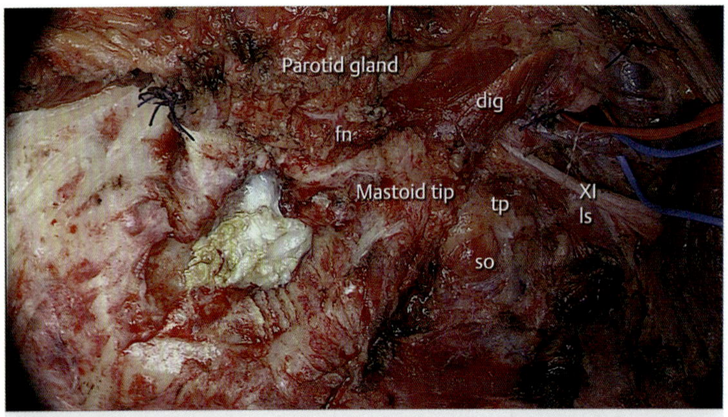

Fig. 6.140 Clinical Case 6, Right ear: The facial nerve is isolated in the parotid gland. The mastoid bone is uncovered and the infiltrative cholesteatoma is seen in the previous surgical cavity. *dig: digastric muscle; fn: facial nerve; ls: levator scapulae muscle; so: oblique capitis superior; tp: transverse process of atlas.*

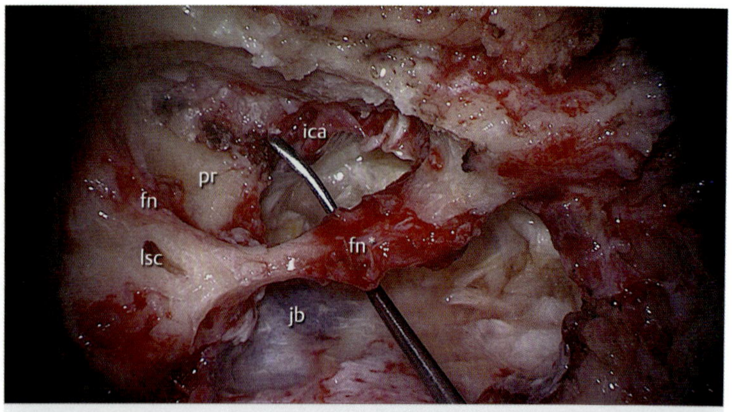

Fig. 6.141 Clinical Case 6, Right ear: A transotic approach is performed; a facial nerve bridge is created. The mastoid tip is removed and the occipital bone is widely drilled, exposing the cholesteatoma with infralabyrinthine extension. *fn: tympanic segment of facial nerve; fn*: mastoid portion of facial nerve; ica: internal carotid artery; jb: jugular bulb; lsc: lateral semicircular canal; pr: promontory.*

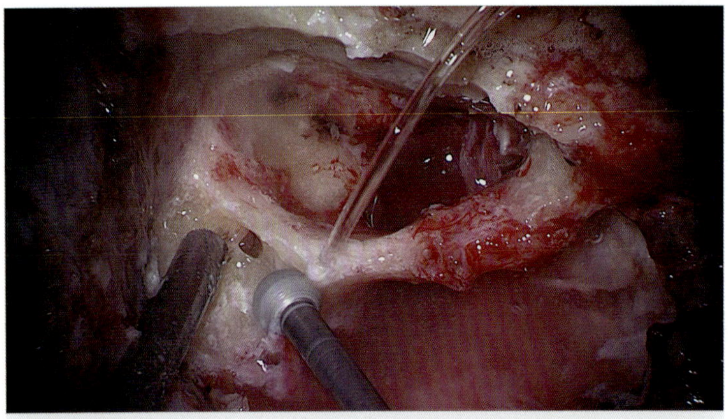

Fig. 6.142 Clinical Case 6, Right ear: A labyrinthectomy is performed. During this step a constant irrigation is mandatory to avoid heat dissipation with consequent facial nerve damage.

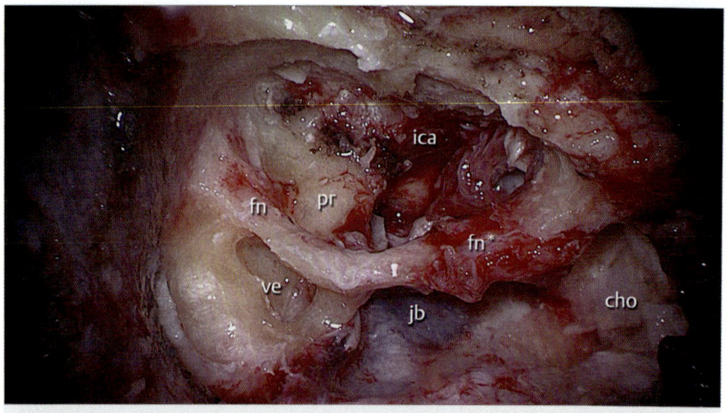

Fig. 6.143 Clinical Case 6, Right ear: The vestibule is opened. *cho: cholesteatoma; fn: tympanic segment of facial nerve; fn*: mastoid portion of facial nerve; ica: internal carotid artery; jb: jugular bulb; pr: promontory; ve: vestibule.*

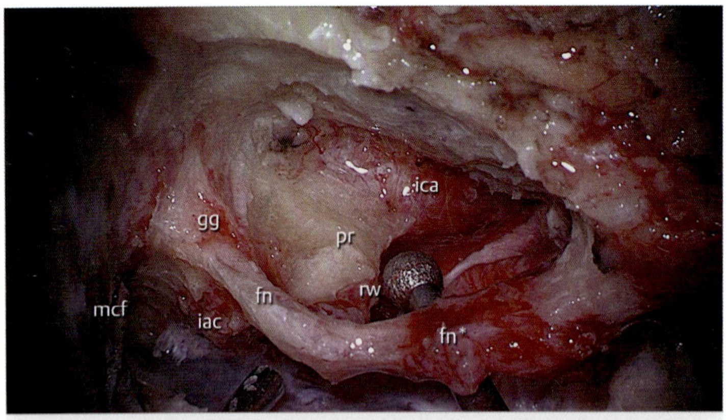

Fig. 6.144 Clinical Case 6, Right ear: The internal auditory canal (IAC) is skeletonized. The vertical portion of internal carotid artery (ICA) is also progressively skeletonized and the promontory is drilled. *fn: tympanic segment of facial nerve; fn*: mastoid portion of facial nerve; gg: geniculate ganglion; iac: internal auditory canal; ica: internal carotid artery; jb: jugular bulb; mcf: middle cranial fossa; pr: promontory; rw: round window.*

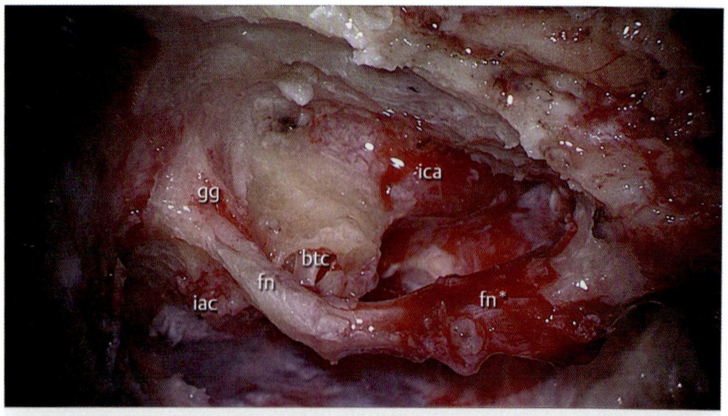

Fig. 6.145 Clinical Case 6, Right ear: The basal turn of the cochlea is opened. *btc: basal turn of cochlea; fn: tympanic segment of facial nerve; fn*: mastoid portion of facial nerve; gg: geniculate ganglion; iac: internal auditory canal; ica: internal carotid artery; mcf: middle cranial fossa.*

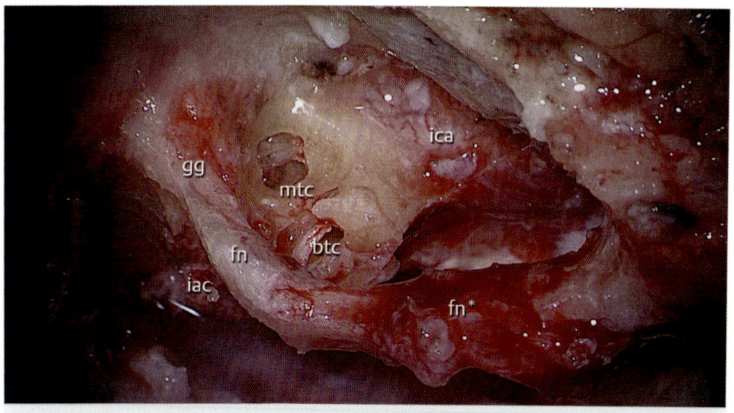

Fig. 6.146 Clinical Case 6, Right ear: The promontory is drilled. All the cochlear turns are opened. *btc: basal turn of cochlea; fn: tympanic segment of facial nerve; fn*: mastoid portion of facial nerve; gg: geniculate ganglion; iac: internal auditory canal; ica: internal carotid artery; mtc: middle turn of the cochlea.*

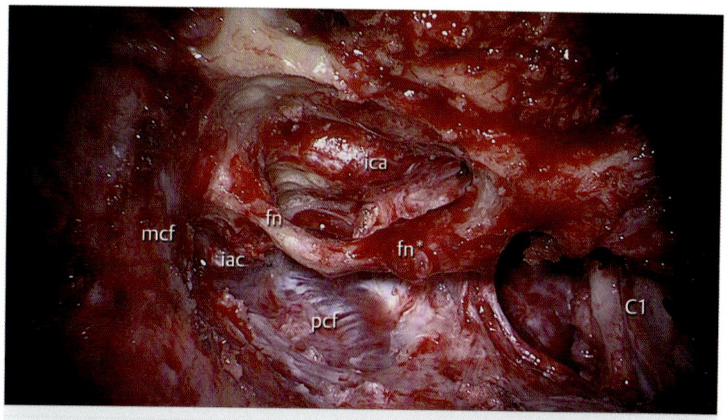

Fig. 6.147 Clinical Case 6, Right ear: Once the cochlea has been removed, the petrous apex under the internal carotid artery (ICA) is reached. The cholesteatoma is progressively removed after the jugular process and the occipital condyle of the occipital bone are drilled out. *fn: tympanic segment of facial nerve; fn*: mastoid portion of facial nerve; iac: internal auditory canal; ica: internal carotid artery; mcf: middle cranial fossa; pcf: posterior cranial fossa.*

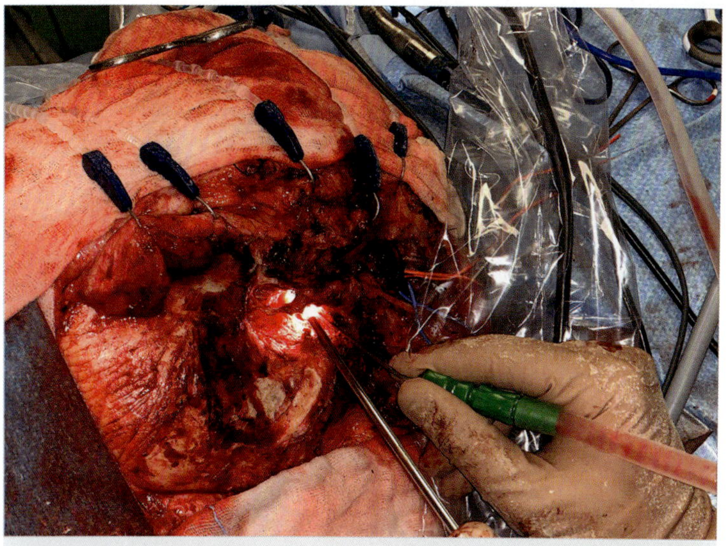

Fig. 6.148 Clinical Case 6, Right ear: Once the cholesteatoma has been removed, after microscopic time, a 0-degree endoscope is introduced into the surgical field to detect any residual disease.

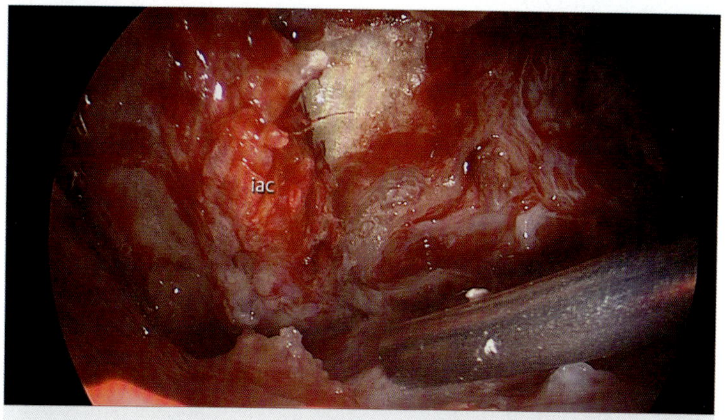

Fig. 6.149 Clinical Case 6, Right ear: Endoscopic view of the internal auditory canal (IAC). *iac: internal auditory canal.*

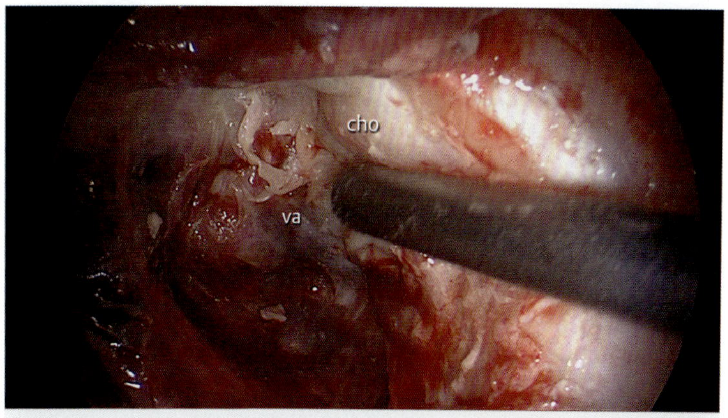

Fig. 6.150 Clinical Case 6, Right ear: A residual cholesteatoma is found deep in the skull base with infralabyrinthine extension close to the vertebral artery. *cho: cholesteatoma; va: vertebral artery.*

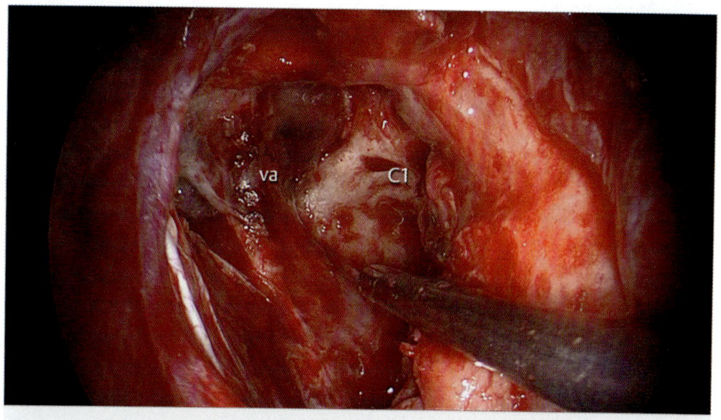

Fig. 6.151 Clinical Case 6, Right ear: The residual cholesteatoma is completely removed under endoscopic view along the skull base. The extraspinal vertebral artery at the exit of the transverse foramen of the C1 is seen. *va: vertebral artery.*

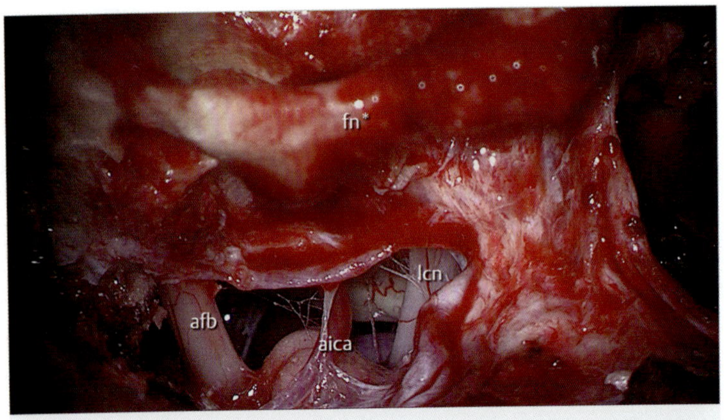

Fig. 6.152 Clinical Case 6, Right ear: The acoustic-facial bundle and the lower cranial nerves are visible through the posterior fossa dural defect. *afb: acoustic-facial bundle; fn*: mastoid segment of facial nerve; lcn: lower cranial nerves.*

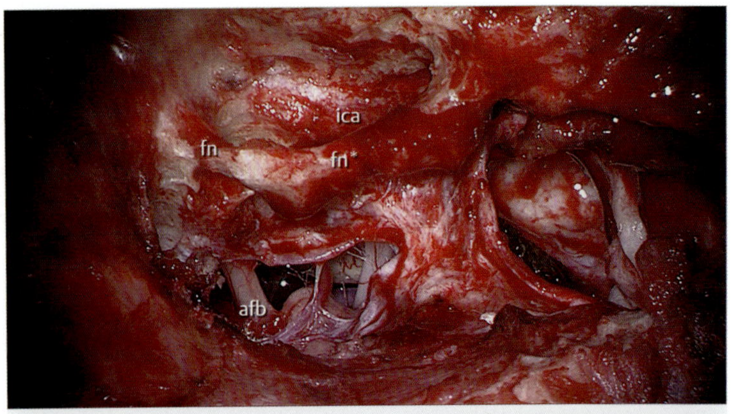

Fig. 6.153 Clinical Case 6, Right ear: General view of the surgical field. *afb: acoustic-facial bundle; fn: tympanic segment of facial nerve; fn*: mastoid segment of facial nerve; ica: internal carotid artery.*

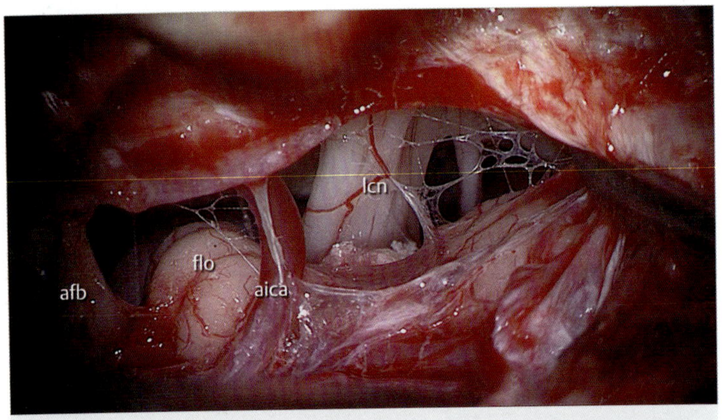

Fig. 6.154 Clinical Case 6, Right ear: Microscopic view of the cerebellopontine angle (CPA) and lower cranial nerves. *afb: acoustic-facial bundle; aica: anterior inferior cerebellar artery; flo: flocculus; lcn: lower cranial nerves.*

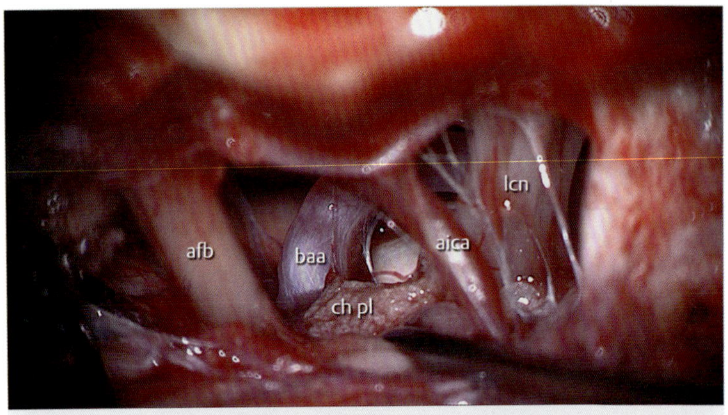

Fig. 6.155 Clinical Case 6, Right ear: The basilar artery and the choroid plexus are seen through the posterior fossa dural defect. *afb: acoustic-facial bundle; aica: anterior inferior cerebellar artery; baa: basilar artery; ch pl: choroid plexus; lcn: lower cranial nerves.*

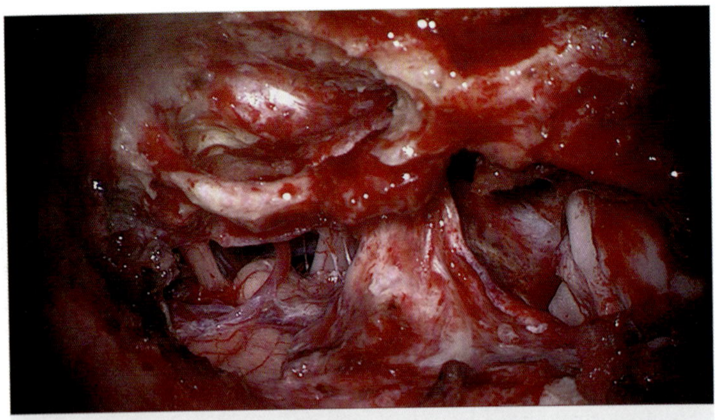

Fig. 6.156 Clinical Case 6, Right ear: Final surgical cavity.

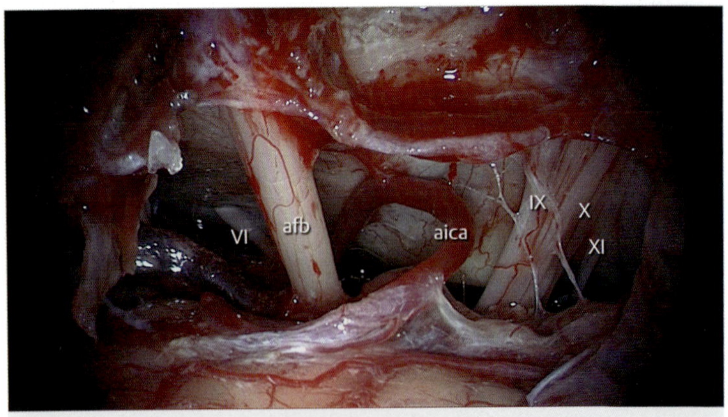

Fig. 6.157 Clinical Case 6, Right ear: Endoscopic check of the cerebellopontine angle (CPA). *afb: acoustic-facial bundle; aica: anterior inferior cerebellar artery.*

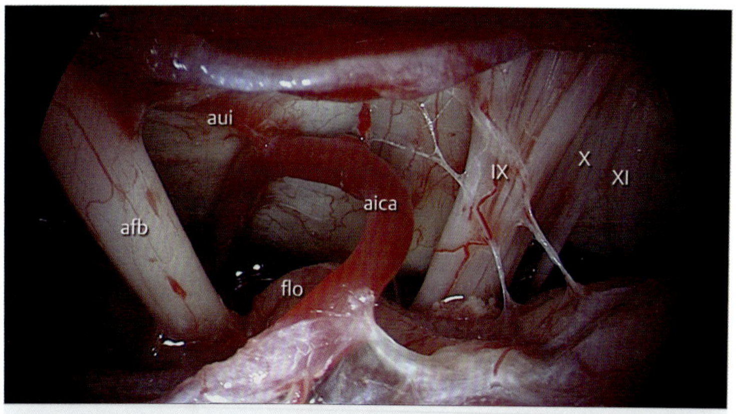

Fig. 6.158 Clinical Case 6, Right ear: The internal auditory artery arising from the anterior inferior cerebellar artery is seen. *afb: acoustic-facial bundle; aica: anterior inferior cerebellar artery; aui: the internal auditory artery; flo: flocculus.*

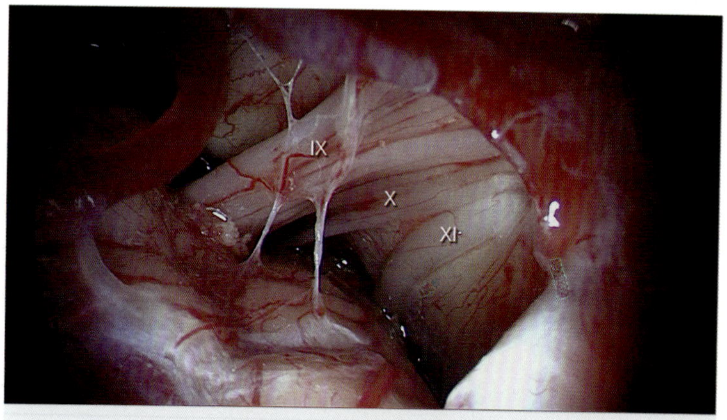

Fig. 6.159 Clinical Case 6, Right ear: Endoscopic magnification of the lower cranial nerves.

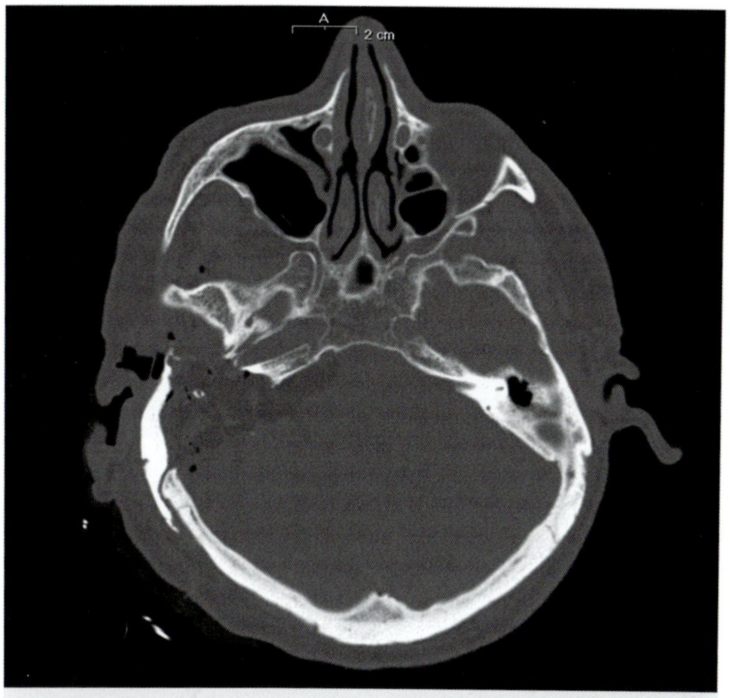

Fig. 6.160 Clinical Case 6, Right ear: Postoperative computed tomography (CT) scan showing the temporal bone dissection.

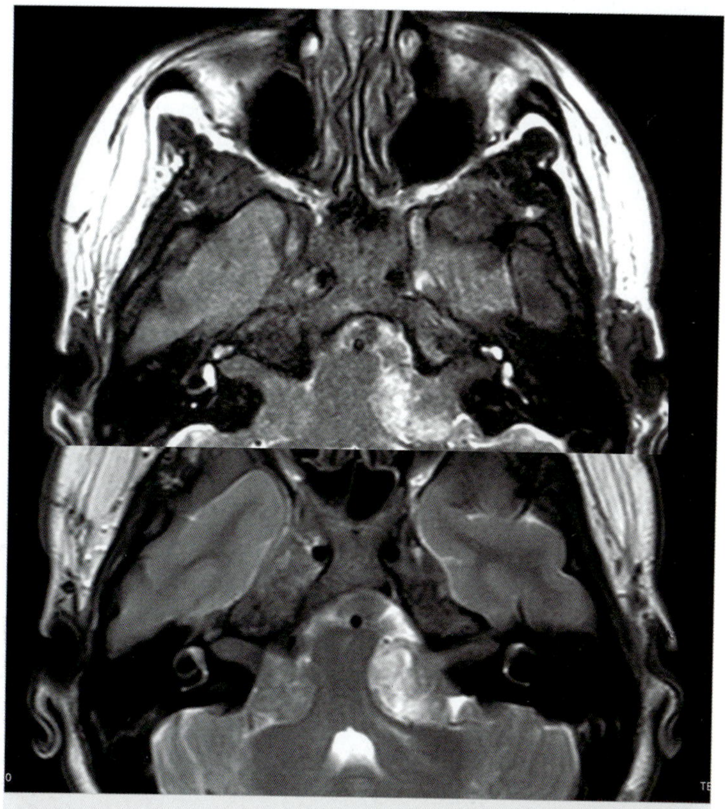

Fig. 6.161 Clinical Case 7, Left ear: Magnetic resonance imaging (MRI) in axial view. A NF2 tumor with bilateral acoustic neuroma compressing the brainstem is seen.

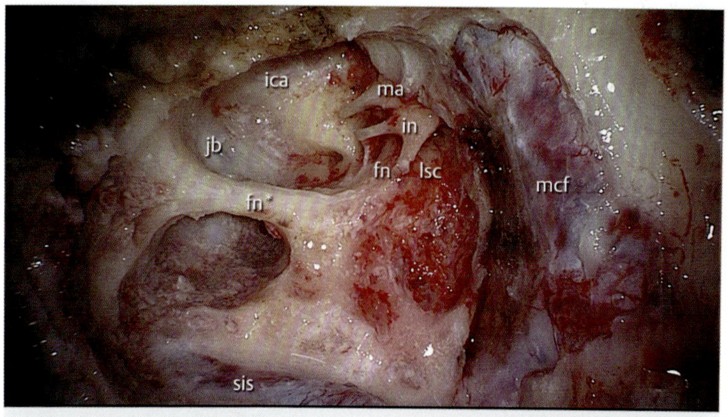

Fig. 6.162 Clinical Case 7, Left ear: A transotic approach is started. *fn: tympanic segment of facial nerve; fn*: mastoid portion of facial nerve; ica: internal carotid artery; in: incus; jb: jugular bulb; lsc: lateral semicircular canal; ma: malleus; mcf: middle cranial fossa; sis: sigmoid sinus.*

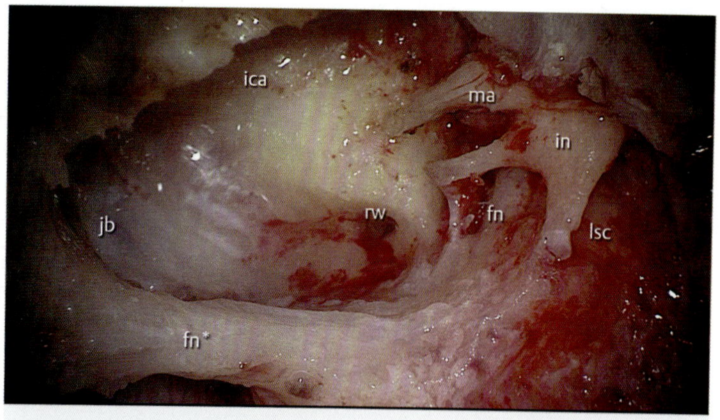

Fig. 6.163 Clinical Case 7, Left ear: Microscopic view of the tympanic cavity. The retrofacial cells are drilled out and the facial nerve bridge is created. *fn: tympanic segment of facial nerve; fn*: mastoid portion of facial nerve; ica: internal carotid artery; in: incus; jb: jugular bulb; lsc: lateral semicircular canal; ma: malleus; rw: round window.*

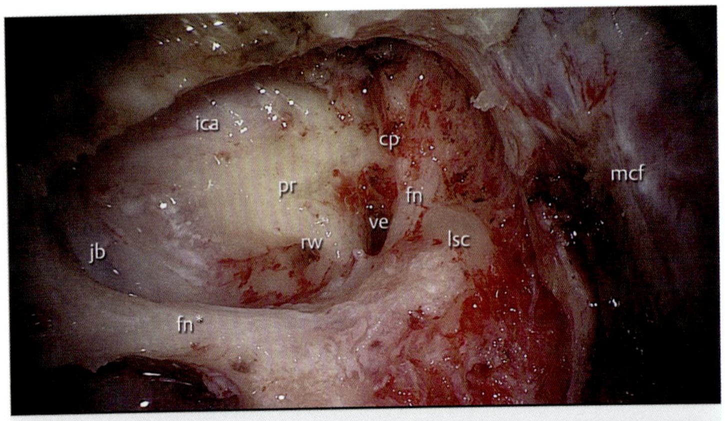

Fig. 6.164 Clinical Case 7, Left ear: The ossicular chain is removed; the vestibule opening is seen. *cp: cochleariform process; fn: tympanic segment of facial nerve; fn*: mastoid portion of facial nerve; ica: internal carotid artery; jb: jugular bulb; lsc: lateral semicircular canal; pr: promontory; rw: round window; ve: vestibule.*

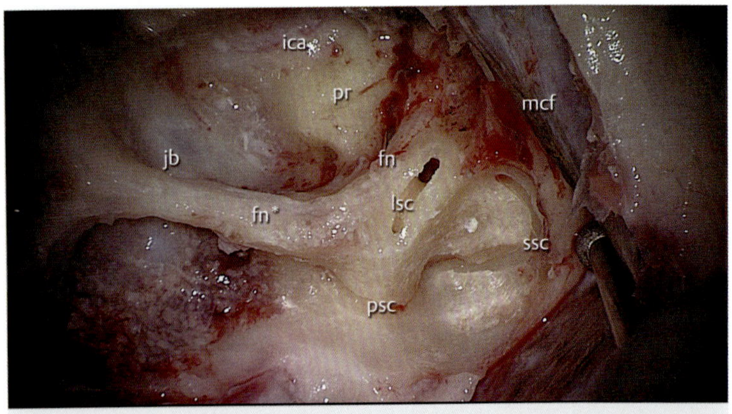

Fig. 6.165 Clinical Case 7, Left ear: A labyrinthectomy is performed. *fn: tympanic segment of facial nerve; fn*: mastoid portion of facial nerve; ica: internal carotid artery; jb: jugular bulb; lsc: lateral semicircular canal; mcf: middle cranial fossa; pr: promontory; psc: posterior semicircular canal; ssc: superior semicircular canal.*

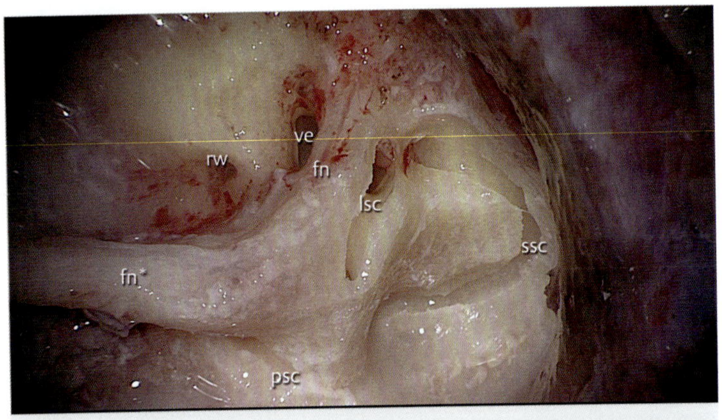

Fig. 6.166 Clinical Case 7, Left ear: Microscopic close view of the labyrinthine block during the labyrinthectomy. *fn: tympanic segment of facial nerve; fn*: mastoid portion of facial nerve; lsc: lateral semicircular canal; psc: posterior semicircular canal; rw: round window; ssc: superior semicircular canal; ve: vestibule.*

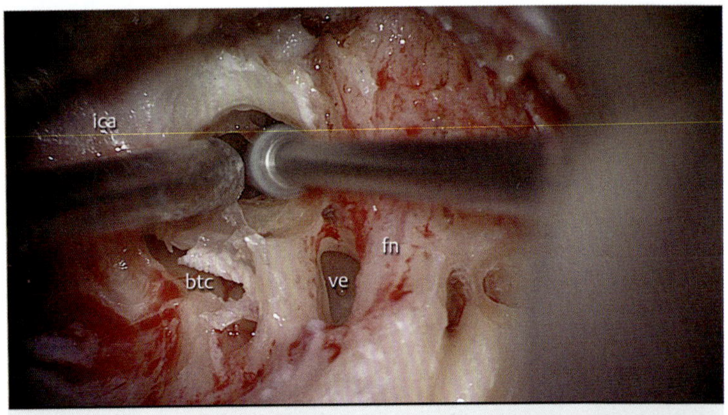

Fig. 6.167 Clinical Case 7, Left ear: The promontory is drilled out. *btc: basal turn of the cochlea; fn: tympanic segment of facial nerve; ve: vestibule.*

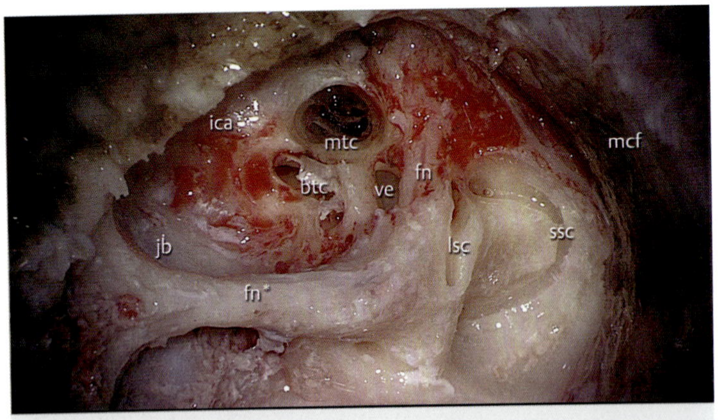

Fig. 6.168 Clinical Case 7, Left ear: Once the promontory has been removed, the anatomical relationship between the cochlea, the internal carotid artery (ICA), and the facial nerve is noted. *btc: basal turn of the cochlea; fn: tympanic segment of facial nerve; fn*: mastoid portion of facial nerve; ica: internal carotid artery; jb: jugular bulb; lsc: lateral semicircular canal; mtc: middle turn of the cochlea; ssc: superior semicircular canal; ve: vestibule.*

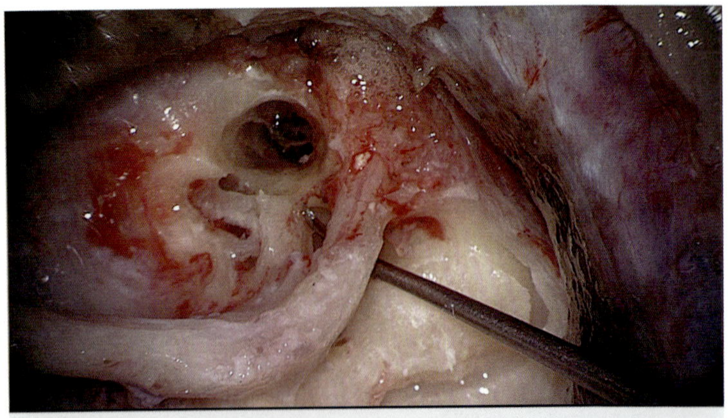

Fig. 6.169 Clinical Case 7, Left ear: The vestibule is opened under the facial nerve, and a facial nerve bridge is created.

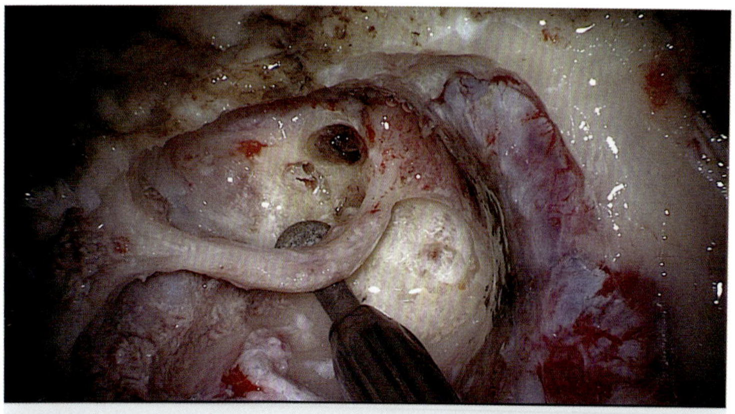

Fig. 6.170 Clinical Case 7, Left ear: A diamond bur is used under the facial nerve bridge to skeletonize the jugular bulb, and to start the dissection of the internal auditory canal (IAC) fundus.

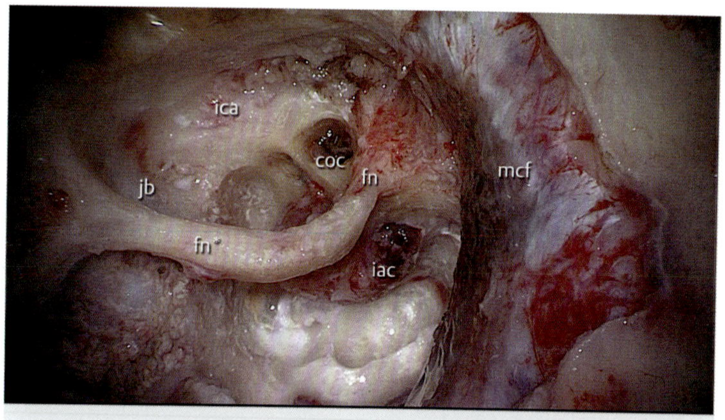

Fig. 6.171 Clinical Case 7, Left ear: The internal auditory canal (IAC) is skeletonized from the fundus; an anterior extension of the tumor under the facial nerve bridge is seen. *coc: cochlea; fn: tympanic segment of facial nerve; fn*: mastoid portion of facial nerve; iac: internal auditory canal; ica: internal carotid artery; jb: jugular bulb; mcf: middle cranial fossa.*

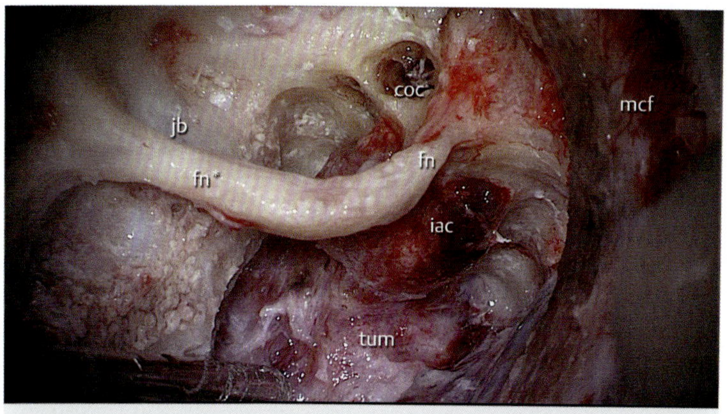

Fig. 6.172 Clinical Case 7, Left ear: The internal auditory canal (IAC) is completely skeletonized, and the tumor in the cerebellopontine angle (CPA) was exposed. *coc: cochlea; fn: tympanic segment of facial nerve; fn*: mastoid portion of facial nerve; iac: internal auditory canal; ica: internal carotid artery; jb: jugular bulb; mcf: middle cranial fossa; tum: tumor in the cerebellopontine angle.*

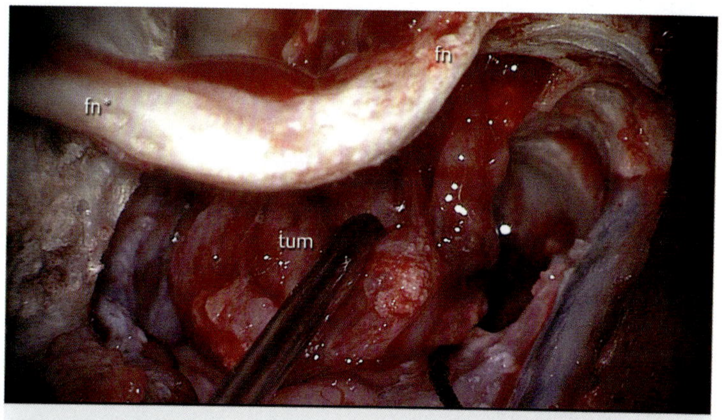

Fig. 6.173 Clinical Case 7, Left ear: The tumor is progressively removed from the internal auditory canal (IAC) and from the cerebellopontine angle (CPA). *fn: tympanic segment of facial nerve; fn*: mastoid portion of facial nerve; tum: tumor.*

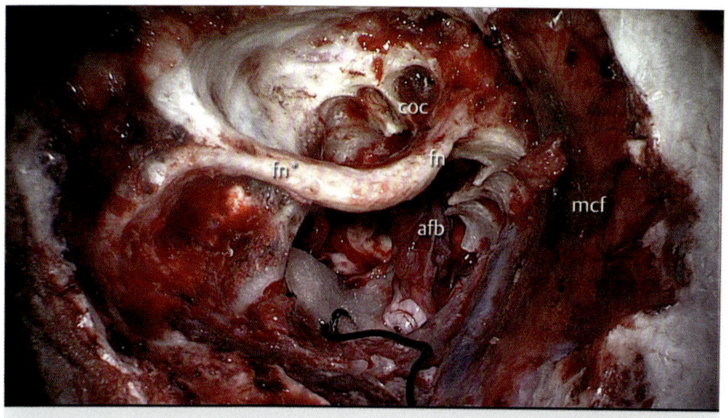

Fig. 6.174 Clinical Case 7, Left ear: Once the tumor has been removed, the cerebellopontine angle (CPA) is decompressed. *afb: acoustic facial bundle; coc: cochlea; fn: tympanic segment of facial nerve; fn*: mastoid portion of facial nerve; mcf: middle cranial fossa.*

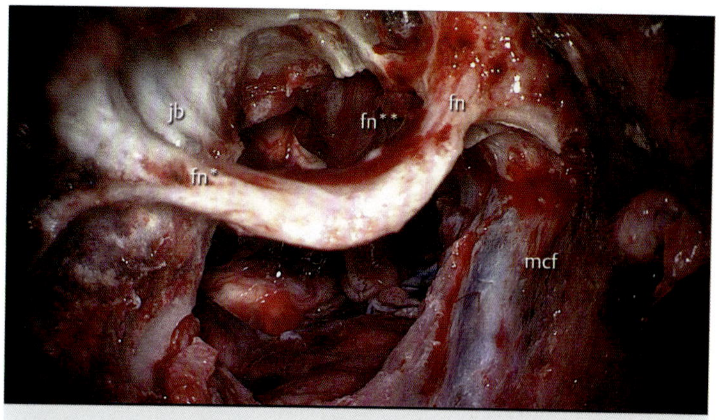

Fig. 6.175 Clinical Case 7, Left ear: A transotic approach is performed. The brainstem is visible; the facial nerve bridge is in the middle of the surgical field. In this case the endoscopic check doesn't detect any residual tumor. *fn: tympanic segment of facial nerve; fn*: mastoid portion of facial nerve; fn**: facial nerve into the IAC; mcf: middle cranial fossa.*

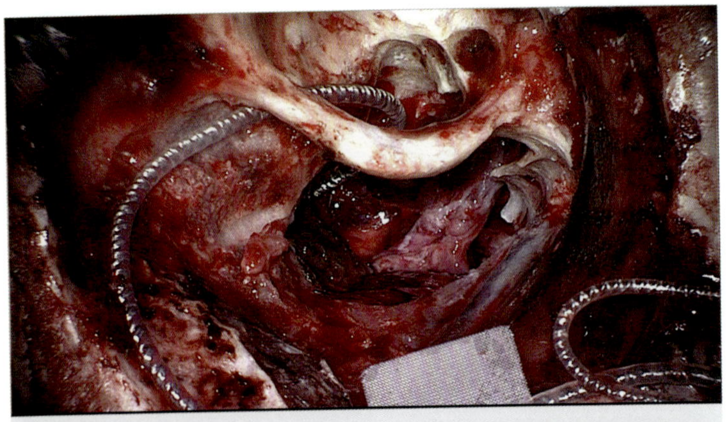

Fig. 6.176 Clinical Case 7, Left ear: A brainstem implant is placed into the Luschka foramen.

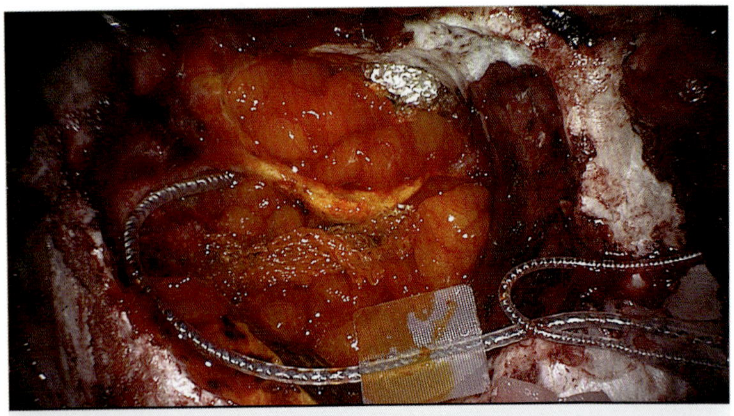

Fig. 6.177 Clinical Case 7, Left ear: The surgical cavity is sealed with abdominal fat.

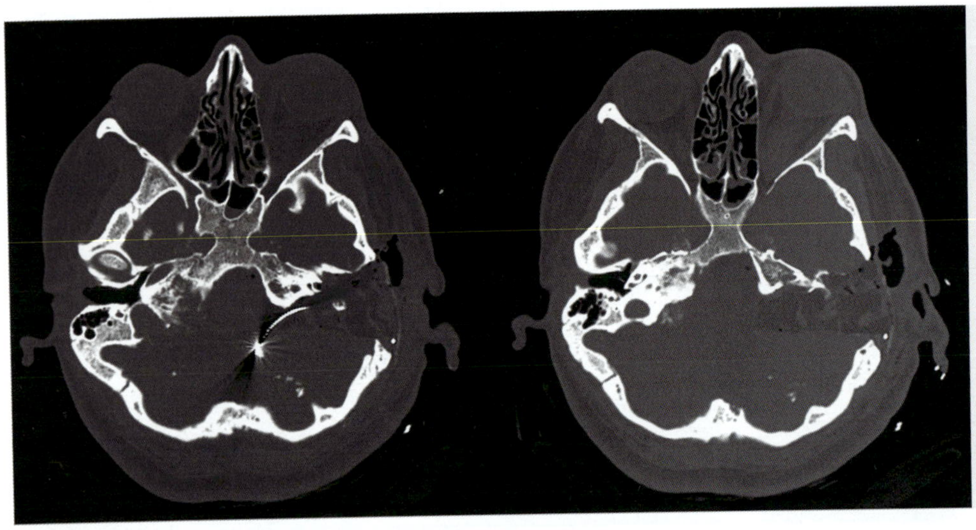

Fig. 6.178 Clinical Case 7, Left ear: Postoperative computed tomography (CT) scan. The transotic dissection and the positioning of brainstem implant can be noticed.

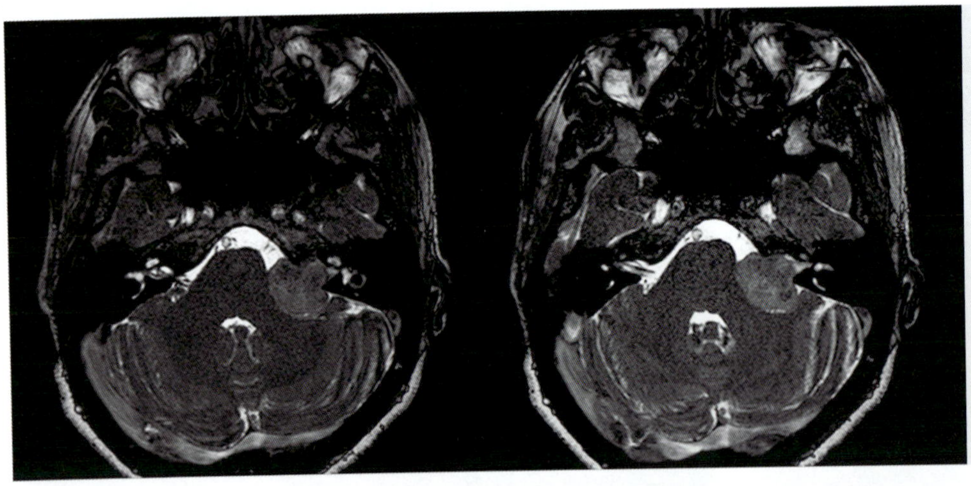

Fig. 6.179 Clinical Case 8, Left ear: Magnetic resonance imaging (MRI) in axial view. An acoustic neuroma with anterior extension in the petrous apex is seen. A transotic approach is planned.

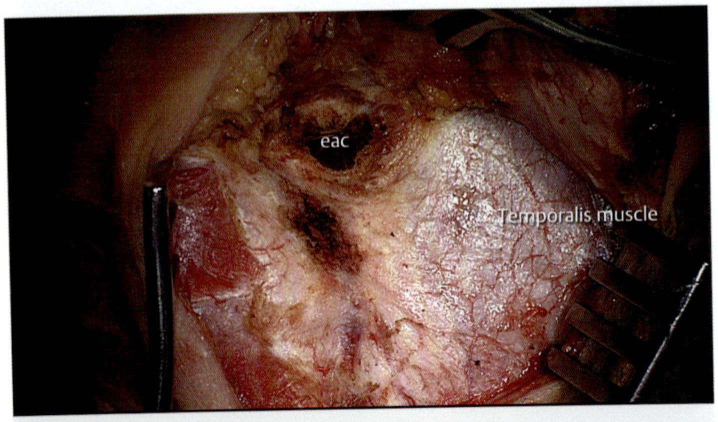

Fig. 6.180 Clinical Case 8, Left ear: The skin flap is elevated and the external auditory canal (EAC) skin is incised. *eac: external auditory canal.*

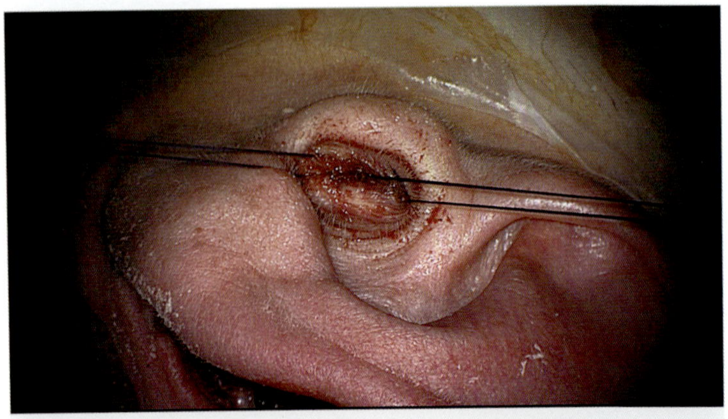

Fig. 6.181 Clinical Case 8, Left ear: The skin of external auditory canal (EAC) is everted and sutured.

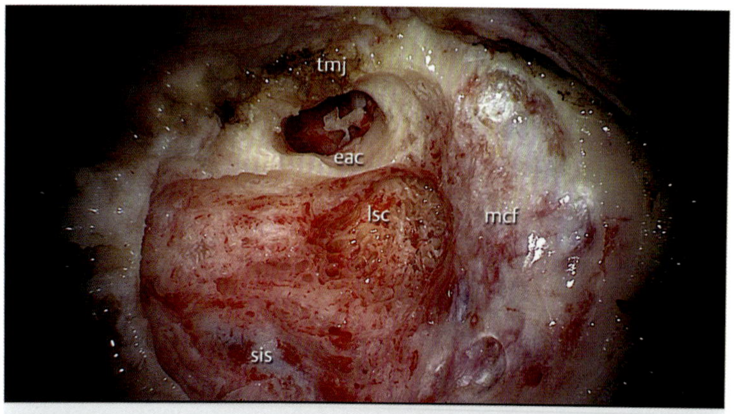

Fig. 6.182 Clinical Case 8, Left ear: A wide mastoidectomy in association with a canal wall down procedure is performed. *eac: external auditory canal; lsc: lateral semicircular canal; mcf: middle cranial fossa; sis: sigmoid sinus; tmj: temporomandibular joint.*

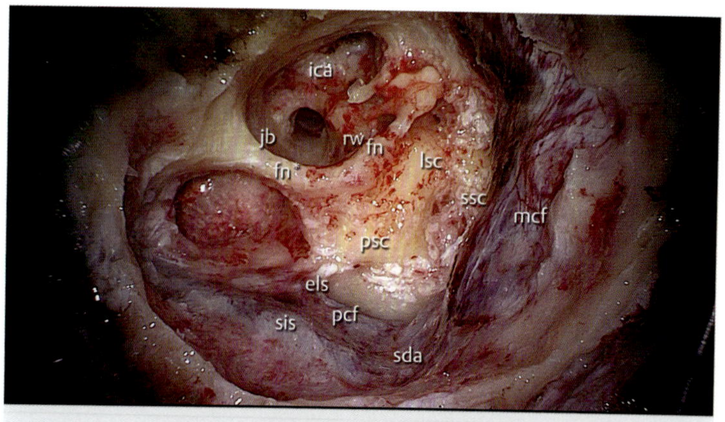

Fig. 6.183 Clinical Case 8, Left ear: The external auditory canal (EAC) is removed; the facial nerve is skeletonized; the retrofacial cells are drilled out and the internal carotid artery (ICA) and jugular bulb are detected. *els: endolymphatic sac; fn: tympanic segment of facial nerve; fn*: mastoid segment of facial neve; ica: internal carotid artery; lsc: lateral semicircular canal; mcf: middle cranial fossa; pcf: posterior cranial fossa; psc: posterior semicircular canal; rw: round window; sda: sinodural angle; sis: sigmoid sinus; ssc: superior semicircular canal.*

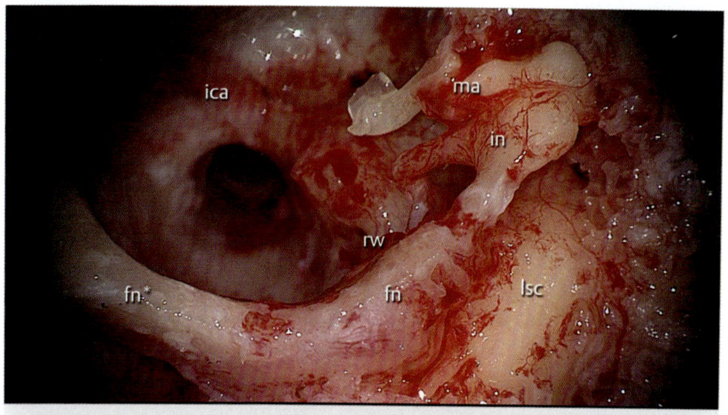

Fig. 6.184 Clinical Case 8, Left ear: Microscopic magnification of the ossicular chain and the tympanic segment of the facial nerve; the retrofacial and infracochlear cells are drilled out. *fn: tympanic segment of facial nerve; ica: internal carotid artery; in: incus; lsc: lateral semicircular canal; ma: malleus; rw: round window.*

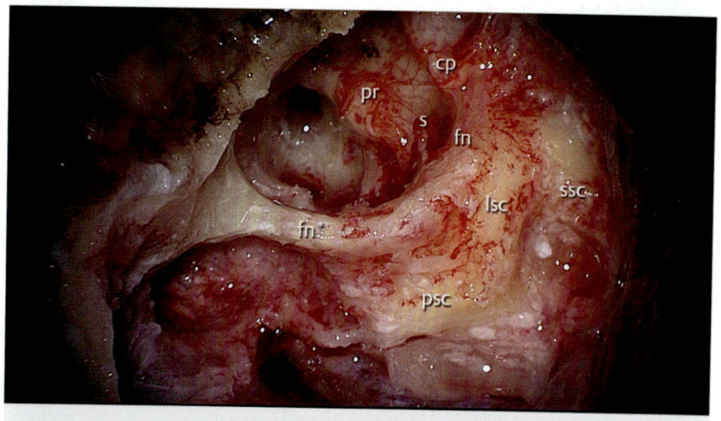

Fig. 6.185 Clinical Case 8, Left ear: The ossicular chain is removed; the tympanic segment of the facial nerve is exposed. *cp: cochleariform process; fn: tympanic segment of facial nerve; fn*: mastoid segment of facial neve; lsc: lateral semicircular canal; pcf: posterior cranial fossa; pr: promontory; psc: posterior semicircular canal; s: stapes; ssc: superior semicircular canal.*

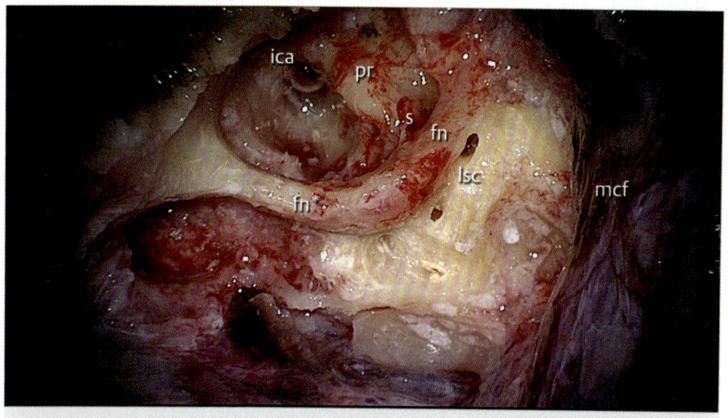

Fig. 6.186 Clinical Case 8, Left ear: The labyrinthectomy is performed. The close anatomical relationship between the lateral semicircular canal and the tympanic facial nerve is noted. *fn: tympanic segment of facial nerve; fn*: mastoid segment of facial neve; ica: internal carotid artery; lsc: lateral semicircular canal; pr: promontory; s: stapes.*

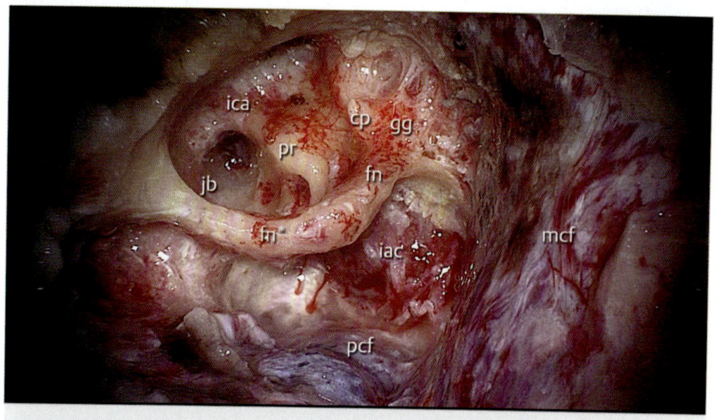

Fig. 6.187 Clinical Case 8, Left ear: The internal auditory canal (IAC) is progressively skeletonized. *cp; cochleariform process; fn: tympanic segment of facial nerve; fn*: mastoid segment of facial nerve; gg: geniculate ganglion; iac: internal auditory canal; ica: internal carotid artery; mcf: middle cranial fossa; pcf: posterior cranial fossa; pr: promontory.*

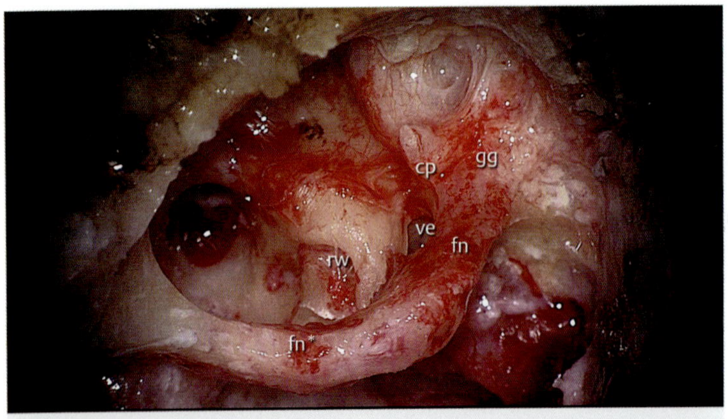

Fig. 6.188 Clinical Case 8, Left ear: The stapes is removed and the vestibule opening is exposed. *cp: cochleariform process; fn: tympanic segment of facial nerve; fn*: mastoid segment of facial neve; gg: geniculate ganglion; rw: round window; ve: vestibule.*

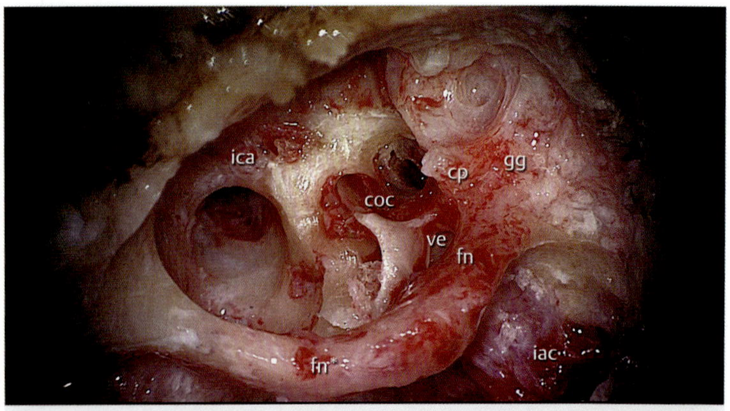

Fig. 6.189 Clinical Case 8, Left ear: The promontory is drilled out and the cochlea detected. *coc: cochlea; cp: cochleariform process; fn: tympanic segment of facial nerve; fn*: mastoid segment of facial neve; gg: geniculate ganglion; iac: internal auditory canal; ica: internal carotid artery; ve: vestibule.*

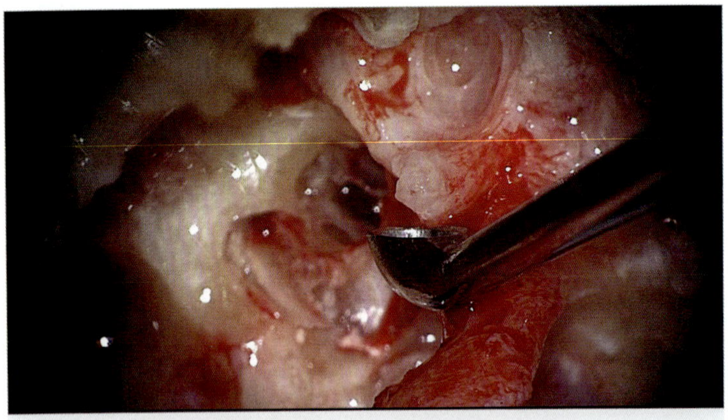

Fig. 6.190 Clinical Case 8, Left ear: The cochleariform process and tympanic tympani muscle are removed.

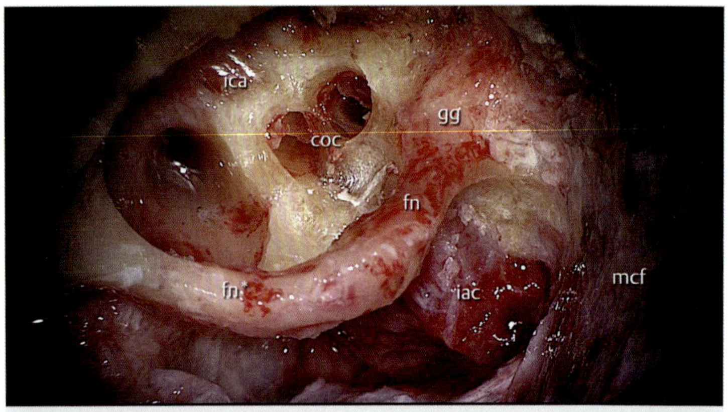

Fig. 6.191 Clinical Case 8, Left ear: Once the cochleariform process has been removed, the geniculate ganglion is detected. *coc: cochlea; fn: tympanic segment of facial nerve; fn*: mastoid segment of facial neve; gg: geniculate ganglion; iac: internal auditory canal; ica: internal carotid artery; mcf: middle cranial fossa.*

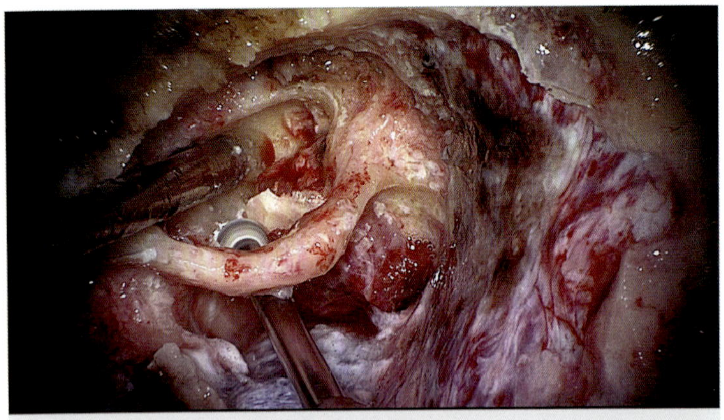

Fig. 6.192 Clinical Case 8, Left ear: The cochlea is removed and the anterior extension of the internal auditory canal (IAC) and the fundus are skeletonized using a diamond bur.

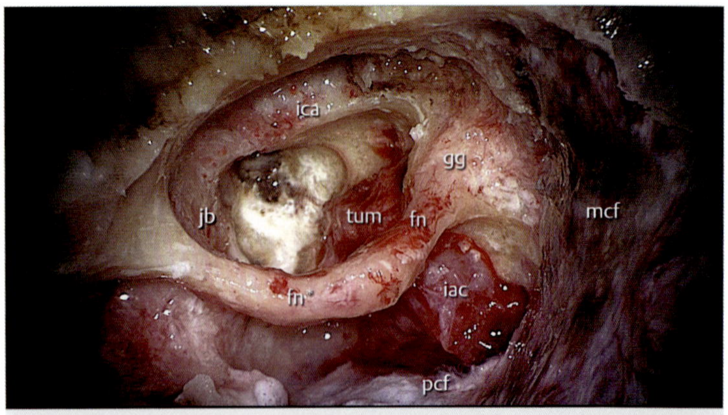

Fig. 6.193 Clinical Case 8, Left ear: The anterior extension of the tumor under the facial nerve bridge is noted. *fn: tympanic segment of facial nerve; fn*: mastoid segment of facial neve; gg: geniculate ganglion; iac: internal auditory canal; ica: internal carotid artery; jb: jugular bulb; mcf: middle cranial fossa; pcf: posterior cranial fossa; tum: tumor.*

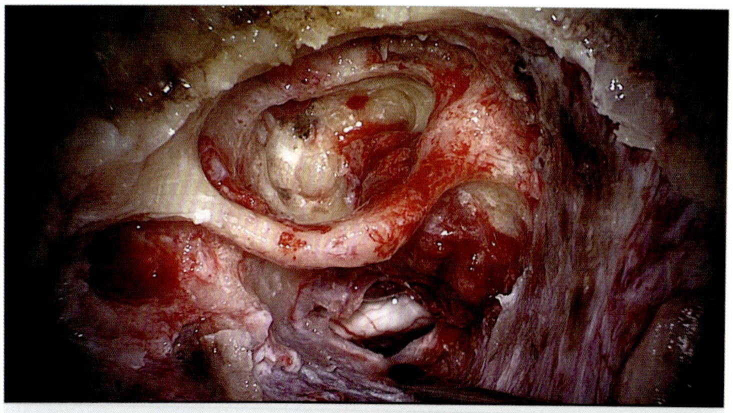

Fig. 6.194 Clinical Case 8, Left ear: The posterior fossa dura is cut; the tumor is isolated from the fundus to the brainstem.

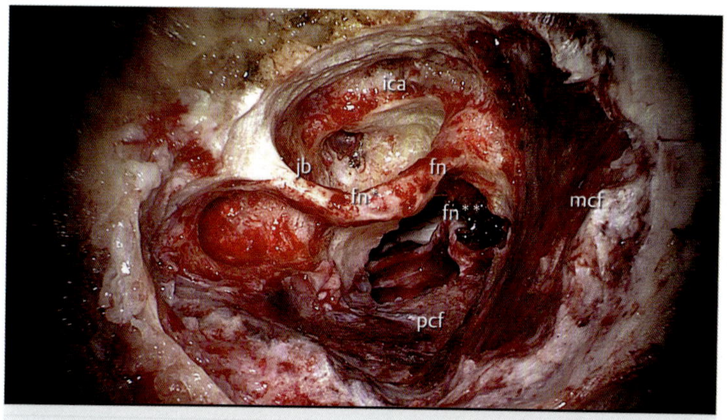

Fig. 6.195 Clinical Case 8, Left ear: Final surgical cavity after microscopic tumor removal. *fn: tympanic segment of facial nerve; fn*: mastoid segment of facial neve; fn**: facial nerve into the IAC; ica: internal carotid artery; jb: jugular bulb; mcf: middle cranial fossa; pcf: posterior cranial fossa.*

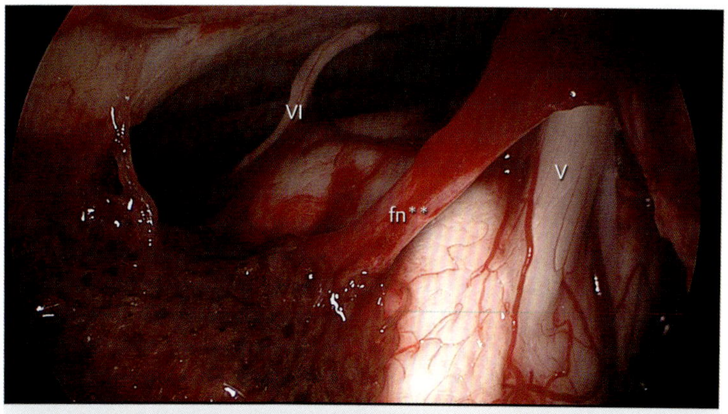

Fig. 6.196 Clinical Case 8, Left ear: Endoscopic check of the cerebellopontine angle (CPA). *fn**: facial nerve.*

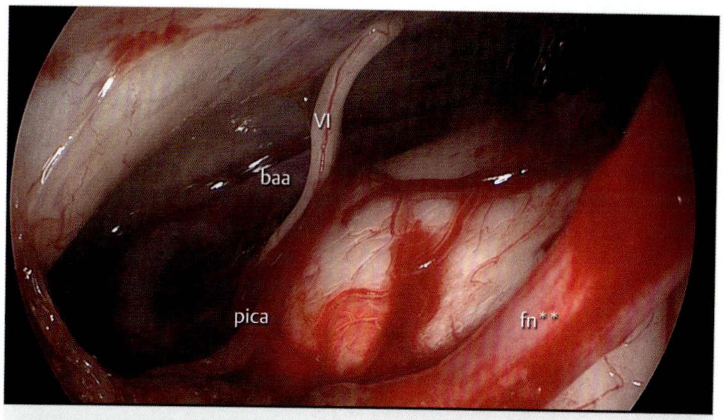

Fig. 6.197 Clinical Case 8, Left ear: The cranial nerve VI is endoscopically detected. *baa: basilar artery; fn**: facial nerve into at the entry zone; pica: posterior inferior cerebellar artery.*

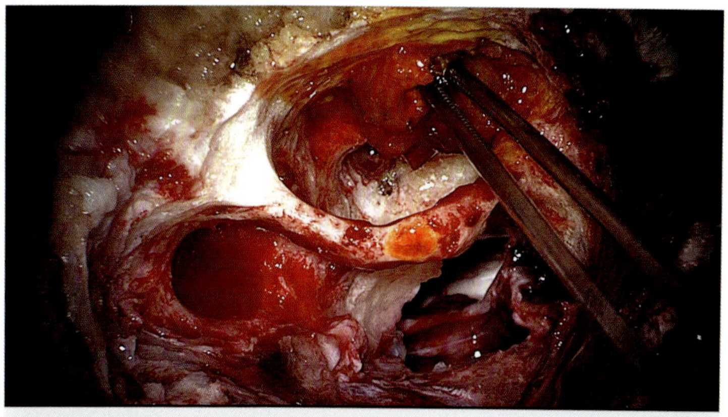

Fig. 6.198 Clinical Case 8, Left ear: A piece of muscle is used to obliterate the eustachian tube orifice.

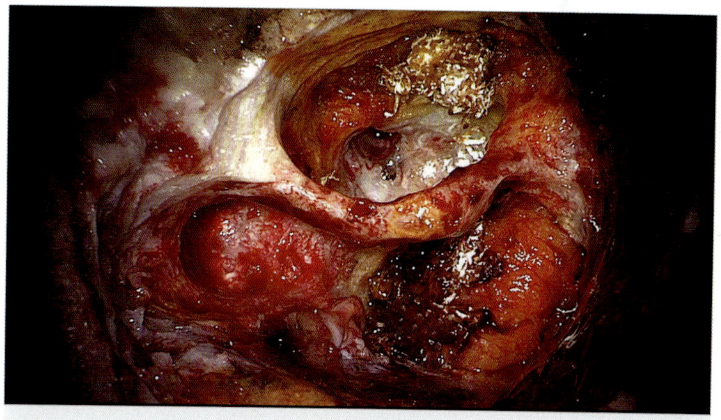

Fig. 6.199 Clinical Case 8, Left ear: Abdominal fat is placed into the dural defect to seal the surgical cavity.

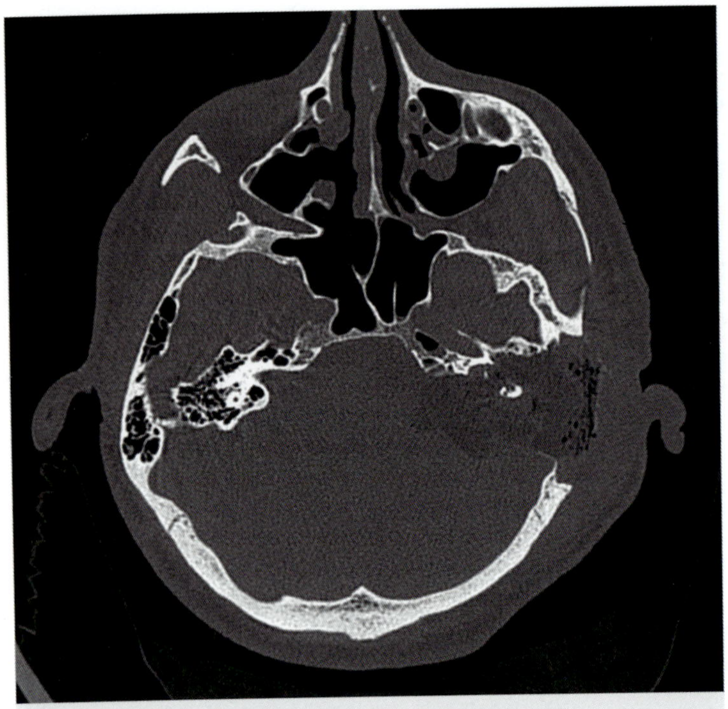

Fig. 6.200 Clinical Case 8, Left ear: Computed tomography (CT) scan in axial view showing the temporal bone dissection. The facial nerve bridge is noted in the middle of the surgical cavity.

Traditionally, the patient is discharged 7 days after surgery; the suture is removed after 10 days. A magnetic resonance imaging (MRI) is planned 1 year after surgery to check the result.

Suggested Readings

Al-Mefty O, Fox JL, Smith RR. Petrosal approach for petroclival meningiomas. Neurosurgery. 1988; 22(3):510–517

Angeli SI, De la Cruz A, Hitselberger W. The transcochlear approach revisited. Otol Neurotol. 2001; 22(5):690–695

Atlas MD, Moffat DA, Hardy DG. Petrous apex cholesteatoma: diagnostic and treatment dilemmas. Laryngoscope. 1992; 102(12 Pt 1):1363–1368

Axon PR, Fergie N, Saeed SR, Temple RH, Ramsden RT. Petrosal cholesteatoma: management considerations for minimizing morbidity. Am J Otol. 1999; 20(4):505–510

Bambakidis NC, Kakarla UK, Kim LJ, et al. Evolution of surgical approaches in the treatment of petroclival meningiomas: a retrospective review. Neurosurgery. 2007; 61(5) Suppl 2:202–209, discussion 209–211

Briggs RJ, Fabinyi G, Kaye AH. Current management of acoustic neuromas: review of surgical approaches and outcomes. J Clin Neurosci. 2000; 7(6):521–526

Browne JD, Fisch U. Transotic approach to the cerebellopontine angle. Otolaryngol Clin North Am. 1992; 25(2):331–346

Chen JM, Fisch U. The transotic approach in acoustic neuroma surgery. J Otolaryngol. 1993; 22(5):331–336

Danesi G, Cooper T, Panciera DT, Manni V, Côté DW. Sanna classification and prognosis of cholesteatoma of the petrous part of the temporal bone: a retrospective series of 81 patients. Otol Neurotol. 2016; 37(6):787–792

De la Cruz A, Teufert KB. Transcochlear approach to cerebellopontine angle and clivus lesions: indications, results, and complications. Otol Neurotol. 2009; 30 (3):373–380

De la Cruz A. The transcochlear approach to meningiomas and cholesteatomas of the cerebellopontine angle. In: Brackmann DE, ed. Neurological Surgery of the Ear and Skull Base. New York, NY: Raven Press; 1982:353–360

De la Cruz A. Transcochlear approach to lesions of the cerebellopontine angle and clivus. Rev Laryngol Otol Rhinol (Bord). 1981; 102(1–2):33–36

Fisch U, Mattox D. Microsurgery of the Skull Base. Stuttgart: Georg Thieme Veriag; 1988:74–135

Fisch U, Pillsbury HC. Infratemporal fossa approach to lesions in the temporal bone and base of the skull. Arch Otolaryngol. 1979; 105(2):99–107

Fournier HD, Mercier P, Velut S, Reigner B, Cronier P, Pillet J. Surgical anatomy and dissection of the petrous and peripetrous area: anatomic basis of the lateral approaches to the skull base. Surg Radiol Anat. 1994; 16(2):143–148

Gantz BJ, Fisch U. Modified transotic approach to the cerebellopontile angle. Arch Otolaryngol. 1983; 109(4):252–256

Glasscock ME, III, Woods CI, III, Poe DS, Patterson AK, Welling DB. Petrous apex cholesteatoma. Otolaryngol Clin North Am. 1989; 22(5):981–1002

Horn KL, Hankinson HL, Erasmus MD, Beauparalant PA. The modified transcochlear approach to the cerebellopontine angle. Otolaryngol Head Neck Surg. 1991; 104 (1):37–41

House JW, Brackmann DE. Facial nerve grading system. Otolaryngol Head Neck Surg. 1985; 93(2):146–147

House WF, De la Cruz A, Hitselberger WE. Surgery of the skull base: transcochlear approach to the petrous apex and clivus. Otolaryngology. 1978; 86(5):ORL-770–ORL-779

House WF, Hitselberger WE. The transcochlear approach to the skull base. Arch Otolaryngol. 1976; 102(6):334–342

House WF. Transcochlear approach to the petrous apex and clivus. Trans Sect Otolaryngol Am Acad Ophthalmol Otolaryngol. 1977; 84(5):ORL927–ORL931

Jackler RK, Sim DW, Gutin PH, Pitts LH. Systematic approach to intradural tumors ventral to the brain stem. Am J Otol. 1995; 16(1):39–51

Javed T, Sekhar LN. Surgical management of clival meningiomas. Acta Neurochir Suppl (Wien). 1991; 53:171–182

Jenkins HA, Fisch U. The transotic approach to resection of difficult acoustic tumors of the cerebellopontine angle. Am J Otol. 1980; 2(2):70–76

King TT, Benjamin JC, Morrison AW. Epidermoid and cholesterol cysts in the apex of the petrous bone. Br J Neurosurg. 1989; 3(4):451–461

Mayberg MR, Symon L. Meningiomas of the clivus and apical petrous bone. Report of 35 cases. J Neurosurg. 1986; 65(2):160–167

Moffat D, Jones S, Smith W. Petrous temporal bone cholesteatoma: a new classification and long-term surgical outcomes. Skull Base. 2008; 18(2):107–115

Pellet W, Cannoni M, Pech A. The widened transcochlear approach to jugular foramen tumors. J Neurosurg. 1988; 69(6):887–894

Profant M, Steno J. Petrous apex cholesteatoma. Acta Otolaryngol. 2000; 120 (2):164–167

Saleh EA, Taibah AK, Achilli V, Aristegui M, Mazzoni A, Sanna M. Posterior fossa meningioma: surgical strategy. Skull Base Surg. 1994; 4(4):202–212

Samii M, Tatagiba M. Experience with 36 surgical cases of petroclival meningiomas. Acta Neurochir (Wien). 1992; 118(1–2):27–32

Sanna M, Zini C, Gamoletti R, et al. Petrous bone cholesteatoma. Skull Base Surg. 1993; 3(4):201–213

Thedinger BA, Glasscock ME, III, Cueva RA. Transcochlear transtentorial approach for removal of large cerebellopontine angle meningiomas. Am J Otol. 1992; 13 (5):408–415

Chapter 7

Endoscopic Assisted Retrosigmoid Approach

7 Endoscopic Assisted Retrosigmoid Approach

Daniele Marchioni, Marco Bonali, Matteo Fermi, Barbara Masotto, Gianpietro Pinna, Matteo Alicandri Ciufelli, Giacomo Pavesi, and Livio Presutti

Abstract

The retrosigmoid route represents one of the traditional surgical approaches to the posterior cranial fossa and, in particular, to the cerebellopontine angle. The indications are neoplasms of the posterior cranial fossa and/or the cerebellopontine angle, like VIII cranial nerve schwannomas, meningiomas, epidermoid cysts, and metastases, with or without internal auditory canal involvement with/without serviceable hearing, symptomatic neurovascular conflicts, or brainstem implant placement. The retrosigmoid approach requires a retromastoid craniotomy (or craniectomy), a microscopic dissection with dural incision behind the sigmoid sinus, in order to expose the cerebellar cisterna and open the arachnoid to enter the subarachnoid space. This maneuver allows cerebrospinal fluid drainage, which is a key step to decompress the anatomical structures inside the cerebellopontine angle and to create enough space to work in this region. At the end of microscopic lesion removal, an angled optics is useful to help the surgeon dissect the pathology and remove the remnants with intrameatal extension inside the fundus of the internal auditory canal. In this way, an extensive drilling of the posterior portion of the internal auditory canal can be avoided. Other important things to consider are the possibility to check the relationship of the pathology with the anatomical structures in the cerebellopontine angle at the beginning of the procedure and the great value of the angled optics (45-degree and 70-degree lenses) during the final check to control the radicality of the excision. Moreover, in case of neurovascular conflict, the endoscope allows the surgeon to directly reach the area. In these cases, the magnification of the image also provides a better visualization of any possible anomalies of the nerve position, and the final check after the surgical procedure also allows the surgeon to be sure about the correct resolution of the conflict and to make an accurate hemostasis.

Keywords: retrosigmoid approach, acoustic neuroma, vestibular schwannoma, neurovascular conflict, cerebellopontine angle, internal auditory canal

7.1 Surgical Anatomy

The retrosigmoid approach requires thorough knowledge of the relationship between the nerves, the cerebellar surface and the vascular structures, the brainstem, and the bony landmarks in the cerebellopontine angle (CPA).

Three neurovascular complexes can be defined:

- The upper complex (III, IV, and V cranial nerves, midbrain, cerebellomesencephalic fissure, superior cerebellar artery, superior cerebellar peduncle, and tentorial surface of cerebellum);
- The middle complex (VI, VII, and VIII cranial nerves, pons, cerebellopontine fissure, anterior inferior cerebellar artery (AICA), middle cerebellar peduncle, and petrosal surface of cerebellum);
- The lower complex (IX, X, and XI cranial nerves, medulla, cerebellomedullary fissure, posterior inferior cerebellar artery, inferior cerebellar peduncle, occipital surface of cerebellum).

The acoustic-facial bundle arises from the brainstem. The VII cranial nerve originates from the supraolivar fossa about 1 to 2 mm anteriorly to the VIII cranial nerve and the intermediate nerve of Wrisberg. These two nerves join the facial nerve in the CPA, getting closer as they approach the internal auditory canal (IAC). In their course toward the posterior section of the petrous bone, the position of these nerves changes. Indeed, the position of the facial nerve with respect to the other nerves is anterior and medial until the IAC is reached, while when the porus is reached it becomes anterosuperior. The relationship of the extrameatal portion of acoustic-facial bundle must be kept in mind during surgery. In particular, as it approaches the IAC, it passes the superior petrosal vein (also known as *Dandy's vein*) and the AICA. Once the opening of the IAC is reached, the acoustic-facial bundle runs laterally toward the porus, where the transverse crest and vertical crest (also known as *Bill's bar*) divide it into four sections (see ▶ Fig. 7.24):

- Facial nerve anteriorly and superiorly
- Cochlear nerve anteriorly and inferiorly
- Superior vestibular nerve posteriorly and superiorly
- Inferior vestibular nerve posteriorly and inferiorly

At this level the variable pneumatization of the temporal bone plays an important role in the surgical planning. A highly pneumatized temporal bone, specifically when its petrous part is pneumatized, puts the patient at higher risk of developing a postoperative cerebrospinal fluid (CSF) leakage due to the extensive connection among the temporal bone cells created by means of drilling. Thus, a thorough preoperative study of the temporal bone is mandatory for this approach in order to evaluate the dimensions of the IAC and the presence of air cells around it.

Another important anatomic detail is the position of the jugular bulb which can be assessed through a preoperative computed tomography (CT) scan and magnetic resonance imaging (MRI). Sometimes it can have a high position in contact with the inferior portion of the IAC, leading the surgeon to the risk of damaging it while drilling.

7.2 Retrosigmoid Endoscopic Assisted Surgery

The retrosigmoid route is a microscopic approach, which allows a good exposure of the cerebellopontine angle, but a poor view of the fundus of the internal auditory canal. In order to optimize this approach to the IAC, several authors have developed this exclusive microscopic technique with endoscopic assistance. Indeed, through the use of the angled optics, it is easier to dissect the pathology and to remove the remnants of the disease with an intrameatal extension inside the fundus of the IAC. In this way, an extensive drilling of the posterior portion of the IAC can be avoided. Other important aspects to consider are the possibility to check the relationship of the pathology with the anatomical structures at the beginning of the procedure and the great value of an angled optics (45- and 70-degree lenses) during the final check to control the radicality of the excision. Therefore, the surgeon has a dynamic tool at his/her disposal to explore and treat a

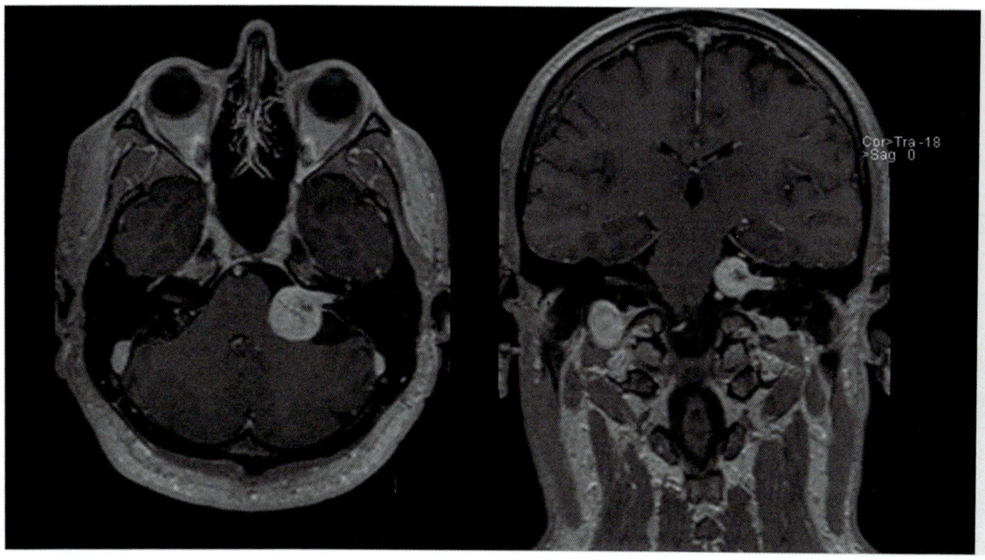

Fig. 7.1 Magnetic resonance imaging (MRI) in axial and coronal views showing an acoustic neuroma located in the cerebellopontine angle (CPA) with internal auditory canal (IAC) involvement. In case of normal hearing function, typically a retrosigmoid endoscopic assisted surgery with hearing preservation should be attempted.

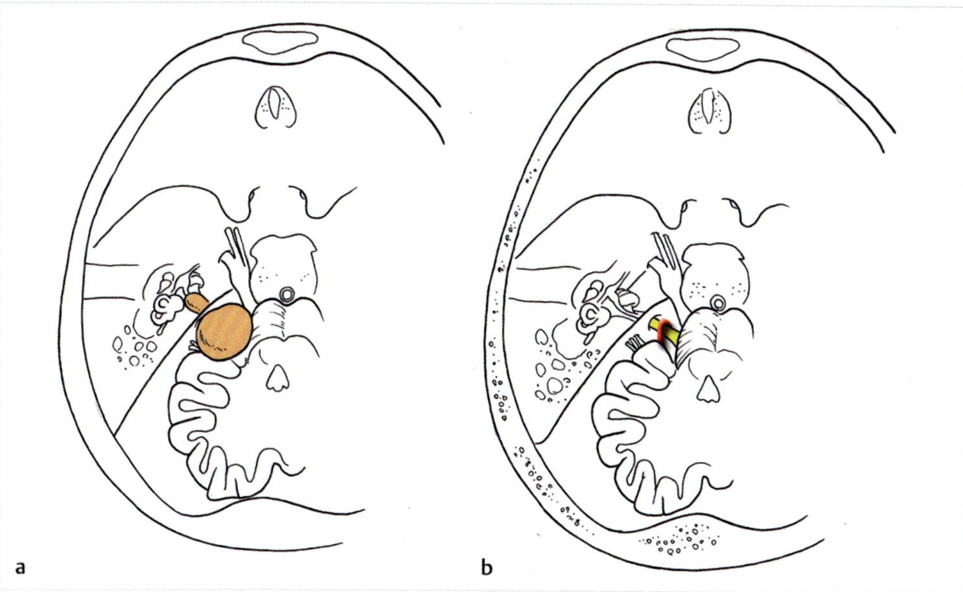

Fig. 7.2 Typical surgical indications for retrosigmoid approach: **(a)** Acoustic neuroma of the cerebellopontine angle (CPA) with internal auditory canal (IAC) involvement; **(b)** Neurovascular conflict between the anterior inferior cerebellar artery (AICA) and the acoustic-facial bundle.

very narrow and complex region, with neurovascular structures to preserve, thus ensuring a faster procedure and preserving the facial nerve and the auditory function as much as possible.

Another important application of this combined micro-endoscopic surgical technique is the treatment of neurovascular conflicts, a group of cranial nerves dysfunctions due to a conflict between a blood vessel and the neural structure. Because of the usual localization of these diseases at the level of the CPA, the most involved cranial nerves are the V, VII, and IX, and the vessels which are often responsible for the compression are mainly arterial. The entry zone represents the most affected region; therefore, the standard microscopic approach would require retractors to manipulate the cerebellum and gain more space to expose this anatomical area, with the risk of damaging the brain tissue during the manipulation. On the contrary, the endoscope enables the surgeon to directly reach the area of the neurovascular conflict. Moreover, the magnification of the image provides a better visualization of possible anomalies of the nerve position or modifications of the neural surface (i.e., color alterations, decubitus, or indentations). The final check after the surgical procedure also allows the surgeon to be sure about the correct resolution of the conflict and to make an accurate hemostasis.

7.3 Indications

- Neoplasms of the posterior cranial fossa and/or the CPA, like VIII cranial nerve schwannomas, or meningiomas (see Clinical Case 6), epidermoids and metastases, with or without IAC involvement with/without serviceable hearing (see ▶ Fig. 7.1 and ▶ Fig. 7.2a);
- Symptomatic neurovascular conflicts (see ▶ Fig. 7.2b and Clinical Cases 8–10);
- Brainstem implant (see Clinical Case 7).

7.4 Contraindications

Because of the additional value of the endoscope combined with the microscope for this surgical approach, there are no major contraindications to this technique. The surgeon must be aware

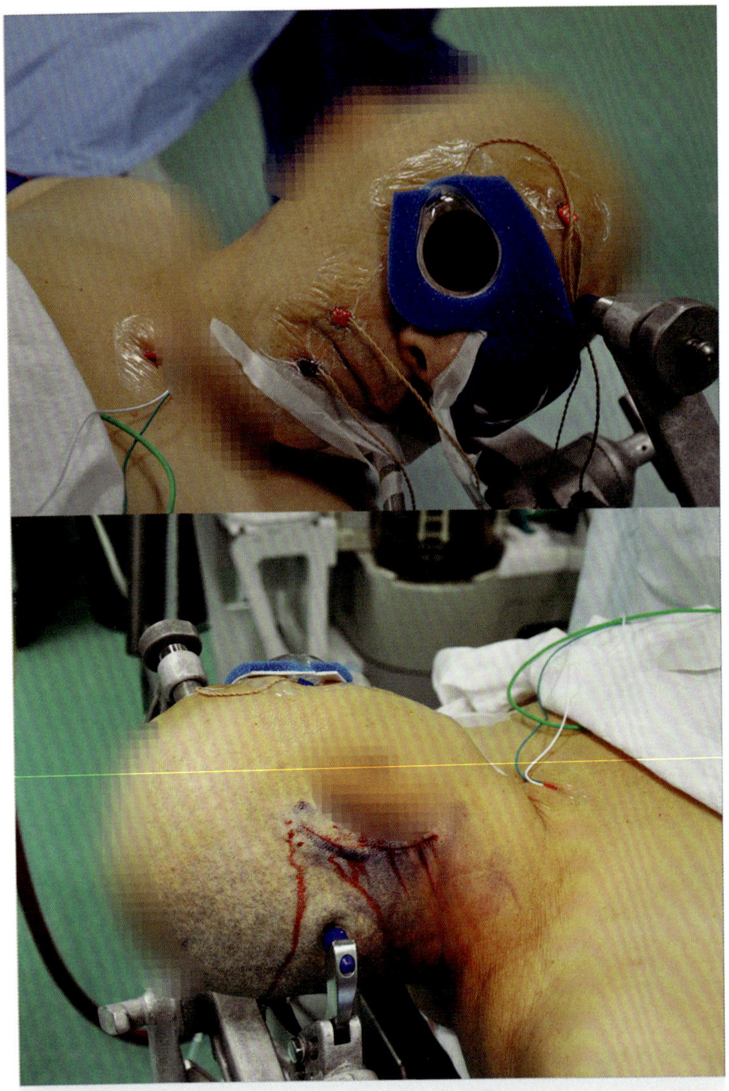

Fig. 7.3 Head is in a supine position during a retrosigmoid approach. The Mayfield head holder is positioned to keep the position of the head constant.

of some relative limitations, especially due to some anatomical variations:

- A high-riding jugular bulb can be a loose limitation for the surgeon if it encroaches on the inferior wall of the IAC.
- In case of pneumatization of the temporal bone, particularly around the IAC, the surgeon must be very careful while drilling through this region. If these air cells are not properly occluded with bone wax, the risk of CSF leak increases.

Finally, in case of a neoplasm with exclusive involvement of the CPA and without extension to the fundus of the IAC, the role of the endoscope can be limited. On the other hand, an initial exploration of the anatomical area and a final check for radicality of the excision are helpful options that go beyond imaging findings.

7.5 Advantages

- Fast access
- No limitation in case of a particularly large jugular bulb
- Safer dissection of the pathology from the facial nerve at the level of the anterior lip of the porus (at this level the nerve is really vulnerable)

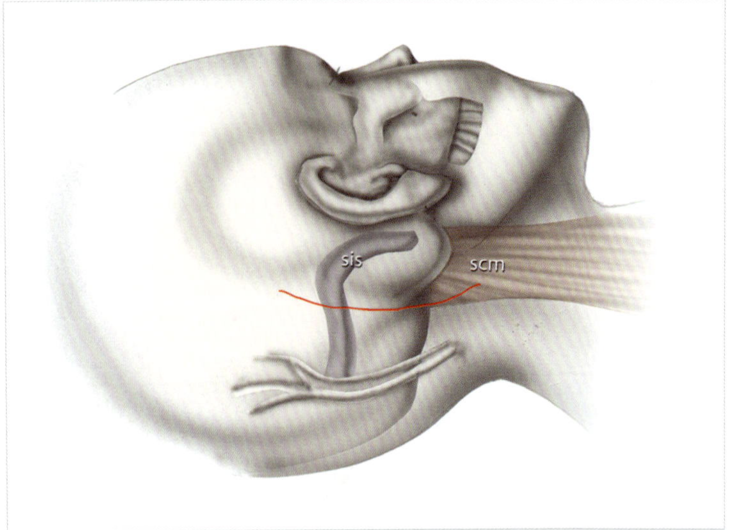

Fig. 7.4 Right ear: Skin incision. The location of the major landmarks of the retrosigmoid approach is also visible. *scm: sternocleidomastoid muscle; sis: sigmoid sinus.*

- Easier repair in case of perimeatal cell dehiscence
- Possibility to expose the fundus of the IAC avoiding extensive drilling of the outer portion of the IAC
- Possible hearing preservation (depending on the size of the tumor)
- Complete control of the posterior cranial fossa
- Low risk of postoperative CSF leakage (watertight closure of the dura)
- Low risk of meningitis

7.6 Surgical Approach for Acoustic Neuroma Removal

The patient is in a supine position with the head rotated away from the surgeon and a flexed neck. A Mayfield holder is placed to maintain a constant position of the head and to prevent decubitus (see ▶ Fig. 7.3). Facial nerve monitoring is needed. A retroauricular incision of the skin is made about 3 cm behind the retroauricular sulcus in order to expose the occipital bone posterior to the sigmoid sinus and inferior to the transverse sinus (see ▶ Fig. 7.4). The temporal muscle is incised until the bone is exposed and then detached with a periosteal elevator until the digastric insertion on the mastoid tip is reached (see ▶ Fig. 7.5 and Clinical Case 1; ▶ Fig. 7.26, ▶ Fig. 7.27, ▶ Fig. 7.28). A 4 cm × 4 cm craniotomy is performed with a cutting bur starting from the inferior margin of the transverse sinus until the posterior portion of the sigmoid sinus is exposed, completing the identification of the anterior and superior landmarks of the surgical access (see ▶ Fig. 7.5 and Clinical Case 1, ▶ Fig. 7.29 and ▶ Fig. 7.30). The last bony layer over the dura is carefully removed by means of a septal dissector; a diamond bur is used to enlarge the opening especially inferiorly to gain a proper access (see ▶ Fig. 7.6). The bone dust and bone island are preserved for the following reconstructive phase. A small (2 mm) dural incision is made just posteriorly to the sigmoid sinus to decompress and limit the cerebellar herniation. During this maneuver a CSF leak from the incision is to be expected. The incision of the dura is completed, forming a half-moon behind the sigmoid sinus (see ▶ Fig. 7.7 and Clinical

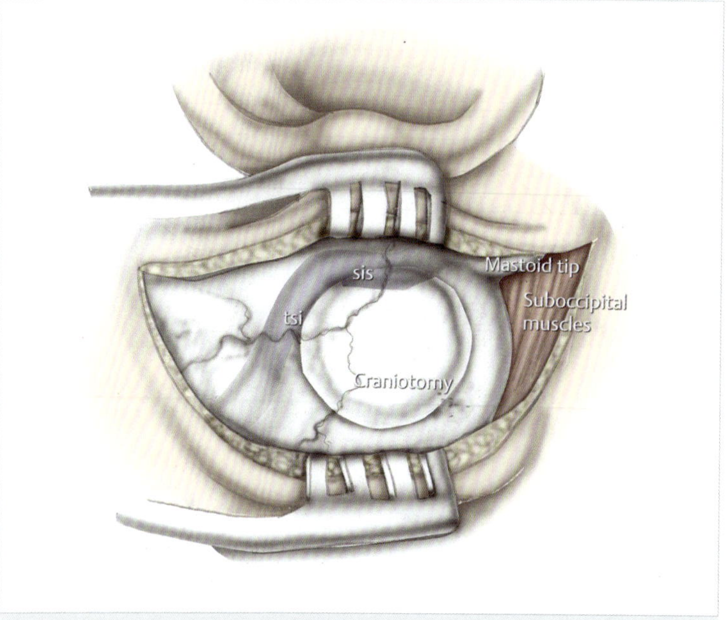

Fig. 7.5 Right ear: The flap is elevated, uncovering the occipital and mastoid bone up to the tip. The 4 cm × 4 cm craniotomy is performed posteriorly to the sigmoid sinus. *sis: sigmoid sinus; tsi: transverse sinus.*

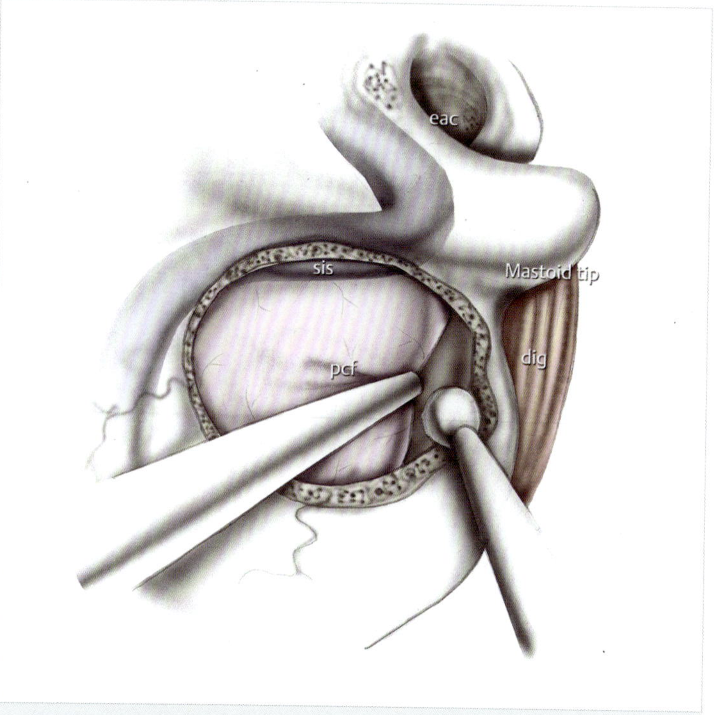

Fig. 7.6 Right ear: Once the craniotomy is performed, the dura of the posterior fossa is elevated, and a diamond bur is used to enlarge the surgical approach inferiorly. *dig: digastric muscle; eac: external auditory canal; pcf: posterior cranial fossa; sis: sigmoid sinus.*

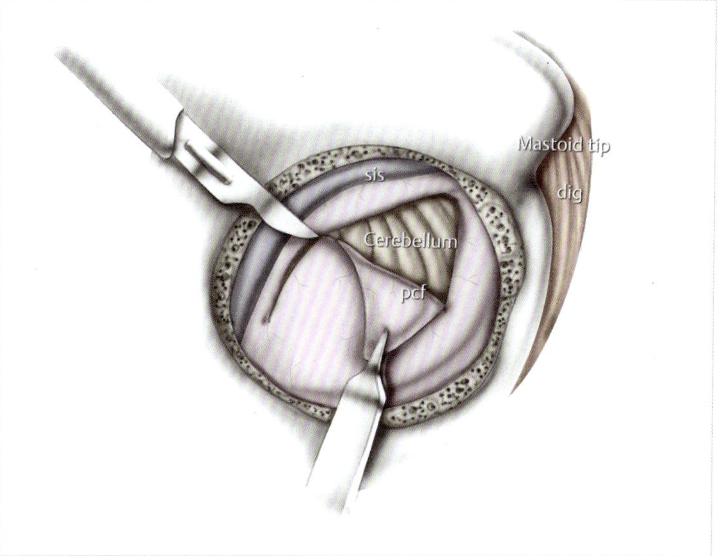

Fig. 7.7 Right ear: A half-moon shape dural incision behind the sigmoid sinus is performed. *dig: digastric muscle; pcf: posterior cranial fossa; sis: sigmoid sinus.*

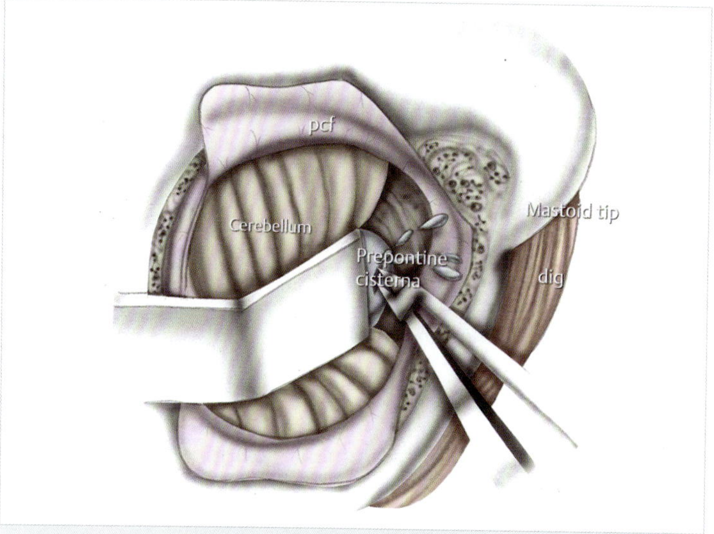

Fig. 7.8 Right ear: The cerebellum is carefully elevated, exposing the cerebellar cisterna; a pair of microscissors is used to remove the arachnoid entering the subarachnoid space where the cerebrospinal fluid (CSF) flows. *dig: digastric muscle; pcf: posterior cranial fossa.*

Case 1, ▶ Fig. 7.31). The surgeon uses a small dissector, carefully elevating the cerebellum in order to expose the cerebellar cisterna and open the arachnoid to enter the subarachnoid space where the CSF flows (see ▶ Fig. 7.8). This maneuver leads to CFS drainage which is a key step to decompress the anatomical structures inside the CPA and to create enough space to work.

The dural flaps are suspended using stay sutures and the cerebellum is exposed. The cerebellum is detached from the arachnoid layer and from the posterior section of the petrous bone avoiding the traditional use of the retractor (see ▶ Fig. 7.9; also see Clinical Case 1, ▶ Fig. 7.32 and ▶ Fig. 7.33). The CPA with the tumor is exposed (see ▶ Fig. 7.10; also see Clinical Case 1, ▶ Fig. 7.34, ▶ Fig. 7.35, ▶ Fig. 7.36, ▶ Fig. 7.37, ▶ Fig. 7.38). A neurosurgical cottonoid is placed on the surface of the cerebellum to protect it throughout the surgery. The arachnoid layers are microscopically dissected from the tumor. An endoscopic exploration of the CPA is carried out with a 0-degree endoscope in order to evaluate the relationship between the tumor and the other important anatomical structures of this area (e.g., facial nerve, cochlear nerve, Dandy's vein, AICA, PICA, trigeminal nerve, lower cranial nerves) (see Clinical Case 1, ▶ Fig. 7.38, ▶ Fig. 7.39, ▶ Fig. 7.40, ▶ Fig. 7.41, ▶ Fig. 7.42). The facial nerve is very often hidden by the neoplasm. An endoscopic detection of the entry zone, where the facial nerve lies more anteriorly and inferiorly to the vestibulocochlear nerve, is recommended. A small dissector is useful to gently displace the mass so that its relationship with the nerve can be understood. Moreover, it might be useful to follow the nerve from the entry point toward the porus of the IAC if

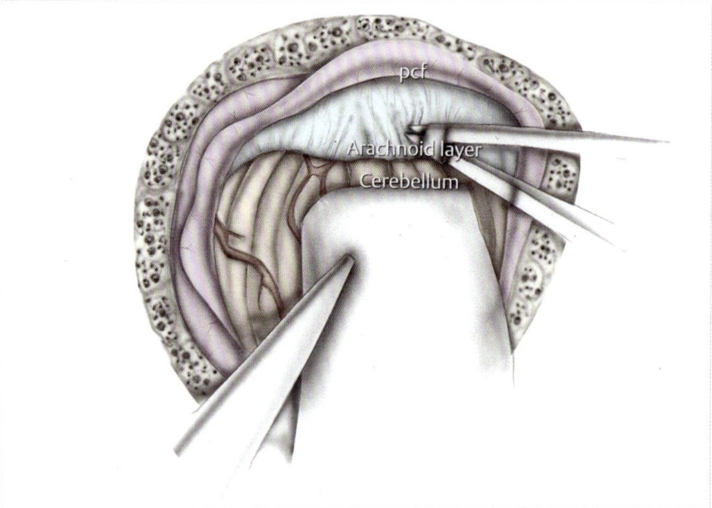

Fig. 7.9 Right ear: A pair of microscissors is used to cut the arachnoid layer entering the prepontine cisterna, exposing the cerebellopontine angle (CPA). *pcf: posterior cranial fossa.*

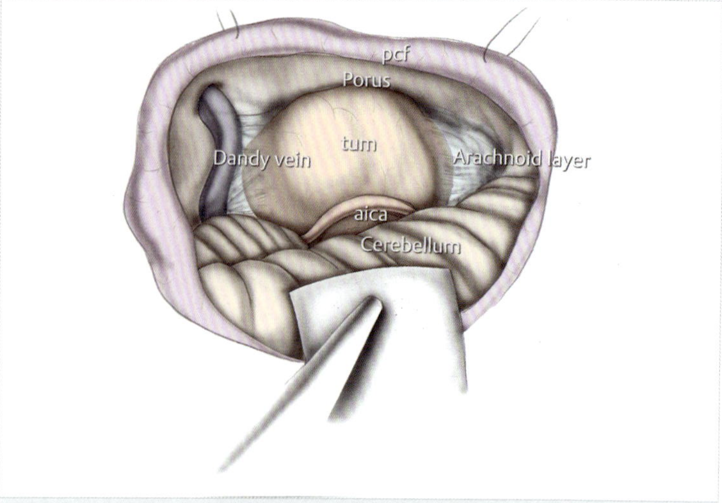

Fig. 7.10 Right ear: Once the cerebellopontine angle (CPA) is microscopically exposed, the acoustic tumor is detected in the middle of the surgical field. *aica: anterior inferior cerebellar artery; pcf: posterior cranial fossa; tum: tumor.*

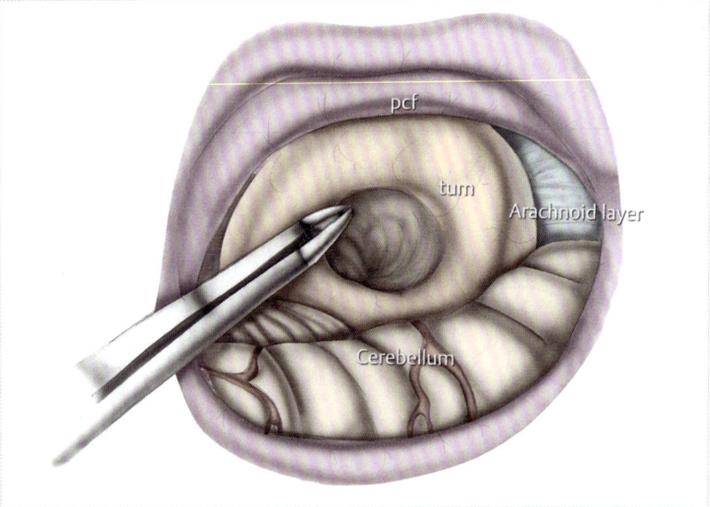

Fig. 7.11 Right ear: A central debulking of the tumor mass is performed. *pcf: posterior cranial fossa; tum: tumor.*

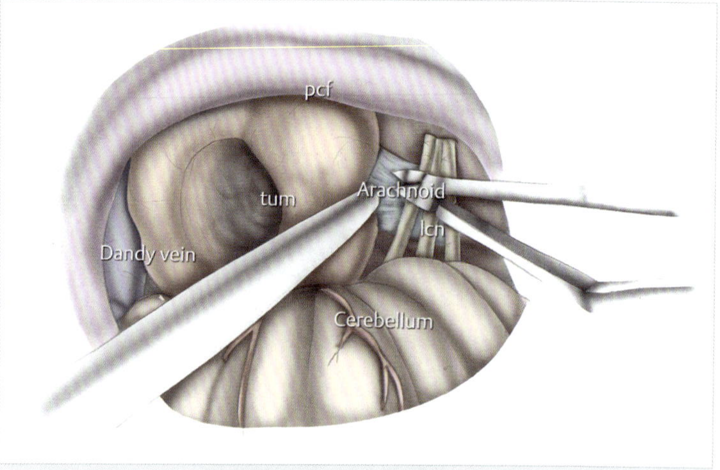

Fig. 7.12 Right ear: Debulking of the tumor is performed, reducing the mass in the middle. This procedure allows the dislocation of the mass and the identification of the lower cranial nerves. A gentle dissection of the tumor from the lower cranial nerve is performed. *lcn: lower cranial nerves; pcf: posterior cranial fossa; tum: tumor.*

possible. The tumor is microscopically reduced in size by means of an ultrasound suction instrument positioned in the middle of the mass to debulk the neoplasm (see ▶ Fig. 7.11). Sometimes this surgical step is needed to mobilize the tumor and to localize the facial nerve at the entry point. Later, a careful dissection of the capsule from the surrounding structures is performed (see ▶ Fig. 7.12, ▶ Fig. 7.13, ▶ Fig. 7.14). Whenever possible the cochlear nerve should be dissected and preserved, especially in patients with residual hearing function (see ▶ Fig. 7.15 and ▶ Fig. 7.16). Once the extrameatal portion of the tumor has been completely excised, the residual tumor at the level of the meatus of the IAC is microscopically visualized (see ▶ Fig. 7.17; also see Clinical Case 1, ▶ Fig. 7.43, ▶ Fig. 7.44, ▶ Fig. 7.45). The porus is microscopically identified and two dural flaps are created exposing the bone around the porus (see ▶ Fig. 7.18). A diamond bur is used to drill and enlarge the opening of the porus (see ▶ Fig. 7.19). In this way the endoscopic time for tumor removal in the IAC is facilitated. When the porus has already been enlarged by the tumor mass, the drilling of the porus may be avoided.

Further surgical steps will be managed endoscopically. A 45-degree endoscope (18 cm length, 4 mm diameter) is gently

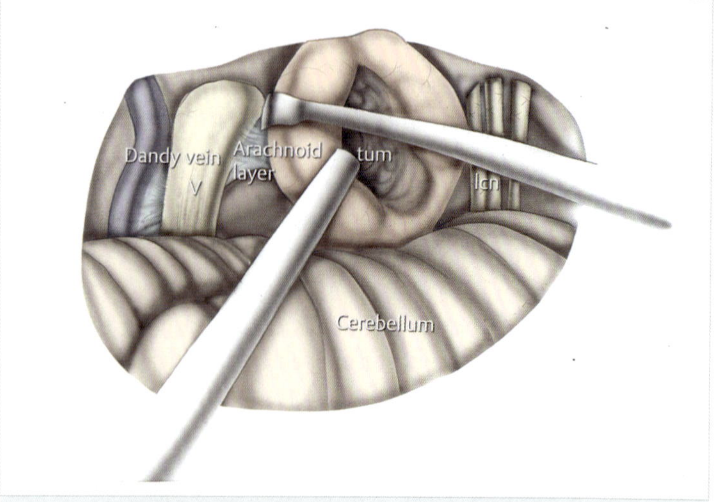

Fig. 7.13 Right ear: The trigeminal nerve is detected, and the surrounding arachnoid layer is cut, permitting the dislocation of the tumor mass from the nerve. *lcn: lower cranial nerves; tum: tumor.*

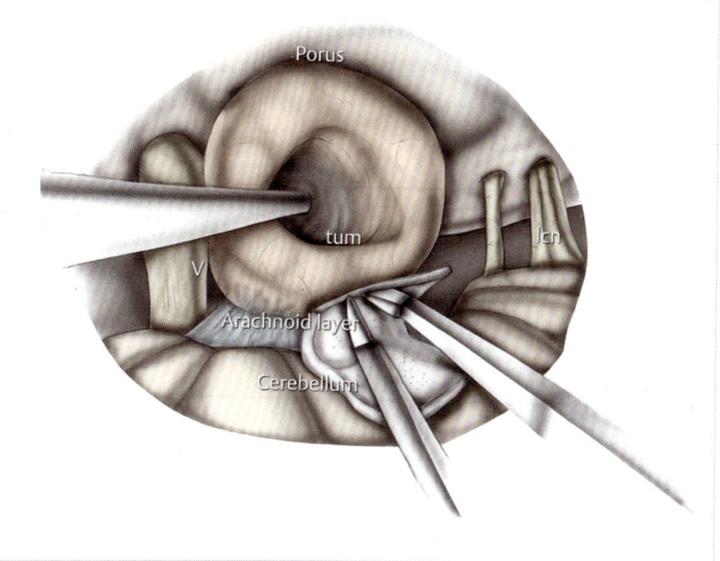

Fig. 7.14 Right ear: A cottonoid is used to gently dissect the tumor mass from the brainstem. *lcn: lower cranial nerves; tum: tumor.*

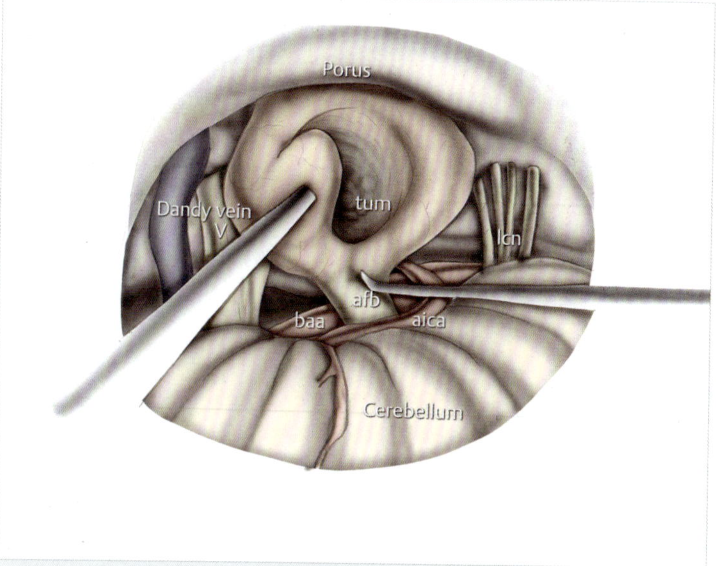

Fig. 7.15 Right ear: The acoustic-facial bundle at the entry zone is identified. *afb: acoustic-facial bundle; aica: anterior inferior cerebellar artery; baa: basilar artery; lcn: lower cranial nerves; tum: tumor.*

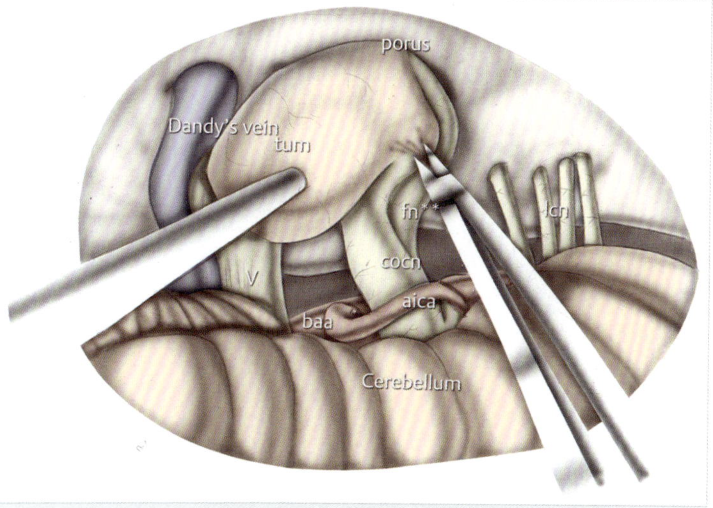

Fig. 7.16 Right ear: The tumor is progressively removed from the cerebellopontine angle (CPA), preserving the cochlear and facial nerves. *aica: anterior inferior cerebellar artery; baa: basilar artery; cocn: cochlear nerve; fn**: facial nerve into the CPA; lcn: lower cranial nerves; tum: tumor.*

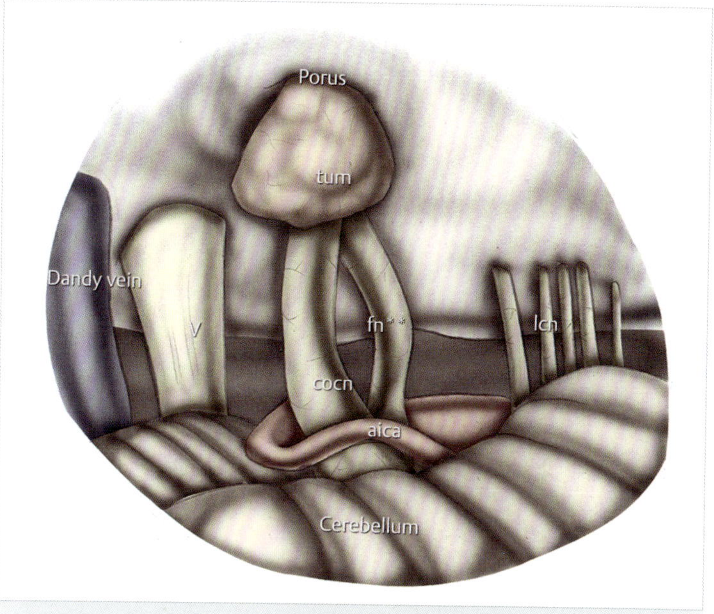

Fig. 7.17 Right ear: A residual tumor in the internal auditory canal (IAC) is found. *aica: anterior inferior cerebellar artery; cocn: cochlear nerve; fn**: facial nerve into the cerebellopontine angle (CPA); lcn: lower cranial nerves; tum: tumor.*

inserted following the neurosurgical cottonoid placed on the cerebellar surface avoiding contact with the adjacent nerves and vessels (see ▶ Fig. 7.20). The facial nerve is detected and followed into the IAC, which can be enlarged by the tumor simplifying the surgical maneuvers (see ▶ Fig. 7.21 and ▶ Fig. 7.22; also see Clinical Case 1 and Clinical Case 2). In this case the residual disease is removed from the fundus using an angulated dissector. On the other hand, when the intrameatal portion of the neoplasm reaches the fundus of the IAC and the porus has not been enlarged by the tumor mass, further drilling of the porus of the IAC may be required to create enough space for the endoscopic removal of the acoustic neuroma from the fundus. During this step the surgeon must be careful not to open the temporal bone cells close to the IAC. If it happens, the endoscope allows the detection of the defect and its immediate repair with bone powder and/or a fragment of muscle fixed with fibrin glue. The lateral portion of the porus is drilled until the dura mater of the IAC is exposed. If needed, the dura of the IAC can be opened to access the IAC. Dissection of the tumor is performed in a medial to lateral direction, being careful to preserve the facial nerve and the internal auditory artery (see ▶ Fig. 7.23 and ▶ Fig. 7.24). If the intrameatal portion of the tumor is encapsulated, its dissection en bloc from the anatomical structures of the IAC is easier to accomplish, because the mass is easily dissociable from other structures. On the other hand, if the intrameatal portion of the tumor is not encapsulated and the surrounding structures are attached to the mass, the dissection can be much harder. Angled dissectors with various shapes and sizes are used to remove the residual neoplasms from the IAC from the fundus to the CPA (see Clinical Case 3 and Clinical Case 4). Facial nerve monitoring is

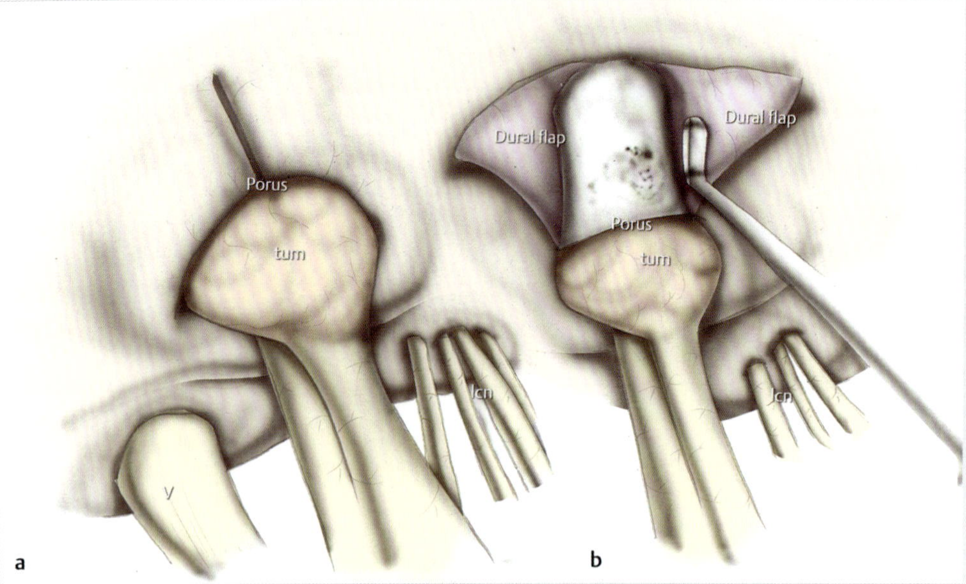

Fig. 7.18 Right ear: Incision of the dural layer on the porus is carried out **(a)** and two dural flaps are created, uncovering the bone of the porus **(b)**. *lcn: lower cranial nerves; tum: tumor.*

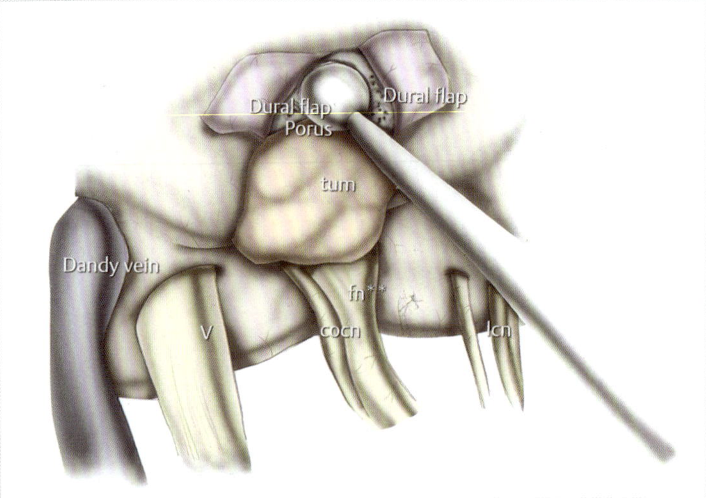

Fig. 7.19 Right ear: A diamond bur is used to drill the bone on the porus, reaching the dura of the internal auditory canal (IAC). *cocn: cochlear nerve; fn**: facial nerve into the cerebellopontine angle (CPA); lcn: lower cranial nerves; tum: tumor.*

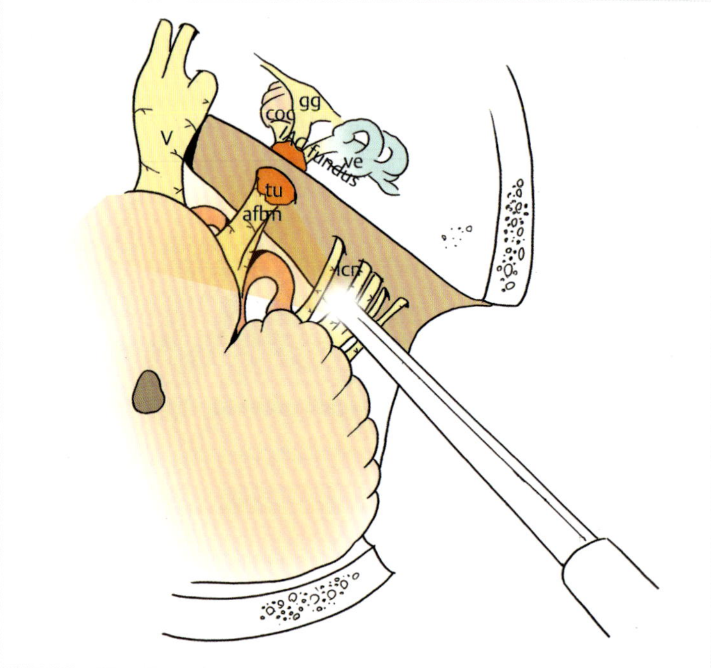

Fig. 7.20 Right ear: A 0-degree endoscope is introduced into the cerebellopontine angle (CPA) through the surgical cavity, detecting the residual tumor in the internal auditory canal (IAC). *afb: acoustic facial bundle; coc: cochlea; gg: geniculate ganglion; lcn: lower cranial nerves; tum: tumor; ve: vestibule.*

crucial in this phase allowing the surgeon to immediately abandon any surgical maneuvers that stress the nerve too much. Ringer solution is used to clean the IAC and/or to avoid depolarization of the nerve fibers. A final endoscopic/microscopic check for bleeding control is needed (see Clinical Case 5). A watertight closure of the dura is performed. A piece of muscle with a transfixion suture is used to repair small defects on the dural flap (see ▶ Fig. 7.25). The bony island is repositioned. Bone dust and Spongostan are used to close the defect around the bone. Muscular, subcutaneous, and cutaneous layers are sutured. After surgery, the patient is kept under observation in the intensive care unit for 24 to 36 hours. A CT is carried out 6 hours after surgery. Antibiotics are used in the immediate postoperative period. Another CT is carried out 48 to 72 hours after surgery.

7.7 Surgical Approach for Neurovascular Conflicts

Some clinical disorders may be the manifestations of neurovascular conflicts in the CPA. These disorders generally cause unbearably painful attacks or involuntary muscular contraction of the face and treatment needs to be found. The following are the major neurovascular disorders located in the CPA.

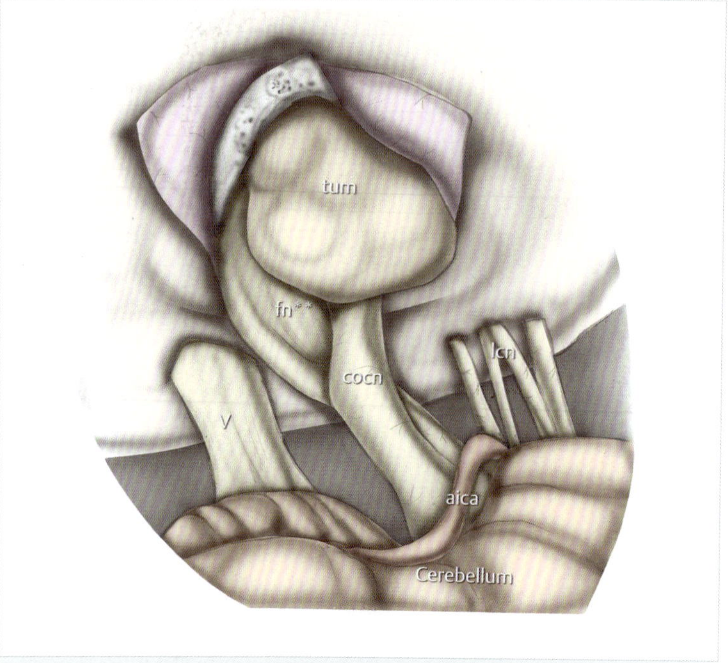

Fig. 7.21 Right ear: The tumor in the internal auditory canal (IAC) is endoscopically exposed. *aica: anterior inferior cerebellar artery; cocn: cochlear nerve; fn**: facial nerve into the cerebellopontine angle (CPA); lcn: lower cranial nerves; tum: tumor.*

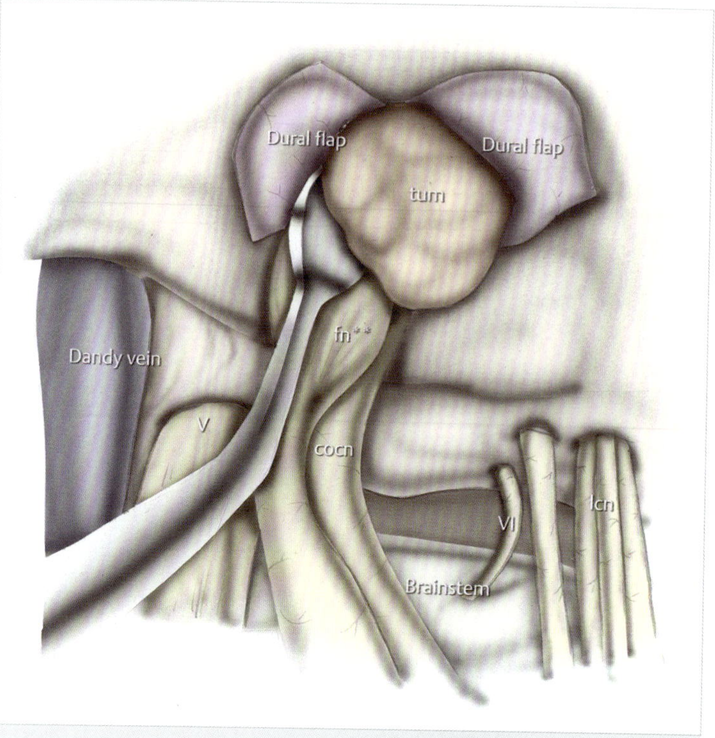

Fig. 7.22 Right ear: Once the dura of the internal auditory canal (IAC) is opened, a curve dissector is used to gently endoscopically dissect the residual tumor from the IAC, carefully preserving the facial nerve. *cocn: cochlear nerve; fn**: facial nerve into the cerebellopontine angle (CPA); lcn: lower cranial nerves; tum: tumor.*

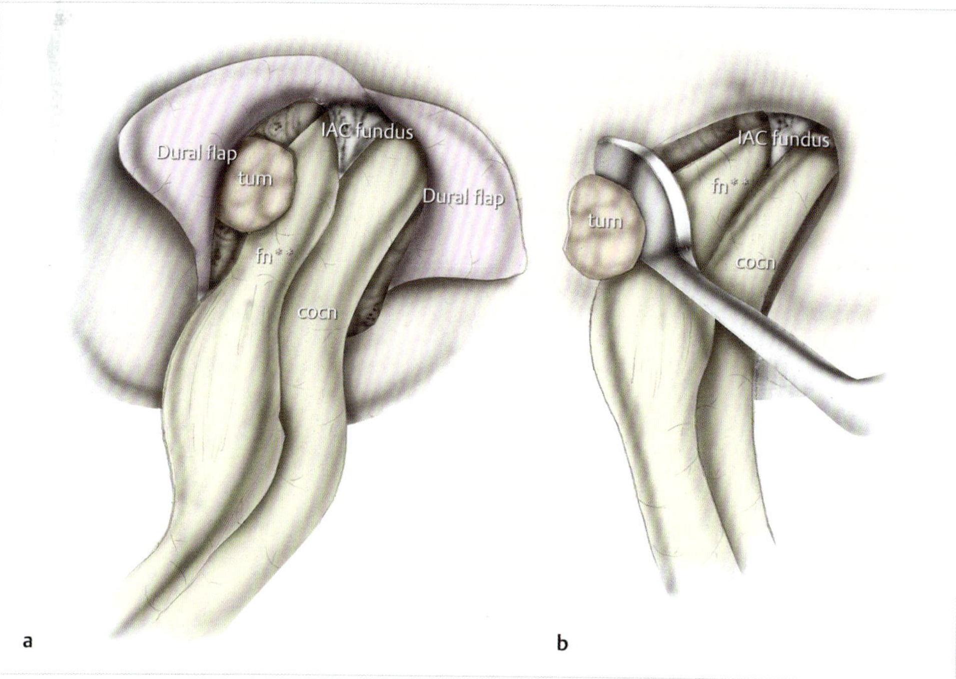

Fig. 7.23 Right ear: Once the tumor has been removed, a 45-degree endoscope is used to detect the fundus of the internal auditory canal (IAC), looking for residual tumor. In case of a remnant, a curve dissector should be used to remove the residual tumor from the fundus using a 45-degree endoscope **(a, b)**. Whenever possible the preservation of the acoustic nerve is attempted. *cocn: cochlear nerve; fn**: facial nerve into the IAC; tum: tumor.*

7.7.1 Trigeminal Neuralgia

This rare disease is characterized by intermittent attacks of severe and debilitating facial pain that occurs along the distribution of the trigeminal branches. In the majority of cases the trigeminal nerve is compressed by an aberrant artery (the superior cerebellar artery) or venous structures at the level of the root entry zone of this nerve (see Clinical Case 8, ▶ Fig. 7.109, ▶ Fig. 7.110, ▶ Fig. 7.111).

7.7.2 Hemifacial Spasm

This is characterized by a unilateral, involuntary, sporadic contraction of the musculature innervated by the facial nerve (bilateral involvement is extremely rare but possible). Most of the times, ectatic blood vessels are found that exert pressure on or keep contact with the facial nerve in the CPA or a loop artery around the facial nerve can cause compression of this nerve. (The inferior cerebellar artery is often involved in this neurovascular contact.)

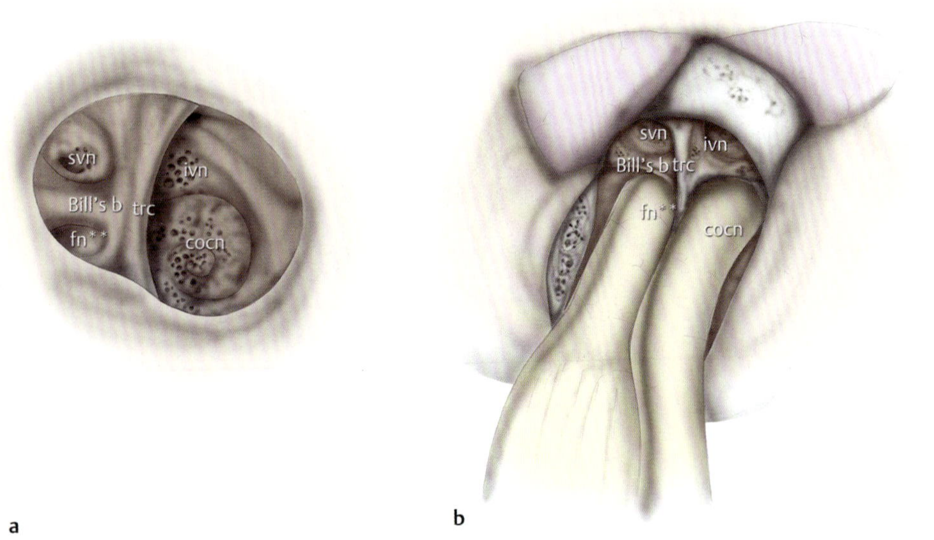

Fig. 7.24 Right ear: Final check of the fundus. A 70-degree endoscope may be used to visualize the anatomy of the fundus of the internal auditory canal (IAC). **(a)** Bony anatomy of the fundus in surgical position; **(b)** Final view of the fundus after tumor removal with preservation of the facial and cochlear nerves. *Bill's b: Bill's bar; cocn: cochlear nerve; fn**: facial nerve into the IAC; ivn: inferior vestibular nerve; svn: superior vestibular nerve; trc: transverse crest.*

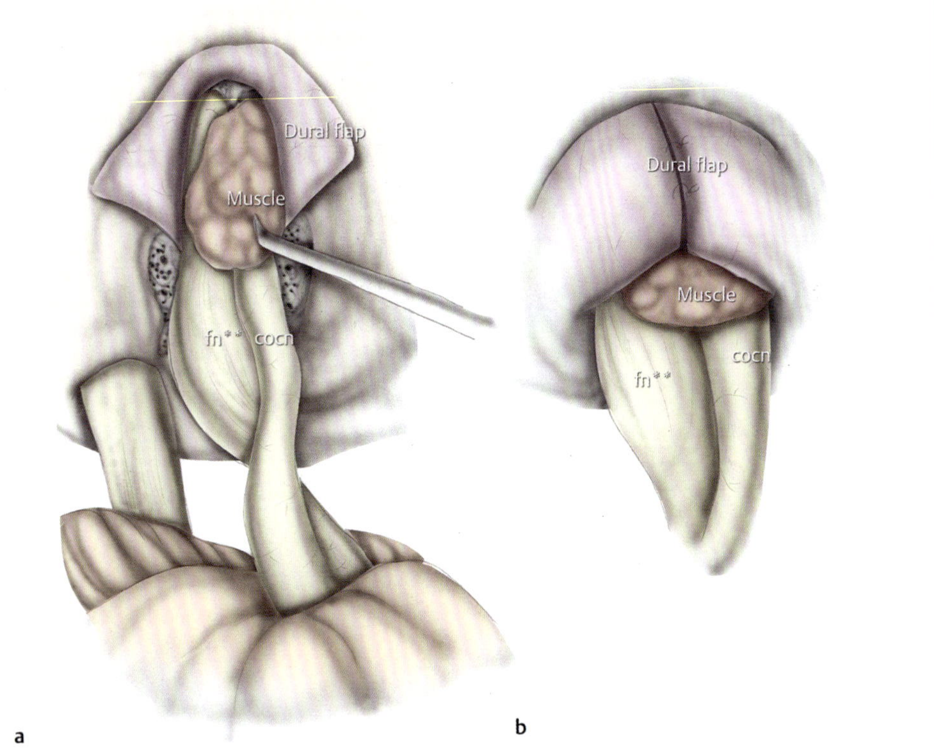

Fig. 7.25 Right ear. **(a)** A piece of muscle is used to obliterate the internal auditory canal (IAC). **(b)** The dural flap is replaced and sutured. *cocn: cochlear nerve; fn**: facial nerve into the IAC.*

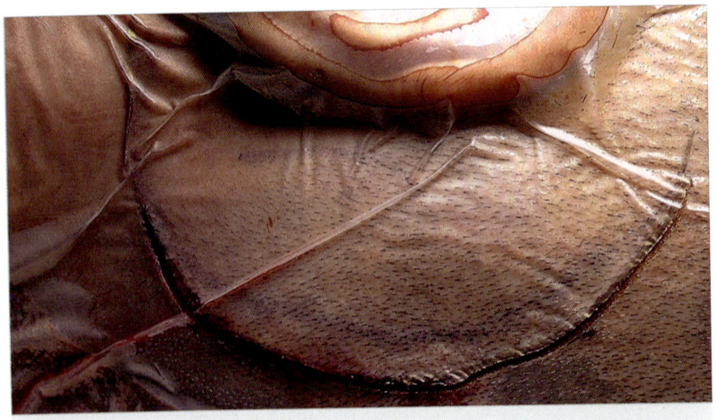

Fig. 7.26 Clinical Case 1, Left ear: The skin incision is performed.

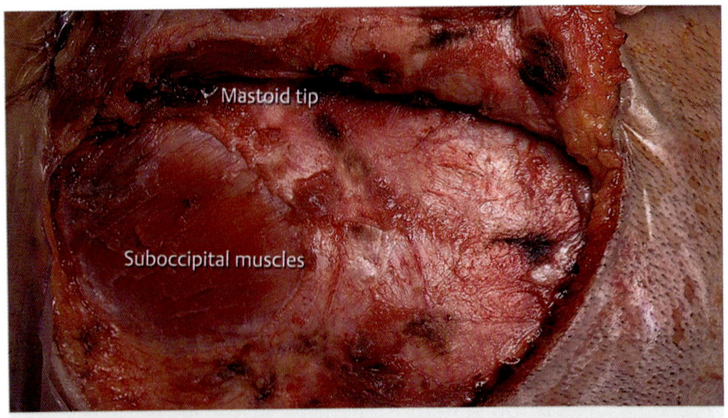

Fig. 7.27 Clinical Case 1, Left ear: The skin flap is elevated and the suboccipital muscles and the mastoid tip are detected.

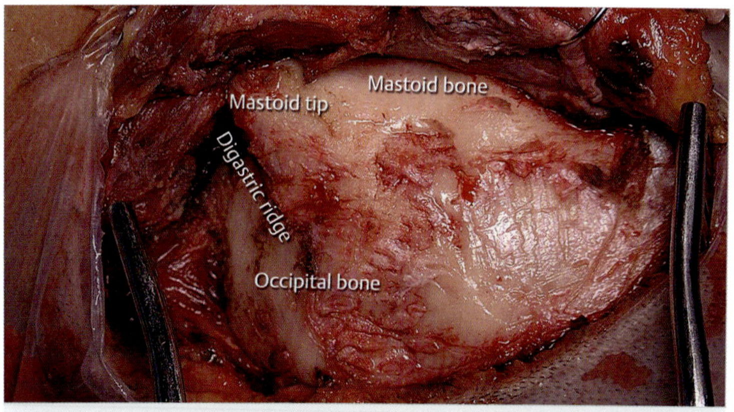

Fig. 7.28 Clinical Case 1, Left ear: The occipitomastoid bone is uncovered; the anatomical bony landmarks are visible.

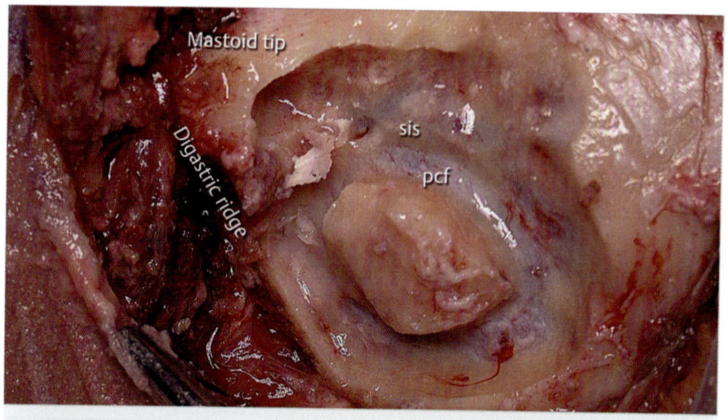

Fig. 7.29 Clinical Case 1, Left ear: The retrosigmoid craniotomy is started; a bony island is created. *pcf: posterior cranial fossa; sis: sigmoid sinus.*

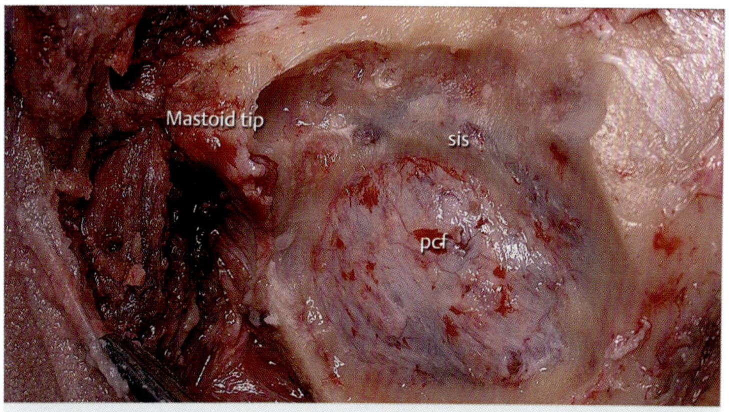

Fig. 7.30 Clinical Case 1, Left ear: The craniotomy is performed, the bony island is removed, and the dura of posterior cranial fossa is exposed. *pcf: posterior cranial fossa; sis: sigmoid sinus.*

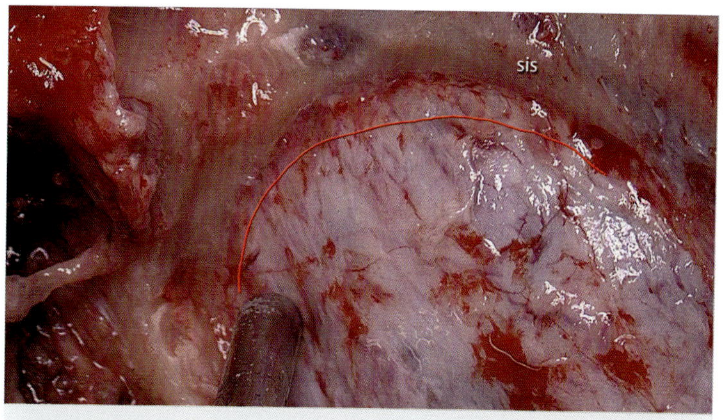

Fig. 7.31 Clinical Case 1, Left ear: The line of incision along the sigmoid sinus is planned. *sis: sigmoid sinus.*

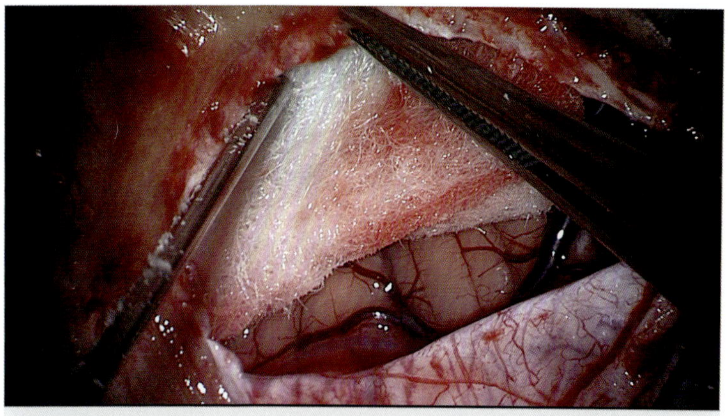

Fig. 7.32 Clinical Case 1, Left ear: The incision of the dura is completed, forming a half-moon shape behind the sigmoid sinus. The dural layer margins are suspended using stay sutures and the cerebellum is thus exposed.

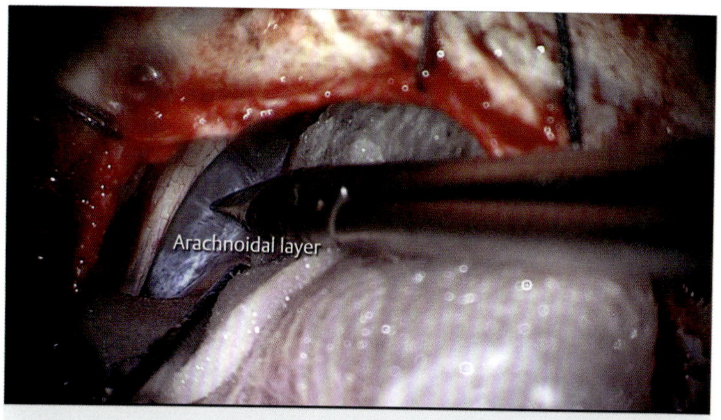

Fig. 7.33 Clinical Case 1, Left ear: To avoid trauma to the cerebellum, neurosurgical cottonoids are placed on the surface of cerebellum. The arachnoid layer is cut using microscissos.

7.7.3 Glossopharyngeal Neuralgia

This extremely rare disease is characterized by paroxysmal attacks associated with severe and debilitating pain along the distribution of the glossopharyngeal branches. (The pain distribution includes the soft palate, the base of the tongue, the pharyngeal pillar and tonsil, the posterior pharyngeal wall, and the inner ear.) Vagal stimulation is also possible, causing hypotension, bradycardia, and syncope. Neurovascular compression is also found to be the cause of this rare clinical entity.

Once the clinical examination has been performed and the suspected disease is confirmed, in all cases MRI is required to visualize the neurovascular conflict before the surgical treatment.

Surgery is proposed when the conflict is visible on MRI, or when it is strongly suspected, and when the symptoms are intolerable and greatly reduce the quality of life of the patient; the retrosigmoid approach is the surgery of choice.

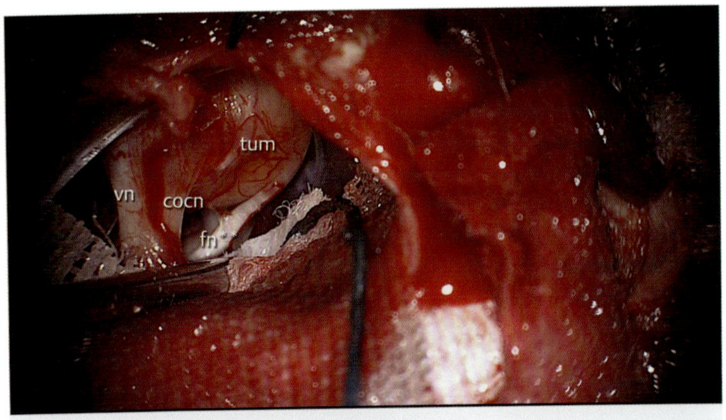

Fig. 7.34 Clinical Case 1, Left ear: The tumor in the cerebellopontine angle (CPA) is exposed. *cocn: cochlear nerve; fn**: facial nerve in the CPA; tum: tumor; vn: vestibular nerve.*

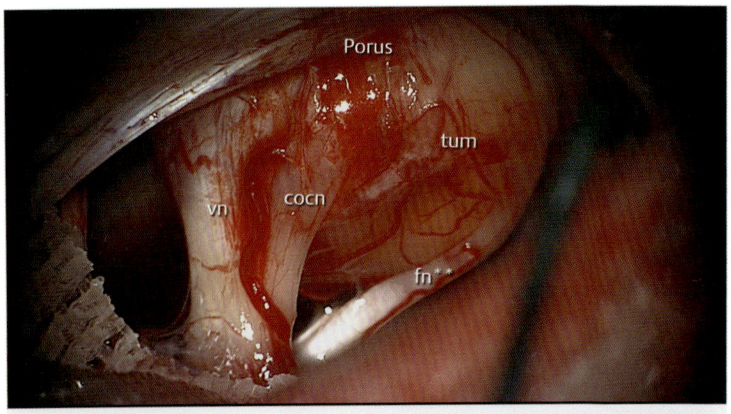

Fig. 7.35 Clinical Case 1, Left ear: Microscopic view of the cerebellopontine angle (CPA); the tumor is visible. An anterior displacement of the facial nerve from the tumor mass is noted. *cocn: cochlear nerve; fn**: facial nerve in the CPA; tum: tumor; vn: vestibular nerve.*

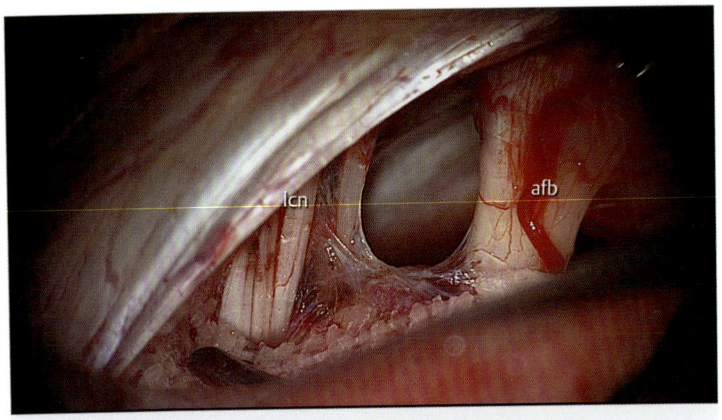

Fig. 7.36 Clinical Case 1, Left ear: The lower cranial nerve is microscopically detected. *afb: acoustic facial bundle; lcn: lower cranial nerves.*

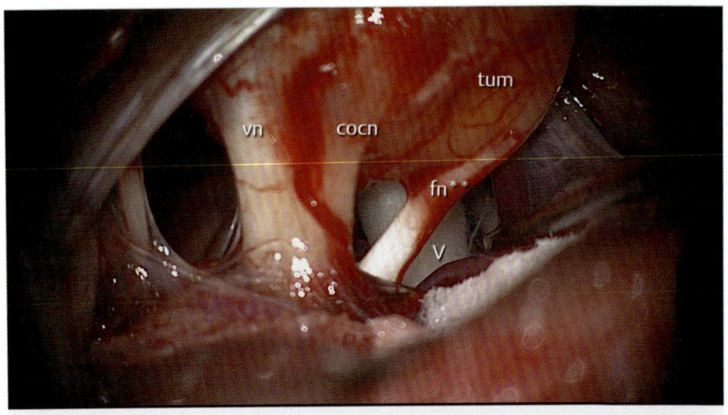

Fig. 7.37 Clinical Case 1, Left ear: The trigeminal nerve is seen under the tumor. *cocn: cochlear nerve; fn**: facial nerve in the cerebellopontine angle (CPA); tum: tumor; vn: vestibular nerve.*

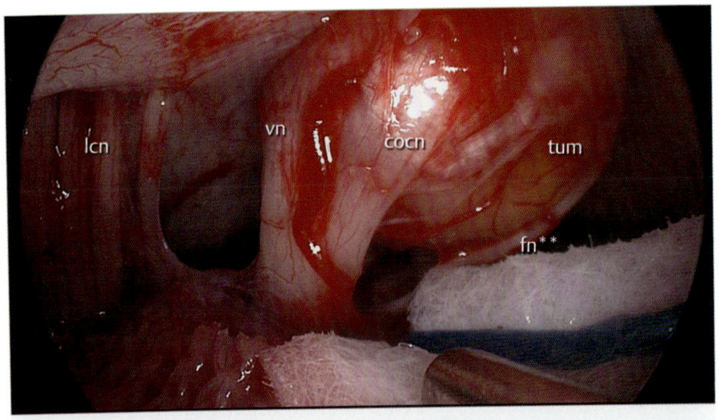

Fig. 7.38 Clinical Case 1, Left ear: A 0-degree endoscope is introduced into the surgical field to detect the position of the facial nerve in relation to the tumor mass. *cocn: cochlear nerve; fn**: facial nerve in the cerebellopontine angle (CPA); lcn: lower cranial nerves; tum: tumor; vn: vestibular nerve.*

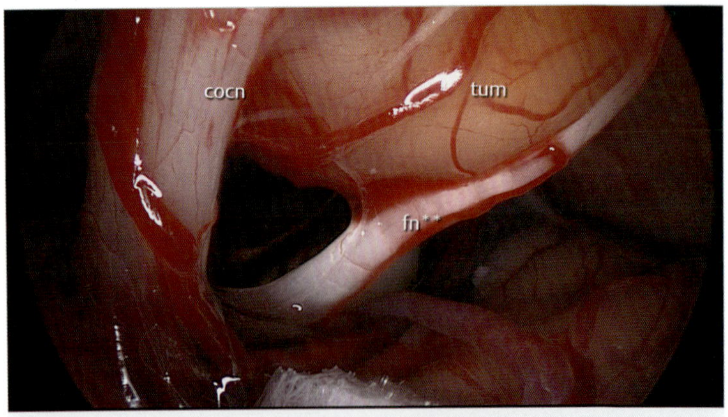

Fig. 7.39 Clinical Case 1, Left ear: The anatomical relationship between the tumor and the facial nerve is appreciated under endoscopic magnification. *cocn: cochlear nerve; fn**: facial nerve in the cerebellopontine angle (CPA).*

7.8 Surgical Approach

The retrosigmoid approach is performed in the same way as the one described earlier in this chapter. The majority of neurovascular conflicts is located at the entry zone close to the brainstem, which implies the use of cerebellar retractor to improve the exposure in that area (see ▶ Fig. 7.104). This can lead to cerebellar compression with possible sequelae. On the other hand, this problem can often be overcome by using the endoscope, which can allow a direct identification of the neurovascular conflict avoiding brain retraction (see ▶ Fig. 7.105).

Once the retrosigmoid route has been opened, some neurosurgical cottonoids can be placed on the cerebellum to protect it and the endoscope is introduced to allow for the evaluation of the whole tract of the involved nerve. When the area of conflict,

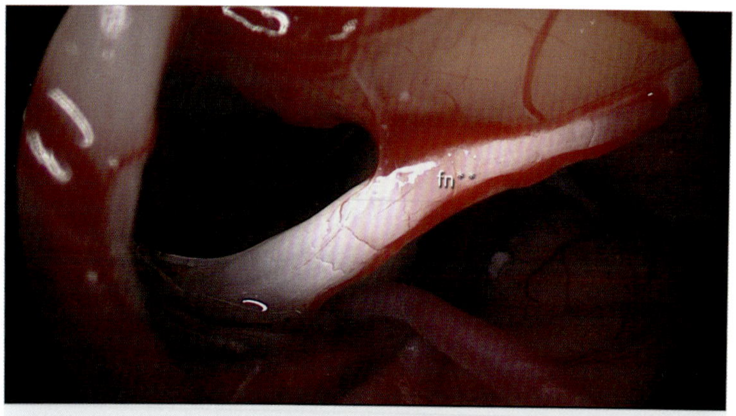

Fig. 7.40 Clinical Case 1, Left ear: Endoscopic magnification of the facial nerve in the cerebellopontine angle (CPA). *fn**: facial nerve in the CPA.*

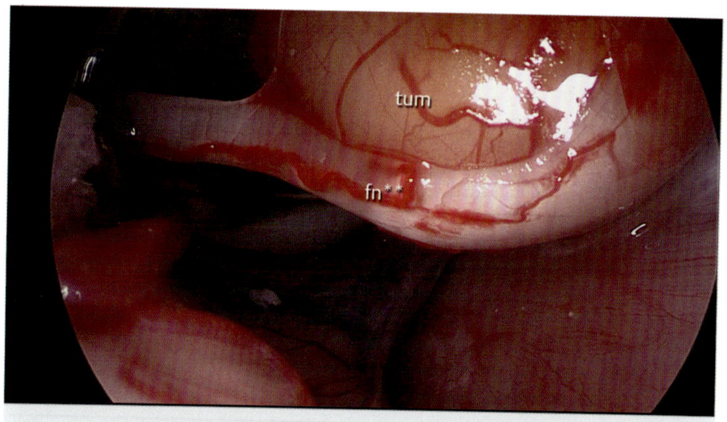

Fig. 7.41 Clinical Case 1, Left ear: A 45-degree endoscopic view shows the displacement of the facial nerve from the tumor mass close to the surface of the temporal bone before entering the internal auditory canal (IAC) porus. *fn**: facial nerve in the cerebellopontine angle (CPA); tum: tumor.*

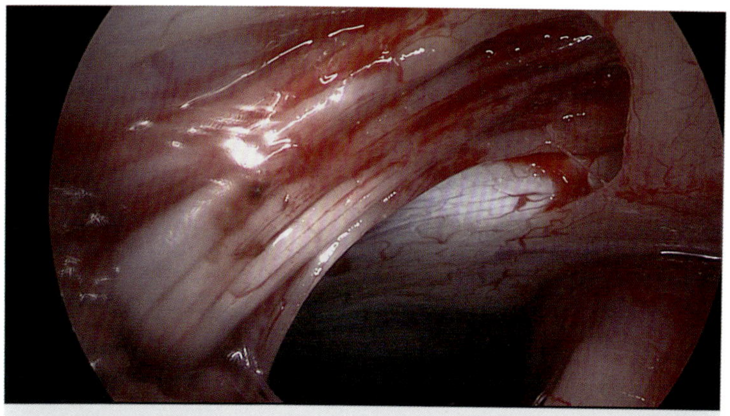

Fig. 7.42 Clinical Case 1, Left ear: Endoscopic magnification of the lower cranial nerves.

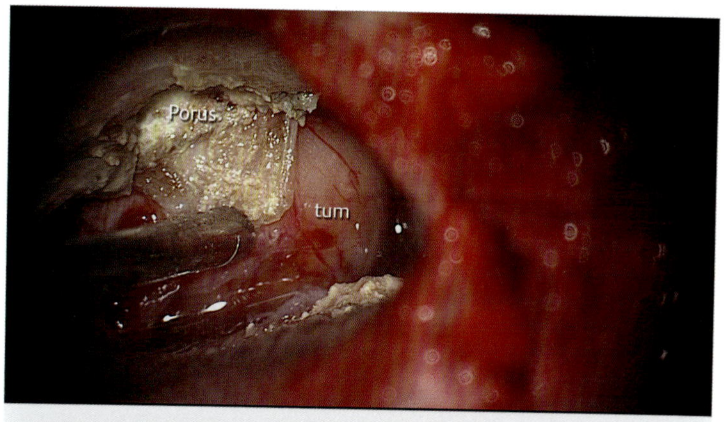

Fig. 7.43 Clinical Case 1, Left ear: Once dural flaps are created, a diamond bur is used to microscopically drill the porus of the internal auditory canal (IAC). *tum: tumor.*

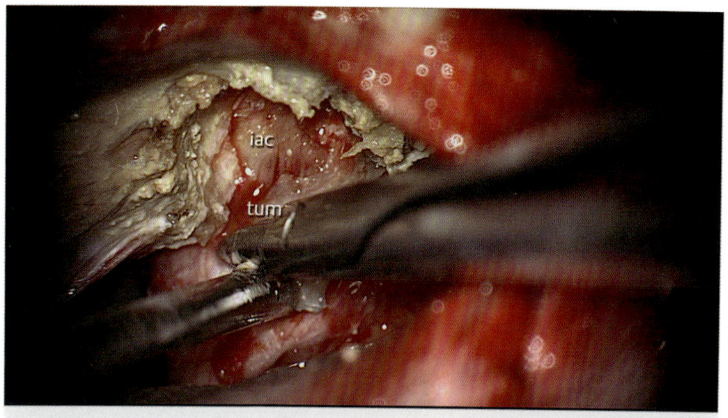

Fig. 7.44 Clinical Case 1, Left ear: The internal auditory canal (IAC) is exposed and the tumor dissection is started performing the central debulking of the tumor mass. *iac: internal auditory canal; tum: tumor.*

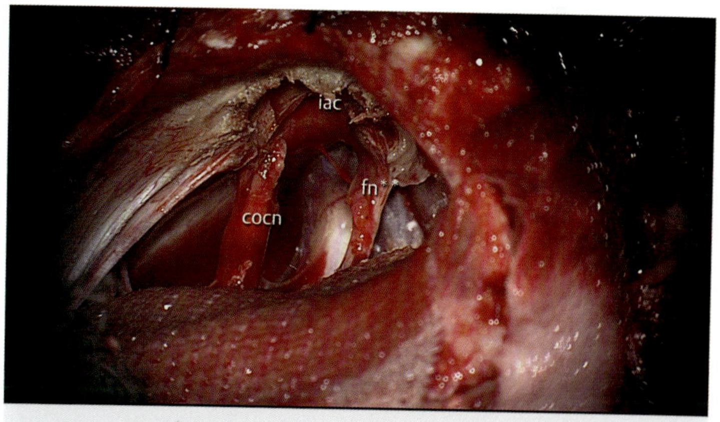

Fig. 7.45 Clinical Case 1, Left ear: Microscopic view of the cerebellopontine angle (CPA) after tumor removal. *cocn: cochlear nerve; fn**: facial nerve in the CPA; iac: internal auditory canal.*

which is usually confirmed by the displacement of the nerve and/or the modification of its surface (e.g., decubitus, alteration of color, indentations), is identified, a careful dissection with blunt instruments is attempted and arachnoidian adhesions are progressively sectioned (see ▶ Fig. 7.106).

Depending on the kind of conflict, after sectioning the arachnoidal adhesions surrounding the conflict, the vascular structure may be gently endoscopically dislocated from the nerve; then, using a dissector, a soft dissection of the conflict is made in order to remove the vascular structure from the compressed nerve.

When a vascular loop is present on the facial nerve, this contact has to be gently dissected to create a space between the vascular and the nervous structures.

Once the vascular structure is detached from the nerve and displaced, a piece of muscle or a teflon pad is inserted between the two structures in order to solve the conflict (see ▶ Fig. 7.107). The interposed material is kept in situ to separate the offending vessel from the nerve and also to decompress the nerve, serving

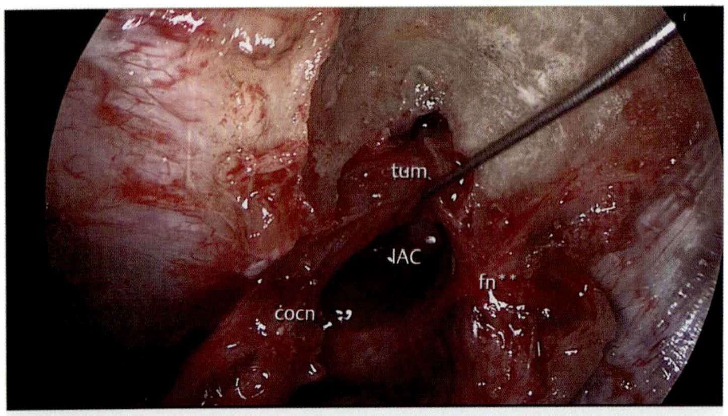

Fig. 7.46 Clinical Case 1, Left ear: A 45-degree endoscope is used to check the internal auditory canal (IAC), looking for any residual tumor. A remnant is seen endoscopically. *cocn: cochlear nerve; fn**: facial nerve in the cerebellopontine angle (CPA); iac: internal auditory canal; tum: tumor.*

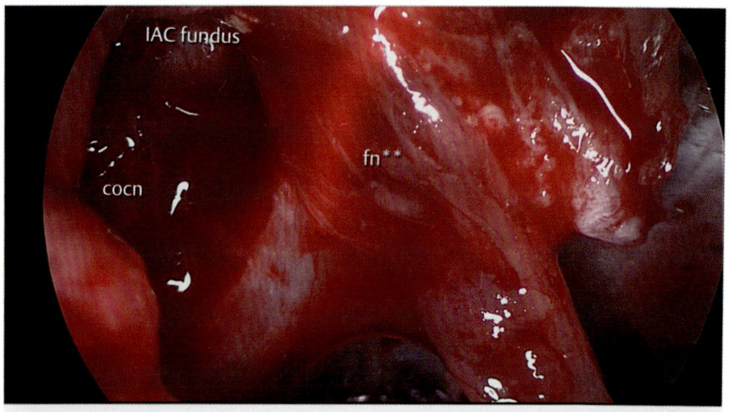

Fig. 7.47 Clinical Case 1, Left ear: Once the residual tumor is removed under endoscopic view, the fundus of the internal auditory canal (IAC) can be detected. *cocn: cochlear nerve; fn**: facial nerve in the cerebellopontine angle (CPA); iac: internal auditory canal.*

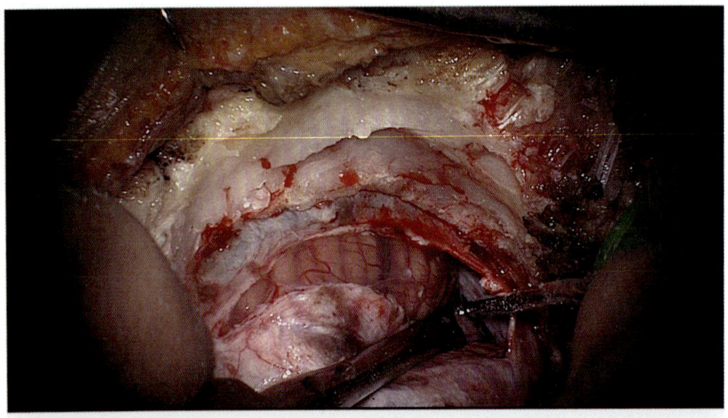

Fig. 7.48 Clinical Case 2, Right ear: A posterior based dural flap is created; the cerebellum is gently elevated to gain access to the cisterna magna; the arachnoid of the cistern is opened allowing the drainage of cerebrospinal fluid (CSF).

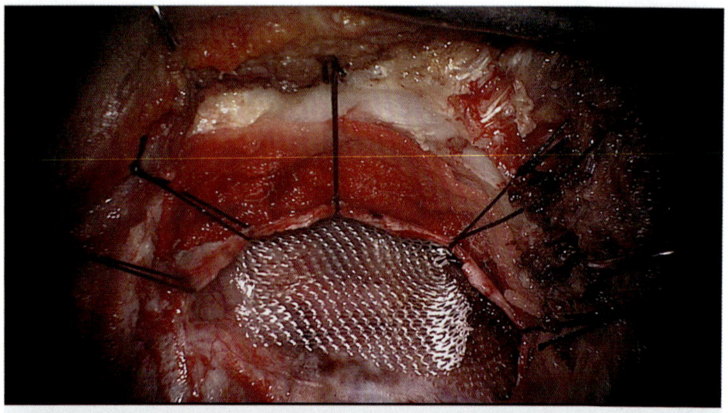

Fig. 7.49 Clinical Case 2, Right ear: The dural layer margins are suspended using stay sutures and the cerebellum is exposed.

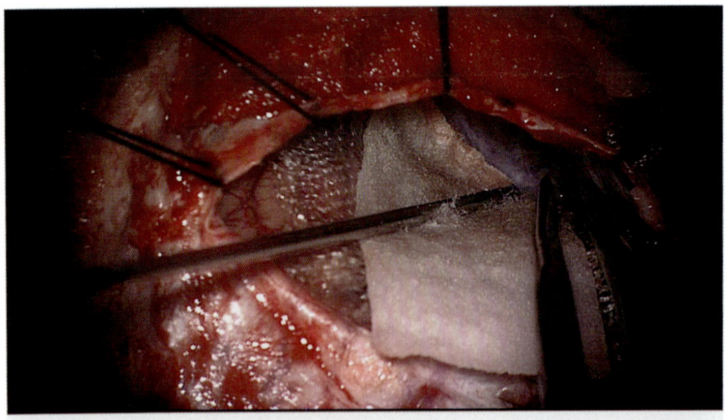

Fig. 7.50 Clinical Case 2, Right ear: A neurosurgical cottonoid is placed on the cerebellum surface to protect it, and the arachnoid layers are cut.

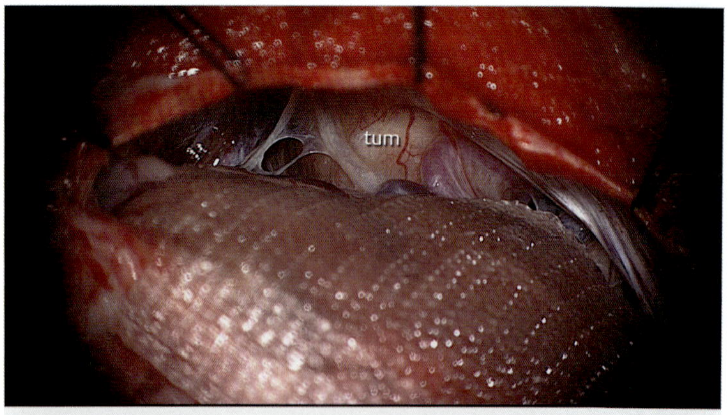

Fig. 7.51 Clinical Case 2, Right ear: The acoustic tumor is exposed in the cerebellopontine angle (CPA). *tum: tumor.*

to "cushion" the nerve from the pulsating artery (see Clinical Case 9).

After the separation of the offending vessel from the nerve, another technique suggests, putting a teflon sheet around the vascular structure and performing a suture of the teflon loop on the dura of the surface of the temporal bone, keeping the artery off the nerve, so that the neurovascular contact can be solved (see ▶ Fig. 7.108; see also Clinical Case 10).

Through an endoscope it is possible to check the correct placement of the material, the integrity of the neural structures as well as the status of the cerebellar lobe. Once a safe hemostasis has been achieved, the dura can be thoroughly closed through a watertight closure. Then, the bony island can be put back to its original position. A piece of Surgicel is used to fill the gap with the surrounding occipital bone, and fibrin glue is added to the surgical region. Muscular and subcutaneous tissues are carefully

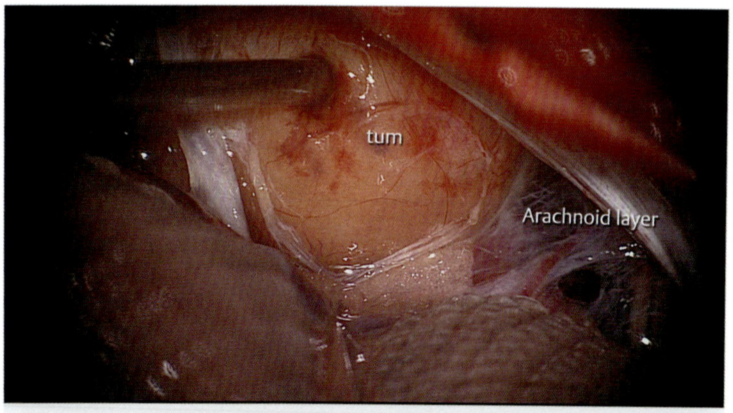

Fig. 7.52 Clinical Case 2, Right ear: The central debulking of the tumor is started and the tumor mass is progressively removed from the cerebellopontine angle (CPA). *tum: tumor.*

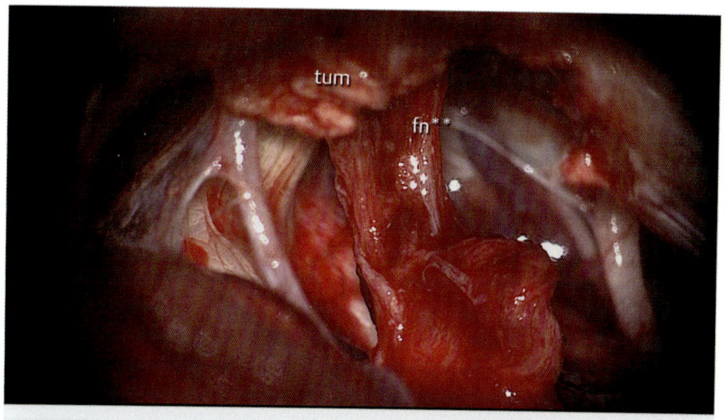

Fig. 7.53 Clinical Case 2, Right ear: Microscopic view of the cerebellopontine angle (CPA) after tumor removal; a residual tumor is seen in the proximity of the porus. *fn**: facial nerve in the CPA; tum: tumor.*

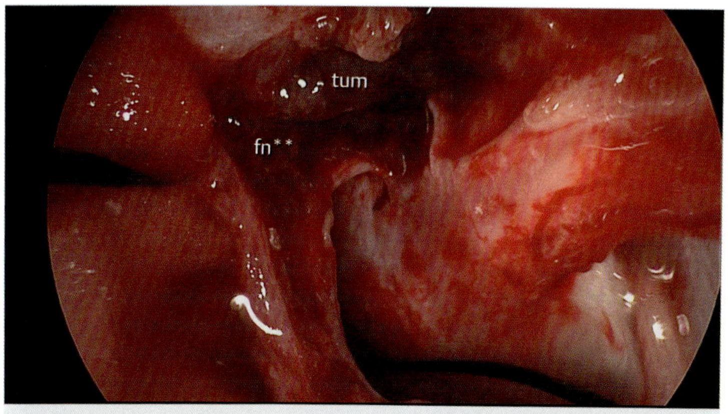

Fig. 7.54 Clinical Case 2, Right ear: A 45-degree endoscope is used to detect the residual tumor in the internal auditory canal (IAC). *fn**: facial nerve in the cerebellopontine angle (CPA); tum: tumor.*

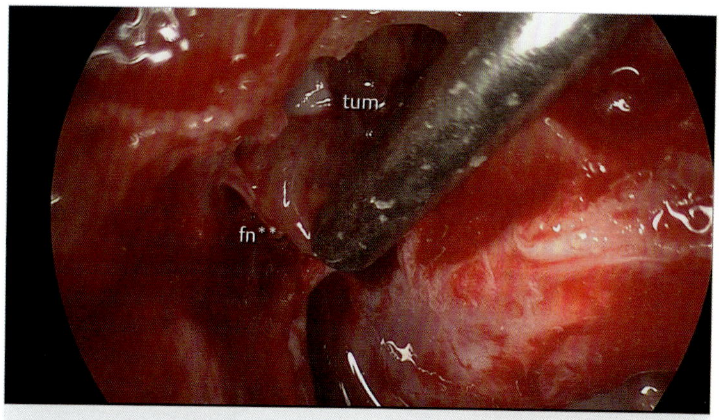

Fig. 7.55 Clinical Case 2, Right ear: The residual tumor is progressively removed from the internal auditory canal (IAC), carefully preserving the facial nerve. *fn**: facial nerve in the cerebellopontine angle; tum: tumor.*

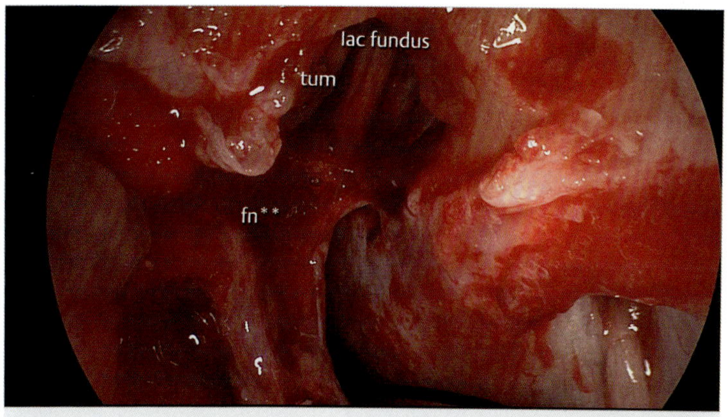

Fig. 7.56 Clinical Case 2, Right ear: The fundus of the internal auditory canal (IAC) is exposed, and a plane of cleavage between the residual tumor and the nerves is found. *fn**: facial nerve in the cerebellopontine angle (CPA); tum: tumor.*

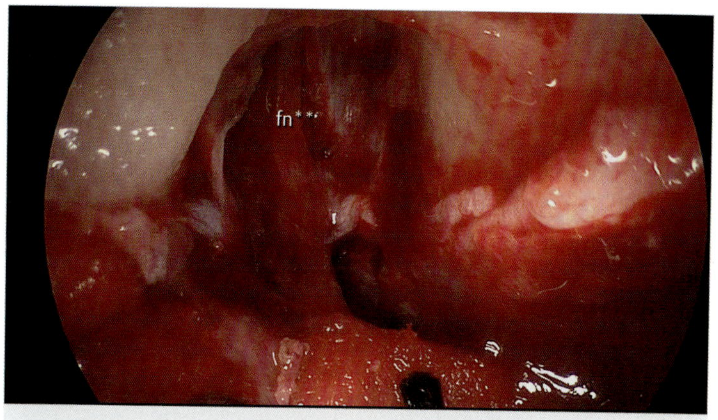

Fig. 7.57 Clinical Case 2, Right ear: Endoscopic view of the internal auditory canal (IAC) after tumor removal. *fn**: facial nerve in the cerebellopontine angle (CPA).*

stitched and the skin closure is performed. The patient is kept in an intensive care unit under observation for 24 hours after surgery. A CT scan is carried out 6 hours after surgery. Antibiotics are used in the immediate postoperative period. Further imaging is carried out 48 to 72 hours after surgery.

7.9 Complications

The retrosigmoid approach is a relatively safe procedure for the majority of patients, especially when endoscopic assistance is used. Nevertheless, there are some potential postoperative complications, which include:

- Brainstem and cerebellar injury with edema and/or hematoma
- CPA hematoma
- Meningitis
- Vascular rupture
- CSF leakage
- Facial palsy (transient or permanent)
- Other cranial nerve impairments
- Postoperative headache
- Equilibrium impairment

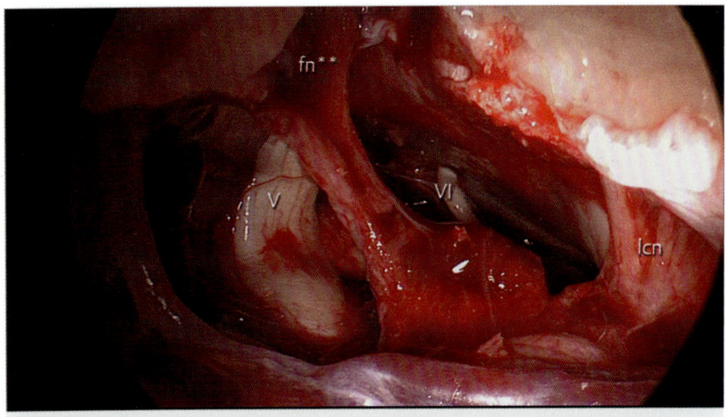

Fig. 7.58 Clinical Case 2, Right ear: Final endoscopic check of the surgical cavity, with a 0-degree endoscope, in the cerebellopontine angle (CPA). *fn**: facial nerve in the CPA; lcn: lower cranial nerves.*

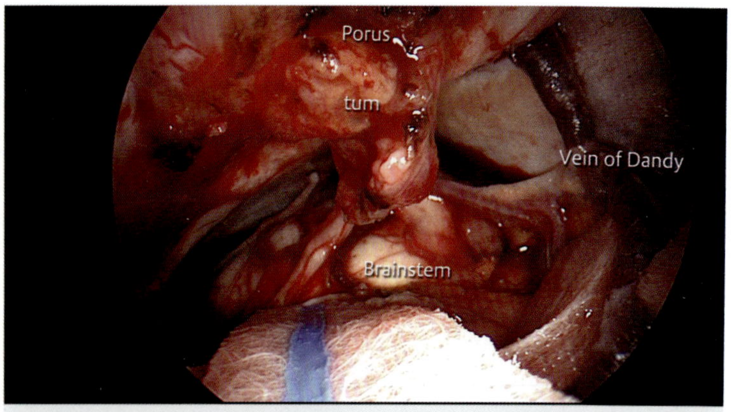

Fig. 7.59 Clinical Case 3, Left ear: The tumor mass has been microscopically removed from the cerebellopontine angle (CPA). A 0-degree endoscope is introduced into the surgical cavity detecting the residual tumor developing in the internal auditory canal (IAC). *tum: tumor.*

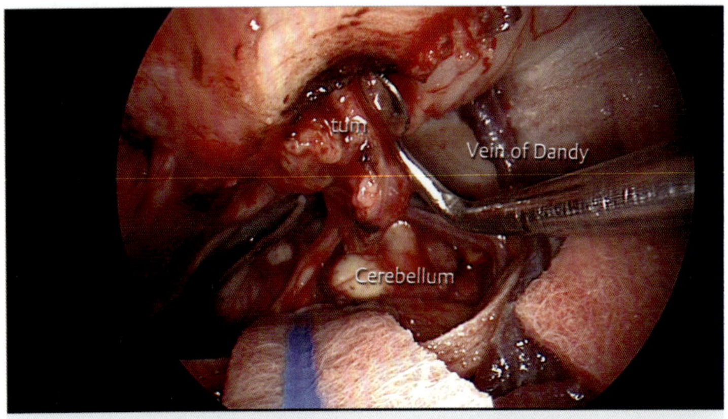

Fig. 7.60 Clinical Case 3, Left ear: A curved dissector is used to gently remove the tumor at the level of the porus, detecting the facial nerve. *tum: tumor.*

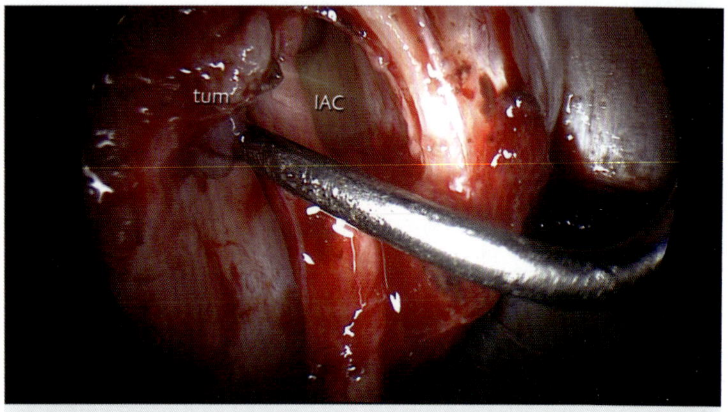

Fig. 7.61 Clinical Case 3, Left ear: A 45-degree endoscope may be useful to remove the tumor from the internal auditory canal (IAC), following the facial nerve into the fundus. *iac: internal auditory canal; tum: tumor.*

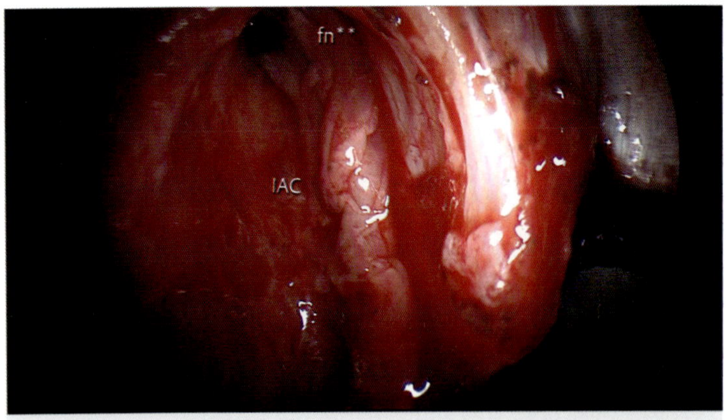

Fig. 7.62 Clinical Case 3, Left ear: Endoscopic view (45-degree endoscope) of the fundus of the internal auditory canal (IAC). *fn**: facial neve into the IAC; iac: internal auditory canal.*

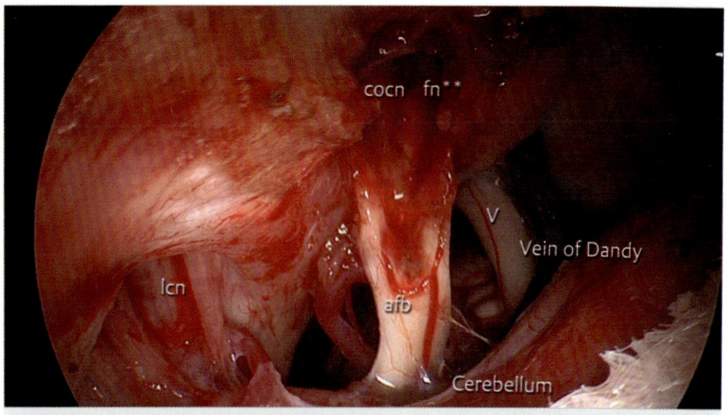

Fig. 7.63 Clinical Case 4, Left ear: Final endoscopic check after tumor removal. *afb: acoustic-facial bundle; cocn: cochlear nerve; fn**: facial neve into the internal auditory canal (IAC); lcn: lower cranial nerves.*

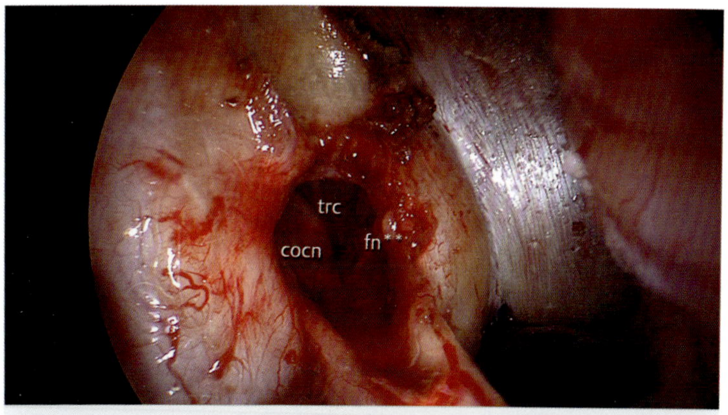

Fig. 7.64 Clinical Case 4, Left ear: A 70-degree endoscope is used to magnify the fundus of the internal auditory canal (IAC). *cocn: cochlear nerve; fn**: facial neve into the IAC; trc: transverse crest.*

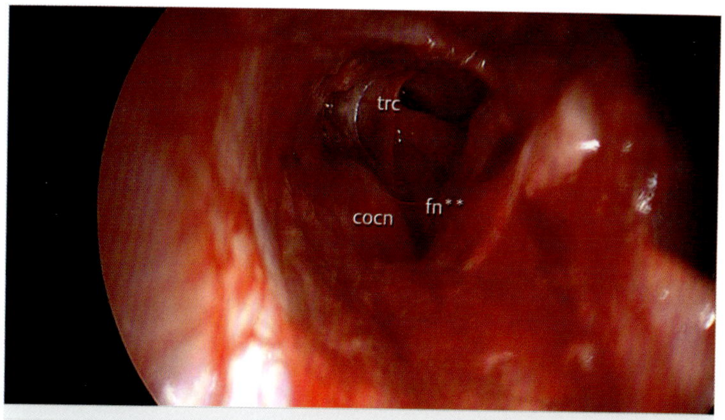

Fig. 7.65 Clinical Case 4, Left ear: Fundus of the internal auditory canal (IAC) (70-degree endoscopic view). *cocn: cochlear nerve; fn**: facial neve into the IAC; trc: transverse crest.*

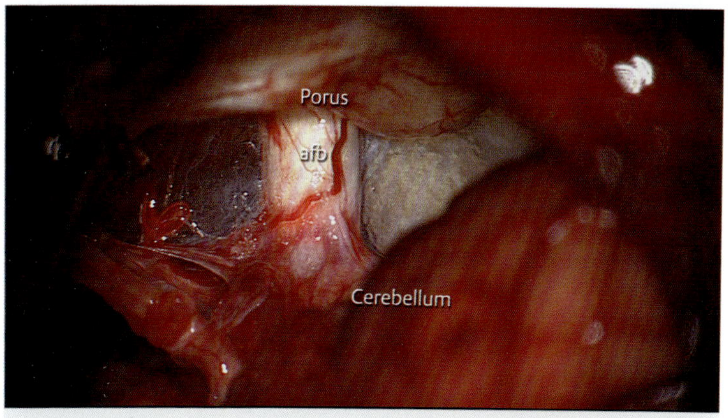

Fig. 7.66 Clinical Case 5, Left ear: Microscopic view of the cerebellopontine angle (CPA) after tumor removal (lower cranial nerve neuroma). *afb: acoustic-facial bundle.*

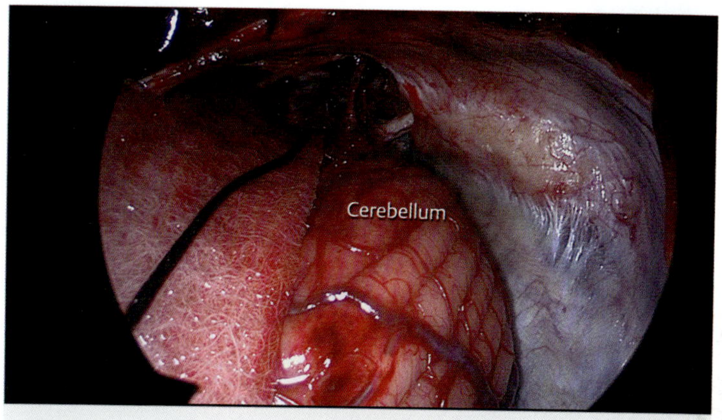

Fig. 7.67 Clinical Case 5, Left ear: Final endoscopic check of the surgical cavity. A cottonoid pad is placed on the cerebellum to protect it; no retractor is necessary. A 0-degree endoscope is carefully inserted through the cavity to inspect the cerebellopontine angle (CPA).

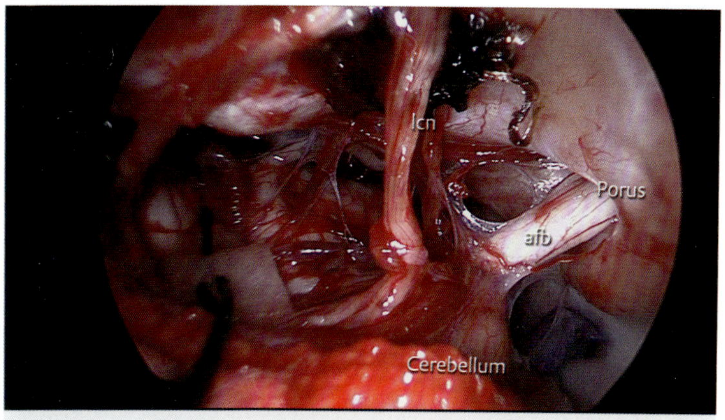

Fig. 7.68 Clinical Case 5, Left ear: The lower cranial nerve and the acoustic-facial bundle are endoscopically detected. *afb: acoustic-facial bundle; lcn: lower cranial nerves.*

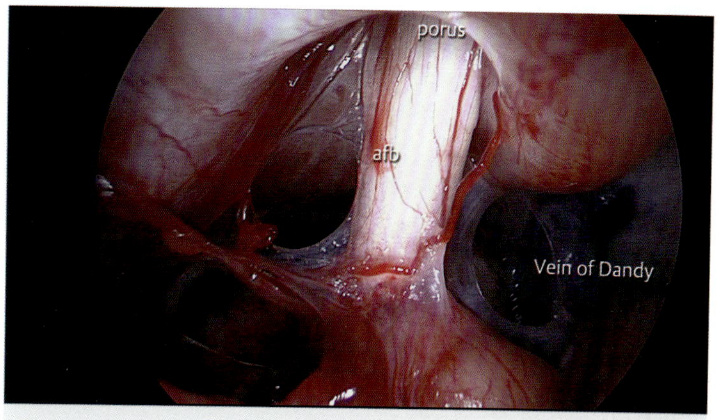

Fig. 7.69 Clinical Case 5, Left ear: Endoscopic magnification of the acoustic-facial bundle from the entry zone to the porus. *afb: acoustic-facial bundle.*

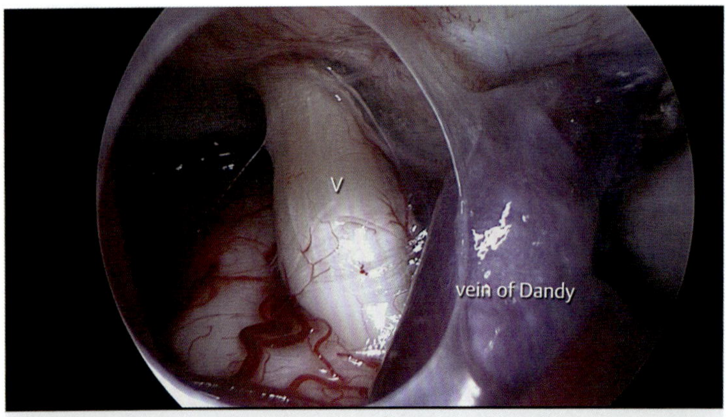

Fig. 7.70 Clinical Case 5, Left ear: Endoscopic view of the trigeminal nerve and Dandy's vein.

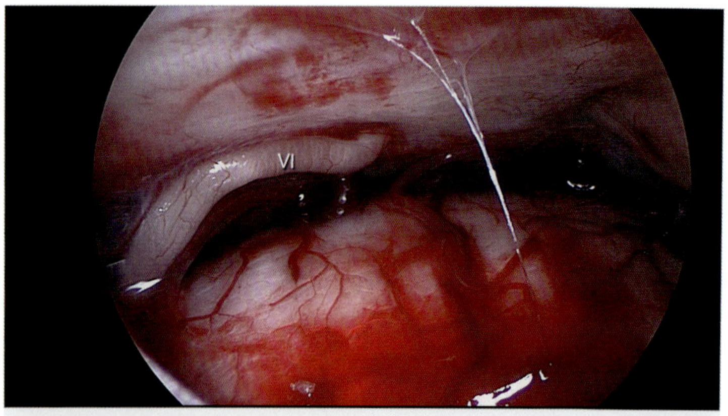

Fig. 7.71 Clinical Case 5, Left ear: Endoscopic view of VI cranial nerve.

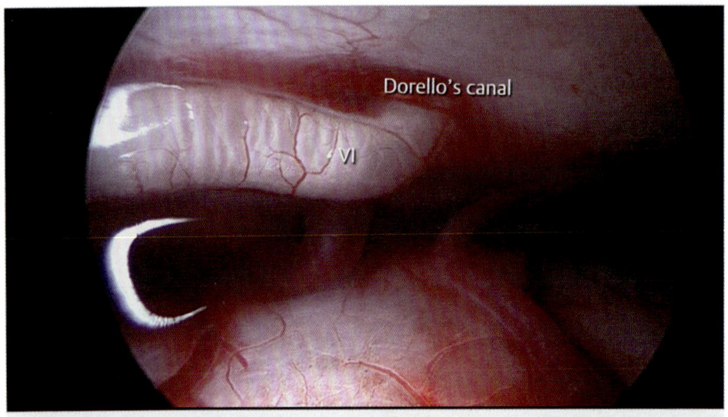

Fig. 7.72 Clinical Case 5, Left ear: The Dorello's canal is seen.

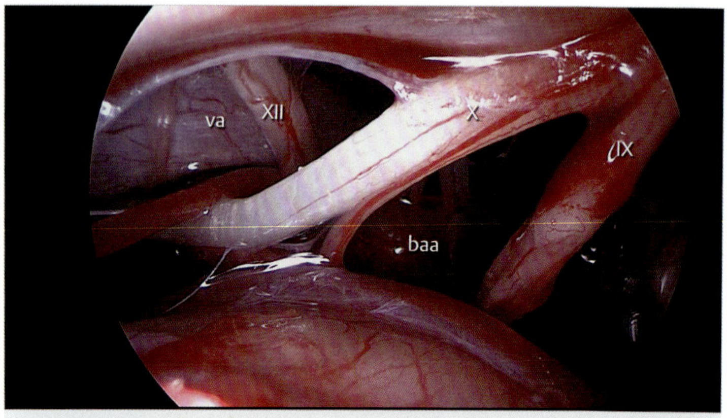

Fig. 7.73 Clinical Case 5, Left ear: Endoscopic view of the lower cranial nerves and hypoglossal nerve; inferomedially to the lower cranial nerves, the vertebral artery enters the skull base through the foramen magnum. *baa: basilar artery; va: vertebral artery.*

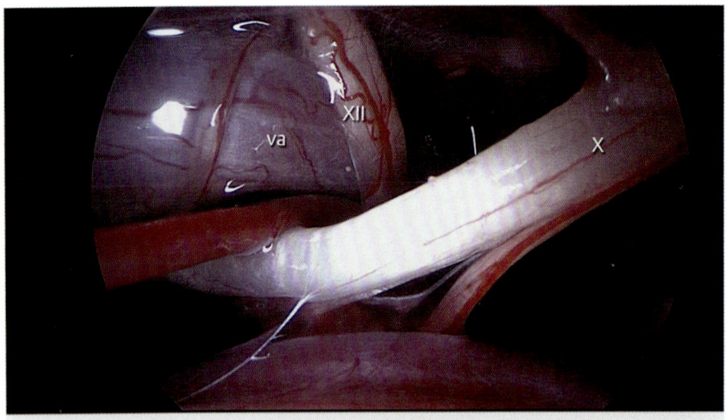

Fig. 7.74 Clinical Case 5, Left ear: The hypoglossal nerve is endoscopically seen running across the vertebral artery. This nerve leaves the ventral surface of the medulla oblongata medially to the lower cranial nerves. The nerve fibers are grouped into two main trunks entering the hypoglossal canal. *va: vertebral artery.*

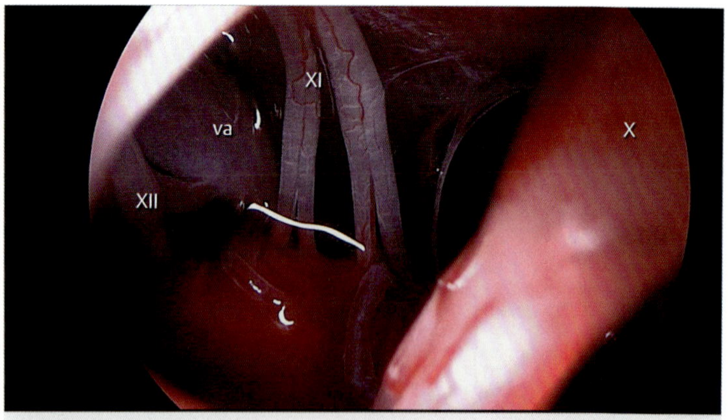

Fig. 7.75 Clinical Case 5, Left ear: The two distinct roots (cranial and spinal roots) of the spinal accessory nerve are endoscopically visible. *va: vertebral artery.*

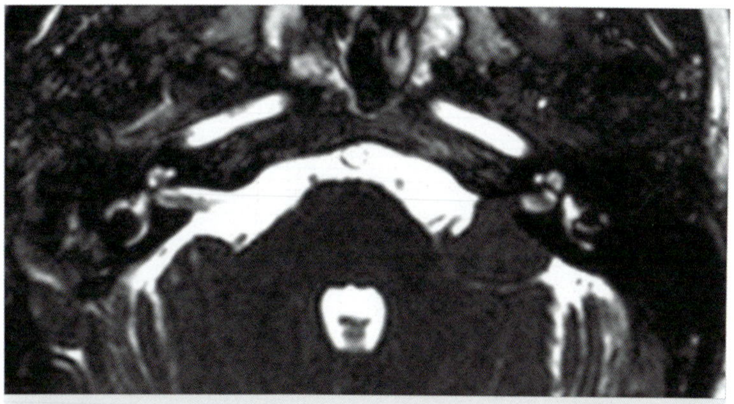

Fig. 7.76 Clinical Case 6: Magnetic resonance imaging (MRI), axial view showing a meningioma on the left side, occupying the cerebellopontine angle (CPA) with internal auditory canal (IAC) involvement.

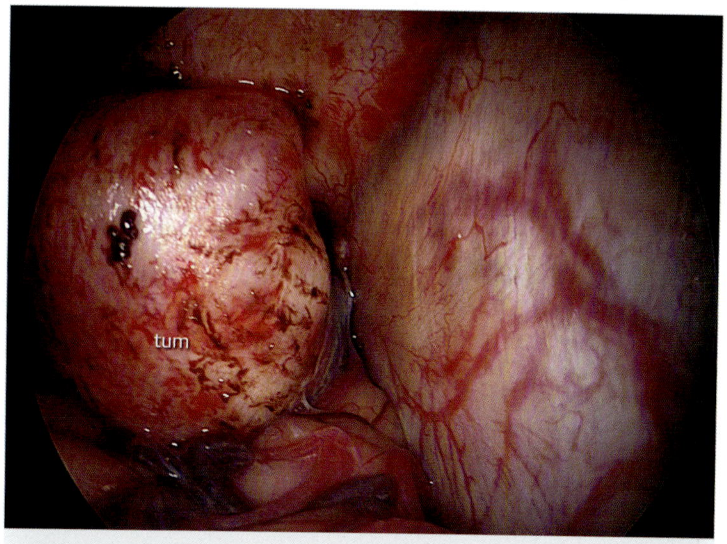

Fig. 7.77 Clinical Case 6, Left ear: A 0-degree endoscope is used to inspect the cerebellopontine angle (CPA) before starting the tumor removal. *tum: tumor.*

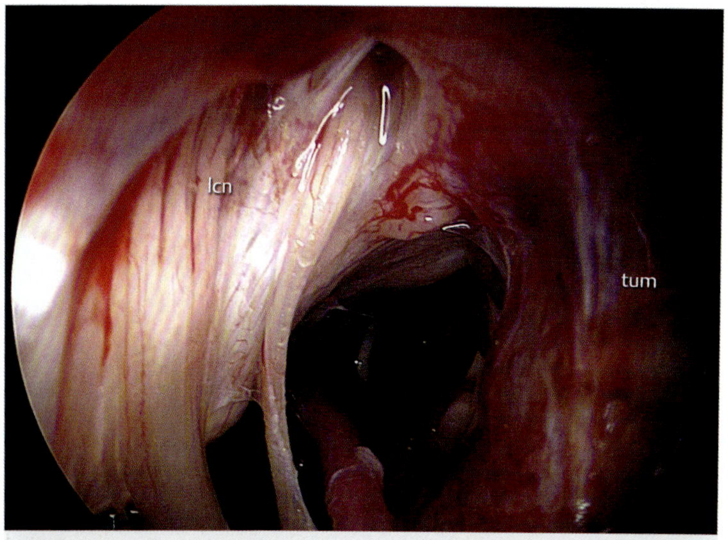

Fig. 7.78 Clinical Case 6, Left ear: The anatomical relationship between the glossopharyngeal, the vagus nerves, and the tumor is endoscopically investigated. *lcn: lower cranial nerves; tum: tumor.*

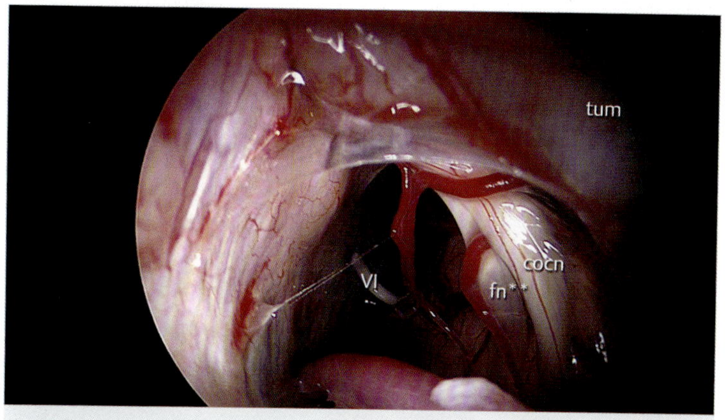

Fig. 7.79 Clinical Case 6, Left ear: The facial nerve and the cochlear nerve are endoscopically detected at the entry zone under the tumor mass. *cocn: cochlear nerve; fn**: facial nerve in the cerebellopontine angle (CPA); tum: tumor.*

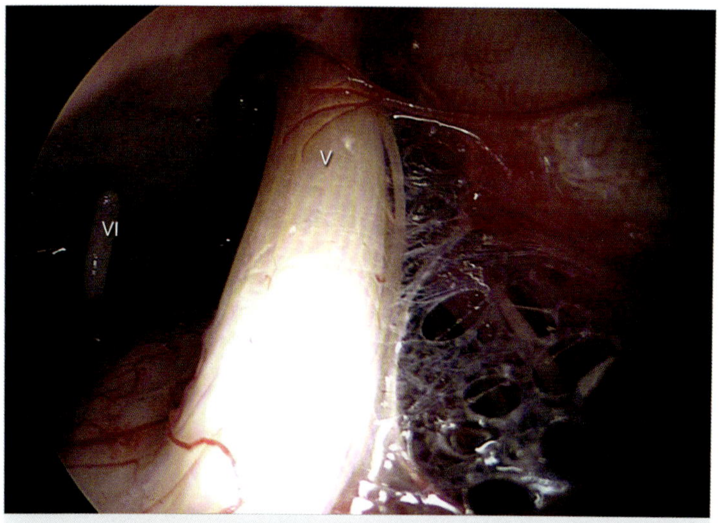

Fig. 7.80 Clinical Case 6, Left ear: The trigeminal nerve is seen.

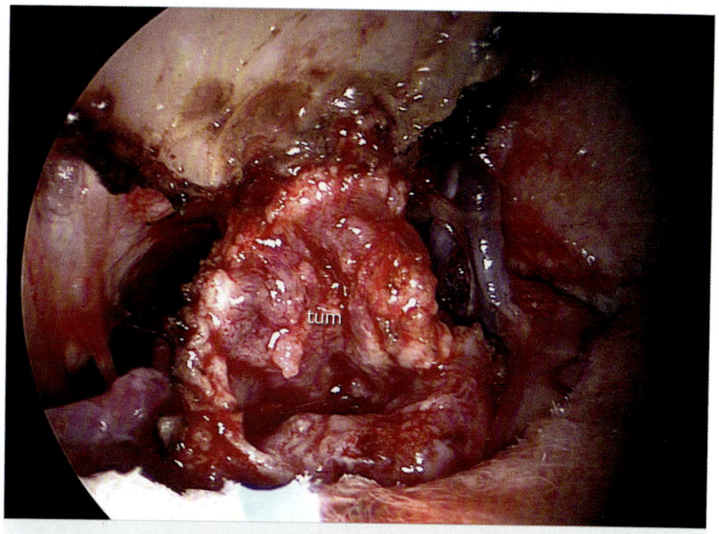

Fig. 7.81 Clinical Case 6, Left ear: A central debulking of the mass is performed; this procedure allows for the mobilization of the tumor and the dissection of the mass from the acoustic-facial bundle microscopically. *tum: tumor.*

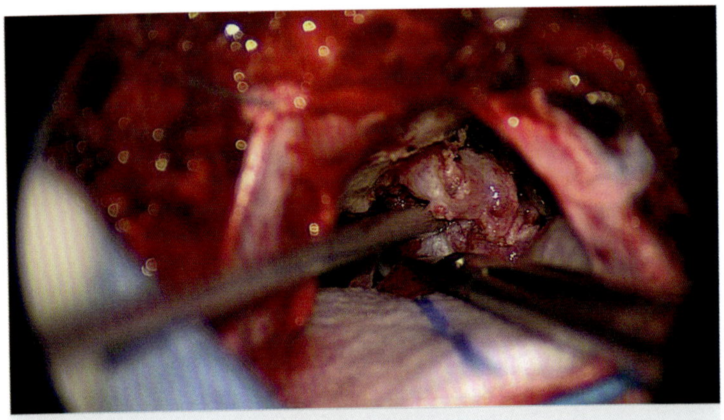

Fig. 7.82 Clinical Case 6, Left ear: The tumor is progressively microscopically removed and separated from the acoustic-facial bundle.

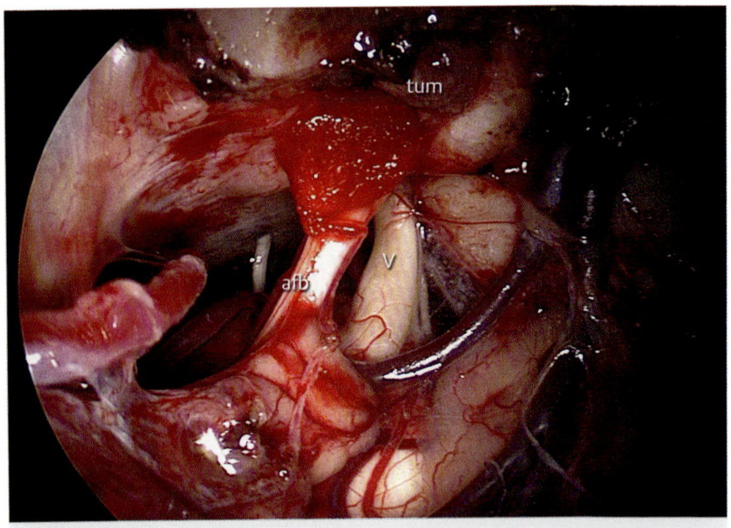

Fig. 7.83 Clinical Case 6, Left ear: Once the microscopical tumor removal is performed, a 0-degree endoscope is used to inspect the presence of any residual tumor in the internal auditory canal (IAC). *afb: acoustic-facial bundle; tum: tumor.*

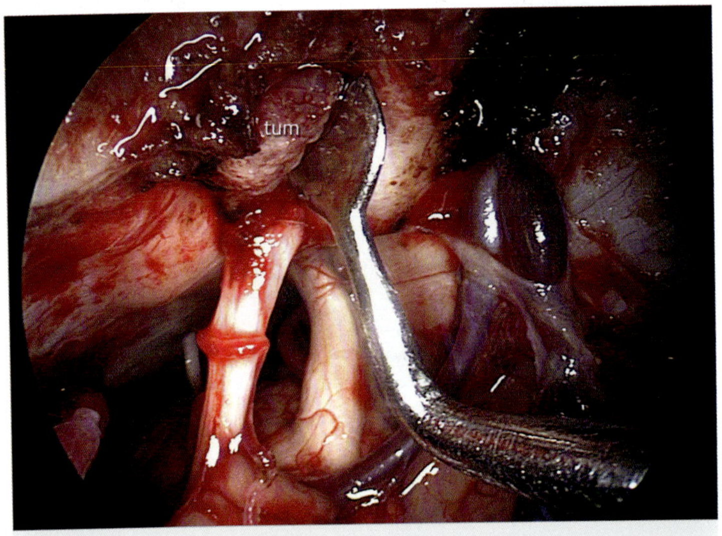

Fig. 7.84 Clinical Case 6, Left ear: A curved dissector is used to gently removed the residual tumor from the internal auditory canal (IAC) under endoscopic view. *tum: tumor.*

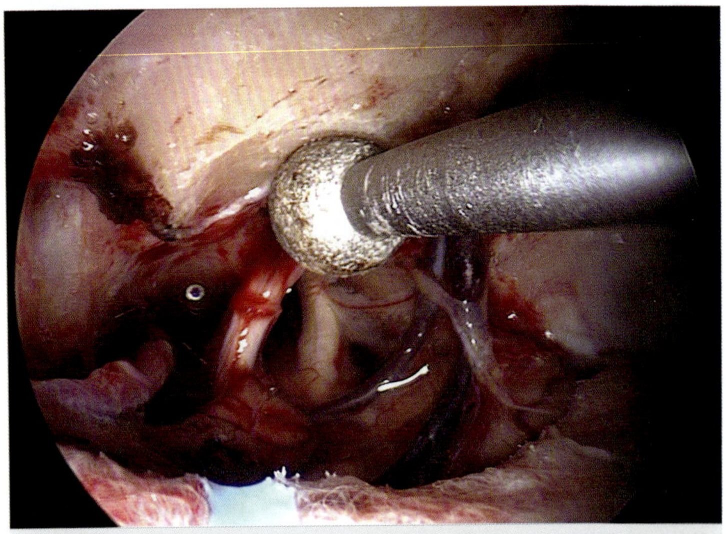

Fig. 7.85 Clinical Case 6, Left ear: Limited drilling of the porus is required to reach the residual tumor in the internal auditory canal (IAC).

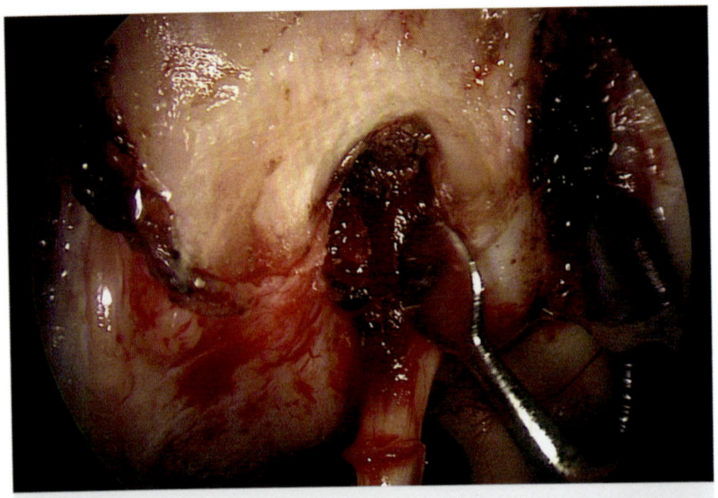

Fig. 7.86 Clinical Case 6, Left ear: The residual tumor is removed from the internal auditory canal (IAC).

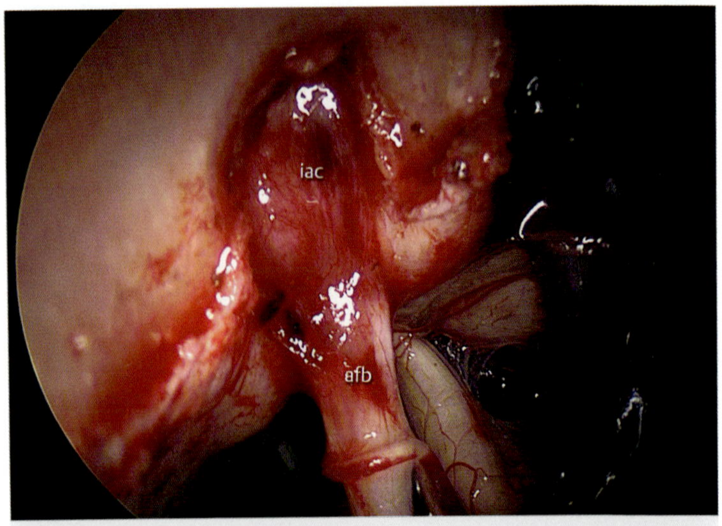

Fig. 7.87 Clinical Case 6, Left ear: Endoscopic view of the internal auditory canal (IAC) after residual tumor removal, preserving the acoustic-facial bundle. *afb: acoustic-facial bundle.*

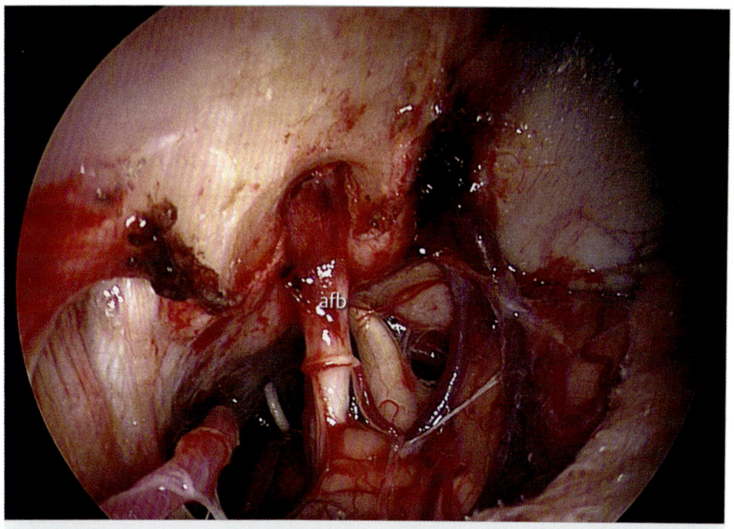

Fig. 7.88 Clinical Case 6, Left ear: Final endoscopic view of the cerebellopontine angle (CPA) after tumor removal. *afb: acoustic-facial bundle.*

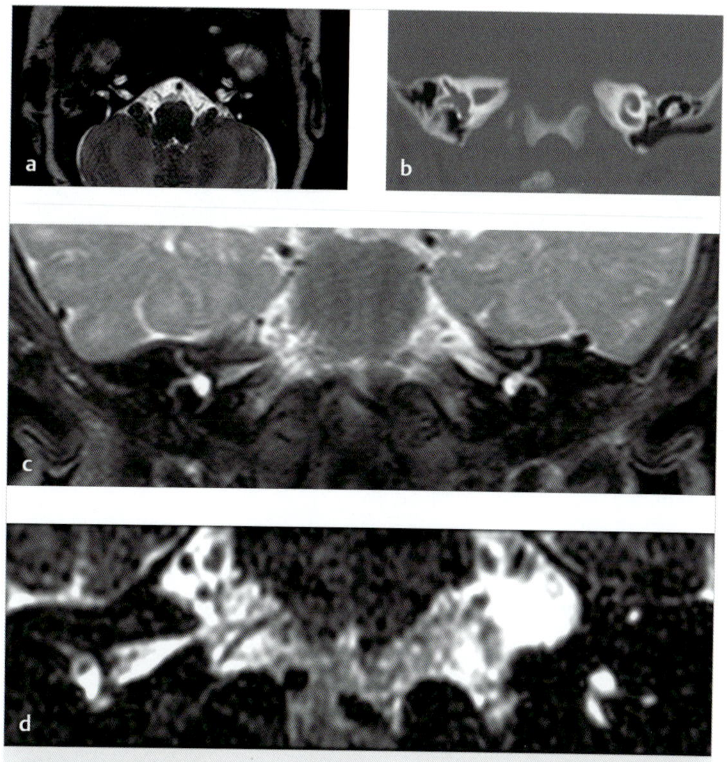

Fig. 7.89 Clinical Case 7, Left ear: Magnetic resonance imaging (MRI) axial view **(a)** and coronal view **(c, d)**. Computed tomography (CT) scan, coronal view **(b)**. Patient with bilateral cochlear nerve aplasia, with congenital malformation of the left internal auditory canal (IAC).

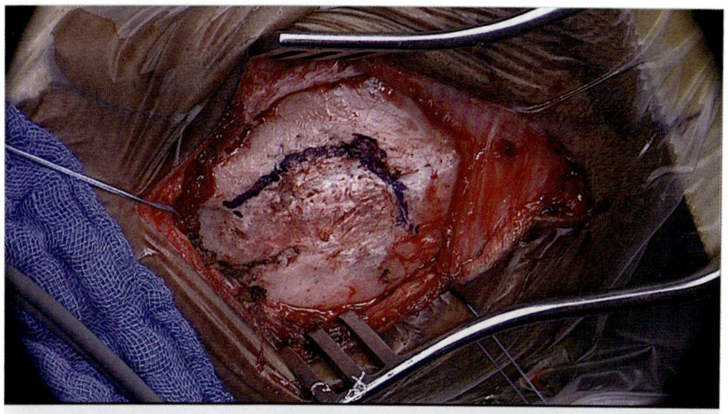

Fig. 7.90 Clinical Case 7, Left ear: The occipital-mastoid bone is exposed. The line of the sigmoid sinus is marked.

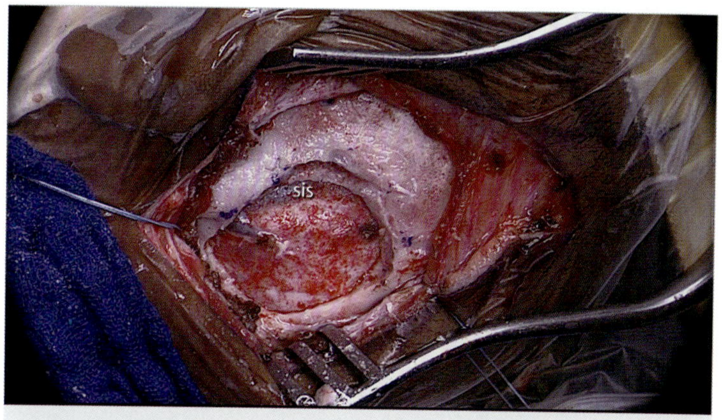

Fig. 7.91 Clinical Case 7, Left ear: The bony flap is created and the posterior fossa dura is exposed. *sis: sigmoid sinus.*

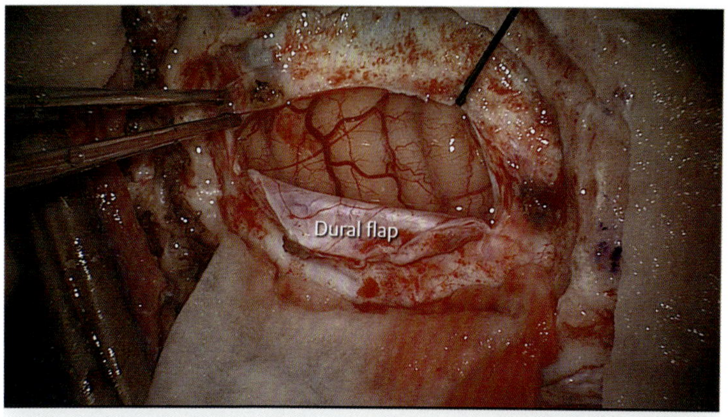

Fig. 7.92 Clinical Case 7, Left ear: A half-moon shaped dural incision behind the sigmoid sinus is performed, and the dural margins are suspended using stay sutures.

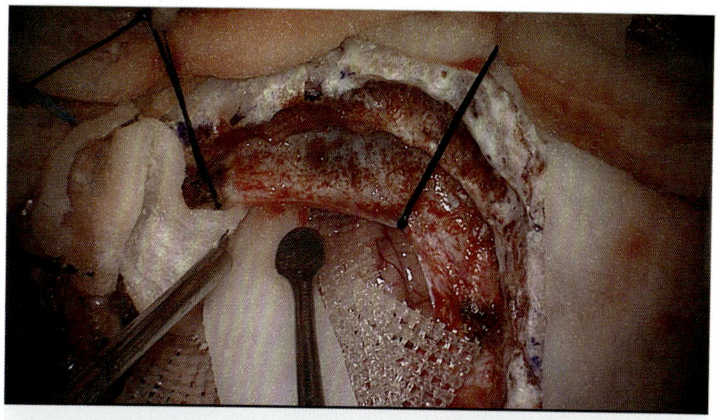

Fig. 7.93 Clinical Case 7, Left ear: Once cerebrospinal fluid (CSF) release has been performed, an Adaptic strip is used on the brain to protect it, and the cerebellum is gently retracted, exposing the prepontine cisterna.

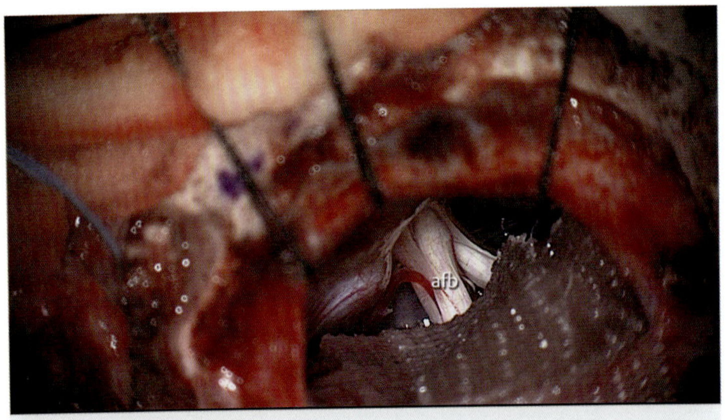

Fig. 7.94 Clinical Case 7, Left ear: Once the cerebellopontine angle (CPA) has been exposed, the acoustic-facial bundle is microscopically detected. *afb: acoustic-facial bundle.*

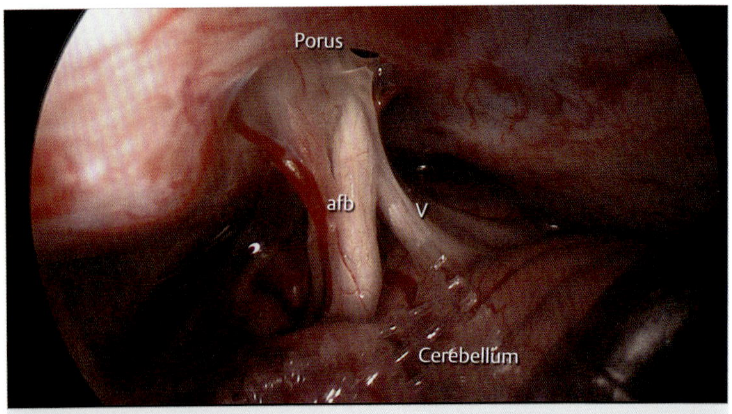

Fig. 7.95 Clinical Case 7, Left ear: A 0-degree endoscope is used through the surgical cavity to investigate the anomalous anatomy. The trigeminal nerve runs close to the acoustic-facial bundle. *afb: acoustic-facial bundle.*

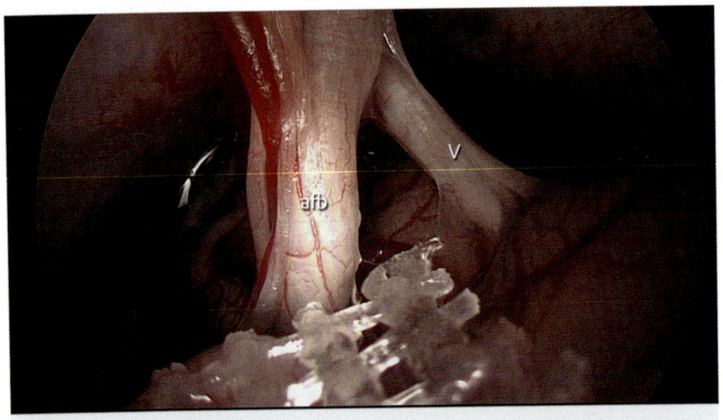

Fig. 7.96 Clinical Case 7, Left ear: An endoscopic investigation of the acoustic-facial bundle at the root exit zone is performed. *afb: acoustic-facial bundle.*

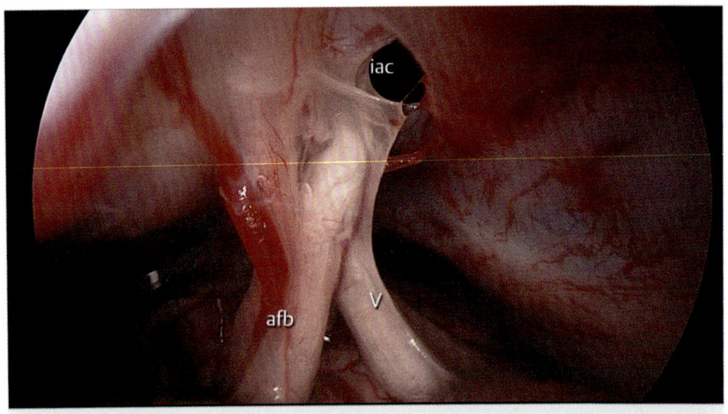

Fig. 7.97 Clinical Case 7, Left ear: The internal auditory canal (IAC) is endoscopically inspected; the anomalous anatomical relationship between the acoustic-facial bundle and the trigeminal nerve is noted. *afb: acoustic-facial bundle; iac: internal auditory canal.*

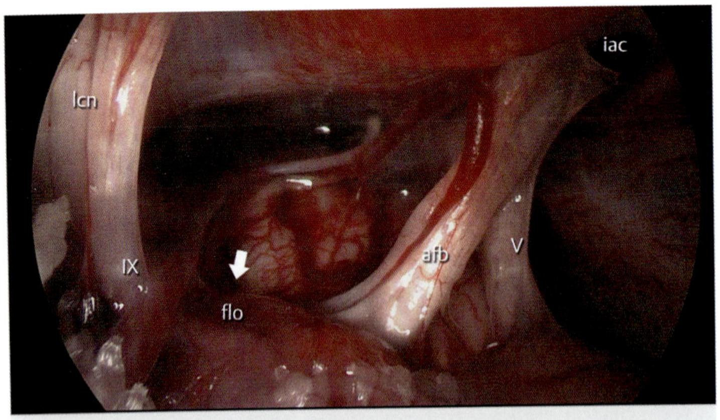

Fig. 7.98 Clinical Case 7, Left ear: The surface of the brainstem between the root exit zone of the glossopharyngeal nerve and the acoustic-facial bundle related to the flocculus is endoscopically investigated. The endoscopic check is especially crucial in case of anomalous anatomy to detect the lateral recess opening and the Luschka foramen (see the *white arrow*). *afb: acoustic-facial bundle; flo: flocculus; iac: internal auditory canal; lcn: lower cranial nerves.*

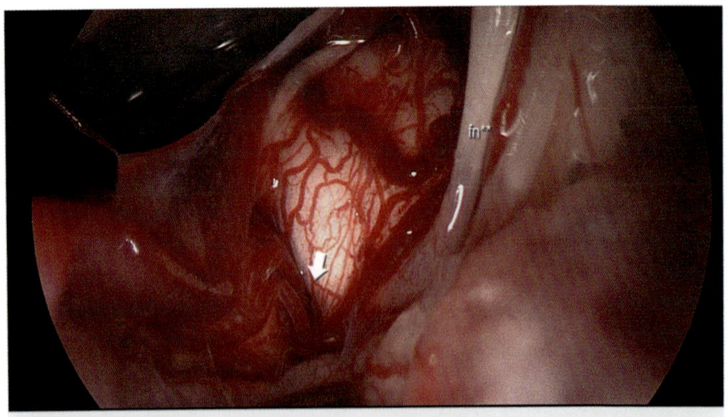

Fig. 7.99 Clinical Case 7, Left ear: The lateral recess is detected (*white arrow*); the root exit zone of the facial nerve is noted. *fn**: root exit zone of facial nerve.*

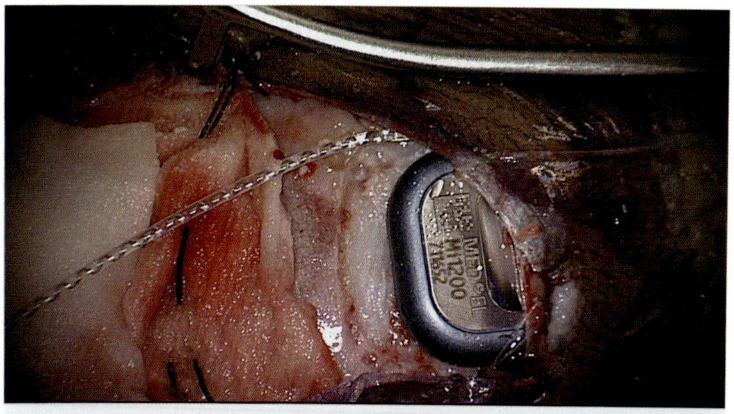

Fig. 7.100 Clinical Case 7, Left ear: The receiver-stimulator is placed under the temporalis muscle.

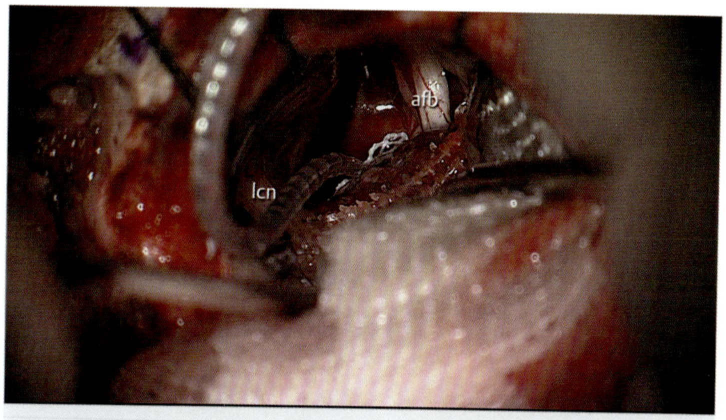

Fig. 7.101 Clinical Case 7, Left ear: The electrode paddle is gently microscopically placed into the Luschka foramen through the lateral recess. *afb: acoustic-facial bundle; lcn: lower cranial nerves.*

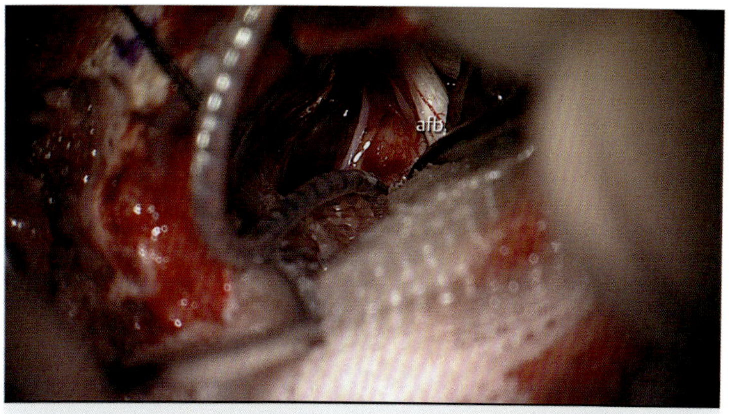

Fig. 7.102 Clinical Case 7, Left ear: The electrode paddle is gently more deeply pushed into the lateral recess to reach the Luschka foramen. *afb: acoustic-facial bundle.*

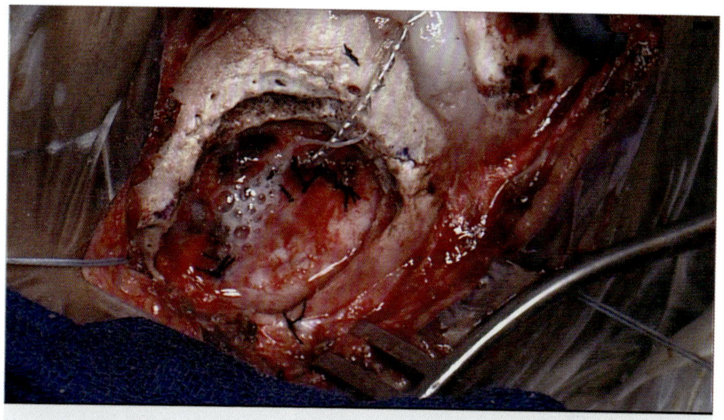

Fig. 7.103 Clinical Case 7, Left ear: When an acceptable positioning is obtained, a muscle plug is inserted into the foramen and fibrin glue is used to fix the electrode. The dura of the posterior fossa is sutured around the electrode.

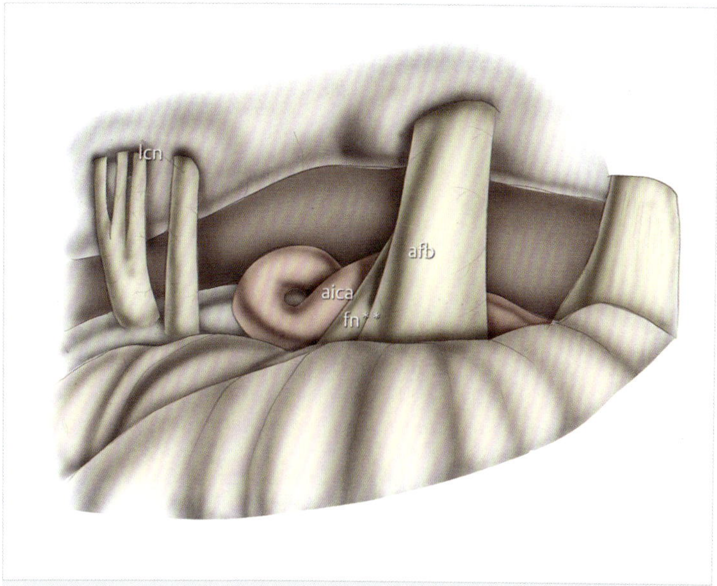

Fig. 7.104 Left ear. Treatment of facial spasm: A loop of the inferior cerebellar artery around the root of the exit zone of the facial nerve causing the compression of the nerve is noted. *afb: acoustic-facial bundle; aica: anterior inferior cerebellar artery; fn**: exit zone of facial nerve; lcn: lower cranial nerves.*

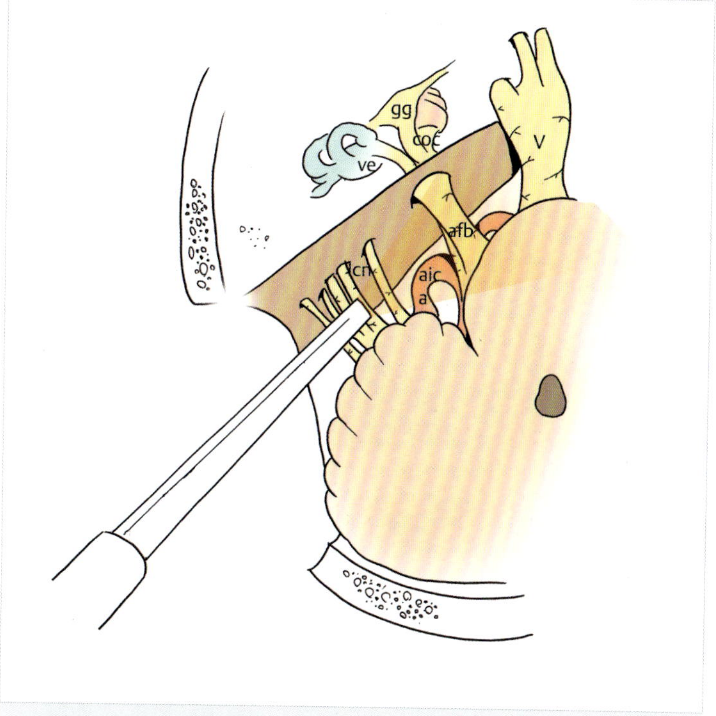

Fig. 7.105 Left ear: Once the retrosigmoid access has been done, a 0-degree endoscope is used to inspect the root of the exit zone of the facial nerve, detecting the offending vessels. *afb: acoustic-facial bundle; aica: anterior inferior cerebellar artery; coc: cochlea; gg: geniculate ganglion; lcn: lower cranial nerves; ve: vestibule.*

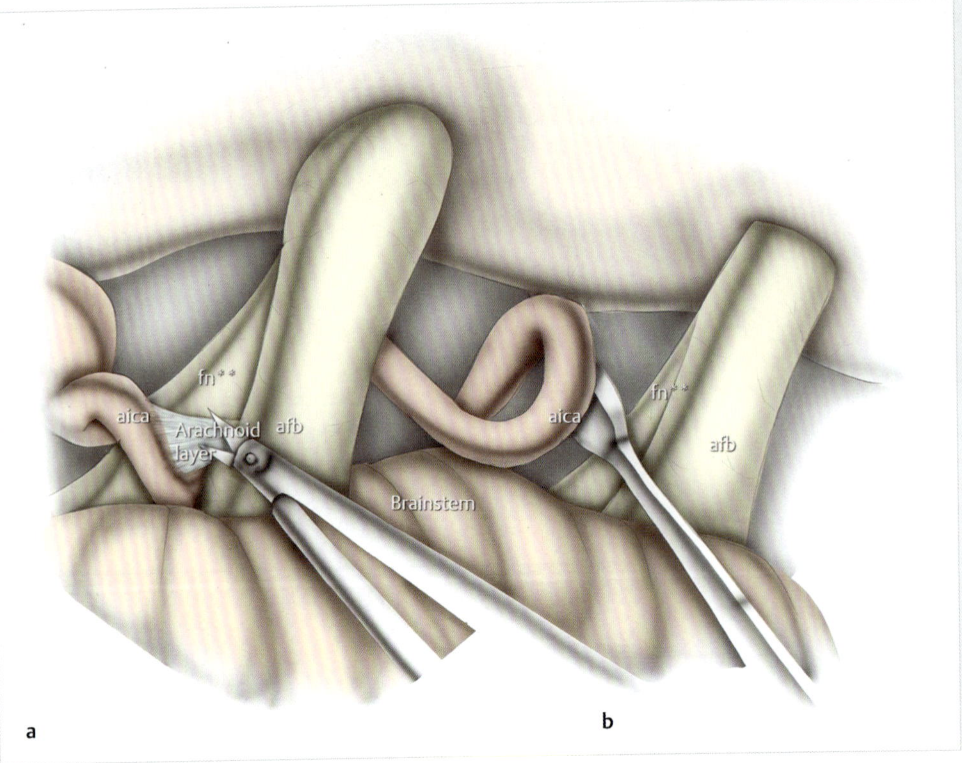

Fig. 7.106 Left ear: The offending artery (anterior inferior cerebellar artery [AICA]) is endoscopically separated from the root of the exit zone of the facial nerve. Microscissors are used to cut the arachnoid layer around the neurovascular structures **(a)**, and a dissector is used to move away the artery from the exit zone of the facial nerve **(b)**. *afb: acoustic-facial bundle; aica: anterior inferior cerebellar artery; fn**: exit-zone of facial nerve; lcn: lower cranial nerves.*

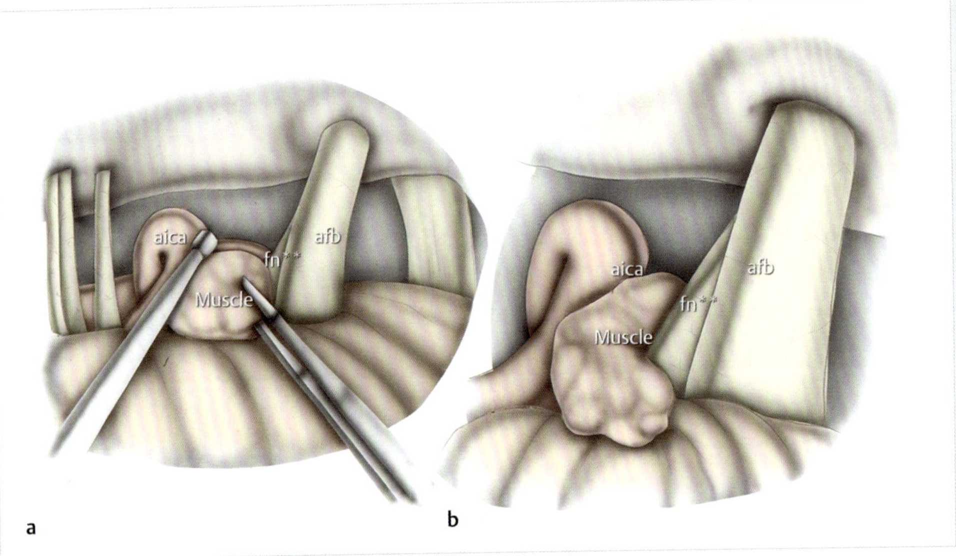

Fig. 7.107 Left ear: A muscle plug is placed between the offending artery and the exit zone of the facial nerve, to separate the two structures and decompress the nerve **(a, b)**. *afb: acoustic-facial bundle; aica: anterior inferior cerebellar artery; fn**: exit zone of facial nerve.*

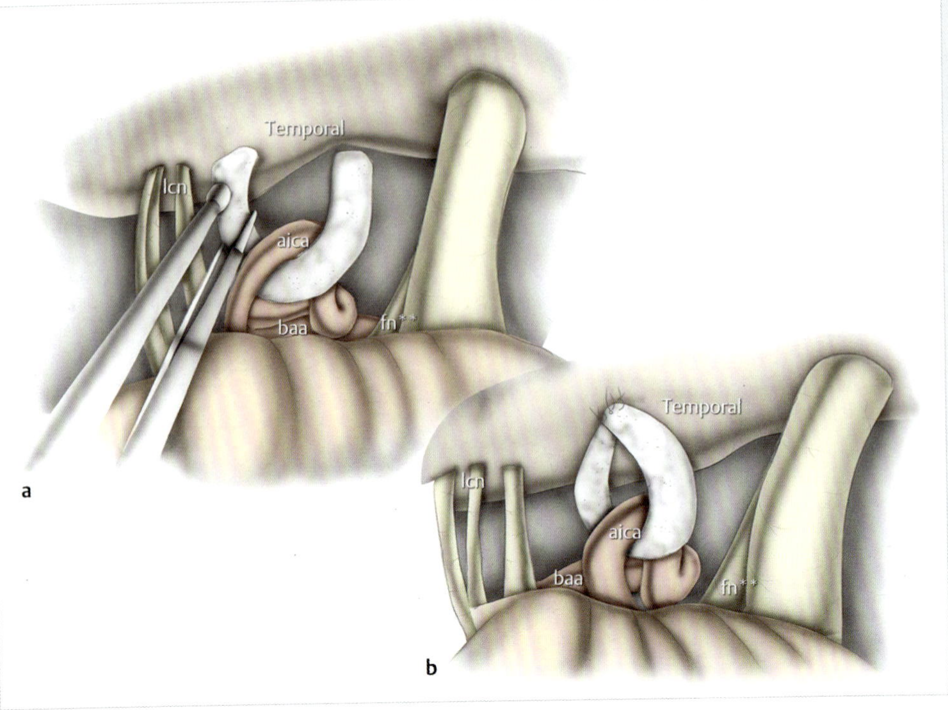

Fig. 7.108 **(a, b)** Left ear: A surgical technique variation: A teflon sheet is placed around the vascular structure and a suture of the teflon loop on the dura of the surface of the temporal bone is performed, keeping the artery off the nerve, so that the neurovascular contact can be solved. *aica: anterior inferior cerebellar artery; baa: basilar artery; fn**: exit zone of facial nerve; lcn: lower cranial nerves.*

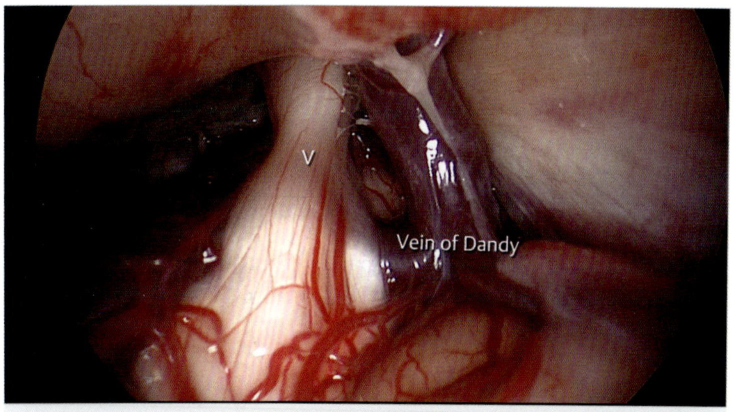

Fig. 7.109 Clinical Case 8, Left ear: Trigeminal neuralgia. An endoscopic check of the cerebellopontine angle (CPA) shows the underlying blood vessel which causes the compression of the trigeminal nerve at the root exit zone. In this case a vein arising from Dandy's vein is the offending vessel.

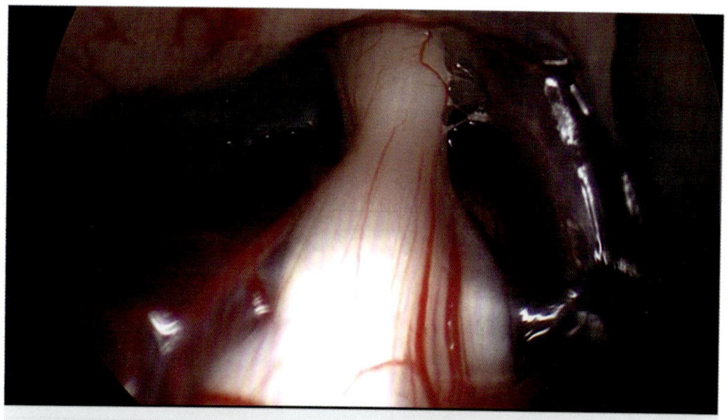

Fig. 7.110 Clinical Case 8, Left ear: Trigeminal neuralgia. Endoscopic magnification of the status of the trigeminal nerve fibers.

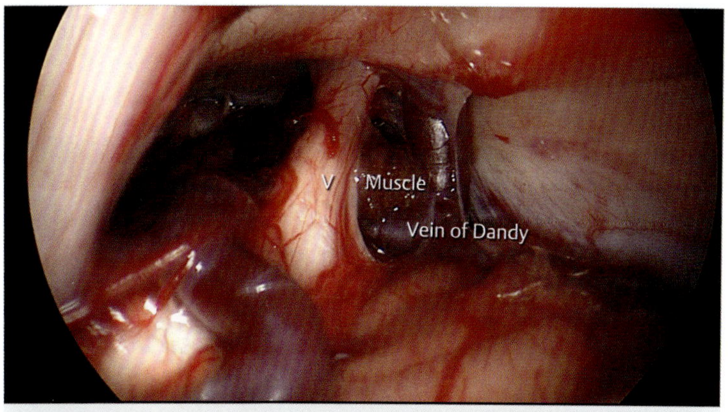

Fig. 7.111 Clinical Case 8, Left ear: Trigeminal neuralgia. A piece of muscle is placed between the trigeminal nerve and the underlying offending vein.

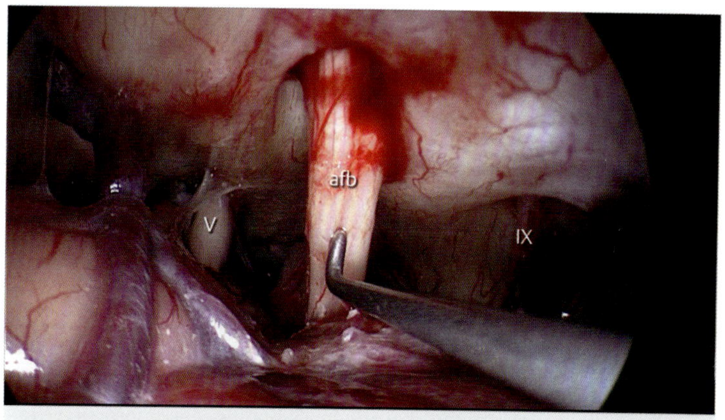

Fig. 7.112 Clinical Case 9, Right ear: Facial nerve spasm. Endoscopic view of the acoustic-facial bundle. *afb: acoustic-facial bundle.*

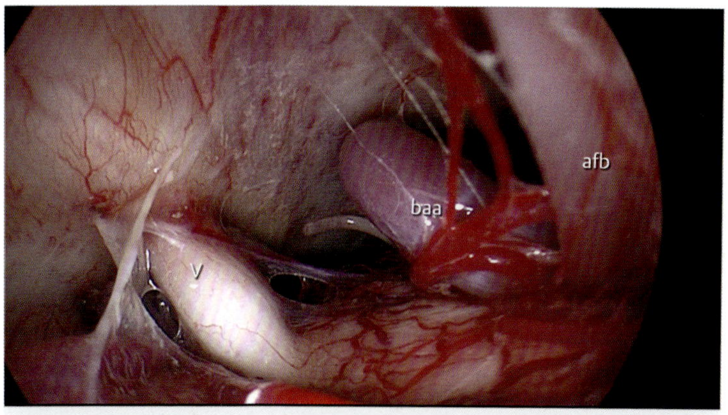

Fig. 7.113 Clinical Case 9, Right ear: The endoscopic check of the acoustic-facial bundle at the exit zone shows a basilar artery loop underlying the facial nerve, causing the offending neurovascular contact. *afb: acoustic-facial bundle; baa: basilar artery.*

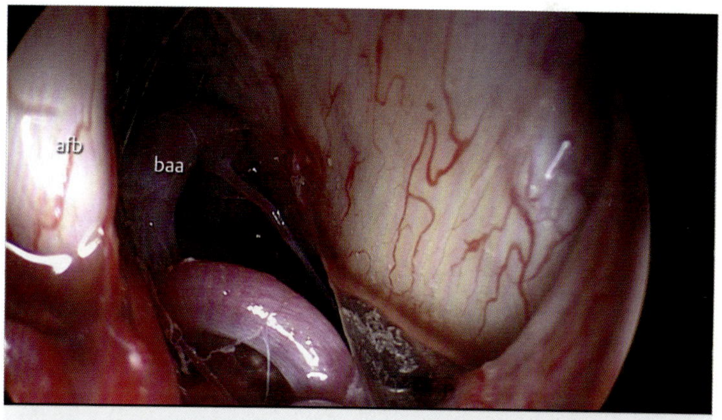

Fig. 7.114 Clinical Case 9, Right ear: The offending vessel is endoscopically seen at the exit zone of the facial nerve. *afb: acoustic-facial bundle; baa: basilar artery.*

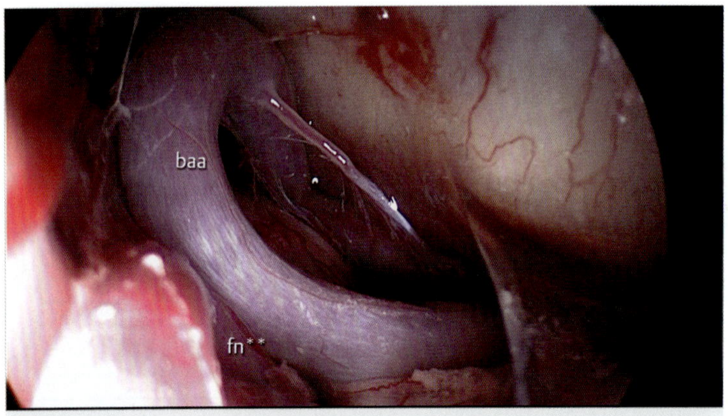

Fig. 7.115 Clinical Case 9, Right ear: Endoscopic magnification of the basilar artery loop underlying the root of the facial nerve at the exit zone. *baa: basilar artery; fn**: facial nerve at the exit zone.*

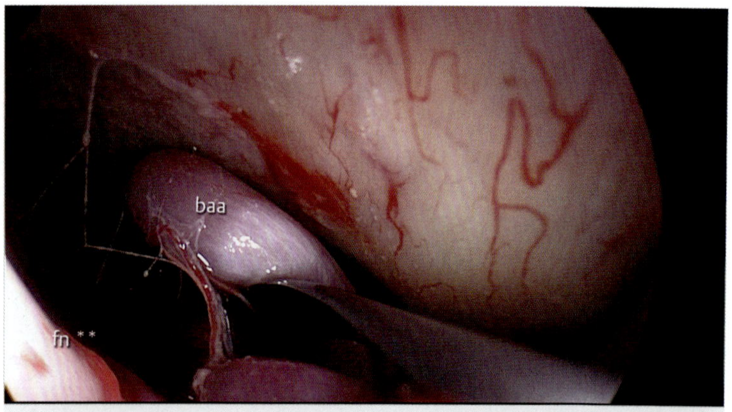

Fig. 7.116 Clinical Case 9, Right ear: A careful dissection of the vascular loop is performed, separating the facial nerve from the offending artery. *baa: basilar artery; fn**: facial nerve at the exit zone.*

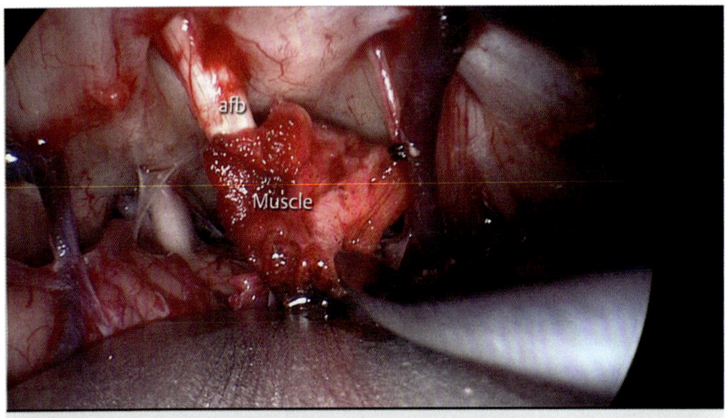

Fig. 7.117 Clinical Case 9, Right ear: A muscular graft is inserted between the artery and the acoustic-facial bundle, decompressing the nerve. *afb: acoustic-facial bundle.*

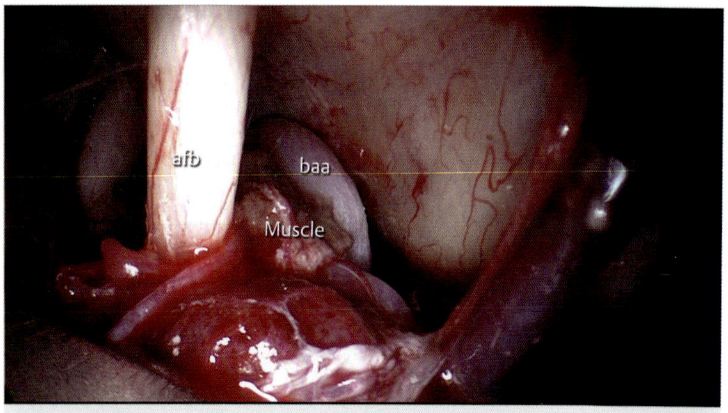

Fig. 7.118 Clinical Case 9, Right ear: Endoscopic view of the decompression. The muscular graft is seen between the nerve and the artery. *baa: basilar artery; fn**: facial nerve at the exit zone.*

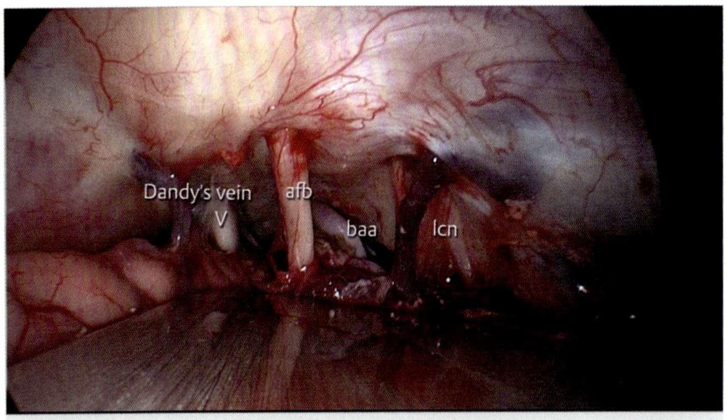

Fig. 7.119 Clinical Case 9, Right ear: General view of the cerebello-pontine angle (CPA) at the end of surgical procedure. *afb: acoustic-facial bundle; baa: basilar artery; lcn: lower cranial nerves.*

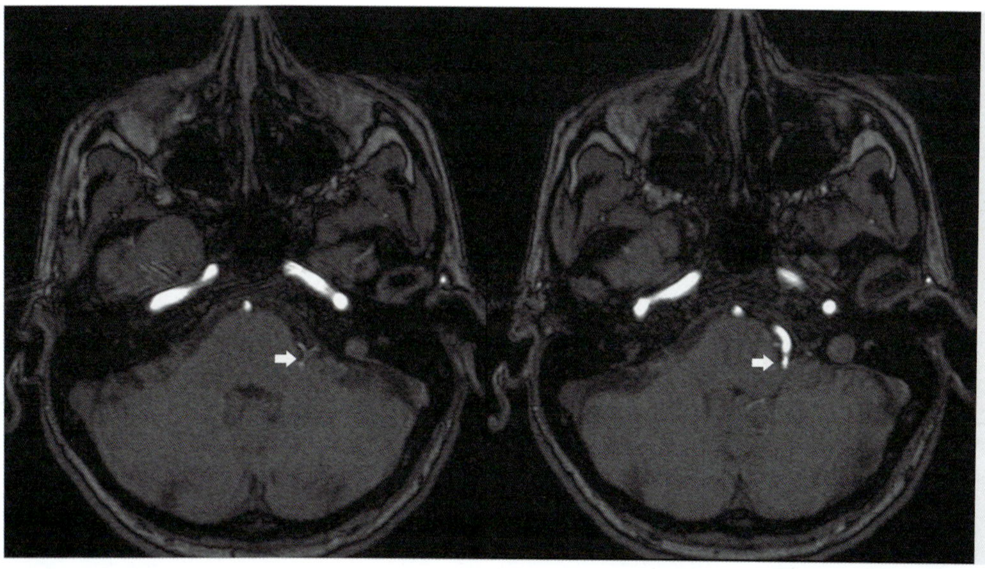

Fig. 7.120 Clinical Case 10, Right ear: Magnetic resonance imaging (MRI) shows the offending vessel (see the *white arrow*: anterior inferior cerebellar artery [AICA]) running at the exit zone of the facial nerve in a patient with facial nerve spasm.

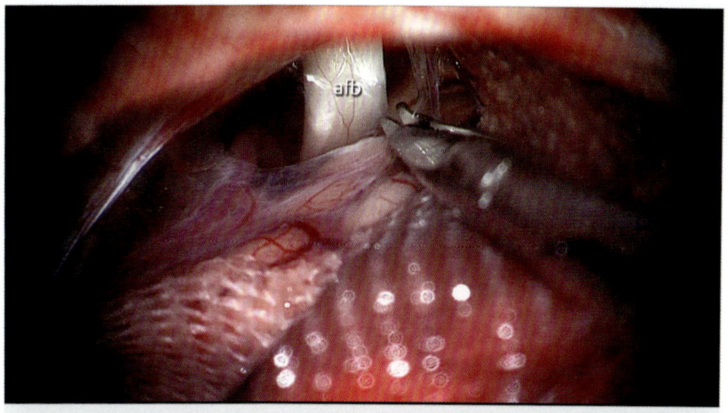

Fig. 7.121 Clinical Case 10; facial nerve spasm; right ear: The acoustic-facial bundle is microscopically exposed through a retrosigmoid approach. *afb: acoustic-facial bundle.*

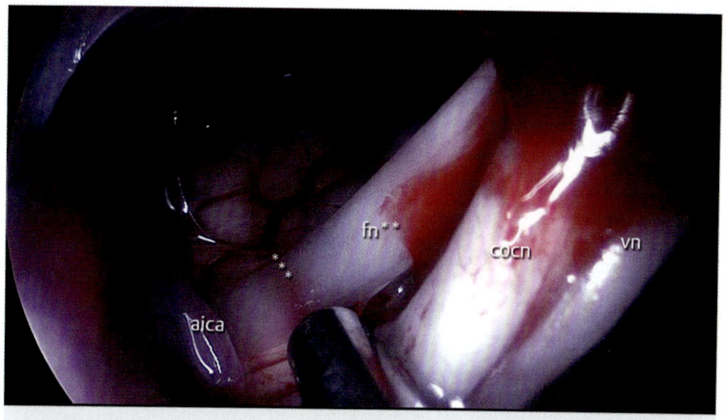

Fig. 7.122 Clinical Case 10, Right ear: A 0-degree endoscope is used to detect the offending vessel (anterior inferior cerebellar artery [AICA]) to the facial nerve; the characteristic color alteration on the surface of the root of the exit zone of the facial nerve, indicating the decubitus, is noted (see the ***). *aica: anterior inferior cerebellar artery; cocn: cochlear nerve; fn**: facial nerve at the exit zone; vn: vestibular nerve.*

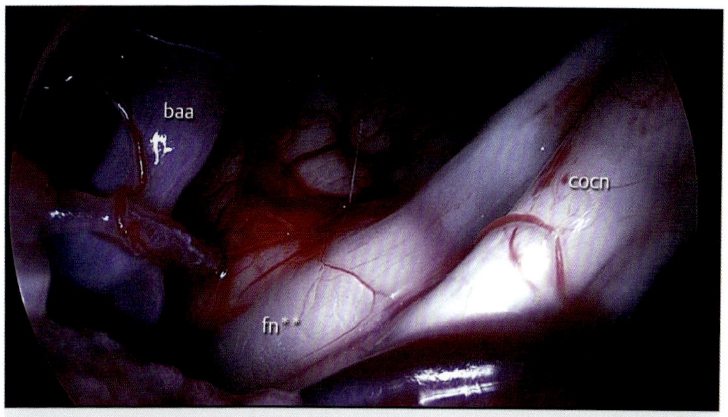

Fig. 7.123 Clinical Case 10, Right ear: The anterior inferior cerebellar artery (AICA) is detached from the exit zone of the facial nerve and moved away, decompressing the nerve. *baa: basilar artery; cocn: cochlear nerve; fn**: facial nerve at the exit-zone.*

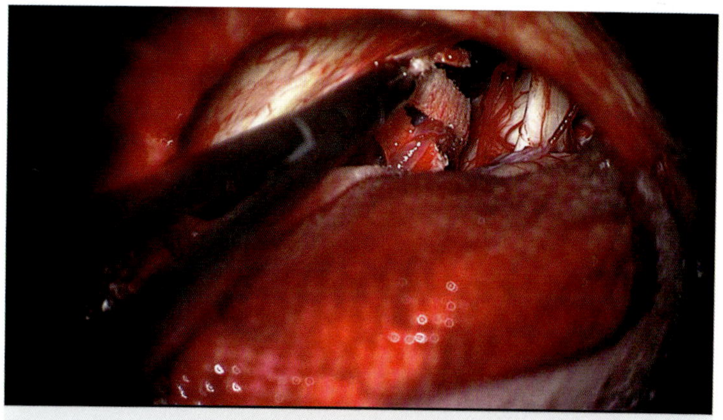

Fig. 7.124 Clinical Case 10, Right ear: A teflon sheet is placed around the anterior inferior cerebellar artery (AICA) using the microscope.

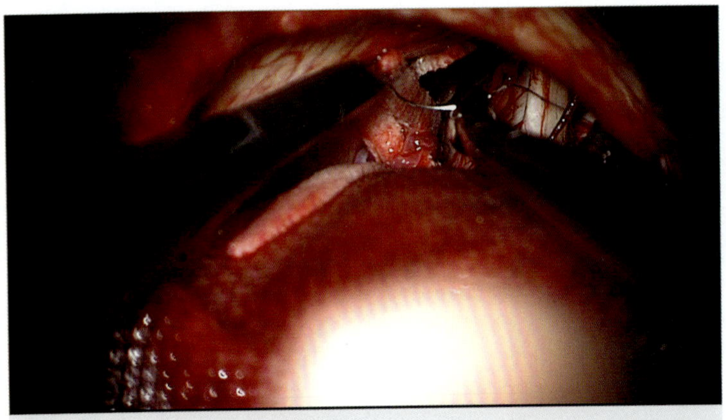

Fig. 7.125 Clinical Case 10, Right ear: The teflon loop is microscopically sutured on the dura of the surface of the temporal bone to keep the artery away from the facial nerve.

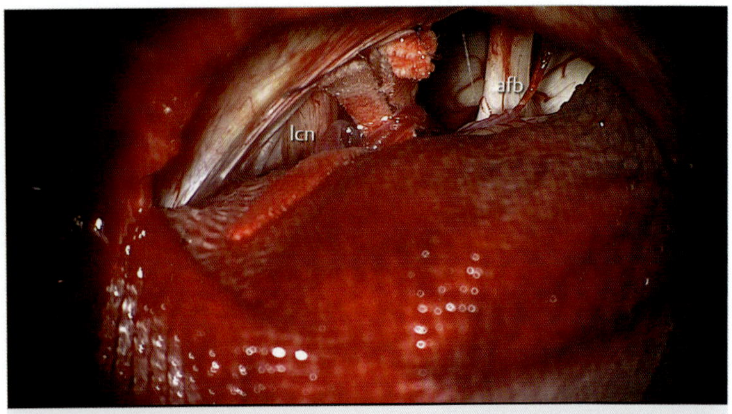

Fig. 7.126 Clinical Case 10, Right ear: Final microscopic view of the cerebellopontine angle (CPA) at the end of the surgical procedure. *afb: acoustic facial bundle; lcn: lower cranial nerves.*

Suggested Readings

Abolfotoh M, Bi WL, Hong CK, et al. The combined microscopic-endoscopic technique for radical resection of cerebellopontine angle tumors. J Neurosurg. 2015; 123(5):1301–1311

Abolfotoh M, Dunn IF, Al-Mefty O. Transmastoid retrosigmoid approach to the cerebellopontine angle: surgical technique. Neurosurgery. 2013; 73(1) Suppl Operative:ons16–ons23, discussion ons23

Betka J, Chovanec M, Zerina E, Profant O, Lukes P, Skrivan J. Minimally invasive endoscopic and endoscopy-assisted microsurgery of vestibular schwannoma. In: Iancu C, ed. Advances in Endoscopic Surgery. Rijeka, Croatia: InTech; 2011:191–216

Broggi M, Acerbi F, Ferroli P, Tringali G, Schiariti M, Broggi G. Microvascular decompression for neurovascular conflicts in the cerebello-pontine angle: which role for endoscopy? Acta Neurochir (Wien). 2013; 155(9):1709–1716

Cappabianca P, Cavallo LM, Esposito F, de Divitiis E, Tschabitscher M. Endoscopic examination of the cerebellar pontine angle. Clin Neurol Neurosurg. 2002; 104 (4):387–391

Chaynes P, Deguine O, Moscovici J, Fraysse B, Becue J, Lazorthes Y. Endoscopic anatomy of the cerebellopontine angle: a study in cadaver brains. Neurosurg Focus. 1998; 5(3):e8

Chovanec M, Zvěřina E, Profant O, et al. Impact of video-endoscopy on the results of retrosigmoid-transmeatal microsurgery of vestibular schwannoma: prospective study. Eur Arch Otorhinolaryngol. 2013; 270(4):1277–1284

Chowdhury FH, Haque MR. Endoscopic assisted microsurgical removal of cerebellopontine angle and prepontine epidermoid. J Neurosci Rural Pract. 2012; 3 (3):414–419

Copeland WR, Mallory GW, Neff BA, Driscoll CL, Link MJ. Are there modifiable risk factors to prevent a cerebrospinal fluid leak following vestibular schwannoma surgery? J Neurosurg. 2015; 122(2):312–316

El-Garem HF, Badr-El-Dine M, Talaat AM, Magnan J. Endoscopy as a tool in minimally invasive trigeminal neuralgia surgery. Otol Neurotol. 2002; 23(2):132–135

Elhammady MS, Telischi FF, Morcos JJ. Retrosigmoid approach: indications, techniques, and results. Otolaryngol Clin North Am. 2012; 45(2):375–397, ix

Fukushima T. Endoscopy of Meckel's cave, cisterna magna, and cerebellopontine angle. Technical note. J Neurosurg. 1978; 48(2):302–306

Göksu N, Bayazit Y, Kemaloğlu Y. Endoscopy of the posterior fossa and dissection of acoustic neuroma. J Neurosurg. 1999; 91(5):776–780

Ho SY, Hudgens S, Wiet RJ. Comparison of postoperative facial nerve outcomes between translabyrinthine and retrosigmoid approaches in matched-pair patients. Laryngoscope. 2003; 113(11):2014–2020

Jarrahy R, Berci G, Shahinian HK. Endoscope-assisted microvascular decompression of the trigeminal nerve. Otolaryngol Head Neck Surg. 2000; 123(3):218–223

Jennings CR, O'Donoghue GM. Posterior fossa endoscopy. J Laryngol Otol. 1998; 112 (3):227–229

Jung S, Kang SS, Kim TS, et al. Current surgical results of retrosigmoid approach in extralarge vestibular schwannomas. Surg Neurol. 2000; 53(4):370–377, discussion 377–378

Kane AJ, Sughrue ME, Rutkowski MJ, Berger MS, McDermott MW, Parsa AT. Clinical and surgical considerations for cerebellopontine angle meningiomas. J Clin Neurosci. 2011; 18(6):755–759

King WA, Wackym PA. Endoscope-assisted surgery for acoustic neuromas (vestibular schwannomas): early experience using the rigid Hopkins telescope. Neurosurgery. 1999; 44(5):1095–1100, discussion 1100–1102

Kumon Y, Kohno S, Ohue S, et al. Usefulness of endoscope-assisted microsurgery for removal of vestibular schwannomas. J Neurol Surg B Skull Base. 2012; 73(1):42–47

Little AS, Almefty KK, Spetzler RF. Endoscopic surgery of the posterior fossa: strengths and limitations. World Neurosurg. 2014; 82(3–4):322–324

Mercier P, Sindou M. The conflicting vessels in hemifacial spasm: literature review and anatomical-surgical implications. Neurochirurgie. 2018; 64(2):94–100

Miyazaki H, Deveze A, Magnan J. Neuro-otologic surgery through minimally invasive retrosigmoid approach: endoscope assisted microvascular decompression, vestibular neurotomy, and tumor removal. Laryngoscope. 2005; 115(9):1612–1617

Nguyen VN, Basma J, Sorenson J, Michael LM, II. Microvascular decompression for geniculate neuralgia through a retrosigmoid approach. J Neurol Surg B Skull Base. 2019; 80 Suppl 3:S322

Nonaka Y, Fukushima T, Watanabe K, et al. Contemporary surgical management of vestibular schwannomas: analysis of complications and lessons learned over the past decade. Neurosurgery. 2013; 72(2) Suppl Operative:ons103–ons115, discussion ons115

O'Donoghue GM, O'Flynn P. Endoscopic anatomy of the cerebellopontine angle. Am J Otol. 1993; 14(2):122–125

Safavi-Abbasi S, Di Rocco F, Bambakidis N, et al. Has management of epidermoid tumors of the cerebellopontine angle improved? A surgical synopsis of the past and present. Skull Base. 2008; 18(2):85–98

Schroeder HW, Hickmann AK, Baldauf J. Endoscope-assisted microsurgical resection of skull base meningiomas. Neurosurg Rev. 2011; 34(4):441–455

Schroeder HW, Oertel J, Gaab MR. Endoscope-assisted microsurgical resection of epidermoid tumors of the cerebellopontine angle. J Neurosurg. 2004; 101 (2):227–232

Takemura Y, Inoue T, Morishita T, Rhoton AL, Jr. Comparison of microscopic and endoscopic approaches to the cerebellopontine angle. World Neurosurg. 2014; 82 (3–4):427–441

Tatagiba M, Matthies C, Samii M. Microendoscopy of the internal auditory canal in vestibular schwannoma surgery. Neurosurgery. 1996; 38(4):737–740

Tuchman A, Platt A, Winer J, Pham M, Giannotta S, Zada G. Endoscopic-assisted resection of intracranial epidermoid tumors. World Neurosurg. 2014; 82(3–4):450–454

Turek G, Cotúa C, Zamora RE, Tatagiba M. Endoscopic assistance in retrosigmoid transmeatal approach to intracanalicular vestibular schwannomas—an alternative for middle fossa approach. Technical note. Neurol Neurochir Pol. 2017; 51 (2):111–115

Xia Y, Li XP, Han DM, Zheng J, Long HS, Shi JF. Anatomic structural study of cerebellopontine angle via endoscope. Chin Med J (Engl). 2007; 120(20):1836–1839

Yuguang L, Chengyuan W, Meng L, et al. Neuroendoscopic anatomy and surgery of the cerebellopontine angle. J Clin Neurosci. 2005; 12(3):256–260

Chapter 8

Middle Cranial Fossa Approaches: Traditional Surgery and Endoscopic Assisted Procedure

8

8 Middle Cranial Fossa Approaches: Traditional Surgery and Endoscopic Assisted Procedure

Daniele Marchioni, Raphaelle A. Chemtob, Elliott D. Kozin, Daniel J. Lee, and Davide Soloperto

Abstract

The middle fossa approach has become a necessary technique for surgeons managing lesions of the petrous apex and the internal auditory canal (IAC) with hearing preservation, but it is surgically challenging because the anatomy of this area is variable, which causes difficulty in identifying landmarks. Moreover, pathologies sometimes cause the encasement of important neurovascular structures. The anterior petrosectomy procedure represents a natural anterior extension of the middle fossa approach designed to expose petrous apex lesions with intradural extension on the ventral and ventrolateral portions of the upper third of the brainstem. Currently, the major surgical indications are represented by inflammatory, malformative or tumoral pathologies, or conditions spreading into or involving the petrous apex, with extension to the IAC, with preserved preoperative hearing; some examples are small vestibular schwannomas of the fundus of the IAC, cholesterol granuloma, petrous bone cholesteatomas, chondrosarcomas, chordomas. Cochlear implantation in middle ear malformation, repair of superior secircular canal (SSC) dehiscence (Minor's syndrome) and decompression for facial nerve palsy are other known indications.

Recently, while performing middle cranial fossa and anterior petrosectomy surgical routes, the use of endoscopic assisted technique is increasing in order to work around the critical anatomical structures such as the horizontal IAC and along hidden areas lying in the petrous apex, removing remnant lesions and minimizing the manipulation of the neurovascular structures surrounding neurovascular structures.

Keywords: middle cranial fossa, petrous apex, acoustic neuroma, endoscopic approach

8.1 Introduction

The middle fossa approach has become a necessary technique for surgeons managing lesions of the petrous apex and the internal auditory canal (IAC), also for the possibility of preserving useful hearing. The recent application of middle fossa labyrinthine facial nerve decompression for Bell's palsy has renewed interest in this approach. The middle fossa approach is surgically challenging because of the proximity of critical structures located within millimeters from each other. For this reason, its popularity has slowly increased, due to the anatomical complexity of the approach and the absence of consistent landmarks on the superior surface of the temporal bone. Since the early 1900s, during middle cranial fossa surgery, the superior aspect of the petrous pyramid has been approached extradurally in order to treat trigeminal neuralgia and petrositis. In 1904, Parry described the section of the VIIIth cranial nerve through middle fossa approach to treat Meniere's disease. In the early 1960s, William House finally developed the modern middle cranial fossa approach, originally trying to decompress the auditory nerve from osteosclerotic foci inside the IAC in highly advanced otosclerosis. House introduced revolutionary concepts, including many of the principles of skull base surgery that are now taken for granted, such as the use of the operating microscope, continuous suction irrigation, diamond stone burs, and a multidisciplinary team approach. Over the years, the main indication for this approach has been the treatment of neurotologic conditions. Some examples are: the removal of small laterally placed vestibular schwannomas, facial nerve decompression with exposure of its labyrinthine and upper tympanic segments, repair of semicircular canal dehiscence, vestibular nerve section, repair of meningoceles, and debridement of inflammatory lesions of the petrous apex. In general, middle cranial fossa surgery is useful for the management of lesions of the petrous apex and the IAC in patients with preoperative usable hearing function.

8.2 Surgical Anatomy

The anatomy of the floor of the middle cranial fossa is variable, which causes difficulty in identifying landmarks. The surgeon must have an accurate knowledge of the three-dimensional anatomy of the temporal bone, and must avoid damage of facial nerve, ampulla of the SSC, and basal turn of the cochlea.

The position of the facial nerve, the cochlear nerve, and both the inferior and superior vestibular nerves in the lateral part of the internal acoustic meatus is crucial, especially during a middle cranial fossa approach. The meatus is divided into a superior and an inferior portion by a horizontal ridge, called either the transverse or the falciform crest (see ▶ Fig. 8.1 and ▶ Fig. 8.2). The facial and the superior vestibular nerves are above the crest. The facial nerve is anterior to the superior vestibular nerve and it is separated from it at the lateral end of the meatus by a vertical ridge of bone called the vertical crest (see ▶ Fig. 8.2 and ▶ Fig. 8.3). The vertical crest is also known as Bill's bar in recognition of William House's role in focusing on the importance of this crest in the identification of the facial nerve in the lateral end of the canal. The cochlear and inferior vestibular nerves run below the transverse crest with the cochlear nerve being located anteriorly. Thus, the lateral meatus can be split into four portions, with the facial nerve lying in an anterior-superior position; the cochlear nerve, anterior-inferior; the superior vestibular nerve, posterior-superior; and the inferior vestibular nerve, posterior-inferior (see ▶ Fig. 8.3). The position of the nerves is most consistent in the lateral portion of the meatus and this concept is really important for surgery involving the IAC and the cerebellopontine angle (CPA). In the middle fossa route, the meatus is approached from above, through a temporal craniotomy performed anterior to the ear and above the zygoma.

Although the middle cranial approach is a well-codified procedure, providing an effective good exposure of the IAC and the petrous apex, there is a lack of consistent anatomical landmarks.

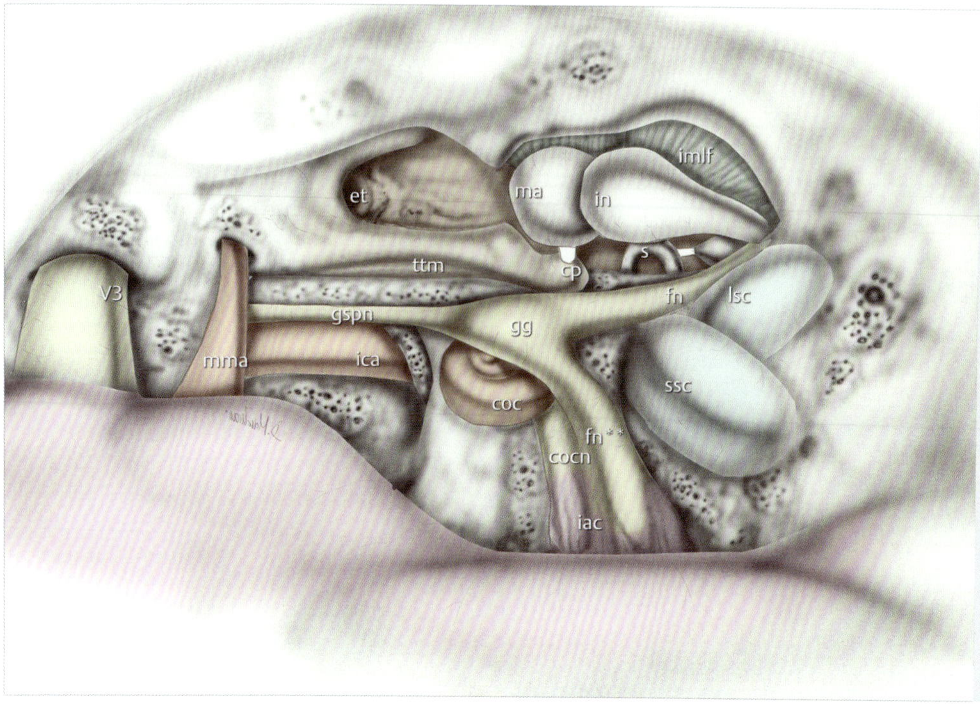

Fig. 8.1 Right side: View of the anatomy of the temporal bone from the middle cranial fossa approach. The relationships between the facial nerve and the surrounding anatomical structures are showed. *coc: cochlea; cocn: cochlear nerve; cp: cochleariform process; et: eustachian tube; fn: tympanic portion of the facial nerve; fn**: intracanalicular portion of the facial nerve; gg: geniculate ganglion; gspn: greater superficial petrosal nerve; iac: internal auditory canal; ica: internal carotid artery; imlf: lateral incudo-malleal fold; in: incus; lsc: lateral semicircular canal; ma: malleus; mma: middle meningeal artery; s: stapes; ssc: superior semicircular canal; ttm: tensor tympani muscle canal; V3: mandibular division of trigeminal nerve.*

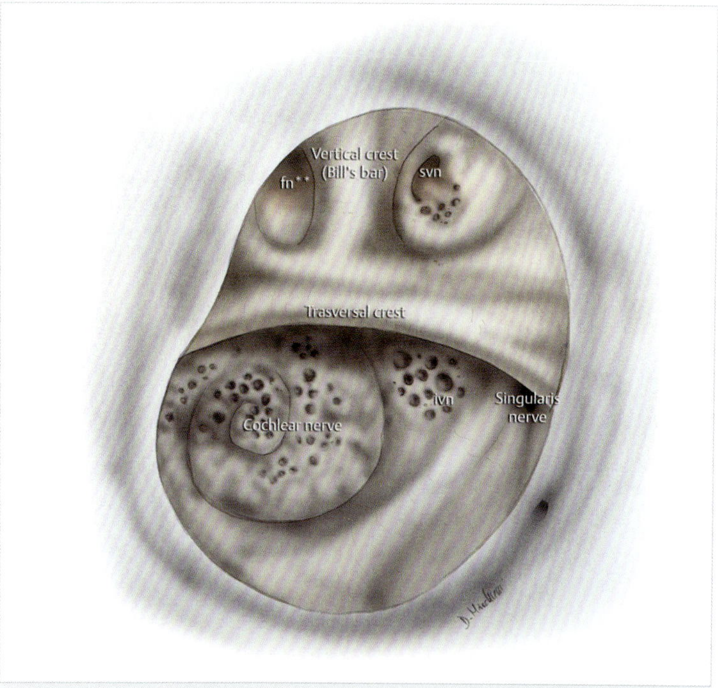

Fig. 8.2 Right side: Anatomy of the bony wall of the internal auditory canal (IAC), viewed from the posterior fossa to the fundus of the IAC. The transverse (falciform) crest, dividing the IAC into superior and inferior portions, is noted. The Bill's bar is located in the superior portion of the canal, dividing it into anterior and posterior portions. *fn**: intracanalicular portion of the facial nerve; ivn: inferior vestibular nerve; svn: superior vestibular nerve.*

In particular, it is difficult to find a proper anatomical way of safely exposing the IAC, and a proper surgical training with this approach is needed. The middle meningeal artery and the trigeminal nerve (V3) are considered the anterior limits of the dissection, while exposing the superior surface of the temporal bone.

One surgical method described by House is currently being used by the present authors due the simplicity. Since the greater superficial petrosal nerve (GSPN) run in the superior surface of the temporal bone, it may be used as a landmark to identify the IAC.

The bone covering the GSPN is progressively removed, following the nerve posteriorly till the geniculate ganglion and the first genu of the facial nerve. After this step the drilling continues in the posterior portion of the geniculate ganglion, detecting the labyrinthine portion of the facial neve and the lateral end of the IAC. In this way the IAC is progressively exposed from a lateral to a medial direction. The bisection line of the angle formed by the GSPN and the arcuate eminence may be used as well in order to identify the orientation of the IAC. In this case drilling can start from the most medial portion of this bisection line, above the porus, away from the fundus of the IAC, avoiding possible damage of the cochlea and the superior labyrinth. In some cases, the exposition of the incudomalleolar joint, after tegmen removal, should be considered in order to gain a better orientation (see Section 8.4.2, Identification of the IAC for Acoustic Neuroma Resection).

The natural extension of the middle fossa approach is the anterior petrosal approach (anterior petrosectomy); this approach is useful especially for the removal of lesions located in the petrous apex in subjects with preserved hearing function. This last approach requires expanded bony resection between the horizontal portion of the internal carotid artery (ICA), the IAC, and the trigeminal nerve (V3) in order to expose the petrous apex and the clivus till the upper petroclival region and the ventrolateral brainstem, if necessary.

8.3 The Middle Cranial Fossa and the Anterior Petrosectomy Approaches

8.3.1 Indications

Currently, the major indications for this surgery are represented by pathologies or conditions in which the patient has a preserved hearing function before surgery, in particular:

- Middle fossa approach; surgical indications:
  - Facial nerve decompression (due to idiopathic paralysis, herpes zoster, or longitudinal fracture of temporal bone)

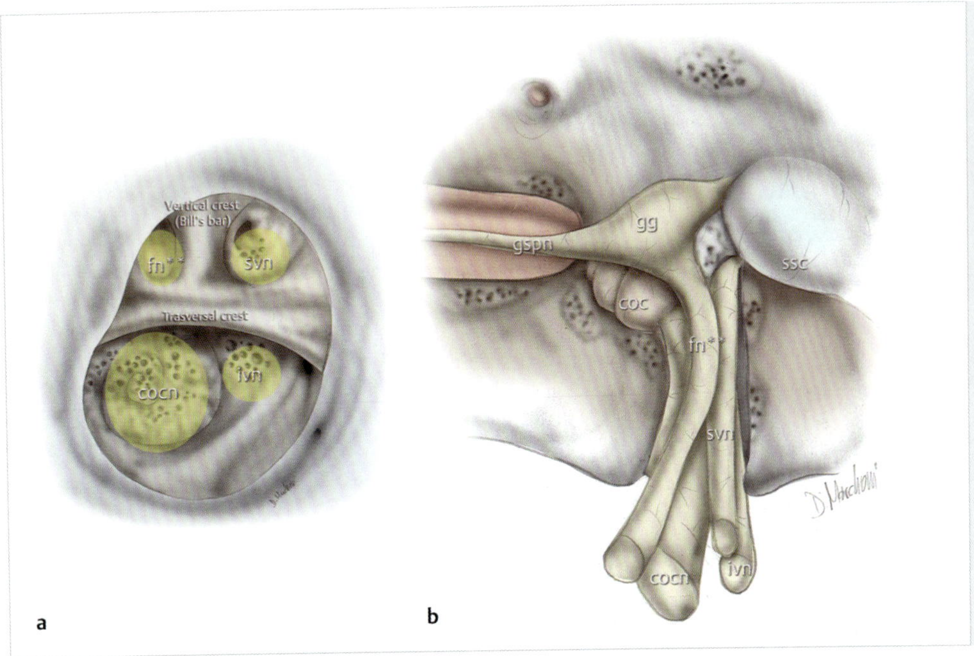

Fig. 8.3 Right side: Anatomy of the internal auditory canal (IAC) and related cranial nerves through the middle cranial fossa approach. **(a)** The fundus of the IAC is showed and the positions of the nerves in this anatomical area are visible. **(b)** View of the IAC from above (middle cranial fossa). The IAC dura is opened, exposing its contents. The position of the nerves is noted. *coc: cochlea; cocn: cochlear nerve; fn**: facial nerve; gg: geniculate ganglion; gspn: greater superficial petrosal nerve; ivn: inferior vestibular nerve; ssc: superior semicircular canal; svn: superior vestibular nerve.*

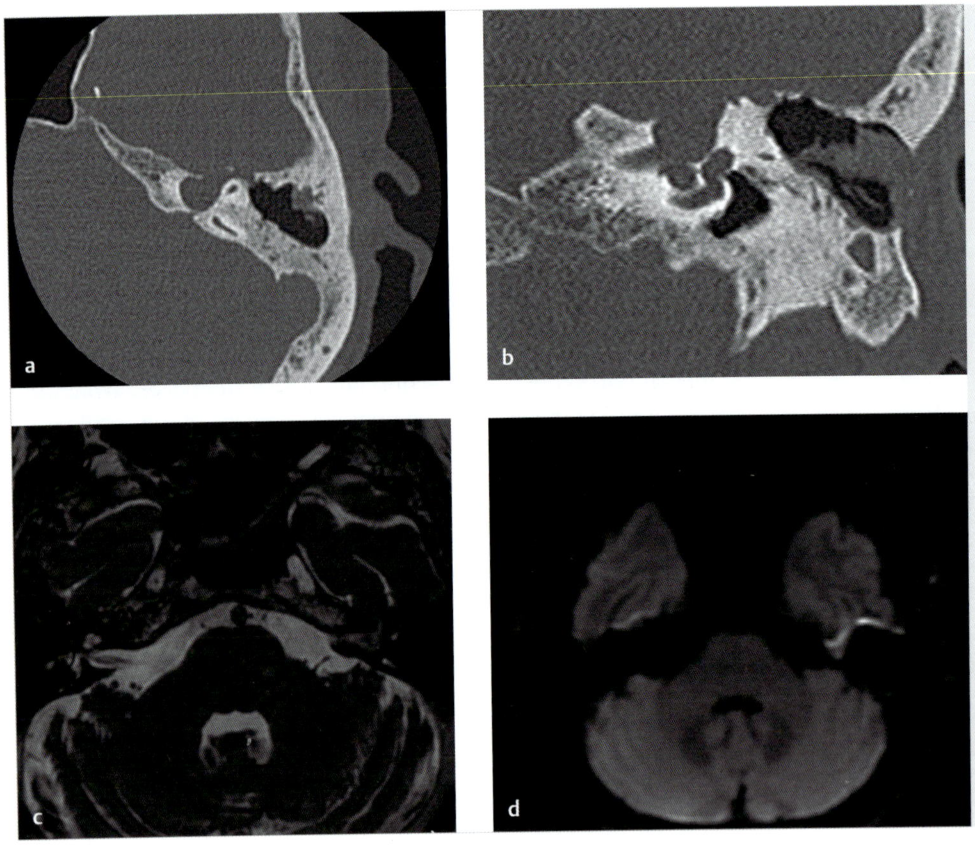

Fig. 8.4 Left supralabyrinthine petrous bone cholesteatoma with internal auditory canal (IAC) involvement, in subject who underwent previous canal wall up procedure. **(a)** Computed tomography (CT) scan, axial view. **(b)** CT scan, coronal view. **(c)** Magnetic resonance imaging (MRI), axial view, that shows the IAC involvement of the cholesteatoma. **(d)** Diffusion-weighted magnetic resonance imaging (DWI or DW-MRI) confirming the presence of cholesteatoma.

  - Small vestibular schwannomas reaching the fundus of the IAC with a CPA extension of less than 0.5 cm, with good hearing function
  - Facial nerve tumors located between the geniculate ganglion and the IAC
  - Supralabyrinthine non-eroding petrous bone cholesteatomas (see ▶ Fig. 8.4 and Clinical Case 2)
  - Cochlear implantation in middle ear malformations
  - Repair of SSC dehiscence (Minor's syndrome) (see Clinical Case 3, ▶ Fig. 8.70 and ▶ Fig. 8.71)
- Anterior petrosectomy approach; surgical indications:
  - Petrous apex lesions, with or without epidural extension, including: anterior petrosal cysts (epidermoid or cholesteatomas), cholesterol granulomas, chordomas and chondrosarcomas (see Clinical Case 4 and Clinical Case 5)
  - Upper petroclival and Meckel's cave tumors (meningiomas, trigeminal schwannomas)
  - Lateral and ventral midbrain and pontine intra-axial lesions

8.3.2 Advantages

- Hearing function preservation
- Good exposure of labyrinthine and tympanic tracts of the facial nerve
- Good exposure of superior aspect of the IAC and petrous apex
- Exposure of the horizontal portion of petrous ICA and gasserian ganglion with V3
- Low incidence of postoperative headache

8.3.3 Limitations

- Limited access to the posterior fossa (in case of traditional middle fossa approach)
- Difficult anatomy with the lack of consistent landmarks
- Unsuitable for large tumors
- Postoperative facial nerve weakness
- Unsuitable in case of active infection of the middle ear as in chronic otitis media

8.3.4 Use of the Endoscope

The endoscopic assisted procedure through the middle cranial fossa and anterior petrosectomy surgical routes has been recently introduced. The endoscope is used after the microscopic based procedure in order to work around the critical anatomical structures such as the horizontal portion of internal carotid artery and along hidden areas lying in the petrous apex, to remove remnant lesions and minimize the manipulation of the neurovascular structures surrounding neurovascular structures.

Indications

- Endoscopic assisted surgery for detection and removal of residual tumor in the fundus of the IAC (especially below the transverse crest)
- Detection and removal of residual disease lying in the hidden areas along the petrous apex while treating supralabyrinthine petrous bone cholesteatomas, cholesterol granulomas, or chondrosarcomas
- Endoscopic assisted surgery for residual disease lying below and lateral to the horizontal portion of the ICA, during anterior petrosectomy procedure
- Minimizing craniotomy and temporal bone retraction during SSC dehiscence repair

8.4 Middle Fossa Approach for IAC Lesions

8.4.1 Surgical Steps

The patient is placed in a supine position with the head turned to the contralateral side of the lesion; facial nerve and cochlear nerve monitoring is placed (see ▶ Fig. 8.5).

The incision starts in front of the tragus and extends superiorly, first heading posteriorly and then anteriorly, describing a curve in a C shape ending in the temporalis area (see ▶ Fig. 8.29, Clinical Case 1). The skin flap is elevated, maintaining the plane of the dissection over the temporalis muscle fascia (see ▶ Fig. 8.6a). The temporalis muscle is thus exposed. The incision of the temporalis muscle is performed in a C shape, parallel to the skin incision, and the muscle is elevated and placed over the skin flap anteriorly until the temporal squama is exposed (see ▶ Fig. 8.6b).

During this step, the zygomatic arch is detected and partially uncovered (see ▶ Fig. 8.7). This bony structure is a crucial landmark defining the level of the middle fossa floor. The soft tissues on the external auditory canal (EAC) are elevated and gently dissected in order to identify the superior portion of the EAC. Based on these two anatomical landmarks the craniotomy should be made close to the zygoma, extending one-third in front and two-thirds behind the EAC (see ▶ Fig. 8.8).

A classical 4 × 4 cm craniotomy is performed. The bone is gently separated from the underlying dura and preserved in a saline solution (see ▶ Fig. 8.9). During the next steps the surgeon and first assistant are positioned at the head of the bed (see ▶ Fig. 8.10a). The dura is gently elevated from the superior face of the temporalis bone, from a posterior direction, at the level of the petrous ridge, to an anterior direction, until the middle meningeal artery is identified. A small incision on the dura of the middle fossa should be considered in order to decompress the temporal lobe, facilitating elevation and retraction of the brain (see ▶ Fig. 8.10b, c). Once the dura of the middle fossa is elevated (see ▶ Fig. 8.11), the middle meningeal artery is detected. This artery is the anterior limit of the dissection. The GSPN (see ▶ Fig. 8.12 and ▶ Fig. 8.13) and the arcuate eminence are identified. A Fisch middle cranial fossa retractor is placed to support the temporal lobe, and cottonoids are placed between the temporal lobe and the retractor, protecting the dural layer (see ▶ Fig. 8.14a). After the exposure of the superior surface of the temporal bone, the middle meningeal artery is coagulated and cut (see ▶ Fig. 8.14b); then the IAC identification is required.

8.4.2 Identification of the IAC for Acoustic Neuroma Resection

Different methods for exposing the IAC are described in literature, and they can be used separately or in combination (see ▶ Fig. 8.15).

- House's original description of the middle cranial fossa approach emphasized the initial identification of the GSPN (facial hiatus) as the only landmark to follow to reach the geniculate ganglion, labyrinthine segment, and IAC (▶ Fig. 8.15b). After the detection of the GSPN on the superior surface of the temporal bone, the bony covering of this nerve is progressively removed. The dissection of this nerve should be performed in a lateral to medial direction, until the geniculate ganglion and the genu of the facial nerve are found. Once the geniculate ganglion is detected, further drilling should be performed posteriorly, finding the labyrinthine portion of the facial nerve and following it till its entrance in the fundus of the IAC. This procedure allows the surgeon to localize the fundus of the IAC; a progressive skeletonization of the IAC is then performed from the medial to the lateral section. During the dissection of the labyrinthine portion of the facial nerve, bone removal must be carried out carefully, since this structure runs just above the cochlea and it is separated from the membranous cochlea just by a very thin bony layer. The disadvantages of House's classical technique are that the geniculate ganglion and the distal labyrinthine facial nerve are exposed to drilling, and that the dissection of the labyrinthine segment of the facial nerve might injure the cochlea and the ampullated end of the SSC. Another anatomical risk should be considered during this surgical approach. The superior tympanic artery and the petrosal artery run along the superior surface of the temporal bone along with the GSPN. This anatomical relationship is important especially because the petrosal artery may supply the labyrinthine

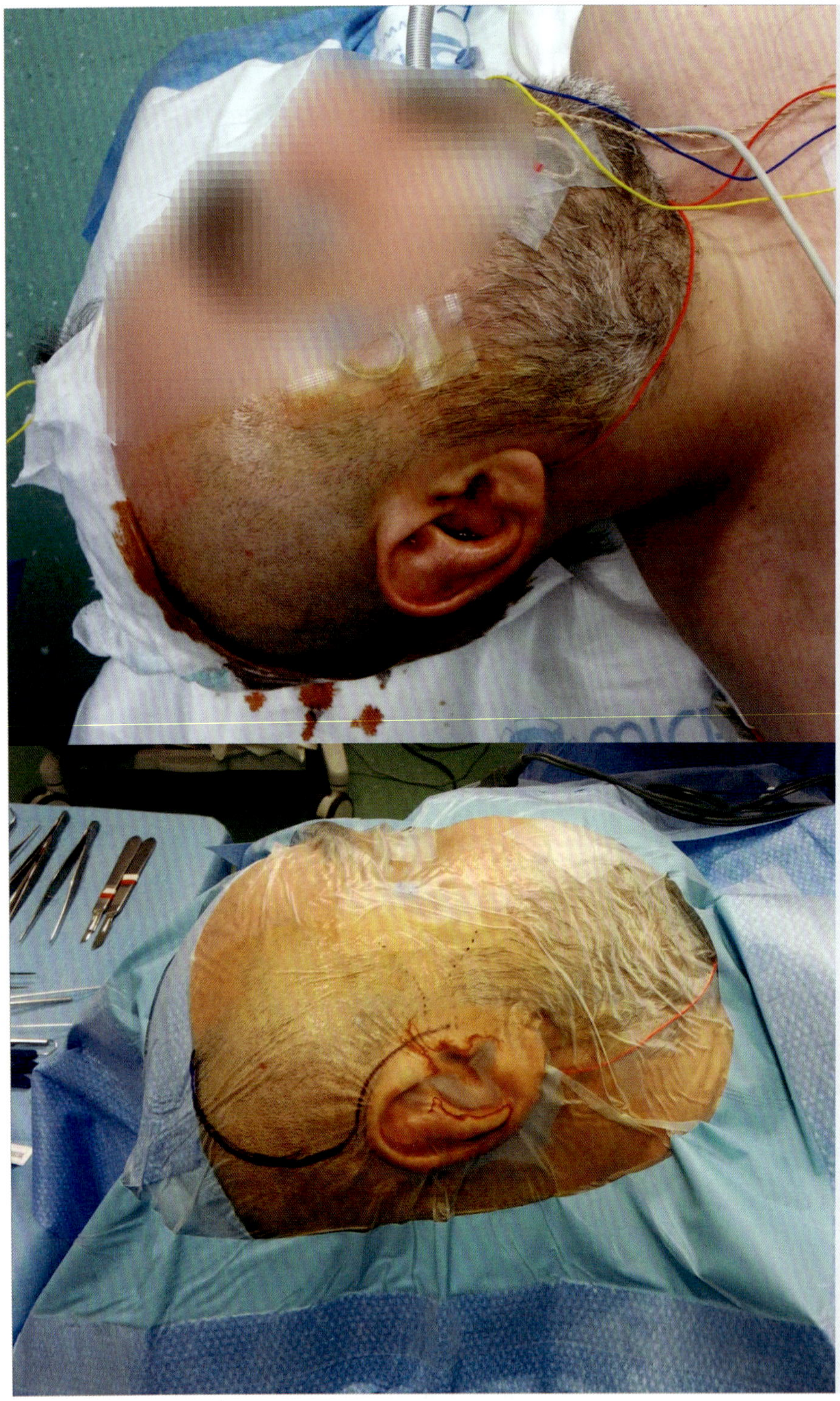

Fig. 8.5 Position of the head of the patient during middle cranial fossa approach.

portion of the facial nerve. For this reason this artery should be preserved during the dissection of the GSPN avoiding compromission of the vascular supply. Furthermore, the labyrinthine portion of the facial nerve is the most fragile portion and a possible damage may be expected since, in this technique, damage to the cochlea, the vestibule, and the SSC is mainly avoided by staying close to the facial nerve.

- Ugo Fisch described the use of the blue line of the SSC as a landmark and noted that the IAC lies within a 60-degree angle from this line (see ▶ Fig. 8.15a). Although this technique avoids the retrograde dissection of the facial nerve through the geniculate ganglion and labyrinthine segment, the obvious disadvantage is that it carries a risk of fenestrating the SSC. A congenital SSC dehiscence can be found in approximately 1% of temporal bones and this finding helps to identity the location of the canal within the arcuate eminence before drilling.
- Garcia Ibanez and Sanna use the bisection line of the angle formed by the imaginary lines that pass through the GSPN and the arcuate eminence (see ▶ Fig. 8.16). This bisection line indicates the location and the anatomical orientation of the IAC. A 20-degree Trendelenburg position of the patient can help exposing the dura at the meatal level, reducing temporal bone retraction. In this way the drilling can start along the bisection line in the proximity of the lateral portion of the IAC (see

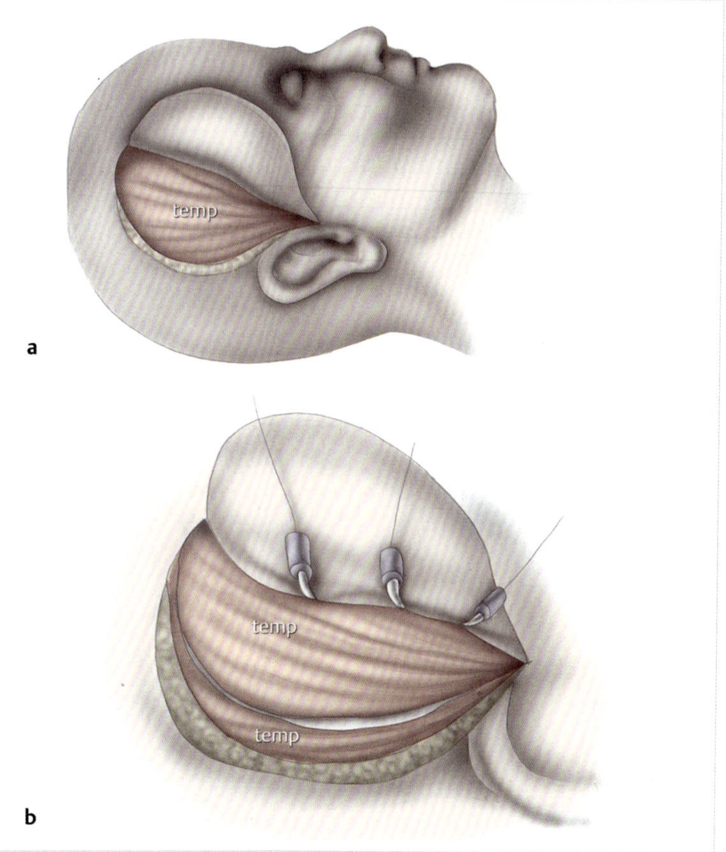

Fig. 8.6 Right side: **(a)** The skin flap is elevated exposing the temporalis fascia. Inferiorly, the zygomatic arch is detected. **(b)** The temporalis muscle is incised posteriorly, following the line of skin incision. *temp: temporalis muscle.*

▶ Fig. 8.15d) or along the bisection line located in the most medial portion of the IAC, which represents the safest area of the superior surface of the temporal bone, as it is located far from the cochlea, semicircular canals, and facial nerve (see ▶ Fig. 8.15c). In this case bone removal is carried out along the porus using a large diamond bur until the dura of the IAC is identified. The dura of the IAC are skeletonized until three-fourths of its circumference should be exposed. In case of tumor with CPA involvement the dura of the posterior fossa may be exposed widely drilling the bone at the level of the medial end of the IAC. The IAC dura is then skeletonized from the most medial portion to the lateral portion until the labyrinthine portion of the facial nerve and Bill's bar are detected in the fundus (see ▶ Fig. 8.16). The lateral portion of the IAC is carefully exposed only on the superior surface avoiding damage to the cochlea and SSC.

- Opening the tegmen tympani during the dissection can be helpful in difficult situations, when the anatomy is not clear and when dealing with facial nerve pathology (see ▶ Fig. 8.17, ▶ Fig. 8.18, ▶ Fig. 8.19, ▶ Fig. 8.20, see Clinical Case 1) (in this situation the tegmen always needs to be unroofed). However, there is no recommendation about which landmarks to use once the tegmen is opened. The use of cochleariform process as a landmark allows the less experienced surgeon to use measurements to relate the underlying anatomical structures. This method is necessary in case of supralabyrinthine cholesteatoma facial nerve decompression, or petrous apex lesion, in order to have the whole control of the facial nerve during disease removal; but the potential risk of cerebrospinal fluid (CSF) leak, brain herniation, and meningitis should be considered (see Clinical Case 2).

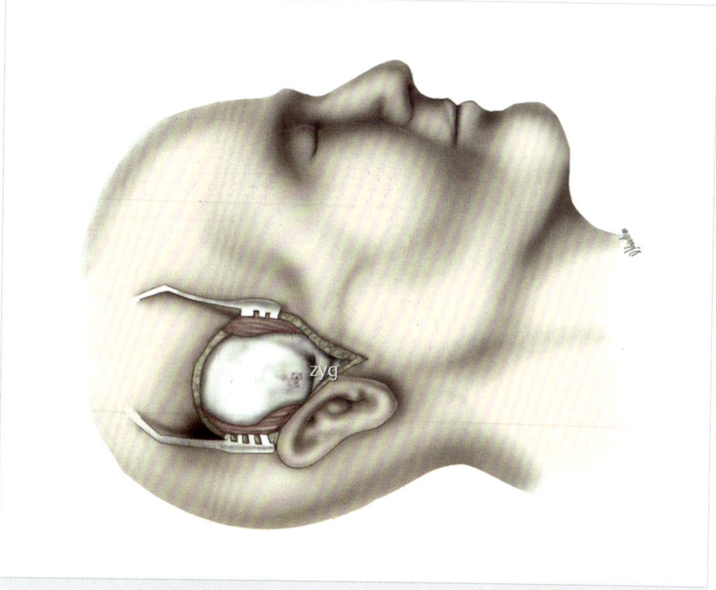

Fig. 8.7 Right side: The squama temporalis is exposed and the zygomatic arch uncovered. *zyg: zygomatic arch.*

8.4.3 Dural Opening and Tumor Dissection

Once the IAC is skeletonized, the dura of the IAC is opened longitudinally, along its posterior border, using a microsurgical blade or hook. The dural flaps are reflected and the content of the IAC is exposed. The separation between the facial nerve and the superior vestibular nerve is identified at the level of the fundus, and the interposed vertical crest (Bill's bar) is also identified. When dealing with an acoustic neuroma, the tumor can be gently rolled from a medial to a lateral or from an anterior to a posterior direction and carefully separated from the facial nerve, the delicate fibers of the cochlear nerve and the labyrinthine artery using a 2-mm hook. The tumor usually originates from the inferior vestibular nerve, pushing the facial nerve superiorly and putting it at greater risk. The superior vestibular nerve is first dislocated using a small hook, and the tumor is then dealt carefully to avoid injury of the facial nerve lying between the surgeon and the tumor (see ▶ Fig. 8.21). In tumors with an extrameatal component, a dissection plane between the tumor pseudocapsule and the structures of the CPA is sought. The tumor can be separated from the anterior-inferior cerebellar artery and its branches to avoid accidental injury.

When the tumor has been separated from the facial nerve, the vestibular nerve is cut distally to its emergence from the main trunk of the VIIIth cranial nerve and removed along with the tumor (see ▶ Fig. 8.21a). During the dissection, the auditory function should be monitored with either cochlear nerve action potential or auditory brainstem response. In order to maintain the cochlear nerve function the internal auditory artery must be preserved. This artery runs between the facial nerve and cochlear nerves. For this reason, a sharp dissection of the tumor in a

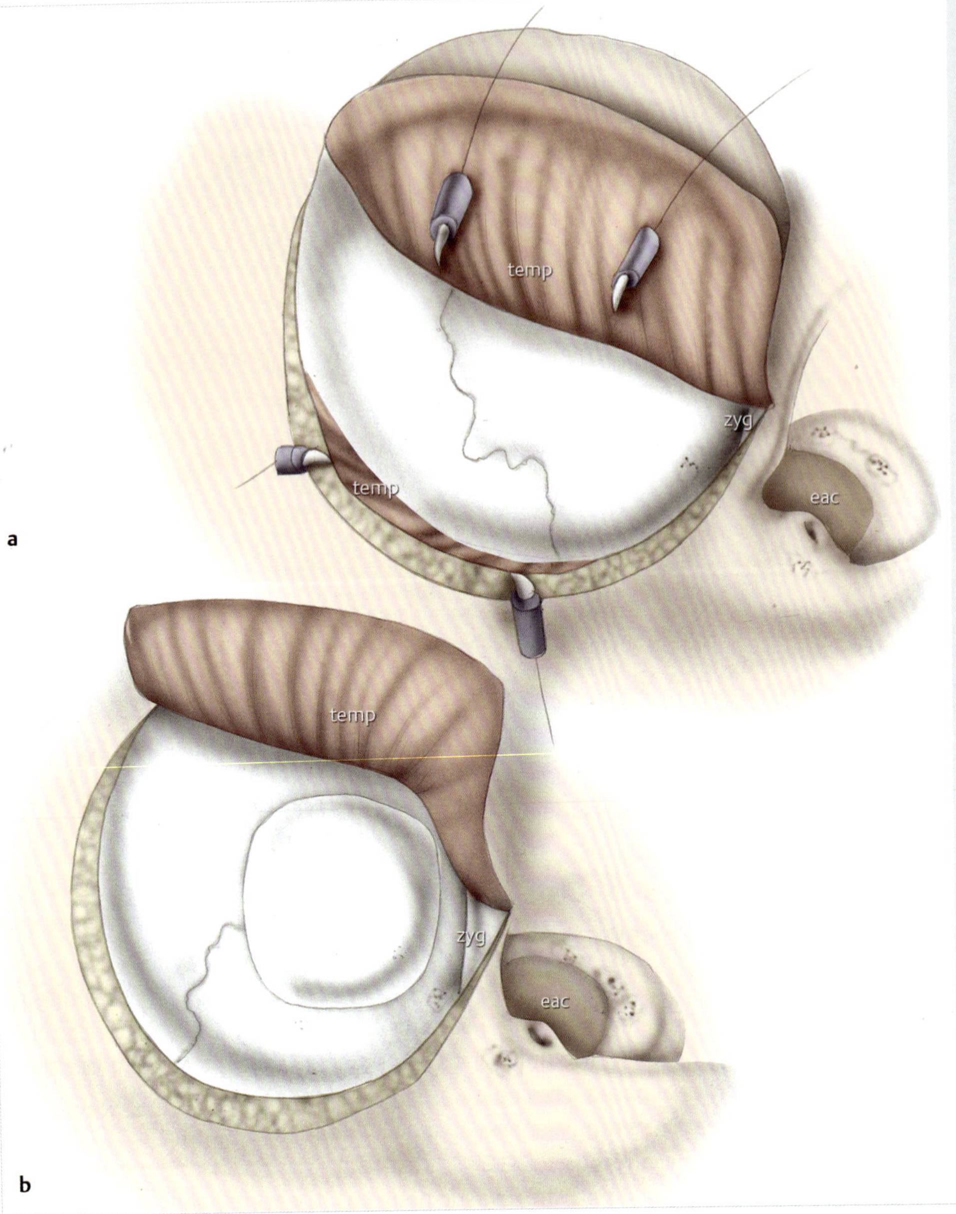

Fig. 8.8 Right side: **(a)** The muscle flap is elevated, the bone of squama temporalis is exposed, and the zygomatic arch is partially visible. **(b)** A 4 cm × 4 cm craniotomy is performed, close to the zygoma, extending one-third in front and two-thirds behind the external auditory canal. *eac: external auditory canal; temp: temporalis muscle; zyg: zygomatic arch.*

medial to lateral direction is mandatory in order to avoid damage of the internal auditory artery.

8.4.4 Endoscopic Assisted Surgery

The use of the surgical endoscope during a middle cranial fossa approach has been proposed to help overcome the technical challenges of tumor dissection, especially in the lateral IAC. As previously reported, the dissection of the lateral IAC toward the fundus is limited by the neighboring cochlea and superior semicircular canal if compared to the 270 degrees of dissection that is possible toward the porus. For this reason, residual tumors can hide in the area vestibularis (area of the fundus where the superior and inferior vestibular nerves enter the vestibule), out of the microscopic direct sight. The microscopic resection of the tumor from the fundus may require a blind dissection, especially if the tumor involves the most lateral portion of the fundus, under the transverse crest and along the vestibular nerves (see ▶ Fig. 8.22). It is well known that the lateral extension of intracanicular tumors, involving the fundus of the IAC, is related to a poor chance of hearing preservation and a high risk of leaving residual disease. In such cases endoscopic assisted surgery may help the surgeon to detect and remove the residual disease, avoiding a blind microscopic surgical dissection. Especially in middle cranial fossa approaches, the use of angled (45 and 70 degrees) endoscopes is recommended to allow a close-up high-definition lateral visualization toward the fundus, in the inferior portion of the transverse crest, which is difficult with traditional microscopy. Standard equipment for endoscopic assisted surgery includes a light source, a rigid endoscope coupled to a three-CCD camera, a high-definition (HD) camera, and an HD video monitor. The HD camera and monitor should be placed opposite to the surgeon, close to sight level to reduce neck strain. The light source should be set at no more than 50% intensity to reduce heat exposure of the surrounding tissues.

After the completion of the microscopic resection of the tumor, a 45-degree 3 or 4mm in diameter and 15 cm long endoscope is introduced through the surgical cavity of the surgical field (see ▶ Fig. 8.23, ▶ Fig. 8.24). During the endoscopic inspection, cottonoids soaked with water are placed over the middle cranial fossa dura and temporal lobe. In order to protect these anatomical areas, a constant irrigation is also necessary to clean the surgical field and to reduce heat dissipation from the tip of the endoscope. The endoscope is held with the nondominant hand, and a dissection instrument is carefully used with the dominant hand. The fundus of the IAC is endoscopically magnified and the transverse crest detected. Particular attention should be paid during

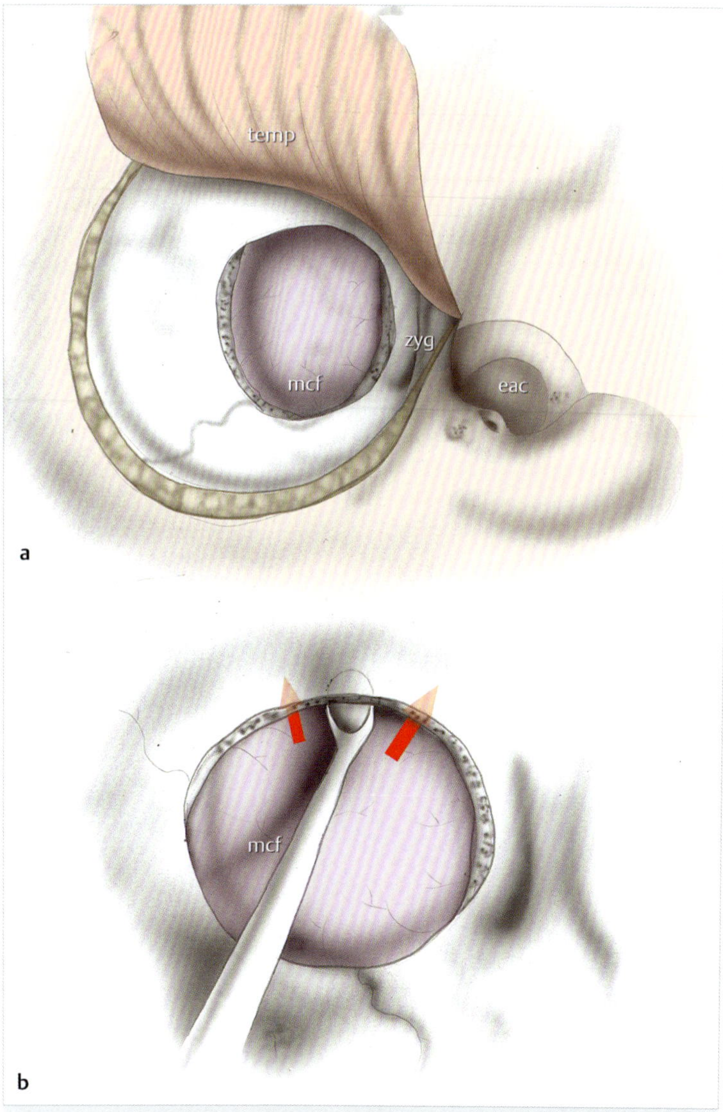

Fig. 8.9 Right side: **(a)** The craniotomy is performed and the middle cranial fossa dura exposed. The bone plate is preserved. **(b)** A dissector is used to gently detach the dura from the edges of craniotomy. *eac: external auditory canal; mcf: middle cranial fossa; temp: temporalis muscle; zyg: zygomatic arch.*

this step to detect the facial and cochlear nerves, located in the anterior portion of the IAC.

Suction instruments should be avoided during this step, because of the high risk of damage to the nervous and vascular structures inside the IAC. If blood covers the residual tumor and the lateral part of the IAC, a gentle irrigation under endoscopic view should be considered in order to clean the IAC before the surgical maneuvers.

In case residual disease is found under the transverse crest, an angulate dissector is gently used to remove the remnant from the most lateral portion of the fundus (see ▶ Fig. 8.25 and ▶ Fig. 8.26). The dissection should be performed from an anterior to a posterior direction as opposed to the direction of the acoustic and facial nerves, avoiding damage to the nerves and to the internal auditory artery. In some cases, a piezosurgery device may be used under endoscopic view in order to remove the most posterior portion of the transversal crest, gaining a better access of this portion of the lateral section of the IAC. In this way the residual tumor may be easily reached and removed. Once the tumor has been removed, further irrigation should be carried out before the final endoscopic check. The facial nerve and the IAC are covered with corticosteroid-soaked Gelfoam.

8.4.5 Closure

After tumor removal, during wound closure, all the exposed air cells are sealed with bone wax, and hemostasis is secured. The dural flaps are approximated with one or two stitches of 6–0 neurolon when possible. A graft of subcutaneous abdominal fat or temporalis muscle is used to obliterate the IAC (see ▶ Fig. 8.27). The graft is placed into the bone defect with care to not disturb the facial and cochlear nerves. When tegmen removal is necessary a bone graft is used to repair the defect in the middle cranial fossa floor to prevent brain herniation; a fascia graft is then placed between the dura of the temporal lobe and the bone graft (see ▶ Fig. 8.20). The original bony plate is put back to his position and fixed with titanium plates. The temporalis muscle is then rotated and sutured; the skin is closed in layers (see ▶ Fig. 8.28). A compressive bandage is performed.

8.4.6 Postoperative Care

Intensive care unit (ICU) observation is necessary for 24 hours, and a computed tomography (CT) scan 6 hours after surgery is planned. Early deambulation of the patient is required, and the hospitalization of the patient usually lasts about 5 to 6 days.

8.4.7 Complications

- Sensorineural hearing loss (accidental opening of the cochlea, damage to cochlear neve) (see ▶ Fig. 8.64, ▶ Fig. 8.65)
- Conductive hearing loss caused by disruption of the ossicular chain or a prolapse of the temporal lobe dura on the incudomalleolar joint
- Extradural hematoma
- Intracranial bleeding
- Facial palsy
- CSF leakage

8.4.8 Endoscopic Middle Fossa Approach to Repair Superior Semicircular Canal Dehiscence

Special consideration should be given regarding SSC repair, since endoscopic assisted surgery was developed by the Harvard group in order to minimize the surgical approach. The middle fossa craniotomy (MFC) is a well-established surgical technique to repair SSC dehiscence. The advantage of the MFC approach is the direct visualization of the superior canal dehiscence (SCD) without the need for labyrinthine bone removal. For patients with a low-lying tegmen, the MFC approach is ideal as it allows a wide exposure of the arcuate eminence without drilling close to the horizontal canal. However, adequate visualization of the surgical anatomy under a binocular intraoperative microscopy may still be challenging. The limited microscopic view often requires larger craniotomies and prolonged retraction of the temporal lobe. In particular, when an arcuate eminence defect is very thin (blue-lined) or a medial arcuate eminence defect lies along a downsloping tegmen (29% of arcuate eminence defects), it may be difficult

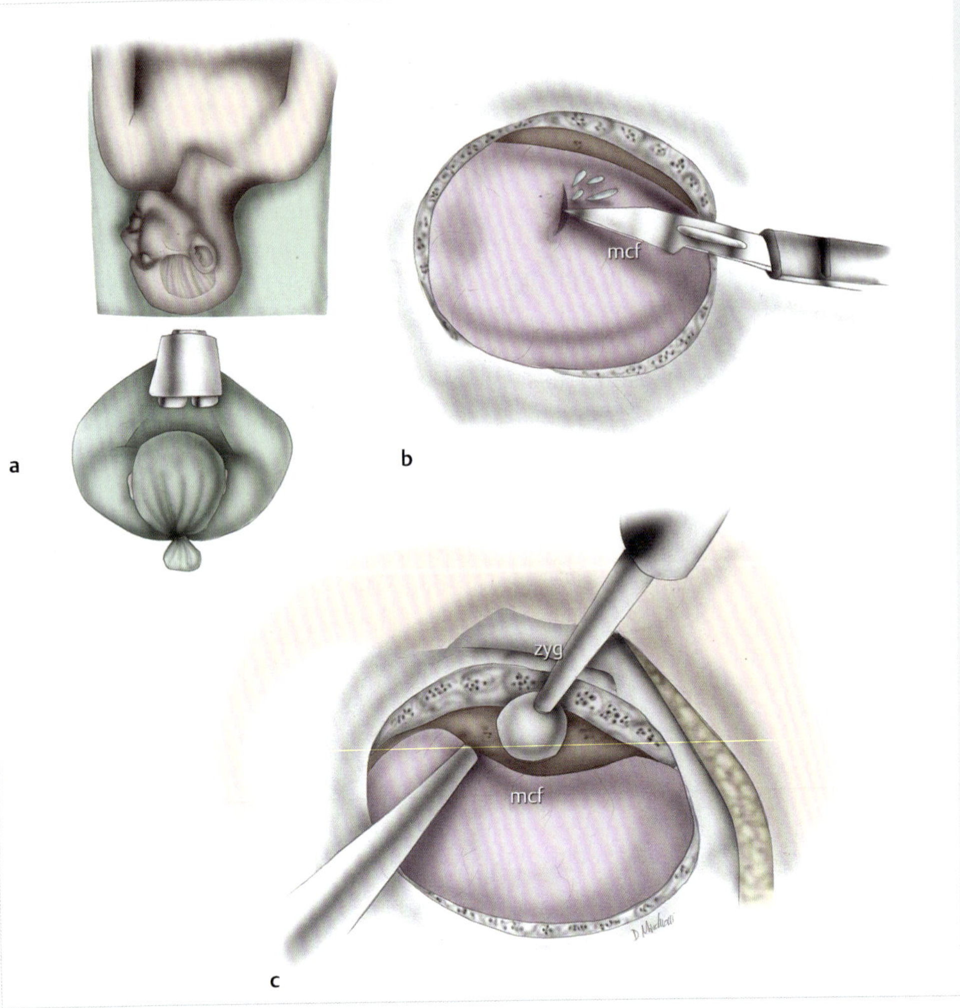

Fig. 8.10 Right side: **(a)** The patient lies in supine position, with the head turned to the contralateral side. The surgeon sits at the patient's head, to permit an adequate view over the middle fossa floor. **(b)** A small incision is made on the dura of the middle cranial fossa. A cerebrospinal fluid (CSF) leakage is expected during this procedure, allowing the decompression and the elevation of the temporal lobe. **(c)** A diamond bur is used to remove bone in the inferior edge of the craniotomy, parallel to the floor of middle cranial fossa. During this step, the dura is protected and retracted using a suction instrument. *mcf: middle cranial fossa dura; zyg: zygomatic arch.*

to be visualized without significant brain retraction or drilling of the overlying skull base (see ▶ Fig. 8.66). Prolonged or significant temporal lobe retraction can lead to dural tearing, CSF leakage or brain contusion. The additional extradural dissection, needed to fully expose the defect increases the risk of facial nerve injury.

The Role of an Endoscopic Assisted MFC Approach for SCD Repair

Binocular microscopy provides a high-resolution, magnified view of the surgical field, but visualization of deeper recesses of the skull base is limited. The goals of endoscopic assisted repair of SCD are to facilitate the exposure of the skull base and to visualize the arcuate eminence while avoiding damage to the brain and facial nerve, as well as exposing the ossicles from an associated tegmental defects. A traditional microscope can be employed for most SCD repairs, but an endoscopic assisted approach is useful in cases with a dehiscence lying along a downsloping tegmen or in the posteromedial nonampullated end of the superior canal (see ▶ Fig. 8.66). Before the incorporation of the endoscope, these cases were often approached with a large craniotomy and an extensive temporal lobe retraction, and the repair with bone wax was blindly applied along the predicted location of the dehiscence. However, a poor visualization of the defect increases the risk of inadequate repair and postoperative complications due to prolonged brain retraction.

Preoperative Planning

The most common subtype of SCD is a defect of the arcuate eminence (95%). In this case, the defect can be medial to the peak of the arcuate eminence, lying along a downsloping tegmen (29% of arcuate eminence defects). For this reason the endoscopic assisted MCF approach is deemed to be most appropriate. The remaining subtype of SCD involves the medial aspect of the SSC in close proximity to the superior petrosus sinus (5%). Radiological classification of the SCD position along the middle fossa floor and the surrounding skull base topography, including the appearance to the tegmen and facial nerve, is important in the preoperative planning of an endoscopic assisted repair to determine the more suitable approach (see ▶ Fig. 8.67).

Surgical Steps

The Massachusetts Eye and Ear institute codified the surgical steps of endoscopic assisted repair of SCD as follows:

During the procedure the patient is kept in a supine position. Following intubation, minimal hair shave and a 3 to 4 cm preauricular curvilinear skin incision is made. Traditionally the skin incisions for an MFC approach consist of a straight or curved pretragal incision (see ▶ Fig. 8.68, ▶ Fig. 8.69). We favor a 3 to 4 cm preauricular skin incision with minimal hair removal and a minimal invasive craniotomy (3 × 2 cm) in order to perform an endoscopic assisted SCD repair. The approach allows a reduction in size of the craniotomy created for the procedure. Despite a

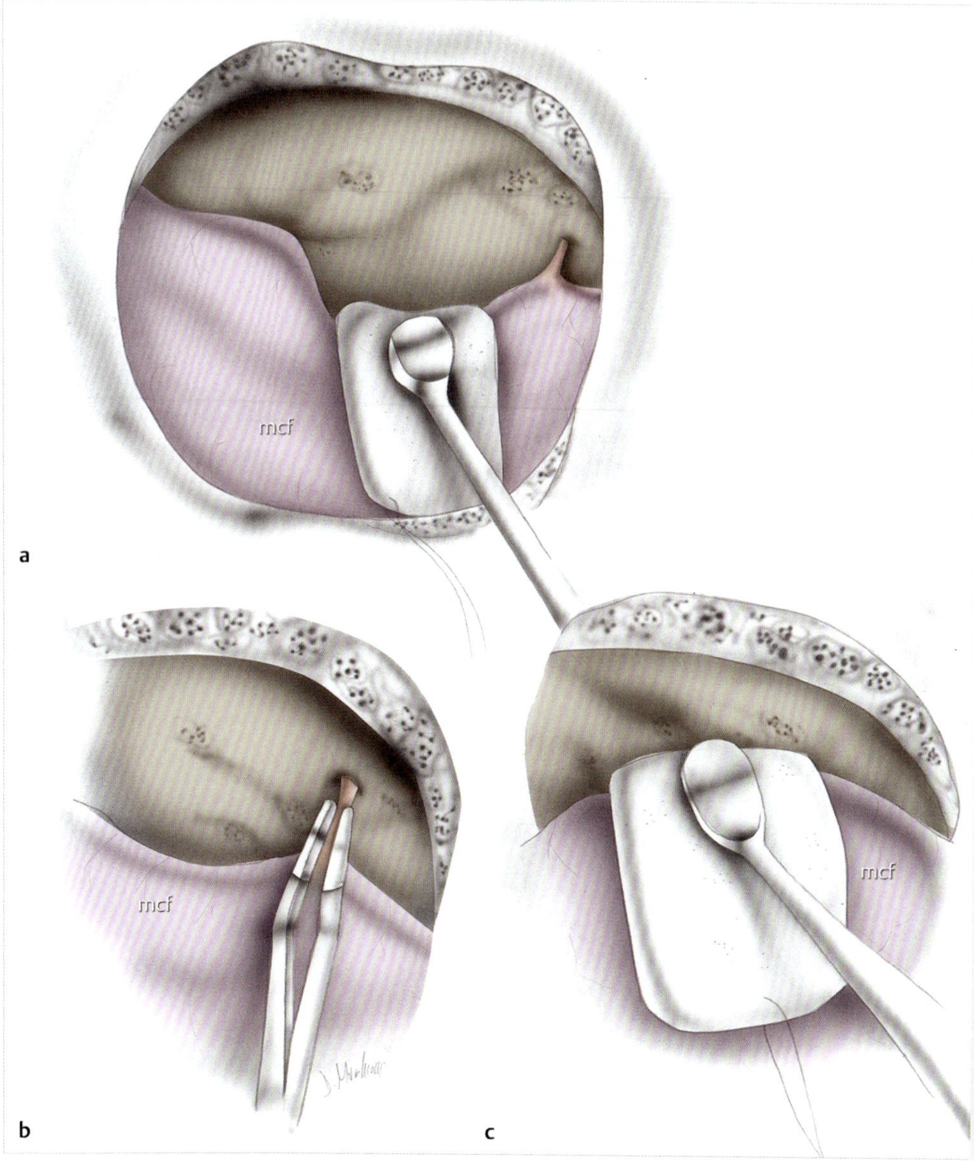

Fig. 8.11 Right side: **(a)** The dura of temporal lobe is gently elevated from the floor of the middle cranial fossa. A cottonoid is used over the dura to gently detach it from the surface of the temporal bone. **(b)** The small vessels that keep the dural plane attached to the temporal bone surface are coagulated and cut. **(c)** A large cottonoid is placed on the dural plane, helping the elevation of the temporal lobe, uncovering progressively the floor of the middle cranial fossa. *mcf: middle cranial fossa dura.*

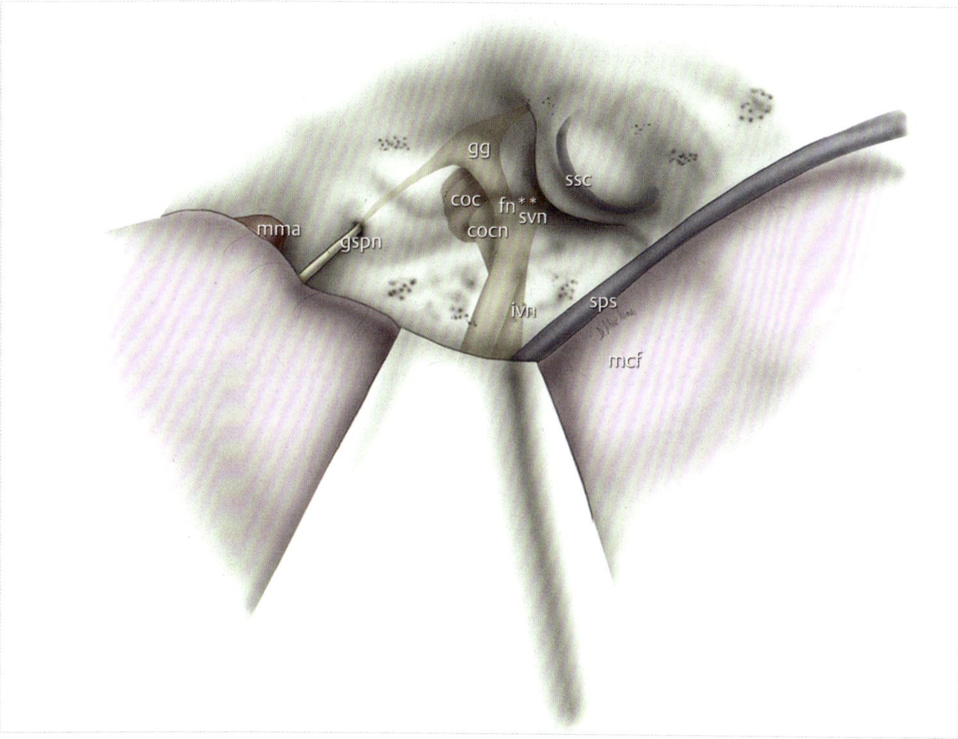

Fig. 8.12 Right side: Anatomy of the floor of middle cranial fossa from above. The anatomical structures in the internal auditory canal are depicted in trasparency along the surface of temporal bone. *coc: cochlea; cocn: cochlear nerve; fn**: intracanalicular portion of the facial nerve; gg: geniculate ganglion; gspn: greater superficial petrosal nerve; ivn: inferior vestibular nerve; mcf: middle cranial fossa dura; mma: middle meningeal artery; sps: superior petrosal sinus; ssc: superior semicircular canal; svn: superior vestibular nerve.*

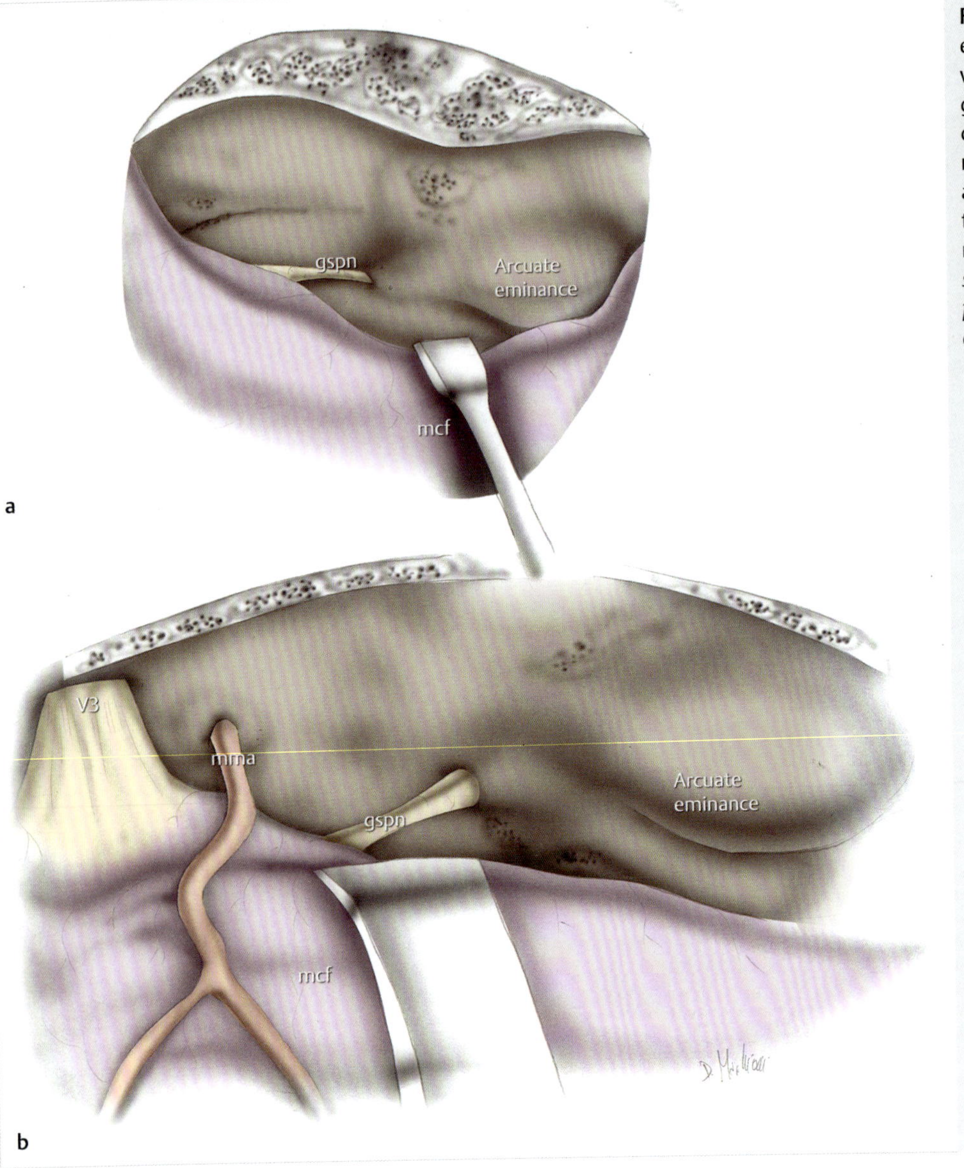

Fig. 8.13 Right side: **(a)** The temporal lobe is elevated and the arcuate eminence exposed, where lies the prominence of the SSC. The greater superficial petrosal nerve (*gspn*) is detected, and the identification of the middle meningeal artery and V3 is performed in the anterior portion of the surgical field (see [**b**]). All the anatomical landmarks to identify the internal auditory canal are exposed. *gspn: greater superficial petrosal nerve; mcf: middle cranial fossa; mma: middle meningeal artery; V3: mandibular division of trigeminal nerve.*

smaller incision with limited brain retraction and drilling close to the inner ear, the angle endoscope allows a visualization beyond the arcuate eminence.

Continuous facial nerve monitoring is employed. A temporalis fascia graft is harvested and a periosteal flap is inferiorly elevated to the level of the EAC. The minimally invasive 3 × 2 cm craniotomy is marked and gently elevated centered on the EAC (see ▶ Fig. 8.70, ▶ Fig. 8.71). Under microscopic view, the middle fossa dura is carefully dissected and detached from the tegmen mastoideum and tegmen tympani until the arcuate eminence is visualized. If the region of the arcuate eminence is not well exposed at this point, the endoscope is introduced into the craniotomy to provide a view of the medial skull base (see ▶ Fig. 8.72). The standard equipment for the endoscopic assisted SCD repair is the one previously described. A 3-mm diameter, 14-cm long, 0-, 30-, or 45-degree endoscope is used during these steps in order to magnify the arcuate eminence and the defect of SCD. The endoscope is stabilized with the nondominant hand while a retractor is used to keep the temporal lobe retracted (see ▶ Fig. 8.73). Under endoscopic view the dura is dissected from the medial portion of the defect. The repair of the dehiscent superior canal can be achieved by either plugging or resurfacing the defect. If a blue-lined or near dehiscence is encountered, a 1.5-mm diamond burr at a low speed (5,000 RPM) is used under endoscopic visualization to unroof the defect to the endosteum layer in order to subsequently close it with bone wax (see ▶ Fig. 8.74). If the tegmen is dehiscent around the arcuate eminence, a split calvarial bone chip, temporalis fascia, or a dural graft can be used to repair the skull base. The wound is closed in a layered fashion and a mastoid dressing is applied for 5 days (see ▶ Fig. 8.75). All patients are hospitalized and monitored in the ICU for the first 24 hours.

8.5 Anterior Petrosectomy or Extended Middle Fossa Approach

8.5.1 Rationale

The middle fossa approach was designed for the removal of small acoustic neuromas limited to the IAC. If we extend the surgical approach anteriorly to the IAC through the same surgical route we are able to remove lesions located in the petrous apex. Using the middle fossa corridor, Kawase and colleagues further expanded its indications, performing an extradural anterior petrosectomy that allows, through opening of the dura mater and division of the superior petrosal sinus (SPS) from the tentorium, the treatment of lower lying basilar artery aneurysms and petroclival meningiomas.

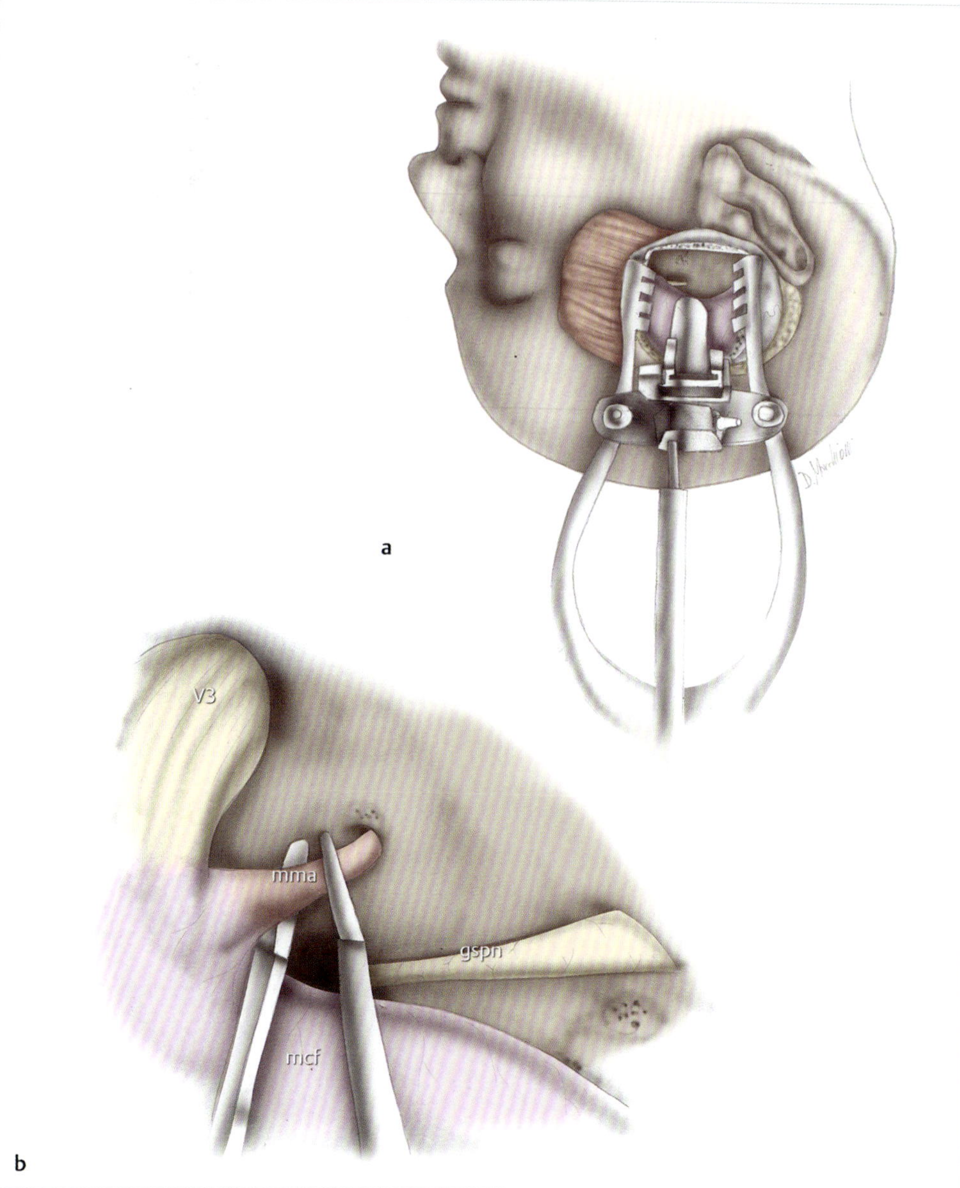

Fig. 8.14 Right side: **(a)** The Fisch middle cranial fossa retractor is placed to keep the temporal lobe elevated. **(b)** The middle meningeal artery is coagulated and cut. *gspn: greater superficial petrosal nerve; mcf: middle cranial fossa; mma: middle meningeal artery; V3: mandibular division of trigeminal nerve.*

The anterior petrosectomy procedure represents a natural anterior extension of the middle fossa approach designed to expose petrous apex lesions with intradural extension to the ventral and ventrolateral portions of the upper third of the brainstem.

The anterior petrosectomy procedure includes the removal of the bone housed in the posteromedial triangle of the middle fossa, also known as Kawase's or quadrilateral triangle. The Kawase's triangle defines a precise area of the petrous apex. The boundaries of this anatomical area are posteriorly defined by the arcuate eminence, laterally by the GSPN, medially by the SPS, and anteriorly by the posterior margin of Meckel's cave containing the mandibular division of the trigeminal nerve (see ▶ Fig. 8.76, ▶ Fig. 8.77).

8.5.2 Surgical Steps

The first surgical steps are the same as the ones previously described for the middle fossa approach.

In this procedure, it is crucial to expose the zygoma, defining the level of the middle fossa floor; the superior portion of the EAC is also identified. Once these two landmarks have been identified, the craniotomy is performed two-thirds anteriorly and one-third posteriorly to the EAC.

If required, the superior edge of the zygomatic arch may also be drilled to gain a better exposure of the floor of the middle fossa. The dura on the floor of the anterior portion of the middle fossa is then gently elevated. The middle meningeal artery, entering through the foramen spinosum, is identified along the anterior part of the bone exposure and cauterized. The artery should be coagulated and cut close to the dura of the middle fossa to avoid retraction of this vascular structure into the spinosum foramen and bleeding, which might be difficult to manage. The greater superficial petrosal nerve (GSPN) and lesser superficial petrosal nerve (LSPN) are detected on the floor of the middle fossa, and carefully dissected, trying to avoid their damage detaching them gently from the dura of middle fossa. During this surgical step, the surgeon should be careful to avoid traction on the geniculate ganglion via the GSPN; this nerve runs from the geniculate ganglion to the pterygopalatine ganglion like the vidian nerve, along with branches from the carotid sympathetic plexus, and cooperates in lacrimal function.

The dura mater propria can now be lifted from the lateral wall of the cavernous sinus, and the mandibular division of the trigeminal nerve (V3) can be exposed as it exits the foramen ovale. Elevation of the dura is carried out medially until till medial petrous ridge.

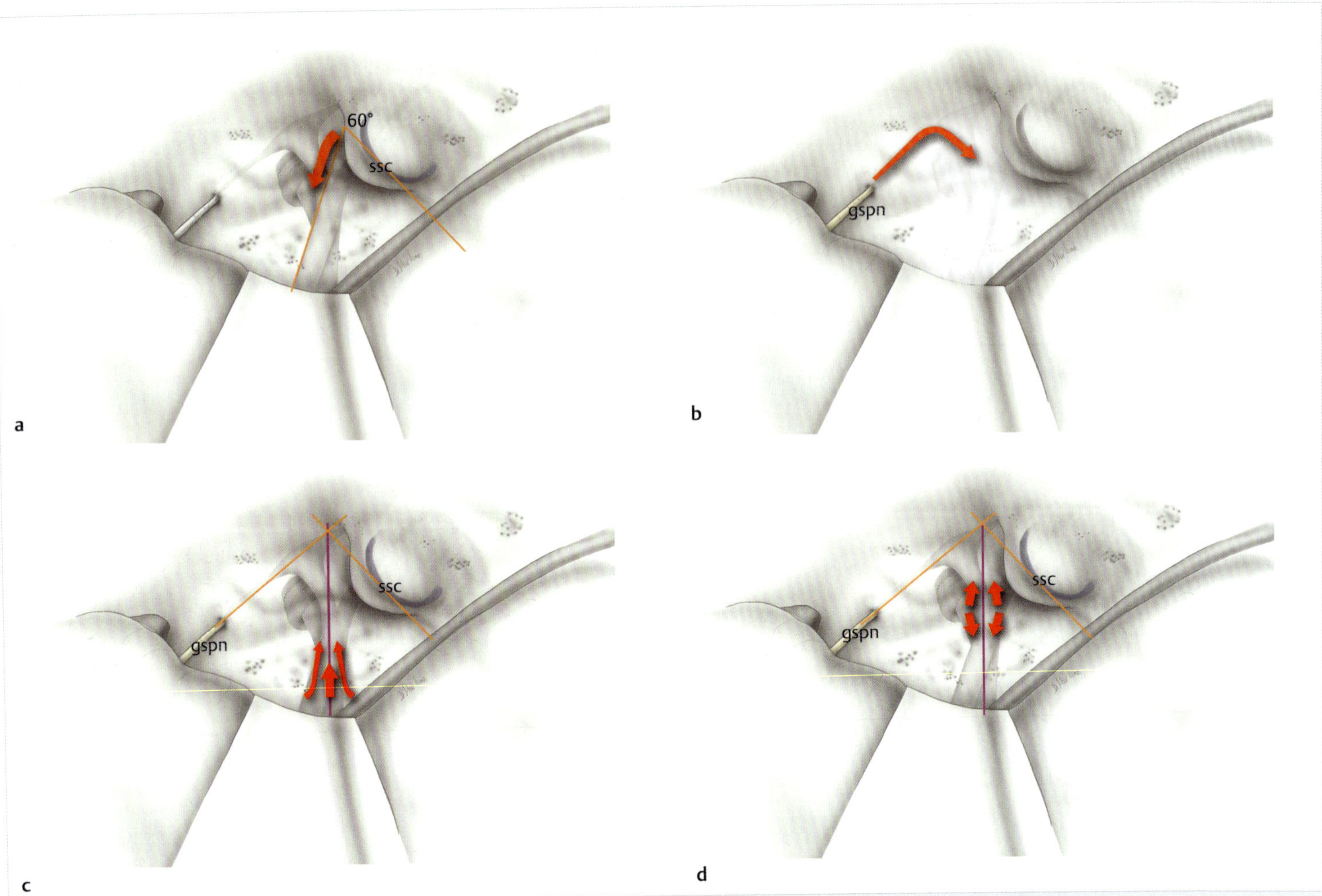

Fig. 8.15 (a–d) Right side: The different methods described in literature to expose the internal auditory canal (see the text). *gspn: greater superficial petrosal nerve; ssc: superior semicircular canal.*

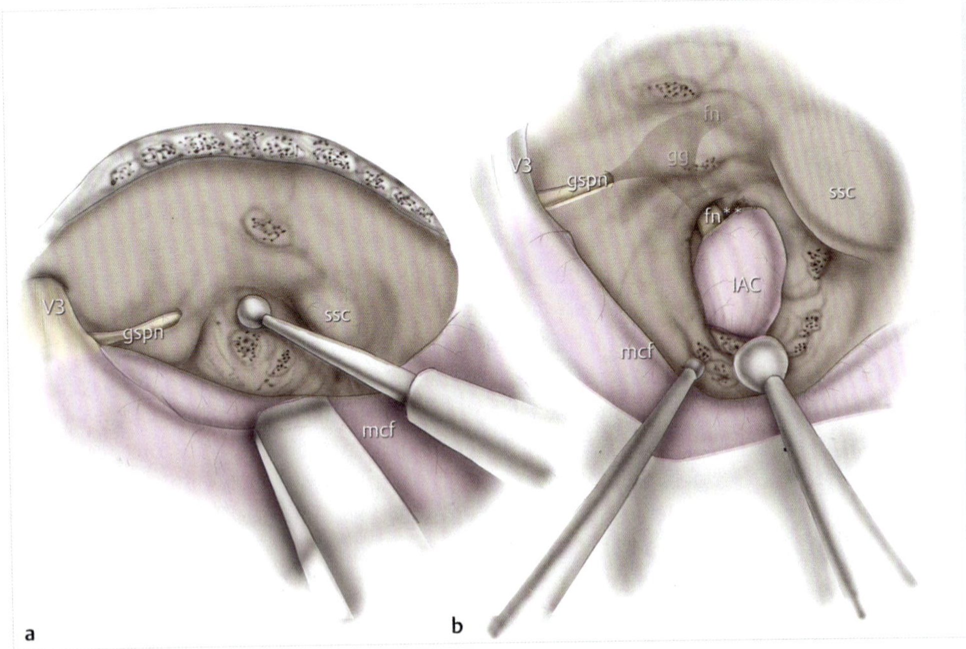

Fig. 8.16 Right side: **(a)** A diamond bur is used to remove the bone at the bisection of the angle formed by the imaginary lines that pass through the greater superficial petrosal nerve and the arcuate eminence. **(b)** The dura of the internal auditory canal (IAC) is progressively exposed, drilling from the porus to the lateral portion. *fn: tympanic portion of the facial nerve; fn**: intra-labyrinthine portion of the facial nerve; gg: geniculate ganglion; gspn: greater superficial petrosal nerve; IAC: internal auditory canal; mcf: middle cranial fossa; ssc: superior semicircular canal; V3: mandibular division of trigeminal nerve.*

The dura of the middle fossa is then carefully detached and elevated from the petrous ridge. The SPS forming the petrosal groove along the superior portion of the petrous ridge is thus detected. The Fisch middle cranial fossa retractor is then placed and used to gently elevate the dura of the floor of the middle fossa.

Once the dura is completely elevated to the level of the petrous ridge, the boundaries of Kawase's triangle/quadrilateral triangle are progressively identified: medially, the petrous ridge; laterally, the GSPN and the horizontal portion of ICA; posteriorly, the arcuate eminence; anteriorly, V3 with the posterior edge of the gasserian ganglion.

The IAC is detected on the plane that bisects the angle between the GSPN and the arcuate eminence as previously described. The cochlea is anteromedial and inferior to the geniculate ganglion. The horizontal portion of ICA must be identified, representing our lateral limit during the drilling of the petrous apex in the deep area (see ▶ Fig. 8.78). In some cases, the horizontal segment of the petrous ICA may be visible through a bone dehiscence in the floor of the middle fossa; the segment runs parallel and deeper than the GSPN.

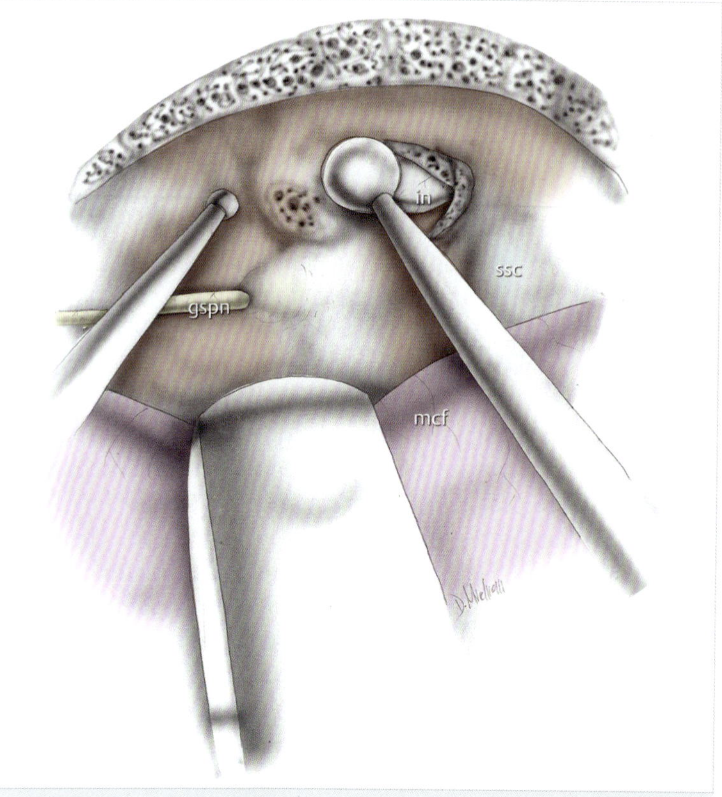

Fig. 8.17 Right side: In difficult anatomical conditions, an opening of the tegmen tympani may be helpful, in order to detect the right orientation of the facial nerve. A diamond bur is used to remove partially the tegmen until the ossicular chain is exposed from above. *gspn: greater superficial petrosal nerve; in: incus; mcf: middle cranial fossa dura; ssc: superior semicircular canal.*

An anterior petrosectomy is performed by removing the rhomboid bone of the middle fossa with care to preserve the neurovascular and otological structures. A high-speed diamond bur is used under copious irrigation to drill the petrous apex. Drilling should start in a mediolateral direction, beginning at the level of the medial petrous edge, to unroof the medial two-thirds of the IAC. The bone is progressively removed between the posterior edge of V3 and the anterior edge of the IAC (see ▶ Fig. 8.79). For lesions located in the petrous apex without intradural extension, it is not necessary to expose the whole dura of the IAC and the cochlea. The identification of the anatomical landmarks showing the IAC orientation may be sufficient to safely reach the lesion. Petrous apex lesions located anteriorly to the IAC, that lie along the horizontal portion of the ICA, are easily detected removing the Kawase triangle (see ▶ Fig. 8.80). Once the bone of the petrous apex is removed and the most superior portion of the lesion is isolated, tumor removal starts under microscopic view. Regardless of the nature of the lesion (cholesteatoma, cholesterol granuloma, chordoma, chondrosarcoma), the dissection of the tumor should be performed carefully around the neurovascular structures. In the majority of cases the dissection is progressively performed in a piecemeal way, using a dissector with the dominant hand and the suction instrument with the other hand (see ▶ Fig. 8.81). Angulated instruments are crucial to remove the lesions from the petrous apex cells and clivus lying under the horizontal portion of the carotid artery (see ▶ Fig. 8.82). To remove fragments of the lesion adherent to the vascular and nervous structures, a cottonoid should be used, gently scratching them from the neurovascular structures. Once the tumor is removed using microscopic view, endoscopic assisted surgery is mandatory to detect and remove residual diseases (see ▶ Fig. 8.83).

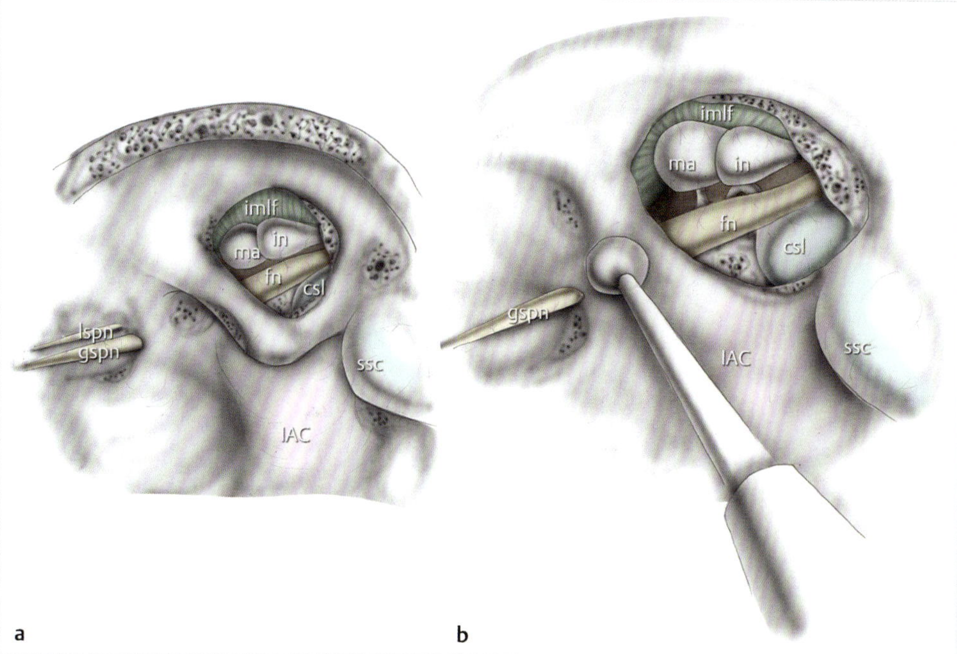

Fig. 8.18 Right side: **(a)** After tegmen removal, the tympanic segment of the facial nerve can be easily detected. A diamond bur is used to remove the bone between the greater superficial petrosal nerve (GSPN) and the arcuate eminence, looking for the internal auditory canal. In case of facial nerve decompression, the bone around the GSPN is removed, uncovering the geniculate ganglion **(b)**. *fn: tympanic portion of the facial nerve; gspn: greater superficial petrosal nerve; IAC: internal auditory canal; imlf: lateral incudo-malleal fold; in: incus; lsc: lateral semicircular canal; lspn: lesser superficial petrosal nerve; ma: malleus; ssc: superior semicircular canal.*

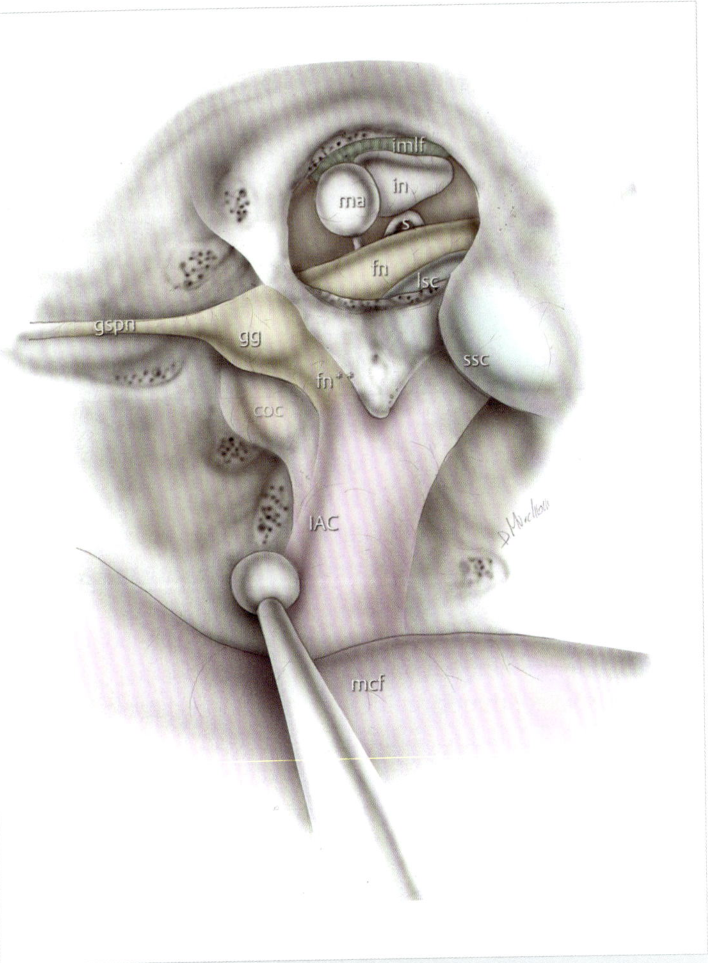

Fig. 8.19 Right side: The geniculate ganglion is exposed, and the intralabyrinthine portion of the facial nerve is detected at the entering point into the fundus of the internal auditory canal (IAC). The IAC is then progressively skeletonized from the porus to the lateral portion. *coc: cochlea; fn: tympanic portion of the facial nerve; fn**: intralabyrinthine portion of the facial nerve; gg: geniculate ganglion; gspn: greater superficial petrosal nerve; IAC: internal auditory canal; imlf: lateral incudomalleolar ligament fold; in: incus; lsc: lateral semicircular canal; ma: malleus; s: stapes; ssc: superior semicircular canal.*

8.5.3 Endoscopic Assisted Anterior Petrosectomy

During the endoscopic steps the room setup is similar to the one of the microscopic middle fossa approach. The surgeon sits behind the patient's head at the head of the bed, and the anesthesiologist at the foot. The surgical bed is pushed down as much as possible, to allow a proper use of the endoscope through the surgical cavity. A high-resolution monitor with an endoscopic tower is placed in front of the surgeon on the left side for right middle fossa approach, and on the right for left middle fossa approach. An HD camera with 0- and 45-degree endoscopes are used (see ▶ Fig. 8.84b).

A 0- to 45-degree endoscope, in 4 mm diameter and 15 cm in length, is introduced through the surgical field, cottonoids are placed on the middle fossa dura in order to protect the dural layer and the temporal lobe during the procedure. A Fisch middle cranial fossa retractor is placed on the temporal lobe in order to facilitate the endoscopic surgery, creating an adequate space for endoscopic maneuvers (see ▶ Fig. 8.84a). The endoscope can magnify the surgical field under the horizontal portion of the ICA, looking for any residual disease (see ▶ Fig. 8.84c). The endoscope is fixed on the Fisch middle cranial fossa retractor and with the dominant hand a dissection instrument is carefully introduced into the surgical cavity. In case of remnant disease, a curved dissector is used to safely remove the disease from the bottom of the petrous apex under the ICA. In case of cholesteatoma, a suction instrument should be used to remove the matrix lying in the petrous apex (see ▶ Fig. 8.85a). If required, a 45-degree endoscope can be used to check the most lateral portion of the petrous apex under the ICA in order to remove remnants eventually located on the inferior surface of the ICA. Once the lesion is removed, a long diamond bur (preferably with just tip rotation) is used to remove the bone tissue around the anterior petrosectomy, to radicalize the cavity (see ▶ Fig. 8.85b).

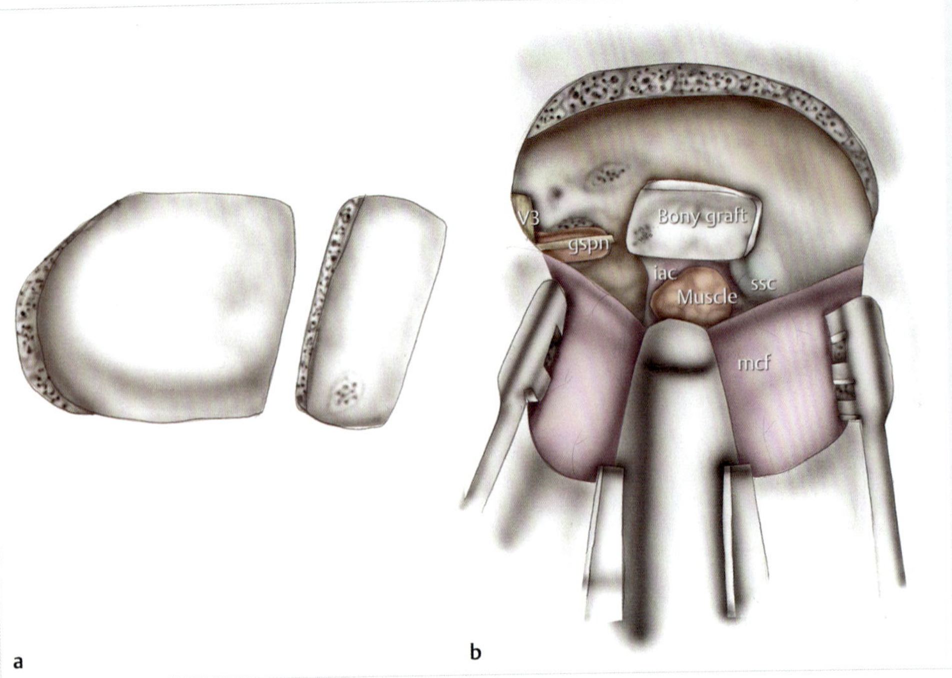

Fig. 8.20 Right side: When a tympanic cavity exposure is performed, a tegmen tympani defect reconstruction is mandatory at the end of surgery to avoid prolapse of the temporal lobe into the tympanic cavity. A bony piece of craniotomy plate is used **(a)**. This piece of bone is modelled to have the right size and thickness and placed over the tegmen defect **(b)**; it is finally fixed with fibrin glue, recreating the roof of the tympanic cavity. A piece of temporalis muscle is placed into the internal auditory canal (iac), covering the dural defect. *gspn: greater superficial petrosal nerve; mcf: middle cranial fossa dura; ssc: superior semicircular canal; V3: mandibular division of trigeminal nerve.*

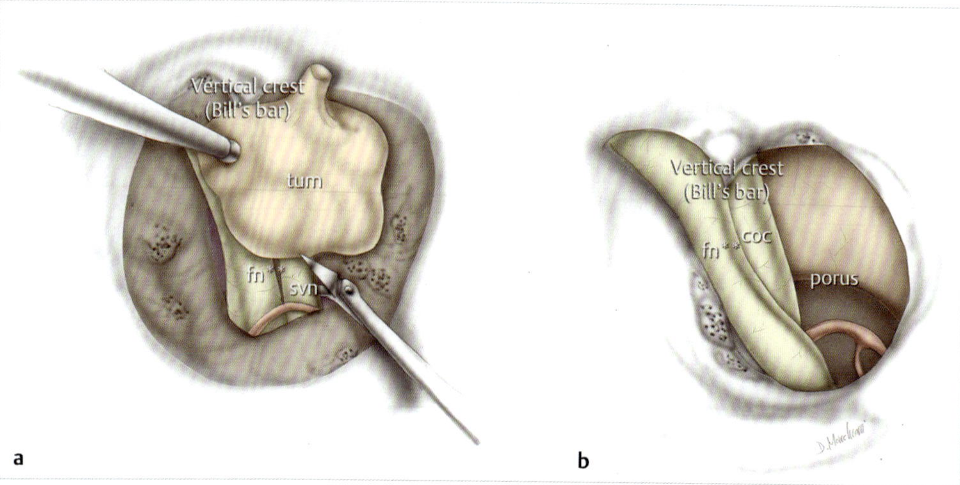

Fig. 8.21 Right side: **(a)** The dura of the internal auditory canal (IAC) is opened and the tumor exposed and dissected. A micro-scissor is used to cut the vestibular nerves, preserving facial and cochlear nerves, allowing tumor removal. **(b)** Microscopic view of the IAC after tumor removal. *coc: cochlear nerve; fn**: intracanalicular portion of the facial nerve; svn: superior vestibular nerve; tum: tumor.*

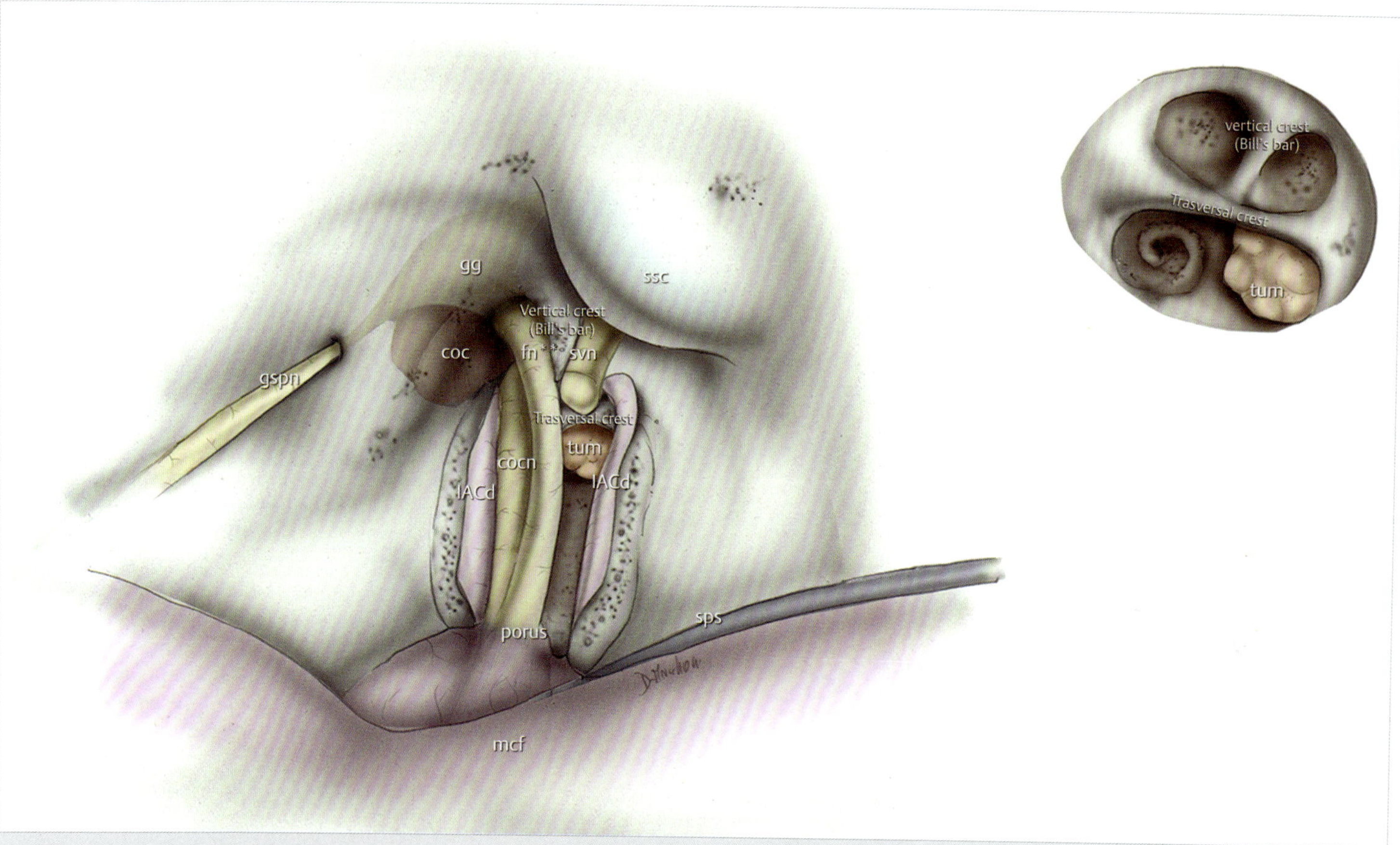

Fig. 8.22 Right side: Residual tumor involving the most lateral portion of the internal auditory canal under the transverse crest, along the vestibular nerves, after microscopic tumor removal. *coc: cochlea; cocn: cochlear nerve; fn**: intracanalicular portion of the facial nerve; gg: geniculate ganglion; gspn: greater superficial petrosal nerve; IACd: dura of internal auditory canal; mcf: middle cranial fossa; sps: superior petrosal sinus; ssc: superior semicircular canal; svn: superior vestibular nerve; tum: tumor.*

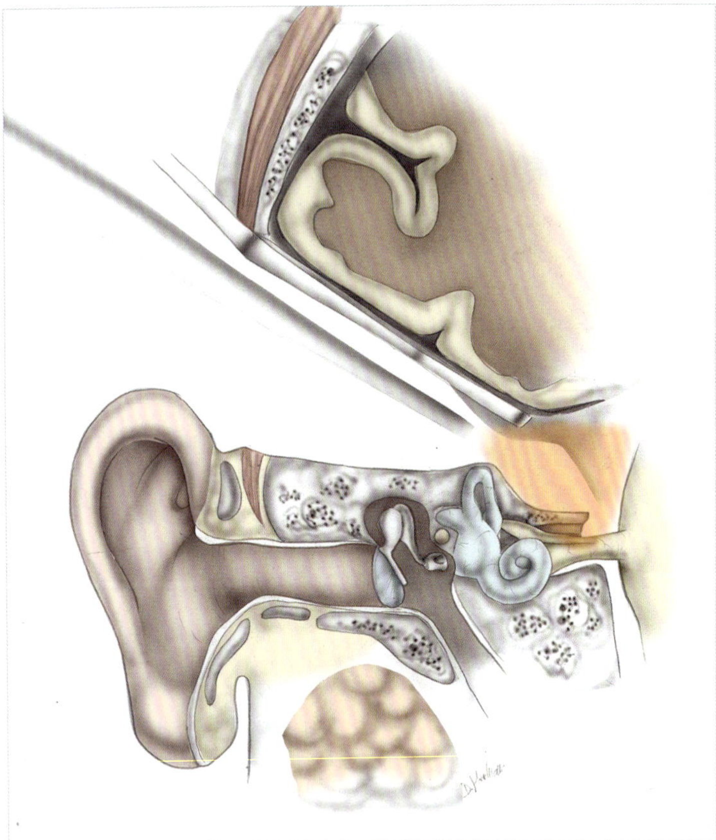

Fig. 8.23 Right side: A 45-degree endoscope of 4 mm diameter and 15 cm length is introduced through the surgical cavity. An inspection of the lateral portion of the internal auditory canal (IAC) is performed.

Closure

Abdominal fat is used to fill the petrous apex defect (see ▶ Fig. 8.86). If necessary, a dural allograft is placed in an onlay fashion to seal the floor of the middle fossa and fibrin glue is used to reinforce the reconstruction.

8.5.4 Lesions with Intradural Extension

The anterior petrosectomy performed for the removal of intradural lesions requires a wide skeletonization of structures located in the middle fossa, such as the dura of the IAC, and the horizontal portion of the ICA, in order to enough surgical space for the management of the intradural neurovascular structures.

The horizontal segment of the petrous ICA must be exposed since it represents the lateral limit of the petrosectomy. If a wide exposure of the petrous ICA is required, the bone overlying the Glasscock triangle can be removed using a diamond bur. This triangle is bordered by the posterior rim of the foramen ovale, the foramen spinosum, the posterior border of V3, and the cochlear apex. During this surgical step, the surgeon should avoid opening the eustachian tube which lies lateral to the horizontal petrous ICA. If the eustachian tube is accidentally violated, an obliteration of the tube is crucial to prevent a CSF fistula.

The superior, anterior, and posterior dura of the IAC is exposed in the same way as previously described for acoustic neuroma removal. The GSPN is posteriorly followed to detect the geniculate ganglion area; subsequently the cochlea should be detected

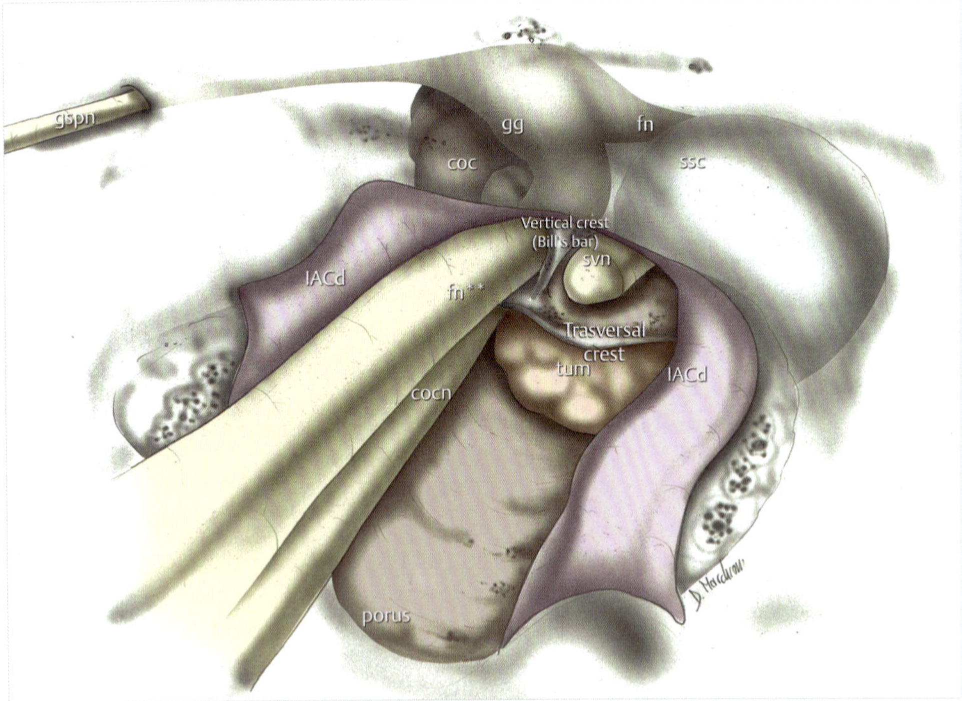

Fig. 8.24 Right side: The endoscopic view of the lateral portion of the internal auditory canal allows detecting residual tumor under the transverse crest along the inferior vestibular nerve. *coc: cochlea; cocn: cochlear nerve; fn: tympanic portion of the facial nerve; fn**: intracanalicular portion of the facial nerve; gg: geniculate ganglion; gspn: greater superficial petrosal nerve; IACd: dura of the internal auditory canal; ssc: superior semicircular canal; svn: superior vestibular nerve; tum: tumor.*

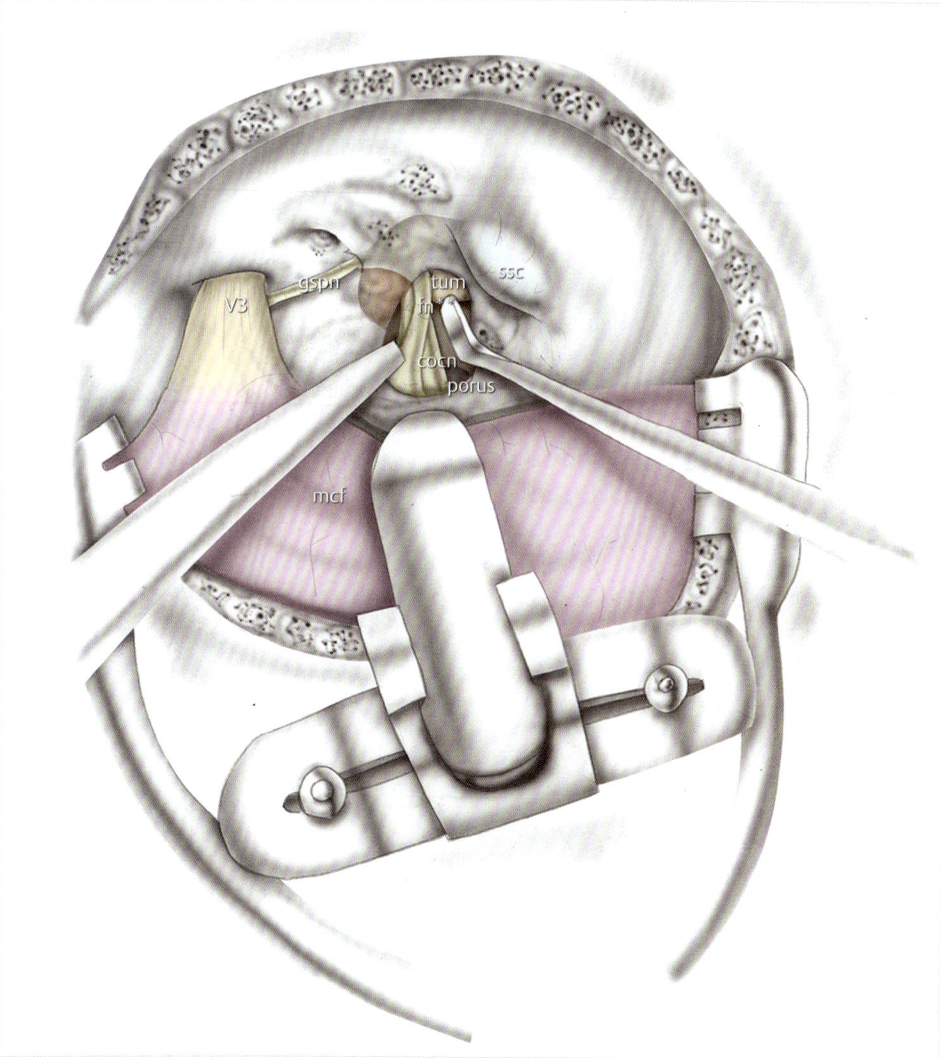

Fig. 8.25 Right side: The endoscope is held with the nondominant hand and gently inserted into the cavity. During this maneuvers the surgeon should pay attention not to damage the temporalis lobe. A curved dissector is used with the dominant hand on the fundus of the internal auditory canal. *cocn: cochlear nerve; fn**: intracanalicular portion of facial nerve; gspn: greater superficial petrosal nerve; mcf: middle cranial fossa dura; ssc: superior semicircular canal; tum: tumor; V3: mandibular division of trigeminal nerve.*

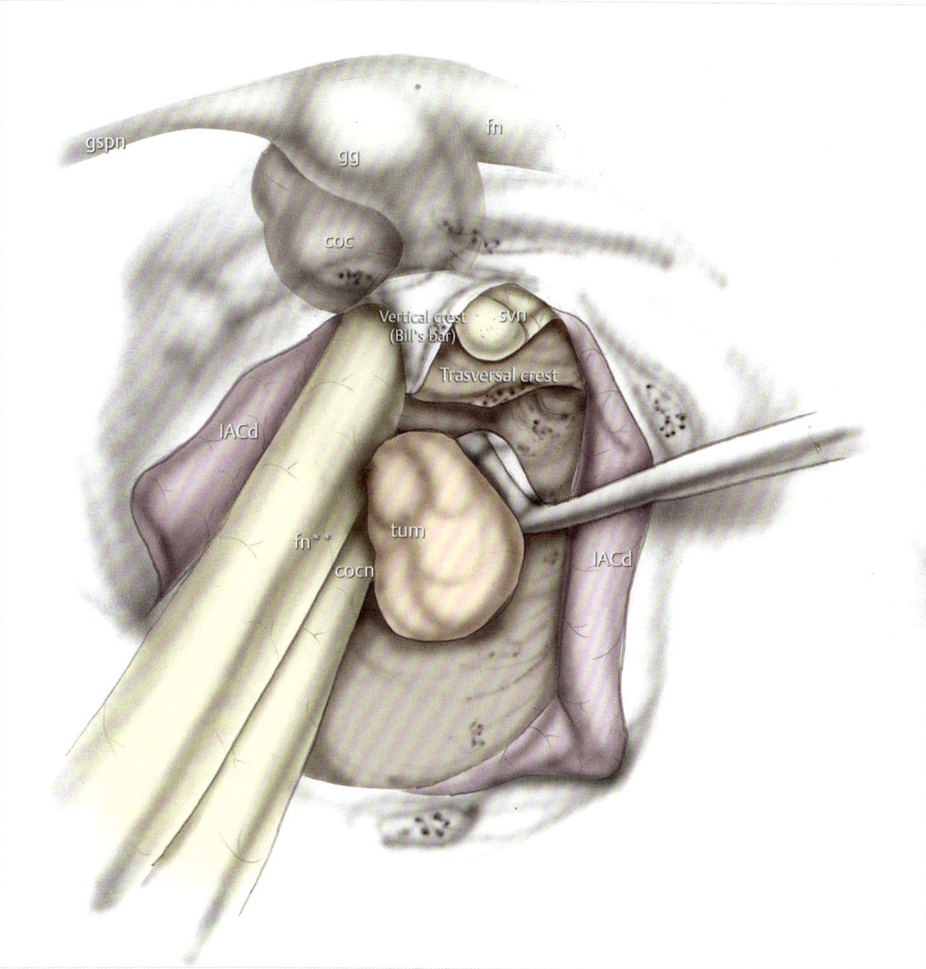

Fig. 8.26 Right side: Under endoscopic magnification, a curved dissector is used to remove the residual tumor from the fundus of the internal auditory canal, under the transverse crest. *coc: cochlea; cocn: cochlear nerve; fn: tympanic portion of the facial nerve; fn**: intracanalicular portion of the facial nerve; gg: geniculate ganglion; gspn: greater superficial petrosal nerve; IACd: dura of the internal auditory canal; svn: superior vestibular nerve; tum: tumor.*

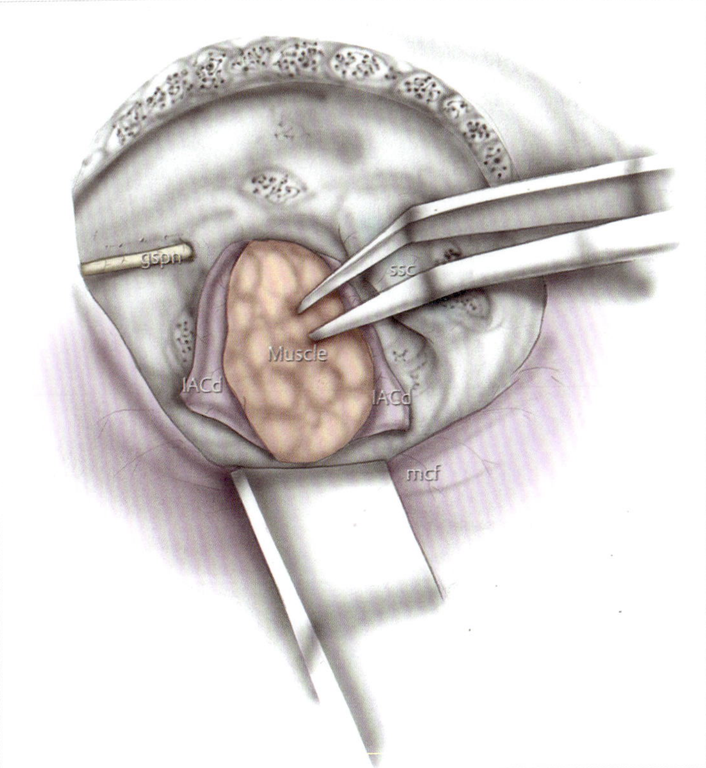

Fig. 8.27 Right side: A temporalis muscle graft is placed into the internal auditory canal (IAC). *gspn: greater superficial petrosal nerve; IACd: internal auditory canal dura; mcf: middle cranial fossa dura; ssc: superior semicircular canal.*

anteromedially and inferiorly to the geniculate ganglion. The petrous bone should be widely removed; especially the inferior and medial portions should be progressively drilled out until the dura of the posterior fossa with the inferior petrosal sinus is visualized. In order to gain space, drilling can be continued under the trigeminal impression downward to the entrance of the abducent nerve in Dorello's canal (see ▶ Fig. 8.76). This landmark is, on average, 7 mm anteroinferior to the trigeminal impression (range, 5–9 mm) and it lies at the level of the inferior petrosal sinus in the petroclival fissure, which represents the deepest point of petrous apex removal.

Once the anterior petrosectomy is completed a careful elevation of the dura of the middle cranial fossa and posterior cranial fossa is performed until the superior and inferior petrosal sinuses become visible in the surgical field (see ▶ Fig. 8.87).

A dural layer incision is needed to access the intradural lesion. The dura is opened adopting a T-shaped incision. The first incision is parallel to the inferior border of the craniotomy along the basal temporal dura. The second incision should be perpendicular to the first, crossing the SPS till the dura of the posterior fossa (see ▶ Fig. 8.88). During the second incision, a metallic clip is used to ligate the SPS. During this step, care must be taken to include the superior petrosal vein (Dandy's vein) in the posterior part of the divided SPS. The tentorium cerebelli is then sharply divided posteriorly from the trochlear nerve as it enters the tentorial edge. During incision and elevation of dural flaps, the trigeminal nerve should be detected and protected, especially as it enters Meckel's cave at the level of the porus trigeminus (see ▶ Fig. 8.89).

Closure

Bone wax is used to close all the petrous bone cells to prevent a connection between the CPA, the mastoid cells, and the petrous bone. The first horizontal dural incision along the temporal base is reapproximated as much as possible. If a transtentorial rhomboid incision of the middle fossa dura is performed, a watertight direct closure will be impossible to achieve. Abdominal fat is used to fill petrous apex defect and empty spaces across the dural opening. A multilayer repair with temporalis fascia and dural allograft is performed in an onlay fashion to seal the floor of the middle fossa after fat interposition. Fibrin glue is used to reinforce the reconstruction.

8.5.5 Postoperative Care

The middle cranial fossa patient requires a 24-hour observation in ICU. A CT scan is performed 6 hours after surgery.

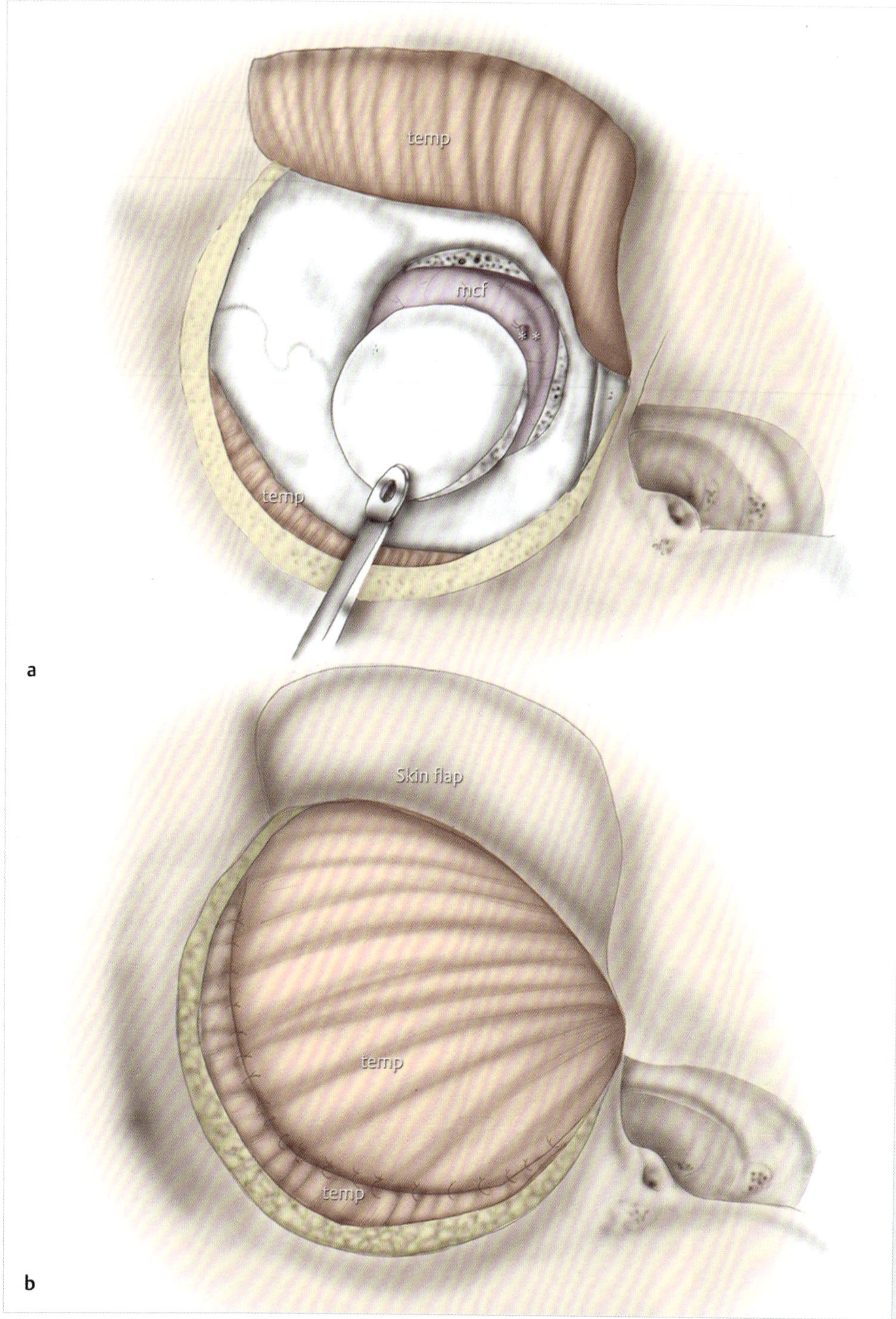

Fig. 8.28 Right side. **(a)** The bone plate is placed back in order to close the craniotomy and fixed using bony dust and fibrin glue. The temporalis muscle flap is repositioned and sutured **(b)**. A meticulous suture of the subcutaneous and skin flaps is then performed. *mcf: middle cranial fossa dura; temp: temporalis muscle; **: defect of the dura sutured.*

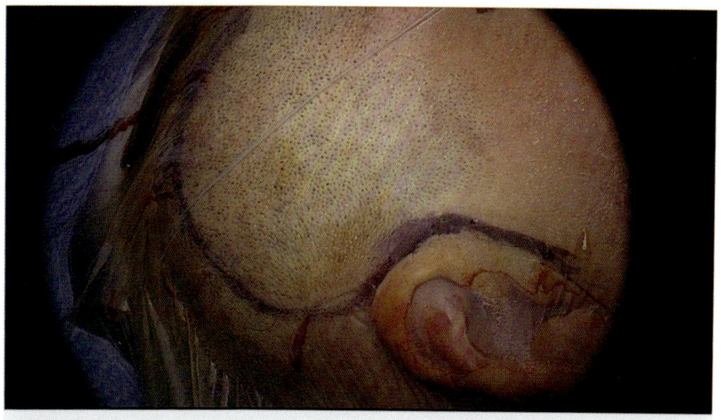

Fig. 8.29 Clinical Case 1, Right side: A C-shaped incision, extended inferiorly along the preauricular sulcus, is performed.

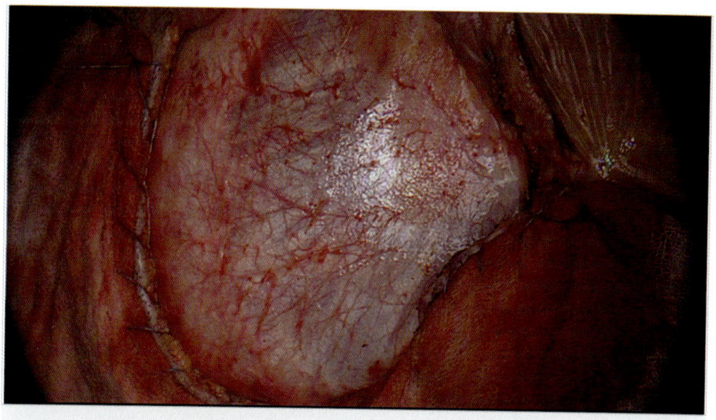

Fig. 8.30 Clinical Case 1, Right side: The skin flap is elevated over the temporalis fascia plane, and the temporalis muscle is incised in the same fashion as the skin flap.

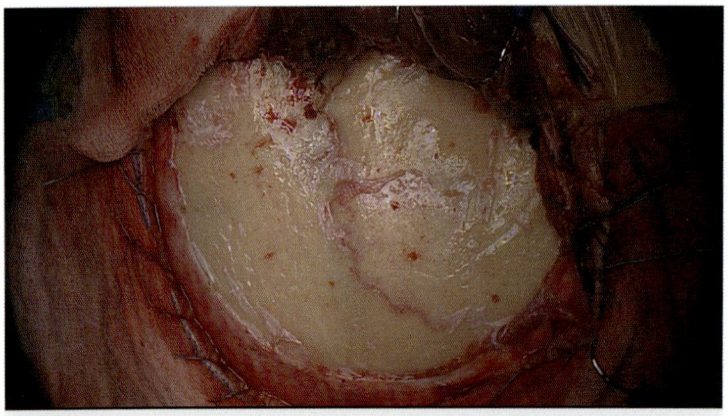

Fig. 8.31 Clinical Case 1, Right side: The temporalis muscle flap is elevated and the bone of squama temporalis is exposed.

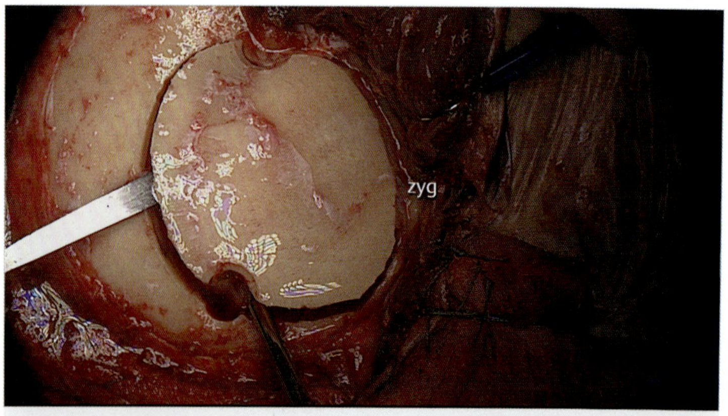

Fig. 8.32 Clinical Case 1, Right side: A craniotomy is performed close to the zygomatic arch. *zyg: zygomatic arch.*

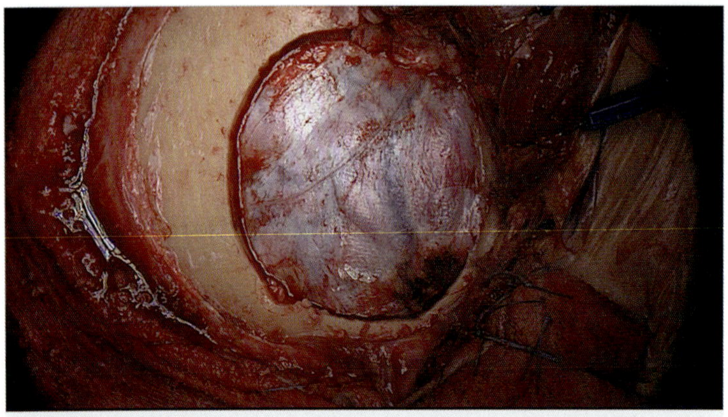

Fig. 8.33 Clinical Case 1, Right side: The dura of the middle cranial fossa is exposed.

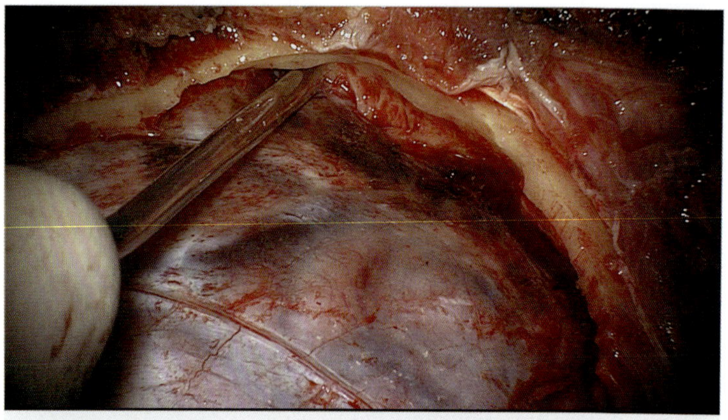

Fig. 8.34 Clinical Case 1, Right side: A diamond bur is used to remove the bone in the inferior border of the craniotomy, allowing the exposure of the floor of the middle cranial fossa.

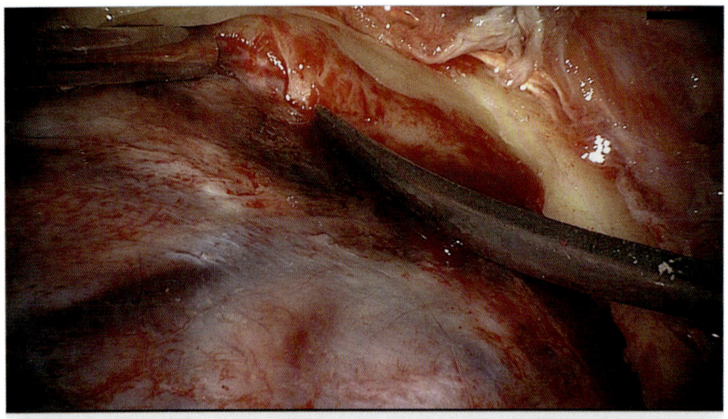

Fig. 8.35 Clinical Case 1, Right side: The temporal lobe is gently separated from the bony floor of the middle cranial fossa using a dissector.

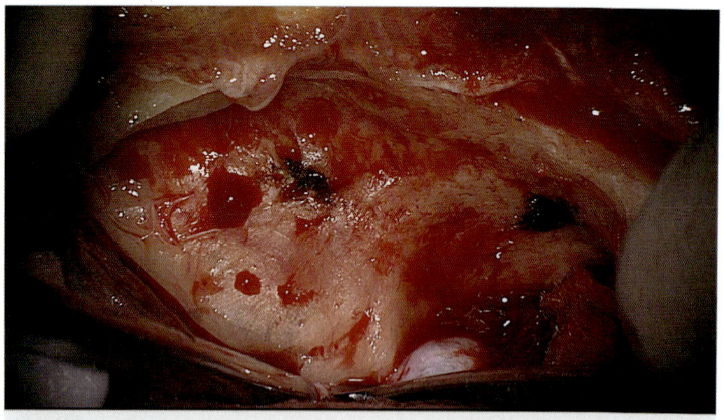

Fig. 8.36 Clinical Case 1, Right side: The superior surface of temporal bone is progressively exposed.

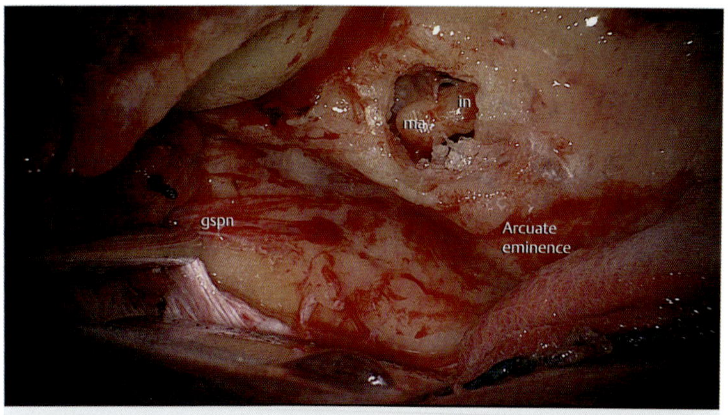

Fig. 8.37 Clinical Case 1, Right side: The greater superficial petrosal nerve and the arcuate eminence are detected; the tegmen of the tympanic cavity is partially drilled exposing the incudomalleolar joint. *gspn: greater superficial petrosal nerve; in: incus; ma: malleus.*

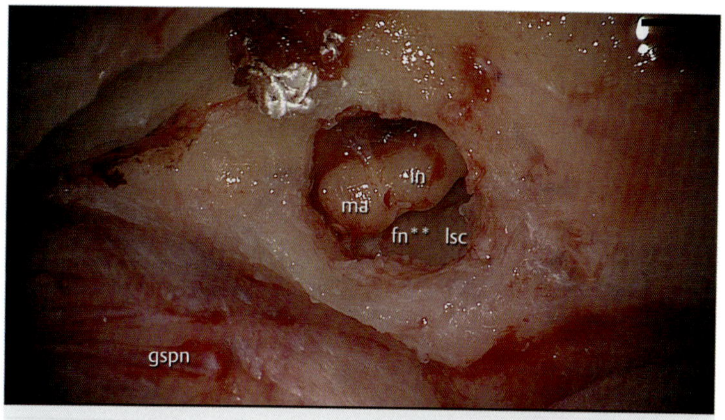

Fig. 8.38 Clinical Case 1, Right side: Microscopic view of the tympanic cavity from above, after partial removal of the tegmen tympani. The tympanic segment of the facial nerve and the prominence of lateral semicircular canal are identified. *fn**: tympanic portion of facial nerve; gspn: greater superficial petrosal nerve; in: incus; lsc: lateral semicircular canal; ma: malleus.*

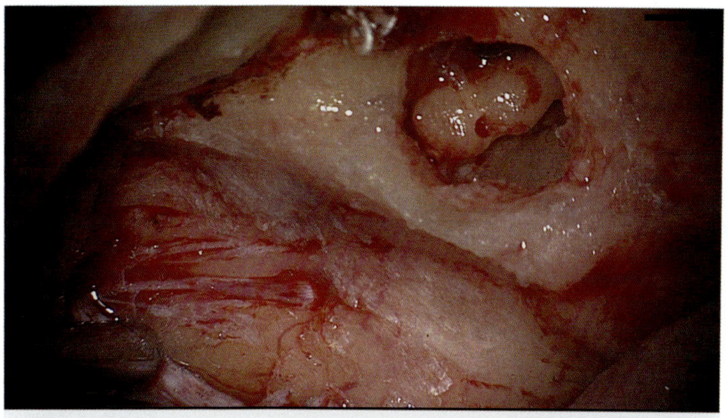

Fig. 8.39 Clinical Case 1, Right side: The greater superficial petrosal nerve and the lesser superficial petrosal nerve are both exposed on the floor of the middle fossa.

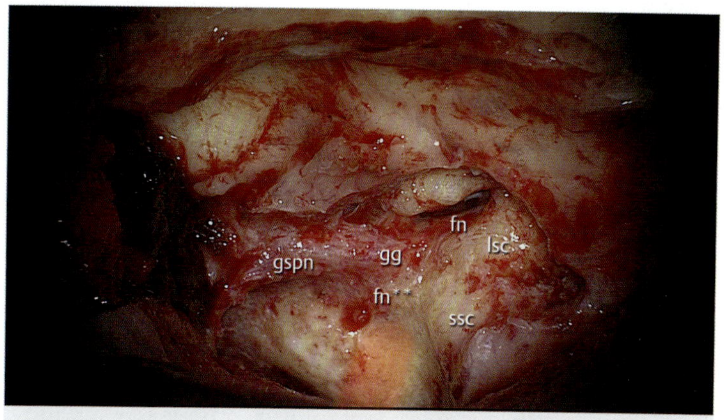

Fig. 8.41 Clinical Case 1, Right side: The bone over the greater superficial petrosal nerve is removed posteriorly to identify the geniculate ganglion and to detect the labyrinthine portion of the facial nerve, entering the internal auditory canal. *fn: tympanic portion of the facial nerve; fn**: labyrinthine portion of the facial nerve; gg: geniculate ganglion; gspn: greater superficial petrosal nerve; lsc: lateral semicircular canal; ssc: superior semicircular canal.*

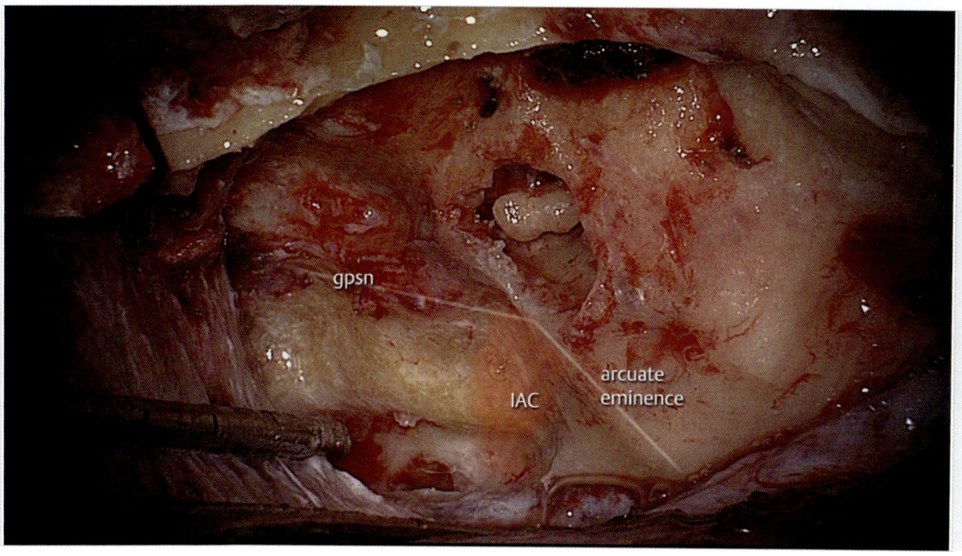

Fig. 8.40 Clinical Case 1, Right side: The floor of the middle cranial fossa is exposed. The bisection line of the angle formed by the imaginary lines that pass through the greater superficial petrosal nerve and the arcuate eminence is used to find the right anatomical orientation of the internal auditory canal (IAC) (*orange shadow*). *gspn: greater superficial petrosal nerve.*

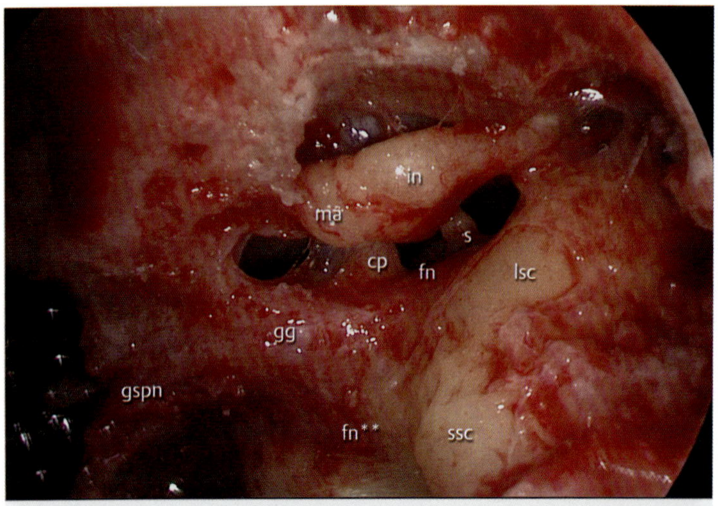

Fig. 8.42 Clinical Case 1, Right side: Endoscopic view through the middle fossa approach showing the anatomy of facial nerve and ossicular chain. The tympanic segment of the facial nerve, the geniculate ganglion, the labyrinthine segment of the facial nerve, the greater superficial petrosal nerve, and the labyrinthine block are seen from above. *cp: cochleariform process; fn: tympanic portion of the facial nerve; fn**: labyrinthine portion of the facial nerve; gg: geniculate ganglion; gspn: greater superficial petrosal nerve; in: incus; lsc: lateral semicircular canal; ma: malleus; s: stapes; ssc: superior semicircular canal.*

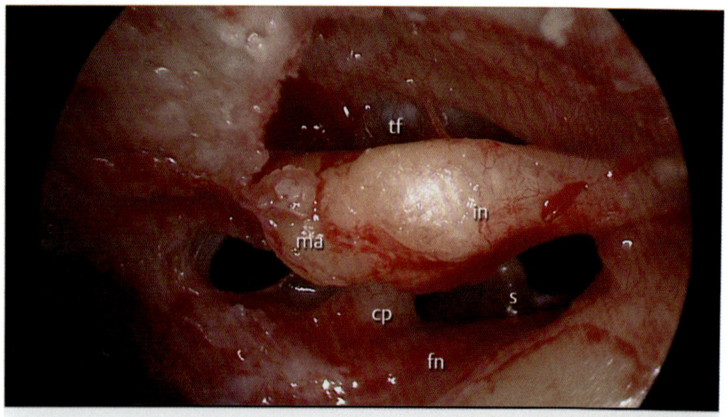

Fig. 8.43 Clinical Case 1, Right side: Endoscopic magnification (with 0-degree endoscope) of the tympanic cavity anatomy from above. *cp: cochleariform process; fn: tympanic portion of the facial nerve; in: incus; ma: malleus; s: stapes; tf: tensor fold.*

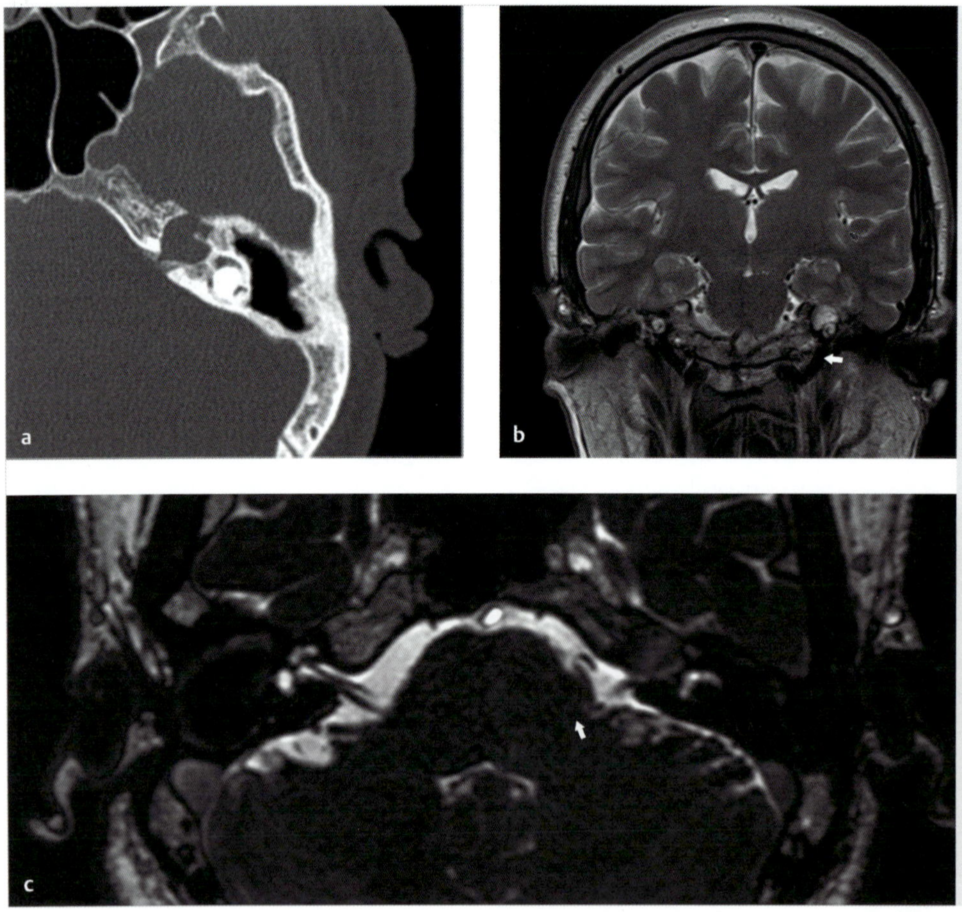

Fig. 8.44 Clinical Case 2, Left side: **(a)** Computed tomography (CT) scan, axial view: A supralabyrinthine cholesteatoma is detected, involving the labyrinthine portion of facial nerve and the internal auditory canal (IAC). **(b)** Magnetic resonance imaging (MRI), coronal view, that shows the cholesteatoma located above the cochlea. **(c)** MRI, axial view, showing the involvement of the left petrous apex and IAC in a patient who underwent a previous bilateral Canal Wall Down procedures.

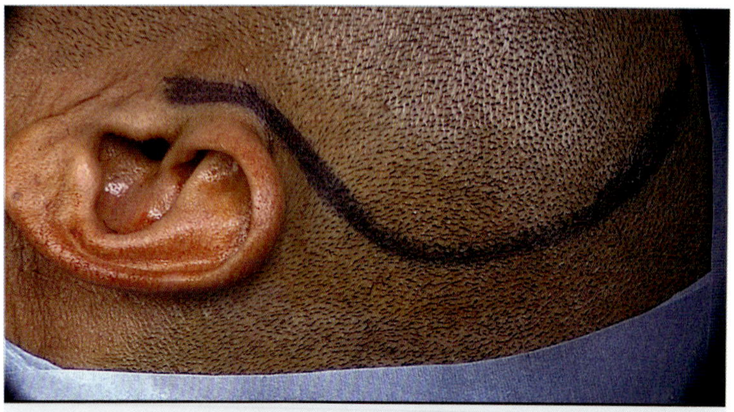

Fig. 8.45 Clinical Case 2, Left side: A C-shaped skin incision, extending inferiorly along the preauricular sulcus, is performed.

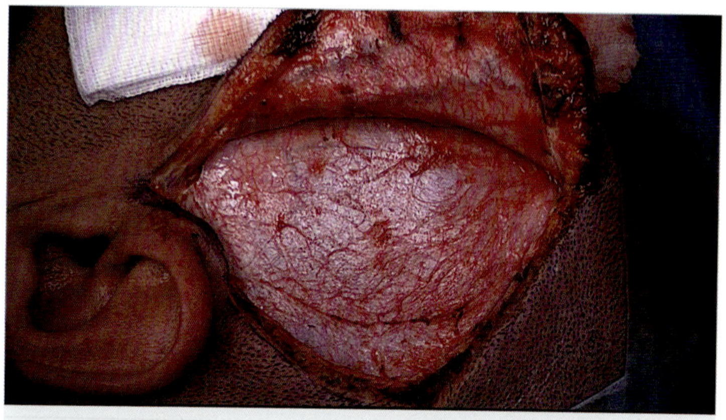

Fig. 8.46 Clinical Case 2, Left side: The skin flap is elevated over the temporalis fascia.

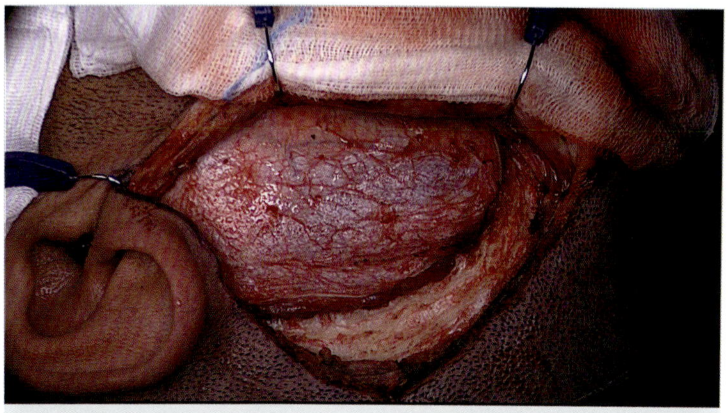

Fig. 8.47 Clinical Case 2, Left side: The temporalis muscle is incised.

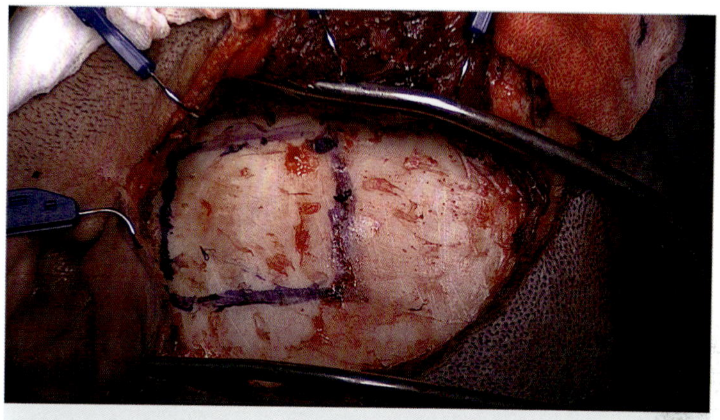

Fig. 8.48 Clinical Case 2, Left side: The craniotomy is drawn over the temporal bone.

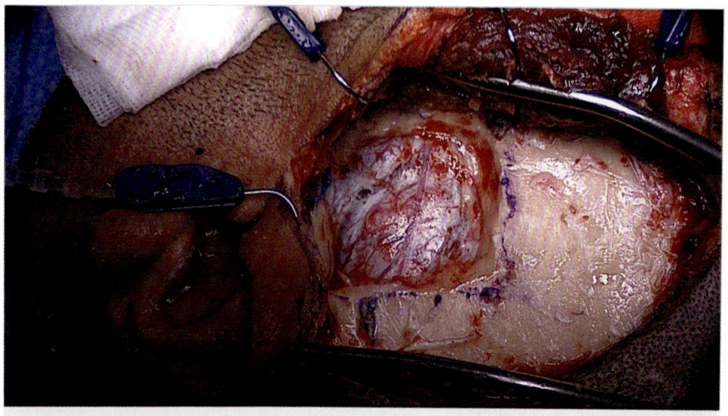

Fig. 8.49 Clinical Case 2, Left side: The craniotomy is performed and the middle cranial fossa dura is exposed.

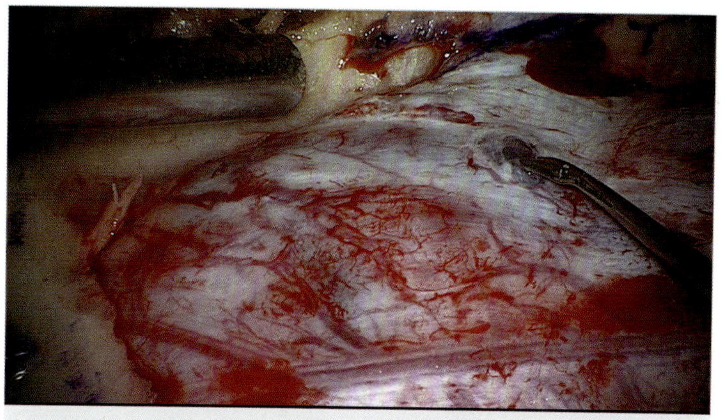

Fig. 8.50 Clinical Case 2, Left side: A small incision of the middle cranial fossa dura is performed. A cerebrospinal fluid (CSF) leakage is expected in order to decompress the temporal lobe.

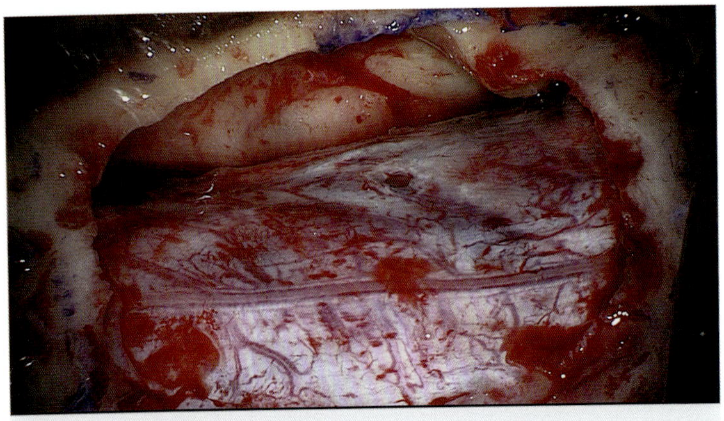

Fig. 8.51 Clinical Case 2, Left side: The temporal lobe is gently elevated and the floor of middle fossa is exposed.

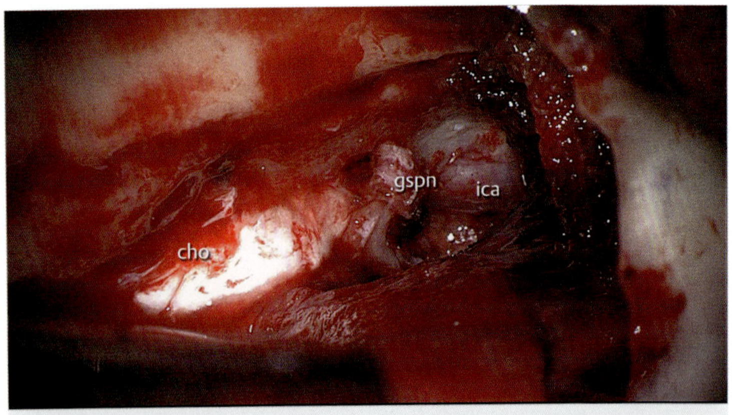

Fig. 8.52 Clinical Case 2, Left side: The greater superficial petrosal nerve (*gspn*) and the horizontal portion of internal carotid artery (*ica*) are detected, and the cholesteatoma is seen lying above the lateral portion of the internal auditory canal. *cho: cholesteatoma; gspn: greater superficial petrosal nerve; ica: internal carotid artery.*

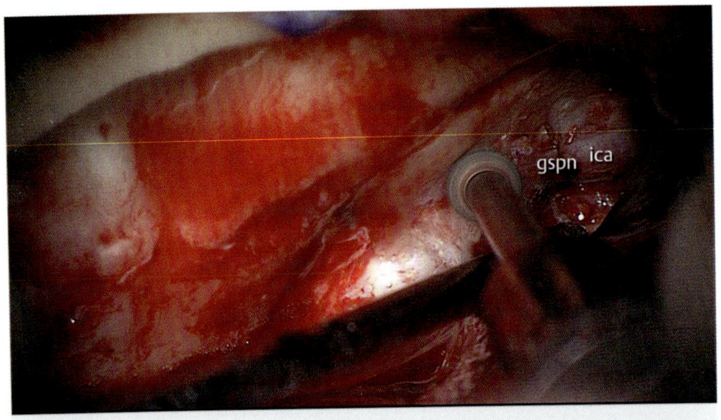

Fig. 8.53 Clinical Case 2, Left side: The greater superficial petrosal nerve (GSPN) is used as landmark to find the geniculate ganglion; a diamond bur is used to remove the bone over the GSPN, following it posteriorly. The cholesteatoma is isolated. *gspn: greater superficial petrosal nerve; ica: internal carotid artery.*

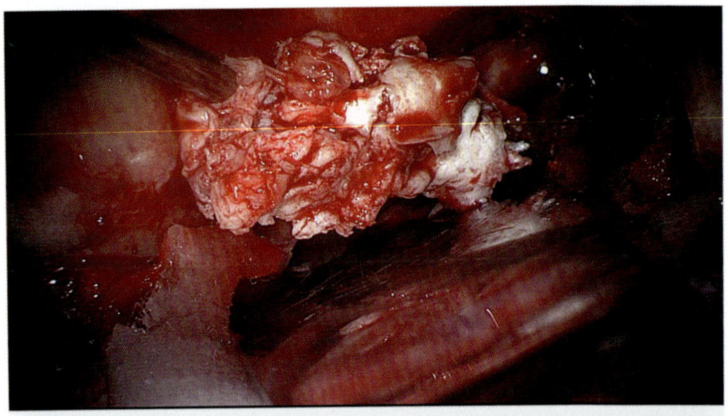

Fig. 8.54 Clinical Case 2, Left side: The cholesteatoma is removed.

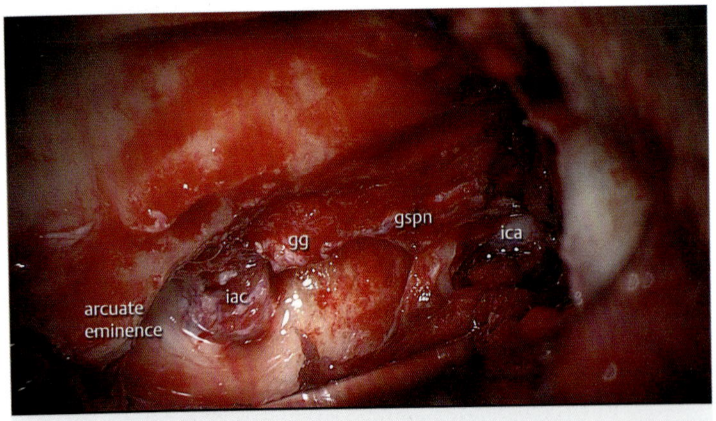

Fig. 8.55 Clinical Case 2, Left side: After cholesteatoma removal, a diamond bur is used to remove the bone between the facial nerve, the geniculate ganglion, the arcuate eminence, and the cochlea, skeletonizing the internal auditory canal. *gg: geniculate ganglion; gspn: greater superficial petrosal nerve; iac: internal auditory canal; ica: internal carotid artery.*

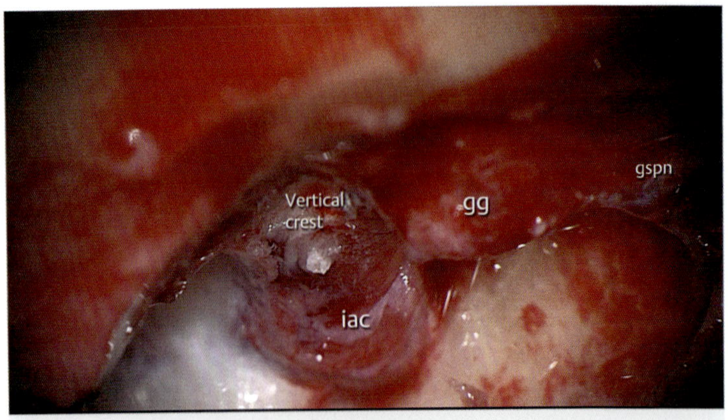

Fig. 8.56 Clinical Case 2, Left side: Microscopic view of the internal auditory canal (IAC) from the middle cranial fossa approach; a residual cholesteatoma is detected around the vertical crest. *gg: geniculate ganglion; gspn: greater superficial petrosal nerve; iac: internal auditory canal.*

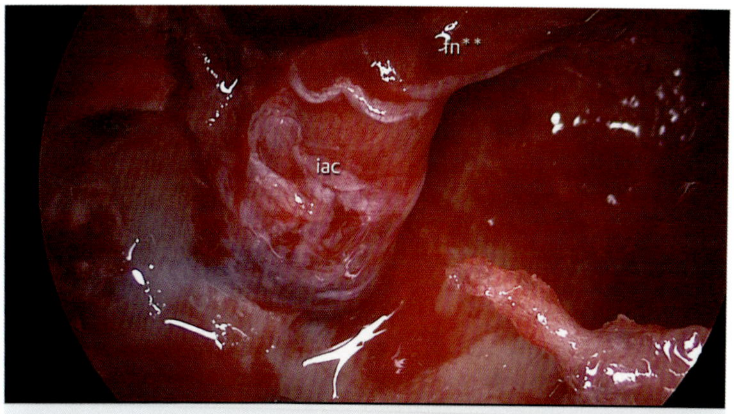

Fig. 8.57 Clinical Case 2, Left side: A 45-degree angled endoscope, is used to remove the residual disease in the lateral aspect of the internal auditory canal (IAC). The dura of the IAC is opened and the facial nerve in the IAC is identified. *fn**: labyrinthine portion of the facial nerve; iac: internal auditory canal.*

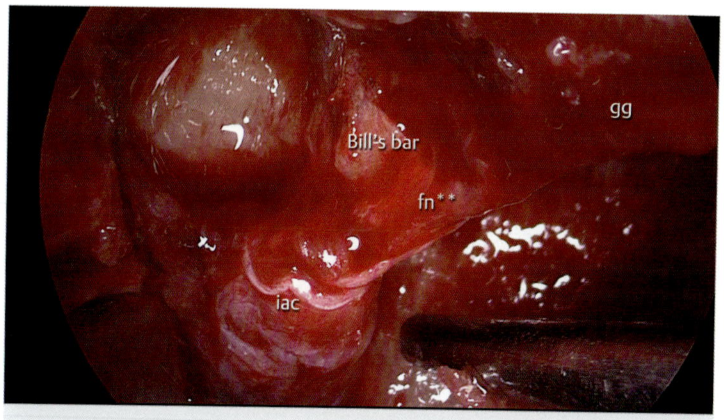

Fig. 8.58 Clinical Case 2, Left side: Endoscopic magnification of vertical crest (Bill's bar) and labyrinthine portion of facial nerve after cholesteatoma removal. *fn**: labyrinthine portion of the facial nerve; gg: geniculate ganglion; iac: internal auditory canal.*

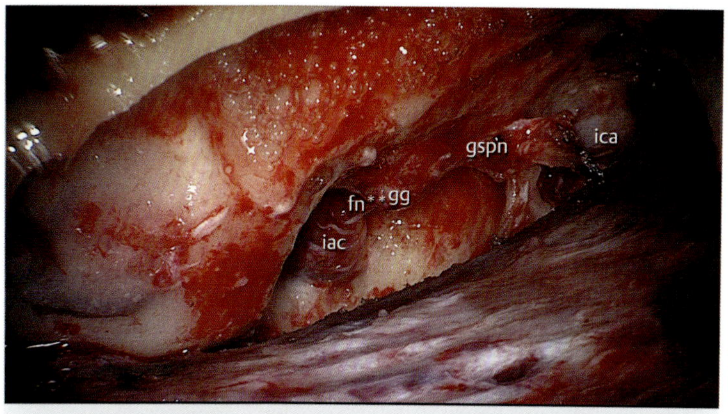

Fig. 8.59 Clinical Case 2, Left side: Final microscopic view from middle cranial fossa approach. *fn**: intralabyrinthine portion of the facial nerve; gg: geniculate ganglion; gspn: greater superficial petrosal nerve; iac: internal auditory canal; ica: internal carotid artery.*

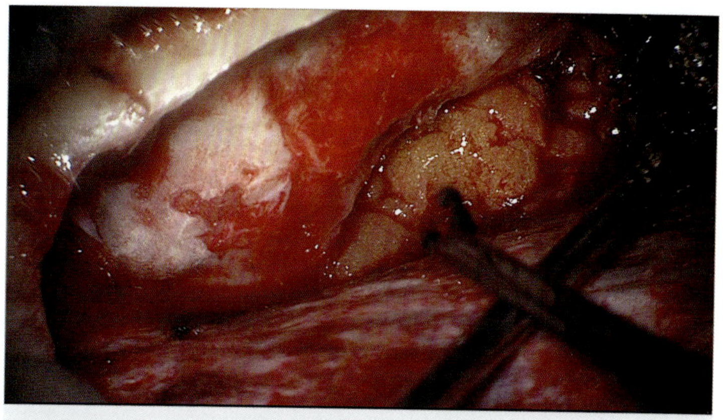

Fig. 8.60 Clinical Case 2, Left side: A fat pad is used to obliterate the petrous apex.

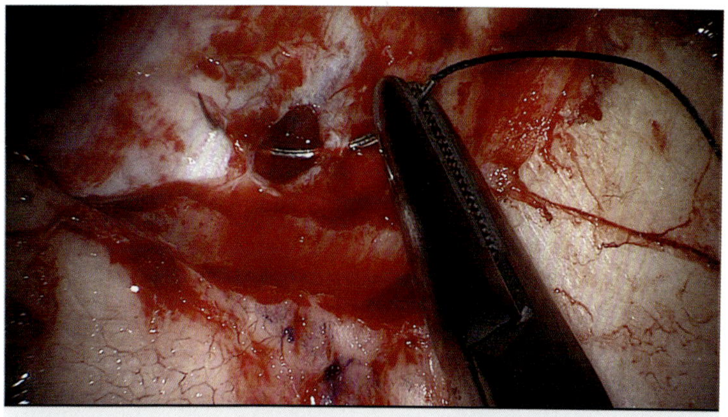

Fig. 8.61 Clinical Case 2, Left side: The small dural defect of the middle cranial fossa dura, previously created, is sutured.

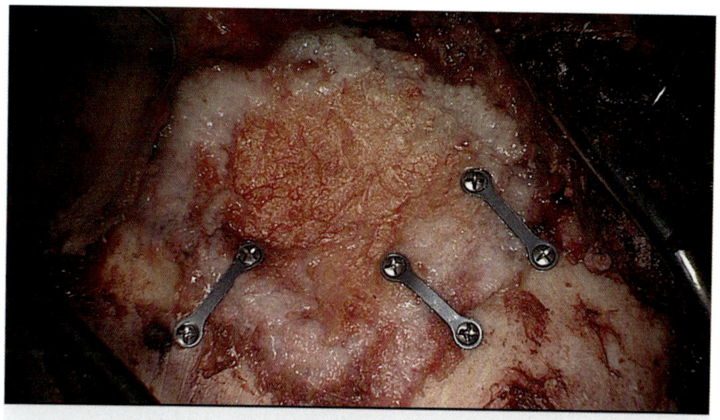

Fig. 8.62 Clinical Case 2, Left side: The craniotomy plate is put back in place and secured using titanium plates and screws.

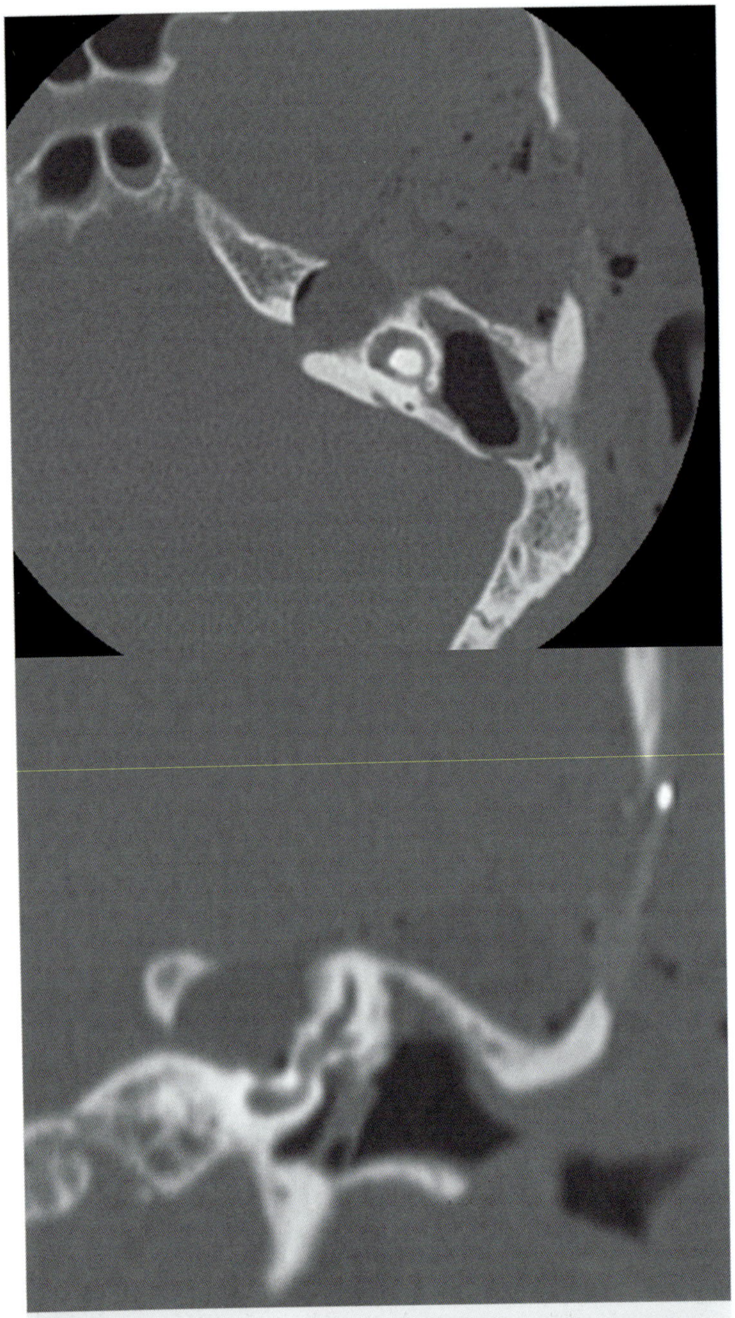

Fig. 8.63 Clinical Case 2, Left side: Postoperative computed tomography (CT) scan, axial and coronal views.

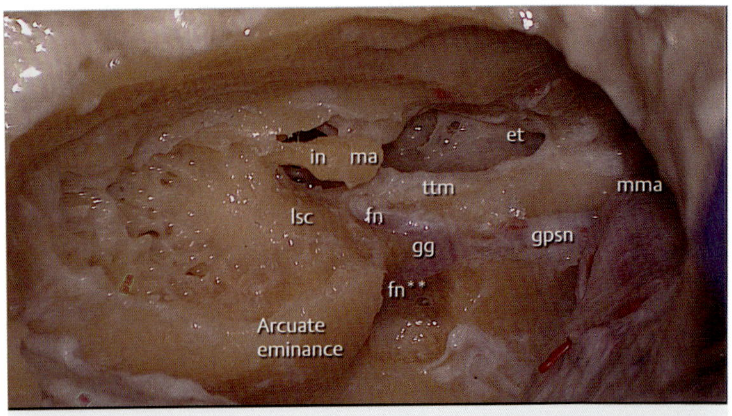

Fig. 8.64 Dissection. Left side: Anatomy of the floor of middle cranial fossa. The tegmen tympani is opened and the ossicular chain and protympanum exposed. The facial nerve is seen running from the tympanic cavity to the lateral portion of the internal auditory canal. *et: eustachian tube; fn: tympanic portion of the facial nerve; fn**: labyrinthine portion of the facial nerve; gg: geniculate ganglion; gspn: greater superficial petrosal nerve; in: incus; lsc: lateral semicircular canal; ma: malleus; mma: middle meningeal artery; ttm: tensor tympani muscle hemicanal.*

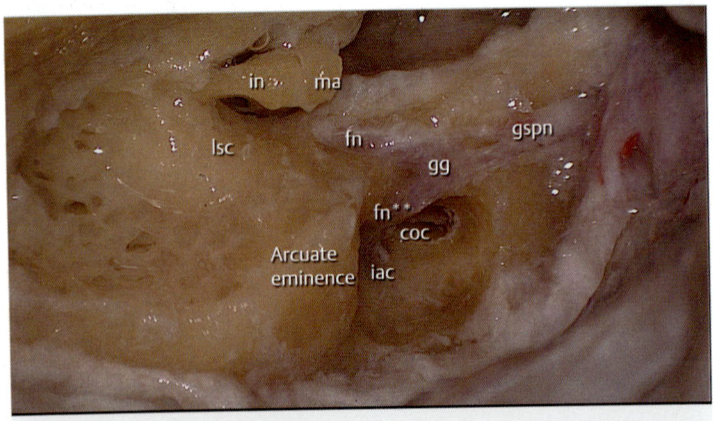

Fig. 8.65 Dissection. Left side: The cochlea is opened. The reader can appreciate the close relationship between the labyrinthine portion of facial nerve and the cochlea, since the nerve runs just above the cochlea, entering the fundus of the internal auditory canal. *coc: cochlea; fn: tympanic portion of the facial nerve; fn**: labyrinthine portion of the facial nerve; gg: geniculate ganglion; gspn: greater superficial petrosal nerve; iac: internal auditory canal; in: incus; lsc: lateral semicircular canal; ma: malleus.*

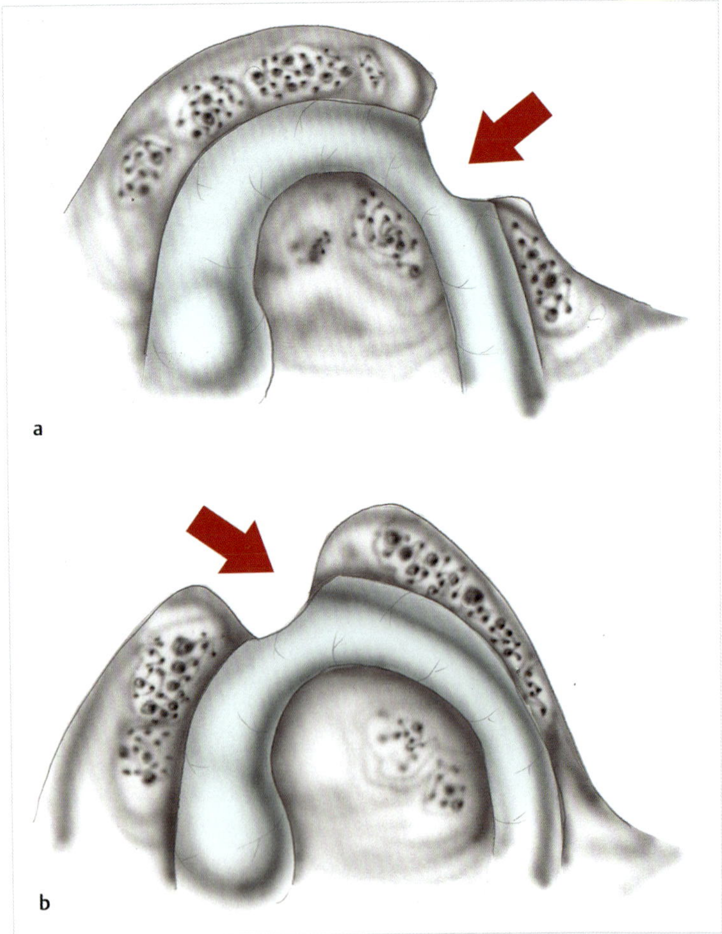

Fig. 8.66 **(a)** Dehiscence of the superior semicircular canal on its medial downslope. **(b)** Dehiscence of superior semicircular canal on its lateral upslope.

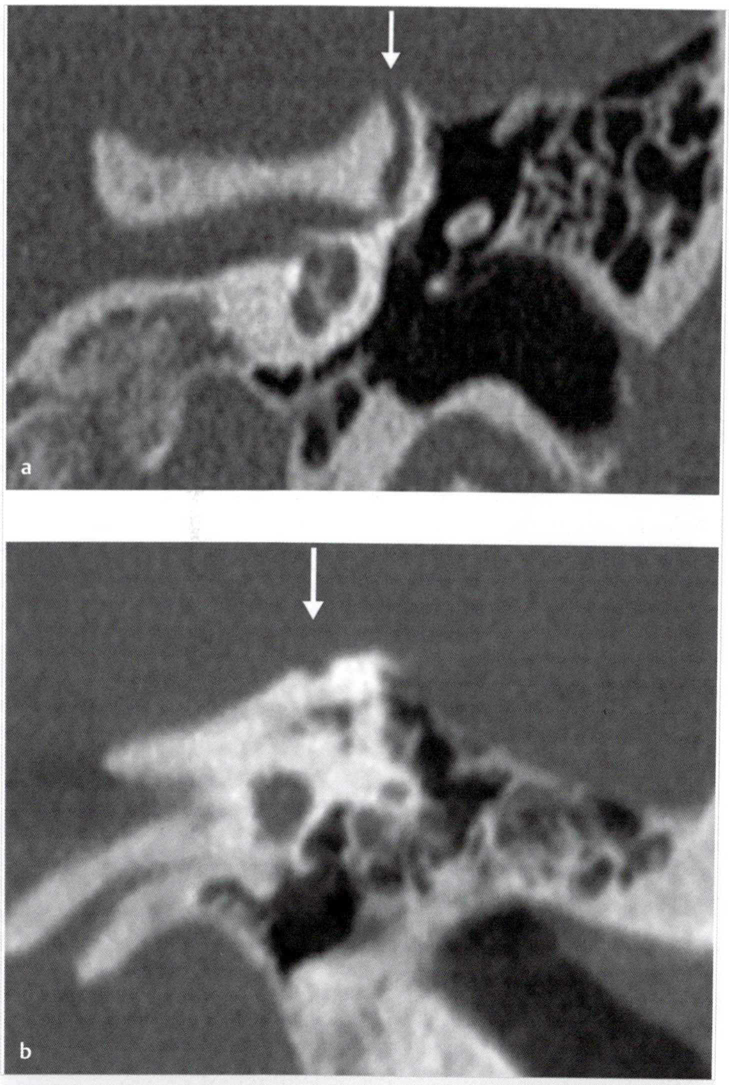

Fig. 8.67 **(a, b)** Clinical Case 3. Preoperative computed tomography (CT) scan; the coronal view shows a left superior semicircular canal defect (*white arrow*).

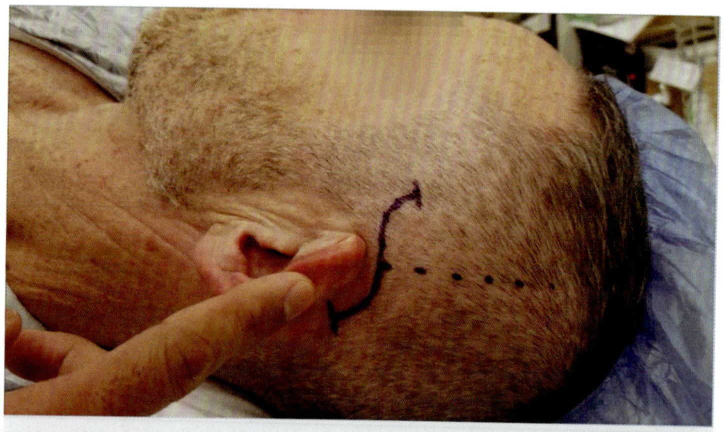

Fig. 8.68 Clinical Case 3, Right side: Endoscopic assisted superior canal dehiscence repair: a 3 to 4 cm preauricular curvilinear skin incision is made.

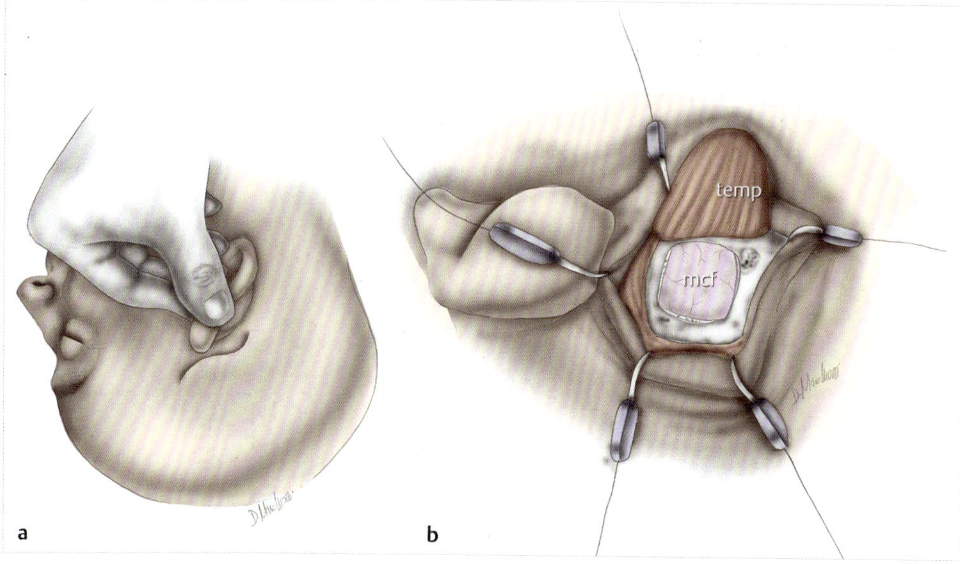

Fig. 8.69 Clinical Case 3, Right side: Endoscopic assisted superior canal dehiscence repair. **(a)** A preauricular curvilinear skin incision is made. **(b)** After skin incision, a temporalis muscle flap is elevated and a minimal invasive craniotomy (3 × 2 cm) is performed, uncovering the dura of middle cranial fossa. *mcf: middle cranial fossa; temp: temporalis muscle.*

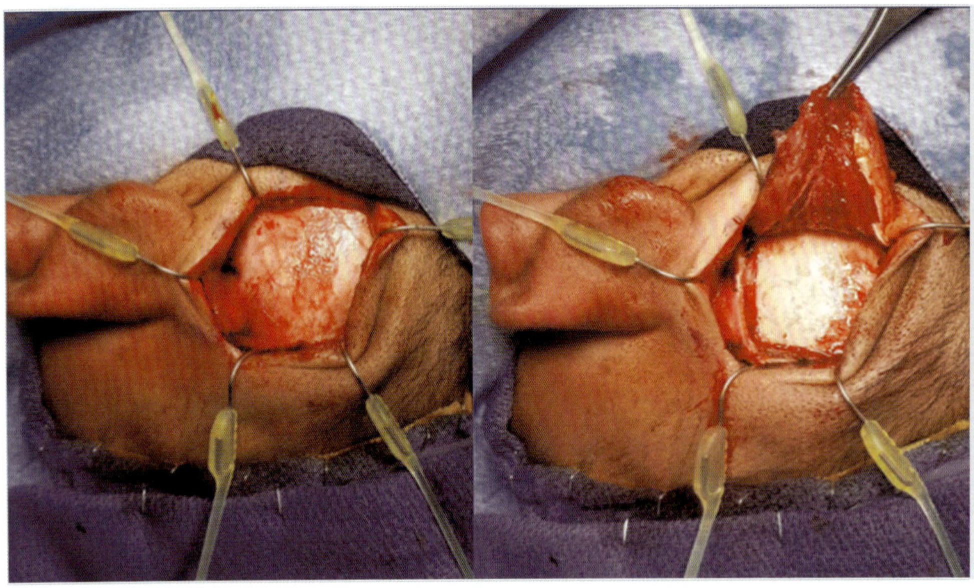

Fig. 8.70 Clinical Case 3, Right side: Endoscopic assisted superior canal dehiscence repair. The skin flap is elevated, and the temporalis fascia is detected. Subsequently the temporalis muscle flap is elevated uncovering the temporalis bone and the zygomatic arch.

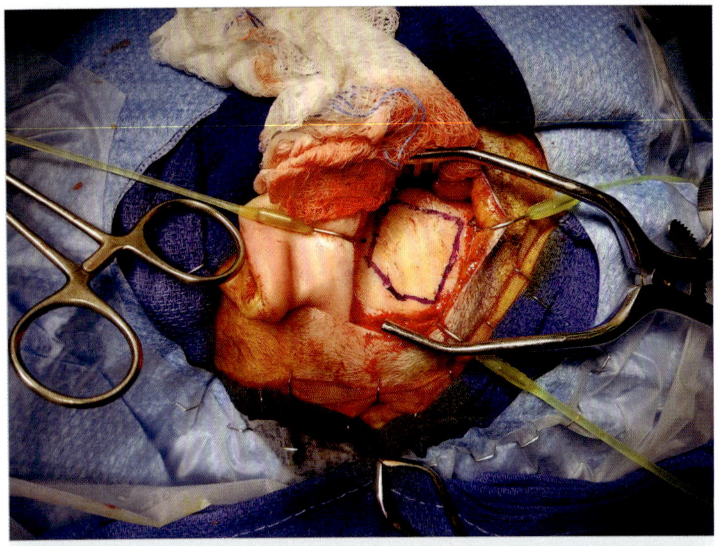

Fig. 8.71 Clinical Case 3, Right side: Endoscopic assisted superior canal dehiscence repair. A craniotomy (3 × 2 cm) is created, centered on the external auditory canal.

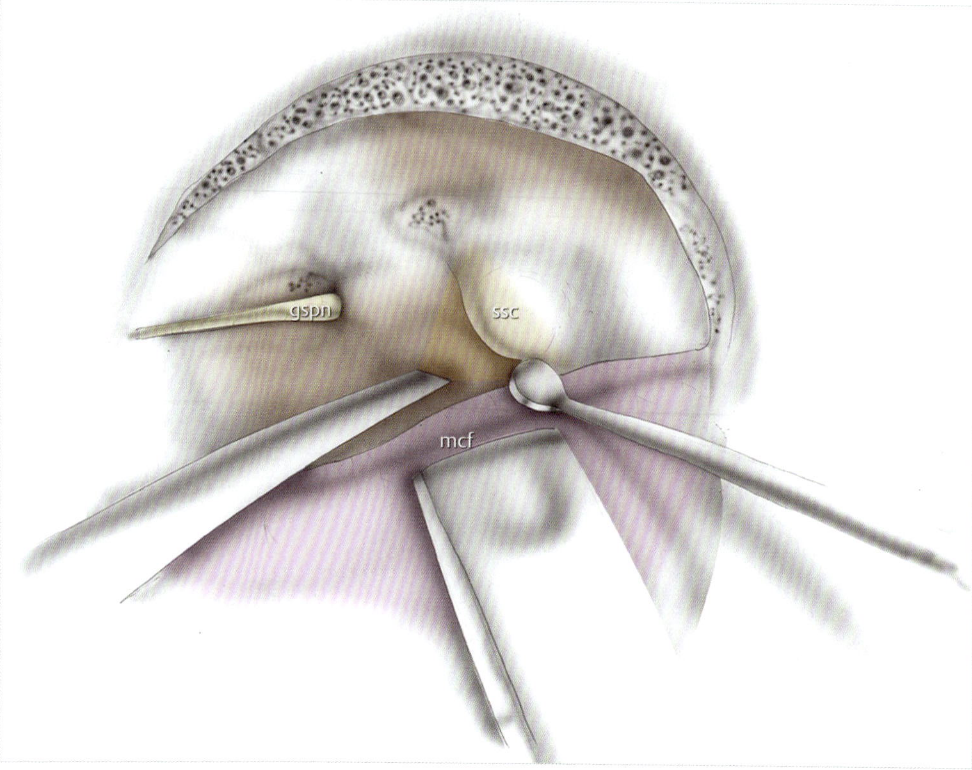

Fig. 8.72 Clinical Case 3, Right side: Endoscopic assisted superior canal dehiscence repair. The temporal lobe is gently elevated, exposing the floor of the middle cranial fossa. An endoscope is introduced into the surgical cavity to detect the defect of the superior semicircular canal (ssc). *gspn: greater superficial petrosal nerve; mcf: middle cranial fossa; ssc: superior semicircular canal.*

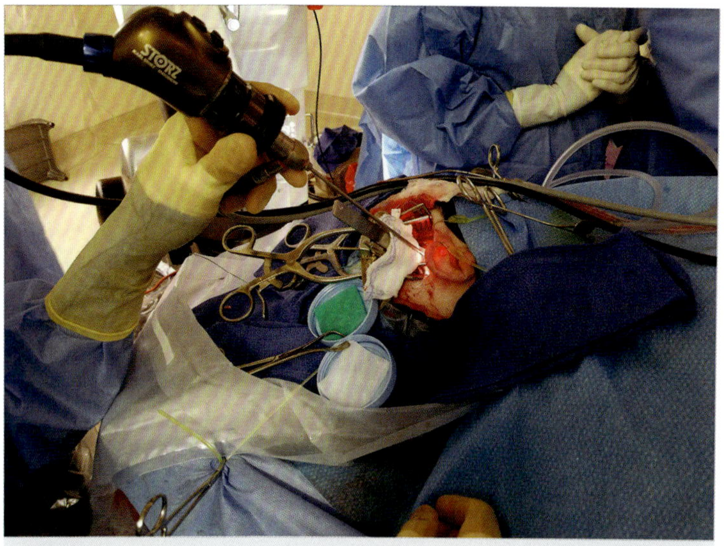

Fig. 8.73 Setting of the operating room and position of the surgeon during the endoscopic procedure.

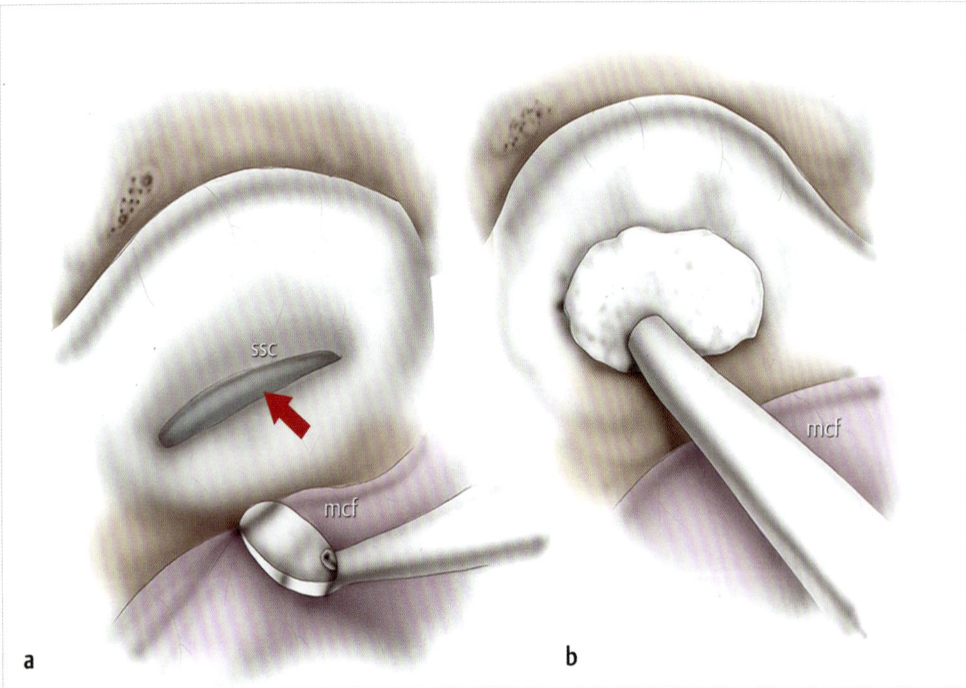

Fig. 8.74 Clinical Case 3, Right side: Endoscopic assisted superior canal dehiscence repair.
(a) Under endoscopic view, a dissector is used to gently detach the dura from the medial aspect of the superior semicircular canal defect.
(b) The repair of the dehiscent superior canal can be achieved plugging the defect with bone wax. *mcf: middle cranial fossa; ssc: superior semicircular canal.*

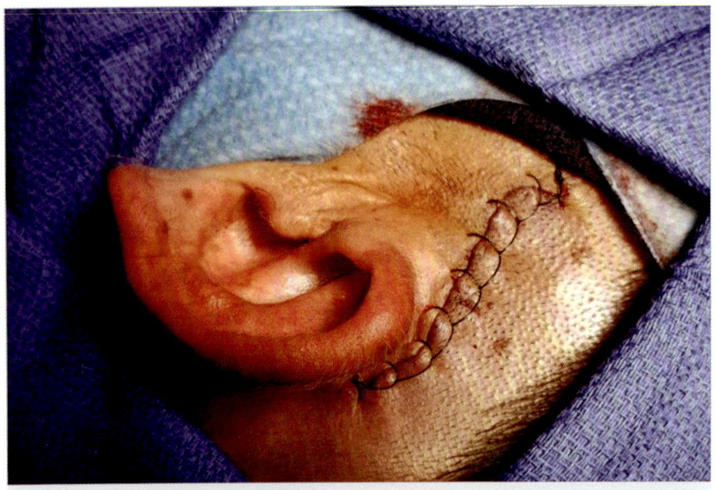

Fig. 8.75 Clinical Case 3, Right side: Final view after suture of the skin.

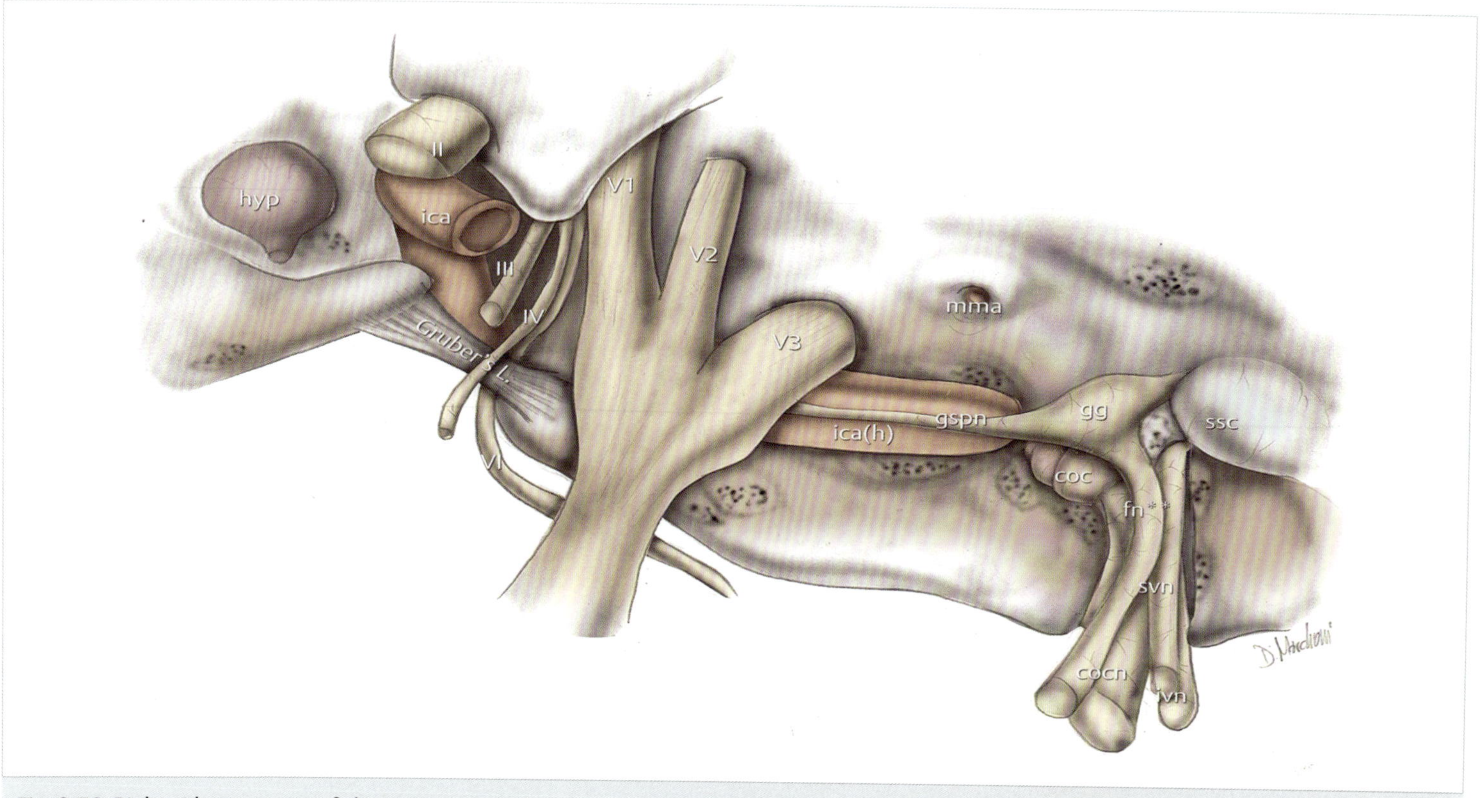

Fig. 8.76 Right side: Anatomy of the petrous apex from above, related to the anterior petrosectomy approach. The Meckel's cave, the oculomotor nerve, the trochlear nerve, the V1 (ophthalmic division of the trigeminal nerve), and the abducens nerve running in the cavernous sinus are seen; especially the position of the abducens nerve running inside the Dorello's canal is noted. *coc: cochlea; cocn: cochlear nerve; fn**: intracanalicular portion of the facial nerve; gg: geniculate ganglion; Gruber's L: Gruber's ligament; gspn: greater superficial petrosal nerve; hyp: hypophysis; ica(h): horizontal segment of intrapetrous carotid artery; ica: internal carotid artery; II: II cranial nerve (optic nerve); III: III cranial nerve (oculomotor nerve); IV: IV cranial nerve (trochlear nerve); ivn: inferior vestibular nerve; mma: middle meningeal artery; ssc: superior semicircular canal; svn: superior vestibular nerve; V1: ophthalmic division of the trigeminal nerve; V2: maxillary division of trigeminal nerve; V3: mandibular division of trigeminal nerve; VI: VI cranial nerve (abducens nerve).*

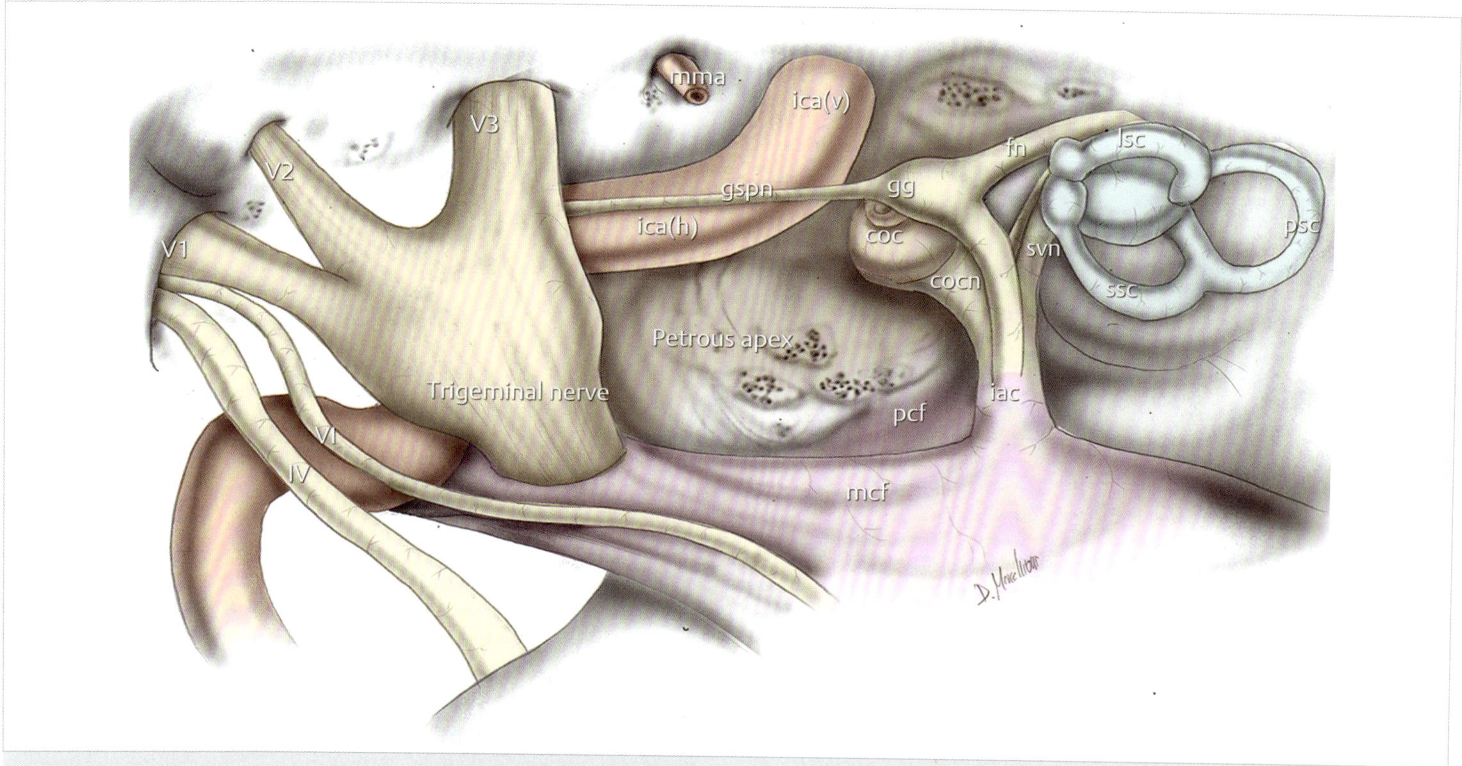

Fig. 8.77 Right side: Anatomical drawing that shows the petrous apex bony removal between the internal auditory canal (*iac*), internal carotid artery (*ica*), V3, and the posterior fossa dura, during anterior petrosectomy. *coc: cochlea; cocn: cochlear nerve; fn: tympanic portion of the facial nerve; gg: geniculate ganglion; gspn: greater superficial petrosal nerve; iac: internal auditory canal; ica(h): horizontal segment of intrapetrous carotid artery; ica(v): vertical segment of intrapetrous carotid artery; IV: IV cranial nerve (trochlear nerve); lsc: lateral semicircular canal; mcf: middle cranial fossa dura; mma: middle meningeal artery; pcf: posterior cranial fossa dura; psc: posterior semicircular canal; ssc: superior semicircular canal; svn: superior vestibular nerve; V1: ophthalmic division of the trigeminal nerve; V2: maxillary division of trigeminal nerve; V3: mandibular division of trigeminal nerve; VI: VI cranial nerve (abducens nerve).*

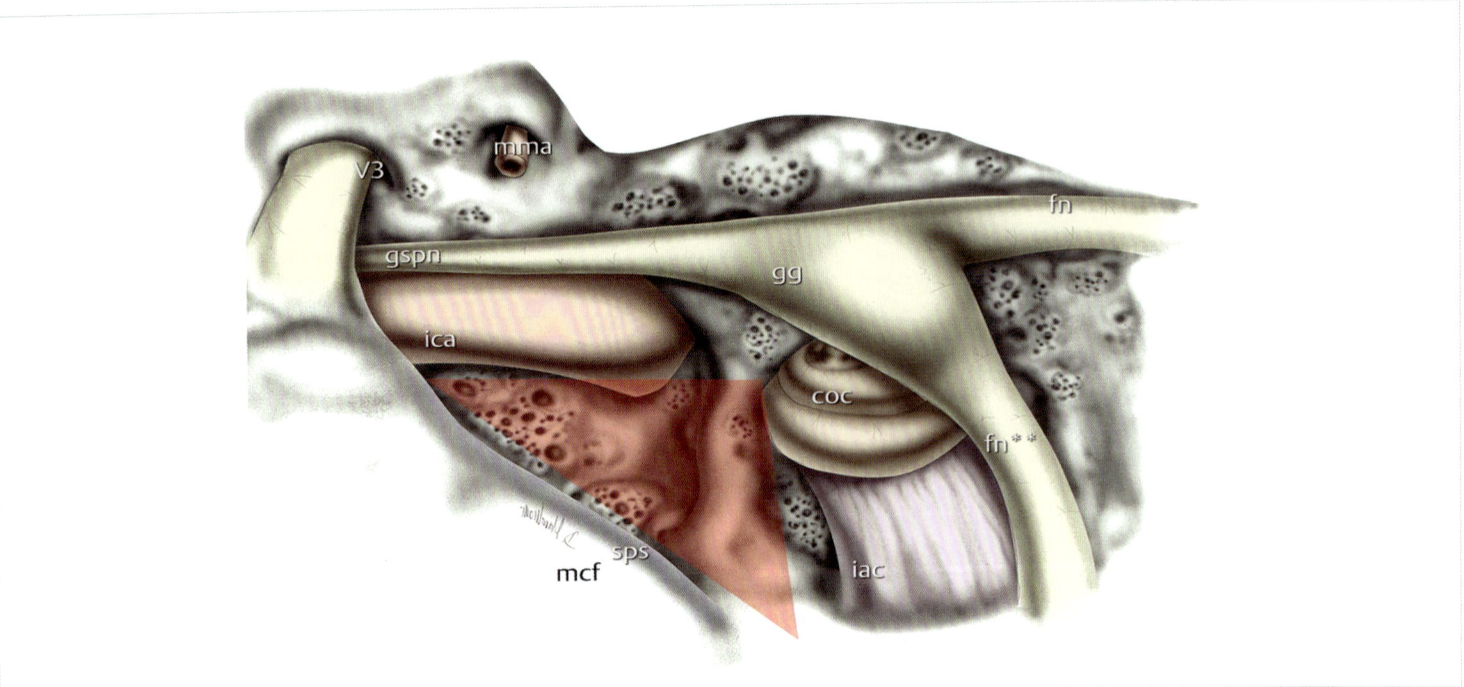

Fig. 8.78 Right side: A schematic drawing shows the limits of Kawase's triangle: medially, the petrous ridge with superior petrosal sinus (*sps*); laterally, the greater superficial petrosal nerve (*gspn*) and the horizontal portion of the internal carotid artery (ICA); anteriorly, V3 and the posterior edge of the gasserian ganglion; and posteriorly, the internal auditory canal (*iac*). The cochlea is located anteromedial and inferior to the geniculate ganglion. *coc: cochlea; fn: tympanic portion of the facial nerve; fn**: intracanalicular portion of the facial nerve; gg: geniculate ganglion; gspn: greater superficial petrosal nerve; iac: internal auditory canal; ica: internal carotid artery (intrapetrous horizontal segment); mcf: middle cranial fossa dura; mma: middle meningeal artery; sps: superior petrosal sinus; V3: mandibular division of trigeminal nerve.*

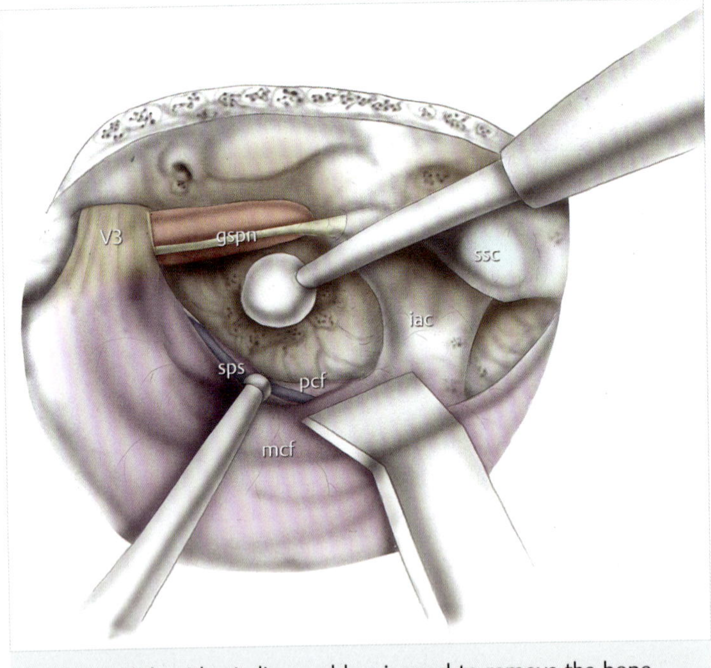

Fig. 8.79 Right side: A diamond bur is used to remove the bone around internal carotid artery, internal auditory canal, trigeminal nerve (V3), and dura of the middle and posterior *cranial fossae*, in order to reach the lesion in the petrous apex. *gspn: greater superficial petrosal nerve; iac: internal auditory canal; mcf: middle cranial fossa dura; pcf: posterior cranial fossa dura; sps: superior petrosal sinus; ssc: superior semicircular canal; V3: mandibular division of trigeminal nerve.*

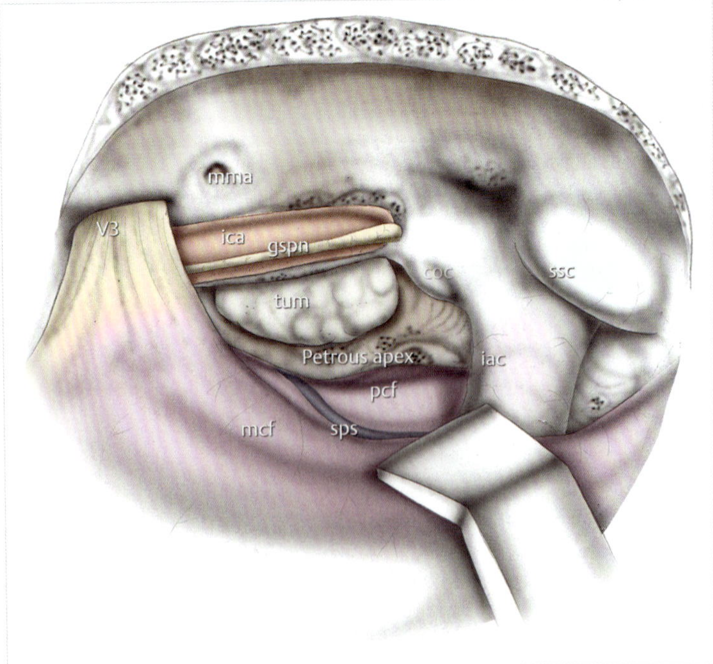

Fig. 8.80 Right side: The bone of the petrous apex is removed and the most superior portion of the lesion is isolated. *coc: cochlea; gspn: greater superficial petrosal nerve; iac: internal auditory canal; ica: internal carotid artery; mcf: middle cranial fossa dura; mma: middle meningeal artery; pcf: posterior cranial fossa dura; sps: superior petrosal sinus; ssc: superior semicircular canal; tum: tumor; V3: mandibular division of trigeminal nerve.*

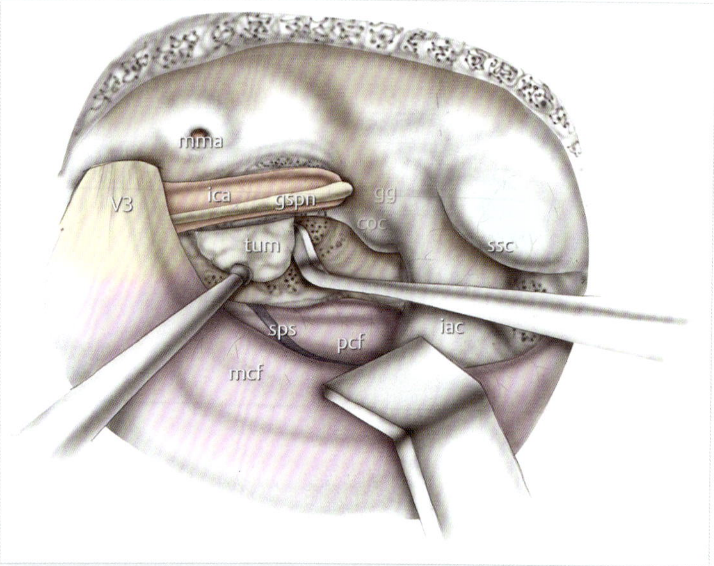

Fig. 8.81 Right side: The tumor dissection starts. A curve dissector is used with the dominant hand to remove the disease, and the suction instrument is held with the contralateral hand to help dissection. *coc: cochlea; gg: geniculate ganglion; gspn: greater superficial petrosal nerve; iac: internal auditory canal; ica: internal carotid artery; mcf: middle cranial fossa dura; mma: middle meningeal artery; pcf: posterior cranial fossa dura; sps: superior petrosal sinus; ssc: superior semicircular canal; tum: tumor; V3: mandibular division of trigeminal nerve.*

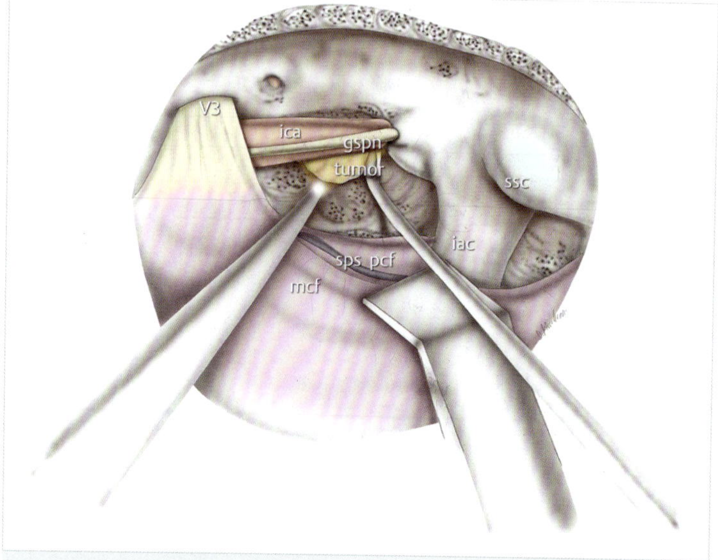

Fig. 8.83 Right side: A 45-degree endoscope is introduced into the surgical cavity, exposing the petrous apex under the horizontal portion of the internal carotid artery; an angulate dissector is used to remove remnant disease, under endoscopic view. *gspn: greater superficial petrosal nerve; iac: internal auditory canal; ica: horizontal segment of the intrapetrous internal carotid artery; mcf: middle cranial fossa dura; pcf: posterior cranial fossa dura; sps: superior petrosal sinus; ssc: superior semicircular canal; V3: mandibular division of trigeminal nerve.*

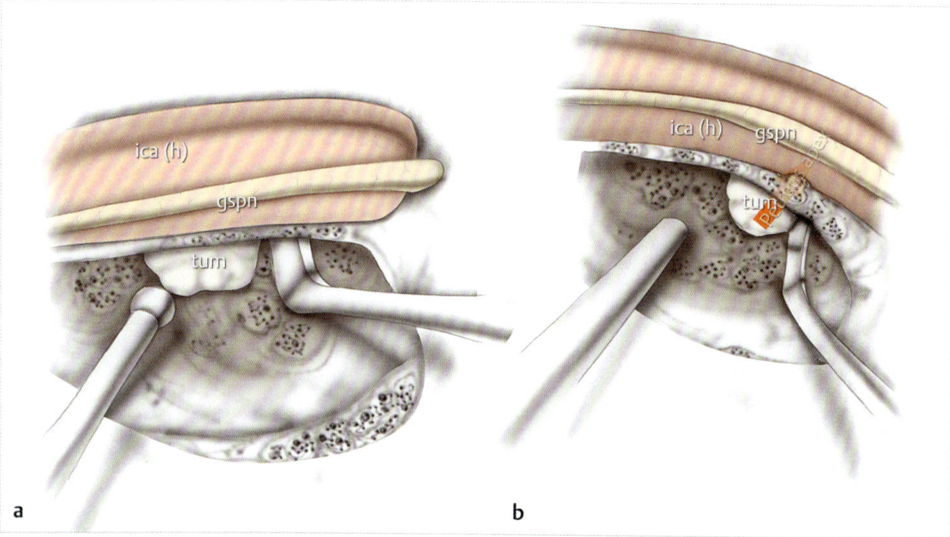

Fig. 8.82 Right side: **(a)** An angulated dissector is used to remove the tumor from the areas inferior and anterior to the horizontal portion of the internal carotid artery (ICA).
(b) The portion of the petrous apex located under the horizontal tract of the ICA is hidden, forcing the surgeon to a microscopic blind dissection. *gspn: greater superficial petrosal nerve; ica(h): horizontal segment of intrapetrous carotid artery; tum: tumor.*

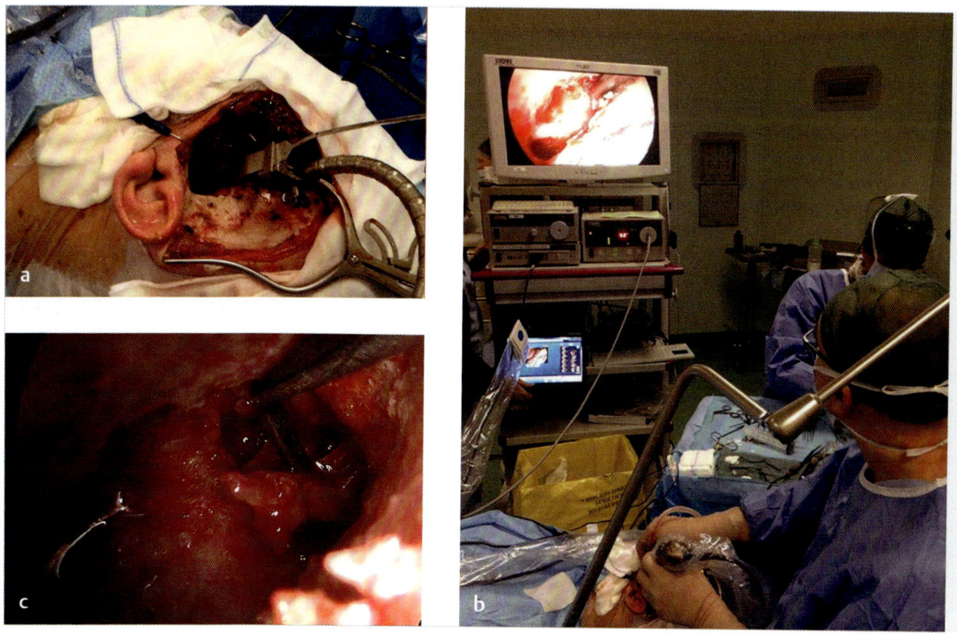

Fig. 8.84 Right side: **(a)** A retractor is placed to gently retract the temporal lobe, exposing the whole petrous apex. **(b)** The surgeon introducing the endoscope in the surgical field.
The monitor is placed in front of the surgeon.
(c) Endoscopic view of the petrous apex, beneath the internal carotid artery. A curve dissector is used to remove remnant disease.

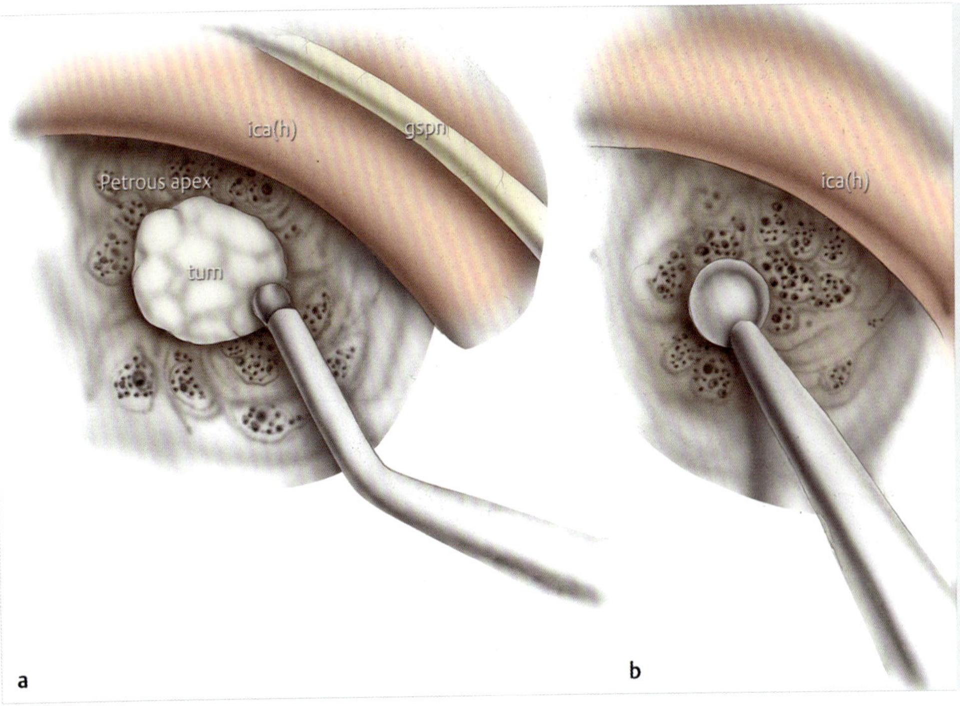

Fig. 8.85 Right side: **(a)** Endoscopic view of the petrous apex; a curved suction instrument is used to remove remnant disease. **(b)** After tumor removal, a diamond bur should be used to drill out petrous apex cells to improve the radicality of the dissection. *gspn: greater superficial petrosal nerve; ica(h): horizontal segment of intrapetrous carotid artery; tum: tumor.*

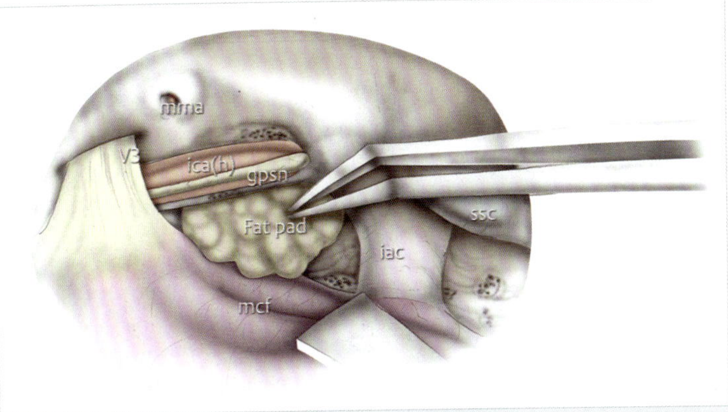

Fig. 8.86 Right side: After tumor removal, the petrous apex cavity is filled with abdominal fat. *gspn: greater superficial petrosal nerve; iac: internal auditory canal; ica(h): horizontal segment of the intrapetrous internal carotid artery; mcf: middle cranial fossa; mma: middle meningeal artery; ssc: superior semicircular canal; V3: mandibular division of trigeminal nerve.*

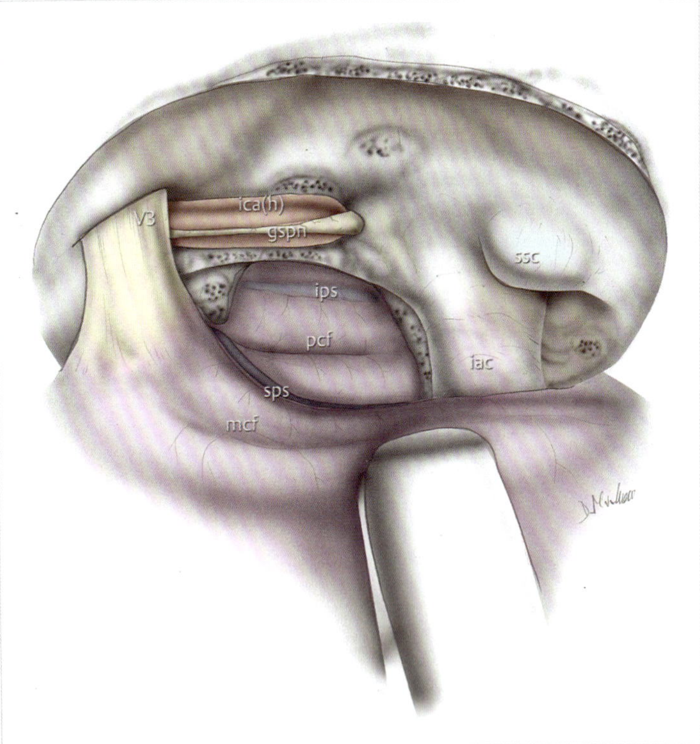

Fig. 8.87 Right side: Anterior petrosectomy for intradural lesion. The entire bone between the internal auditory canal, the horizontal portion of internal carotid artery, and V3 is removed, exposing the dura of the posterior cranial fossa. The superior and inferior petrosal sinuses are identified. *gspn: greater superficial petrosal nerve; iac: internal auditory canal; ica(h): horizontal segment of the intrapetrous internal carotid artery; ips: inferior petrosal sinus; mcf: middle cranial fossa; pcf: posterior cranial fossa; sps: superior petrosal sinus; ssc: superior semicircular canal; V3: mandibular division of trigeminal nerve.*

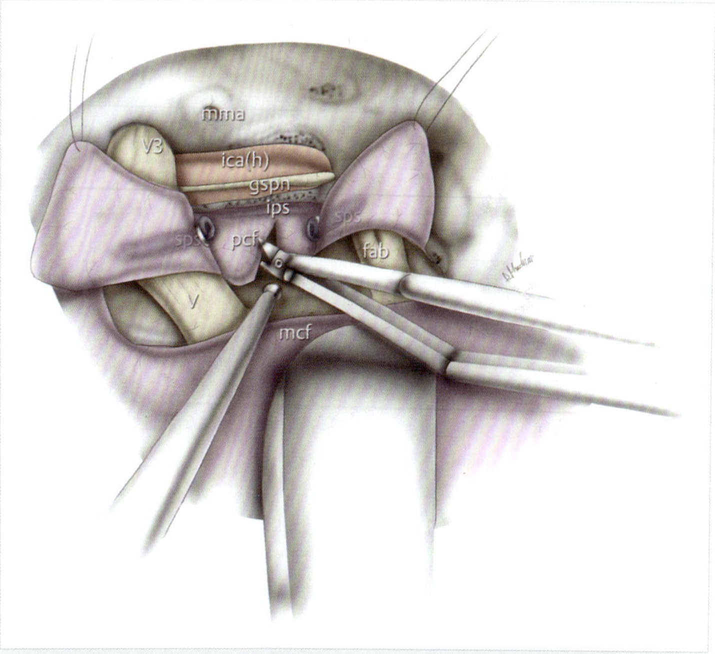

Fig. 8.88 Right side: Anterior petrosectomy for intradural lesion. The first incision of the dura of the middle cranial fossa is parallel to the long axis of the petrous apex. The superior petrosal sinus (*sps*) is clipped, and the dura of the posterior fossa is incised in a perpendicular way to the major axis of the petrous apex. *fab: acoustic-facial bundle; gspn: greater superficial petrosal nerve; ica(h): horizontal segment of the intrapetrous internal carotid artery; ips: inferior petrosal nerve; mcf: middle cranial fossa dura; mma: middle meningeal artery; pcf: posterior cranial fossa; sps: superior petrosal sinus; V: V cranial nerve (trigeminal nerve); V3: mandibular division of trigeminal nerve.*

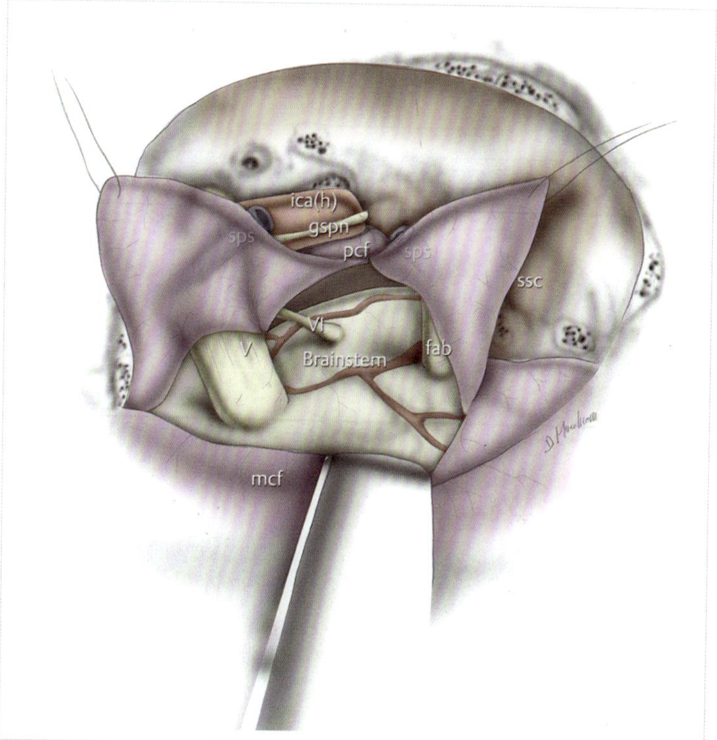

Fig. 8.89 Right side: Anterior petrosectomy for intradural lesion. The intradural anatomy exposed through this approach is showed. The trigeminal nerve (V cranial nerve) and the abducens nerve (VI cranial nerve) are easily identified; the acoustic-facial bundle is also visible. *fab: acoustic-facial bundle; gspn: greater superficial petrosal nerve; ica(h): horizontal segment of the intrapetrous internal carotid artery; mcf: middle cranial fossa; pcf: posterior cranial fossa dura; sps: superior petrosal sinus; ssc: superior semicircular canal; V: trigeminal nerve; VI: abducens nerve.*

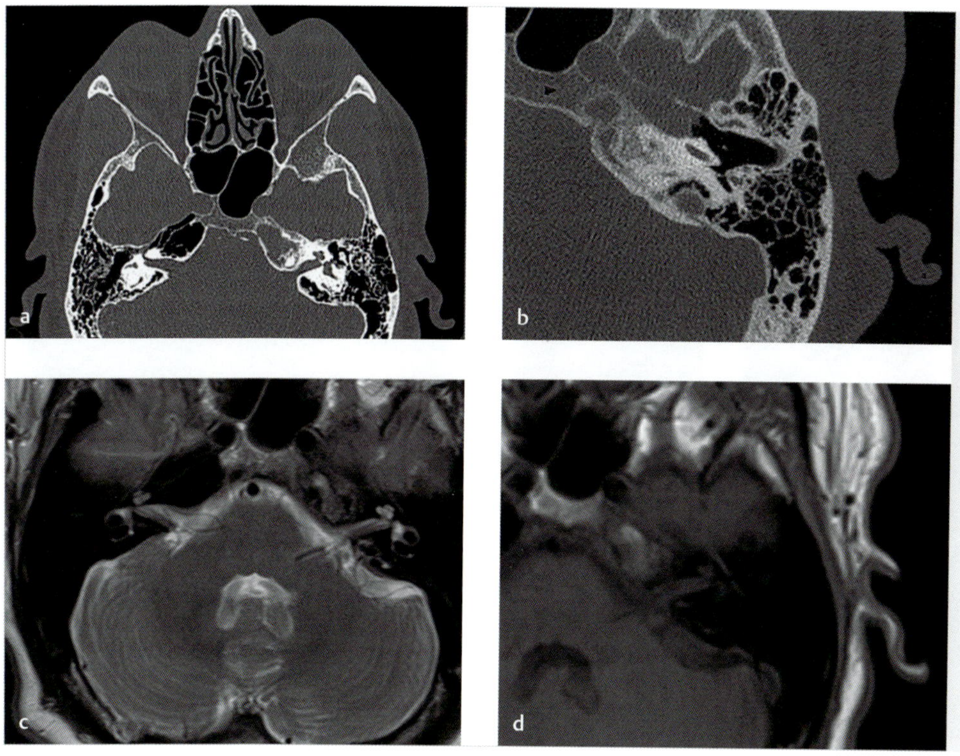

Fig. 8.90 Clinical Case 4: **(a, b)** Computed tomography (CT) scan, axial view: a coalescence of air cells, associated with bony erosion, is visible in the left petrous apex. **(c, d)** Magnetic resonance imaging (MRI), T1- and T2-weighted axial view, showing a lesion with hyperintense signal, compatible with cholesterol granuloma.

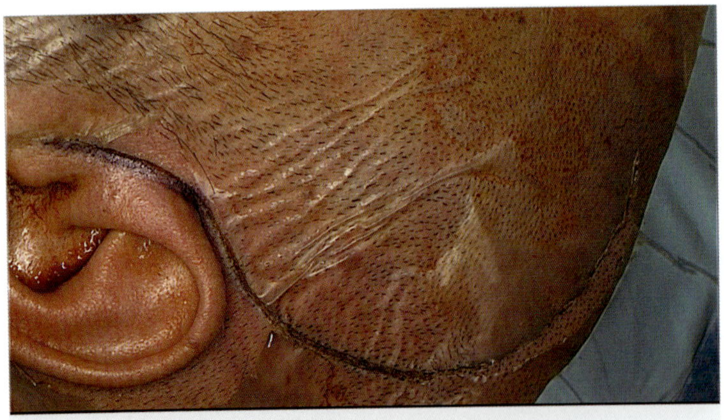

Fig. 8.91 Clinical Case 4, Left side: A preauricular C-shaped incision extended superiorly in the temporal area is performed.

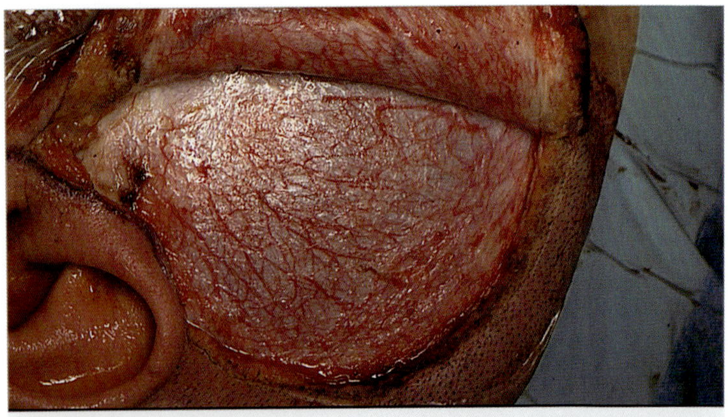

Fig. 8.92 Clinical Case 4, Left side: The skin flap is elevated and the temporalis fascia is exposed.

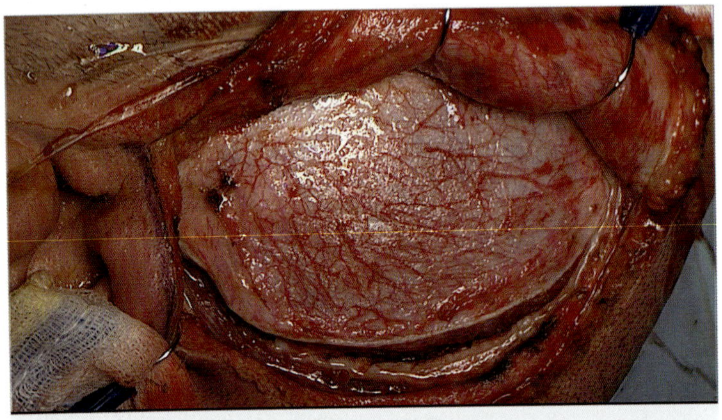

Fig. 8.93 Clinical Case 4, Left side: Incision of the temporalis muscle is performed.

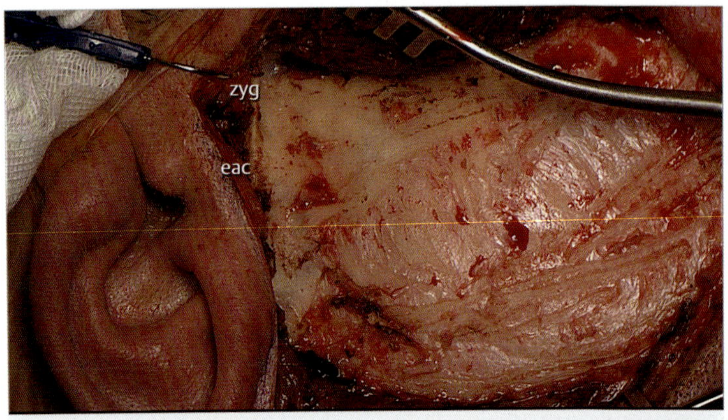

Fig. 8.94 Clinical Case 4, Left side: The squama temporalis is exposed and the zygomatic arch is identified. *eac: external auditory canal; zyg: zygomatic arch.*

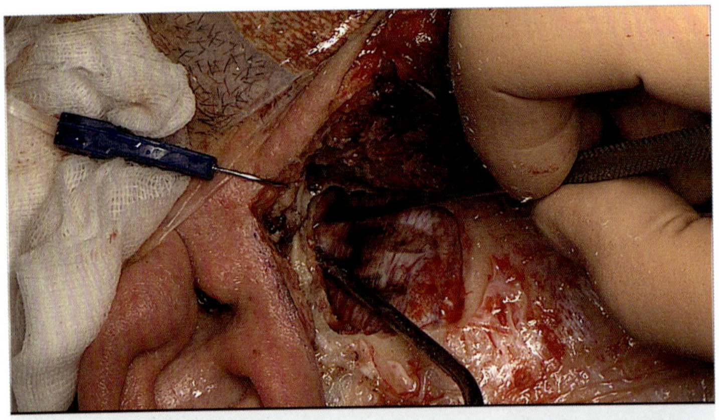

Fig. 8.95 Clinical Case 4, Left side: A craniotomy is performed. The dura of temporal lobe is exposed and gently detached from the floor of the middle cranial fossa.

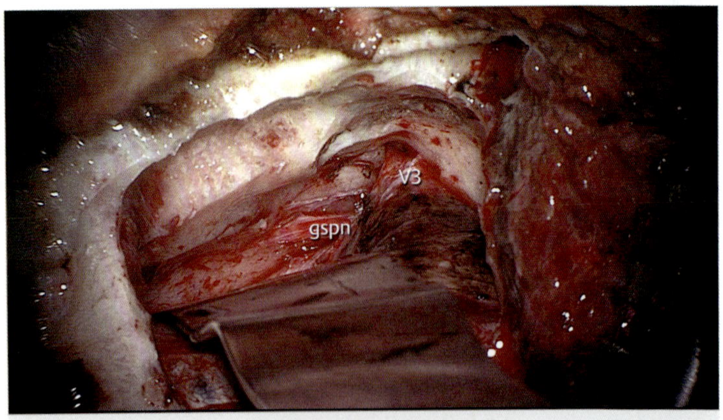

Fig. 8.96 Clinical Case 4, Left side: Once the middle meningeal artery is coagulated and cut, the greater superficial petrosal nerve and the trigeminal nerve (V3) entering the foramen ovale are identified. *gspn: greater superficial petrosal nerve; V3: mandibular division of trigeminal nerve.*

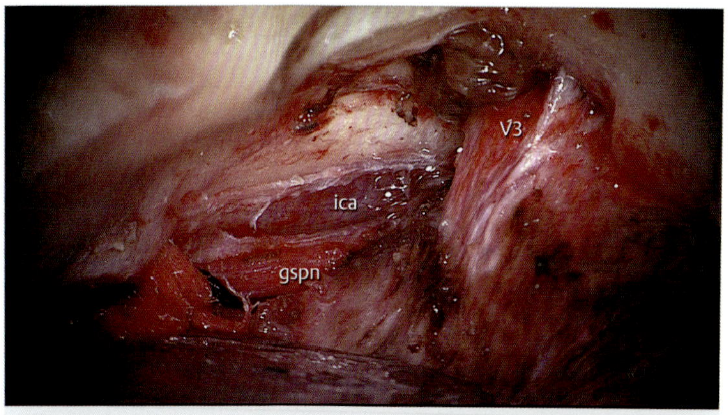

Fig. 8.97 Clinical Case 4, Left side: The horizontal portion of the intrapetrous internal carotid artery is exposed inferiorly to the greater superficial petrosal nerve. These two anatomical structures run in a parallel axes. *gspn: greater superficial petrosal nerve; ica: internal carotid artery; V3: mandibular division of trigeminal nerve.*

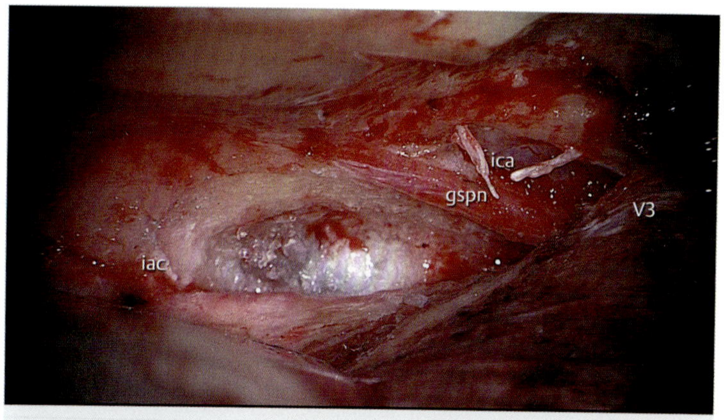

Fig. 8.98 Clinical Case 4, Left side: Once the bone of Glasscock triangle is removed using a diamond bur, the cholesterol granuloma is progressively exposed. *gspn: greater superficial petrosal nerve; iac: internal auditory canal; ica: internal carotid artery; V3: mandibular division of trigeminal nerve.*

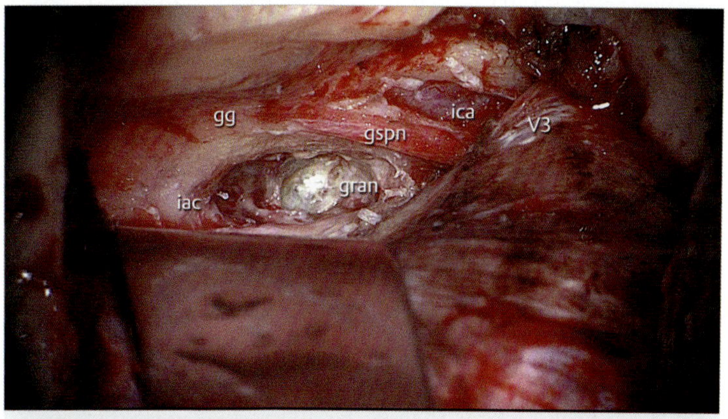

Fig. 8.99 Clinical Case 4, Left side: The lesion is progressively isolated and removed microscopically. *gg: geniculate ganglion; gran: cholesterol granuloma; gspn: greater superficial petrosal nerve; iac: internal auditory canal; ica: internal carotid artery; V3: mandibular division of trigeminal nerve.*

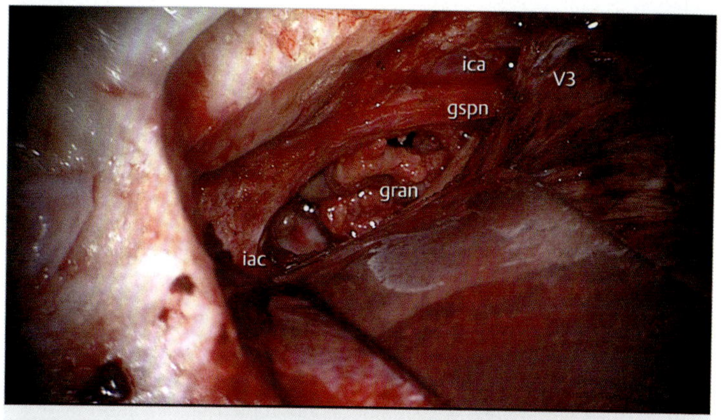

Fig. 8.100 Clinical Case 4, Left side: Using an angulated instrument, the cholesterol granuloma is detached from the bone walls of the petrous apex. *gran: cholesterol granuloma; gspn: greater superficial petrosal nerve; iac: internal auditory canal; ica: internal carotid artery; V3: mandibular division of trigeminal nerve.*

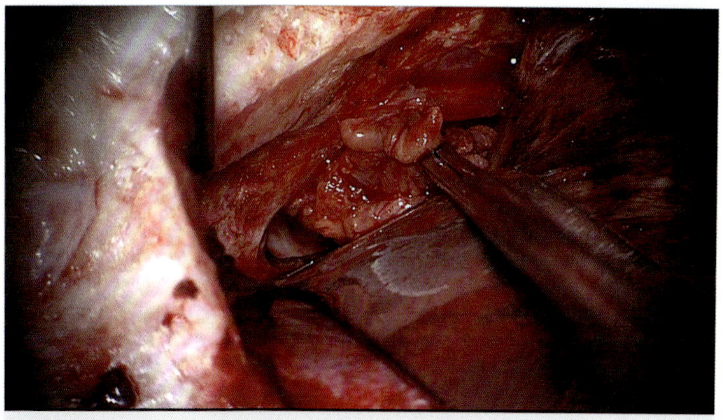

Fig. 8.101 Clinical Case 4, Left side: The lesion is removed from the petrous apex.

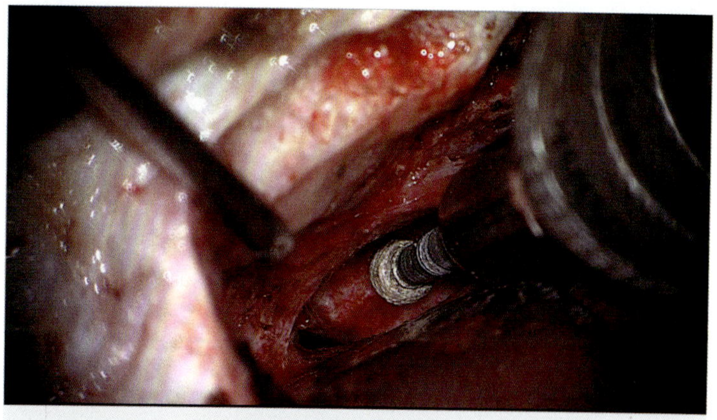

Fig. 8.102 Clinical Case 4, Left side: A diamond bur is used to remove the bone of the petrous apex, visible under microscopic view.

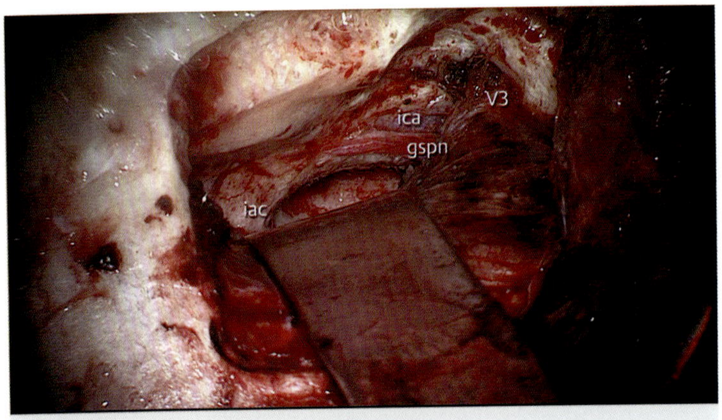

Fig. 8.103 Clinical Case 4, Left side: Final surgical cavity after microscopic procedure. *gspn: greater superficial petrosal nerve; iac: internal auditory canal; ica: internal carotid artery; V3: mandibular division of trigeminal nerve.*

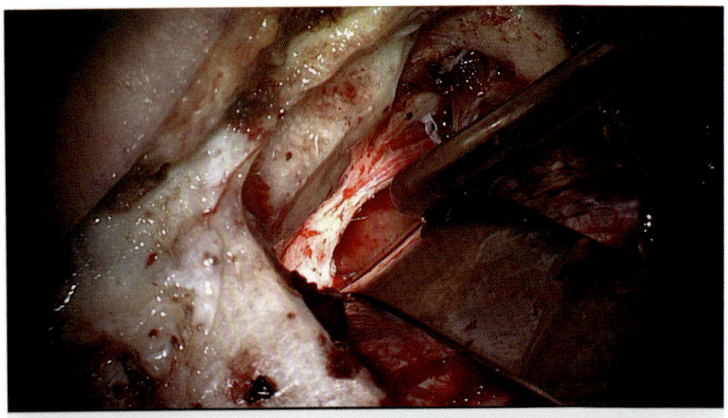

Fig. 8.104 Clinical Case 4, Left side: A 0-degree endoscope is introduced into the final surgical cavity to explore the petrous apex beneath the internal carotid artery, checking for remnant disease.

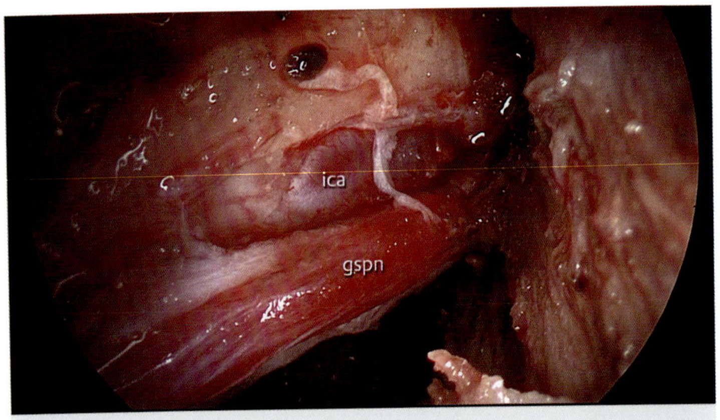

Fig. 8.105 Clinical Case 4, Left side: Endoscopic magnification of the horizontal segment of intrapetrous internal carotid artery and the greater superficial petrosal nerve. *gspn: greater superficial petrosal nerve; ica: internal carotid artery.*

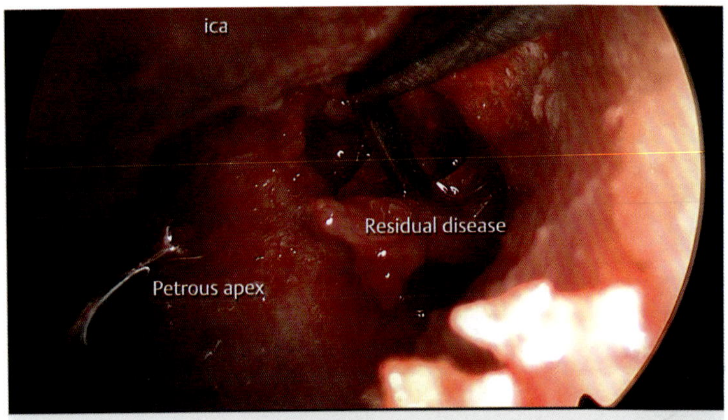

Fig. 8.106 Clinical Case 4, Left side: A remnant lesion is endoscopically detected into the petrous apex under the internal auditory canal. An angulate dissector is used to remove the lesion. *ica: internal carotid artery.*

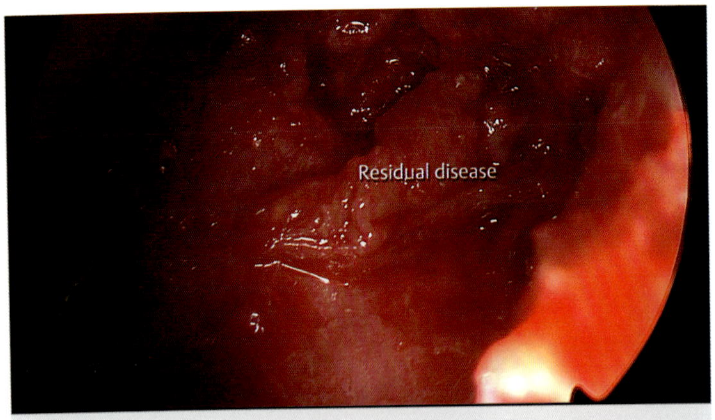

Fig. 8.107 Clinical Case 4, Left side: Endoscopic magnification of a remnant cholesterol granuloma.

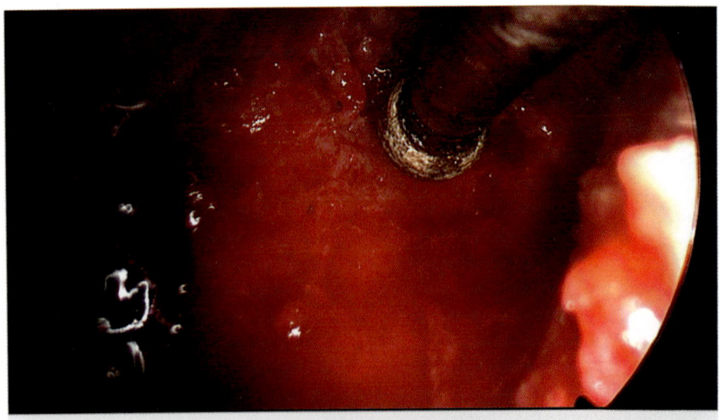

Fig. 8.108 Clinical Case 4, Left side: The surgical cavity is drilled using a diamond bur under endoscopic view for radicalization.

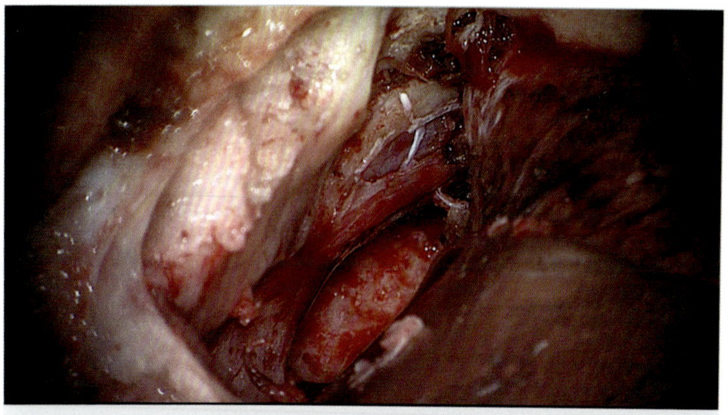

Fig. 8.109 Clinical Case 4, Left side: Final cavity after lesion removal.

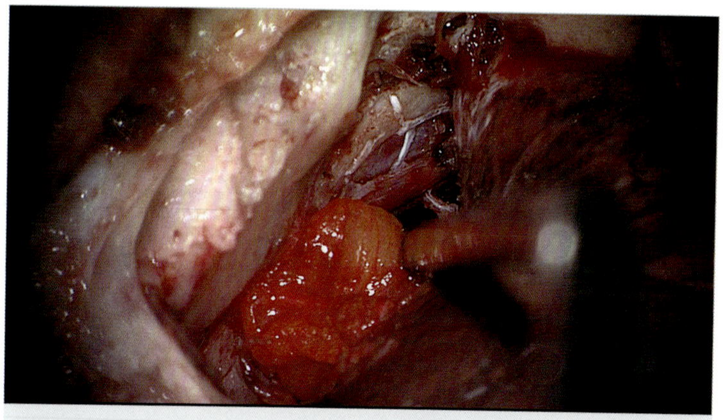

Fig. 8.110 Clinical Case 4, Left side: Abdominal fat is used to fill the petrous apex cavity.

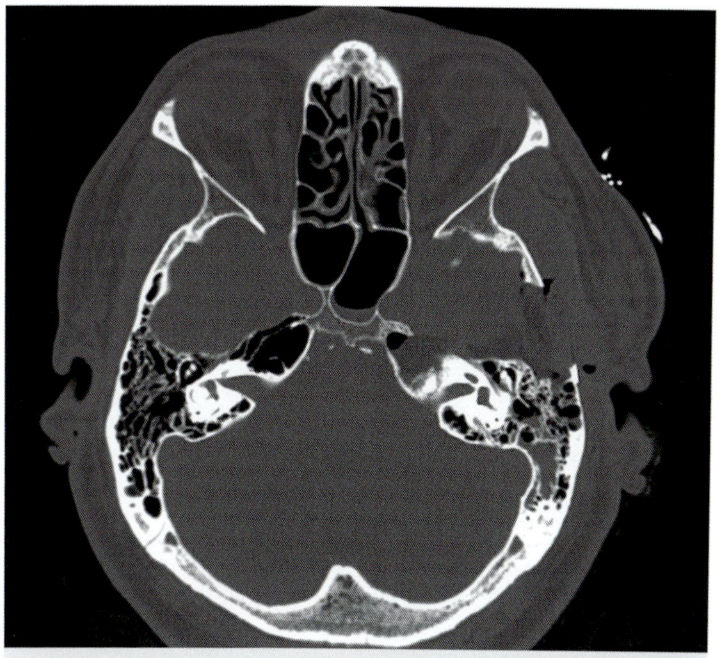

Fig. 8.111 Clinical Case 4, Left side: Computed tomography (CT) scan, axial view, immediately after surgery.

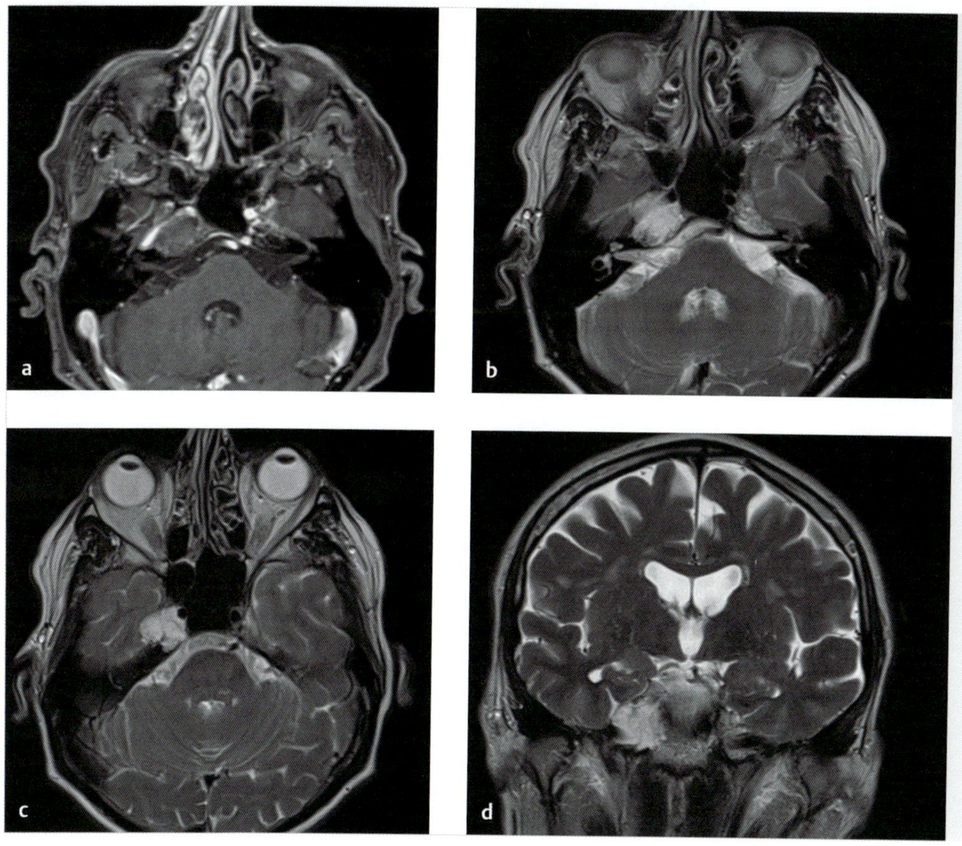

Fig. 8.112 Clinical Case 5: Magnetic resonance imaging (MRI), axial view **(a–c)** and coronal view **(d)**, that shows a chondrosarcoma growing along the right petrous apex, following the horizontal potion of the intrapetrous internal carotid artery with involvement of the cavernous sinus and the clivus.

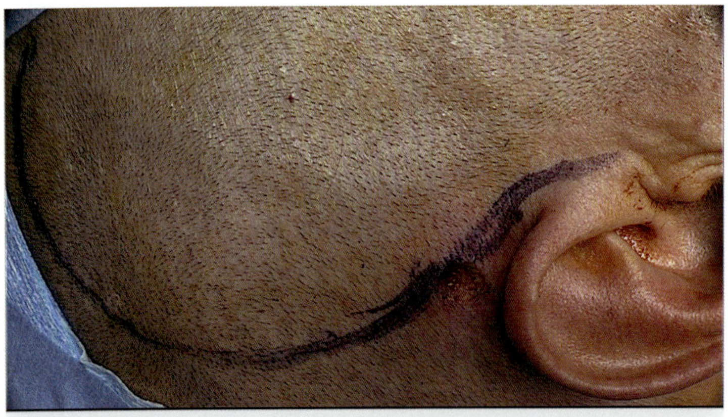

Fig. 8.113 Clinical Case 5, Right side: A C-shaped incision, extending inferiorly along the preauricular sulcus, is performed.

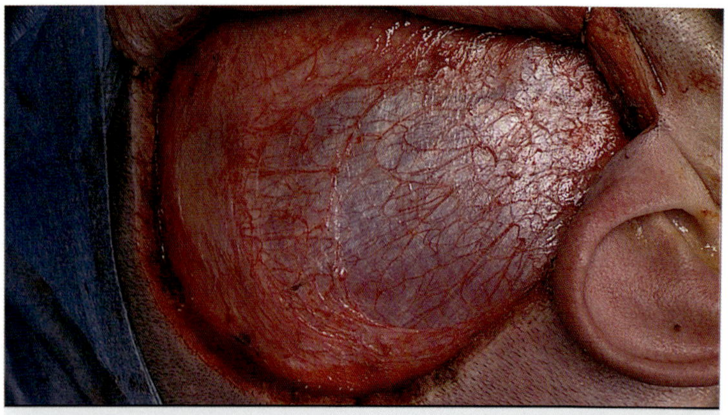

Fig. 8.114 Clinical Case 5, Right side: The skin flap is elevated and the temporalis fascia plane is identified.

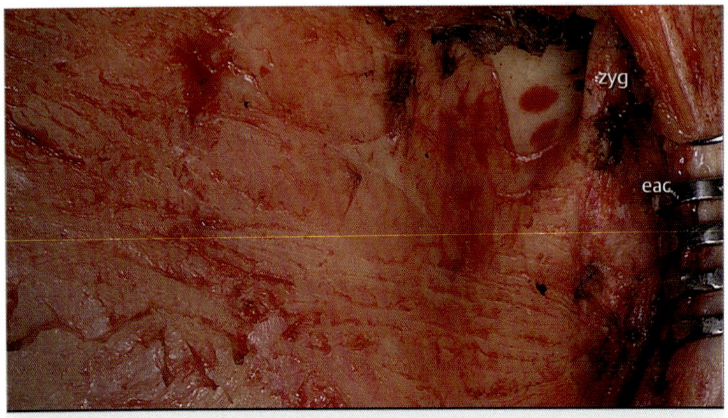

Fig. 8.115 Clinical Case 5, Right side: Squama temporalis and zygomatic arch are exposed. *eac: external auditory canal; zyg: zygomatic arch.*

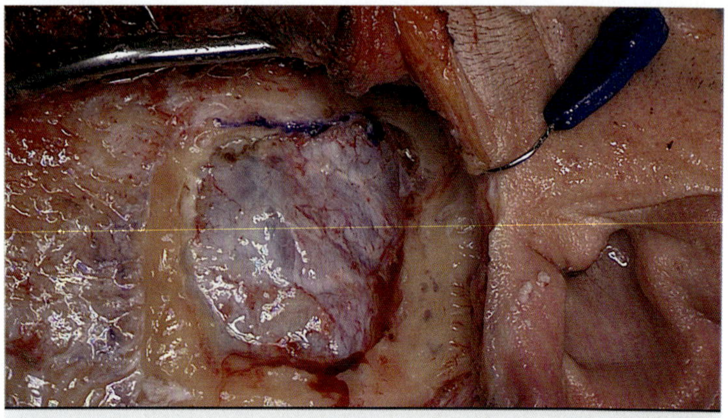

Fig. 8.116 Clinical Case 5, Right side: A craniotomy is performed. The dura of the middle cranial fossa is exposed.

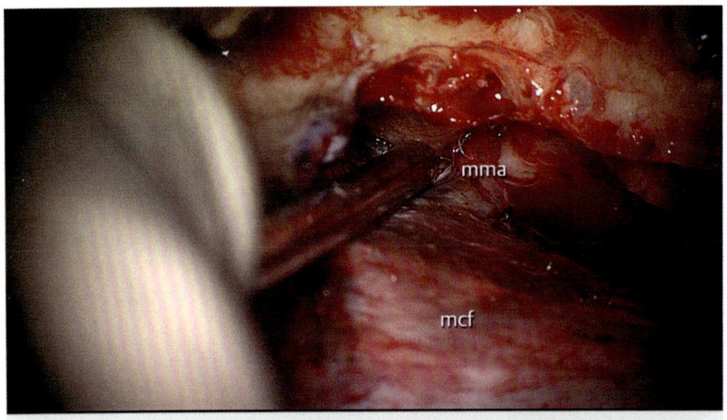

Fig. 8.117 Clinical Case 5, Right side: The temporal lobe is gently elevated and the middle meningeal artery entering the foramen spinosum is identified. *mcf: middle cranial fossa dura; mma: middle meningeal artery.*

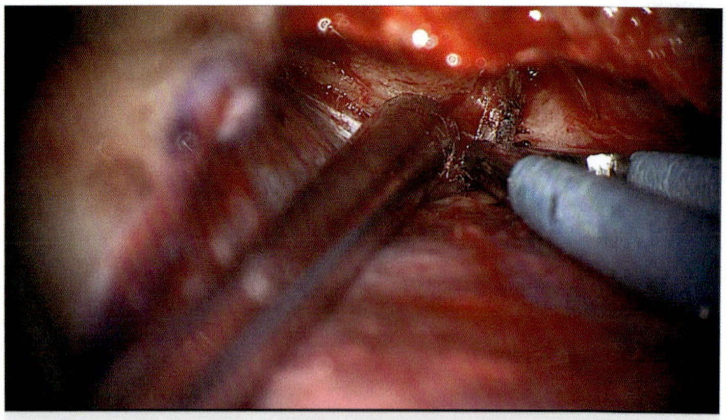

Fig. 8.118 Clinical Case 5, Right side: The middle meningeal artery is coagulated.

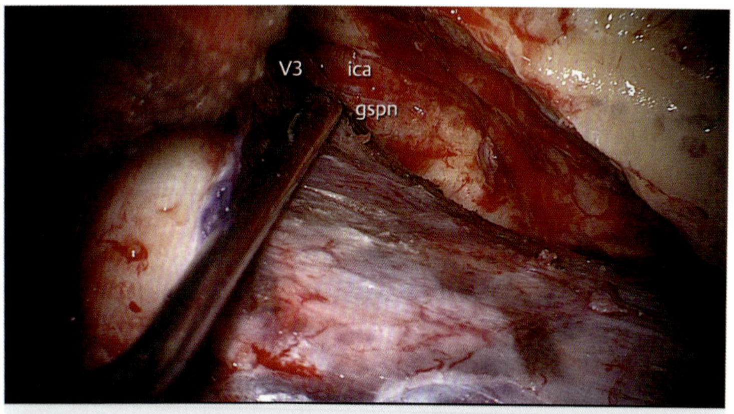

Fig. 8.119 Clinical Case 5, Right side: The trigeminal nerve (V3) entering the foramen ovale, the greater superficial nerve, and the horizontal intrapetrous internal carotid artery are identified. *gspn: greater superficial petrosal nerve; ica: horizontal intrapetrous internal carotid artery; V3: mandibular division of trigeminal nerve.*

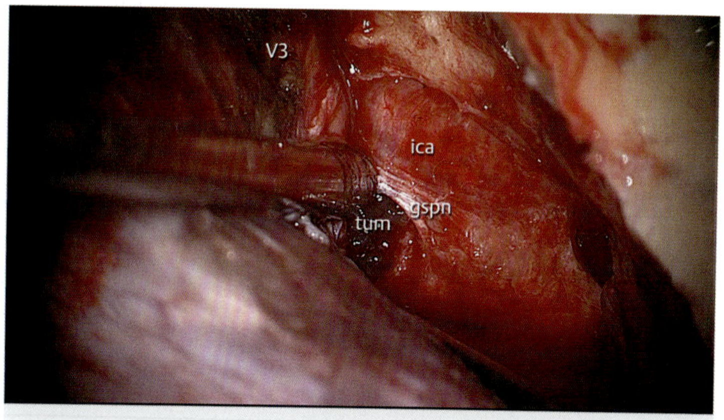

Fig. 8.120 Clinical Case 5, Right side: Once the bone of Glasscock triangle is removed using a diamond bur, the chondrosarcoma is progressively exposed. *gspn: greater superficial petrosal nerve; ica: horizontal intrapetrous internal carotid artery; tum: tumor; V3: mandibular division of trigeminal nerve.*

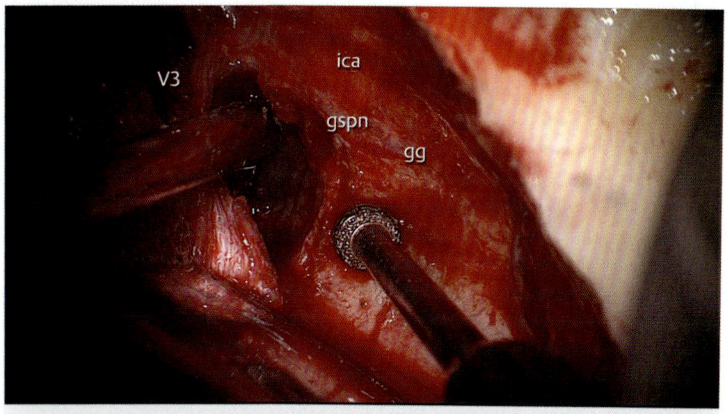

Fig. 8.121 Clinical Case 5, Right side: The drilling is progressively performed from an anterior to a posterior direction, using the greater superficial petrosal nerve as landmark to find the geniculate ganglion and the internal auditory canal. *gg: geniculate ganglion; gspn: greater superficial petrosal nerve; ica: horizontal intrapetrous internal carotid artery; V3: mandibular division of trigeminal nerve.*

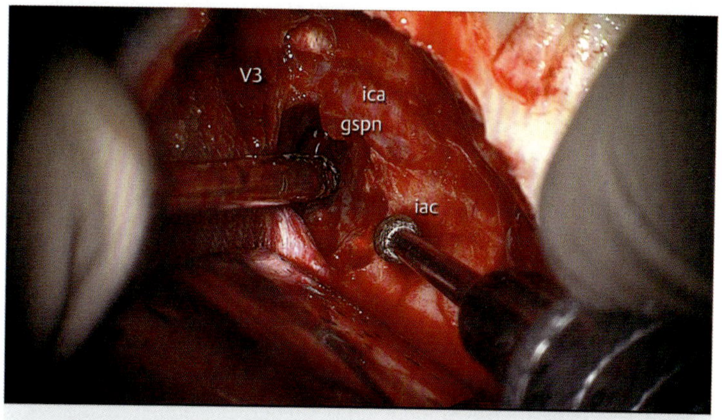

Fig. 8.122 Clinical Case 5, Right side: The bone around the internal auditory canal (IAC) is gently drilled to identify the anterior border of the IAC, that represent the posterior limit of the dissection. The tumor is thus exposed in the petrous apex. *gspn: greater superficial petrosal nerve; iac: internal auditory canal; ica: internal carotid artery; V3: mandibular division of trigeminal nerve.*

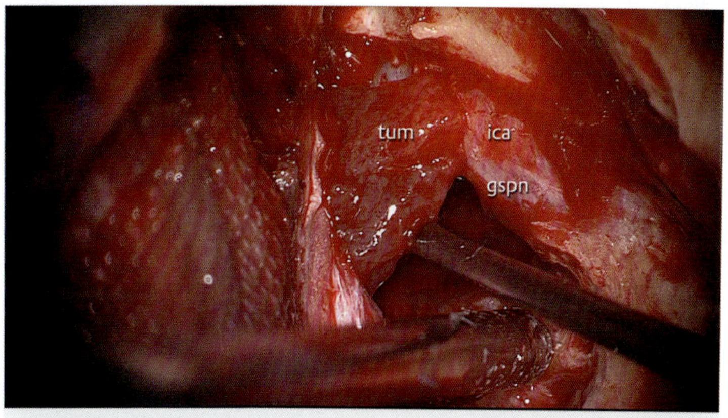

Fig. 8.123 Clinical Case 5, Right side: The tumor is microscopically removed. *gspn: greater superficial petrosal nerve; ica: internal carotid artery; tum: tumor.*

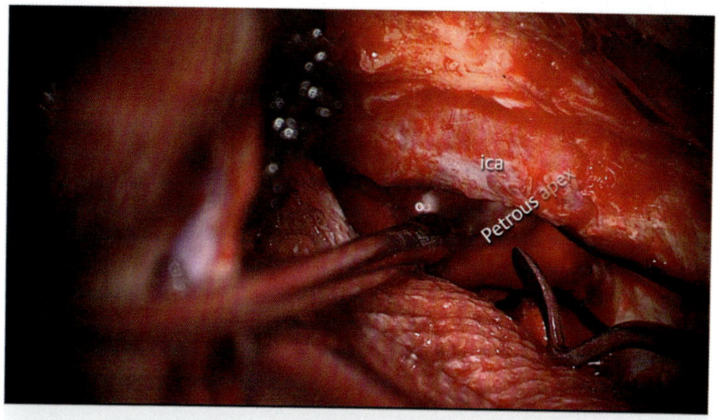

Fig. 8.124 Clinical Case 5, Right side: Microscopic view of the horizontal segment of the intrapetrous internal carotid artery, after tumor removal. *ica: horizontal segment of the internal carotid artery.*

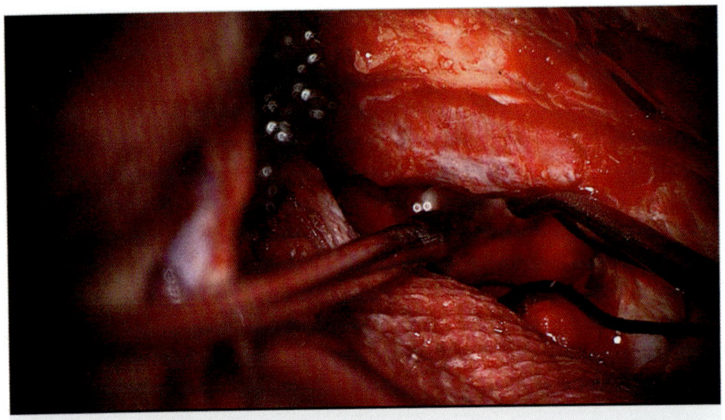

Fig. 8.125 Clinical Case 5, Right side: A long angled dissector shows the depth of the petrous apex cells located under the horizontal portion of the internal carotid artery. These air cells are not visible under microscopic view.

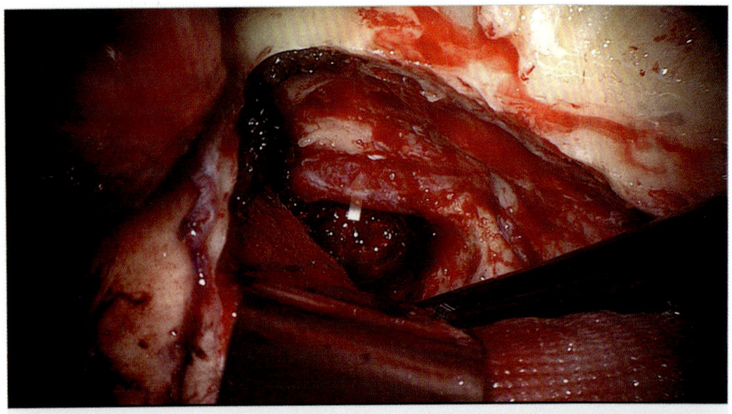

Fig. 8.126 Clinical Case 5, Right side: The *white arrow* shows the hidden anatomical area lying under the horizontal internal carotid artery.

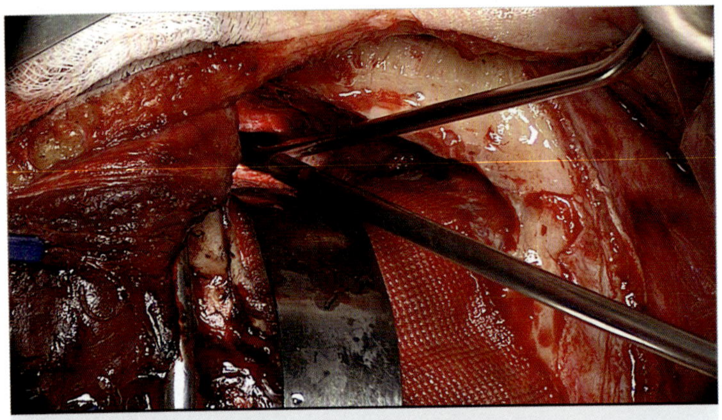

Fig. 8.127 Clinical Case 5, Right side: A 0-degree endoscope is inserted into the surgical cavity to expose the petrous apex cells under the internal carotid artery, checking for remnant tumor.

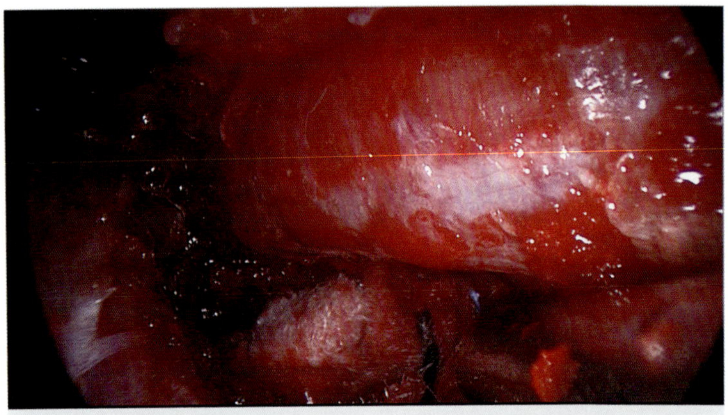

Fig. 8.128 Clinical Case 5, Right side: Endoscopic magnification of horizontal segment of the intrapetrous internal carotid artery.

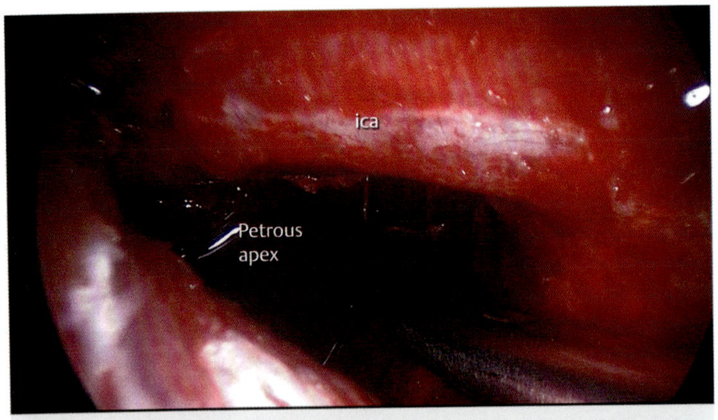

Fig. 8.129 Clinical Case 5, Right side: A curved suction instrument is held with the dominant hand under endoscopic view. *ica: horizontal segment of the internal carotid artery.*

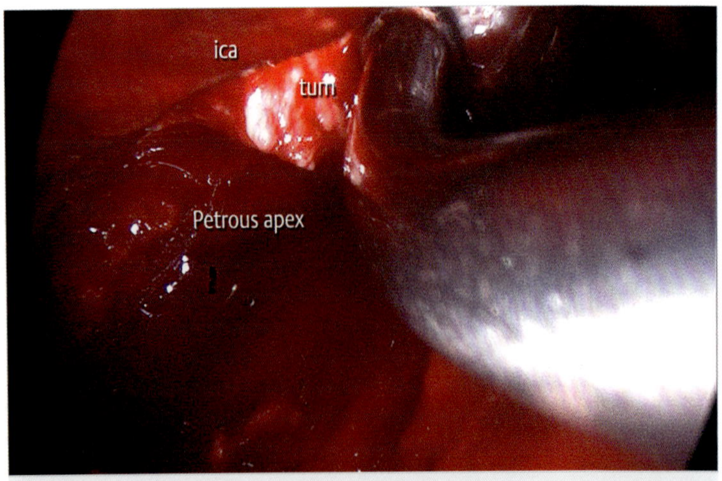

Fig. 8.130 Clinical Case 5, Right side: The petrous apex below the internal carotid artery (ICA) is endoscopically exposed. A curved suction instrument is used to remove remnant tumor beneath the ICA. *ica: horizontal intrapetrous internal carotid artery; tum: tumor.*

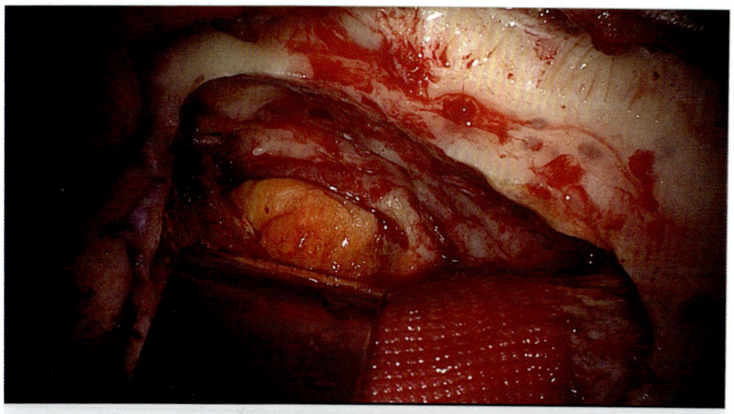

Fig. 8.131 Clinical Case 5, Right Side: A fat pad is used to close the cavity of petrous apex after tumor removal.

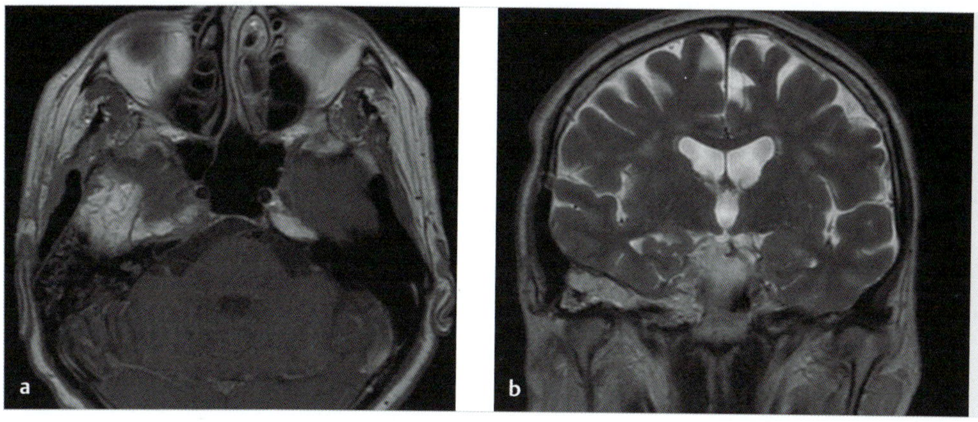

Fig. 8.132 Clinical Case 5. Postoperative magnetic resonance imaging (MRI) showing complete removal of the tumor; the abdominal fat is used to fill petrous apex and clivus defect.

Suggested Readings

Bento RF, Pirana S, Sweet R, Castillo A, Brito Neto RV. The role of the middle fossa approach in the management of traumatic facial paralysis. Ear Nose Throat J. 2004; 83(12):817–823

Bochenek Z, Kukwa A. An extended approach through the middle cranial fossa to the internal auditory meatus and the cerebello-pontine angle. Acta Otolaryngol. 1975; 80(5–6):410–414

Day JD, Fukushima T, Giannotta SL. Microanatomical study of the extradural middle fossa approach to the petroclival and posterior cavernous sinus region: description of the rhomboid construct. Neurosurgery. 1994; 34(6):1009–1016, discussion 1016

Dutt SN, Mirza S, Irving RM. Middle cranial fossa approach for the repair of spontaneous cerebrospinal fluid otorrhoea using autologous bone pate. Clin Otolaryngol Allied Sci. 2001; 26(2):117–123

Fisch U, Mattox D. Microsurgery of the Skull Base. New York: Thieme; 1988

Fournier HD, Mercier P, Roche PH. Surgical anatomy of the petrous apex and petroclival region. Adv Tech Stand Neurosurg. 2007; 32:91–146

Fournier HD, Mercier P, Velut S, Reigner B, Cronier P, Pillet J. Surgical anatomy and dissection of the petrous and peripetrous area: anatomic basis of the lateral approaches to the skull base. Surg Radiol Anat. 1994; 16(2):143–148

Gantz BJ, Parnes LS, Harker LA, McCabe BF. Middle cranial fossa acoustic neuroma excision: results and complications. Ann Otol Rhinol Laryngol. 1986; 95(5 Pt 1):454–459

Garcia-Ibanez E, Garcia-Ibanez JL. Middle fossa vestibular neurectomy: a report of 373 cases. Otolaryngol Head Neck Surg. 1980; 88(4):486–490

Gjurić M, Wigand ME, Wolf SR. Enlarged middle fossa vestibular schwannoma surgery: experience with 735 cases. Otol Neurotol. 2001; 22(2):223–230, discussion 230–231

Gonzales FL, Ferreira MAT, Zabramski JM, et al. The middle fossa approach. BNI Q. 2000; 16:1–7

Hoang S, Ortiz Torres MJ, Rivera AL, Litofsky NS. Middle cranial fossa approach to repair tegmen defects with autologous or alloplastic graft. World Neurosurg. 2018; 118:e10–e17

House WF, Shelton C. Middle fossa approach for acoustic tumor removal. Otolaryngol Clin North Am. 1992; 25(2):347–359

House WF. Middle cranial fossa approach to the petrous pyramid: report of 50 cases. Arch Otolaryngol. 1963; 78(4):460–469

House WF. Surgical exposure of the internal auditory canal and its contents through the middle, cranial fossa. Laryngoscope. 1961; 71:1363–1385

Kanzaki J, Kawase T, Sano K, Shiobara R, Toya S. A modified extended middle cranial fossa approach for acoustic tumors. Arch Otorhinolaryngol. 1977; 217(1):119–121

Kawase T, Shiobara R. Extended middle cranial fossa approaches to the clivus and acoustic meatus. In: Torrens M, Al-Mefty O, Kobayashi S, eds. Operative Skull Base Surgery. New York: Churchill Livingstone; 1997:263–278

Kojima H, Tanaka Y, Yaguchi Y, Miyazaki H, Murakami S, Moriyama H. Endoscope-assisted surgery via the middle cranial fossa approach for a petrous cholesteatoma. Auris Nasus Larynx. 2008; 35(4):469–474

Kosty JA, Stevens SM, Gozal YM, et al. Middle fossa approach for resection of vestibular schwannomas: a decade of experience. Oper Neurosurg (Hagerstown). 2019; 16(2):147–158

Mangham CA, Jr. Retrosigmoid versus middle fossa surgery for small vestibular schwannomas. Laryngoscope. 2004; 114(8):1455–1461

Master AN, Roberts DS, Wilkinson EP, Slattery WH, Lekovic GP. Endoscope-assisted middle fossa craniotomy for resection of inferior vestibular nerve schwannoma extending lateral to transverse crest. Neurosurg Focus. 2018; 44(3):E7

Monfared A, Mudry A, Jackler R. The history of middle cranial fossa approach to the cerebellopontine angle. Otol Neurotol. 2010; 31(4):691–696

Parisier SC. The middle cranial fossa approach to the internal auditory canal—an anatomical study stressing critical distances between surgical landmarks. Laryngoscope. 1977; 87(4 Pt 2) Suppl 4:1–20

Rhoton AL, Jr. The temporal bone and transtemporal approaches. Neurosurgery. 2000; 47(3) Suppl:S211–S265

Rigante L, Herlan S, Tatagiba MS, Stanojevic M, Hirt B, Ebner FH. Petrosectomy and topographical anatomy in traditional Kawase and posterior intradural petrous apicectomy (PIPA) approach: an anatomical study. World Neurosurg. 2016; 86:93–102

Tanriover N, Sanus GZ, Ulu MO, et al. Middle fossa approach: microsurgical anatomy and surgical technique from the neurosurgical perspective. Surg Neurol. 2009; 71(5):586–596, discussion 596

Weber PC, Gantz BJ. Results and complications from acoustic neuroma excision via middle cranial fossa approach. Am J Otol. 1996; 17(4):669–675

Chapter 9

Classification and Indications of Transcanal Lateral Skull Base Surgery

9

9 Classification and Indications of Transcanal Lateral Skull Base Surgery

Daniele Marchioni, Brandon Isaacson, Alessia Rubini, Antonio Gulino, and Livio Presutti

Abstract

Nowadays the endoscope is mostly used in the treatment of middle ear pathology such as cholesteatoma. All over the world endoscopic ear surgery is evolving and has been spreading. Based on experiences of endoscopic approaches to the middle ear and the spatial relationship between the external auditory canal (EAC) and the internal auditory canal (IAC), the authors have gradually considered the medial wall of the tympanic cavity as a surgical window to reach the structures that lie beyond the middle ear such as the lateral skull base and inner ear. Therefore, the concept of a minimally invasive approach to the inner ear and the lateral skull base using the natural corridor of the EAC has been developed, in the same fashion as the nasal surgical corridor is used to manage the anterior skull base and sellar lesions. Based on our experience these approaches are characterized by lower intra- and perioperative morbidity, decreased postoperative complications, reduction of hospitalization, and no need of intensive care unit (ICU) support compared to traditional techniques. Transcanal lateral skull base approaches are classified according to their anatomical relation to the otic capsule: the transcanal transpromontorial passing through the otic capsule, the transcanal suprageniculate passing above the otic capsule, and the transcanal infracochlear passing under the otic capsule.

Keywords: transcanal endoscopic approach, vestibular schwannoma, cerebellopontine angle, internal auditory canal, petrous apex, transpromontorial, infracochlear, suprageniculate

9.1 Introduction

The skull base, including both anterior and lateral region, is an anatomical boundary between the fields of neurosurgery and otolaryngology. Even now, surgical management of lesions located in these areas represents a challenge for both disciplines because of the complexity of the anatomy.

The endoscope is a valuable and well-established instrument in management of anterior skull base (ASB) diseases through nasal natural corridors. Traditional craniofacial open approach was the gold standard technique for resection of sinonasal tumors with ASB extension over the past decades, since the first surgery described by Ketcham et al in 1963. From the last 1990s, thanks to surgeons' improvement in endoscopic management of sinonasal pathologies, endoscopic approaches have been progressively extended to malignancies involving ASB, showing similar rates of gross total resection and perioperative mortality than classical craniofacial approaches. At once, development of high-definition technology has provided a clear visualization of anatomical details, thus allowing a better comprehension of surgical landmarks and targets of this complex area. Ventral midline approach through natural corridors also avoids complications related to brain retraction and neurovascular manipulation typically required during traditional neurosurgical procedures. Furthermore, the introduction of pedicled intranasal flaps, thanks to description of the Hadad-Bassagasteguy flap in 2006, resulted in a considerable reduction of postoperative cerebrospinal fluid (CSF) leak rate associated with endoscopic endonasal approach. Therefore, transnasal endoscopic approach is actually considered as a minimally invasive and safe technique to treat a variety of intra-dural and extra-dural lesions of midline cranial base (see ▶ Fig. 9.1).

As for the ASB, many approaches have been described to reach diseases located in the lateral skull base, including the fundus of the internal auditory canal (IAC), the cerebellopontine angle (CPA), and the petrous apex. Despite the benign nature and limited dimensions of the lesions involving these anatomical regions, extensive approaches are often required to reach the disease. These "open" approaches are based on the use of a microscope; they require a wide external incision, a variable degree of bone removal, and often a significant amount of brain retraction and neurovascular manipulation. Three main routes can be identified: the transpetrous (including translabyrinthine, transcochlear, and transotic) are lateral surgical corridors, the retrosigmoid is posterior surgical corridor, and the middle cranial fossa route is superior. Of these, transpetrous-translabyrinthine, retrosigmoid, and middle fossa approaches are the most widely used to reach the IAC, especially in treatment of the acoustic neuroma. The choice about the approach to perform depends on factors related to the surgeon's preferences and habits, dimensions, location and extent of the pathology, goal of hearing preservation, risk of damage to facial nerve, and postoperative complications.

The first endoscopic application for IAC surgery was introduced in combination with the retrosigmoid approach: after the removal of the CPA portion of the neoplasm, the intracanalicular extension was managed under endoscopic view, in order to avoid wide drilling of the posterior portion of the petrous bone. At once, the use of endoscope was progressively introduced for the treatment of middle ear diseases in the 1990s. Endoscopy was used primarily to better recognize the hidden areas such as the posterior epitympanum during classic microscopic tympanoplasties. Gradually it has become widely used in middle ear surgery replacing the microscope as the primary surgical tool. Actually, endoscopic approach is mostly used for the treatment of middle ear cholesteatoma, but as the technique has evolved, advantages for its use in lateral skull base surgery have been realized as well.

Based on experience of endoscopic approaches to the middle ear and the spatial relationship between the external auditory canal (EAC) and the IAC, the present authors have gradually come to the opinion that the medial wall of the tympanic cavity could represent a surgical corridor to reach the structures "beyond" the middle ear, lateral skull base, and inner ear (vestibule, fundus of the IAC, suprageniculate area, petrous apex).

Therefore, the concept of a direct route with a minimally invasive approach to the inner ear and the lateral skull base using the natural corridor of the EAC has been developed, in the same fashion as the nasal surgical corridor is used to manage the ASB and sellar lesions.

Due to the orientation of the EAC with respect to the IAC it is possible to access the lateral skull base through a direct route and

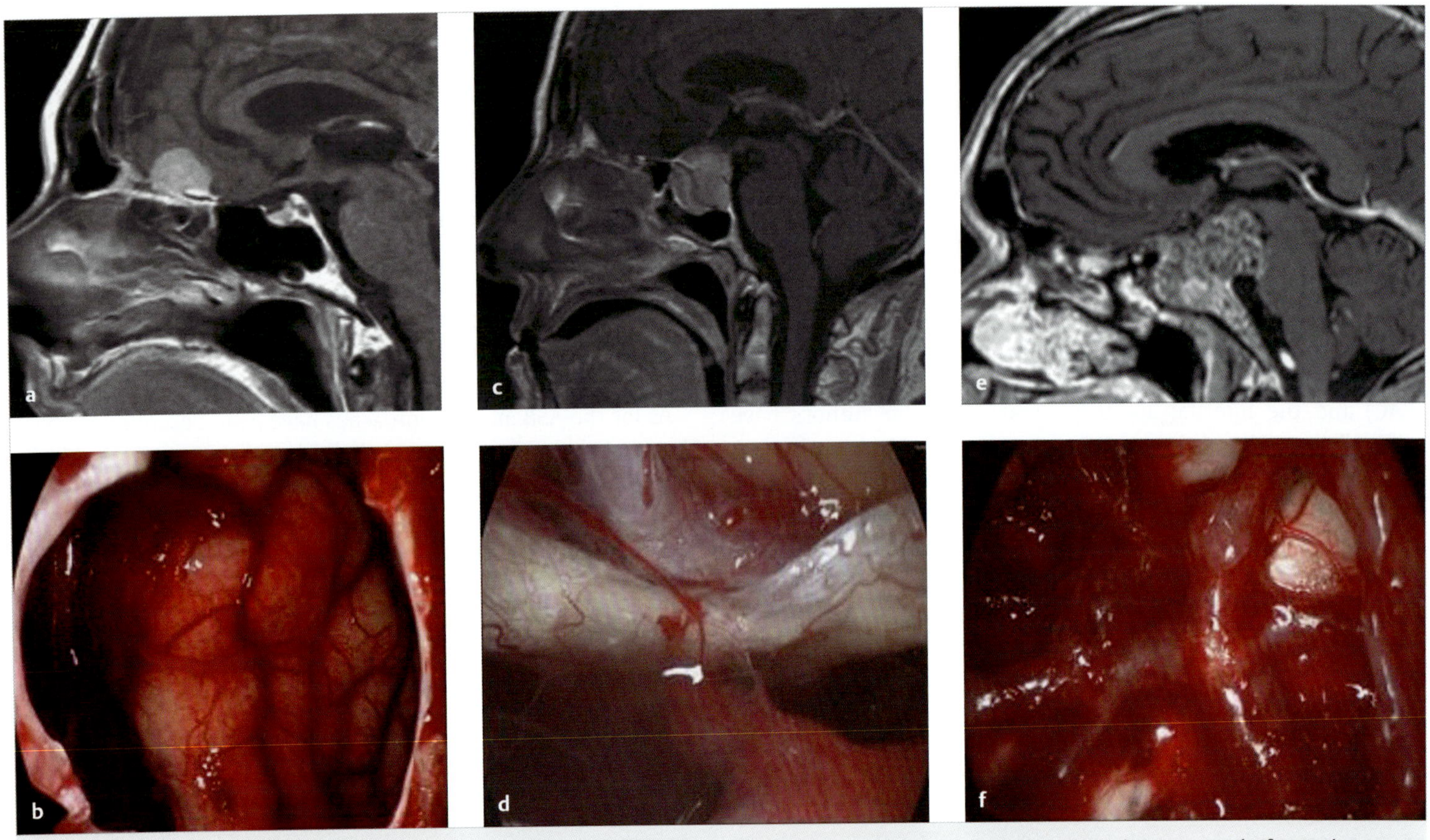

Fig. 9.1 Transnasal endoscopic approaches for three different pathologies. **(a)** Magnetic resonance imaging (MRI) showing a cribriform plate meningioma. **(b)** Dural opening exposing frontal lobes after removal of the meningioma through a transcribriform approach. **(c)** MRI showing a sellar adenoma. **(d)**. Optic chiasm completely exposed and preserved after transnasal trans-sphenoidal trans-sellar approach. **(e)** Upper clival chordoma, with posterior extension to the brainstem. **(f)** The basilar and superior cerebellar arteries (SCA) exposed after tumor removal.

minimally invasive approaches using the natural orifice of the EAC. Endoscope allows a very good visualization of anatomical areas in the petrous bone, petrous apex, and IAC and diseases could be removed from these areas without brain or meningeal manipulations and with short and safe patients' postoperative courses.

Although the group of transcanal approaches to lateral skull base were recently introduced in the clinical practice, and only the first experiences are published in literature, these approaches seem to be characterized by a lower morbidity compared with traditional surgery, because they work in the middle and posterior cranial fossa, avoiding temporal lobe and cerebellum traction. The purpose of these approaches compared to traditional approaches is to obtain a decreased postoperative morbidity by reducing the days of hospitalization, and avoiding the ICU.

Several dissections have been performed to better understand the anatomy, to define the landmarks of the middle and inner ear, and to set up appropriate instruments for this approach. An appropriate procedure was recorded and therefore ready to be clinically applied.

The endoscopic dissection allowed to codify the group of transcanal approaches.

9.2 The Group of Transcanal Approaches

Transcanal lateral skull base approaches can be classified according to the surgical route related to the otic capsule, distinguishing approaches passing through the otic capsule, and approaches with a conservative attitude with respect to the otic capsule:

- Transcanal approaches passing through the otic capsule
  - Transcanal transpromontorial approach
- Transcanal approaches conserving the otic capsule
  - Transcanal suprageniculate approach (passing above the otic capsule)
  - Transcanal infracochlear approach (passing inferiorly to the otic capsule)

9.3 Transcanal Suprageniculate Corridor

In this approach the EAC is used as a natural corridor to reach the suprageniculate fossa. This anatomical region is located between the geniculate ganglion and the second portion of the facial nerve inferiorly, the middle cranial fossa (MCF) lying superiorly, and the labyrinthine bloc posteriorly (see ▶ Fig. 9.2 and ▶ Fig. 9.3). Working above the cochlea and labyrinth, sensorineural hearing function was preserved, although the incus and head of the malleus removal is mandatory in order to have an access to this anatomical area. An ossiculoplasty was required after disease removal; for this reason a variable postoperative conductive hearing loss is expected.

9.3.1 Indications

The correct indication for this approach requires disease with limited extension into an anatomical triangle composed of the

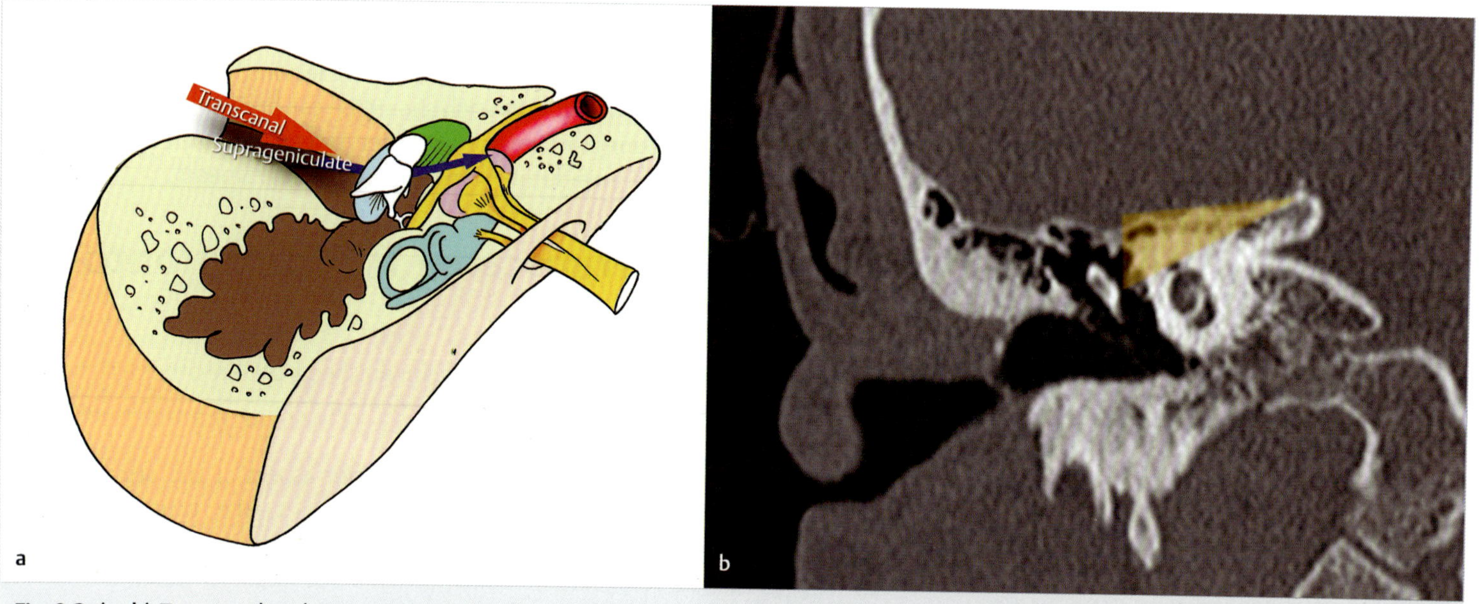

Fig. 9.2 (a, b) Transcanal endoscopic suprageniculate approach. In yellow the suprageniculate fossa, reached with this approach.

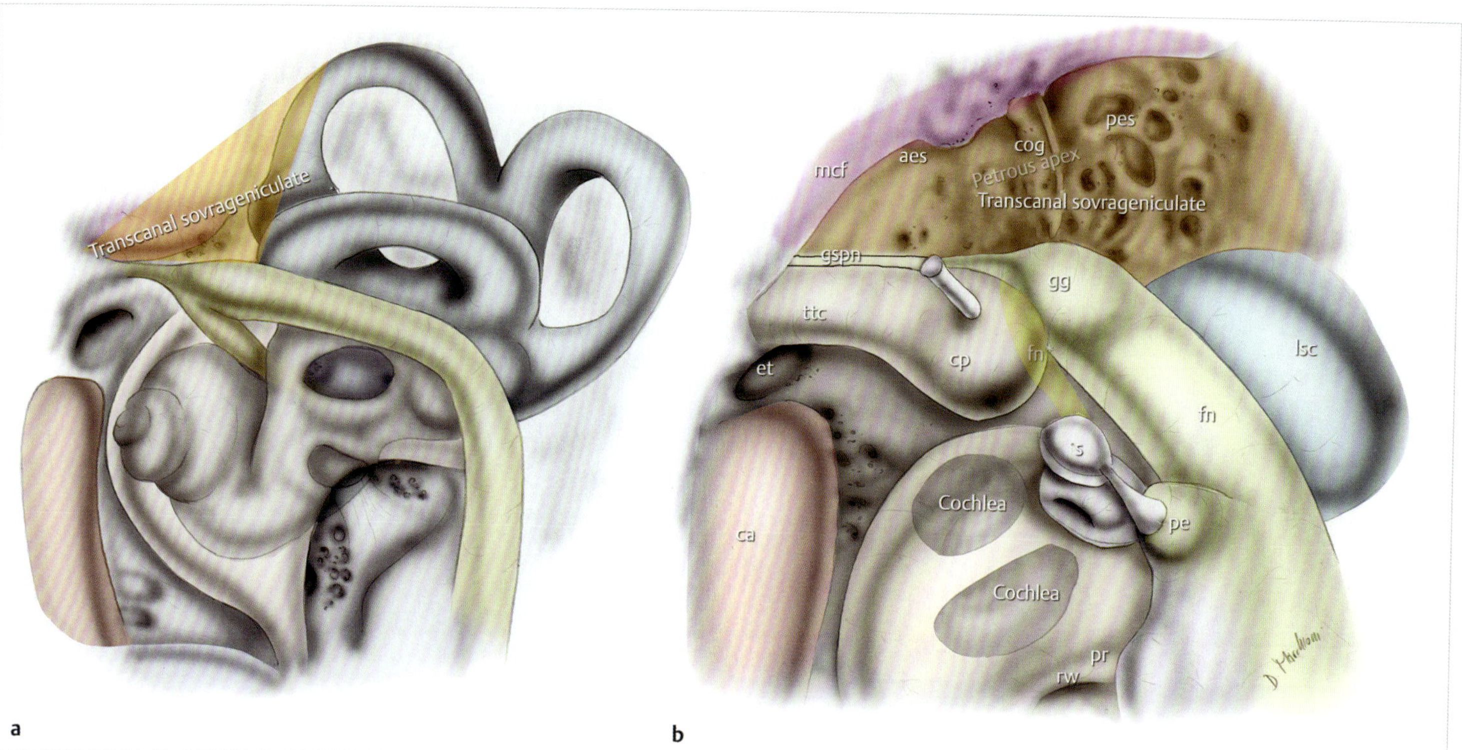

Fig. 9.3 (a, b) Left side: Limits of the suprageniculate area. It is located between the geniculate ganglion and the second portion of the facial nerve inferiorly, the middle cranial fossa (MCF) lying superiorly, and the labyrinthine bloc posteriorly. *aes: anterior epitympanic space; ca: carotid artery; cp: cochleariform process; et: eustachian tube; fn: facial nerve; fn*: labyrinthine segment of the facial nerve; gg: geniculate ganglion; gspn: greater superficial petrosal nerve; lsc: lateral semicircular canal; mcf: middle cranial fossa; pe: pyramidal eminence; pes: posterior epitympanic space; pr: promontory; rw: round window; s: stapes; ttc: tensor tympani canal.*

MCF, facial nerve, and labyrinthine bloc as shown in ► Fig. 9.2 and ► Fig. 9.3. This area can be reached endoscopically by a transcanal route avoiding an MCF approach.

- Facial nerve tumor such as schwannoma or hemangioma with limited extension into the suprageniculate area, without meningeal infiltration in patient with stable facial palsy grades IV–VI HB scale
- Supralabyrinthine petrous bone cholesteatoma limited to the suprageniculate area, in between the cochlea and the middle cranial fossa (see ► Fig. 9.4 and ► Fig. 9.5)
- Facial nerve decompression in patient with facial palsy due a fracture of temporal bone and a spicula compressing the geniculate ganglion

9.3.2 Advantages

- Sensorineural hearing function is preserved.
- They are minimal invasive surgery, avoiding meningeal and brain manipulation.

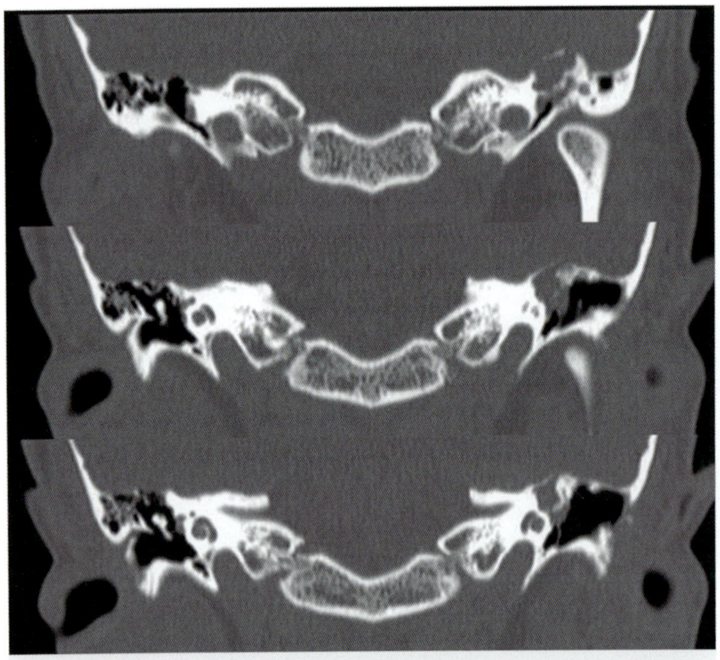

Fig. 9.4 Computed tomography (CT) scan of cholesteatoma located to the suprageniculate fossa. Note the extension between the cochlea inferiorly and the middle cranial fossa (MCF) superiorly, with ossicular chain erosion.

9.3.3 Limitations

- They are not suitable for extensive lesions.
- A microscopic approach should be considered when dural resection is mandatory in order to repair the defect (such as in case of intradural extension, dural involvement).

9.4 Transcanal Transpromontorial Corridor

This approach should be distinguished from the other transtemporal approaches such as transcochlear approaches, where the whole sacrifice of the otic capsule is planned, and the translabyrinthine approach, where only the posterior aspect of the otic capsule is sacrificed (labyrinthine block). In fact, the transpromontorial approach is a labyrinthine sparing approach, passing anteriorly with respect to the third portion of the facial nerve, and preserving the labyrinthine block, removing only the anterior portion of the otic capsule (see ▶ Fig. 9.6, ▶ Fig. 9.7, ▶ Fig. 9.8).

We can distinguish two kinds of transpromontorial approaches:

- Exclusive endoscopic transcanal transpromontorial approach
- Expanded transcanal transpromontorial approach

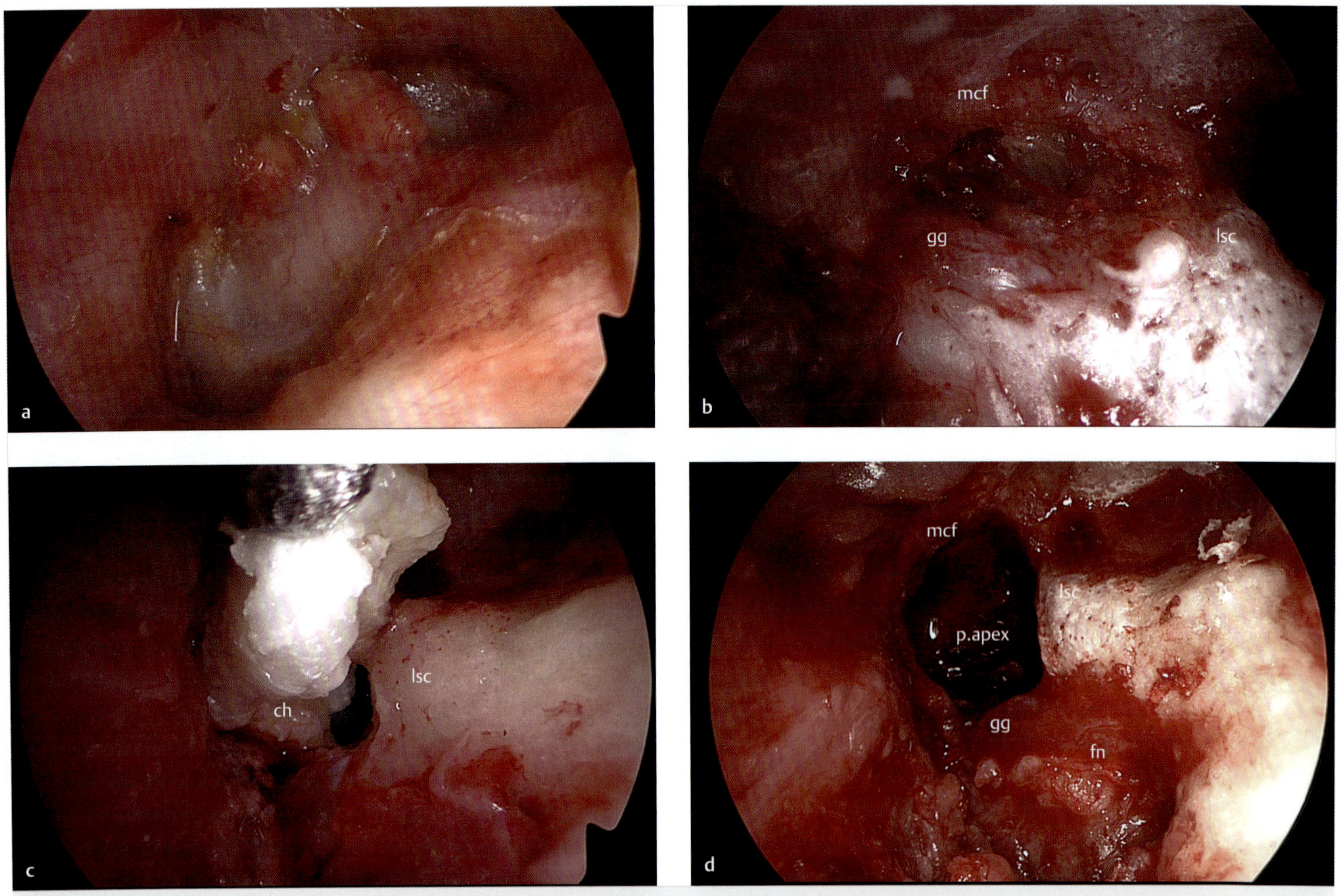

Fig. 9.5 Endoscopic view of suprageniculate cholesteatoma (left ear). (a) Attical erosion with cholesteatoma inside. (b) Suprageniculate area exposed. (c) Cholesteatoma removal. (d) Endoscopic anatomy of suprageniculate fossa and its relationship with petrous apex, endoscopic view. *ch: cholesteatoma; fn: facial nerve; gg: geniculate ganglion; mcf: middle cranial fossa; lsc: lateral semicircular canal; p. apex: petrous apex.*

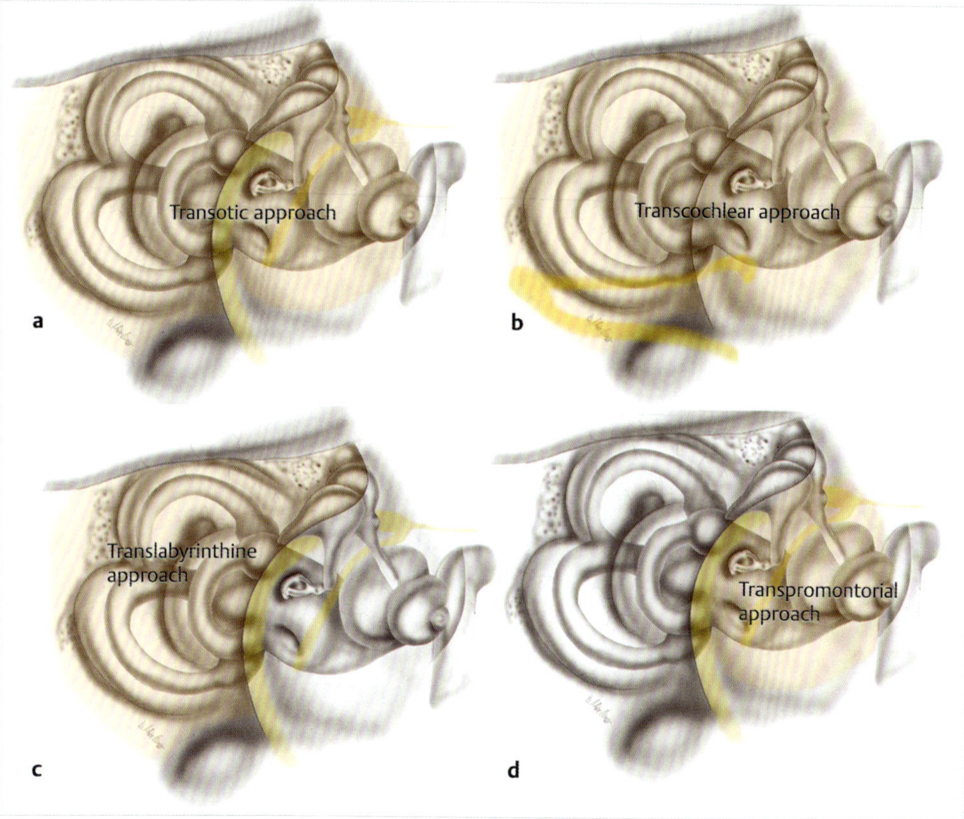

Fig. 9.6 Right side: Schematic drawing of lateral skull base approaches, according to the surgical route related to the otic capsule. The transotic **(a)** and transcochlear **(b)** approaches pass through the whole otic capsule. The translabirynthine **(c)** approach passes through the posterior portion of the otic capsule. The transcanal transpromontorial **(d)** approach passes through the anterior portion of the otic capsule. Yellow area: facial nerve position related to the surgical approach. Brown area: bone demolition related to the surgical approach.

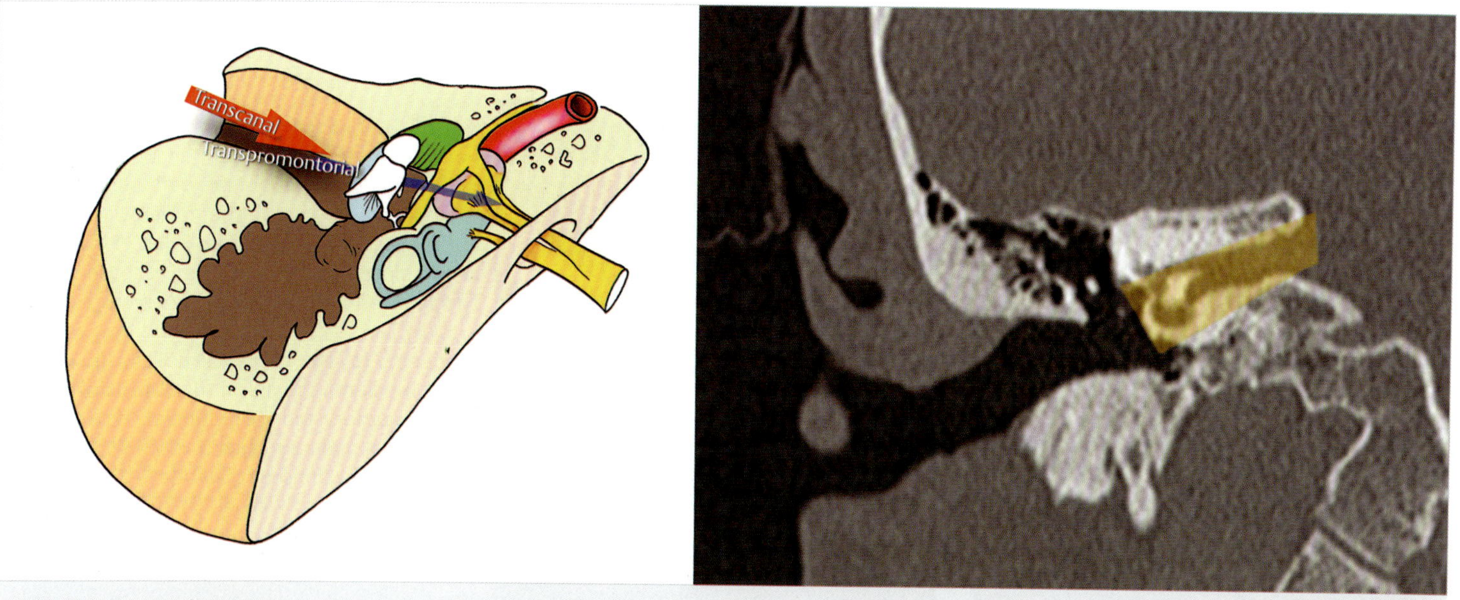

Fig. 9.7 Transcanal endoscopic transpromontorial approach. In yellow the surgical corridor from the external auditory canal to the internal auditory canal, passing through the promontory.

9.4.1 Exclusive Endoscopic Transcanal Transpromontorial Approach

In this approach the EAC is used as a natural corridor to reach the cochlea, vestibule, and fundus of the IAC by passing through the promontory. With this surgical approach, hearing loss is expected, since the promontorial and cochlear removal is necessary to reach the IAC. A cochlear implant should be considered in limited cases when a partial cochlear preservation and cochlear nerve sparing surgery is suitable.

A blind sac closure of the EAC is required at the end of the procedure.

Indications

- Symptom-producing or growing intralabyrinthine schwannomas (cochlea, vestibule), with or without extension to the fundus of the IAC, in patient with no servable hearing function.
- Symptom-producing or growing acoustic neuromas located in the fundus of the IAC, with or without minimal extension to the CPA, in patient with no servable hearing function (see ▶ Fig. 9.9, ▶ Fig. 9.10, ▶ Fig. 9.11).
- Mesotympanic cholesteatomas, with medial extension to the inner ear into the cochlea and vestibule.

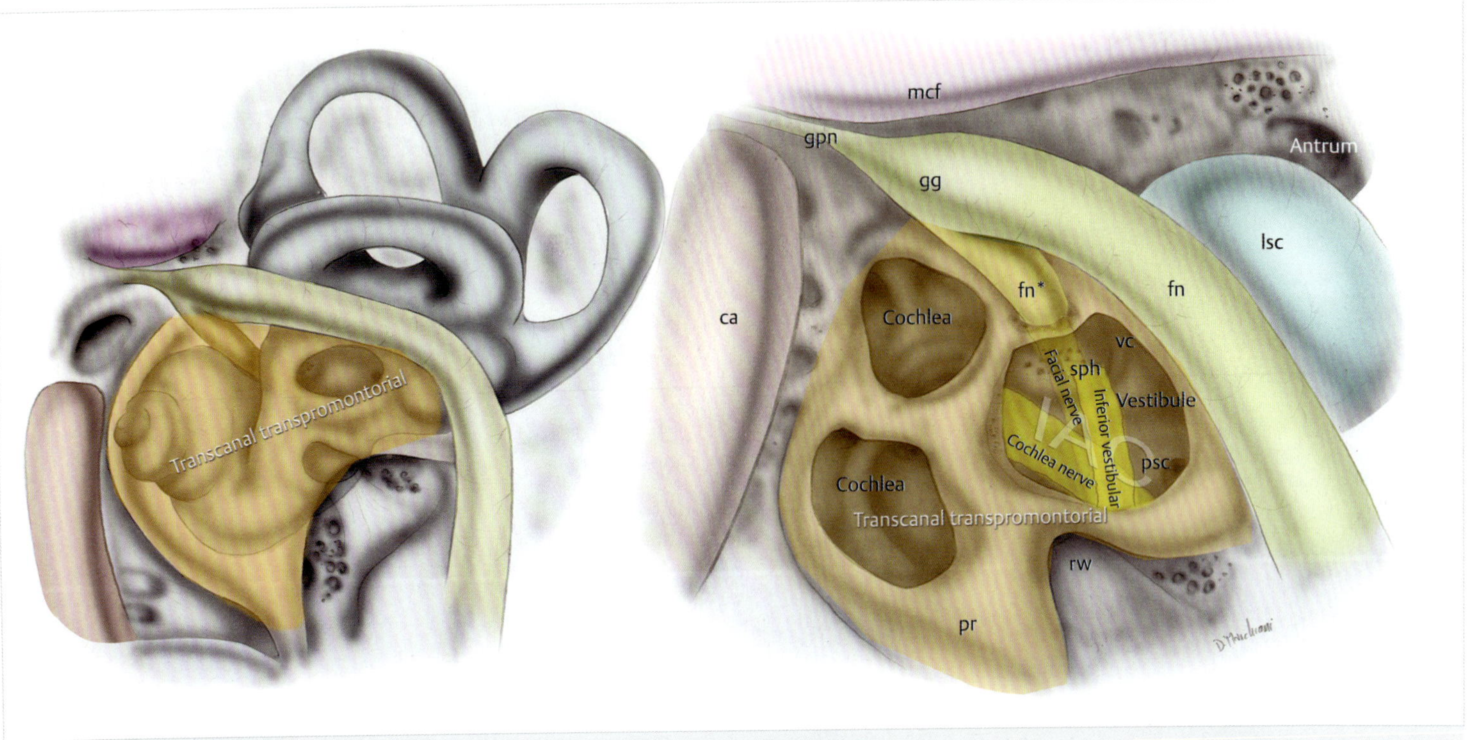

Fig. 9.8 Left side: The transcanal endoscopic transpromontorial approach is a labyrinthine sparing approach, passing anteriorly with respect to the third portion of the facial nerve, and preserving the labyrinthine block, removing only the anterior portion of the otic capsule (yellow area). *ca: carotid artery; fn: facial nerve; fn*: labyrinthine segment of the facial nerve; gg: geniculate ganglion; gpn: greater superficial petrosal nerve; IAC: internal auditory canal; lsc: lateral semicircular canal; mcf: middle cranial fossa; pr: promontory region; psc: posterior semicircular canal; rw: round window; sph: spherical recess; vc: vertical crest.*

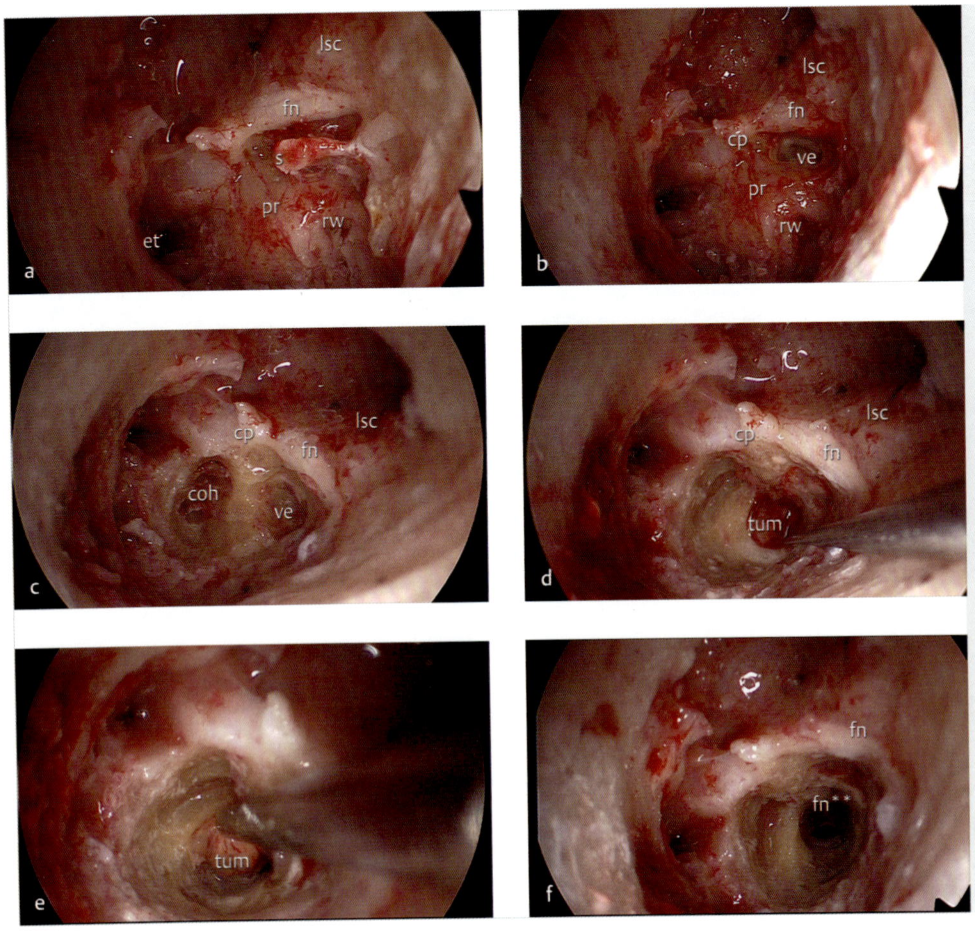

Fig. 9.9 Left side: The transcanal endoscopic transpromontorial approach: endoscopic view. **(a)** The tympanic membrane with the skin of the external auditory canal, the malleus, and incus are removed. Only the stapes is left in place. The attic is drilled and the antrum is exposed. The tympanic portion of the facial nerve is exposed too. **(b)** The stapes is removed and the vestibule is opened. **(c)** The cochlea is drilled, showing basal, medium, and apical turns. **(d)** Drilling of the promontory and the vestibule. The fundus of the internal auditory canal is reached. **(e)** The vestibular schwannoma is gently dissected from the internal auditory canal. **(f)** The intrameatal tract of the facial nerve into the internal auditory canal is perfectly exposed and preserved. *coh: cochlea; cp: cochleariform process; et: eustachian tube; fn: facial nerve tympanic tract; fn**: facial nerve intrameatal tract; lsc: lateral semicircular canal; pe: pyramidal eminence; pr: promontory region; rw: round window; s: stapes; tum: tumor; ve: vestibule.*

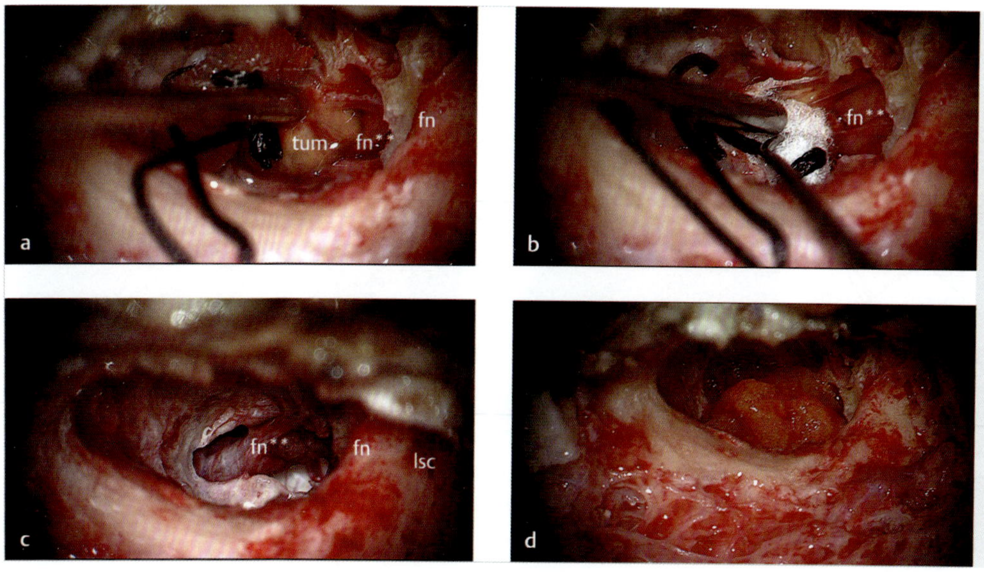

Fig. 9.10 Left side: The expanded transcanal transpromontorial approach. In this technique the dissection is more extensive than in endoscopic approach and an external incision of the skin with soft tissues dissection is required to gain the access. **(a)** The acoustic neuroma is exposed into the fundus, after drilling the vestibule and the cochlea. **(b)** The tumor is dissected, preserving the labyrinthine and intrameatal portions of the facial nerve. **(c)** High magnification view of the facial nerve into the internal auditory canal. Cochlear and vestibular nerves were not preserved, due to the extension of the acoustic neuroma. **(d)** Obliteration of the surgical cavity with fat pad. *cp: cochleariform process; fn: facial nerve; fn**: facial nerve intrameatal tract; lsc: lateral semicircular canal; pr: promontory region; tum: tumor.*

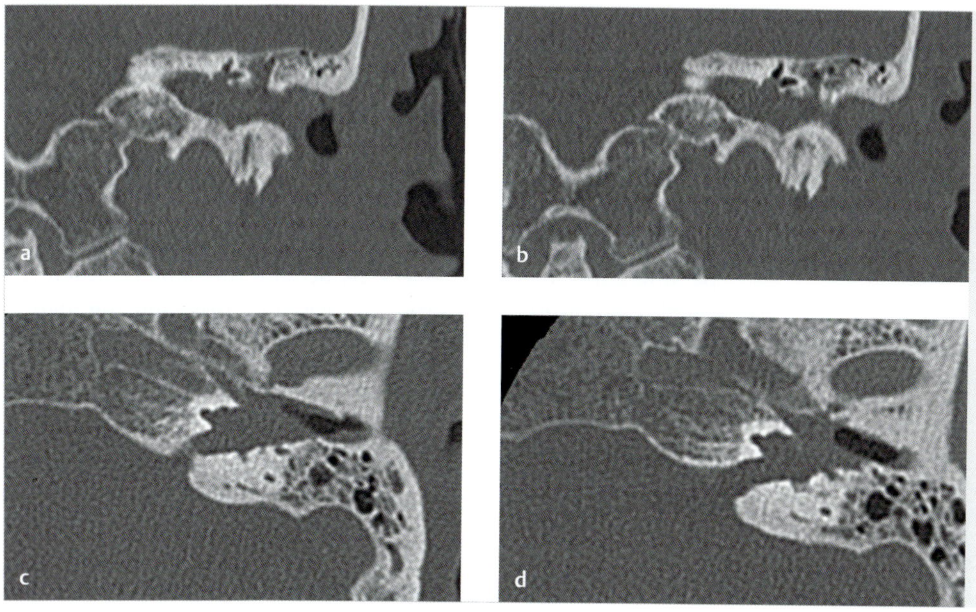

Fig. 9.11 Radiologic aspect of the transcanal endoscopic transpromontorial approach. Note the surgical corridor from the external auditory canal (EAC), to the internal auditory canal (IAC); in coronal view (**a**, **b**) and in axial view (**c**, **d**).

Owing to the postoperative hearing loss on the treated ear, patients who are selected for this procedure should present with profound hearing loss or anacusia on the side of the lesion with a stable contralateral normal hearing function.

Advantages

- Direct surgical route to cochlea, vestibule, and IAC
- Minimal invasive surgery, avoiding external incision, and no brain and meningeal manipulation

Limitation

- Not suitable for extensive lesions, and in case of lesions with extended CPA involvement
- Sacrifice of hearing function
- Poor control of the vascular structures in the CPA

9.4.2 Expanded Transcanal Transpromontorial Approach

The expanded transcanal transpromontorial approach is derived from the formerly described exclusive endoscopic transcanal transpromontorial approach to the CPA and the IAC and it is conducted with the microscope. The endoscope may help the surgeon in some steps of the surgery. In this technique the dissection is more extensive than in endoscopic approach and an external incision of the skin with soft tissues dissection is required to gain access.

Due to the possibility to work under the microscopic view with two hands, tumor removal is easier, with a better management of the surgical instruments, allowing to remove tumor of the IAC with CPA involvement in a straight line with the IAC. The CPA extension of the lesion is removed with further bone drilling to

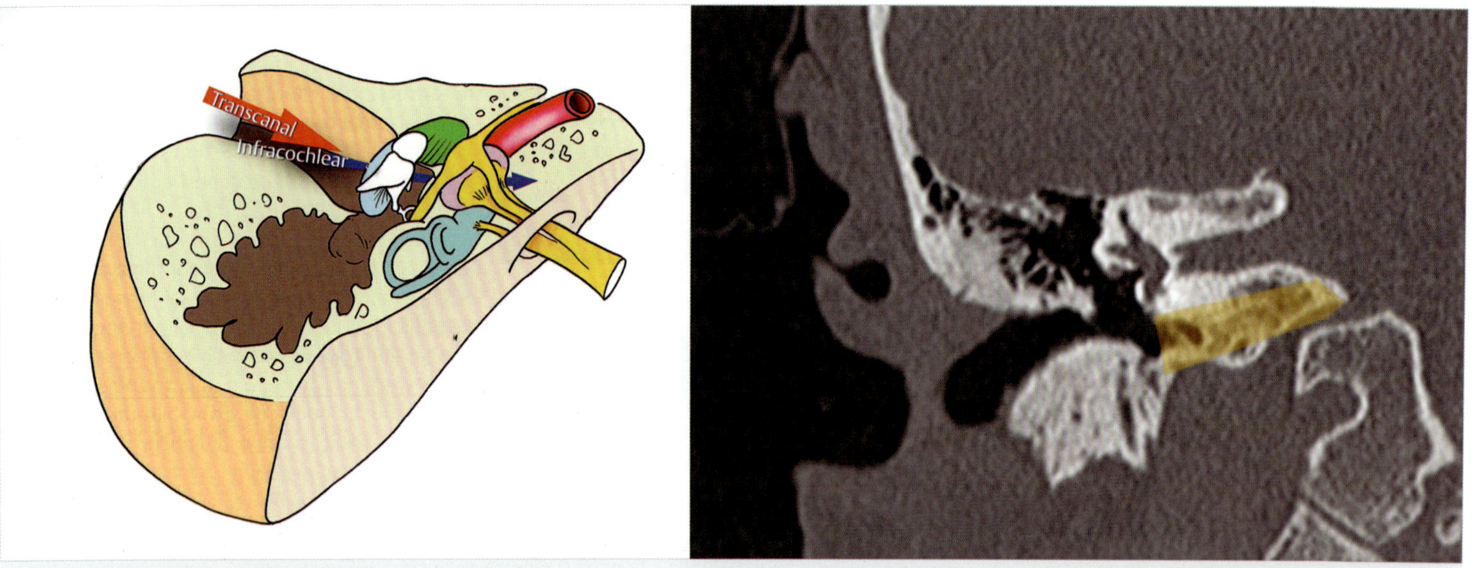

Fig. 9.12 Transcanal endoscopic infracochlear approach. In yellow the surgical corridor from the external auditory canal to the petrous apex, passing below the cochlea.

enlarge the opening of the IAC porus, uncovering the dura of the posterior fossa. At the end of the tumor excision, the endoscope allows us to check the radicality of the procedure and to have a wider view of the vascular and nervous structures in the IAC.

As in the previous technique, because of removal of the cochlea, a postoperative hearing loss is expected in all cases.

Indications

- As in the previous technique it is for acoustic neuroma limited to the IAC with minimal involvement of the CPA, in patient with no servable hearing function.
- It is also suitable for acoustic neuroma growing into the petrous apex under the internal carotid artery.
- It is suitable for medium size acoustic neuroma growing into the CPA in a straight line with the IAC until the entry zone of the acoustic-facial bundle.

Advantages

- Direct access to the IAC and the CPA until the entry zone of acoustic-facial bundle
- No brain retraction and manipulation, while working over the tumor
- Control of the CPA vascular structures

Limitation

- Not suitable for tumor extending in proximity of lower cranial nerves and trigeminal nerve
- Hearing function sacrifice

9.5 Transcanal Infracochlear Corridor

In this approach the EAC is used as a natural corridor to reach the petrous apex portion located below the cochlea and the IAC, passing under the promontory, by drilling the bone between the cochlea superiorly, the carotid artery anteriorly, and the jugular bulb inferiorly, using this opening as a surgical endoscopic corridor to reach the disease in the inferior part of the petrous apex which lies below the IAC and medially compared to the vertical portion of the internal carotid artery. The ossicular chain and the cochlea are preserved, and in this case a postoperative hearing function preservation is expected (see ▶ Fig. 9.12, ▶ Fig. 9.13).

9.5.1 Indications

- Pathologies located inferiorly with respect to the IAC in the petrous apex with limited extent
- Surgical drainage of petrous apex cholesterol granulomas providing and maintaining an outflow pathway to allow for continued drainage of the cholesterol granuloma (see ▶ Fig. 9.14)
- Cholesteatoma with subcochlear canaliculus and lower portion of petrous apex involvement

9.5.2 Advantages

- Hearing function and ossicular chain preservation
- Direct approach to the lower portion of the petrous apex

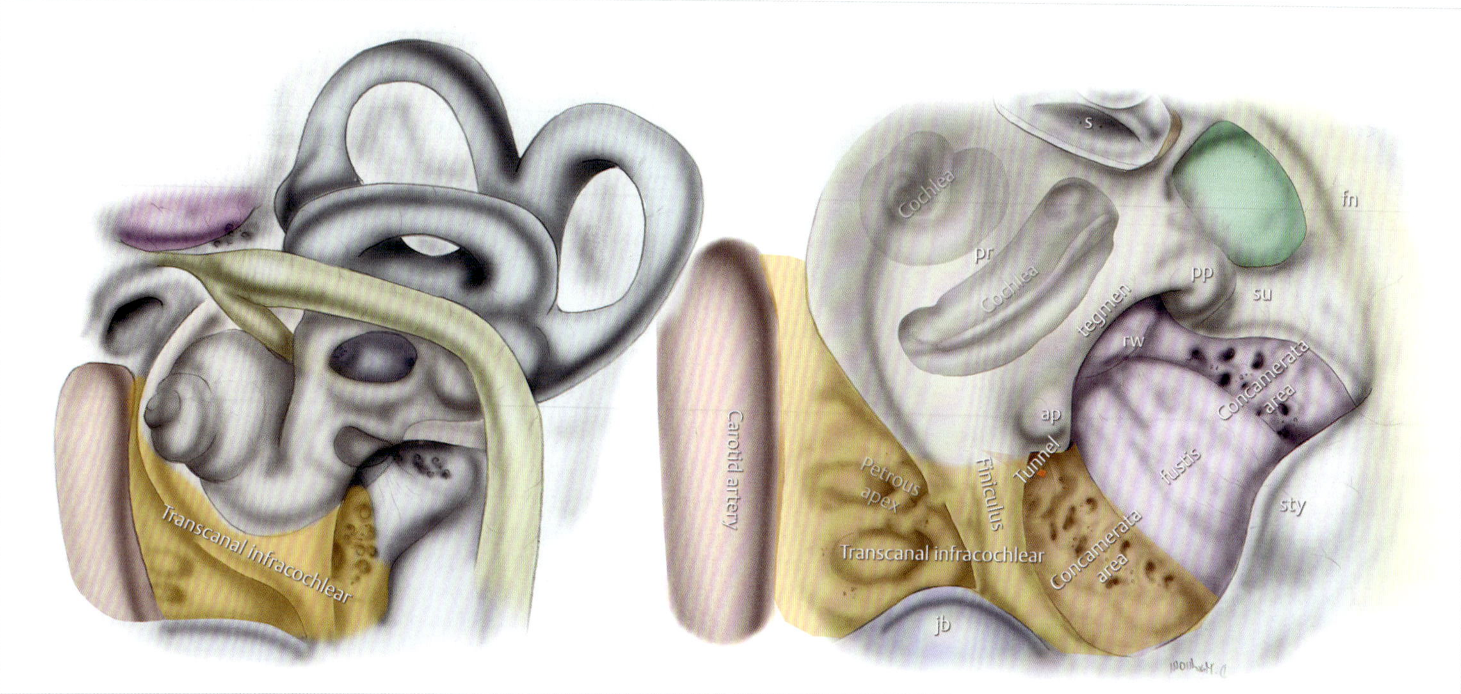

Fig. 9.13 Left side: Transcanal endoscopic infracochlear approach. In yellow the portion of the petrous apex reached with this approach. It is located below the cochlea and internal auditory canal (IAC), passing under the promontory, by drilling the bone between the cochlea superiorly, the carotid artery anteriorly, and the jugular bulb inferiorly. The ossicular chain and the cochlea are preserved. Note the tunnel between the finiculus and the fustis, connecting directly with the petrous apex. *ap: anterior pillar; fn: facial nerve tympanic tract; jb: jugular bulb; pp: posterior pillar; pr: promontory; rw: round window; s: stapes; sty: styloid prominence; su: subiculum.*

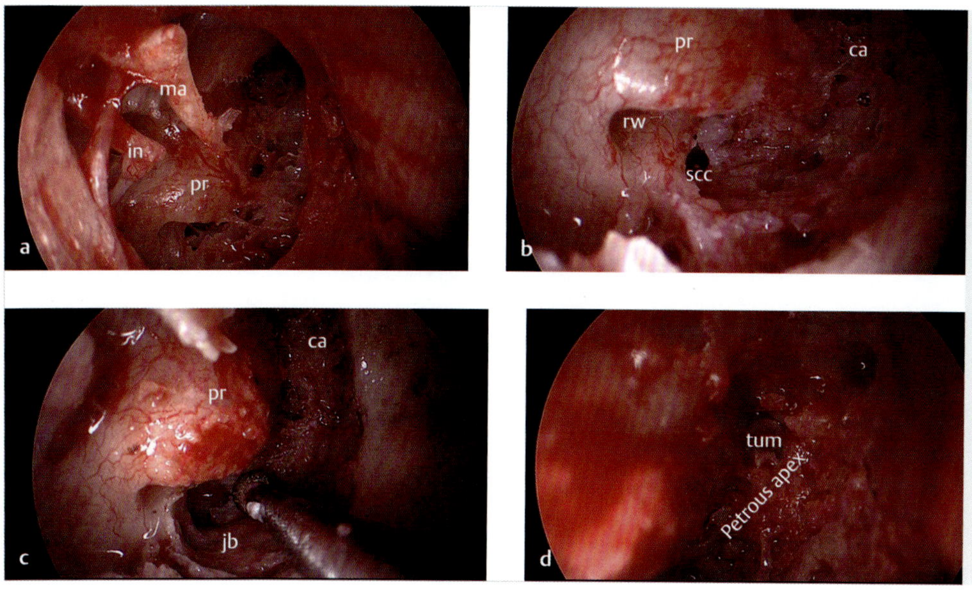

Fig. 9.14 (a–d) Transcanal infracochlear approach. Endoscopic view. Right ear. After exposing surgical limits (carotid artery vertical tract anteriorly and jugular bulb inferiorly), the corridor to the petrous apex is realized, preserving the cochlea superiorly. The petrous apex is opened and the pathology is removed. *ca: carotid artery vertical tract; in: incus; jb: jugular bulb; ma: malleus; pr: promontory; rw: round window; scc: subcochlear canaliculus or tunnel; tum: tumor.*

- Suitable for infralabyrinthine cholesteatoma with limited dimension located in the inferior portion of the petrous apex

9.5.3 Limitations

- This approach is not suitable for extensive infralabyrinthine or infralabyrinthine-apical cholesteatoma.
- This approach is not feasible in case of high jugular bulb.

Suggested Readings

Batra PS, Luong A, Kanowitz SJ, et al. Outcomes of minimally invasive endoscopic resection of anterior skull base neoplasms. Laryngoscope. 2010; 120(1):9–16

Bennett M, Haynes DS. Surgical approaches and complications in the removal of vestibular schwannomas. Otolaryngol Clin North Am. 2007; 40(3):589–609, ix–x

Bennett M, Haynes DS. Surgical approaches and complications in the removal of vestibular schwannomas. Otolaryngol Clin North Am. 2007; 40(3):589–609, ix–x

Cannady SB, Batra PS, Sautter NB, Roh HJ, Citardi MJ. New staging system for sinonasal inverted papilloma in the endoscopic era. Laryngoscope. 2007; 117 (7):1283–1287

Day JD, Chen DA, Arriaga M. Translabyrinthine approach for acoustic neuroma. Neurosurgery. 2004; 54(2):391–395, discussion 395–396

Graffeo CS, Dietrich AR, Grobelny B, et al. A panoramic view of the skull base: systematic review of open and endoscopic endonasal approaches to four tumors. Pituitary. 2014; 17(4):349–356

Hadad G, Bassagasteguy L, Carrau RL, et al. A novel reconstructive technique after endoscopic expanded endonasal approaches: vascular pedicle nasoseptal flap. Laryngoscope. 2006; 116(10):1882–1886

Harvey RJ, Parmar P, Sacks R, Zanation AM. Endoscopic skull base reconstruction of large dural defects: a systematic review of published evidence. Laryngoscope. 2012; 122(2):452–459

Ketcham AS, Wilkins RH, Vanburen JM, Smith RR. A combined intracranial facial approach to the paranasal sinus. Am J Surg. 1963; 106:698–703

Komotar RJ, Starke RM, Raper DMS, Anand VK, Schwartz TH. Endoscopic skull base surgery: a comprehensive comparison with open transcranial approaches. Br J Neurosurg. 2012; 26(5):637–648

Leng LZ, Brown S, Anand VK, Schwartz TH. "Gasket-seal" watertight closure in minimal-access endoscopic cranial base surgery. Neurosurgery. 2008; 62(5) Suppl 2: E342–E343, discussion E343

Magnan J, Chays A, Lepetre C, Pencroffi E, Locatelli P. Surgical perspectives of endoscopy of the cerebellopontine angle. Am J Otol. 1994; 15(3):366–370

Marchioni D, Alicandri-Ciufelli M, Mattioli F, et al. From external to internal auditory canal: surgical anatomy by an exclusive endoscopic approach. Eur Arch Otorhinolaryngol. 2013; 270(4):1267–1275

Marchioni D, Alicandri-Ciufelli M, Molteni G, Genovese E, Presutti L. Endoscopic tympanoplasty in patients with attic retraction pockets. Laryngoscope. 2010; 120 (9):1847–1855

Marchioni D, Alicandri-Ciufelli M, Rubini A, Presutti L. Endoscopic transcanal corridors to the lateral skull base: initial experiences. Laryngoscope. 2015; 125 Suppl 5:S1–S13

Presutti L, Alicandri-Ciufelli M, Rubini A, Gioacchini FM, Marchioni D. Combined lateral microscopic/endoscopic approaches to petrous apex lesions: pilot clinical experiences. Ann Otol Rhinol Laryngol. 2014; 123(8):550–559

Presutti L, Marchioni D, Mattioli F, Villari D, Alicandri-Ciufelli M. Endoscopic management of acquired cholesteatoma: our experience. J Otolaryngol Head Neck Surg. 2008; 37(4):481–487

Pryor SG, Moore EJ, Kasperbauer JL. Endoscopic versus traditional approaches for excision of juvenile nasopharyngeal angiofibroma. Laryngoscope. 2005; 115 (7):1201–1207

Schwartz TH, Fraser JF, Brown S, Tabaee A, Kacker A, Anand VK. Endoscopic cranial base surgery: classification of operative approaches. Neurosurgery. 2008; 62 (5):991–1002, discussion 1002–1005

Staecker H, Nadol JB, Jr, Ojeman R, Ronner S, McKenna MJ. Hearing preservation in acoustic neuroma surgery: middle fossa versus retrosigmoid approach. Am J Otol. 2000; 21(3):399–404

Tarabichi M. Endoscopic management of limited attic cholesteatoma. Laryngoscope. 2004; 114(7):1157–1162

Thomassin JM, Korchia D, Doris JM. Endoscopic-guided otosurgery in the prevention of residual cholesteatomas. Laryngoscope. 1993; 103(8):939–943

Thorp BD, Sreenath SB, Ebert CS, Zanation AM. Endoscopic skull base reconstruction: a review and clinical case series of 152 vascularized flaps used for surgical skull base defects in the setting of intraoperative cerebrospinal fluid leak. Neurosurg Focus. 2014; 37(4):E4

Chapter 10

Endoscopic Transcanal Suprageniculate Approach

10 Endoscopic Transcanal Suprageniculate Approach

Daniele Marchioni, Nirmal Patel, Nicholas Jufas, Alexander J. Saxby, and Jonathan H.K. Kong

Abstract

The suprageniculate area is a pyramid-shaped anatomical area inferiorly bordered by the geniculate ganglion (GG), superiorly by the dura of the middle cranial fossa (MCF), posteriorly by the lateral semicircular canal, and medially there are the petrous apex cells extending to the internal auditory canal (IAC).

The endoscopic transcanal suprageniculate approach is an endoscopic minimally invasive approach to the suprageniculate region, which avoids brain and dural manipulation.

Indications for this approach are tumors involving the suprageniculate fossa (SGF), such as petrous apex supralabyrinthine cholesteatomas limited to the SGF or attic cholesteatomas with suprageniculate ganglion area involvement, and decompression of the GG and the tympanic facial nerve (FN).

This procedure requires partial drilling of the scutum and the removal of the incus and the head of the malleus, in order to obtain a direct and minimally invasive exposure of the SGF and the tympanic FN. Thus, a suprageniculate corridor is created between the GG, the dura of the MCF, and the lateral semicircular canal, to reach the SGF.

This approach has a lower morbidity rate in comparison to traditional surgery, such as a MCF approach. It allows the preservation of serviceable hearing, even though an ossicular chain disarticulation (incus and malleus head removal) and ossiculoplasty are necessary, with a variable postoperative conductive hearing loss. Among the disadvantages, it is important to keep in mind that in case of FN tumor removal and tympanic FN interruption during surgery, a FN reconstruction with end-to-end anastomosis is not suitable, and a cable graft interposition is not always possible. Moreover, when dural repair is needed, a transmastoid approach is required.

Keywords: suprageniculate area, geniculate ganglion, facial nerve, supralabyrinthine pathology, cholesteatoma, facial nerve tumor, facial nerve decompression

10.1 Introduction

The suprageniculate fossa (SGF) is a pyramid-shaped anatomical area inferiorly bordered by the geniculate ganglion (GG), superiorly by the dura of the middle cranial fossa (MCF), posteriorly by the lateral semicircular canal, and medially where the petrous apex cells extend to the internal auditory canal (IAC) (see ▶ Fig. 10.1, ▶ Fig. 10.2).

Although lesions involving this region are uncommon, the most frequently described are cholesteatomas, meningiomas, and perigeniculate facial nerve (FN) tumors such as schwannomas and hemangiomas (see Clinical Case 2, ▶ Fig. 10.34). Symptoms and signs vary according to tumor location. The most common clinical presentation is facial paresis which usually occurs with a progressive or occasionally relapsing/remitting development, often ending in facial paralysis. Conductive, sensorineural, or mixed-type

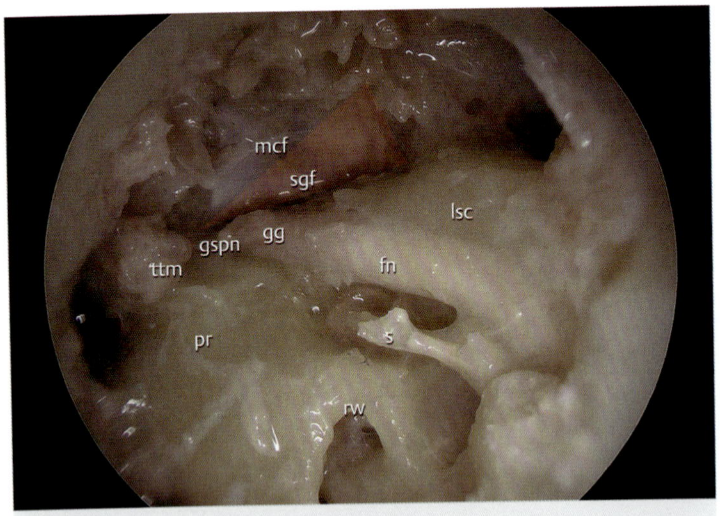

Fig. 10.1 Left ear: Anatomical transcanal endoscopic dissection. The ossicular chain is removed and a wide atticotomy is performed detecting the dural plane of the middle cranial fossa (MCF). The tympanic segment of the facial nerve (FN) with the geniculate ganglion (GG) are exposed. The suprageniculate fossa (SGF) is a pyramid-shaped anatomical area (orange area) bordered inferiorly by the GG, superiorly by the dura of the MCF, posteriorly by the lateral semicircular canal, and medially where the petrous apex cells extend to the internal auditory canal. *fn: facial nerve; gg: geniculate ganglion; gspn: greater superficial petrosal nerve; lsc: lateral semicircular canal; mcf: middle cranial fossa; pr: promontory; rw: round window; s: stapes; sgf: suprageniculate fossa; ttm: tensor tympani muscle.*

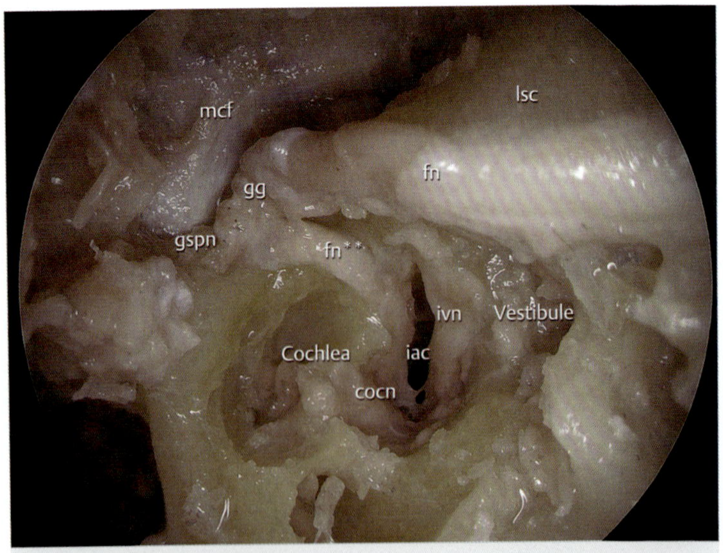

Fig. 10.2 Left ear: Anatomical transcanal endoscopic dissection. The stapes is removed entering the vestibule. The cochlea is opened and the fundus of the internal auditory canal with its content is exposed. The geniculate ganglion (GG), the labyrinthine portion of the facial nerve (FN) with the cochlear nerve, and the inferior vestibular nerve are visible in the surgical cavity. *cocn: cochlear nerve; fn**: facial nerve (labyrinthine portion); fn: facial nerve; gg: geniculate ganglion; gspn: greater superficial petrosal nerve; iac: internal auditory canal; ivn: inferior vestibular nerve; lsc: lateral semicircular canal; mcf: middle cranial fossa.*

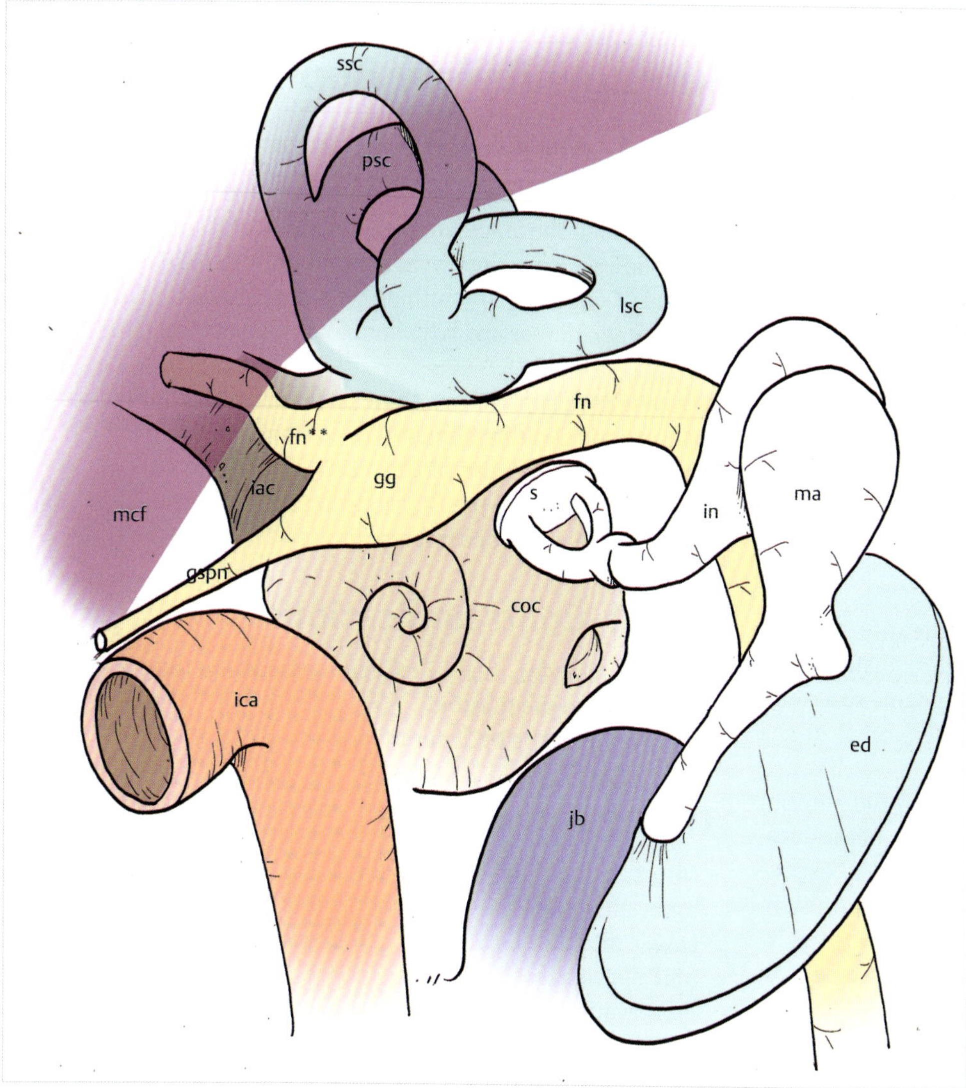

Fig. 10.3 Left ear: Schematic drawing representing the anatomical relationship between the facial nerve (FN), the middle cranial fossa (MCF), internal auditory canal (IAC), and the cochlea, in relation to the suprageniculate fossa. *coc: cochlea; ed: eardrum; fn: facial nerve (tympani portion); fn**: facial nerve (labyrinthine portion); gg: geniculate ganglion; gspn: greater superficial petrosal nerve; iac: internal auditory canal; ica: internal carotid artery; in: incus; jb: jugular bulb; lsc: lateral semicircular canal; ma: malleus; mcf: middle cranial fossa; psc: posterior semicircular canal; s: stapes; ssc: superior semicircular canal.*

hearing loss is the second most common symptom. Specifically, a conductive hearing loss is usually seen in case of ossicular chain involvement, but normal hearing levels are also frequently observed in case of GG tumors.

The surgical treatment aims at the complete removal of the lesion from the SGF, preserving the hearing and FN function when possible. In accessing a disease located in this area, especially in patients with a good hearing function, the MCF is the most frequently used surgical procedure, despite the often-limited dimensions of the lesion. A MCF approach requires an extended temporal craniotomy, as well as the elevation and retraction of the temporal lobe (see Chapter 8). At present, the main application of transcanal endoscopic surgery is the surgical treatment of middle ear cholesteatoma, but with the development of endoscopic anatomy, there has been significant advancement in endoscopic inner ear and lateral skull base surgery.[1,2,3]

It has allowed for the development of minimally invasive surgical approaches to certain lesions located in the SGF through the external auditory canal (EAC), working in a lateral to medial direction within the anatomical boundaries of this area. The great advantage is the possibility to remove lesions from this area without either dural or brain manipulation.

10.2 Surgical Anatomy

The SGF is a pyramid-shaped space inferiorly bordered by the GG and the second portion of the FN, superiorly by the MCF dura, and posteriorly by the ampullated ends of the lateral and superior semicircular canals.

The tympanic segment of the FN begins at the level of the GG and ends at the level of the stapes, where the nerve turns downward below the lateral semicircular canal (see ▶ Fig. 10.1, ▶ Fig. 10.2, ▶ Fig. 10.3). The tegmen is anteriorly grooved by the greater superficial petrosal nerve (GSPN) extending anteriorly and medially from the area in front of the arcuate eminence and crossing the floor of the middle fossa toward the foramen lacerum. The GSPN can be identified medial to the arcuate eminence as it leaves the GG by passing through the facial hiatus to reach the middle cranial fossa floor. It runs beneath the dura of the middle cranial fossa in the sphenopetrosal groove formed by the junction of the petrous and sphenoid bones, immediately superiorly and anterolaterally to the horizontal segment of the petrous carotid artery. From an endoscopic point of view, it is possible to divide the tympanic FN into two portions in relation to the cochleariform process (CP): the precochleariform and the postcochleariform segments.

10.2.1 Precochleariform Segment of the Tympanic Portion of the Facial Nerve

The precochleariform segment is the portion of the tympanic FN lying superiorly and anteriorly to the posterior bony limit of the CP. This segment of the FN is composed by the GG and the GSPN and it has a parallel orientation and lies superiorly to the semicanal of the tensor tympani muscle. It is necessary to remove the malleus head to obtain a good transcanal visualization of the precochleariform segment and the GG area. Traditionally, a microscopic access to the anterior epitympanum requires a mastoidectomy, a posterior atticotomy, and the removal of the incus and the head of the malleus. Conversely, an exclusive endoscopic transcanal route offers the advantage of an adequate visualization and access while obviating the need for a mastoidectomy and posterior atticotomy.

10.2.2 Geniculate Ganglion

The CP represents an excellent landmark to identify the GG, which is located just anteriorly, superiorly, and medially to the CP. The GG lies on the floor of the anterior epitympanic space and it has a horizontal orientation parallel to the semicanal of the tensor tendon of the malleus.

In 67% of cases, the GG is covered by the bone of the anterior epitympanic space cells, so in these cases the air cells of the anterior epitympanic space need to be removed in order to expose the GG. In the remaining 33% of cases, the precochleariform tympanic FN is partially dehiscent.

Another anatomical landmark for the GG is the transverse crest —also known as the "cog"—a bony ridge extending inferiorly from the tegmen tympani of the anterior epitympanic space, just anterior to the CP. The transverse crest is not always clearly described in literature and frequent variability of this structure is noted. It has different conformations and relationships to the GG, the tensor fold, and the supratubal recess. The cog is a complete bony crest in around 60% of endoscopic cases, having a transverse inclination anteriorly and superiorly attached to the most anterior portion of the tegmen tympani. In these cases, the crest points posteriorly and inferiorly to the CP and can be used as a landmark for the GG during a transcanal endoscopic approach. In the remaining 40% of cases, an incomplete or rudimental transverse crest can be found, in close relationship to the tegmen of the anterior epitympanic space. In these cases, the crest cannot reliably be used as a landmark for the GG.

10.2.3 Greater Superficial Petrosal Nerve

An endoscopic access to the greater superficial petrosal nerve (GSPN) can be obtained by removing the head of the malleus in order to identify the anterior bone wall of the anterior epitympanic space. It is necessary to remove the transverse crest and the bone in the medial supratubal recess (when present), anteriorly to the GG, in order to expose the GSPN.

In 40% of cases, there is a dehiscence of the MCF dura at the level of the anterior epitympanic space and the dura of the MCF is in close relationship to both the GG and the GSPN. On the contrary, in 60% of cases, drilling is necessary in order to find the dura of the MCF.

10.3 Endoscopic Transcanal Suprageniculate Approach

10.3.1 Indications

- Tumors involving the SGF, located between the GG, the dura of the MCF and the ampullated end of the lateral semicircular canal with limited extension to the petrous apex cells lying superiorly to the GG, and the labyrinthine FN, in patients with facial palsy (FN hemangiomas and schwannomas) (see Clinical Case 1 and Clinical Case 2).
- Petrous apex supralabyrinthine cholesteatomas limited to the SGF or attic cholesteatomas with suprageniculate ganglion area involvement (see Clinical Cases 3–5).
- Traumatic injury to the GG requiring the removal of bone spicules or hematoma decompression (see Clinical Cases 6–7).

10.3.2 Contraindications

- Lesions involving the SGF extending medial to the cochlea or extending to the mastoid
- Infiltration of the MCF dura

10.3.3 Advantages

- Direct and minimally invasive exposure of the tympanic FN, especially of the most anterior portion
- Lower morbidity in comparison to traditional surgery, such as a MCF approach
- Preservation of serviceable hearing

The endoscopic transcanal suprageniculate approach (ETSA) is a minimally invasive approach to the GG region which allows for the complete removal of lesions in this area, avoiding brain/dural manipulations and the risk of hearing loss. The method may also have a shorter and safer postsurgery time than the open MCF approach.

The possibility of managing a pathology lying in the SGF using an endoscopic approach through the EAC may avoid brain tissue retraction and manipulation, which are required in a MCF craniotomy as well as in large translabyrinthine approaches. Additionally, patients who have undergone ETSA surgery to date have not required admission to an intensive care unit (ICU) after the operation, which also implies a safer and quicker postoperative recovery and may decrease the overall financial burden of the surgery.

10.3.4 Disadvantages

- Ossicular chain disarticulation (incus and malleus head removal) may require an ossiculoplasty which may cause a variable postoperative conductive hearing loss.
- When dural repair is associated, a combined microscopic approach may be necessary.
- In case of intraoperative FN interruption an end-to-end coaptation FN reconstruction is not suitable and a cable graft interposition is not always possible.

The main disadvantage of ETSA, in addition to those related specifically to the endoscopic technique, is the removal of the head of the malleus and the incus which is always necessary.

This surgical step is important to obtain a wide access to the whole SGF and therefore completely extirpate tumors located in this anatomical area. If a significant preoperative sensorineural hearing loss or conductive hearing loss is already present, then this certainly would make removal of the malleus head and incus less of a concern. In most cases, an ossiculoplasty can be performed if ETSA is undertaken.

10.3.5 Preoperative Assessment

A radiological assessment in the form of a high-resolution computed tomography (HRCT) of the temporal bone and cerebral magnetic resonance imaging (MRI) scan is performed in all patients, to allow for preoperative decision-making about the surgical route and the possible access. The hearing function is evaluated before and after surgery using Pure Tone Average (PTA). PTA is calculated using the mean value, in decibels, of pure tone hearing thresholds at frequencies of 500, 1,000, 2,000, and 4,000 Hz. The FN function is assessed by means of the House-Brackmann (HB) grading system before and after surgery in all subjects.

10.4 ETSA for Tumors of the Geniculate Ganglion (see Clinical Case 1 and Clinical Case 2)

Facial nerve tumors are a rare subset. The GG represents one of the most common sites of involvement (about 53.9% of FN tumors). Tumors involving the GG or/and the tympanic segment of the FN are suitable for ETSA.

Although ETSA is a minimally invasive technique for the treatment of GG and tympanic FN tumors, some considerations should be made:

- The most delicate aspect of the treatment of these tumors is deciding when to perform surgery; this decision is especially related to the dimension of the tumor and the function of the FN.
- In patients suffering from a small GG tumor with good FN function (HB grades I–II), a wait and scan policy should be followed as a first choice, since this tumor grows slowly.
- In patients with HB grade III or higher facial palsy, surgery should be considered.
- In case of fast-growing tumors, temporal bone compression or large dimension, surgery is recommended, regardless of the HB scale.

10.4.1 Reconstruction of the Facial Nerve

Also for ETSA a simultaneous reconstruction of the nerve should be considered, since during tumor removal the involved FN is obviously intraoperatively interrupted, and an immediate FN reconstruction is mandatory to obtain the best results.

If the ETSA approach is selected, the surgeon should consider some limitations regarding FN reconstruction:

- Primary end-to-end coaptation is not possible with this surgical technique.
- Only in case of preservation of the most anterior portion of the GG is a cable graft interposition (with great auricular nerve) between the residual GG and the tympanic/mastoid segment of the FN recommended.
- When the whole GG is removed with the tumor, a cable graft interposition is not always possible due to the anatomical position of the labyrinthine portion of the FN. In these cases, a hypoglossal-FN anastomosis should be considered as the first choice.

10.4.2 Surgical Technique

Surgery is conducted under intraoperative FN monitoring (NIM, Medtronic).

Various 0-, 30-, and 45-degree, 3- or 4-mm diameter and 15-cm length endoscopes are used during surgery. A 0-degree endoscope is used through the EAC; an incision of the EAC skin is made with the superior limb at approximately 11 o'clock and the inferior limb at 6 o'clock. The incision should be made in a triangular shape to create a wide space in the epitympanum (▶ Fig. 10.4a). These incisions are then connected at their lateral end, thus creating a standard tympanomeatal flap that is medially elevated toward the tympanic annulus. The fibrous annulus is then lifted from the osseous annular sulcus exposing the posterior mesotympanum. The tympanic membrane is then carefully dissected from the lateral process of the malleus, the handle (▶ Fig. 10.4b). If necessary, the eardrum is dissected from the umbo using a sharp dissector and a cupped forceps. The tympanic membrane is then anteriorly retracted exposing the entire middle ear. A diamond bar or a piezosurgery device is used to perform an atticotomy (see ▶ Fig. 10.5a). The scutum removal is continued until the incudomalleolar joint is completely visible (see ▶ Fig. 10.5b). The tympanic segment of the FN is seen under the incus and inspected. In case of a tumor involving the second portion of the FN, a lateralization of the incus could be visible. Once the attic has been exposed and the tumor has been detected, the incudostapedial joint is carefully detached using a small hook over the joint. The incus is removed. During this maneuver the surgeon should avoid damage to the stapes (see ▶ Fig. 10.6a). The head of the malleus is also cut and removed (see ▶ Fig. 10.6b). After this surgical maneuver the precochleariform and postcochleariform FN portions are well visible, from the second genu to the GG area, and obviously the tumor is also exposed in this anatomical area (see ▶ Fig. 10.7a). In most cases, the tumor of the GG is well visible, after the ossicular chain removal, since it extrudes into the attic, remodeling the perilabyrinthine cells (see ▶ Fig. 10.7b).

In case of a GG tumor without extension to the second portion of the FN, it may be covered by the bony cells around the GG area. In this case, the cog should be detected, and the bony cells around the GG must be removed using a diamond bur, or a piezosurgery device in order to expose the tumor on the deepest

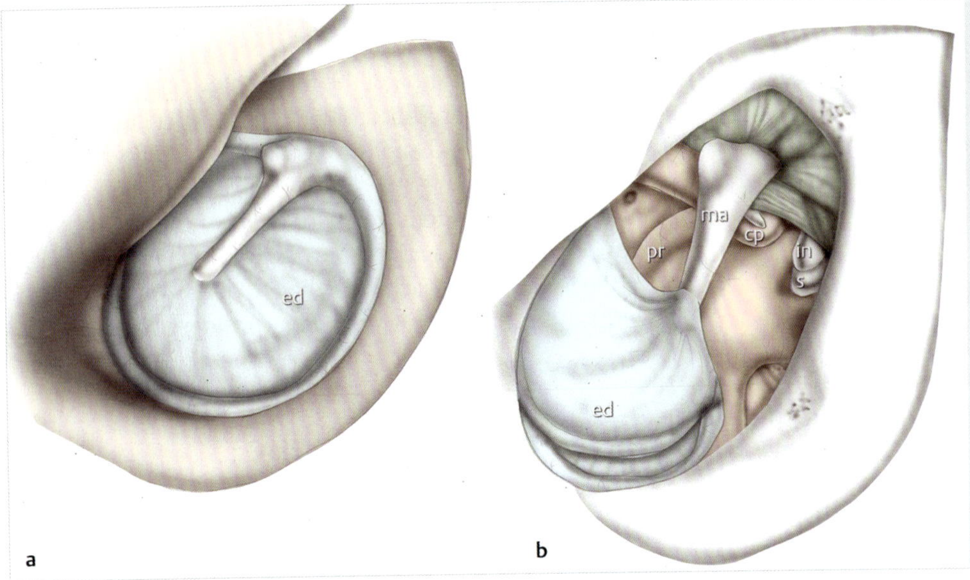

Fig. 10.4 Left ear: **(a)** A triangular shaped incision of the external auditory canal (EAC) skin is made with the superior limb at approximately 11 o'clock and the inferior limb at 6 o'clock. **(b)** The tympanomeatal flap is elevated and dissected from the handle of the malleus, exposing the tympanic cavity. *cp: cochleariform process; ed: eardrum; in: incus; ma: malleus; pr: promontory; s: stapes.*

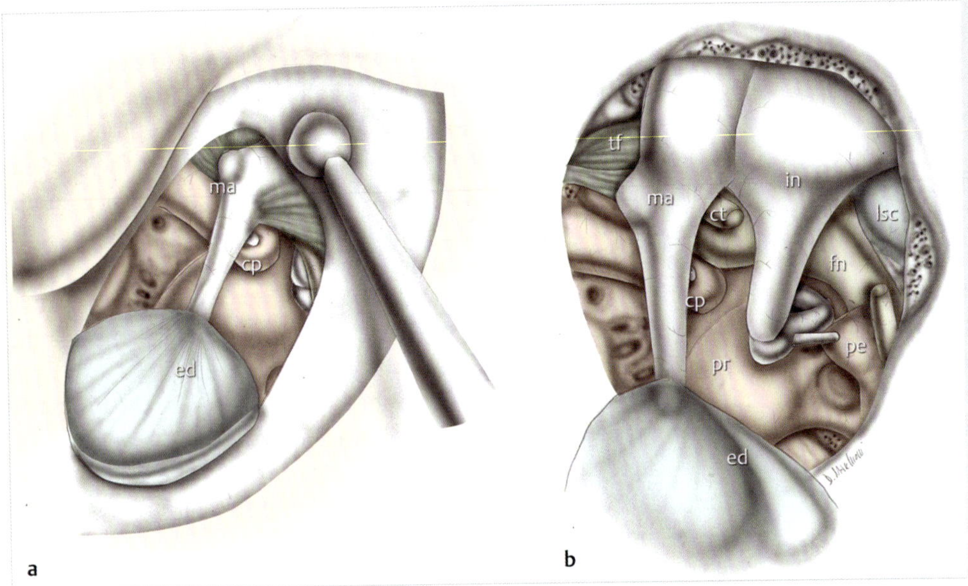

Fig. 10.5 Left ear: **(a)** A small diamond bur is used to remove the scutum. **(b)** The incudo-malleolar joint is progressively exposed. *cp: cochleariform process; ct: chorda tympani; ed: eardrum; fn: facial nerve; in: incus; lsc: lateral semicircular canal; ma: malleus; pe: pyramidal eminence; pr: promontory; tf: tensor fold.*

surgical plane (see ▶ Fig. 10.8a, b and ▶ Fig. 10.9a). During this step, it is crucial to detect the three anatomical landmarks' boundaries of the SGF:

- The line of the MCF dura: The MCF can be superiorly detected following the cog. During this maneuver, it is mandatory to respect the dural plane. Anatomically, the dural plane descends from the posterior epitympanum to the anterior epitympanum where it joins the GSPN in the most anterior portion of the attic.
- The labyrinthine block, in particular the ampullated end of the lateral semicircular canal, should be identified as it serves as the superior and posterior border of the SGF of the bone. This bone wall of the lateral semicircular canal has a superior and just posterior location in relation to the second genu of the FN.
- The tympanic segment of the FN and the GG: In some patients, to uncover the GG, the bony cells around the GG fossa should be removed.

Once the three anatomical landmarks have been detected, the bony cells of the suprageniculate area between these anatomical structures are removed exposing the tumor inside the fossa.

In this way, the FN is endoscopically exposed from the second genu to the GG and GSPN (see ▶ Fig. 10.9a, b). This surgical exposure provides adequate access to completely remove the tumor from the GG fossa and the petrous apex. When a lesion/tumor is intimately associated with the FN, a gentle dissection is performed, looking for a plane between the FN and the lesion, trying to preserve the integrity of the nerve.

Whenever possible, the integrity of the FN should be preserved. In cases in which the FN fibers are involved by the lesion, no clear plane is established, and a preoperative weakness is present, then the sacrifice of the involved portion of the nerve is mandatory (see ▶ Fig. 10.10a, b and ▶ Fig. 10.12, ▶ Fig. 10.13, ▶ Fig. 10.14). Once the lesion has been removed, an endoscopic inspection of the whole geniculate fossa is performed, looking for any residual disease.

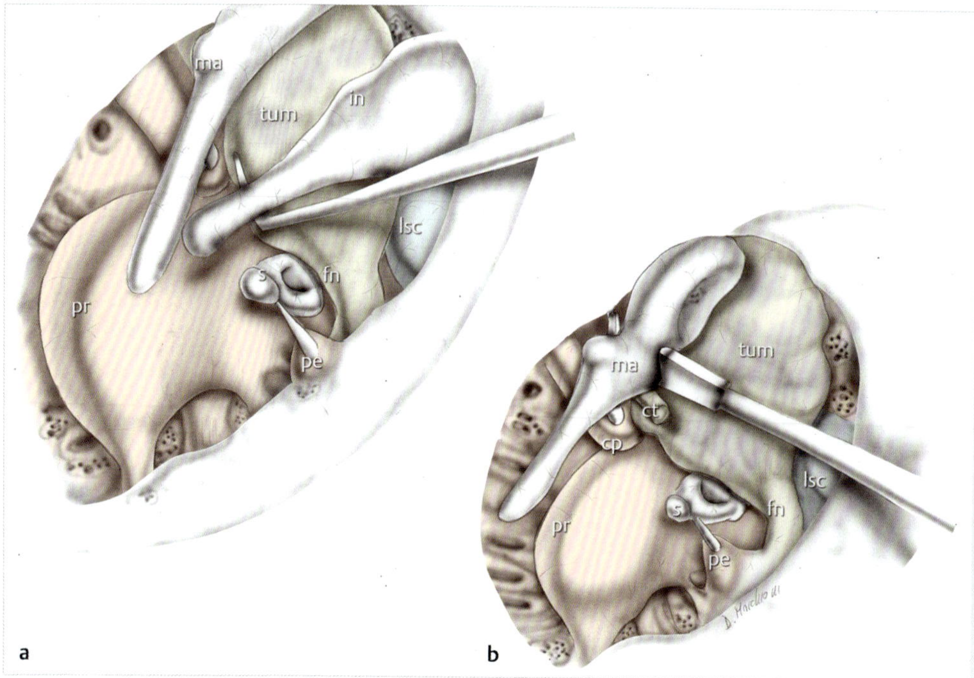

Fig. 10.6 Left ear: **(a)** The incus is endoscopically removed. **(b)** The head of the malleus is cut and removed. *cp: cochleariform process; ct: chorda tympani; fn: facial nerve; in: incus; lsc: lateral semicircular canal; ma: malleus; pe: pyramidal eminence; pr: promontory; s: stapes; tum: tumor.*

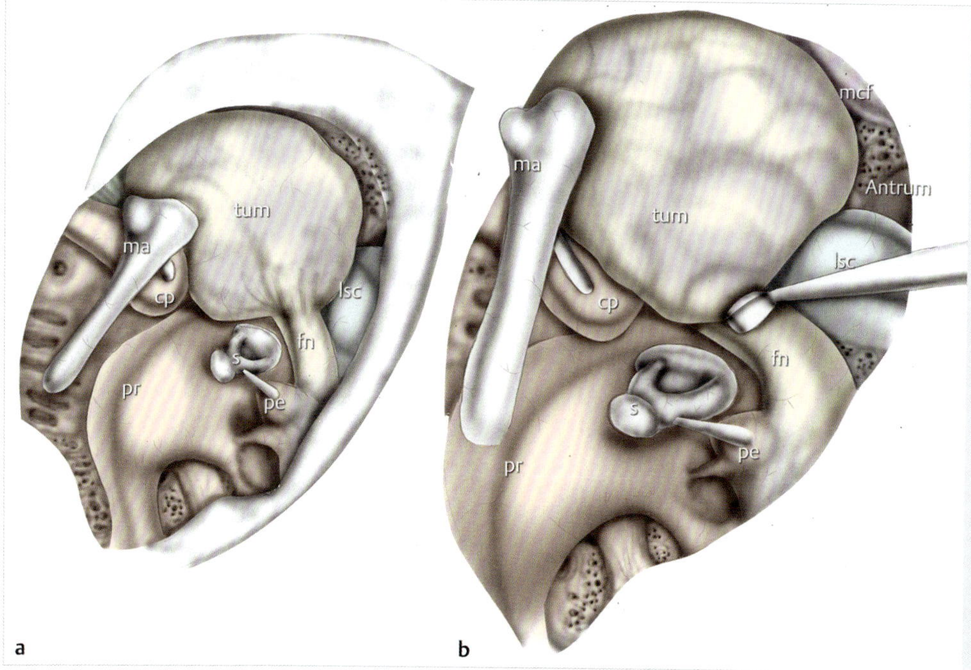

Fig. 10.7 Left ear: **(a)** After the incus and head of the malleus' removal the facial nerve (FN) tumor is visible. **(b)** The dissection of the tumor from the FN is started. *cp: cochleariform process; fn: facial nerve; lsc: lateral semicircular canal; ma: malleus; mcf: middle cranial fossa; pe: pyramidal eminence; pr: promontory; s: stapes; tum: tumor.*

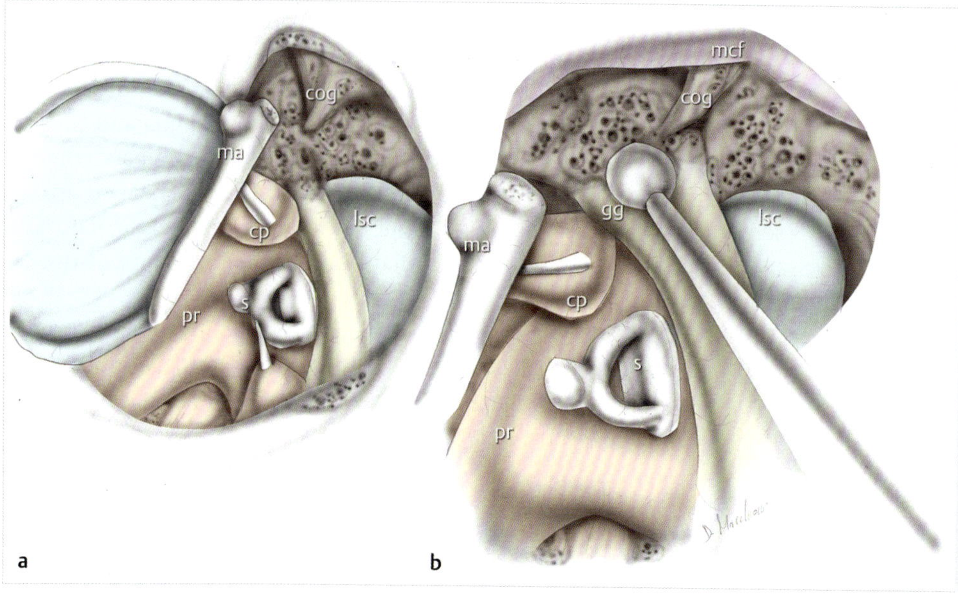

Fig. 10.8 Left ear: **(a)** After the ossicular chain removal, the cog and the middle cranial fossa (mcf) plane are detected. **(b)** A diamond bur is used to remove the bone over the geniculate ganglion (gg) in order to expose the tumor in the suprageniculate fossa. *cp: cochleariform process; gg: geniculate ganglion; lsc: lateral semicircular canal; ma: malleus; mcf: middle cranial fossa; pr: promontory; s: stapes.*

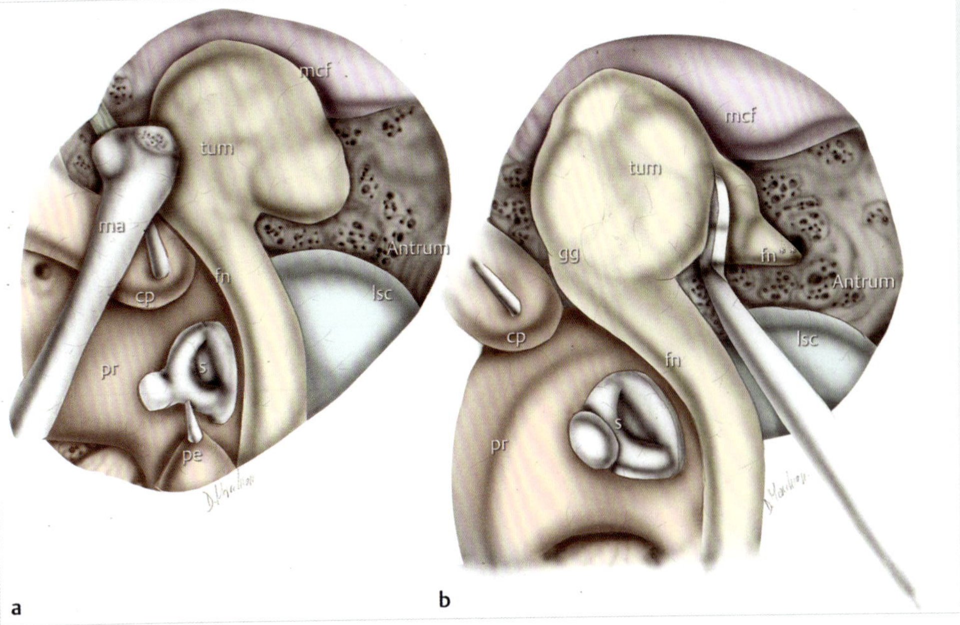

Fig. 10.9 Left ear: **(a)** After drilling the attical bone cells in proximity to the cog, the geniculate ganglion (*gg*) and the tumor are exposed on the deepest surgical plane. **(b)** The dissection of the posterior portion of the tumor is started using a curved dissector, detecting the labyrinthine portion of the facial nerve (*fn***). *cp: cochleariform process; fn: facial nerve; fn**: facial nerve (labyrinthine portion); lsc: lateral semicircular canal; ma: malleus; mcf: middle cranial fossa; pe: pyramidal eminence; pr: promontory; s: stapes; tum: tumor.*

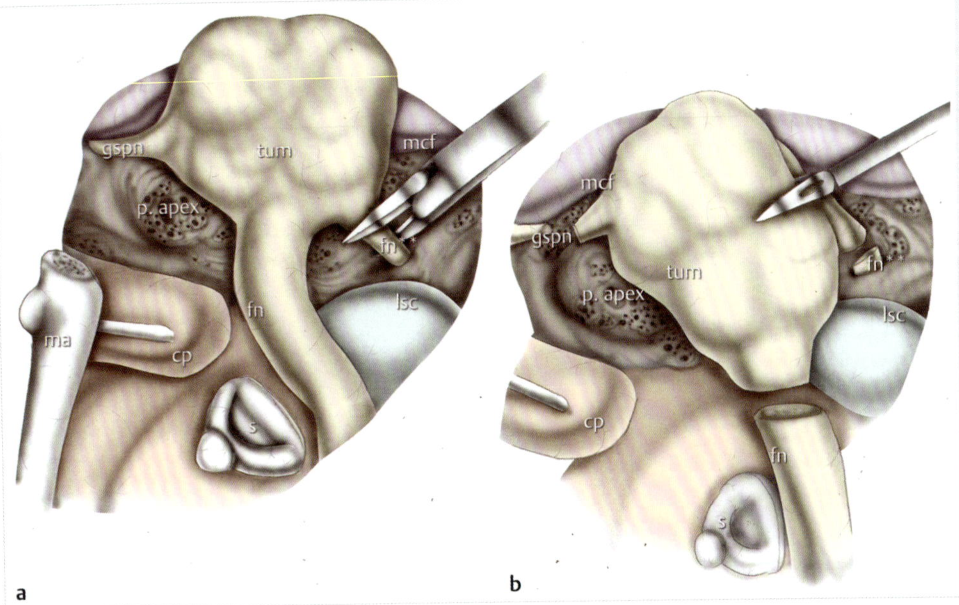

Fig. 10.10 Left ear: **(a, b)** The tumor is exposed and the anatomical landmarks are detected. When a clear cleavage plane between the tumor and the nerve is not found, the sacrifice of the facial nerve (FN) is mandatory. The tumor is detached from the labyrinthine portion and the tympanic portion of the FN using microscissors. *cp: cochleariform process; fn: tympanic portion of facial nerve; fn**: labyrinthine portion of facial nerve; gspn: greater superficial petrosal nerve; lsc: lateral semicircular canal; ma: malleus; mcf: middle cranial fossa; p. apex: petrous apex; s: stapes; tum: tumor.*

In case a nerve is interrupted, an immediate reconstruction of the nerve is recommended. As previously described, the reconstruction depends on the defect of the FN after tumor removal. In case of preservation of a portion of the GG, a cable graft interposition using the great auricular nerve is suggested to reconstruct the nerve defect (see ▶ Fig. 10.15, ▶ Fig. 10.16). The residual FN is exposed until the second genu. Microscissors are used to sharply cut and regularize the residual portion of the GG and the residual FN at the level of the second genu. The great auricular nerve is harvested from an incision along the neck, and the graft is placed and interposed between the residual GG and the FN (see ▶ Fig. 10.16b). Epineurial or perineurial suturing is not necessary. Instead, it is mandatory to have proper contact between the cable graft and the residual FN. Once the cable graft has been placed, a fibrin glue drop is put on the connections between the nerves, to help the coaptation. Then a small temporalis fascia graft is used to cover the interposition, to help the adhesion of the nerves. In case of GG sacrifice a hypoglossal-FN anastomosis should be considered (▶ Fig. 10.11). When necessary the middle fossa dura is covered with a cartilage graft harvested from the tragus (see ▶ Fig. 10.17a).

During the preoperative assessment if serviceable hearing is found, then an ossiculoplasty is mandatory at the end of the procedure and in this case the incus and the head of the malleus are removed, preserving the handle of the malleus and the stapes (see ▶ Fig. 10.17b, c and ▶ Fig. 10.18). In subjects where a preoperative severe or profound sensorineural hearing loss is found, an ossiculoplasty is not necessary and the ossicular chain can be totally removed, to have an optimal exposure of the GG area.

An ossiculoplasty with an incus interposition is then performed. The scutum is reconstructed with a tragal cartilage graft before replacing the tympanomeatal flap. The EAC is then filled with gelfoam. The tympanomeatal flap is then replaced (see ▶ Fig. 10.19).

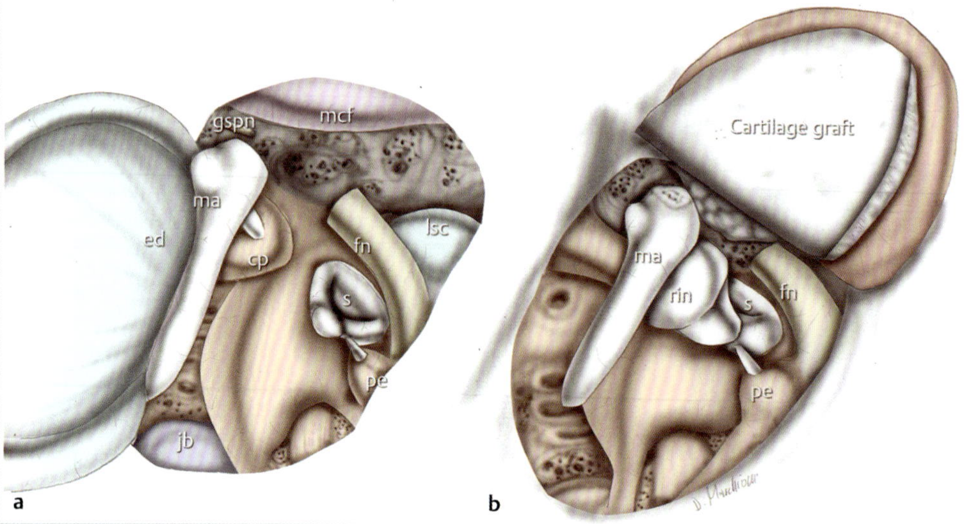

Fig. 10.11 Left ear: **(a)** The tumor is removed with the geniculate ganglion (GG) and the tympanic portion of the facial nerve. In this case, since the defect involves the whole GG, a transcanal cable graft reconstruction is not possible, due to the anatomical position of the labyrinthine portion of the facial nerve. A hypoglossal-facial anastomosis is suggested. **(b)** A remodeled autologous incus is placed between the stapes and the malleus. A cartilage graft is used to reconstruct the attical defect. *cp: cochleariform process; ed: eardrum; fn: facial nerve; gspn: greater superficial petrosal nerve; jb: jugular bulb; lsc: lateral semicircular canal; ma: malleus; mcf: middle cranial fossa; pe: pyramidal eminence; rin: remodeled autologous incus; s: stapes.*

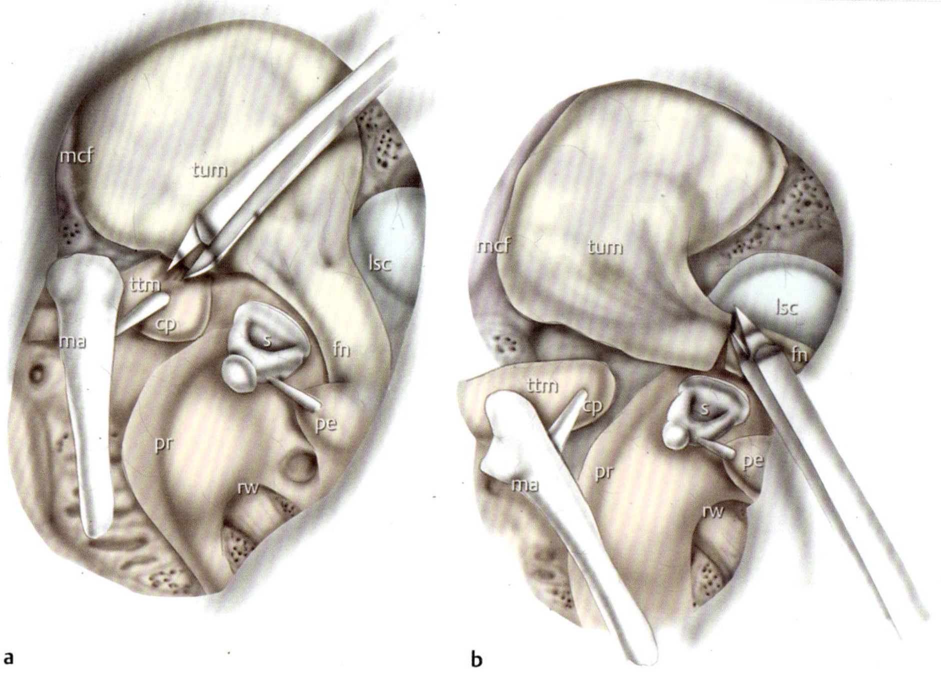

Fig. 10.12 Left ear: In this case the tumor involves the tympanic segment of the facial neve. The dissection starts to detach the tumor from the hemicanal of the tensor tympani muscle **(a)**. After this step, due to the absence of a clear cleavage plane, the tympanic segment of the facial nerve is cut in proximity to the second genu **(b)**. *cp: cochleariform process; fn: facial nerve; lsc: lateral semicircular canal; ma: malleus; mcf: middle cranial fossa; pe: pyramidal eminence; pr: promontory; rw: round window; s: stapes; ttm: hemicanal of the tensor tympani muscle; tum: tumor.*

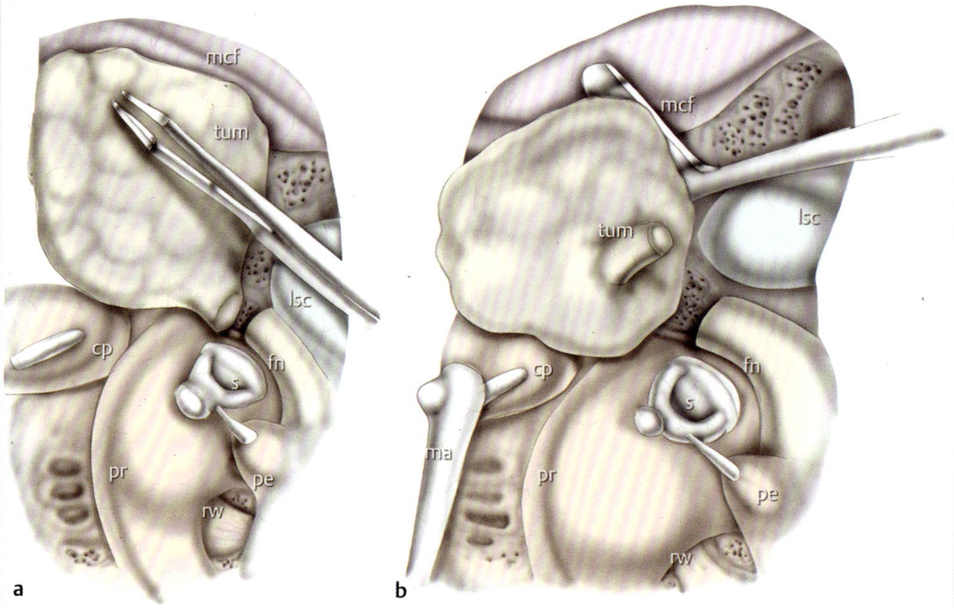

Fig. 10.13 Left ear: **(a)** In case of hemangioma, a micro-bipolar instrument may be used to reduce the bleeding and to coarct the tumor. **(b)** Once the tumor is coarcted, the plane of middle cranial fossa is endoscopically detected and a curved dissector is used to detach the tumor from the middle fossa plane. *cp: cochleariform process; fn: facial nerve; lsc: lateral semicircular canal; ma: malleus; mcf: middle cranial fossa; pe: pyramidal eminence; pr: promontory; rw: round window; s: stapes; tum: tumor.*

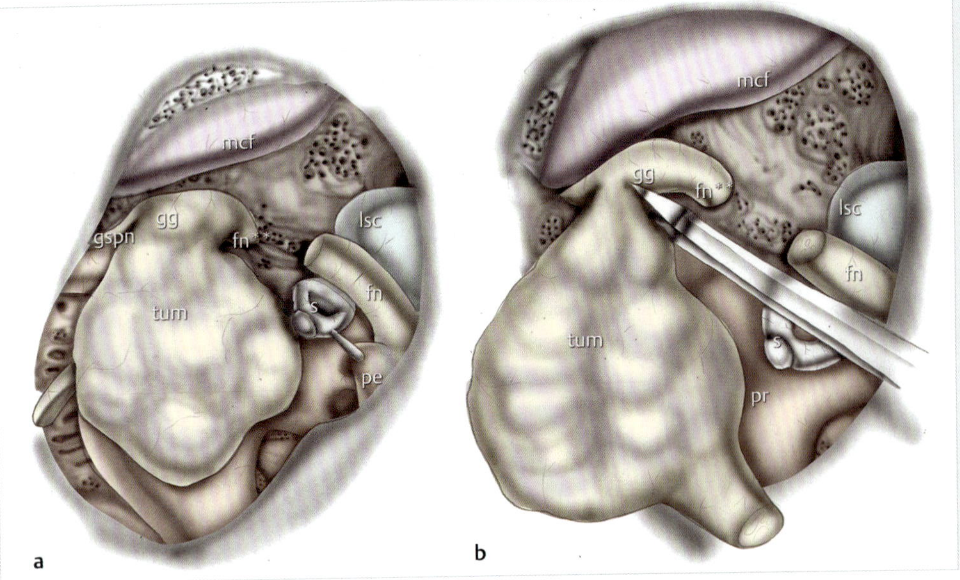

Fig. 10.14 Left ear: **(a)** Once the tumor has been detached from the middle cranial fossa plane, the geniculate ganglion (GG) is visible. **(b)** The tumor is removed. In this case, a preservation of the GG is possible since the tumor involves only the tympanic segment of the facial nerve. *fn**: labyrinthine portion of facial nerve; fn: tympanic portion of facial nerve; gspn: greater superficial petrosal nerve; lsc: lateral semicircular canal; mcf: middle cranial fossa; pe: pyramidal eminence; pr: promontory; s: stapes; tum: tumor.*

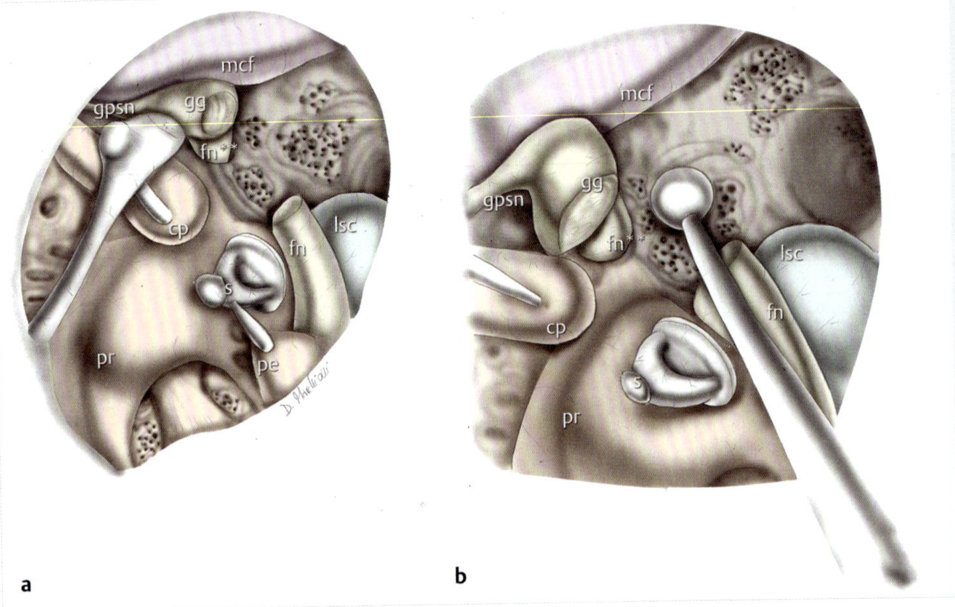

Fig. 10.15 Left ear: **(a, b)** Once the tumor has been removed, a diamond bur is used to drill the cells around the suprageniculate fossa. In case of hemangioma, to avoid a residual tumor, this step is mandatory due to the infiltration of the tumor in this anatomical area. *cp: cochleariform process; fn**: labyrinthine portion of facial nerve; fn: tympanic portion of facial nerve; gg: geniculate ganglion; gspn: greater superficial petrosal nerve; lsc: lateral semicircular canal; mcf: middle cranial fossa; pe: pyramidal eminence; pr: promontory; s: stapes.*

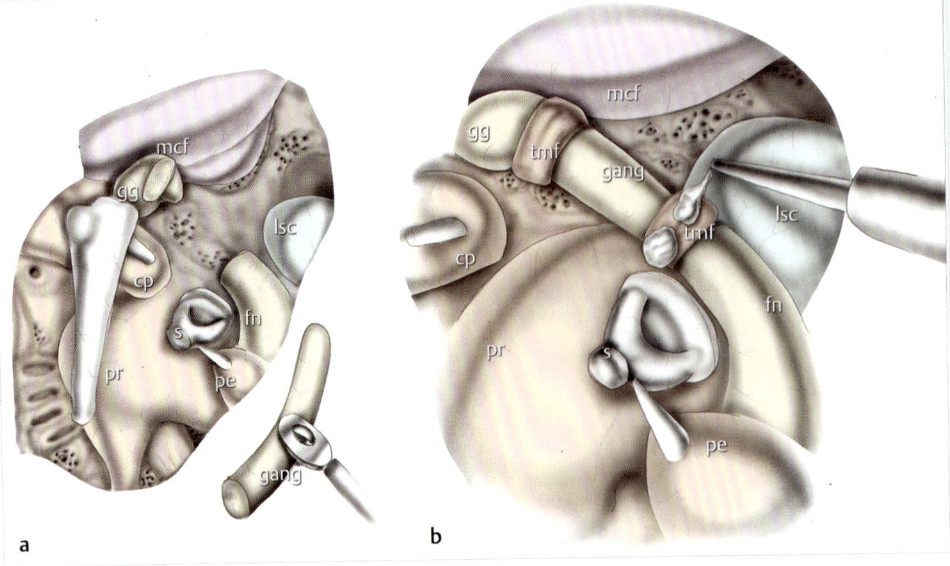

Fig. 10.16 Left ear: **(a, b)** A great auricular nerve cable graft is used to repair the facial nerve (FN) defect, placing the cable graft between the second genu of the FN and the geniculate ganglion. Pieces of temporalis fascia are used to cover the connection between the graft and the FN. Fibrin glue is used to reinforce the nerves' connections. *cp: cochleariform process; fn: facial nerve; gang: great auricular nerve graft; gg: geniculate ganglion; lsc: lateral semicircular canal; mcf: middle cranial fossa; pe: pyramidal eminence; pr: promontory; s: stapes; tmf: temporalis muscle fascia.*

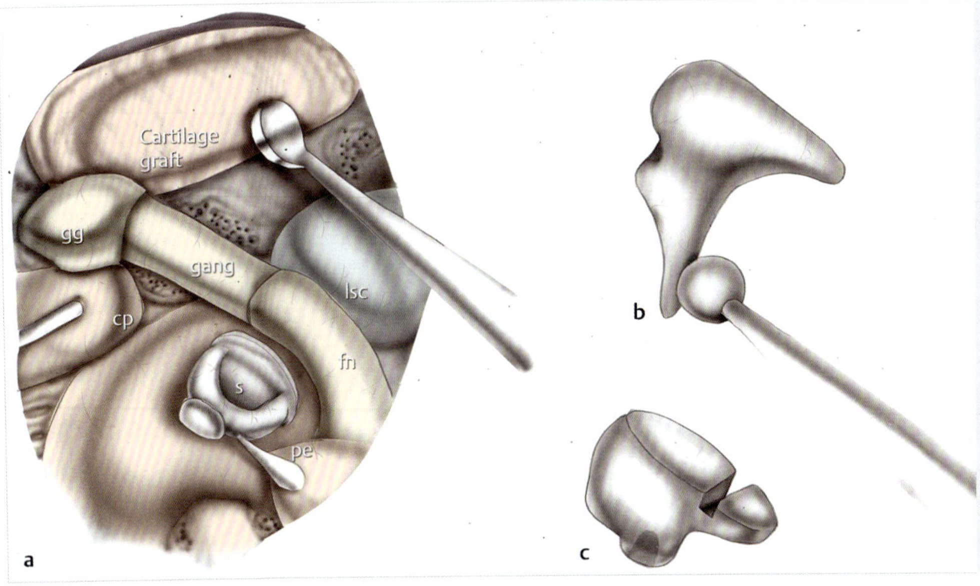

Fig. 10.17 Left ear: **(a)** A cartilage graft is placed over the middle cranial fossa dura to reconstruct the tegmen tympani defect. **(b, c)** Remodeling of the incus is performed. *cp: cochleariform process; fn: facial nerve; gang: great auricular nerve graft; gg: geniculate ganglion; lsc: lateral semicircular canal; pe: pyramidal eminence; s: stapes.*

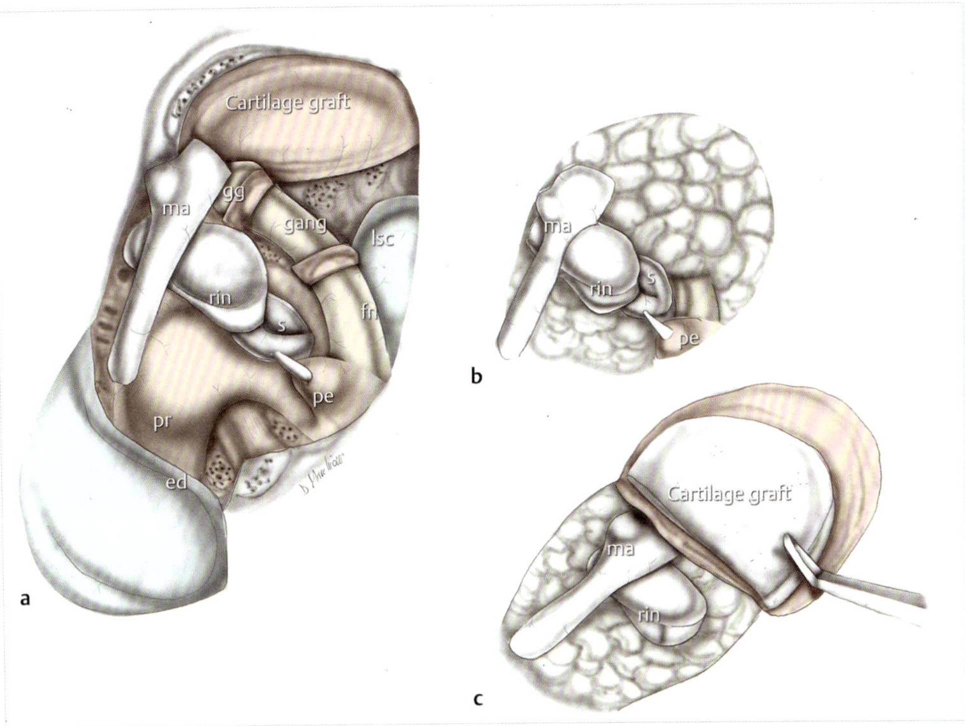

Fig. 10.18 Left ear: **(a)** A remodeled incus is placed between the stapes and the malleus. **(b)** Absorbable gelatine sponge (i.e., Gelfoam) is used to fill the cavity stabilizing the ossiculoplasty. **(c)** A cartilage graft is used to reconstruct the attical defect. *ed: eardrum; fn: facial nerve; gang: great auricular nerve graft; gg: geniculate ganglion; lsc: lateral semicircular canal; ma: malleus; pe: pyramidal eminence; pr: promontory; rin: remodeled autologous incus; s: stapes.*

10.5 ETSA for Cholesteatoma Involving the Suprageniculate Ganglion Area

The ETSA is also used in case of cholesteatoma involving the SGF, or a supralabyrinthine cholesteatoma with limited anterior extension.

10.5.1 Surgical Steps

A wide triangular shape incision around the attic is performed and a large tympanomeatal flap is created (see ▶ Fig. 10.53).

A diamond bur is used to perform a wide canaloplasty and a wide atticotomy exposing the incudomalleolar joint (see ▶ Fig. 10.54). Drilling continues until the whole attic and the antrum are exposed and the middle fossa dura plane is detected (see ▶ Fig. 10.55). The incus and malleus are removed and the cholesteatoma is exposed in the SGF (see ▶ Fig. 10.56 and ▶ Fig. 10.57). Further drilling of the posterior portion of the EAC is mandatory to expose the lateral semicircular canal (see ▶ Fig. 10.57 and ▶ Fig. 10.58). Once the lateral semicircular canal and the dura of the MCF have been detected, the tympanic segment of the facial neve should be detected and the GG decompressed using a microcurette or a diamond bur (see ▶ Fig. 10.59). Once all the anatomical landmarks have been endoscopically detected, the SGF is drilled exposing the cholesteatoma between the FN, the lateral semicircular canal, and the MCF (see ▶ Fig. 10.60, ▶ Fig. 10.61, ▶ Fig. 10.62). A cottonoid soaked with saline solution should be gently used on the FN and GG to detach the cholesteatoma from the nerve (see ▶ Fig. 10.61); a curved dissector may be helpful to remove the cholesteatoma from the SGF (see Clinical Case 4, ▶ Fig. 10.106, ▶ Fig. 10.107, ▶ Fig. 10.108, ▶ Fig. 10.109). Once the cholesteatoma has been removed, a piece of muscle is used to obliterate the attic and antrum (see ▶ Fig. 10.63). A temporalis fascia is used to cover the obliterated tissue (see

▸ Fig. 10.64). To possibly obtain a good hearing result an ossiculoplasty is performed using a remodeled incus and a cartilage graft is used to reconstruct the attical defect. A temporalis fascia is also used to cover the cartilage graft and the eardrum is replaced (see ▸ Fig. 10.65).

10.5.2 Inner Ear Involvement (see Clinical Case 3 and Case 5)

In case of a supralabyrinthine cholesteatoma or a cholesteatoma involving the inner ear, an obliteration of the cavity with an EAC blind sac closure is preferable.

A circumferential incision with progressive EAC skin and eardrum removal is performed.

Once the tympanic cavity, the attic, and the antrum with the semicircular canal and middle cranial fossa have been exposed, a total decompression of the GG is performed. The CP is removed and the muscle of the tensor tendon is anteriorly pulled. The stapes is removed exposing the vestibule (see ▸ Fig. 10.66). The lateral semicircular canal should be drilled in order to expose the vestibule in the superior portion, and in order to gain enough surgical space to remove the cholesteatoma lying in the suprageniculate space (see ▸ Fig. 10.67, ▸ Fig. 10.68). Once the cholesteatoma has been removed, a piece of muscle is used to obliterate the eustachian tube (see ▸ Fig. 10.68b). The cavity is filled with abdominal fat and the skin of the EAC is reversed and a blind sac closure of the EAC is performed (see ▸ Fig. 10.69).

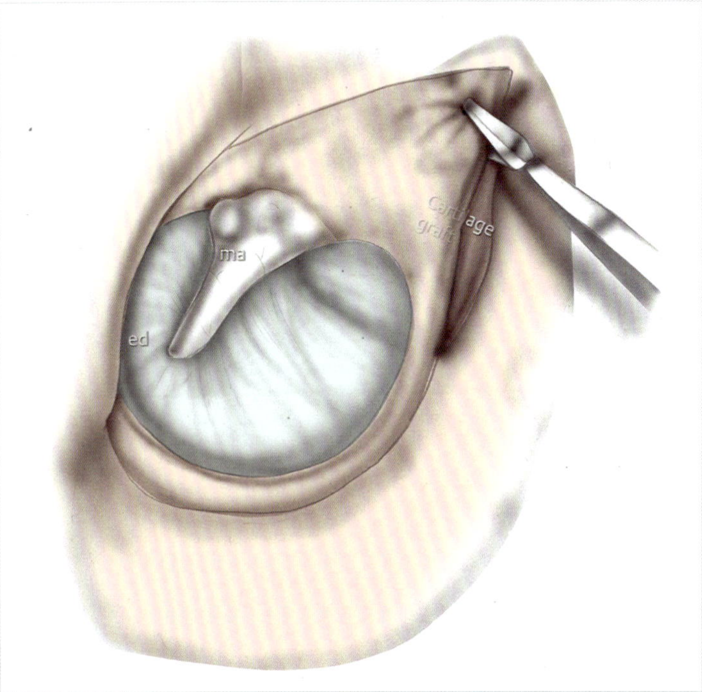

Fig. 10.19 Left ear: The tympanomeatal flap is replaced over the cartilage graft. *ed: eardrum; ma: malleus.*

10.6 ETSA for Decompression of the Geniculate Ganglion and of the Tympanic Facial Nerve

The transcanal endoscopic decompression of the tympanic segment of the FN allows a good exposure of the second genu and the most anterior portion of the nerve, in particular, the region lying anterior to the CP, in close proximity to the GG. The anterior epitympanum and the supratubal recess are correctly shown, without a transmastoid posterior atticotomy (see Clinical Case 6 and Clinical Case 7).

10.6.1 Surgical Steps

Under a 0-degree endoscopic view, a skin incision of the posterior wall of the EAC is performed with a round knife from 11 o'clock to 6 o'clock (see ▸ Fig. 10.115a). An anteriorly and posteriorly based tympanomeatal flap is endoscopically elevated. The tympanic membrane is gently detached from the malleus, cutting the adhesion located in the umbus between the eardrum and the handle of the malleus (see ▸ Fig. 10.115b). The tympanomeatal flap is gently inferiorly pulled in order to uncover the whole scutum and the rim of the fracture involving the pregeniculate area. The scutum is partially drilled, allowing for an adequate access to the anterior epitympanum. The bony fragments from the fracture involving the pregeniculate area and the anterior epitympanum are carefully removed preserving the integrity of the ossicular chain. When an interruption of the incudomalleolar joint is found, the incus and the head of the malleus are removed exposing the FN and the GG area (see ▸ Fig. 10.116). The CP and the cog are endoscopically detected, representing important landmarks for the identification of the GG. Then the bony spicule compressing the GG is detected and removed using a microcurette (see ▸ Fig. 10.117). When required, the CP is removed using a microcurette and the tensor tendon muscle is detached from the GG and anteriorly pulled in order to improve the decompression of the GG (see ▸ Fig. 10.118).

Alternatively, instead of removing the incus, the malleus may be disarticulated from the incus, and then gently pulled down,

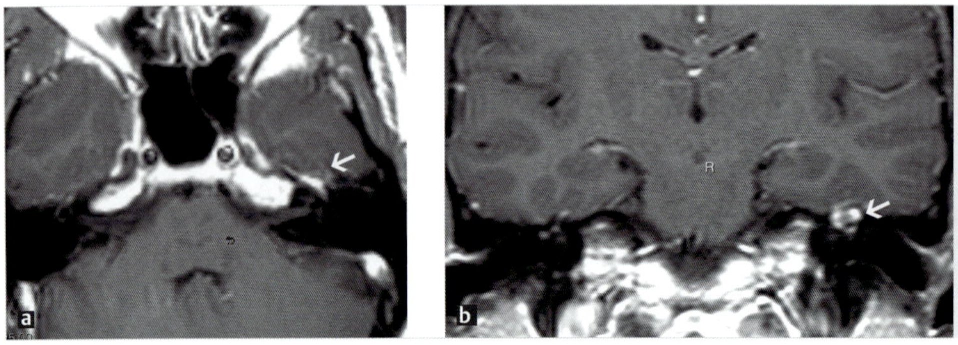

Fig. 10.20 Clinical Case 1: Magnetic resonance imaging (MRI) in axial **(a)** and coronal **(b)** views, showing a tumor of the geniculate ganglion (*white arrow*).

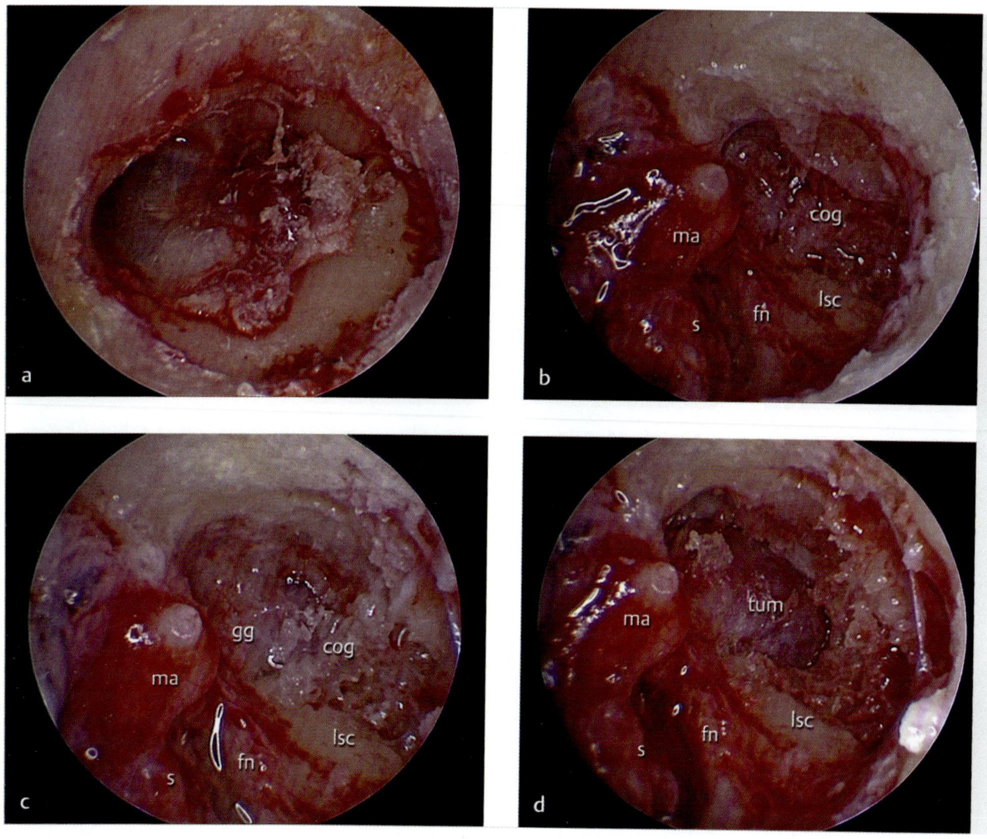

Fig. 10.21 Clinical Case 1, Left ear: Geniculate ganglion (GG) schwannoma. **(a)** A tympanomeatal flap is created and elevated. **(b)** The scutum is removed exposing the attic. The lateral semicircular canal, the tympanic segment of facial nerve, and the cog are endoscopically detected. **(c)** A diamond bur is used to remove the cells over the GG area. **(d)** The tumor of the GG is exposed. *fn: facial nerve; gg: geniculate ganglion; lsc: lateral semicircular canal; ma: malleus; s: stapes; tum: tumor.*

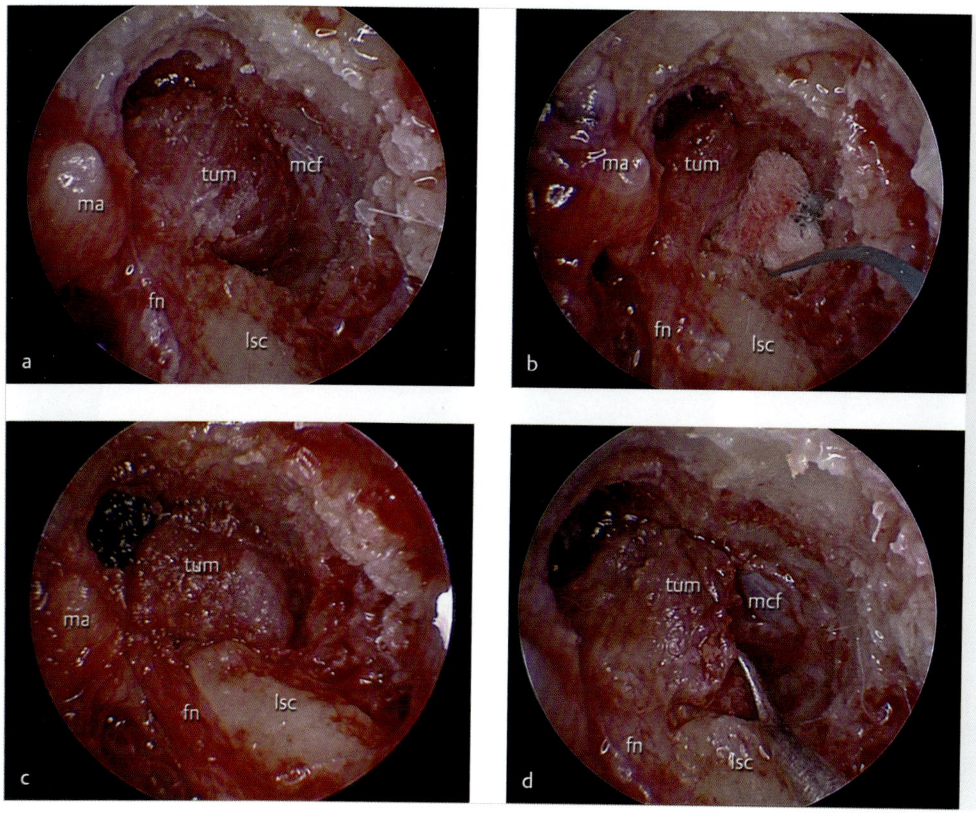

Fig. 10.22 Clinical Case 1, Left ear: Geniculate ganglion schwannoma. **(a)** Endoscopic magnification of the geniculate ganglion. **(b)** A cottonoid is used to dissect the tumor avoiding bleeding. **(c)** Absorbable hemostatic material (i.e., Surgicel) is used to prevent bleeding between the middle fossa dura and the tumor. **(d)** A curved dissector is used to detach the tumor from the dural plane of the middle cranial fossa (MCF). *fn: facial nerve; ma: malleus; lsc: lateral semicircular canal; mcf: middle cranial fossa; tum: tumor.*

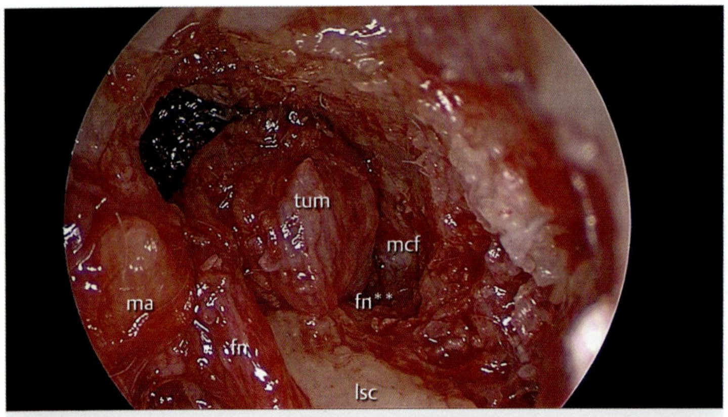

Fig. 10.23 Clinical Case 1, Left ear: Geniculate ganglion schwannoma. Once the tumor has been detached from the dura of the middle cranial fossa, the labyrinthine portion of the facial nerve and the posterior portion of the tumor are endoscopically visible. *fn: tympanic portion of facial nerve; fn**: labyrinthine portion of facial nerve; lsc: lateral semicircular canal; ma: malleus; tum: tumor; mcf: middle cranial fossa.*

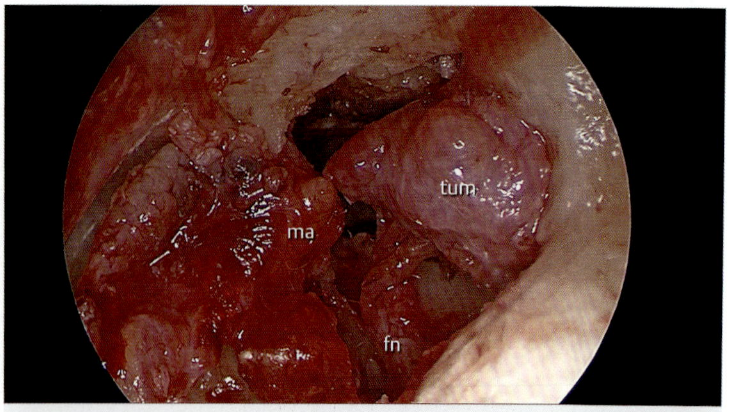

Fig. 10.24 Clinical Case 1, Left ear: Geniculate ganglion schwannoma. The labyrinthine portion of the facial nerve and the greater superficial petrosal nerve are cut. The tumor is thus mobilized. *fn: facial nerve; ma: malleus; tum: tumor.*

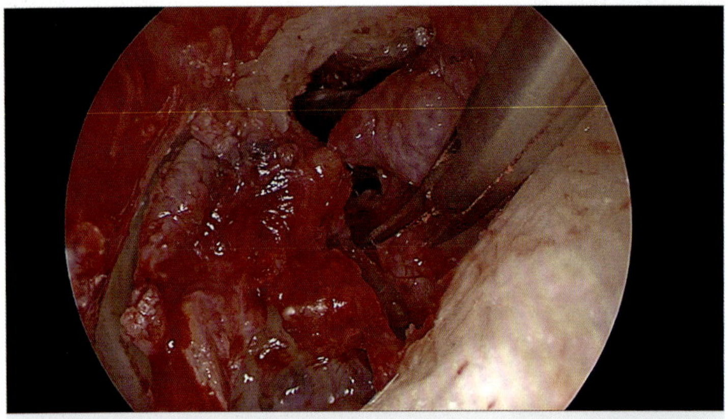

Fig. 10.25 Clinical Case 1, Left ear: Geniculate ganglion schwannoma. The facial nerve is cut in proximity to the second genu.

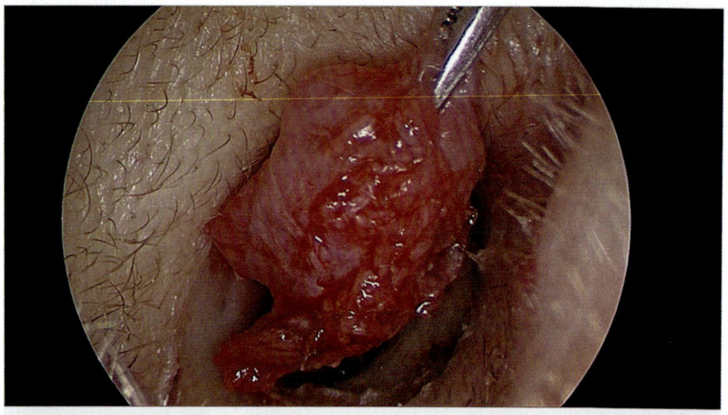

Fig. 10.26 Clinical Case 1, Left ear: Geniculate ganglion schwannoma. The tumor is removed.

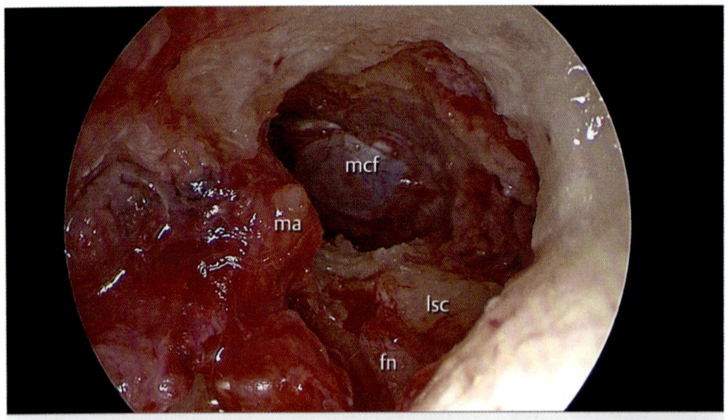

Fig. 10.27 Clinical Case 1, Left ear: Geniculate ganglion schwannoma. In this case, the whole geniculate ganglion with the tumor is removed; the middle cranial fossa dura is exposed and well visible. *fn: tympanic portion of facial nerve; lsc: lateral semicircular canal; ma: malleus; mcf: middle cranial fossa.*

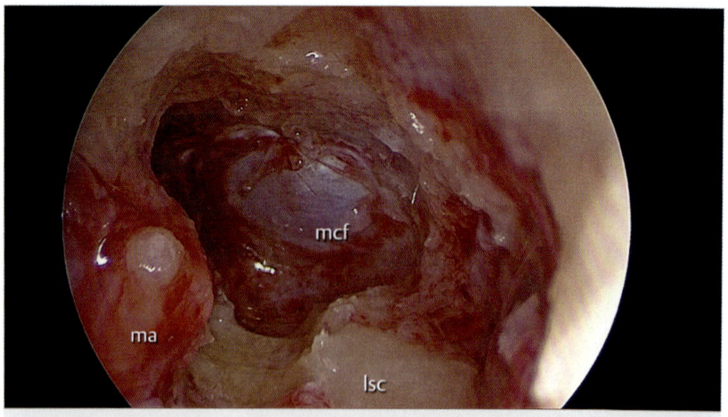

Fig. 10.28 Clinical Case 1, Left ear: Geniculate ganglion schwannoma. The suprageniculate fossa between the dura of middle cranial fossa and the lateral semicircular canal is drilled to perform the radicalization of tumor removal. *lsc: lateral semicircular canal; ma: malleus; mcf: middle cranial fossa.*

without removing it from the tensor tympani tendon (see Clinical Case 6, ▶ Fig. 10.140, ▶ Fig. 10.141, ▶ Fig. 10.142). After this procedure, the tympanic segment of the FN with the GG area is endoscopically visible, allowing for a wide working area. The decompression of the whole tympanic segment is easily performed under an endoscopic view. The fracture on the GG is detected and the bony fragments pressing on the GG are carefully removed using a small dissector. The decompression of the GG is performed until the GSPN is reached. After this procedure, some absorbable gelatin sponge (i.e., Gelfoam) soaked with a corticosteroid solution is placed in the surgical field, close to the FN. The incus is remodeled and gently placed between the stapes and the malleus, restoring the integrity of the ossicular chain. In case of tegmen defect, it is possible to reconstruct the defect with a

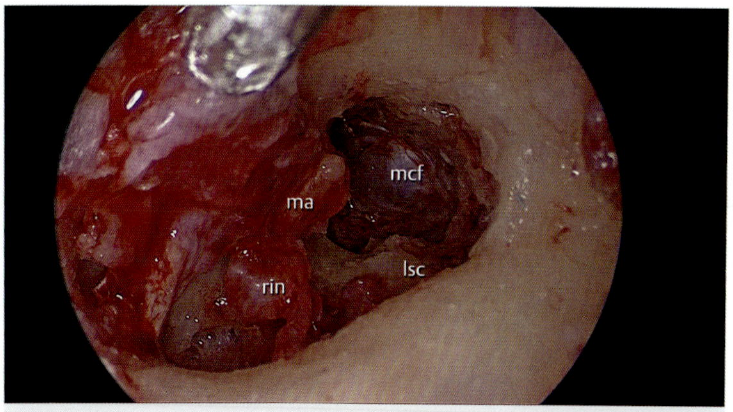

Fig. 10.29 Clinical Case 1, Left ear: Geniculate ganglion schwannoma. A remodeled incus is placed between the stapes and the malleus. *lsc: lateral semicircular canal; ma: malleus; mcf: middle cranial fossa; rin: autologous remodeled incus.*

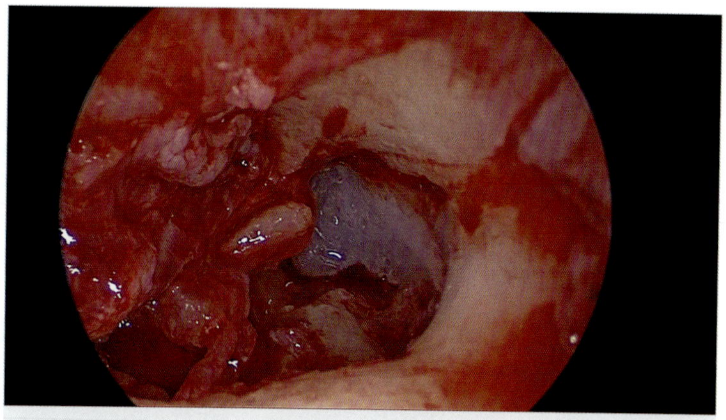

Fig. 10.30 Clinical Case 1, Left ear: Geniculate ganglion schwannoma. A cartilage graft is placed over the tegmen defect, and fibrin glue is used to reinforce the reconstruction.

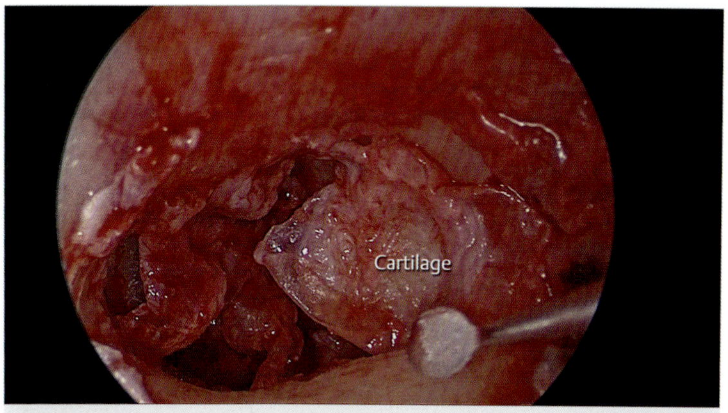

Fig. 10.31 Clinical Case 1, Left ear: Geniculate ganglion schwannoma. A tragal cartilage is used to reconstruct the scutum defect.

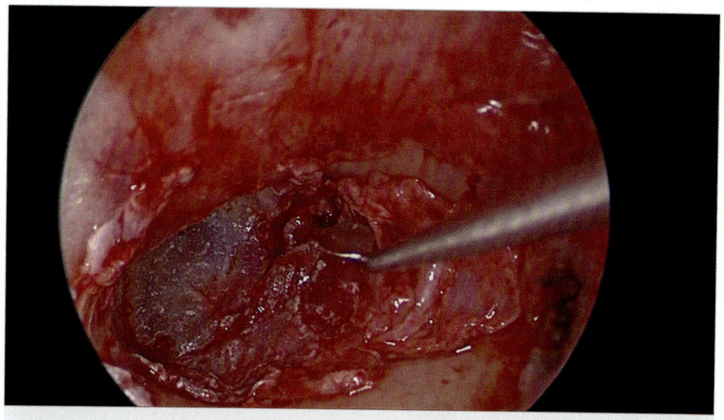

Fig. 10.32 Clinical Case 1, Left ear: Geniculate ganglion schwannoma. The tympanomeatal flap is replaced on the cartilage graft.

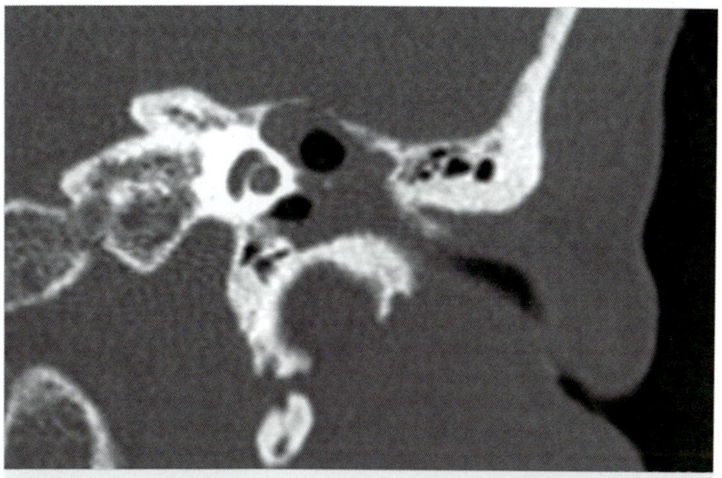

Fig. 10.33 Clinical Case 1, Left ear: Geniculate ganglion schwannoma. Computed tomography (CT) scan in coronal view after surgery. The defect of the attic in the suprageniculate fossa is noted.

cartilage graft harvested from the tragus (see ▶ Fig. 10.119a). The tympanomeatal flap is repositioned, and the EAC is filled with absorbable gelatin sponge (see ▶ Fig. 10.119b).

10.6.2 Postoperative Care and Follow-up

All the patients should undergo a brain CT scan on the first postoperative day to rule out complications. Intravenous antibiotic therapy (third generation—cephalosporin) is administered for 48 hours after surgery. Postoperative pain is well controlled using intravenous analgesics.

The FN function (HB scale) is rated both immediately after surgery and during the follow-up time.

In case of decompression of of the FN and the GG during hospital stay, intravenous corticosteroids and antibiotics (third generation—cephalosporine) are administered, followed by antibiotic and corticosteroid oral therapy when the patient is discharged.

The FN function (according to HB scale[4]) is evaluated immediately after surgery and during the follow-up time. An otoendoscopic evaluation is performed 1 month after surgery. Other otoendoscopic and audiologic examinations are performed 4, 6, and 12 months after surgery.

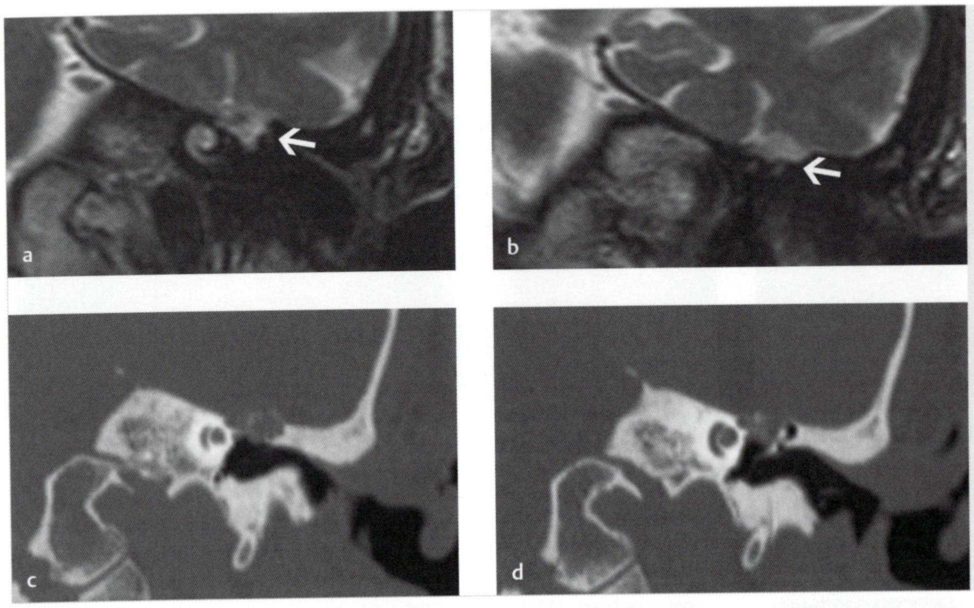

Fig. 10.34 Clinical Case 2: Magnetic resonance imaging (MRI) in coronal view **(a, b)** showing a left facial nerve tumor growing in the suprageniculate fossa with dural involvement. Computed tomography (CT) scan in coronal view **(c, d)** showing the typical features of a facial nerve hemangioma with bony erosion around the tumor.

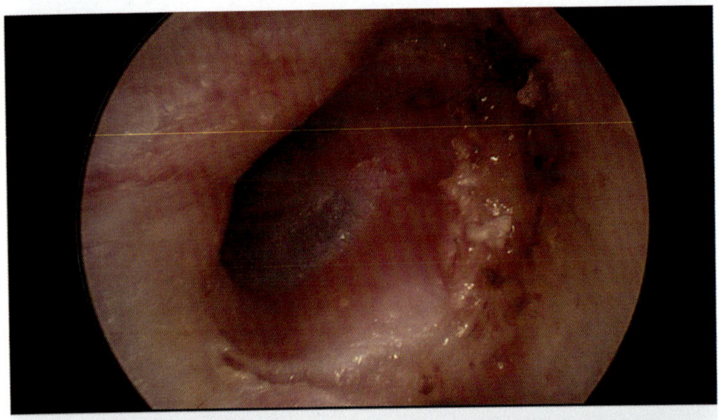

Fig. 10.35 Clinical Case 2, Left ear: Facial nerve hemangioma. The incision of the skin of the external auditory canal is performed.

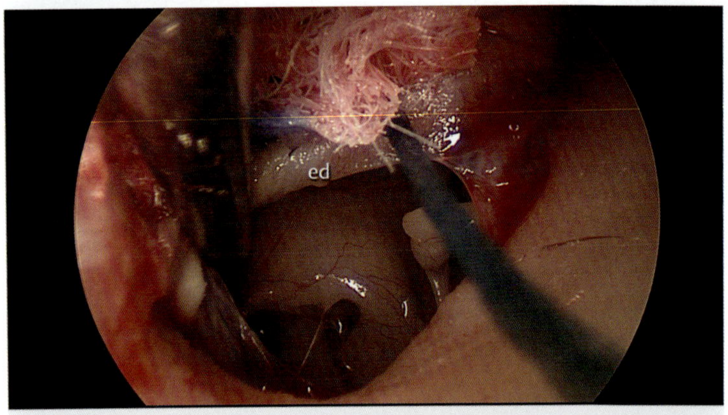

Fig. 10.36 Clinical Case 2, Left ear: Facial nerve hemangioma. The tympanomeatal flap is elevated entering the tympanic cavity. *ed: eardrum.*

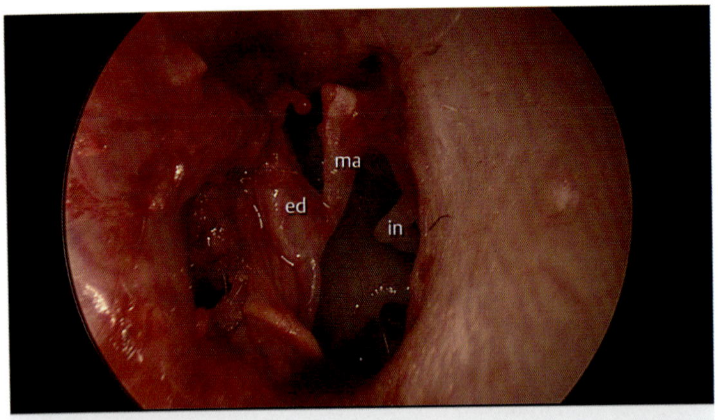

Fig. 10.37 Clinical Case 2, Left ear: Facial nerve hemangioma. The tympanomeatal flap is partially detached from the malleus, maintaining just the umbo's adherences. *ed: eardrum; in: incus; ma: malleus.*

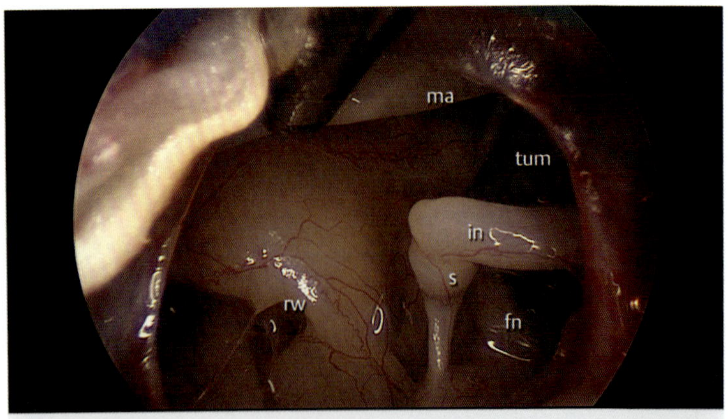

Fig. 10.38 Clinical Case 2, Left ear: Facial nerve (FN) hemangioma. The FN hemangioma is endoscopically visible, arising from the tympanic segment of the FN, medial to the ossicular chain. *fn: facial nerve; in: incus; ma: malleus; rw: round window; s: stapes; tum: tumor.*

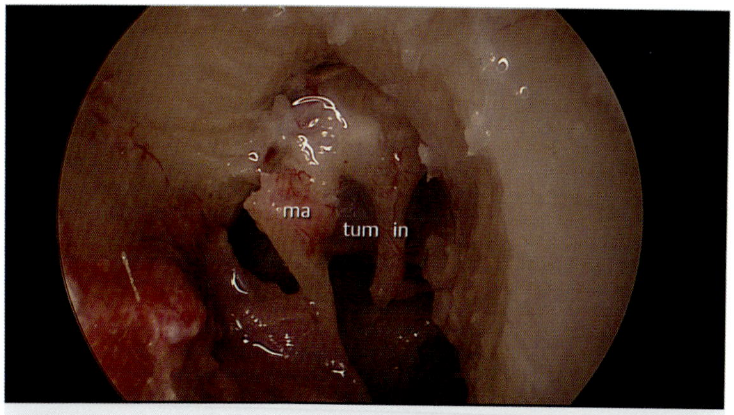

Fig. 10.39 Clinical Case 2, Left ear: Facial nerve hemangioma. The atticotomy is performed using piezosurgery. *in: incus; ma: malleus; tum: tumor.*

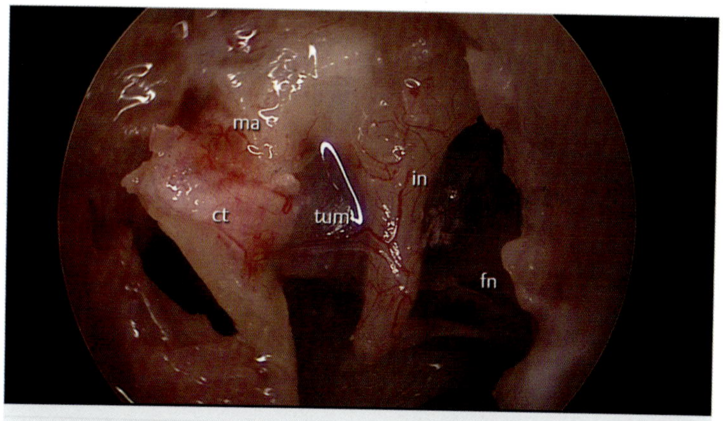

Fig. 10.40 Clinical Case 2, Left ear: Facial nerve (FN) hemangioma. The chorda tympani is cut and the FN hemangioma is endoscopically magnified. *ct: chorda tympani; fn: facial nerve; in: incus; ma: malleus; tum: tumor.*

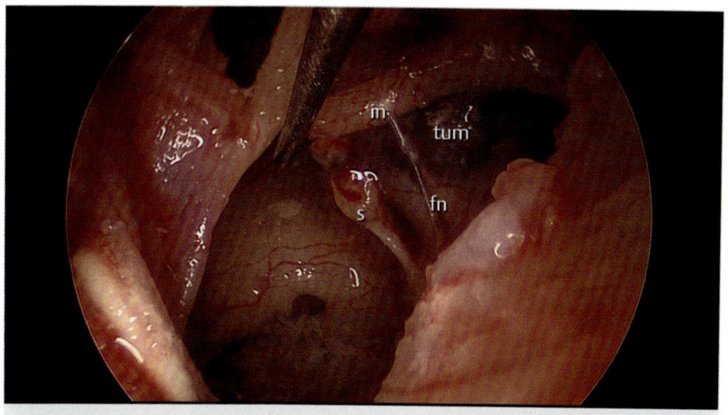

Fig. 10.41 Clinical Case 2, Left ear: Facial nerve hemangioma. The incus is removed, carefully detaching the incudostapedial joint with a micro-hook. *fn: facial nerve; in: incus; s: stapes; tum: tumor.*

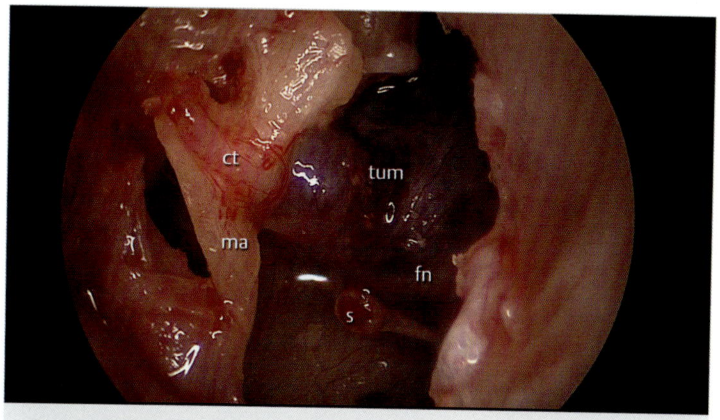

Fig. 10.42 Clinical Case 2, Left ear: Facial nerve (FN) hemangioma. After the incus removal, the FN hemangioma is exposed. *ct: chorda tympani; fn: facial nerve; ma: malleus; s: stapes; tum: tumor.*

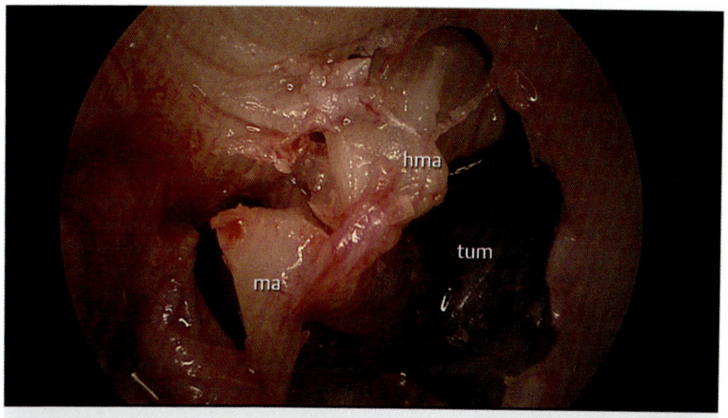

Fig. 10.43 Clinical Case 2, Left ear: Facial nerve hemangioma. The head of the malleus is cut and removed. *hma: head of malleus; ma: malleus; tum: tumor.*

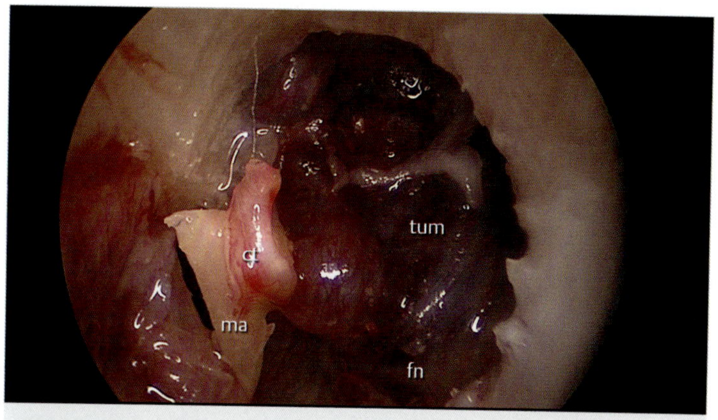

Fig. 10.44 Clinical Case 2, Left ear: Facial nerve (FN) hemangioma. After the head of the malleus removal, the tumor is progressively isolated. *ct: chorda tympani; fn: facial nerve; ma: malleus; tum: tumor.*

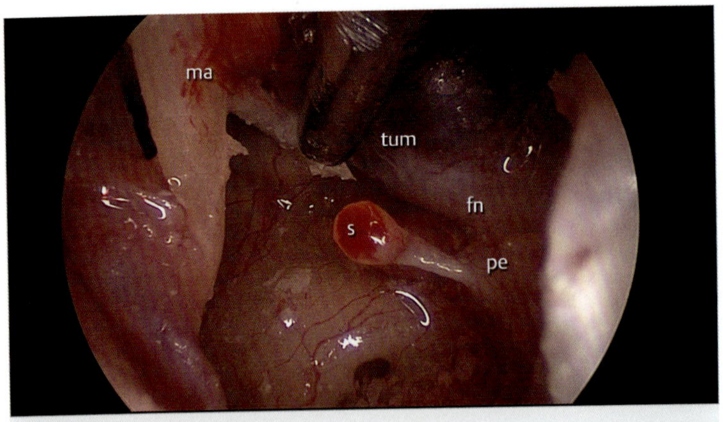

Fig. 10.45 Clinical Case 2, Left ear: Facial nerve (FN) hemangioma. No clear plane of cleavage is found between the tympanic segment of the FN and the tumor. *fn: facial nerve; ma: malleus; pe: pyramidal eminence; s: stapes; tum: tumor.*

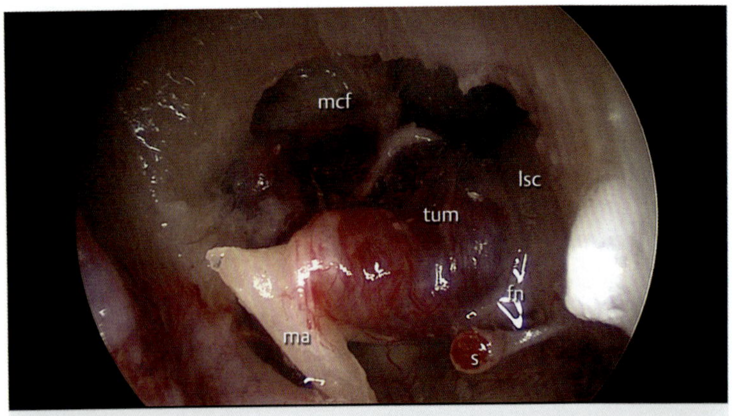

Fig. 10.46 Clinical Case 2, Left ear: Facial nerve hemangioma. Using a 45-degree endoscope the tumor is progressively detached from the middle fossa dural plane and from the lateral semicircular canal. *fn: facial nerve; lsc: lateral semicircular canal; ma: malleus; mcf: middle cranial fossa; s: stapes; tum: tumor.*

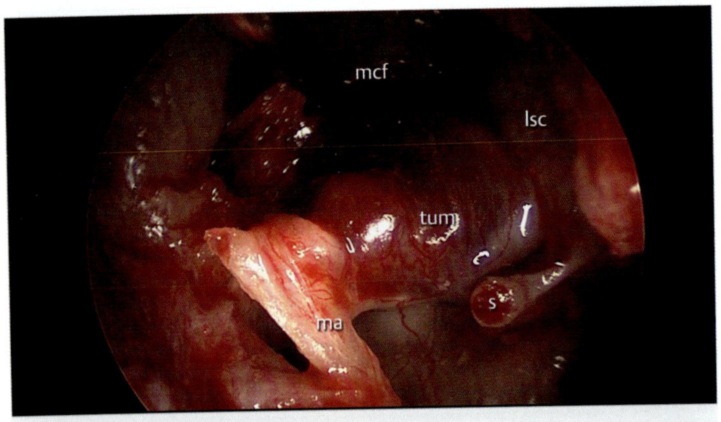

Fig. 10.47 Clinical Case 2, Left ear: Facial nerve (FN) hemangioma. The FN hemangioma is progressively coarcted in a posterior to anterior, and a superior to inferior direction using a micro-bipolar instrument. *lsc: lateral semicircular canal; ma: malleus; mcf: middle cranial fossa; s: stapes; tum: tumor.*

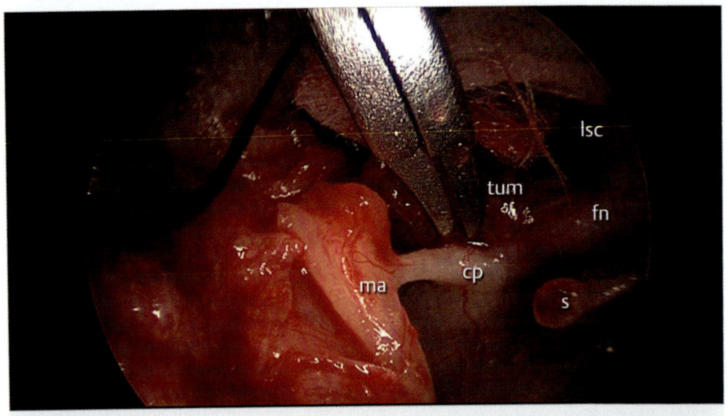

Fig. 10.48 Clinical Case 2, Left ear: Facial nerve hemangioma. A microscissor is used to cut the adhesion between the tumor and the tensor tympani muscle over the cochleariform process. *cp: cochleariform process; fn: facial nerve; lsc: lateral semicircular canal; ma: malleus; s: stapes; tum: tumor.*

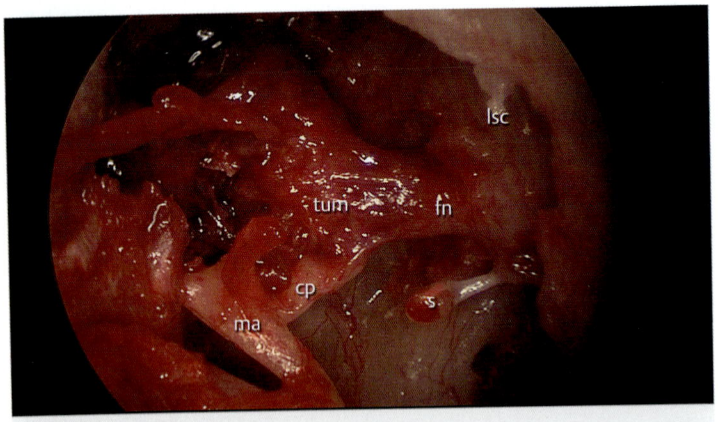

Fig. 10.49 Clinical Case 2, Left ear: Facial nerve (FN) hemangioma. The tumor dissection from the tympanic FN is started. *cp: cochleariform process; fn: facial nerve; lsc: lateral semicircular canal; ma: malleus; s: stapes; tum: tumor.*

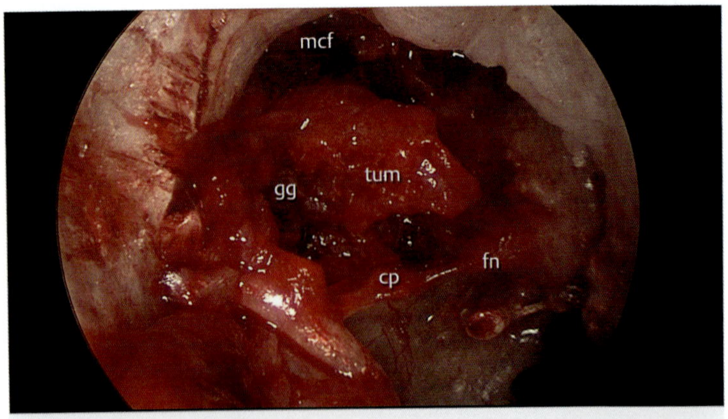

Fig. 10.50 Clinical Case 2, Left ear: Facial nerve (FN) hemangioma. The tympanic segment of the FN is cut in proximity to the second genu. *cp: cochleariform process; fn: facial nerve; gg: geniculate ganglion; mcf: middle cranial fossa; tum: tumor.*

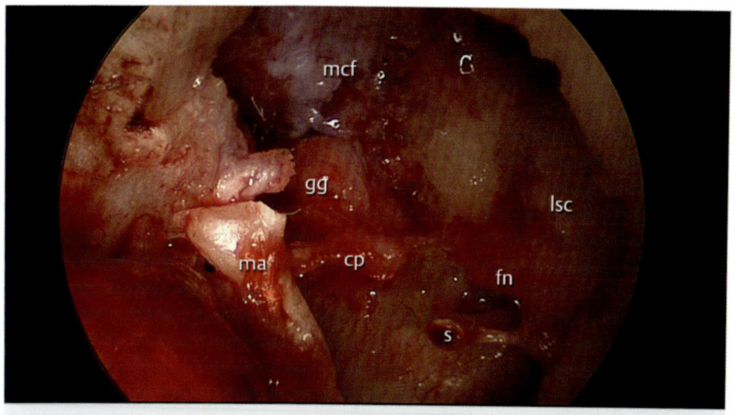

Fig. 10.51 Clinical Case 2, Left ear: Facial nerve (FN) hemangioma. The tumor is removed with the tympanic segment of the FN. In this case the geniculate ganglion is preserved. A reconstruction of the FN with a nerve cable graft can be attempted. *cp: cochleariform process; fn: facial nerve; gg: geniculate ganglion; lsc: lateral semicircular canal; mcf: middle cranial fossa; s: stapes.*

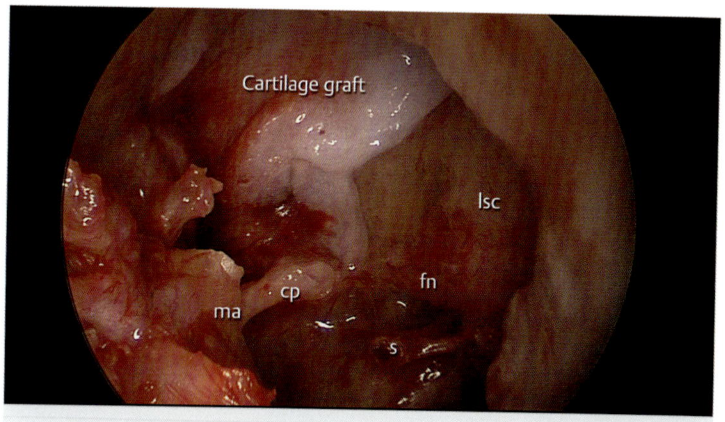

Fig. 10.52 Clinical Case 2, Left ear: Facial nerve hemangioma. A cartilage graft fixed with fibrin glue is used to reconstruct the tegmen tympani defect. *cp: cochleariform process; fn: facial nerve; lsc: lateral semicircular canal; ma: malleus; s: stapes.*

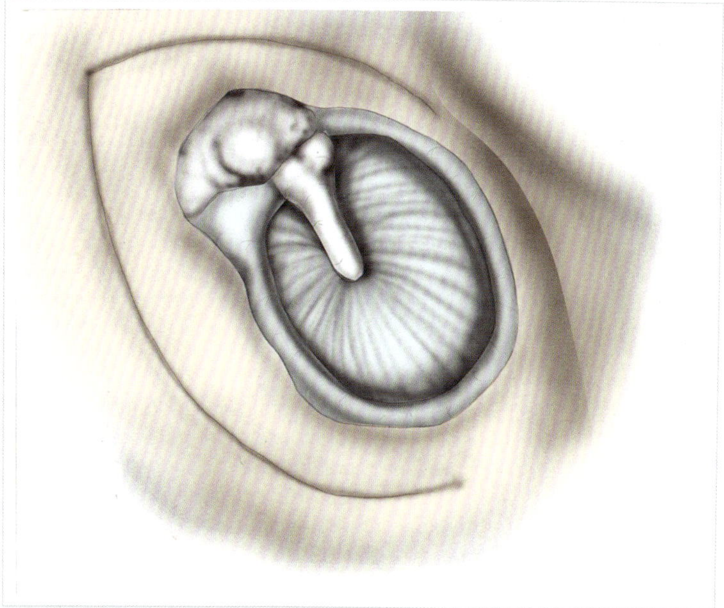

Fig. 10.53 Right ear: A triangular incision of the skin of the external auditory canal around the attic is made.

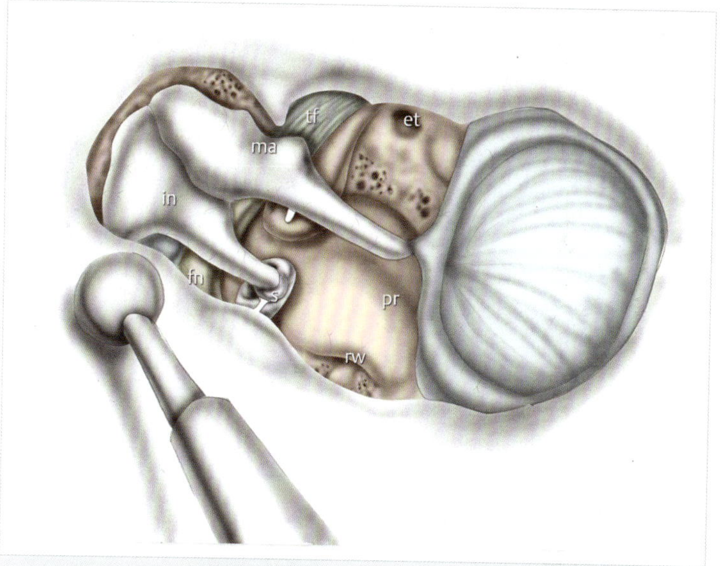

Fig. 10.54 Right ear: A diamond bur is used to remove the scutum and uncover the incudomalleolar joint in the attic. *et: eustachian tube; fn: facial nerve; in: incus; ma: malleus; pr: promontory; rw: round window; s: stapes; tf: tensor fold.*

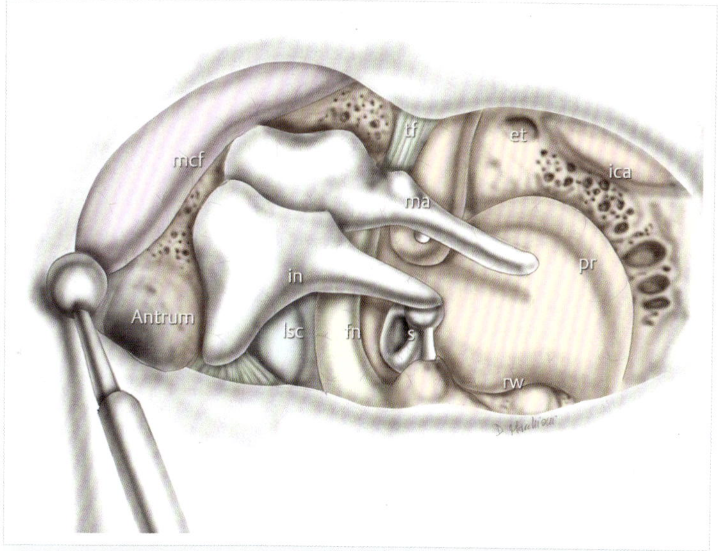

Fig. 10.55 Right ear: Using a diamond bur, the line of the middle cranial fossa dura is endoscopically detected from the antrum to the anterior attic. *et: eustachian tube; fn: facial nerve; ica: internal carotid artery; in: incus; lsc: lateral semicircular canal; ma: malleus; mcf: middle cranial fossa; pr: promontory; rw: round window; s: stapes; tf: tensor fold.*

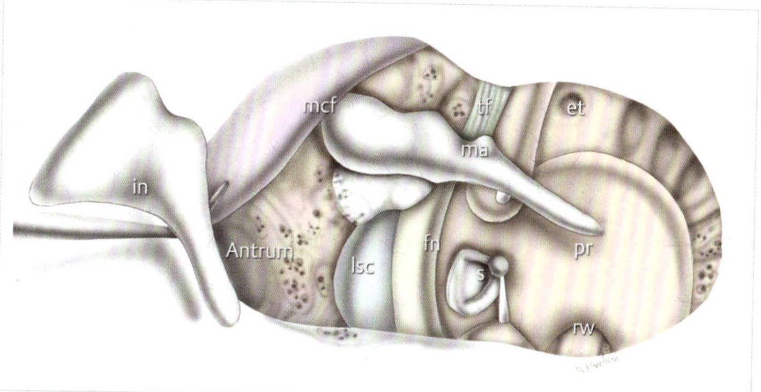

Fig. 10.56 Right ear: The incus is removed, and the perilabyrinthine cholesteatoma is seen in the suprageniculate fossa. *et: eustachian tube; fn: facial nerve; in: incus; lsc: lateral semicircular canal; ma: malleus; mcf: middle cranial fossa; pr: promontory; rw: round window; s: stapes; tf: tensor fold.*

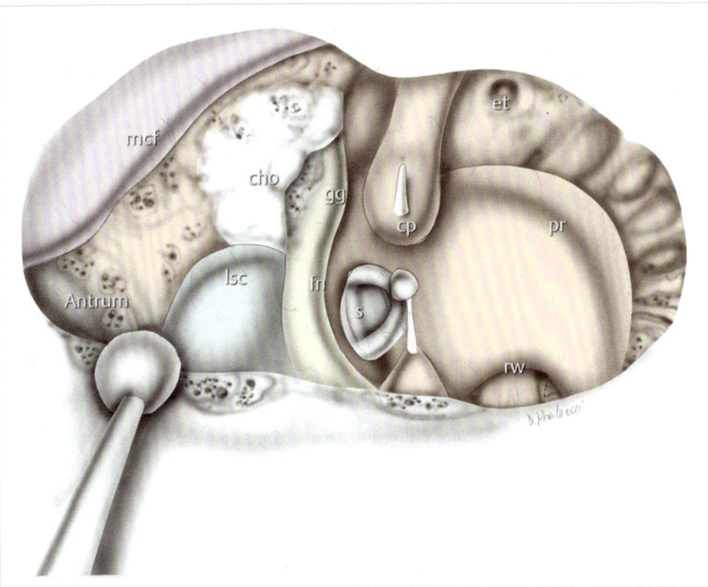

Fig. 10.57 Right ear: The malleus is removed; the cholesteatoma involving the suprageniculate fossa is endoscopically visible. Using a diamond bur, the suprageniculate approach is started endoscopically looking for the anatomical landmarks, such as lateral semicircular canal, facial nerve, geniculate ganglion, and middle cranial fossa dura. *cho: cholesteatoma; cp: cochleariform process; et: eustachian tube; fn: facial nerve; gg: geniculate ganglion; lsc: lateral semicircular canal; mcf: middle cranial fossa; pr: promontory; rw: round window; s: stapes.*

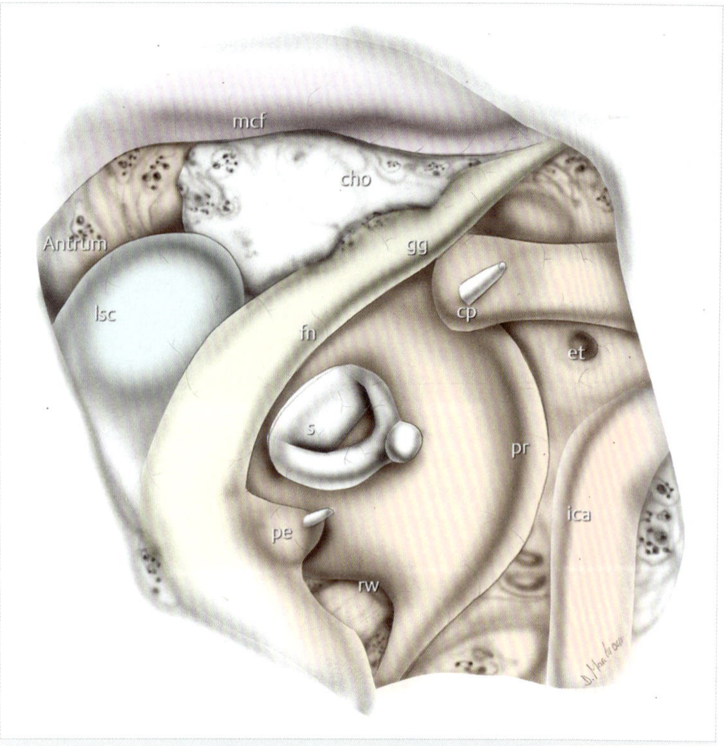

Fig. 10.58 Right ear: Drilling the triangular-shaped bone between the middle cranial fossa dura, the lateral semicircular canal, and the facial nerve, the cholesteatoma is progressively exposed in the suprageniculate fossa. *cho: cholesteatoma; cp: cochleariform process; et: eustachian tube; fn: facial nerve; gg: geniculate ganglion; ica: internal carotid artery; lsc: lateral semicircular canal; mcf: middle cranial fossa; pe: pyramidal eminence; pr: promontory; rw: round window; s: stapes.*

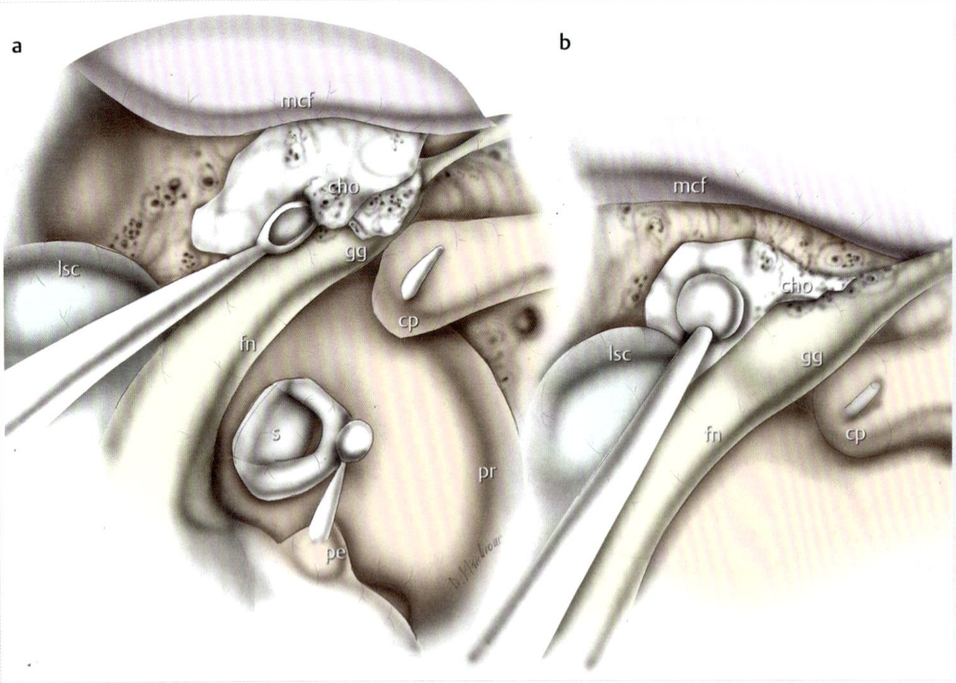

Fig. 10.59 Right ear: **(a)** A micro curette is used to remove the newly formed bone over the geniculate ganglion (GG). **(b)** Once the GG has been detected, a diamond bur is used to remove the bony cells in the suprageniculate fossa in order to remove the cholesteatoma. *cho: cholesteatoma; cp: cochleariform process; fn: facial nerve; gg: geniculate ganglion; lsc: lateral semicircular canal; mcf: middle cranial fossa; pe: pyramidal eminence; pr: promontory; s: stapes.*

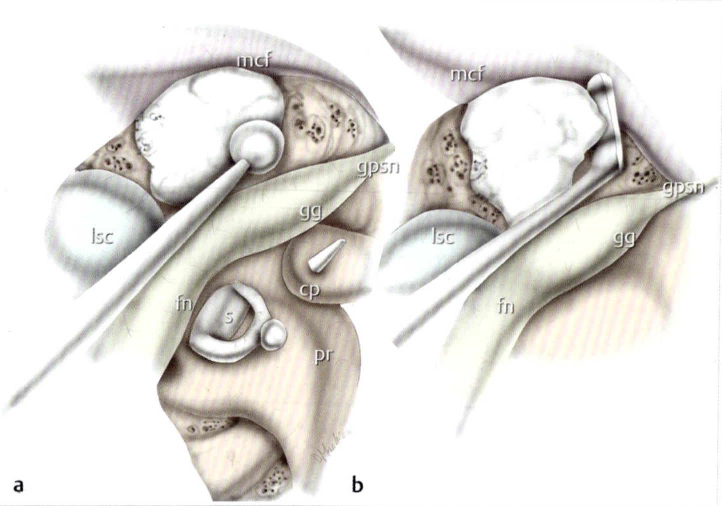

Fig. 10.60 Right ear: **(a, b)** Once the petrous apex in the supra-geniculate fossa has been reached, a curved dissector is used to remove the cholesteatoma from the middle fossa dura. *cp: cochleari-form process; fn: facial nerve; gg: geniculate ganglion; gspn: greater superficial petrosal nerve; lsc: lateral semicircular canal; mcf: middle cranial fossa; pr: promontory; s: stapes.*

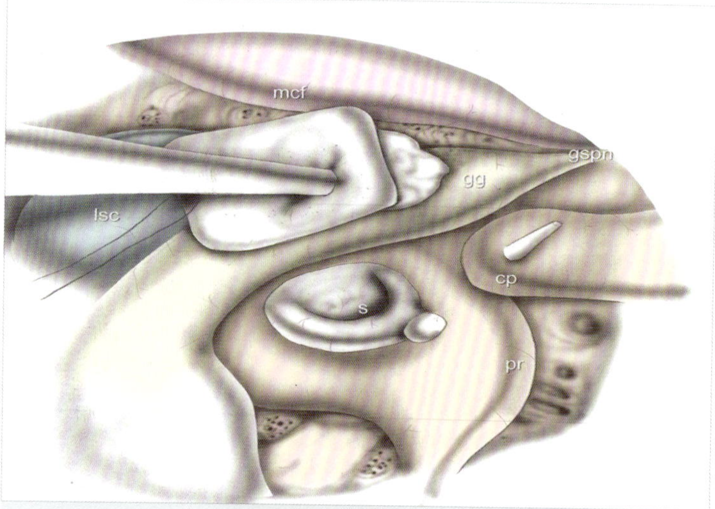

Fig. 10.61 Right ear: In case of facial nerve (FN) cholesteatoma infiltration, a cottonoid soaked with a saline solution is gently pulled over the FN using a suction tube to remove the matrix from the nerve. *cp: cochleariform process; gg: geniculate ganglion; gspn: greater superficial petrosal nerve; lsc: lateral semicircular canal; mcf: middle cranial fossa; pr: promontory; s: stapes.*

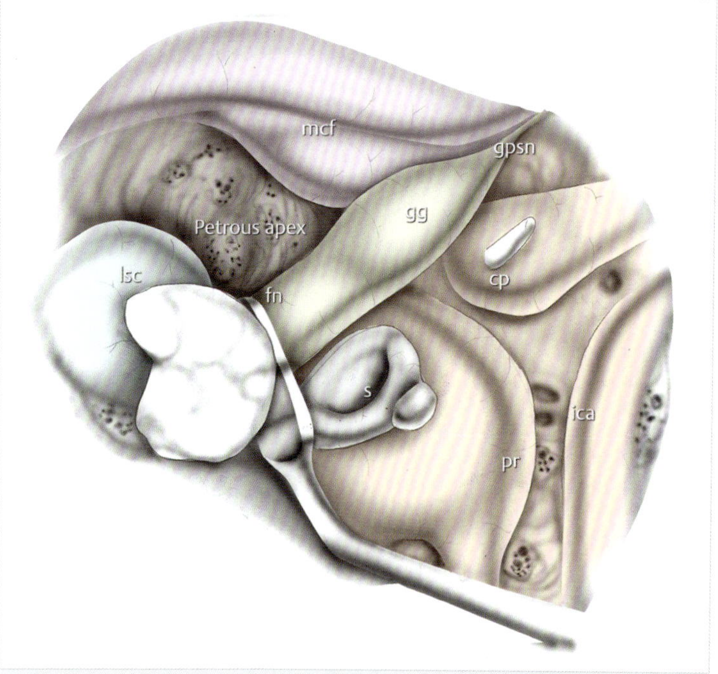

Fig. 10.62 Right ear: A curved dissector is used to remove the remnant cholesteatoma from the facial nerve. *cp: cochleariform process; fn: facial nerve; gg: geniculate ganglion; gspn: greater superficial petrosal nerve; ica: internal carotid artery; lsc: lateral semicircular canal; mcf: middle cranial fossa; pr: promontory; s: stapes.*

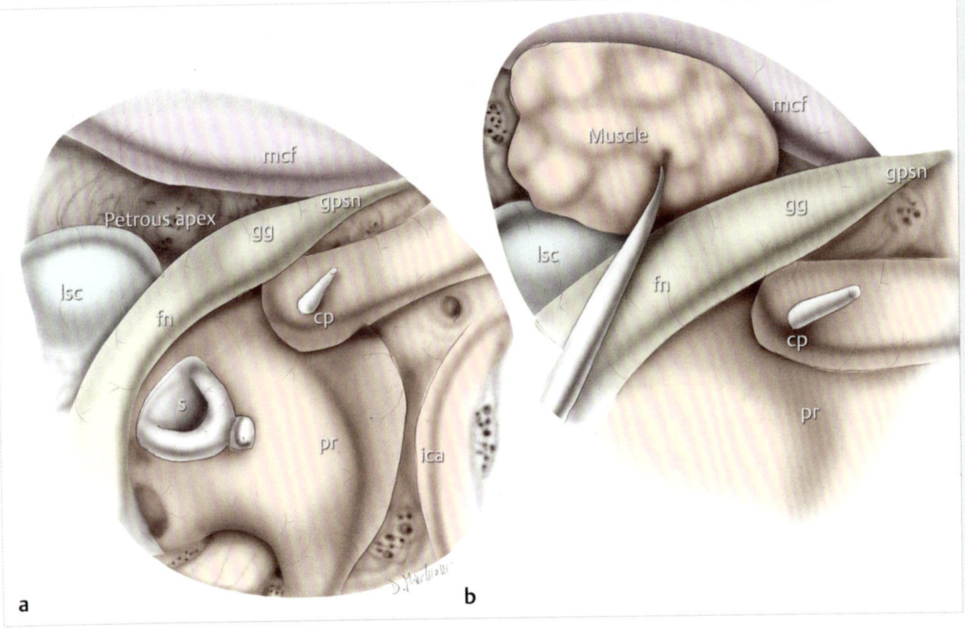

Fig. 10.63 Right ear: **(a)** Final cavity, once the cholesteatoma has been removed. **(b)** A fragment of muscle is placed in the petrous apex inside the suprageniculate fossa to obliterate the suprageniculate defect. *cp: cochleariform process; fn: facial nerve; gg: geniculate ganglion; gspn: greater superficial petrosal nerve; ica: internal carotid artery; lsc: lateral semicircular canal; mcf: middle cranial fossa; pr: promontory; s: stapes.*

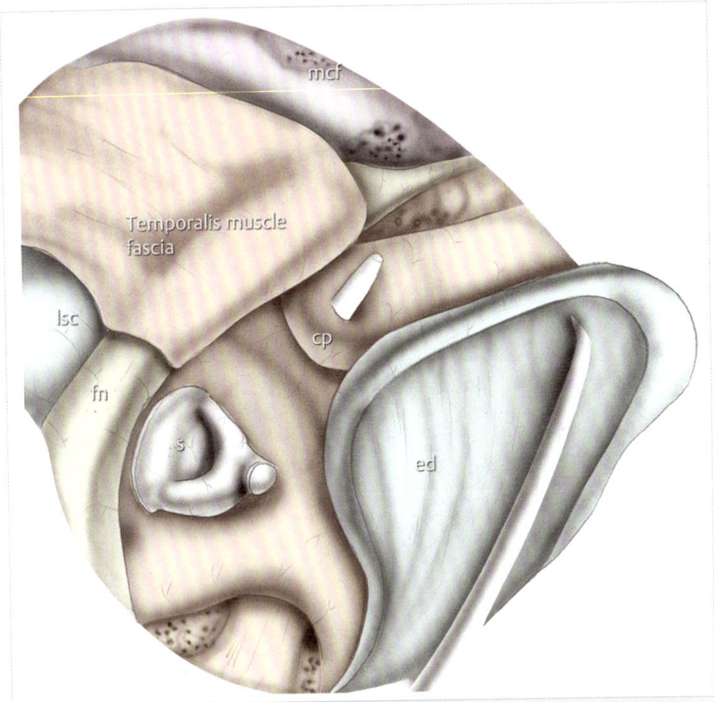

Fig. 10.64 Right ear: A temporalis muscle fascia is placed to cover the obliteration of the suprageniculate fossa. *cp: cochleariform process; ed: eardrum; fn: facial nerve; lsc: lateral semicircular canal; mcf: middle cranial fossa; s: stapes.*

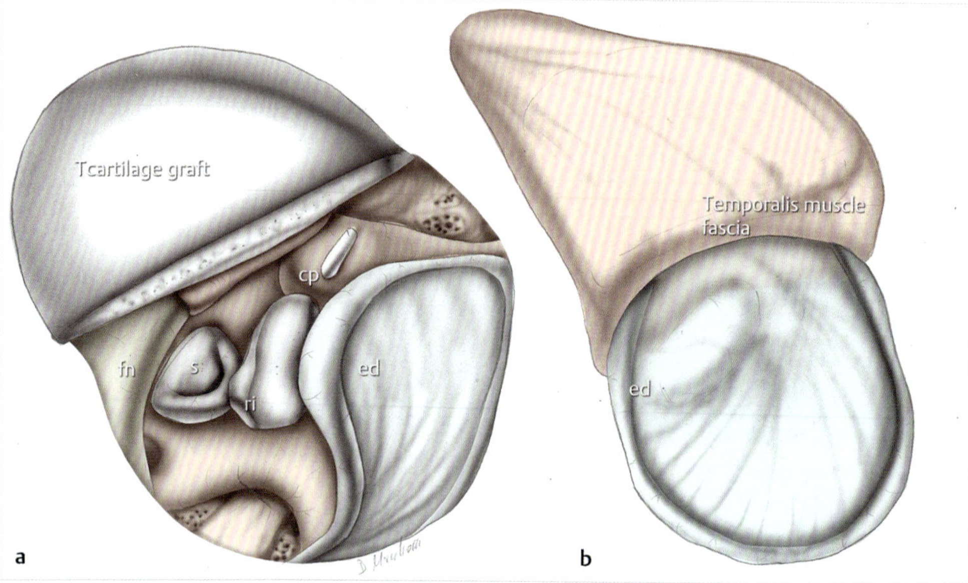

Fig. 10.65 Right ear: **(a)** An ossiculoplasty is performed placing a remodeled incus over the stapes. A cartilage graft is used to reconstruct the scutum defect. **(b)** A temporalis fascia is used to cover the cartilage and the eardrum is replaced. *cp: cochleariform process; ed: eardrum; fn: facial nerve; ri: autologous remodeled incus; s, stapes.*

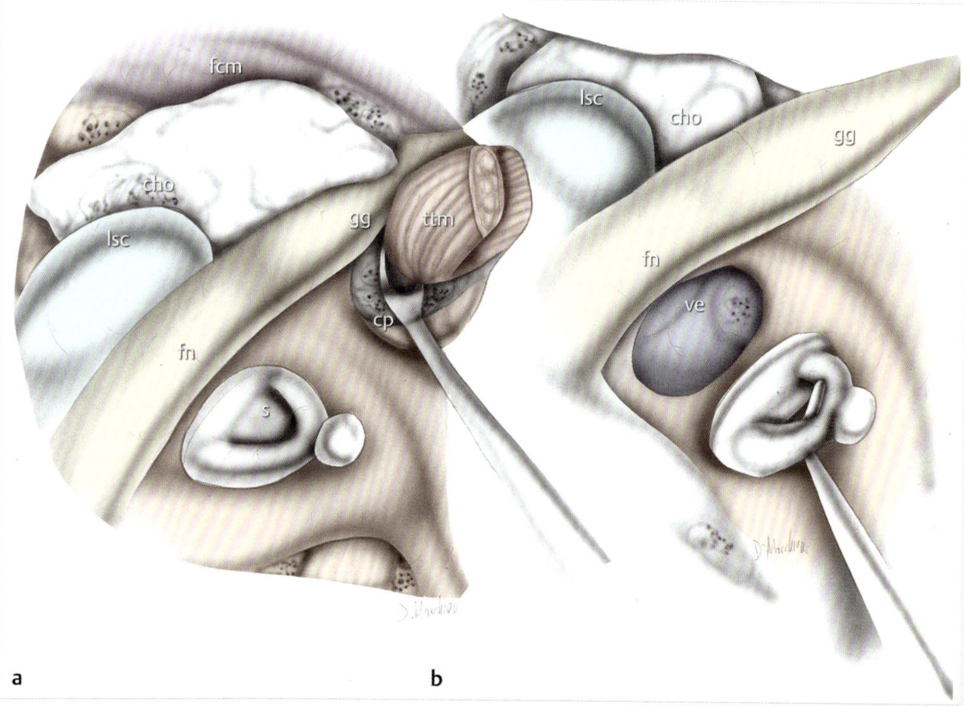

Fig. 10.66 Right ear: **(a)** In case of cholesteatoma extension around the facial nerve and to the labyrinth and the vestibule, the cochleariform process is removed through a microcurette, and the tensor tympani muscle is anteriorly pushed uncovering the geniculate ganglion (GG). During this maneuver, attention must be paid to the close relationship between the GG and the muscle. **(b)** The stapes is removed entering the vestibule. *cho: cholesteatoma; cp: cochleariform process; fn: facial nerve; gg: geniculate ganglion; lsc: lateral semicircular canal; mcf: middle cranial fossa; s: stapes; ttm: tensor tympani muscle; ve: vestibule.*

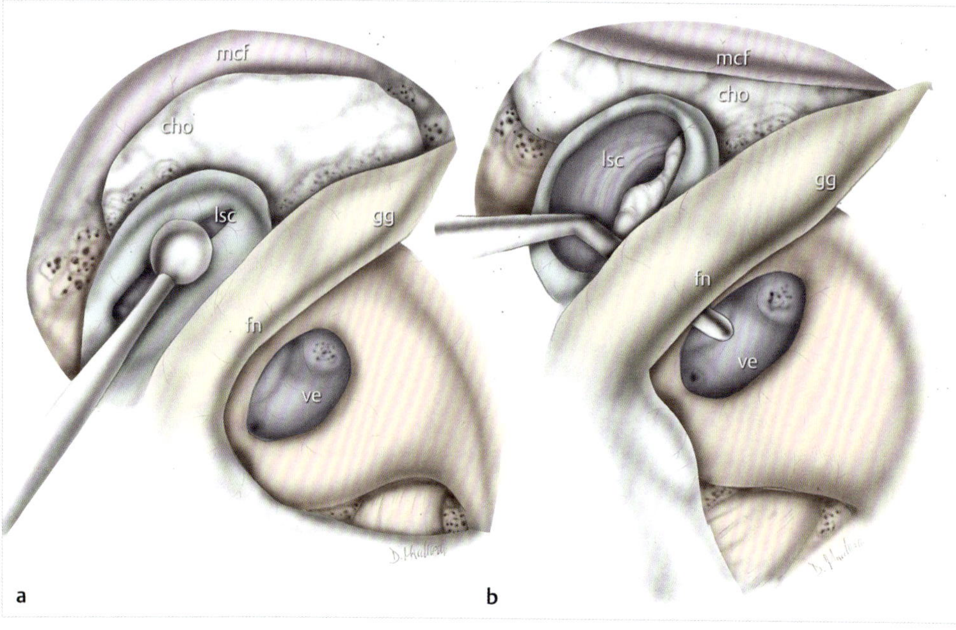

Fig. 10.67 Right ear: **(a)** A diamond bur is used to open the lateral semicircular canal entering the superior part of the vestibule. **(b)** A curved dissector is used to remove the cholesteatoma occupying the labyrinth, medial to the facial nerve. *cho: cholesteatoma; fn: facial nerve; gg: geniculate ganglion; lsc: lateral semicircular canal; mcf: middle cranial fossa; ve: vestibule.*

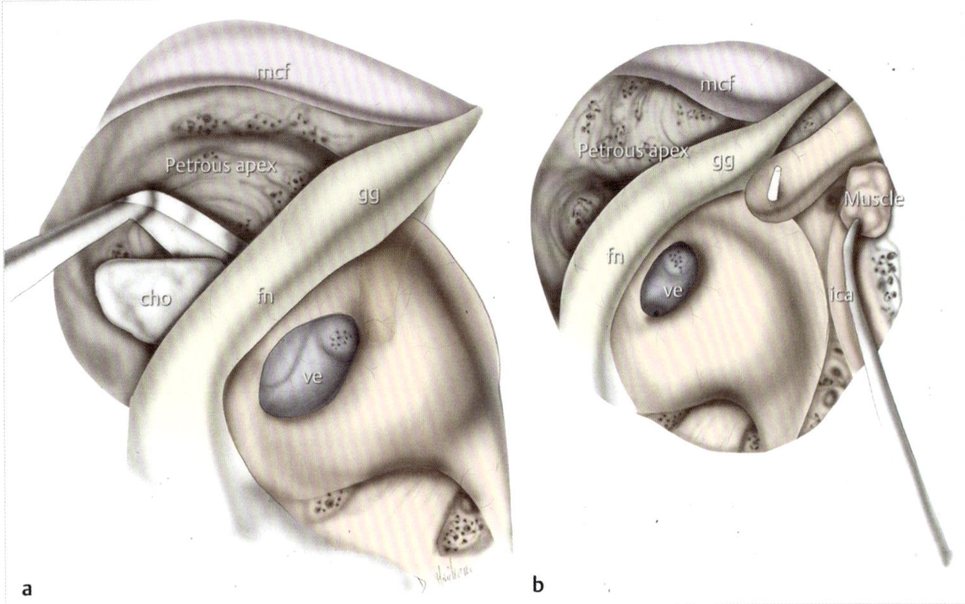

Fig. 10.68 Right ear: **(a)** Once the vestibule has been opened, the cholesteatoma is completely removed. **(b)** A piece of muscle is placed into the eustachian tube obliterating its orifice. *cho: cholesteatoma; fn: facial nerve; gg: geniculate ganglion; ica: internal carotid artery; mcf: middle cranial fossa; ve: vestibule.*

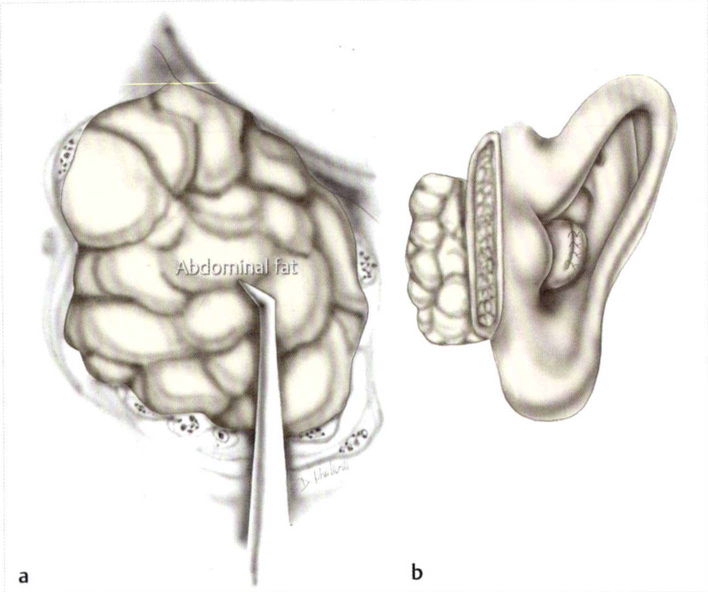

Fig. 10.69 Right ear: **(a)** Abdominal fat is used to fill the surgical cavity. **(b)** The external auditory canal skin is reversed and sutured in a blind sac fashion.

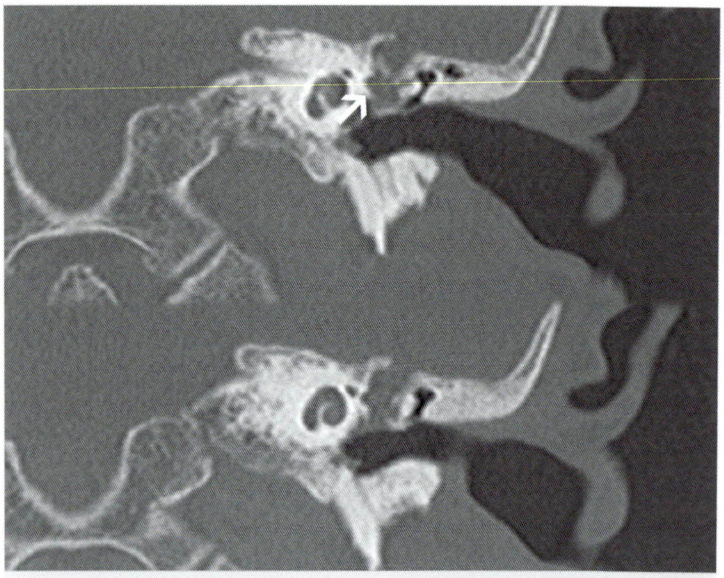

Fig. 10.70 Clinical Case 3: Computed tomography (CT) scan in coronal view showing a cholesteatoma involving the suprageniculate fossa extending between the geniculate ganglion (*white arrow*) and the middle cranial fossa.

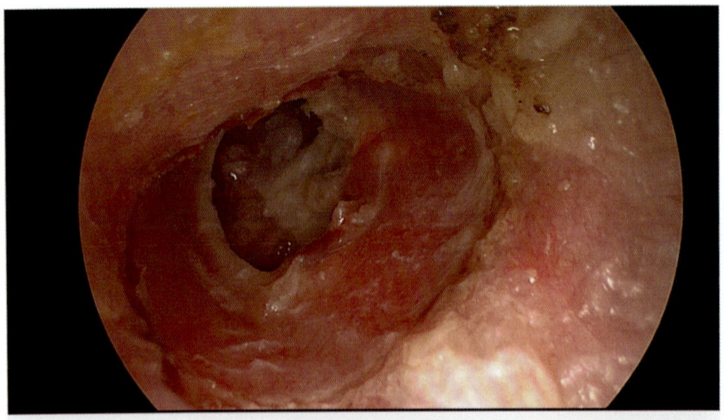

Fig. 10.71 Clinical Case 3, Left ear: Due to the extension of the cholesteatoma and the poor hearing function, a circumferential incision of the skin of the external auditory canal is performed.

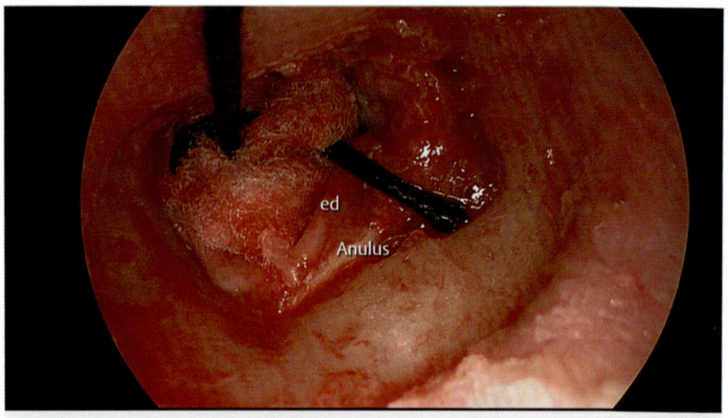

Fig. 10.72 Clinical Case 3, Left ear: The skin of the external auditory canal is circumferentially elevated with the anulus and the residual eardrum using cottonoid, maintaining a clean surgical field. *ed: eardrum.*

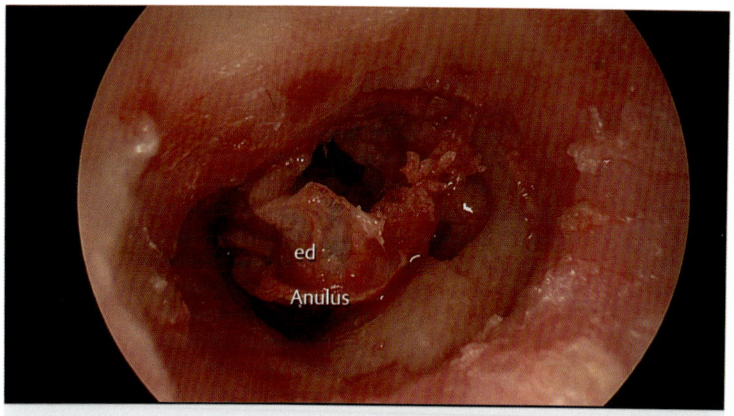

Fig. 10.73 Clinical Case 3, Left ear: The skin of the external auditory canal with the eardrum is progressively detached. *ed: eardrum.*

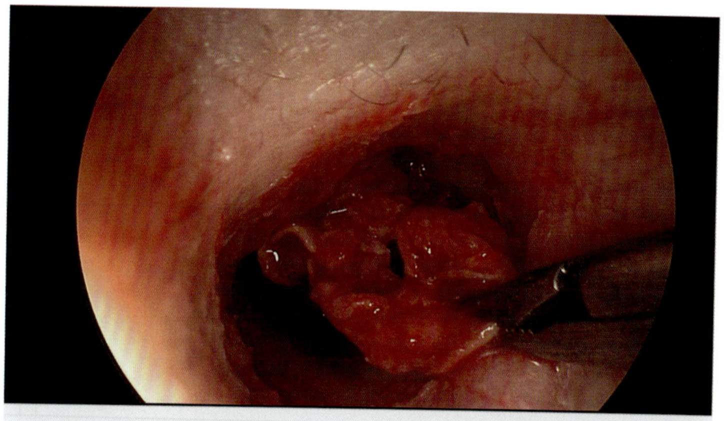

Fig. 10.74 Clinical Case 3, Left ear: The external auditory canal skin and the eardrum are removed.

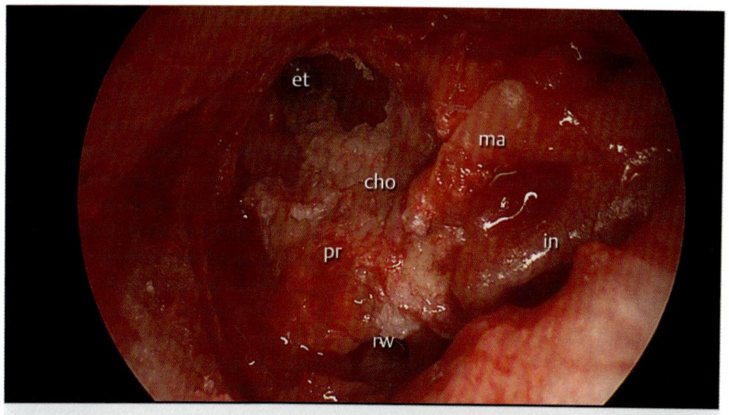

Fig. 10.75 Clinical Case 3, Left ear: An infiltrative matrix cholesteatoma is endoscopically found with promontory erosion, extending to the eustachian tube and medial to the ossicular chain. *cho: cholesteatoma; et: eustachian tube; in: incus; ma: malleus; pr: promontory; rw: round window.*

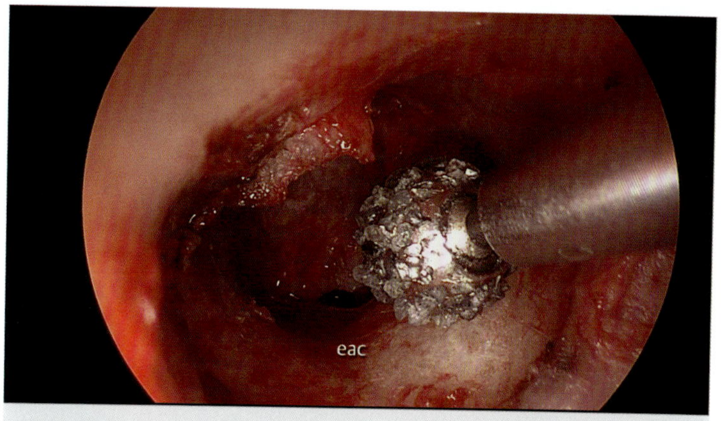

Fig. 10.76 Clinical Case 3, Left ear: A diamond bur is used to circumferentially enlarge the external auditory canal. *eac: external auditory canal.*

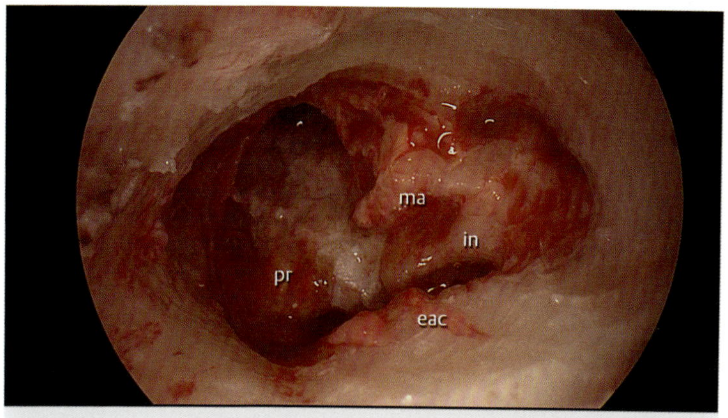

Fig. 10.77 Clinical Case 3, Left ear: The external auditory canal is progressively drilled uncovering the medial wall of the tympanic cavity. *eac: external auditory canal; in: incus; ma: malleus; pr: promontory.*

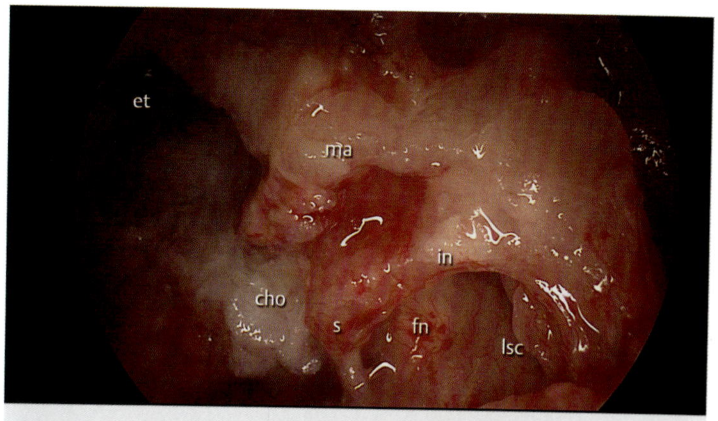

Fig. 10.78 Clinical Case 3, Left ear: Endoscopic magnification of the ossicular chain; an isthmus block is present, and a cholesteatoma extending medially to the ossicular chain is noted. *cho: cholesteatoma; et: eustachian tube; fn: facial nerve; in: incus; lsc: lateral semicircular canal; ma: malleus; s: stapes.*

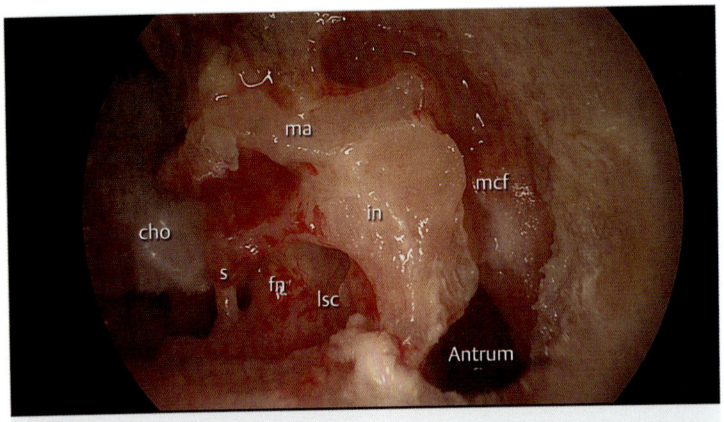

Fig. 10.79 Clinical Case 3, Left ear: Further drilling allows for the exposure of the antrum. The plane of the middle cranial fossa is detected. *cho: cholesteatoma; fn: facial nerve; in: incus; lsc: lateral semicircular canal; ma: malleus; mcf: middle cranial fossa; s: stapes.*

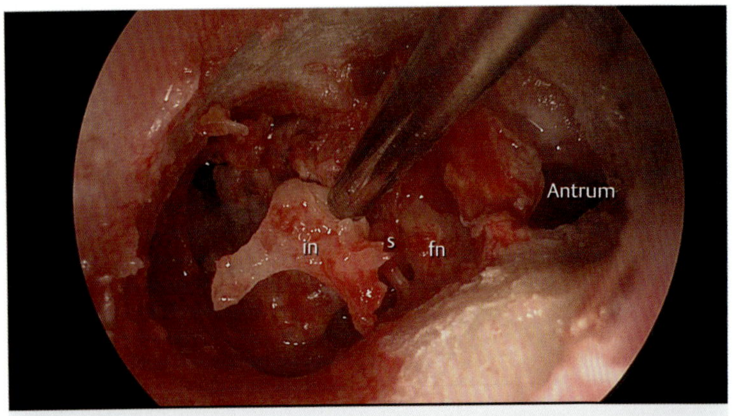

Fig. 10.80 Clinical Case 3, Left ear: The incus is removed. *fn: facial nerve; in: incus; s: stapes.*

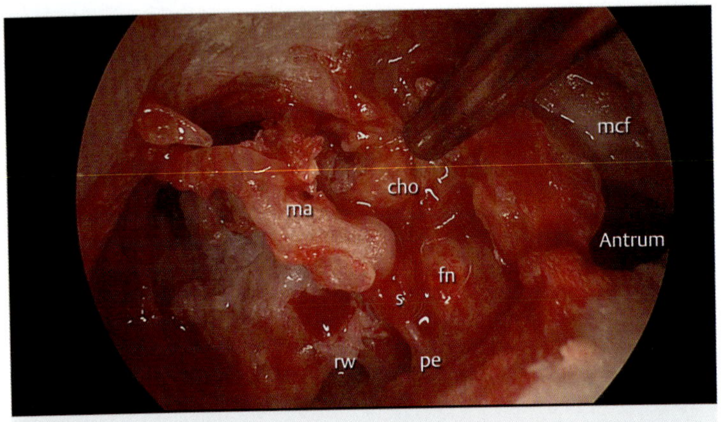

Fig. 10.81 Clinical Case 3, Left ear: The malleus is removed. The cholesteatoma invading the geniculate ganglion area is visible. *cho: cholesteatoma; fn: facial nerve; ma: malleus; mcf: middle cranial fossa; pe: pyramidal eminence; rw: round window; s: stapes.*

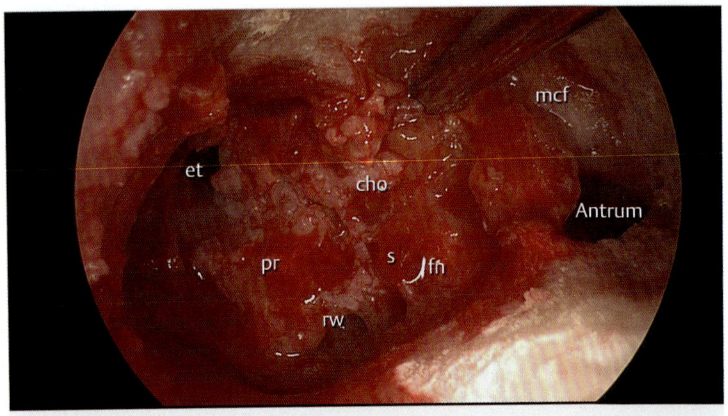

Fig. 10.82 Clinical Case 3, Left ear: Once the ossicular chain has been removed, the extension of the cholesteatoma is endoscopically appreciated. A cholesteatoma with a wide erosion of the medial wall of the tympanic cavity, extending to the suprageniculate fossa, is noted. *cho: cholesteatoma; et: eustachian tube; fn: facial nerve; mcf: middle cranial fossa; pr: promontory; rw: round window; s: stapes.*

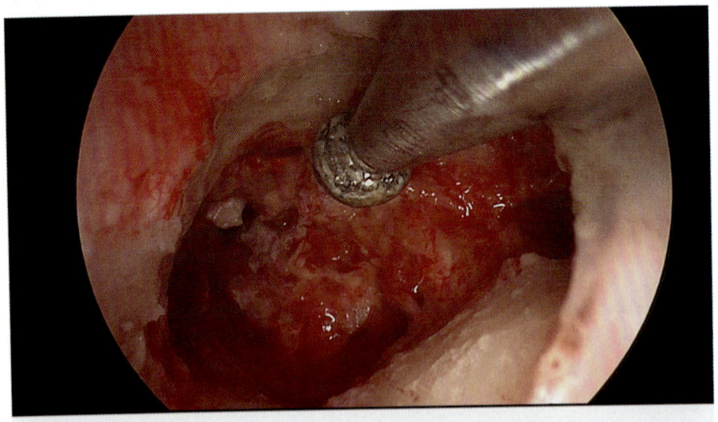

Fig. 10.83 Clinical Case 3, Left ear: A diamond bur is used to enlarge the attic and remove the bone of the suprageniculate fossa, bordering the middle fossa plane.

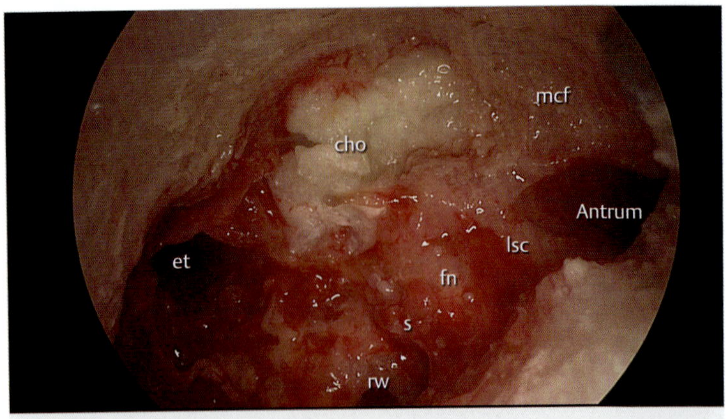

Fig. 10.84 Clinical Case 3, Left ear: A cholesteatoma with a supra-labyrinthine extension is progressively exposed. *cho: cholesteatoma; et: eustachian tube; fn: facial nerve; lsc: lateral semicircular canal; mcf: middle cranial fossa; rw: round window; s: stapes.*

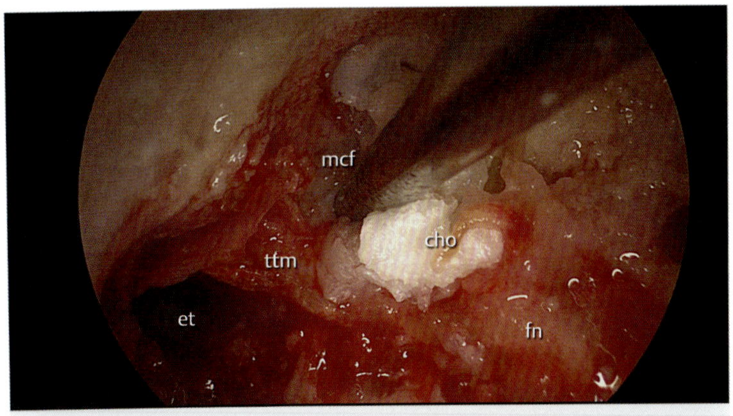

Fig. 10.85 Clinical Case 3, Left ear: A suction instrument is gently used to detect the plane of the middle cranial fossa dura. *cho: cholesteatoma; et: eustachian tube; fn: facial nerve; mcf: middle cranial fossa; ttm: tensor tympani muscle.*

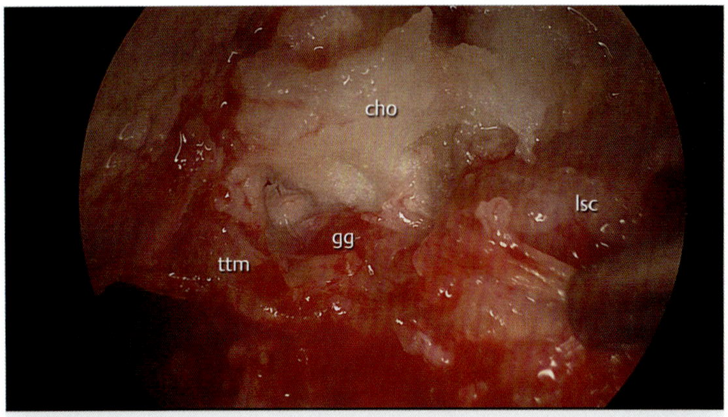

Fig. 10.86 Clinical Case 3, Left ear: The geniculate ganglion and the lateral semicircular canal are endoscopically detected. *cho: cholesteatoma; gg: geniculate ganglion; lsc: lateral semicircular canal; ttm: tensor tympani muscle.*

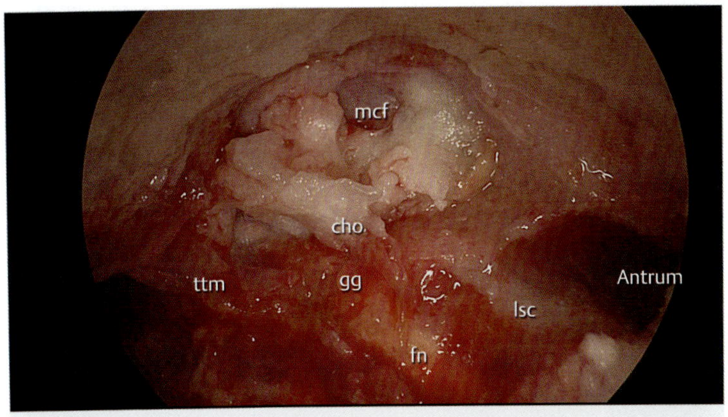

Fig. 10.87 Clinical Case 3, Left ear: All the anatomical landmarks of the suprageniculate fossa are detected (the middle cranial fossa, the facial nerve, the geniculate ganglion, and the lateral semicircular canal). *cho: cholesteatoma; fn: facial nerve; gg: geniculate ganglion; lsc: lateral semicircular canal; mcf: middle cranial fossa; ttm: tensor tympani muscle.*

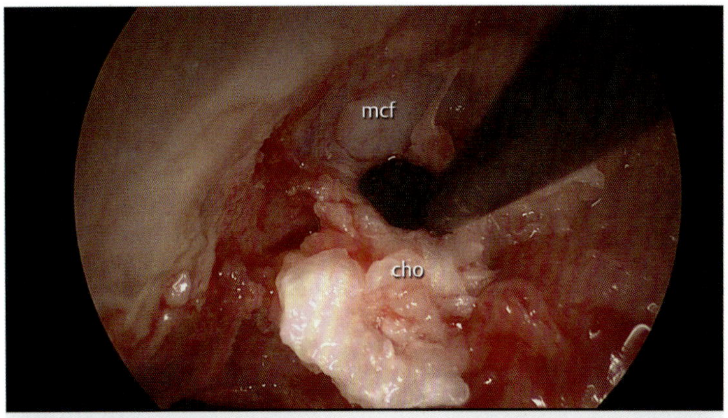

Fig. 10.88 Clinical Case 3, Left ear: The cholesteatoma is detached from the plane of the dura of the middle cranial fossa. *cho: cholesteatoma; mcf: middle cranial fossa.*

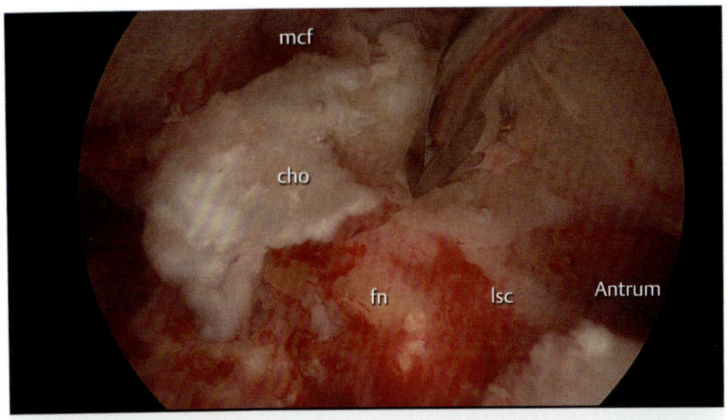

Fig. 10.89 Clinical Case 3, Left ear: Through piezosurgery the bone cells between the facial nerve, the middle cranial fossa, and the lateral semicircular canal are removed, exposing the cholesteatoma lying in the suprageniculate fossa. *cho: cholesteatoma; fn: facial nerve; lsc: lateral semicircular canal; mcf: middle cranial fossa.*

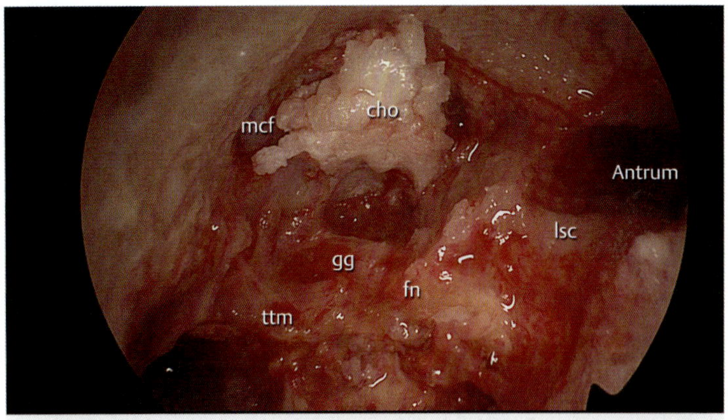

Fig. 10.90 Clinical Case 3, Left ear: The cholesteatoma is progressively removed. *cho: cholesteatoma; fn: facial nerve; gg: geniculate ganglion; lsc: lateral semicircular canal; mcf: middle cranial fossa; ttm: tensor tympani muscle.*

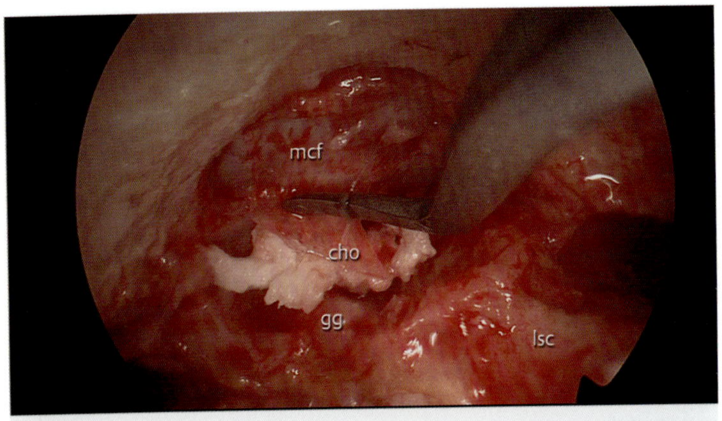

Fig. 10.91 Clinical Case 3, Left ear: Using a curved dissector the last piece of cholesteatoma lying in the suprageniculate fossa is removed. *cho: cholesteatoma; gg: geniculate ganglion; lsc: lateral semicircular canal; mcf: middle cranial fossa.*

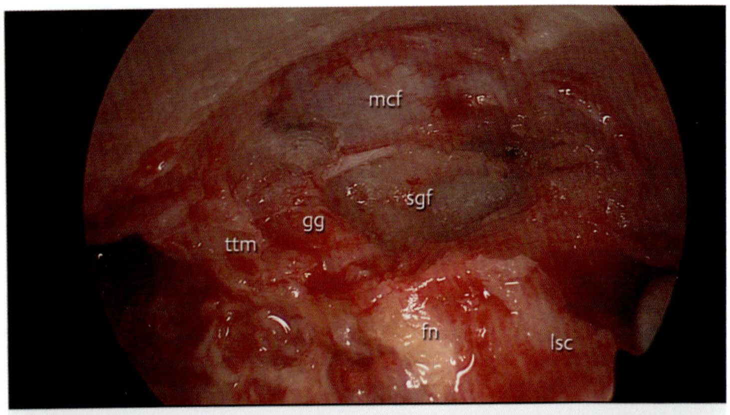

Fig. 10.92 Clinical Case 3, Left ear: The suprageniculate fossa is endoscopically exposed. *fn: facial nerve; gg: geniculate ganglion; lsc: lateral semicircular canal; mcf: middle cranial fossa; sgf: suprageniculate fossa; ttm: tensor tympani muscle.*

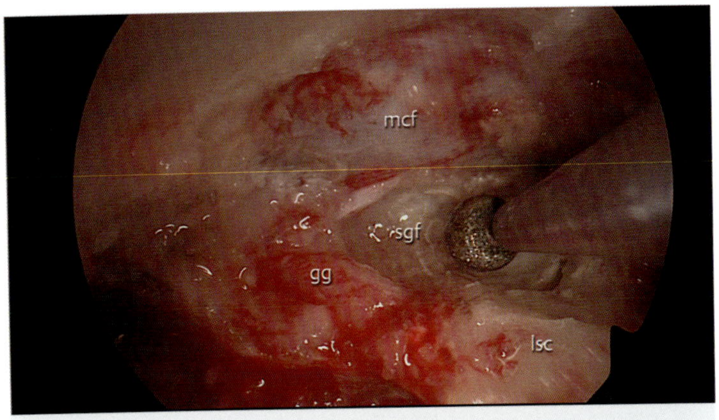

Fig. 10.93 Clinical Case 3, Left ear: A diamond bur is used to remove remnant disease from the fossa. *gg: geniculate ganglion; lsc: lateral semicircular canal; mcf: middle cranial fossa; sgf: soprageniculate fossa.*

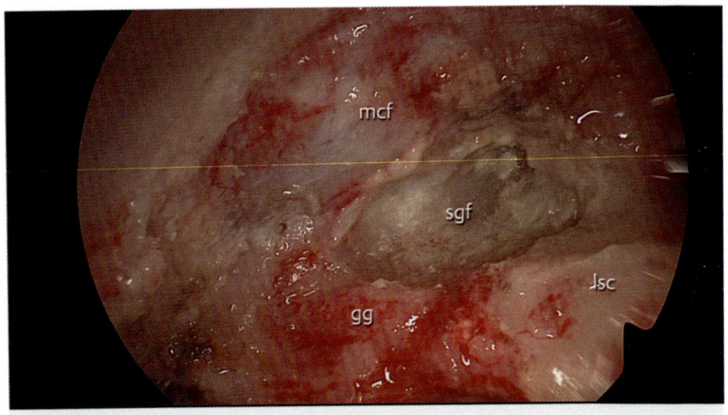

Fig. 10.94 Clinical Case 3, Left ear: Final view of the suprageniculate fossa after drilling. *gg: geniculate ganglion; lsc: lateral semicircular canal; mcf: middle cranial fossa; sgf: suprageniculate fossa.*

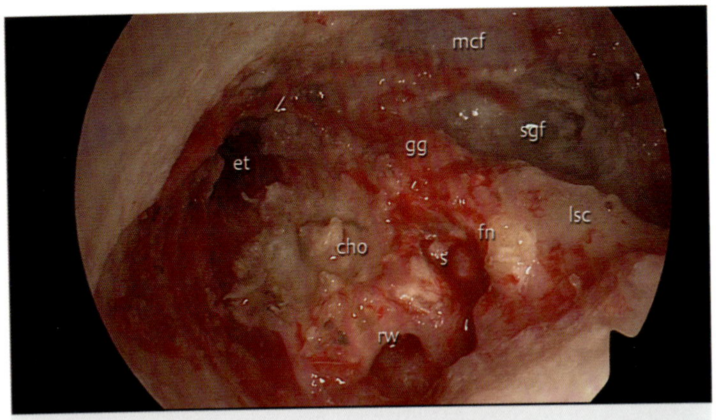

Fig. 10.95 Clinical Case 3, Left ear: Once the cholesteatoma occupying the suprageniculate fossa (SGF) has been removed, the promontory should be drilled due to the presence of infiltrative cholesteatoma involving the cochlea. *cho: cholesteatoma; et: eustachian tube; fn: facial nerve; gg: geniculate ganglion; lsc: lateral semicircular canal; mcf: middle cranial fossa; rw: round window; s: stapes; sgf: soprageniculate fossa.*

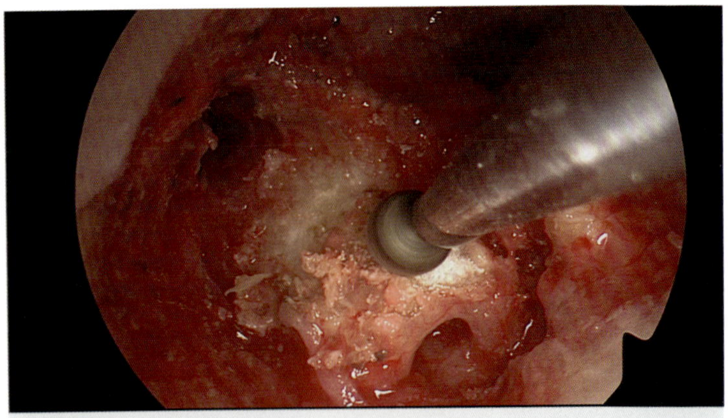

Fig. 10.96 Clinical Case 3, Left ear: The promontory is endoscopically drilled using a diamond bur.

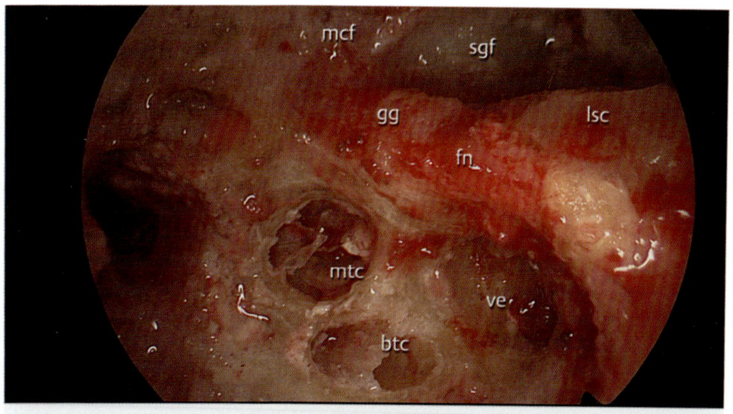

Fig. 10.97 Clinical Case 3, Left ear: Once the cholesteatoma has been removed, the cochlear turns and the vestibule are exposed. *btc: basal turn of the cochlea; fn: facial nerve; gg: geniculate ganglion; lsc: lateral semicircular canal; mcf: middle cranial fossa; mtc: middle turn of the cochlea; sgf: suprageniculate fossa; ve: vestibule.*

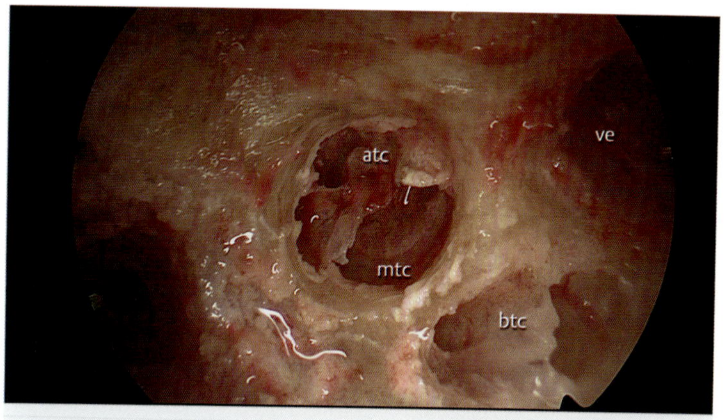

Fig. 10.98 Clinical Case 3, Left ear: Endoscopic view of the cochlea and the vestibule. *atc: apical turn of the cochlea; btc: basal turn of the cochlea; mtc: middle turn of the cochlea; ve: vestibule.*

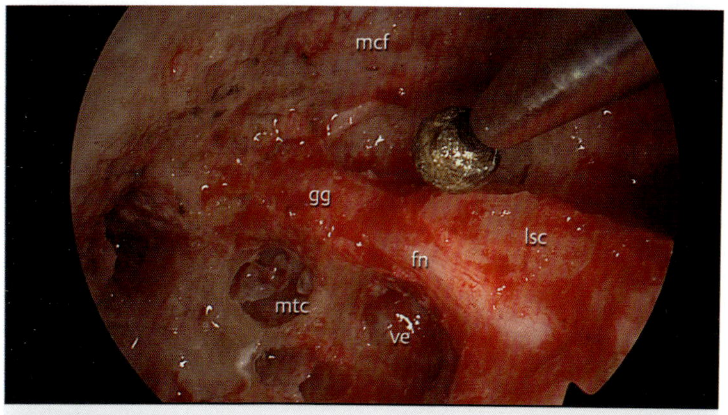

Fig. 10.99 Clinical Case 3, Left ear: Further drilling is performed to make the cavity regular. *fn: facial nerve; gg: geniculate ganglion; lsc: lateral semicircular canal; mcf: middle cranial fossa; mtc: middle turn of the cochlea; ve: vestibule.*

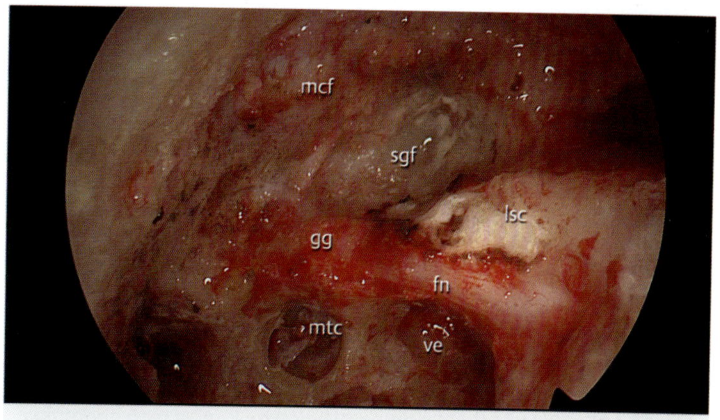

Fig. 10.100 Clinical Case 3, Left ear: The cholesteatoma is completely removed. *fn: facial nerve; gg: geniculate ganglion; lsc: lateral semicircular canal; mcf: middle cranial fossa; mtc: middle turn of the cochlea; sgf: suprageniculate fossa; ve: vestibule.*

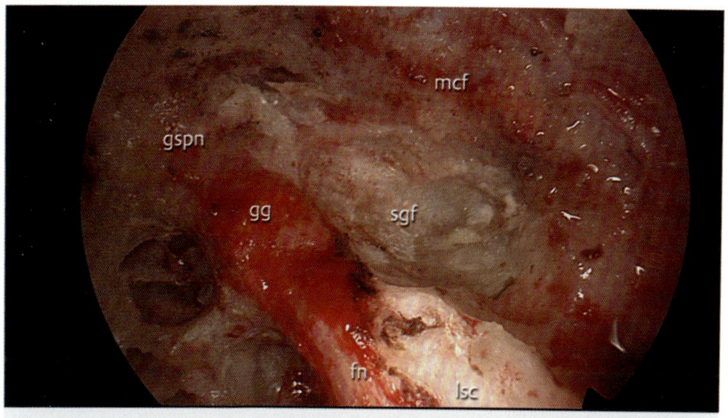

Fig. 10.101 Clinical Case 3, Left ear: Endoscopic view of the suprageniculate fossa. *fn: facial nerve; gg: geniculate ganglion; gspn: greater superficial petrosal nerve; lsc: lateral semicircular canal; mcf: middle cranial fossa; sgf: suprageniculate fossa.*

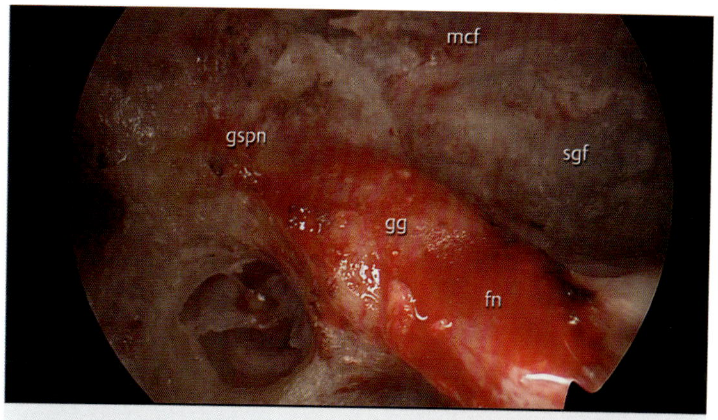

Fig. 10.102 Clinical Case 3, Left ear: Endoscopic magnification of the geniculate ganglion. *fn: facial nerve; gg: geniculate ganglion; gspn: greater superficial petrosal nerve; mcf: middle cranial fossa; sgf: suprageniculate fossa.*

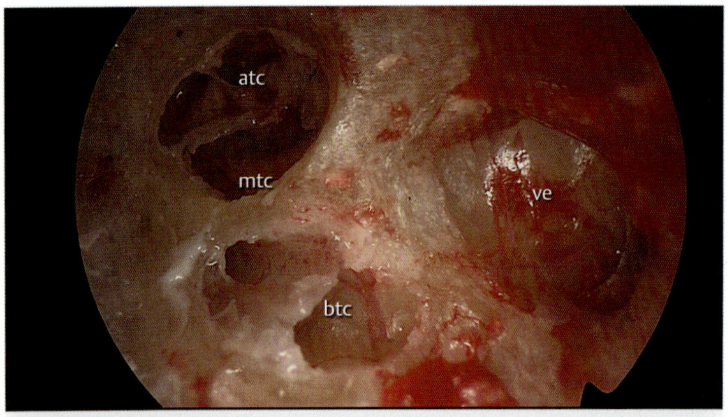

Fig. 10.103 Clinical Case 3, Left ear: The cochlea and the vestibule are endoscopically investigated before closing the cavity. *atc: apical turn of the cochlea; btc: basal turn of the cochlea; mtc: middle turn of the cochlea; ve: vestibule.*

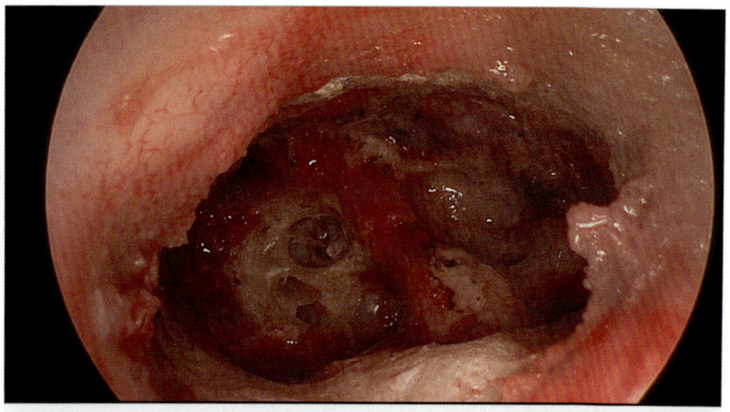

Fig. 10.104 Clinical Case 3, Left ear: Final surgical cavity.

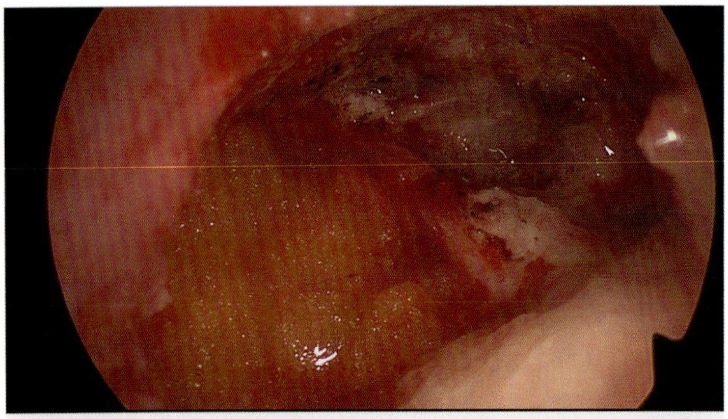

Fig. 10.105 Clinical Case 3, Left ear: The cavity is filled with abdominal fat and the external auditory canal is closed in a blind sac fashion.

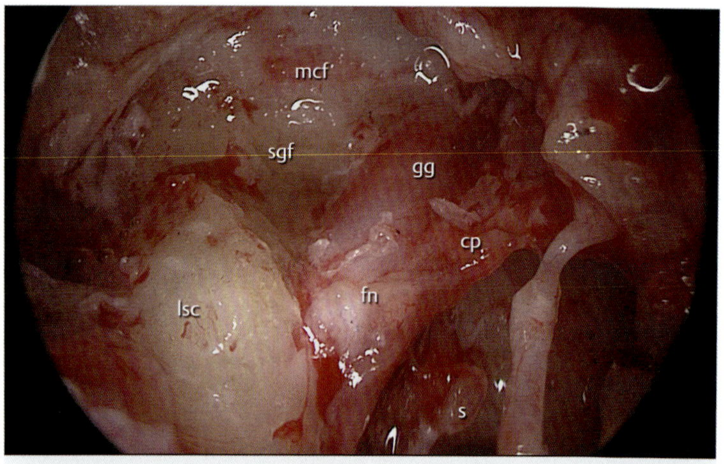

Fig. 10.106 Clinical Case 4, Right ear: Endoscopic view of the suprageniculate fossa after cholesteatoma removal. *cp: cochleariform process; fn: facial nerve; gg: geniculate ganglion; lsc: lateral semicircular canal; mcf: middle cranial fossa; s: stapes; sgf: suprageniculate fossa.*

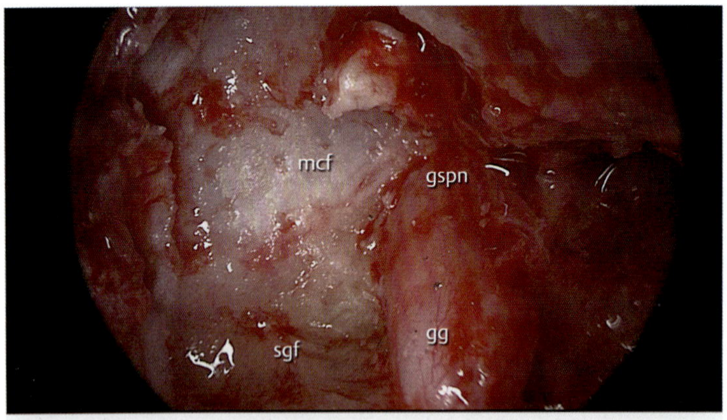

Fig. 10.107 Clinical Case 4, Right ear: Endoscopic magnification of the geniculate ganglion. *gg: geniculate ganglion; gspn: greater superficial petrosal nerve; mcf: middle cranial fossa; sgf: suprageniculate fossa.*

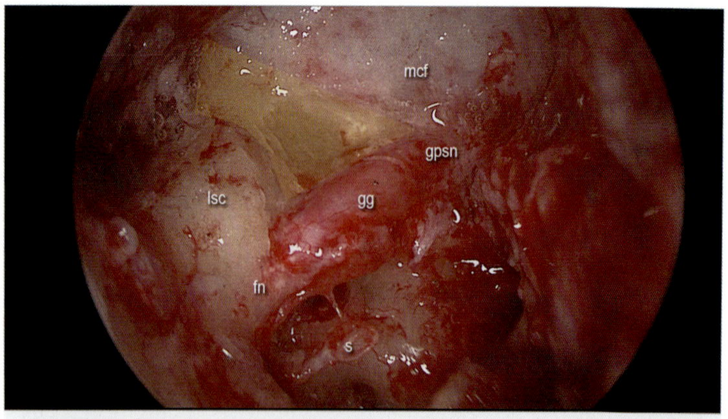

Fig. 10.108 Clinical Case 4, Right ear: Final surgical cavity showing the triangular shape of the suprageniculate fossa (*yellow area*) between the lateral semicircular canal, the dura of the middle cranial fossa, and the facial nerve (FN). *fn: facial nerve; gg: geniculate ganglion; gspn: greater superficial petrosal nerve; lsc: lateral semicircular canal; mcf: middle cranial fossa; s: stapes.*

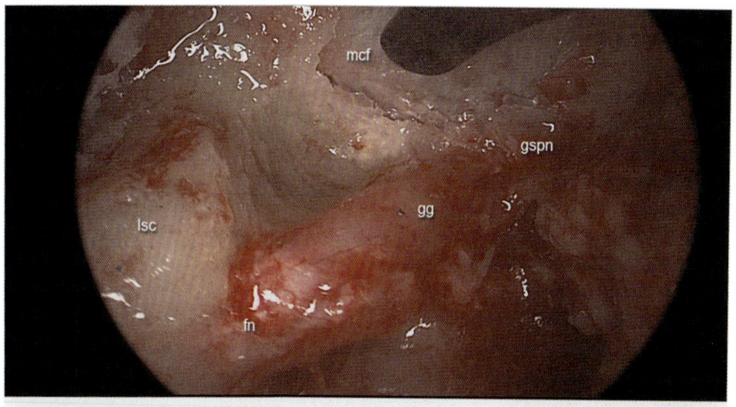

Fig. 10.109 Clinical Case 4, Right ear: The plane of the middle cranial fossa dura is noted. *fn: facial nerve; gg: geniculate ganglion; gspn: greater superficial petrosal nerve; lsc: lateral semicircular canal; mcf: middle cranial fossa.*

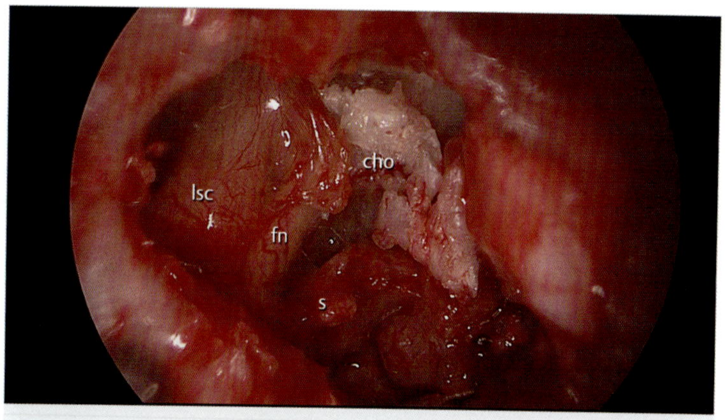

Fig. 10.110 Clinical Case 5, Right ear: Cholesteatoma involving the suprageniculate fossa and the labyrinth. *cho: cholesteatoma; fn: facial nerve; lsc: lateral semicircular canal; s: stapes.*

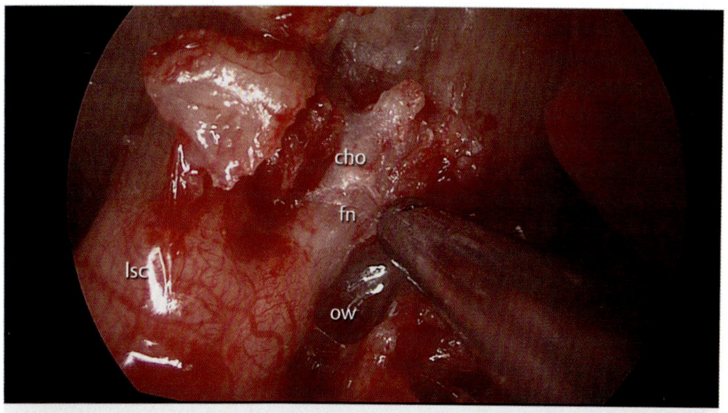

Fig. 10.111 Clinical Case 5, Right ear: The cholesteatoma matrix is progressively removed from the tympanic segment of the facial nerve. *cho: cholesteatoma; fn: facial nerve; lsc: lateral semicircular canal; ow: oval window.*

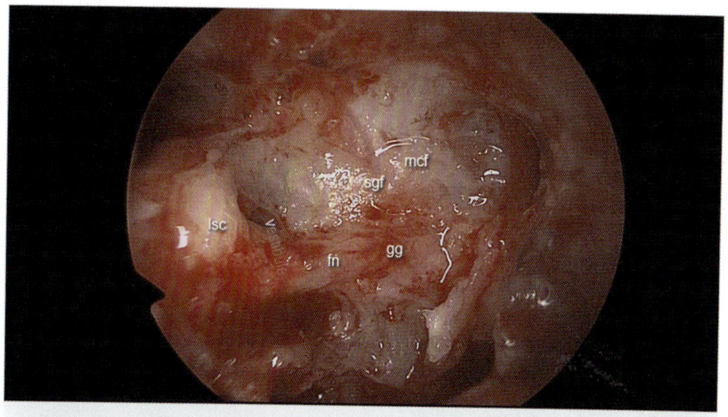

Fig. 10.112 Clinical Case 5, Right ear: The vestibule is opened, removing the last piece of cholesteatoma. *fn: facial nerve; gg: geniculate ganglion; lsc: lateral semicircular canal; mcf: middle cranial fossa; sgf: suprageniculate fossa.*

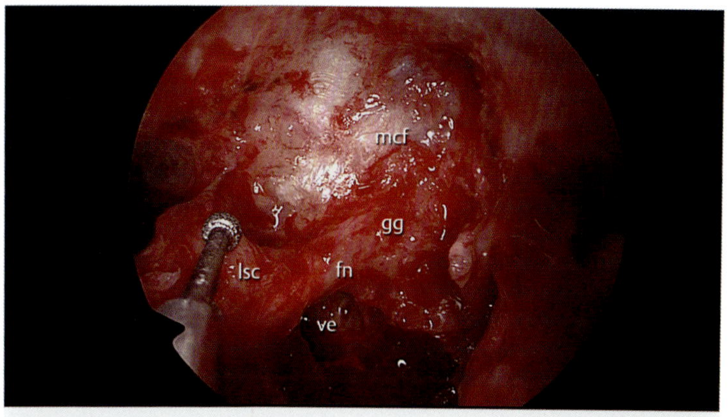

Fig. 10.113 Clinical Case 5, Right ear: A diamond bur is used to radicalize the cavity. *fn: facial nerve; gg: geniculate ganglion; lsc: lateral semicircular canal; mcf: middle cranial fossa; ve: vestibule.*

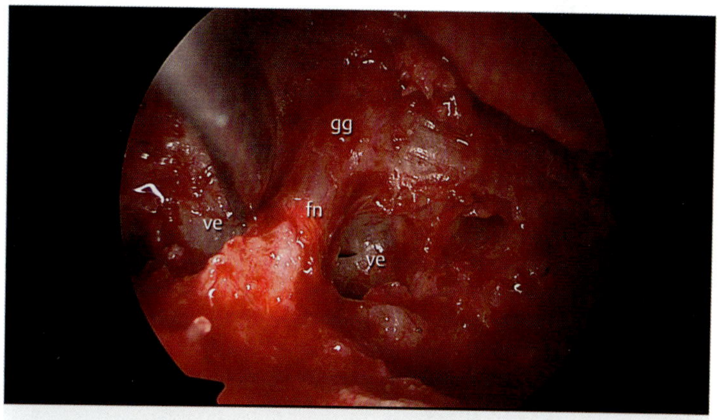

Fig. 10.114 Clinical Case 5, Right ear: Final view after cholesteatoma removal. A curved dissector is placed under the tympanic segment of the facial nerve through the vestibule. *fn: facial nerve; gg: geniculate ganglion; ve: vestibule.*

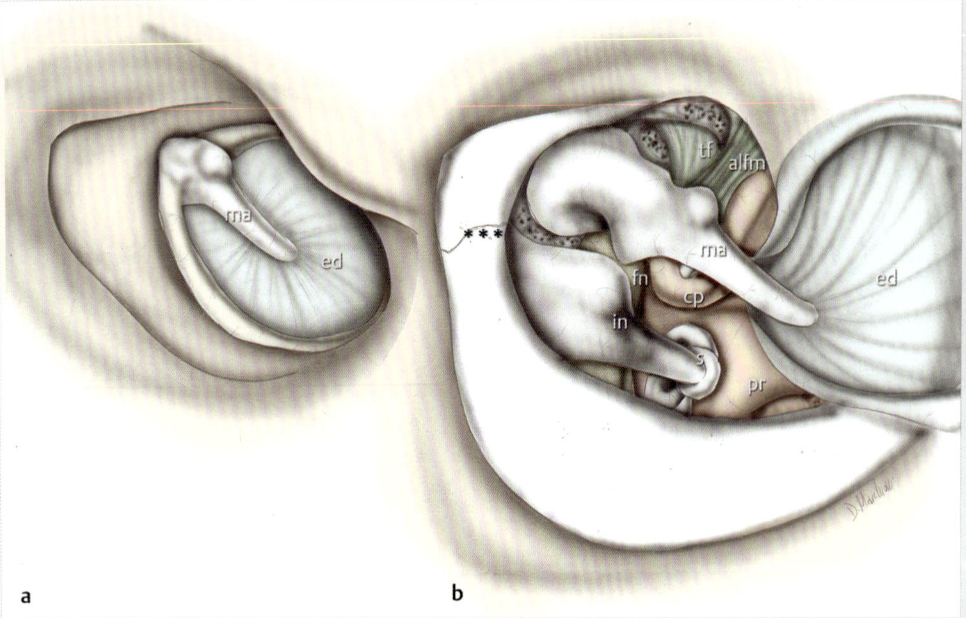

Fig. 10.115 Right ear. **(a)** The incision of the skin of the external auditory canal is made. **(b)** A tympanomeatal flap is elevated; the flap is detached from the malleus uncovering the attic; a dislocation of the malleus with a fracture of the EAC is noted (***). *alfm: anterior ligamental fold of malleus; cp: cochleariform process; ed: eardrum; fn: facial nerve; in: incus; ma: malleus; pr: promontory; s: stapes; tf: tensor fold.*

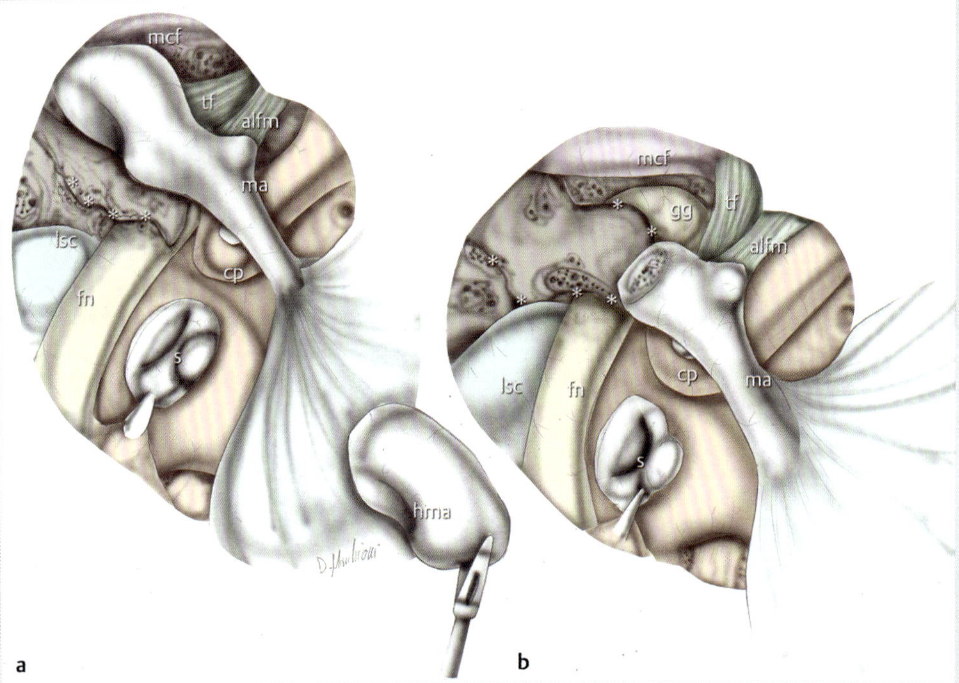

Fig. 10.116 Right ear. **(a)** The incus is removed. **(b)** The head of the malleus is removed to expose the attic and the geniculate ganglion (GG); a fracture with a bony spicule involving the GG is detected (*****). *alfm: anterior ligamental fold of malleus; cp: cochleariform process; fn: facial nerve; gg: geniculate ganglion; hma: head of the malleus; lsc: lateral semicircular canal; ma: malleus; mcf: middle cranial fossa; s: stapes; tf: tensor fold.*

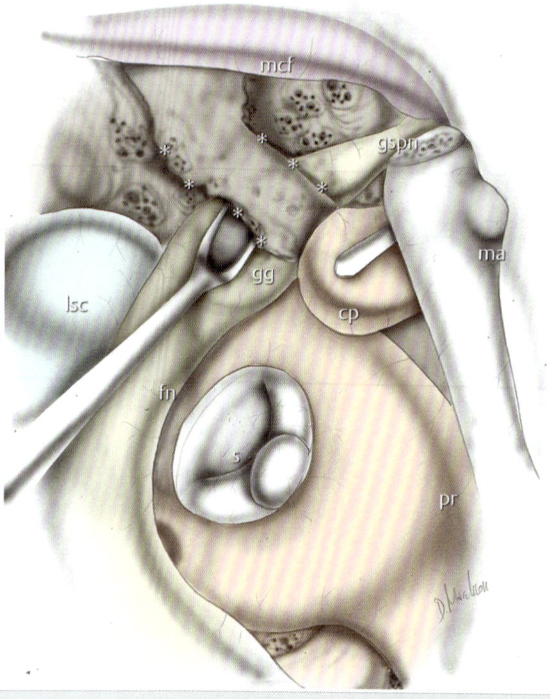

Fig. 10.117 Right ear: A microcurette is used to remove the bone spicule from the geniculate ganglion, decompressing the nerve. *cp: cochleariform process; fn: facial nerve; gg: geniculate ganglion; gspn: greater superficial petrosal nerve; lsc: lateral semicircular canal; ma: malleus; mcf: middle cranial fossa; pr: promontory; s: stapes; *****: bony spicula (fracture).*

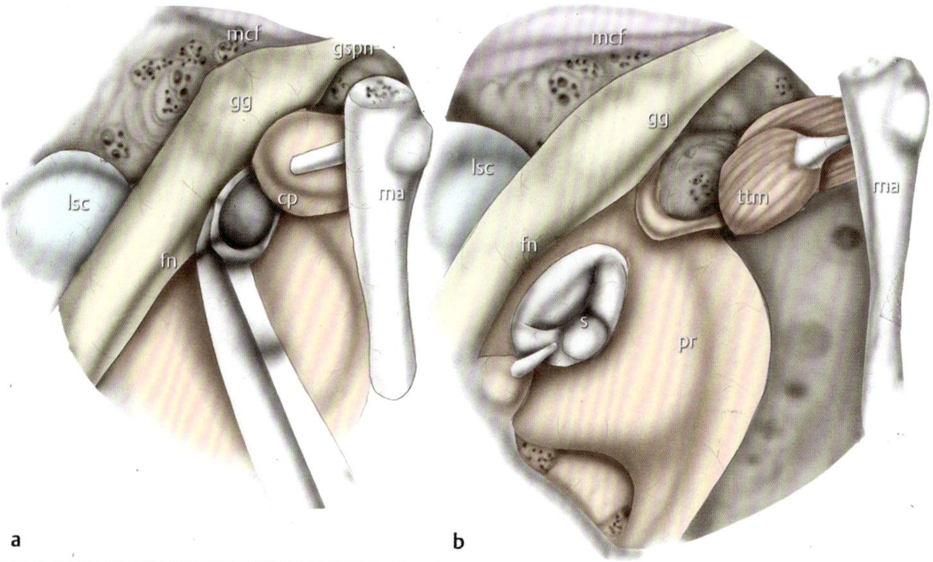

Fig. 10.118 Right ear: **(a, b)** If required, in order to improve the decompression of the geniculate ganglion, the cochleariform process is removed using a microcurette, maintaining the muscle and tendon connection to the malleus. *cp: cochleariform process; fn: facial nerve; gg: geniculate ganglion; gspn: greater superficial petrosal nerve; lsc: lateral semicircular canal; ma: malleus; mcf: middle cranial fossa; pr: promontory; s: stapes; ttm: tensor tympani muscle.*

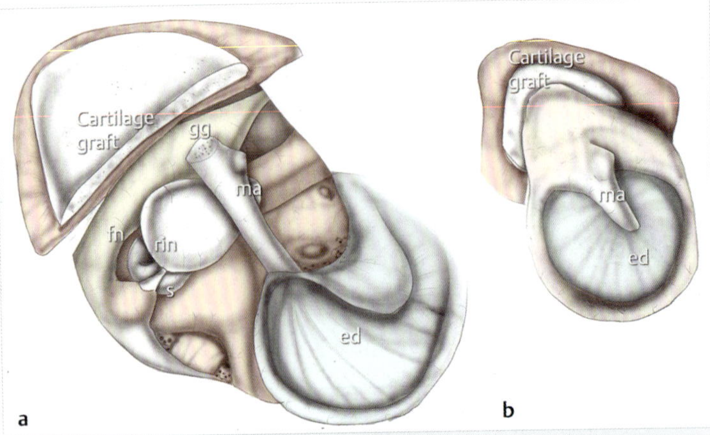

Fig. 10.119 Right ear: **(a)** An ossiculoplasty with a remodeled incus is performed. A cartilage graft is used to reconstruct the attical defect. **(b)** The tympanomeatal flap is replaced. *ed: eardrum; fn: facial nerve; gg: geniculate ganglion; ma: malleus; rin: remodeled incus; s: stapes.*

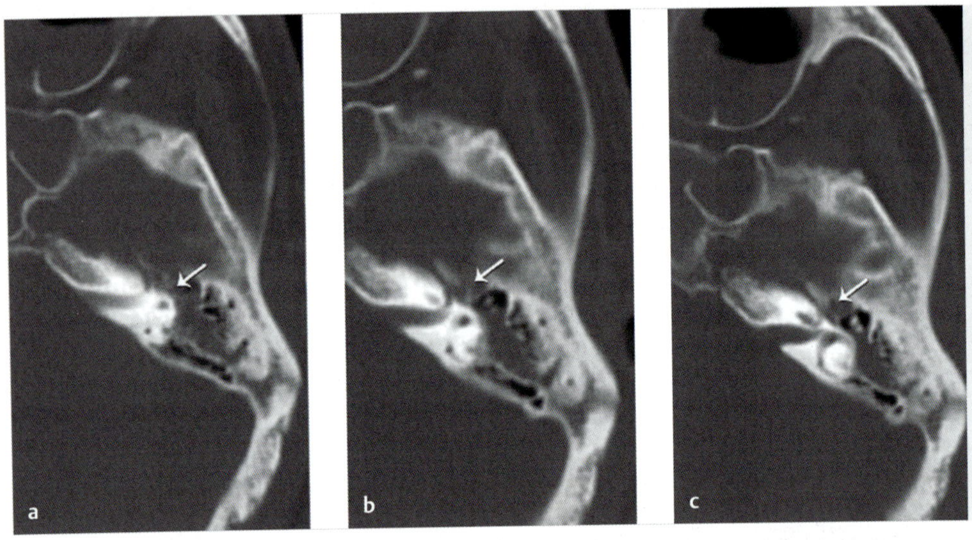

Fig. 10.120 (a–c) Clinical Case 6: Computed tomography (CT) scan in axial view showing a fracture of the temporal bone with a bony spicule involving the geniculate ganglion (*white arrow*).

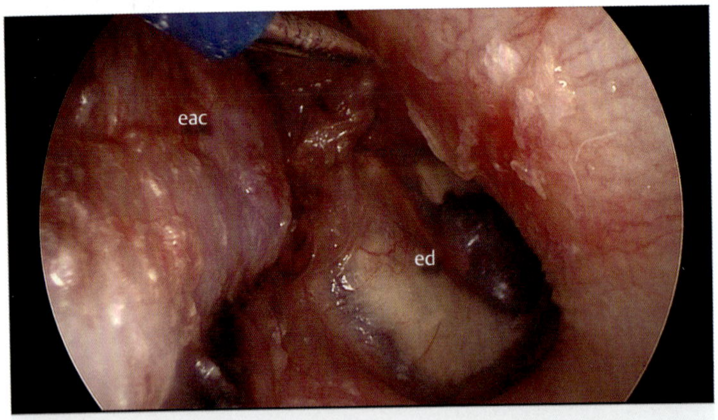

Fig. 10.121 Clinical Case 6, Right ear: A tympanomeatal flap is performed. *eac: external auditory canal; ed: eardrum.*

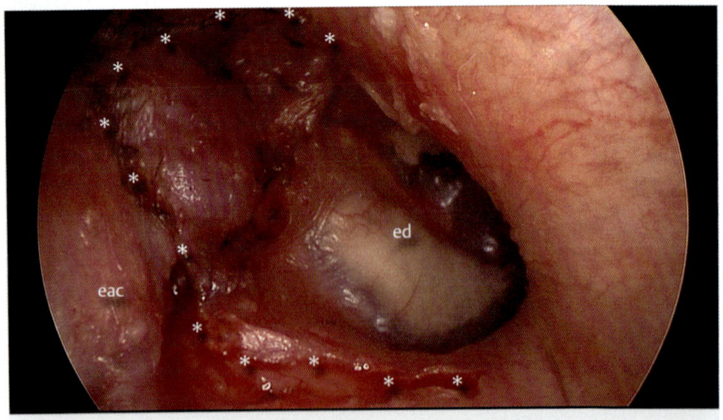

Fig. 10.122 Clinical Case 6, Right ear: A triangle-shaped incision (* * *) is designed on the external auditory canal. *eac: external auditory canal; ed: eardrum.*

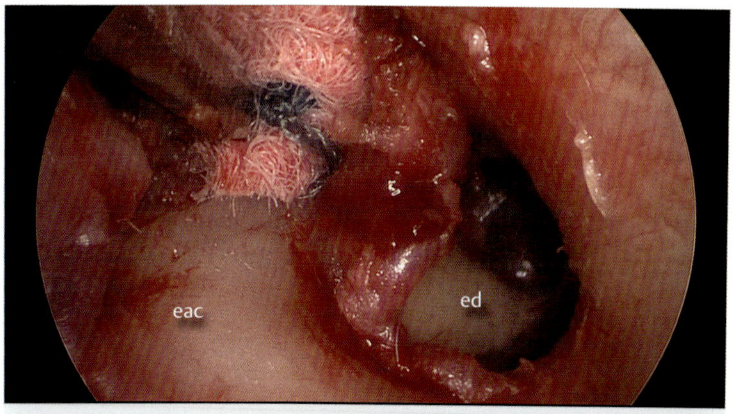

Fig. 10.123 Clinical Case 6, Right ear: A cottonoid is used to raise the flap. *eac: external auditory canal; ed: eardrum.*

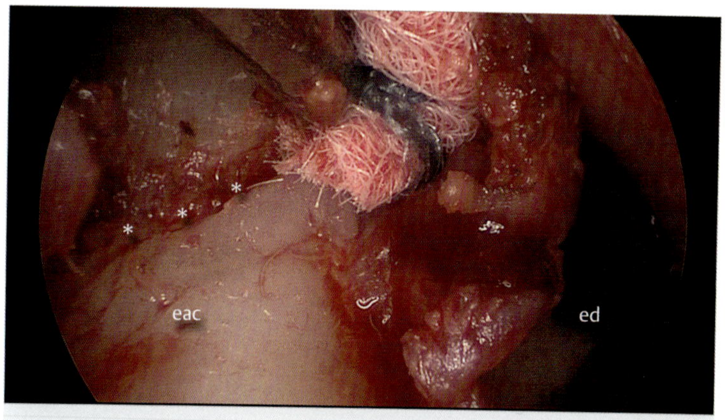

Fig. 10.124 Clinical Case 6, Right ear: A fracture of the external auditory canal is noted (****). *eac: external auditory canal; ed: eardrum.*

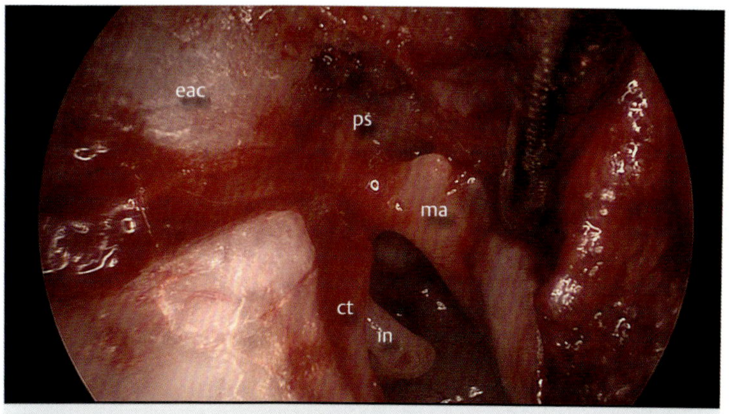

Fig. 10.125 Clinical Case 6, Right ear: The tympanomeatal flap is detached progressively from the malleus. *ct: chorda tympani; eac: external auditory canal; in: incus; ma: malleus; ps: prussak space.*

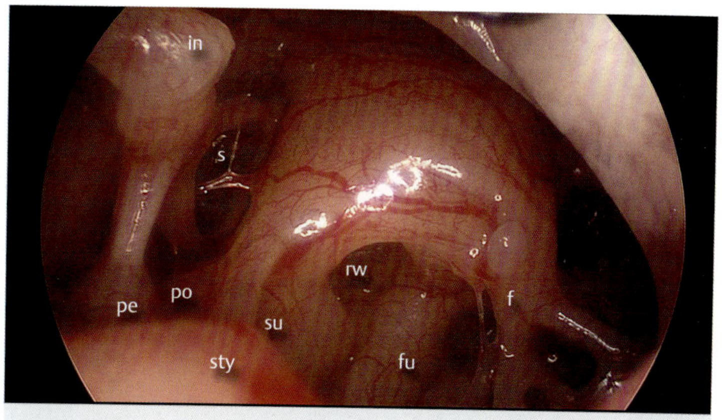

Fig. 10.126 Clinical Case 6, Right ear: Endoscopic magnification of the tympanic cavity. *f: finiculus; fu: fustis; in: incus; pe: pyramidal eminence; po: ponticulus; rw: round window; s: stapes; sty: styloid eminence; su: subiculum.*

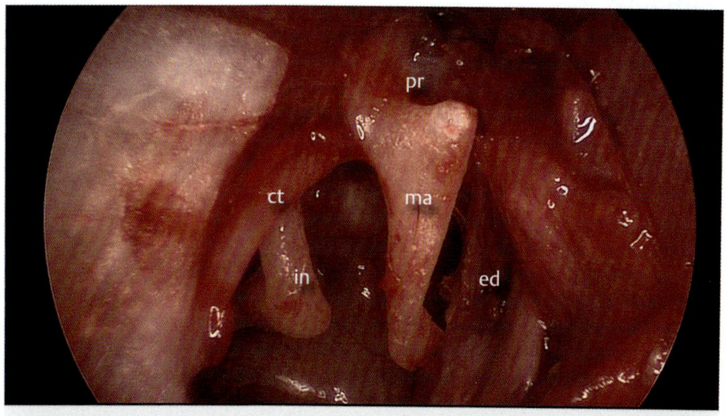

Fig. 10.127 Clinical Case 6, Right ear: The eardrum is detached from the malleus. *ct: chorda tympani; ed: eardrum; in: incus; ma: malleus; pr: Prussak space.*

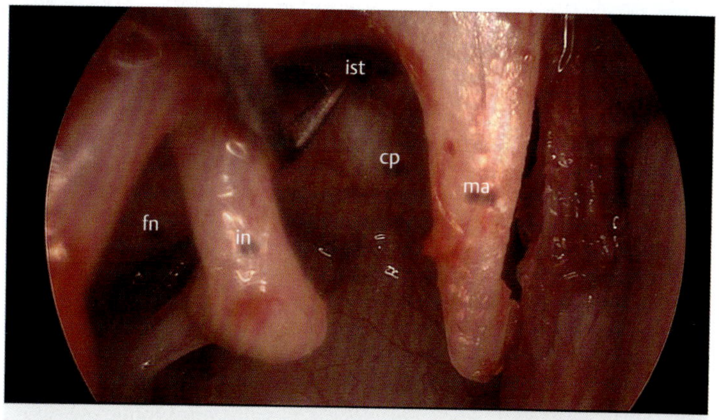

Fig. 10.128 Clinical Case 6, Right ear: An isthmus blockage is found and removed. *cp: cochleariform process; fn: facial nerve; in: incus; ist: epitympanic tympanic; ma: malleus.*

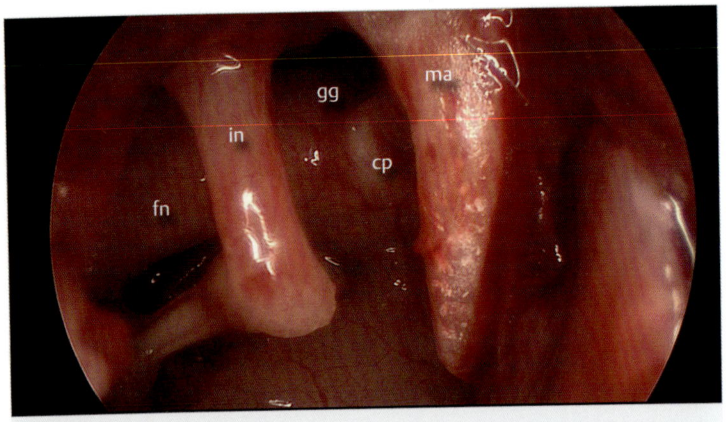

Fig. 10.129 Clinical Case 6, Right ear: The geniculate ganglion is visualized through the isthmus. *cp: cochleariform process; fn: facial nerve; gg: geniculate ganglion; in: incus; ma: malleus.*

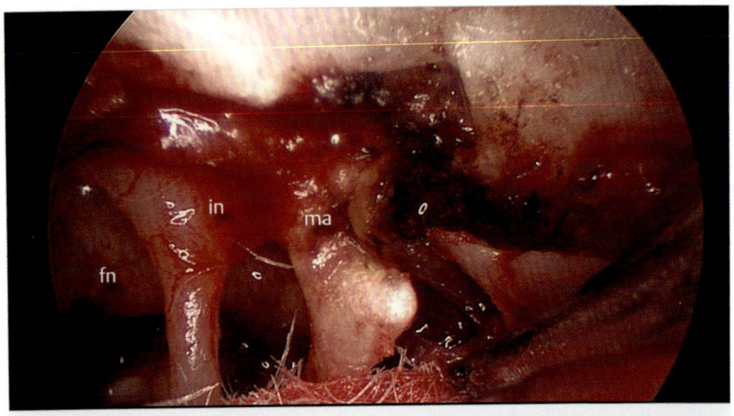

Fig. 10.130 Clinical Case 6, Right ear: A bony fracture anterior to the malleus is detected. *fn: facial nerve; in: incus; ma: malleus.*

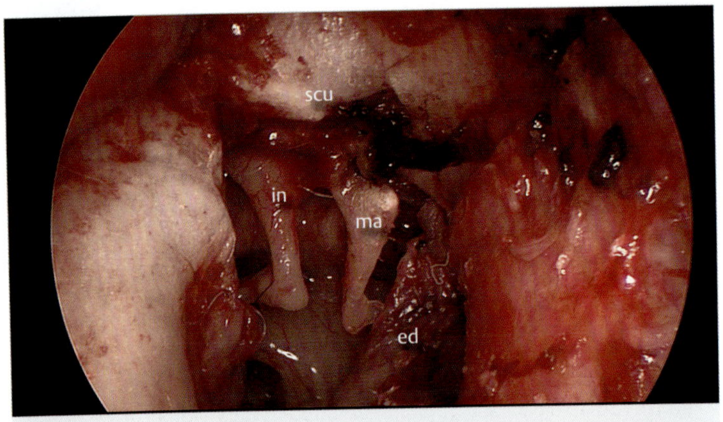

Fig. 10.131 Clinical Case 6, Right ear: Global view of the tympanic cavity. *ed: eardrum; in: incus; ma: malleus; scu: scutum.*

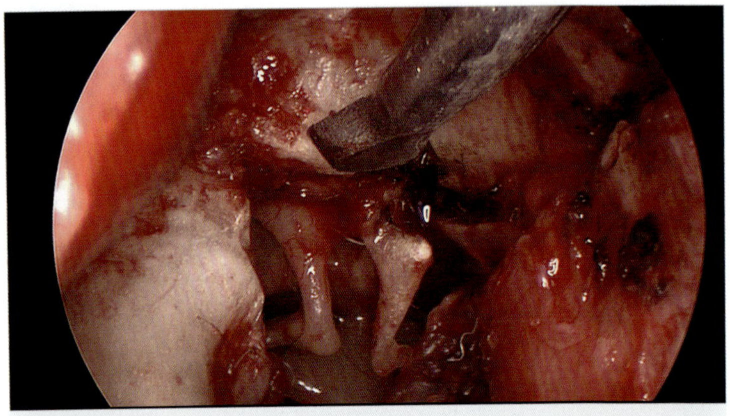

Fig. 10.132 Clinical Case 6, Right ear: Piezosurgery is used to perform the atticotomy.

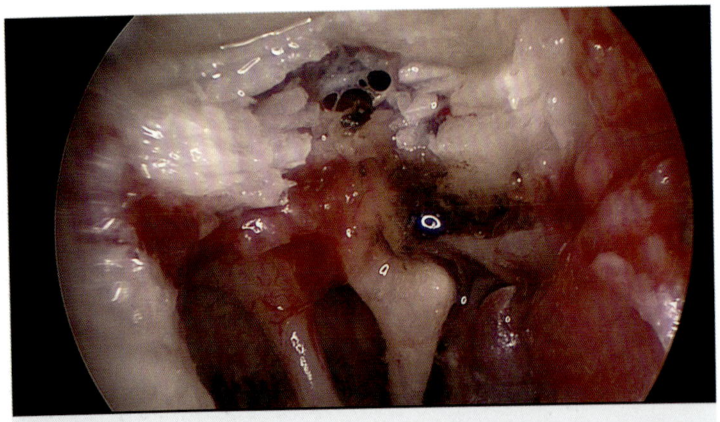

Fig. 10.133 Clinical Case 6, Right ear: The scutum is progressively removed.

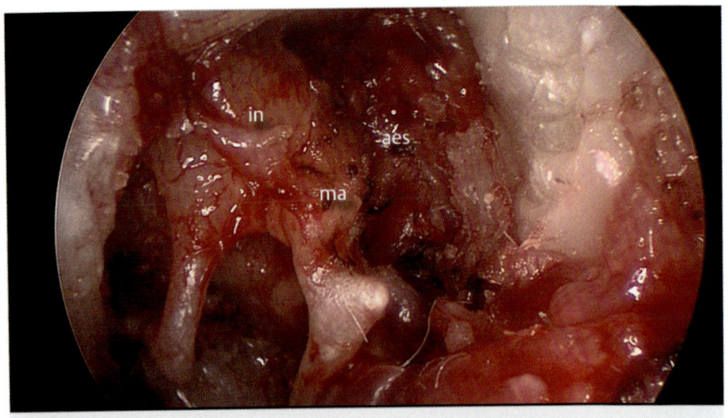

Fig. 10.134 Clinical Case 6, Right ear: The incudomalleolar joint and the attic are endoscopically exposed. *aes: anterior epitympanic space; in: incus; ma: malleus.*

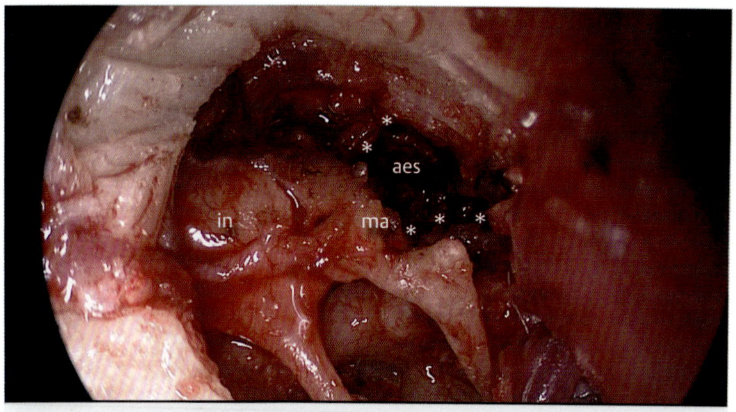

Fig. 10.135 Clinical Case 6, Right ear: The fracture lines are visible (* * *). *aes: anterior epitympanic space; in: incus; ma: malleus.*

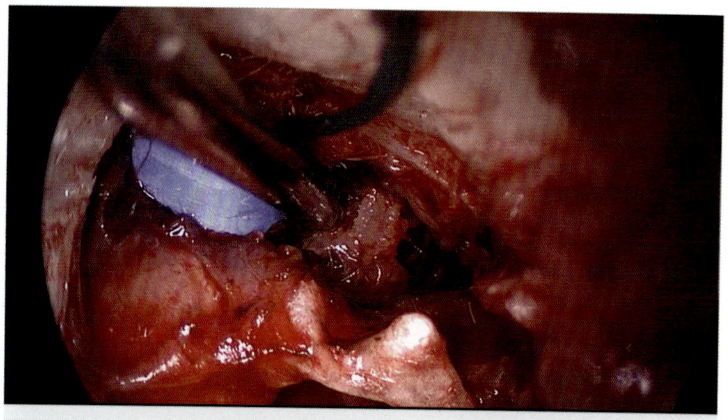

Fig. 10.136 Clinical Case 6, Right ear: The bone spicule is detected.

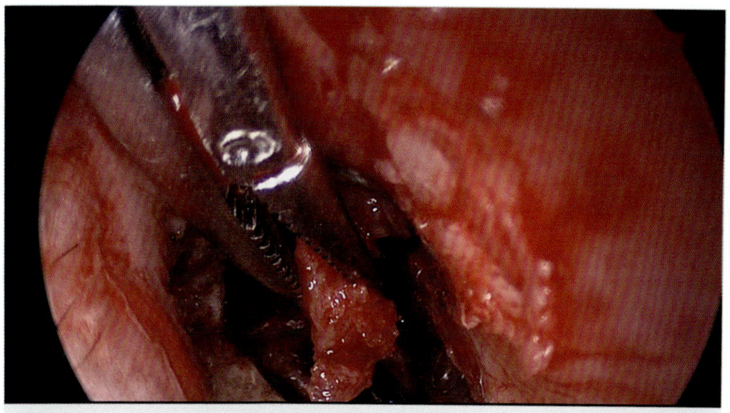

Fig. 10.137 Clinical Case 6, Right ear: The bone spicule is removed.

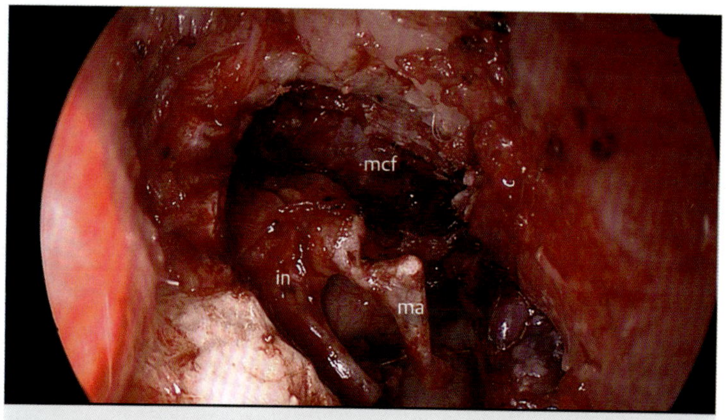

Fig. 10.138 Clinical Case 6, Right ear: The dura of the middle cranial fossa is detected. *in: incus; ma: malleus; mcf: middle cranial fossa.*

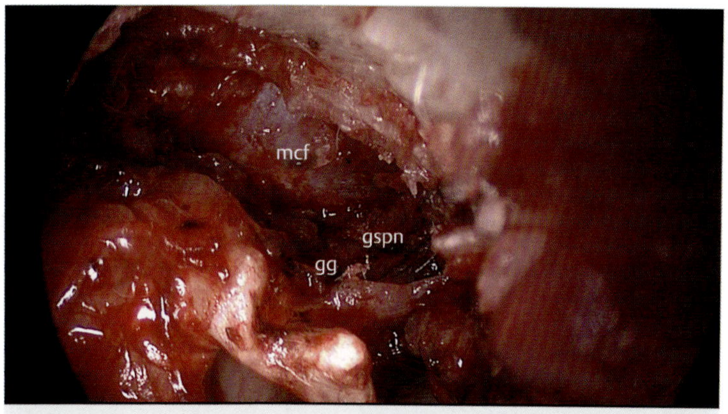

Fig. 10.139 Clinical Case 6, Right ear: The geniculate ganglion and the greater petrosal superficial nerve are visible. *gg: geniculate ganglion; gspn: greater petrosal superficial nerve; mcf: middle cranial fossa.*

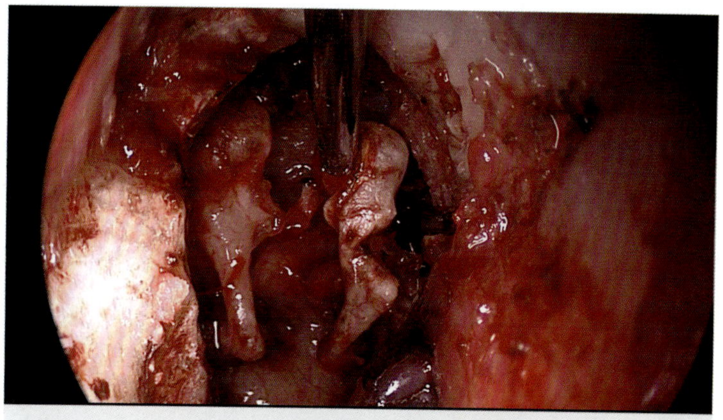

Fig. 10.140 Clinical Case 6, Right ear: The malleus is detached from the incus.

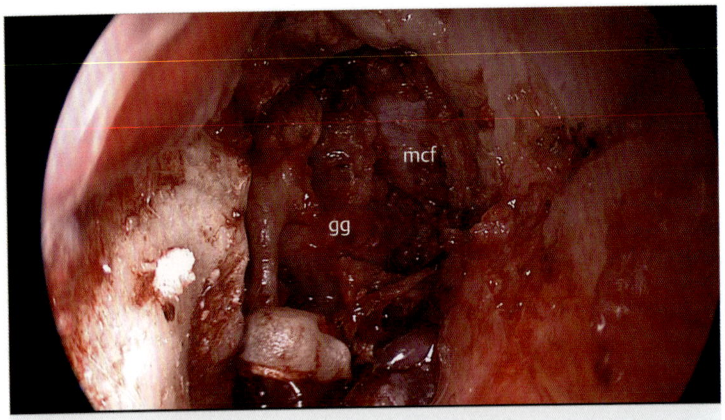

Fig. 10.141 Clinical Case 6, Right ear: The malleus is gently inferiorly pulled, exposing the suprageniculate fossa. *gg: geniculate ganglion; mcf: middle cranial fossa.*

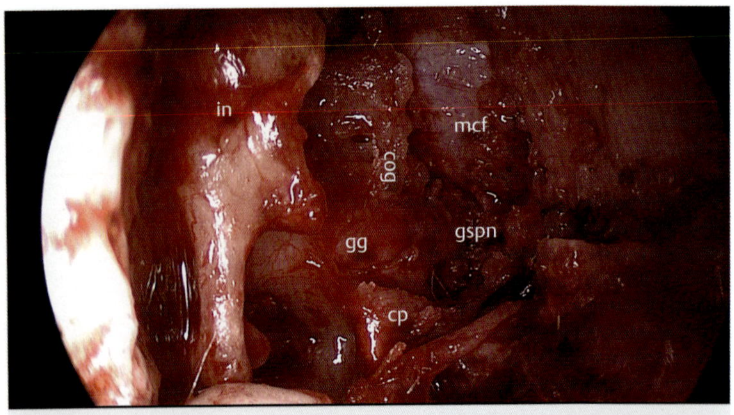

Fig. 10.142 Clinical Case 6, Right ear: The geniculate ganglion is progressively decompressed between the cog and the cochleariform process. *cp: cochleariform process; gg: geniculate ganglion; gspn: greater petrosal superficial nerve; in: incus; mcf: middle cranial fossa.*

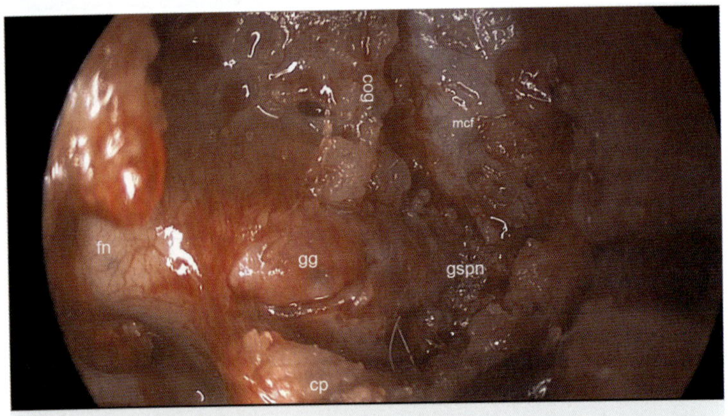

Fig. 10.143 Clinical Case 6, Right ear: Endoscopic magnification of the geniculate ganglion (GG). The relationship among the GG, the cog, and the cochleariform process is noted. *cp: cochleariform process; fn: facial nerve; gg: geniculate ganglion; gspn: greater petrosal superficial nerve; mcf: middle cranial fossa.*

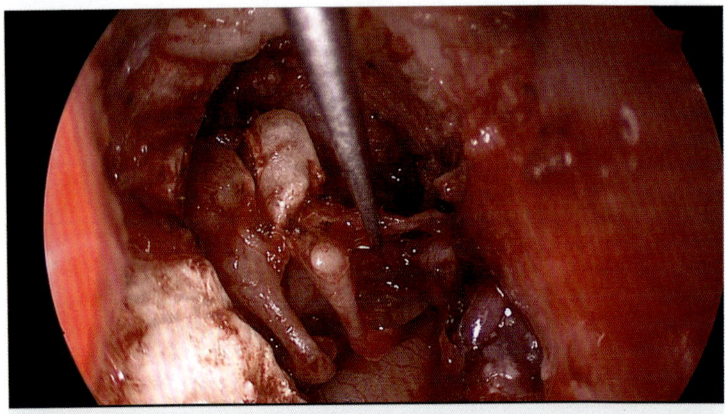

Fig. 10.144 Clinical Case 6, Right ear: The malleus is replaced.

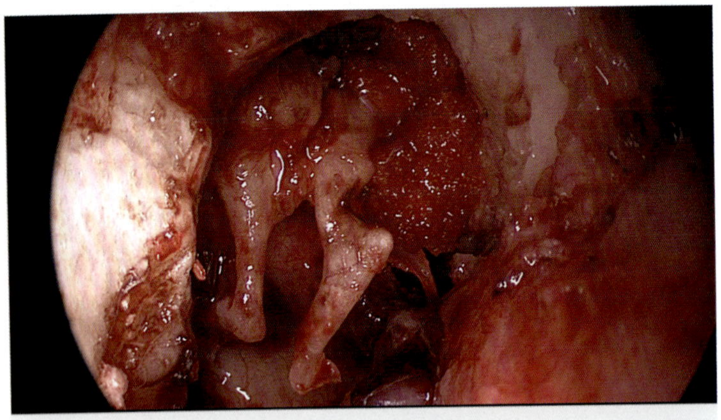

Fig. 10.145 Clinical Case 6, Right ear: The malleus is replaced. A sterile sponge (e.g., Gelfoam) is placed in order to stabilize the incudomalleolar joint.

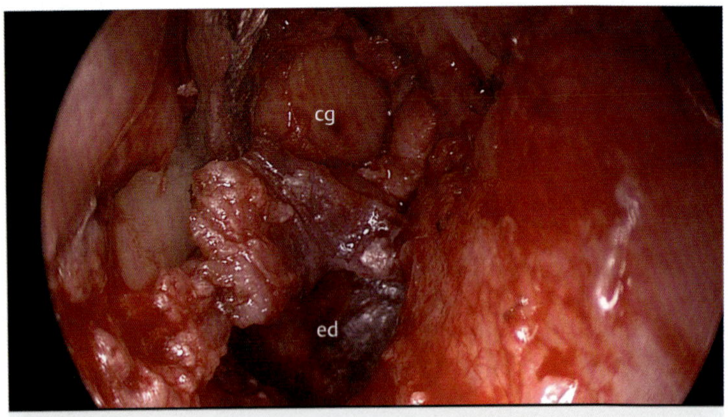

Fig. 10.146 Clinical Case 6, Right ear: A cartilage graft is used to reconstruct the attical defect. *cg: cartilage graft; ed: eardrum.*

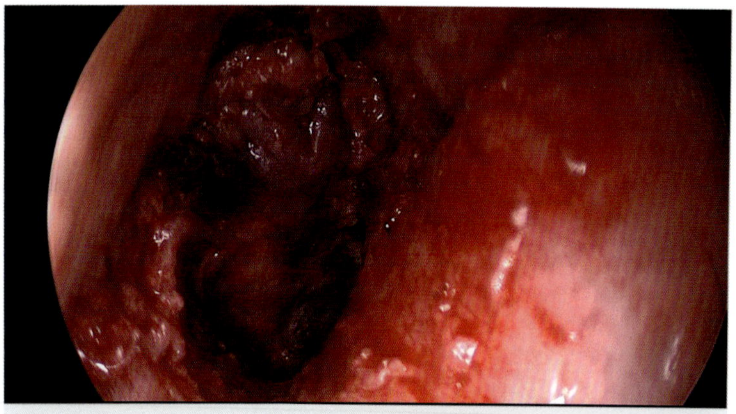

Fig. 10.147 Clinical Case 6, Right ear: Final view after tympano-meatal flap repositioning.

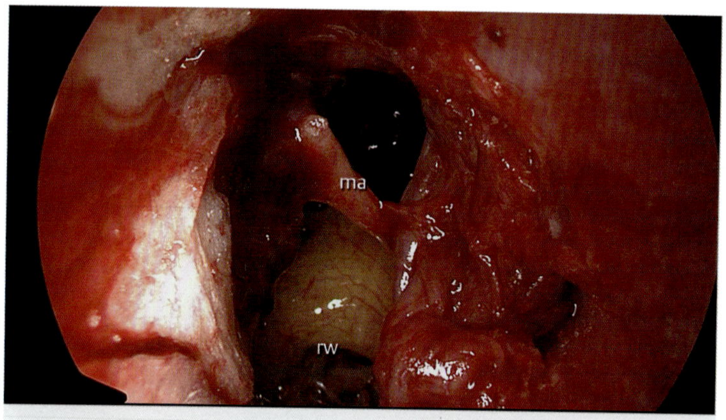

Fig. 10.148 Clinical Case 7, Right ear: Subject with right peripheral facial palsy and right conductive hearing loss after a temporal bone fracture. The tympanomeatal flap is elevated; a blood clot is noted in the tympanic cavity. *ma: malleus; rw: round window.*

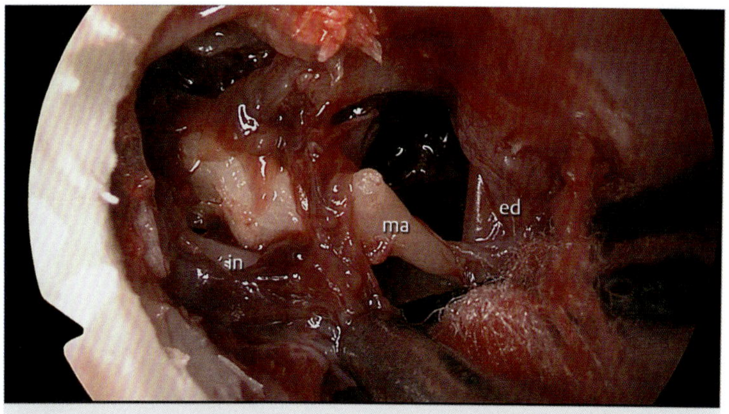

Fig. 10.149 Clinical Case 7, Right ear: The atticotomy is performed. The incus disjointed malleus can be noticed. *ed: eardrum; in: incus; ma: malleus.*

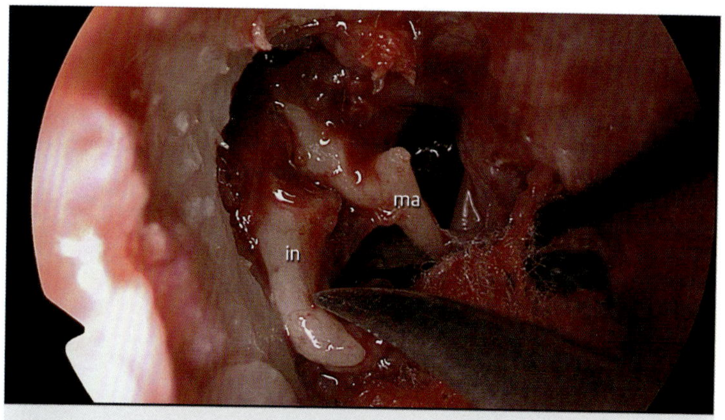

Fig. 10.150 Clinical Case 7, Right ear: The incus is removed. *in: incus; ma: malleus.*

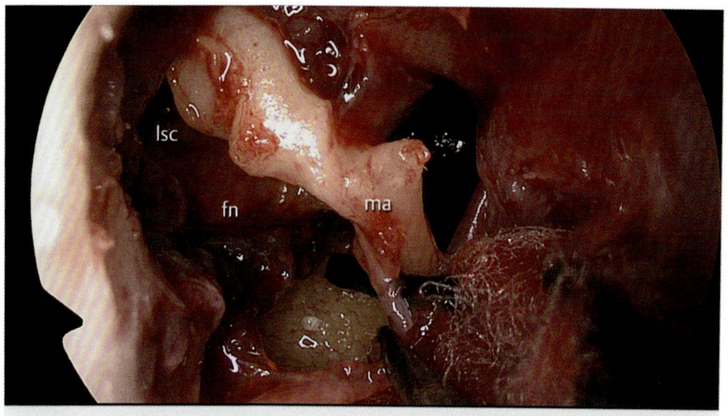

Fig. 10.151 Clinical Case 7, Right ear: The facial nerve is detected. *fn: facial nerve; lsc: lateral semicircular canal; ma: malleus.*

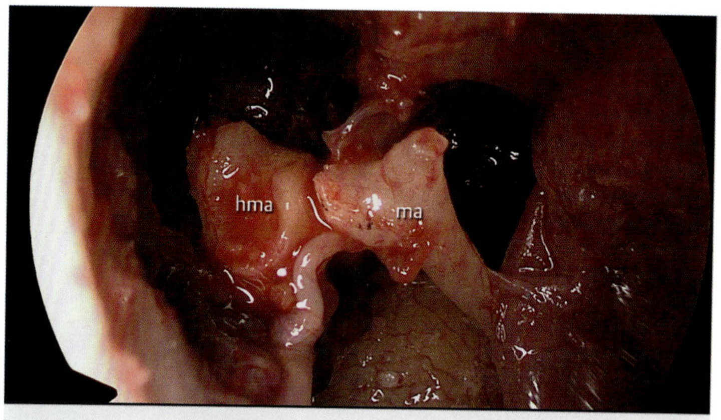

Fig. 10.152 Clinical Case 7, Right ear: The head of the malleus is cut. *hma: head of malleus; ma: malleus.*

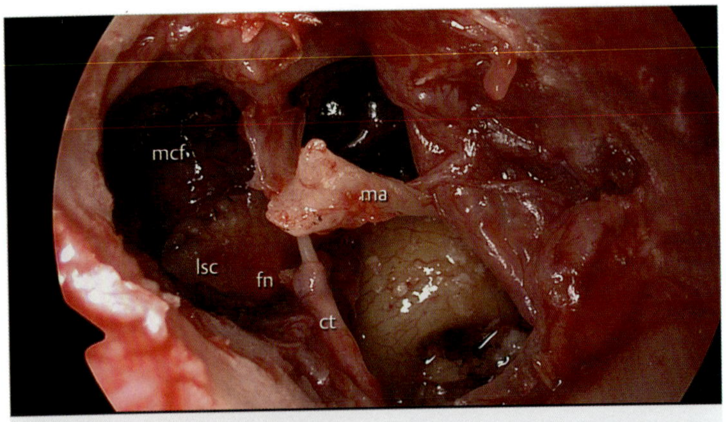

Fig. 10.153 Clinical Case 7, Right ear: The attic with the tympanic segment of the facial nerve is endoscopically exposed. *ct: chorda tympani; fn: facial nerve; lsc: lateral semicircular canal; ma: malleus; mcf: middle cranial fossa.*

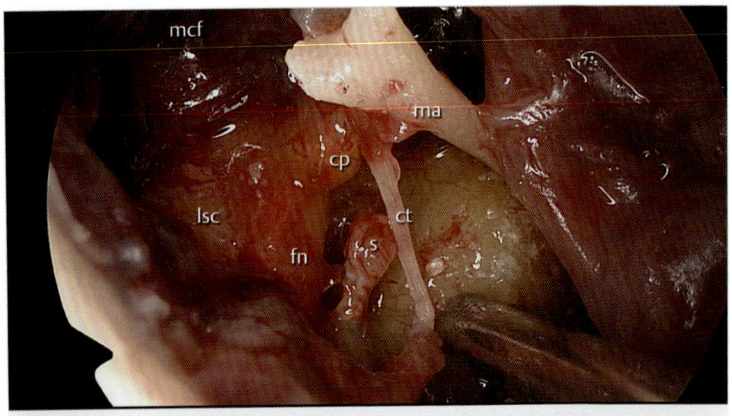

Fig. 10.154 Clinical Case 7, Right ear: The anatomical relationship between the tympanic facial nerve and the cochleariform process is noted. *cp: cochleariform process; ct: chorda tympani; fn: facial nerve; lsc: lateral semicircular canal; ma: malleus; mcf: middle cranial fossa; s: stapes.*

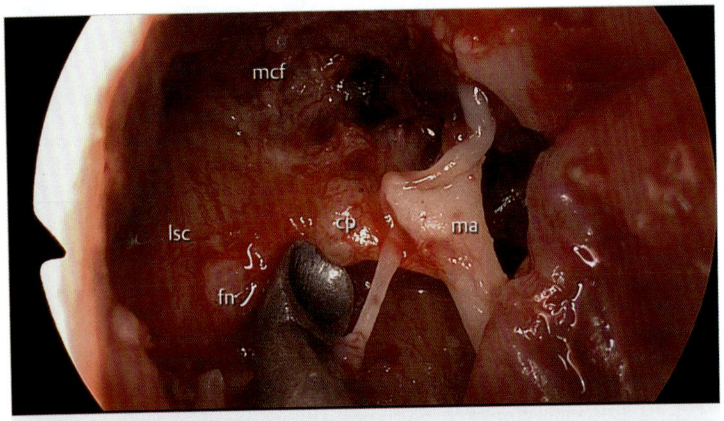

Fig. 10.155 Clinical Case 7, Right ear: A microcurette is used to remove the cochleariform process in order to decompress the geniculate ganglion. *cp: cochleariform process; fn: facial nerve; lsc: lateral semicircular canal; ma: malleus; mcf: middle cranial fossa.*

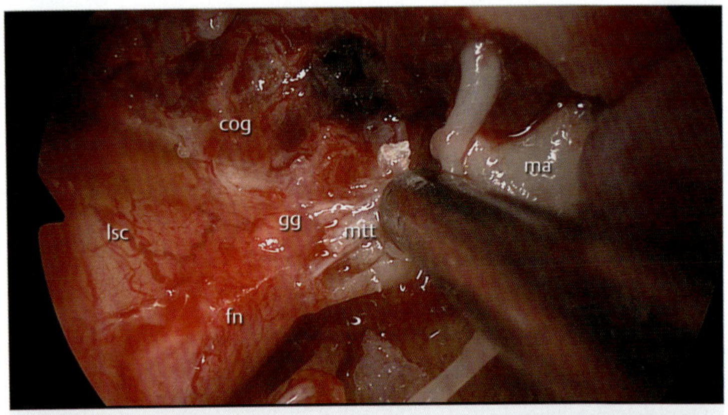

Fig. 10.156 Clinical Case 7, Right ear: During the cochleariform process removal, the surgeon should pay attention to the close relationship between the tensor tympani muscle and the geniculate ganglion. *fn: facial nerve; gg: geniculate ganglion; lsc: lateral semicircular canal; ma: malleus; mtt: tensor tympani muscle.*

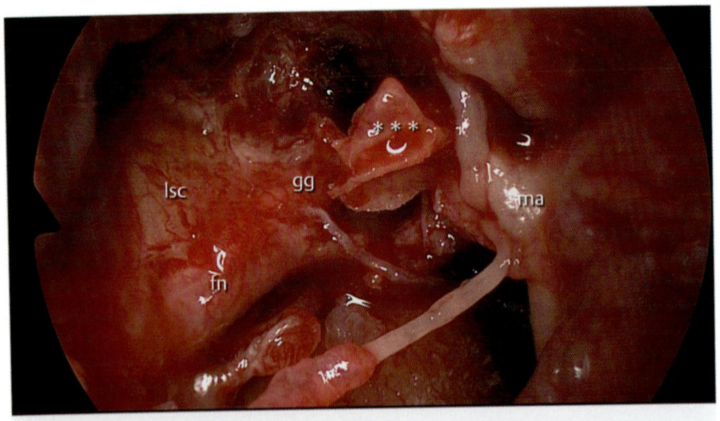

Fig. 10.157 Clinical Case 7, Right ear: The bone spicule (***) compressing the geniculate ganglion is removed. *fn: facial nerve; gg: geniculate ganglion; lsc: lateral semicircular canal; ma: malleus.*

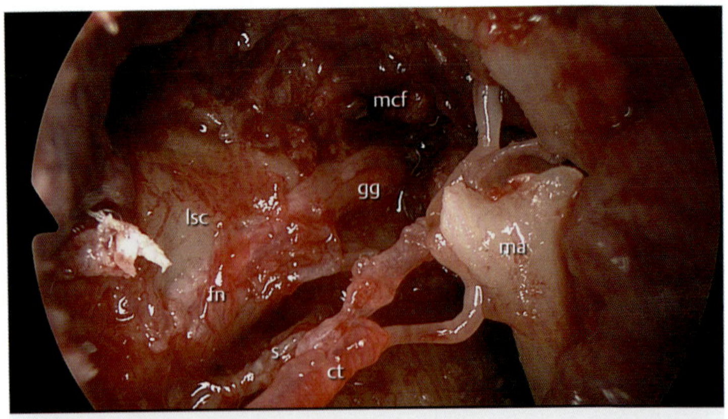

Fig. 10.158 Clinical Case 7, Right ear: The geniculate ganglion is decompressed. *ct: chorda tympani; fn: facial nerve; gg: geniculate ganglion; lsc: lateral semicircular canal; ma: malleus; mcf: middle cranial fossa; s: stapes.*

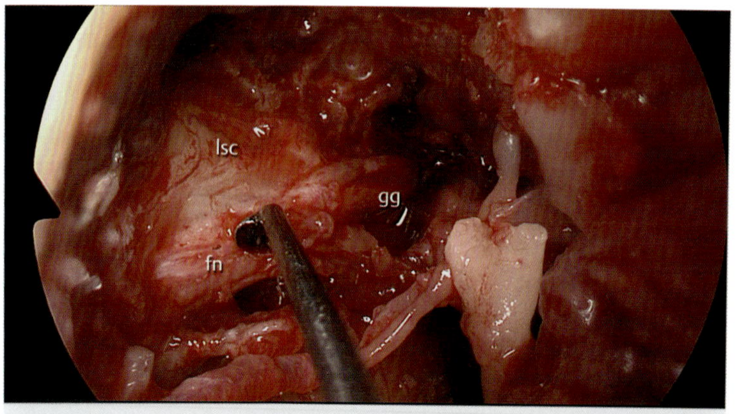

Fig. 10.159 Clinical Case 7, Right ear: The tympanic segment of the facial nerve is decompressed using a small dissector. *fn: facial nerve; gg: geniculate ganglion; lsc: lateral semicircular canal.*

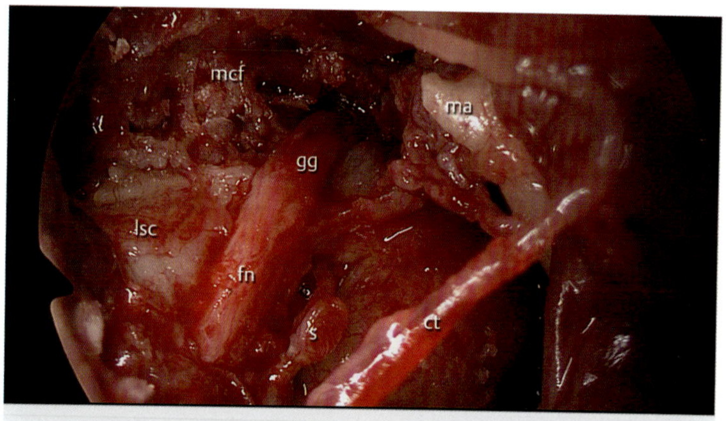

Fig. 10.160 Clinical Case 7, Right ear: Endoscopic view after facial nerve decompression. *ct: chorda tympani; fn: facial nerve; gg: geniculate ganglion; lsc: lateral semicircular canal; ma: malleus; mcf: middle cranial fossa; s: stapes.*

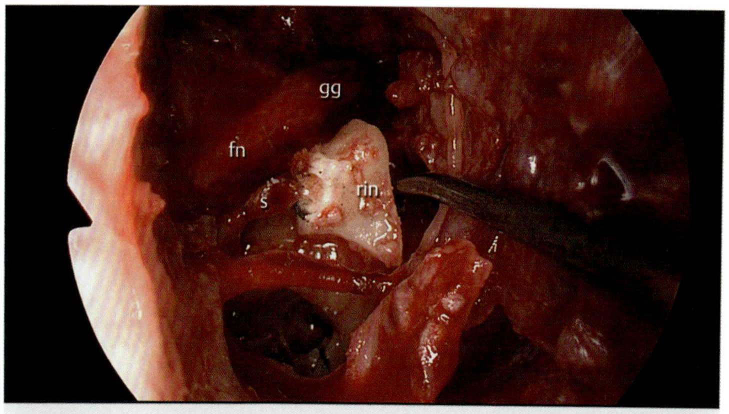

Fig. 10.161 Clinical Case 7, Right ear: An ossicular chain reconstruction is performed using a remodeled incus on the stapes. *fn: facial nerve; gg: geniculate ganglion; rin: remodeled incus; s: stapes.*

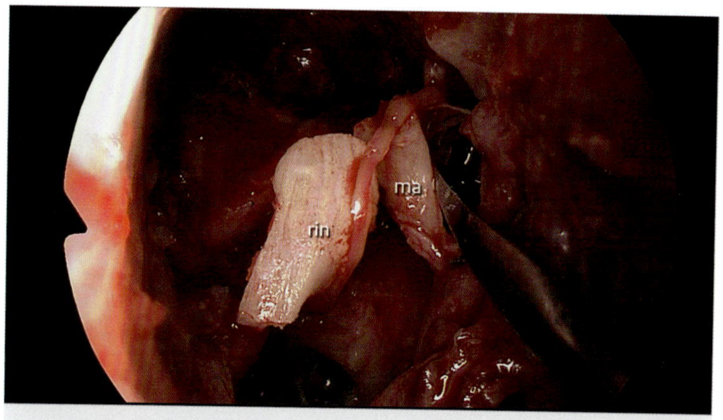

Fig. 10.162 Clinical Case 7, Right ear: Endoscopic view after ossicular chain reconstruction. *ma: malleus; rin: remodeled incus.*

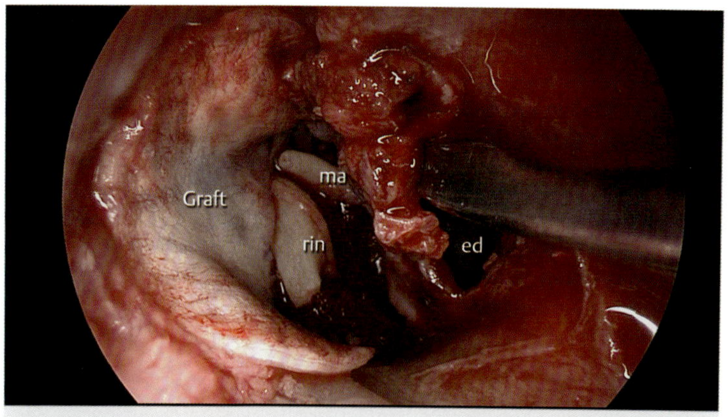

Fig. 10.163 Clinical Case 7, Right ear: A cartilage and perichondrium graft is used to reconstruct the attic. *ed: eardrum; ma: malleus; rin: remodeled incus.*

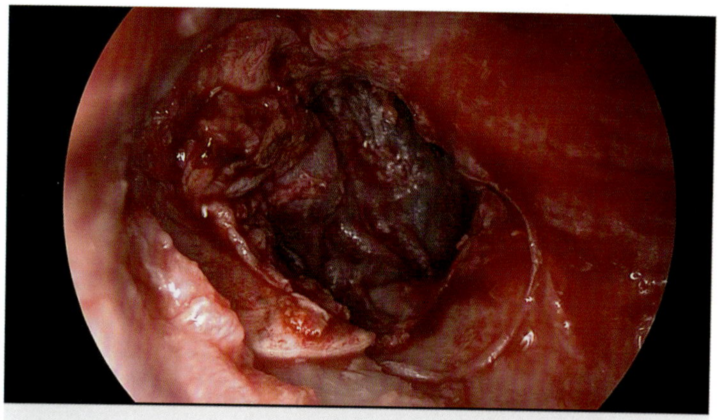

Fig. 10.164 Clinical Case 7, Right ear: The tympanomeatal flap is replaced.

References

[1] Marchioni D, Alicandri-Ciufelli M, Mattioli F, et al. From external to internal auditory canal: surgical anatomy by an exclusive endoscopic approach. Eur Arch Otorhinolaryngol. 2013; 270(4):1267–1275

[2] Marchioni D, Alicandri-Ciufelli M, Rubini A, Presutti L. Endoscopic transcanal corridors to the lateral skull base: Initial experiences. Laryngoscope. 2015; 125 Suppl 5:S1–S13

[3] Presutti L, Alicandri-Ciufelli M, Rubini A, Gioacchini FM, Marchioni D. Combined lateral microscopic/endoscopic approaches to petrous apex lesions: pilot clinical experiences. Ann Otol Rhinol Laryngol. 2014; 123(8):550–559

[4] Marchioni D, Alicandri-Ciufelli M, Piccinini A, et al. Surgical anatomy of transcanal endoscopic approach to the tympanic facial nerve. Laryngoscope. 2011; 121(7):1565–1573

Suggested Readings

Jenkins HA, Ator GA. Traumatic facial paralysis. In: Brackmann DE, Shelton C, Arriaga MA, eds. Otologic Surgery (Chapter 30). 2nd ed. Philadelphia, PA: Saunders; 2001:329

Sanna M, Sunose H, Mancini F, et al. Anatomy of temporal bone. In: Middle Ear and Mastoid Microsurgery (Chapter 1). Stuttgart, Germany: Georg Thieme Verlag; 2003

Marchioni D, Alicandri-Ciufelli M, Mattioli F, et al. From external to internal auditory canal: surgical anatomy by an exclusive endoscopic approach. Eur Arch Otorhinolaryngol. 2013; 270(4):1267–1275

Marchioni D, Mattioli F, Alicandri-Ciufelli M, Presutti L. Endoscopic approach to tensor fold in patients with attic cholesteatoma. Acta Otolaryngol. 2009; 129 (9):946–954

Marchioni D, Alicandri-Ciufelli M, Molteni G, Genovese E, Presutti L. Endoscopic tympanoplasty in patients with attic retraction pockets. Laryngoscope. 2010; 120 (9):1847–1855

Marchioni D, Alicandri-Ciufelli M, Molteni G, Villari D, Monzani D, Presutti L. Ossicular chain preservation after exclusive endoscopic transcanal tympanoplasty: preliminary experience. Otol Neurotol. 2011; 32(4):626–631

Chapter 11

Transcanal Transpromontorial Approaches to the Internal Auditory Canal and the Cerebellopontine Angle

11

11 Transcanal Transpromontorial Approaches to the Internal Auditory Canal and the Cerebellopontine Angle

Daniele Marchioni, Barbara Masotto, Alejandro Rivas, Lukas Anschütz, and Livio Presutti

Abstract

The transcanal transpromontorial approach is an innovative and minimally invasive surgical procedure for the treatment of tumors limited to the inner ear, the internal auditory canal (IAC), with a minimal extension to cerebellopontine angle (CPA).

This approach requires the removal of the promontory region, to reach the inner ear, and the removal of the cochlear-vestibular bone, to reach the internal auditory canal, using a surgical corridor between the following landmarks: the vertical tract of the petrous internal carotid artery anteriorly, the tympanic portion of the facial nerve (FN) superiorly, the mastoid portion of the FN posteriorly, and the jugular bulb inferiorly.

Two different transpromontorial approaches can be distinguished: an endoscopic transcanal transpromontorial approach and a microscopic enlarged transcanal transpromontorial approach.

The endoscopic transcanal transpromontorial approach is a totally endoscopic procedure for the removal of small lesions located in the inner ear and the IAC.

The microscopic enlarged transcanal transpromontorial approach is a microscopic endoscopic assisted procedure for the surgical treatment of larger lesions involving the IAC and the CPA.

In this approach the skeletonization of the meningeal plane and the manipulation of the cerebellum are not required. Therefore, it has a low morbidity rate and it is considered a minimally invasive surgical approach.

Keywords: vestibular schwannoma, internal auditory canal, cerebellopontine angle, acoustic neuroma, minimally invasive

11.1 Introduction

The traditional approaches to the internal auditory canal (IAC) can be classified according to the surgical route in relation to the otic capsule (see ▶ Table 11.1). We distinguish approaches that pass through the otic capsule like the translabyrinthine, transotic, and transcochlear approaches, and approaches that preserve the otic capsule reaching the IAC superiorly like the middle cranial fossa (MCF), and posteriorly like retrosigmoid and retrolabyrinthine. All these approaches require a lot of bone removal with an extensive skeletonization and manipulation of the middle and posterior cranial fossa meninges and manipulation of the brainstemal regions. These procedures are also indicated in case of lesions with exclusive development within the IAC. The recent introduction of the endoscopic surgery of the middle ear has enabled the surgeon to improve the anatomical knowledge of the tympanic cavity and the endoscopic dissection has also allowed for the establishment of a new surgical route directed to the IAC toward the external auditory canal (EAC) as a natural surgical corridor (▶ Fig. 11.1). This surgical route is classified according to the surgical pathways that pass through the otic capsule, and it is characterized by a direct exposure of the fundus of the IAC, the cochlea, and the vestibule. In this approach the skeletonization of the meningeal plane and the manipulation of the encephalic trunk structures is not required; therefore, it is considered a minimally invasive surgical approach to lesions with exclusive localization in the IAC. The result is a type of approach that focuses on the tumor without encephalic trunk and meningeal retraction, sharing the same rationale as the endoscopic transnasal approaches for anterior cranial base lesions.

Table 11.1 A summary of the indications, advantages, and disadvantages of the main surgical approaches to the lateral skull base.

	Indications	Advantages	Disadvantages
Middle cranial fossa	• Tumors inside the IAC	• Hearing preservation • Good control of lateral IAC tumors	• Large craniotomy • Large myocutaneous flap • Access to the FN from above • Retraction of the temporal lobe
Translabyrinthine	• Tumors inside the IAC and with limited extension to the CPA	• Good control of tumors in the posterior part of the IAC	• Demolition of the labyrinth • Demolition of the mastoid
Retrosigmoid	• Tumors at the CPA • Large tumors	• Hearing preservation • Good control of CPA structures and vessels • Possibility to use an endoscope inside the IAC	• Craniotomy • Limited acces to the IAC • Morbidity (headache)
EndoTTA	• Tumors in the fundus of the IAC	• Sraight access • Endoscopic magnification and overview • Minimally invasive access • Low morbidity • Excellent control of the FN	• Demolition of the cochlea
ExpTTA	• Tumors in the IAC with extension to the IAC porus	• Straight access • Endoscopic magnification and overview • Minimally invasive access • Low morbidity • Excellent control of the FN	• Demolition of the cochlea

Abbreviations: CPA, cerebellopontine angle; EndoTTA, exclusively endoscopic transcanal transpromontorial approach; ExpTTA, enlarged transcanal transpromontorial approach; FN, facial nerve; IAC, internal auditory canal.

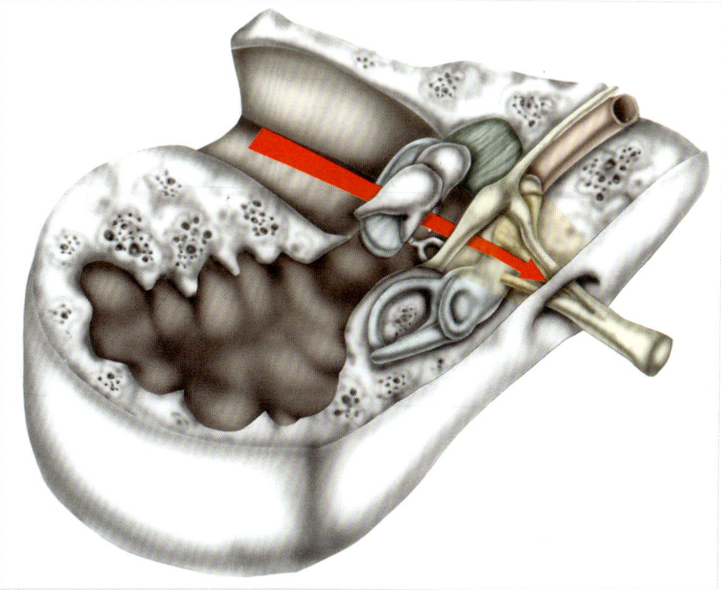

Fig. 11.1 Schematic drawing representing the surgical route to the internal auditory canal (IAC) of the transcanal transpromontorial approach.

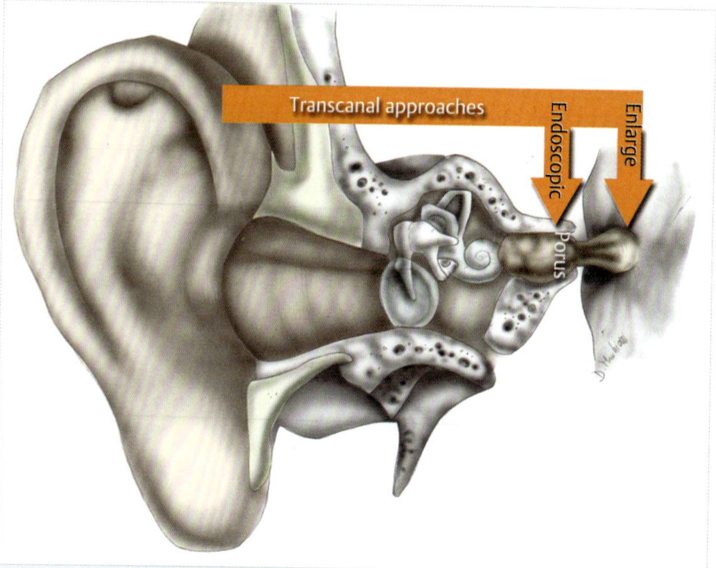

Fig. 11.2 The two transcanal transpromontorial approaches, with relative indications based on the extension of the tumor.

To perform this surgical method, it is necessary to remove the ossicular chain and the promontory with the sacrifice of the cochlea. Therefore, the transpromontoral transcanal pathway is classified as one of the surgical pathways that sacrifice the patient's auditory function (see ▶ Table 11.1). The approach from the EAC to the IAC allows for the skeletonization of the IAC from the fundus to the porus in a lateral to medial direction, from superiorly to inferiorly, exposing the anterior, inferior, and posterior walls of the IAC. Although this surgical approach represents an innovation with minimally invasive characteristics for the treatment of tumors limited to the IAC, lesions that involve the cerebellopontine angle (CPA) represent its relative limitation.

We will deal with different approaches:

- The endoscopic transcanal transpromontorial approach whose indications are lesions located exclusively in the IAC (see ▶ Fig. 11.2)
- The microscopic enlarged transcanal transpromontorial approach whose indications are lesions involving the IAC and the CPA (see ▶ Fig. 11.2)

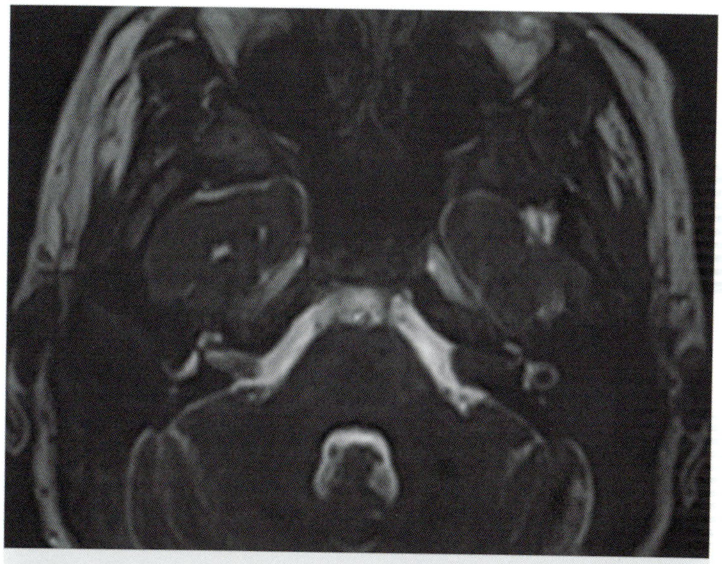

Fig. 11.3 Magnetic resonance imaging (MRI) of the brain, axial view: Typical indication for an endoscopic transcanal transpromontorial approach. A residual tumor growing inside the left internal auditory canal (IAC) in a patient with no hearing function on the same side who underwent a retrosigmoid approach 5 years before.

11.2 Exclusively Endoscopic Transcanal Transpromontorial Approach (EndoTTA)

This surgical procedure is considered an exclusively transcanal pathway that does not require incisions outside the EAC. It requires the exclusive use of endoscopy in the management of the lesion. It is a one-hand technique exactly like traditional endoscopic middle ear surgery and for this reason, the indications are lesions limited to the fundus of the IAC, to the cochlea, and to the vestibule without involvement of the porus.

11.2.1 Indications

- Growing masses located in the IAC discovered during a magnetic resonance imaging (MRI) radiological follow-up;
- Simptomatic vestibular schwannomas of the IAC with intractable vertigo;
- Residual tumors growing inside the IAC after a retrosigmoid approach (see ▶ Fig. 11.3);
- Vestibular schwannomas, Koos scale grade I: mainly located in the fundus of the IAC;
- Intralabyrinthine schwannomas and cochlear schwannomas with or without IAC involvement (see Clinical Case 7);
- American Academy of Otolaryngology–Head and Neck Surgery (AAO-HNS) Class D hearing status (severe to profound hearing loss).

11.2.2 Contraindications

- Tumors with exclusive location in the CPA, or involving the CPA. In these cases, the presence of a larger surgical window with the possibility of two-handed management is considered safer.

- Vascular anomalies of the anterior inferior cerebellar artery (AICA) with loops at the level of the IAC can be a relative contraindication, which might lead to a hemorrhagic risk that would need to convert the intervention to a standard approach.
- A relative contraindication is the anatomical conformation of a high jugular bulb, which would prevent an adequate surgical access to the porus and it would lead to possible bleeding from the jugular bulb during the surgical maneuvers of tumor removal from the IAC.

11.2.3 Advantages

- No external incision, no craniotomy;
- Magnification and excellent view of the delicate anatomical structures, especially the facial nerve (FN);
- Easy postoperative care, no intensive care unit (ICU) is required;
- Short operating time, short hospital stay, low morbidity.

11.2.4 Disadvantages

- One-hand surgical technique, longer learning curve;
- Limited indications in terms of tumor size and location;
- Difficult management in case of unexpected bleeding;
- Complete hearing loss.

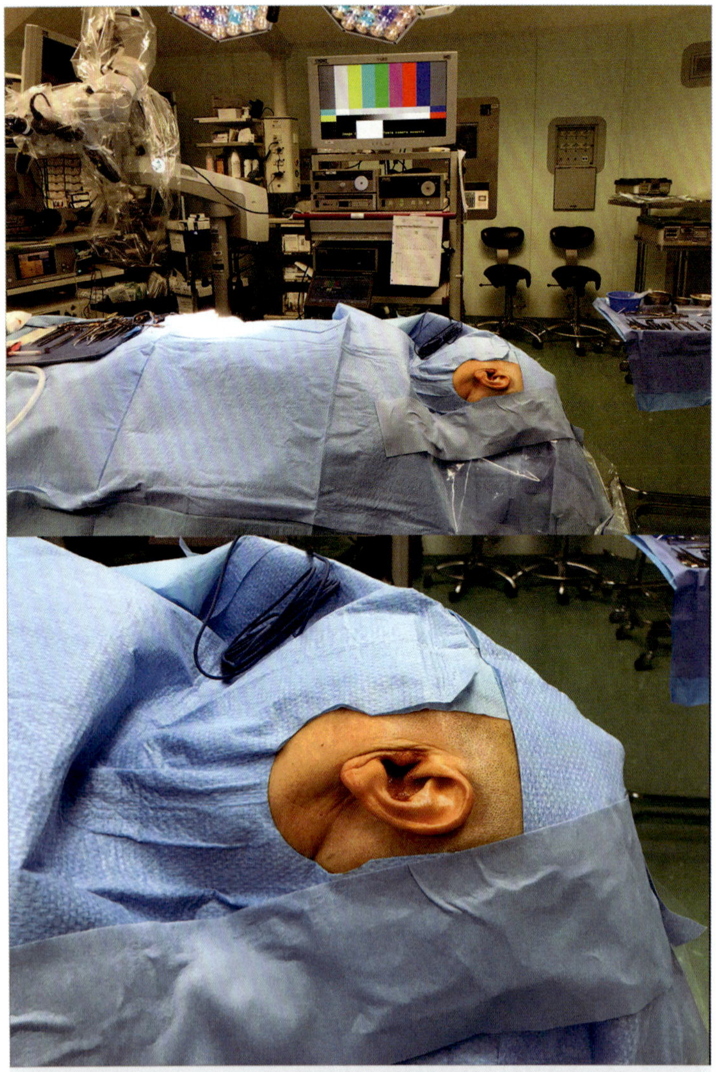

Fig. 11.4 Left side: The patient lies in supine position, with the head contralaterally rotated and extended. The microscope and the monitor for the endoscopic procedures are positioned on the other side with respect to the surgeon.

11.2.5 Preoperative Assessment

- Computed tomography (CT) and MRI with gadolinium contrast, and angiography in selected cases;
- Speech and pure tone audiometry;
- Otoneurological examination.

11.2.6 Surgical Technique (see Clinical Case 1; Clinical Case 2; Clinical Case 3; Clinical Case 4)

The patient lies in a supine position, with the head contralaterally rotated and extended. FN monitoring is installed and tested. The endoscope (0 degrees, 4 mm diameter, and 15 cm length) is held with the left hand and the instrument with the other. The whole surgery is carried out through the EAC; no external incisions are required (▶ Fig. 11.4).

First Step: Access to the Middle Ear

The EAC is circumferentially incised at the level of the osteocartilaginous junction using a monopolar cautery instrument and the skin is elevated until the annulus is reached (▶ Fig. 11.5). During this procedure, cottonoids soaked with an adrenaline solution are placed between the skin and the bone of the EAC to reduce beeding, and the skin flap is progressively and circumferentially elevated and the fibrous annulus in all its circumferential extension is reached (▶ Fig. 11.6). While cutting the skin, particular attention must be paid to the execution of this maneuver to avoid leaving any skin fragments. The annulus is elevated to get into the tympanic cavity and the tympanic membrane is progressively detached from the malleus and lifted along with the skin of the EAC (▶ Fig. 11.7). The skin and the tympanic membrane are removed en bloc allowing for the access to the tympanic cavity (▶ Fig. 11.8).

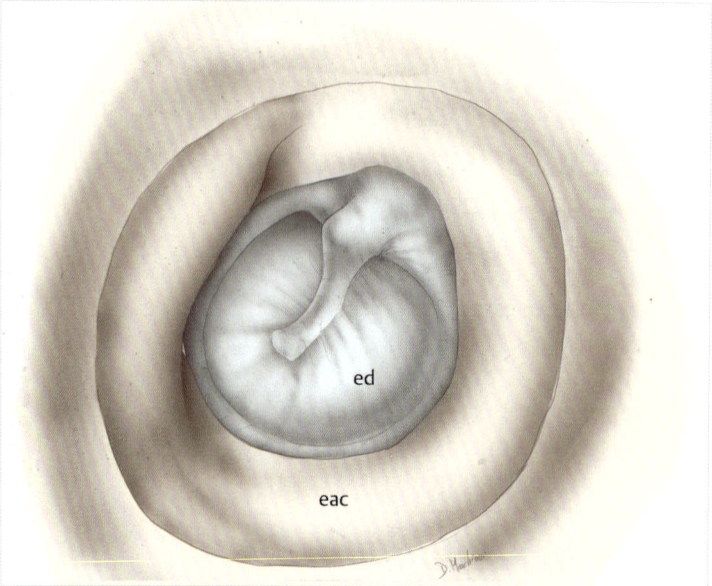

Fig. 11.5 Left side: A circumferential incision of the external auditory canal (EAC) is made. *eac: external auditory canal; ed: eardrum.*

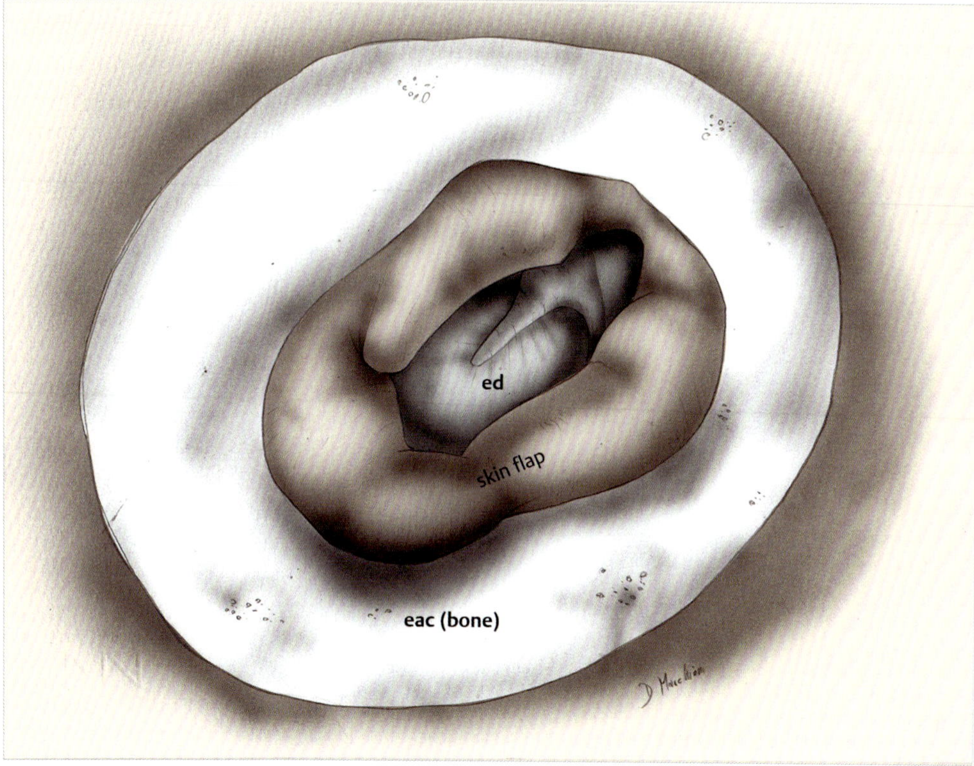

Fig. 11.6 Left side: The skin flap is circumferentially elevated until the annulus is identified. *ed: eardrum; eac: external auditory canal.*

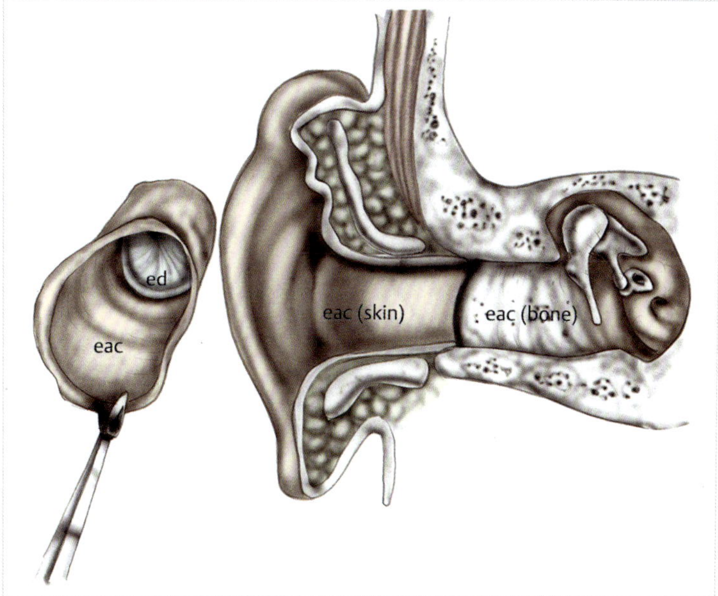

Fig. 11.7 Left side: The skin and the tympanic membrane are removed en bloc to gain access to the tympanic cavity. *eac: external auditory canal; ed: eardrum.*

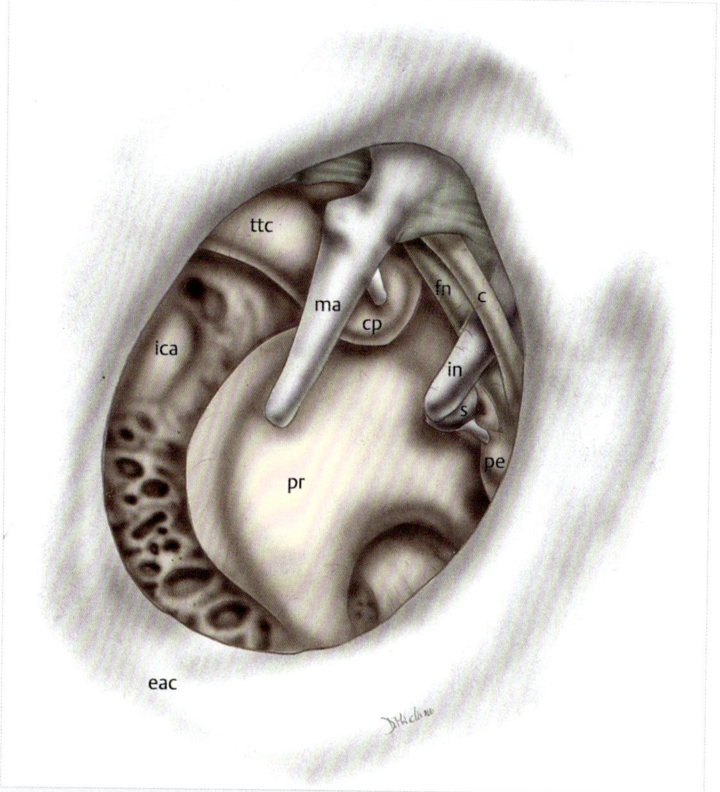

Fig. 11.8 Left side: Endoscopic view of the tympanic cavity after external auditory canal (EAC) skin and eardrum removal. *c: chorda tympani; cp: cochleariform process; fn: facial nerve; ica: internal carotid artery; in: incus; ma: malleus; pe: pyramidal eminence; pr: promontory; s: stapes; ttc: tensor tendon canal.*

The access is enlarged by drilling the bony annulus and the circumference of the EAC, trying not to damage the third intrapetrous portion of the FN (▶ Fig. 11.9). In this phase, it is advisable to use a diamond bur and to perform a circumferential drilling of the whole bony EAC. Drilling makes the use of the instruments through the EAC more comfortable during the phase of tumor removal. It must extend anteriorly to identify the temporomandibular joint, which constitutes the anterior limit of the dissection. It is then continued on the bony annulus to expose the epitympanic, protymanic, hypotympanic, and retrotympanic spaces. The scutum must be progressively removed to uncover the incudomalleolar joint and the entire epitympanum, and the posterior bony annulus is drilled near the third portion of the FN (▶ Fig. 11.10). During this phase it is extremely important to follow the nerve from its tympanic tract up to the second genu, which indicates the level of the third portion of the FN. The hypotympanic and protympanic regions are progressively cut, inferiorly exposing the bulb of the jugular vein and the region of the vertical tract of the internal carotid artery, below the eustachian tube orifice (▶ Fig. 11.11). Once the tympanic cavity has been

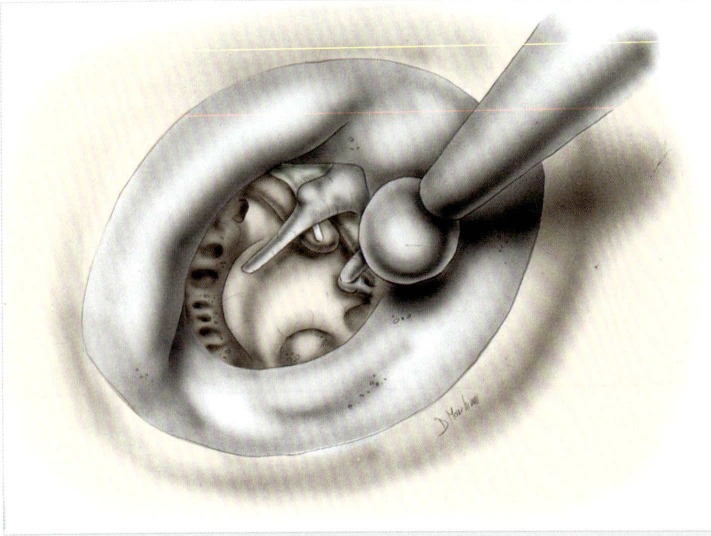

Fig. 11.9 Left side: Under endoscopic view, a diamond bur is used to enlarge the external auditory canal (EAC).

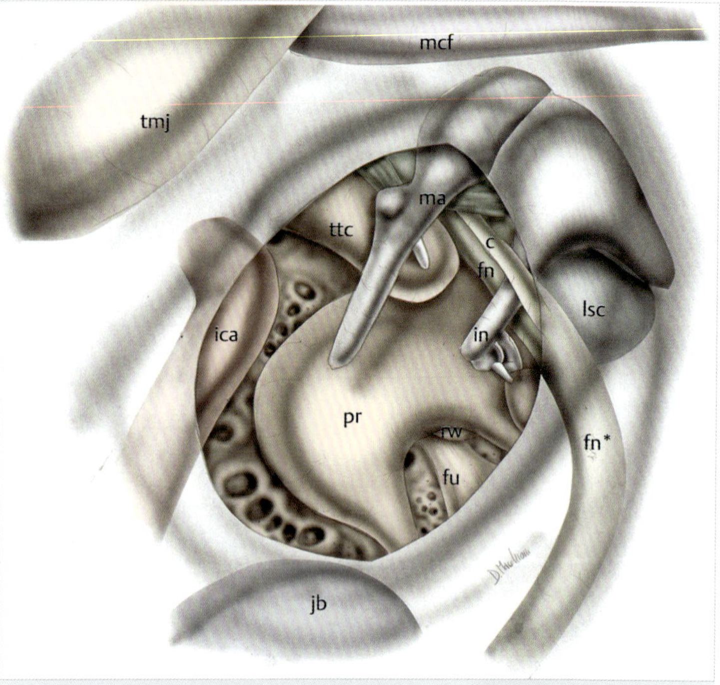

Fig. 11.10 Left side: Endoscopic view of the tympanic cavity. The anatomical boundaries of the endoscopic transcanal transpromontorial approach must be considered during the drilling step of the external auditory canal (EAC). *c: chorda tympani; fn: facial nerve; fn*: mastoid portion of facial nerve; fu: fustis; ica: internal carotid artery; in: incus; jb: jugular bulb; lsc: lateral semicircular canal; ma: malleus; mcf: middle cranial fossa; pr: promontory; rw: round window; tmj: temporomandibular joint; ttc: tensor tendon canal.*

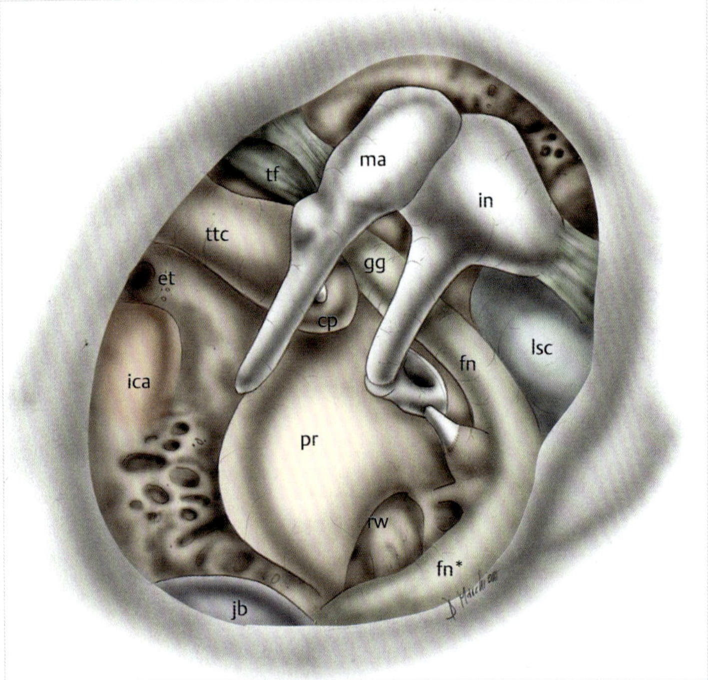

Fig. 11.11 Left side: The tympanic cavity is progressively exposed after the external auditory canal (EAC) drilling; the chorda tympani is cut. *et: eustachian tube; fn: facial nerve; fn* mastoid portion of facial nerve; ica: internal carotid artery; in: incus; jb: jugular bulb; lsc: lateral semicircular canal; ma: malleus; pr: promontory; rw: round window; tf: tensor fold; ttc: tensor tendon canal.*

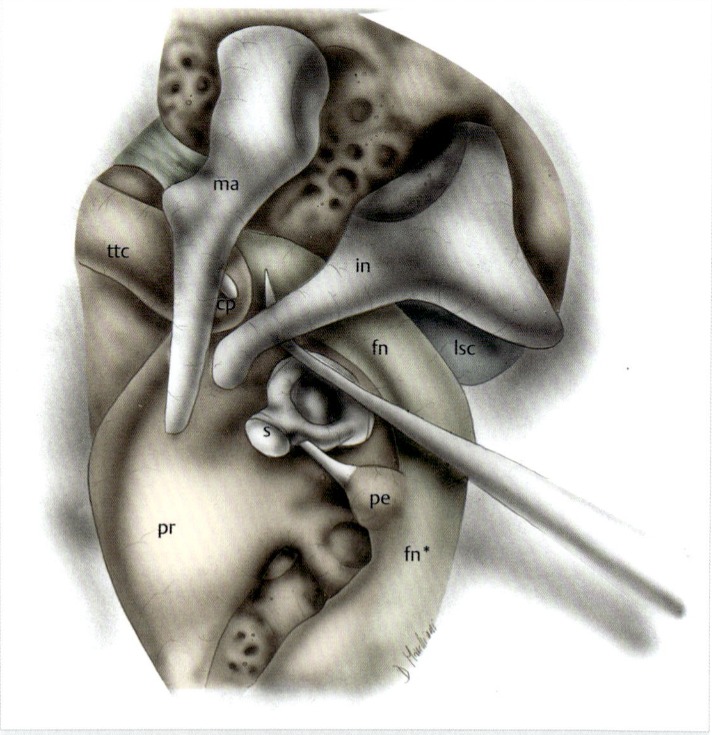

Fig. 11.12 Left side: The incus is removed from the tympanic cavity. *fn: facial nerve; fn* mastoid portion of facial nerve; in: incus; lsc: lateral semicircular canal; ma: malleus; pe: pyramidal eminence; pr: promontory; s: stapes; ttc: tensor tendon canal.*

exposed, the ossicular chain is removed detecting the medial wall of the tympanic cavity.

A hook is used to identify the joint between the incus and the stapes. By gently moving the hook between the joint it is possible to identify the separation plane between the two ossicular structures and detach the incus, which is gently displaced from a medial to a lateral direction and then removed (▶ Fig. 11.12). The excision of the incus allows for the exposure of the tympanic tract of the FN and of the lateral semicircular canal (LSC) posterosuperiorly. The tendon of the tensor tympani muscle is cut at the level of the cochleariform process. The anterior ligament of the malleus is cut off and then the malleus is removed. After this step, it is possible to fully identify the second intrapetrous portion of the FN, from the geniculate ganglion between the cochleariform process and the COG to the LSC (▶ Fig. 11.13).

The oval window, the stapes, and the round window are identified along with the retrotympanic bony crests, the ponticulus, the subiculum, and the finiculus.

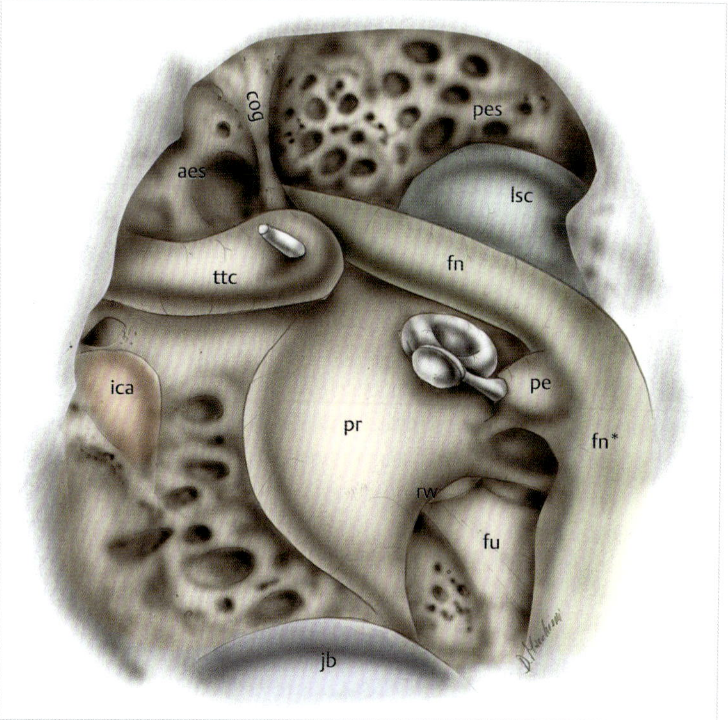

Fig. 11.13 Left side: The malleus is removed, allowing for the access to the medial wall of the tympanic cavity. The tympanic segment of the facial nerve (FN) is detected from the second genu to the geniculate ganglion. *aes: anterior epitympanic space; fn: facial nerve; fn* mastoid portion of facial nerve; fu: fustis; ica: internal carotid artery; jb: jugular bulb; lsc: lateral semicircular canal; pe: pyramidal eminence; pes: posterior epitympanic space; pr: promontory; rw: round window; ttc: tensor tendon canal.*

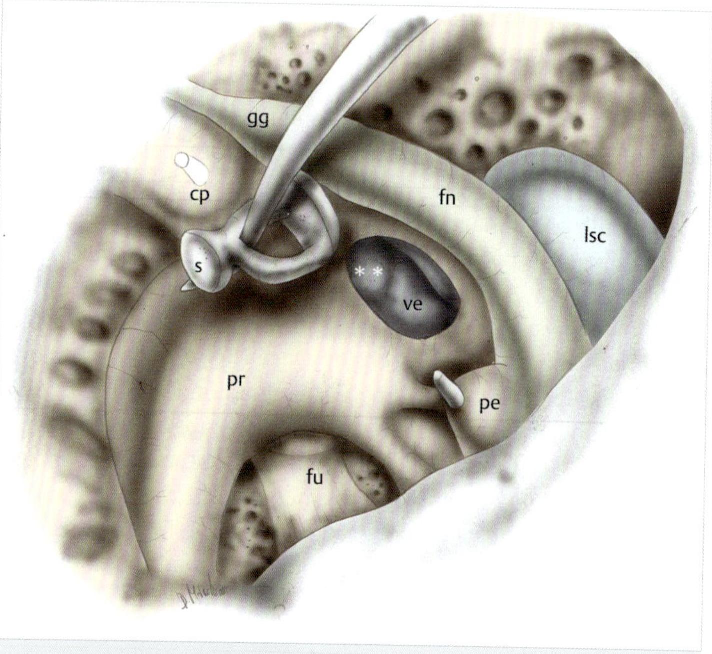

Fig. 11.14 Left side: The stapes is removed, exposing the vestibule. *cp: cochleariform process; fn: facial nerve; fu: fustis; lsc: lateral semicircular canal; pe: pyramidal eminence; pr: promontory; s: stapes; ve: vestibule; **: spherical recess.*

The stapes is then removed, uncovering the vestibule (▶ Fig. 11.14).

Second Step: Identification of the Landmarks and Middle Ear Dissection

Once the ossicular chain has been removed, the tympanic cavity is exposed and the hypotympanic, protympanic, retrotymanic, and epitympanic regions are merged with the EAC. The identification of the intrapetrous vascular structures that represent the anatomical limits of the approach is paramount. The vertical intrapetrous portion of the internal carotid artery is identified beneath the eustachian tube orifice. A medium-sized diamond bur is used to remove the protympanic cellularity with extreme care, until the course of the internal carotid artery is clearly identified. It is strongly recommended not to expose the vessel wall, but only what is necessary to identify its course inside the petrous bone. The anatomy of the protympanic bone close to the internal carotid artery might be variable. In fact, in some subjects we found a bony dehiscence so that the internal carotid artery is more superficial below the eustachian tube, where the vertical portion of the artery becomes horizontal. In other patients, the internal carotid artery is deeper, covered by a greater quantity of bone. This conformation requires a deeper and more accurate drilling until the vascular structure is found. Once the internal carotid artery, which represents the anterior limit of the dissection, has been identified, the jugular bulb is detected. This venous vessel is the lower limit of our dissection (▶ Fig. 11.15). A medium-sized diamond bur is used to drill the hypotympanic cellularity below the promontory region. We should bear in mind

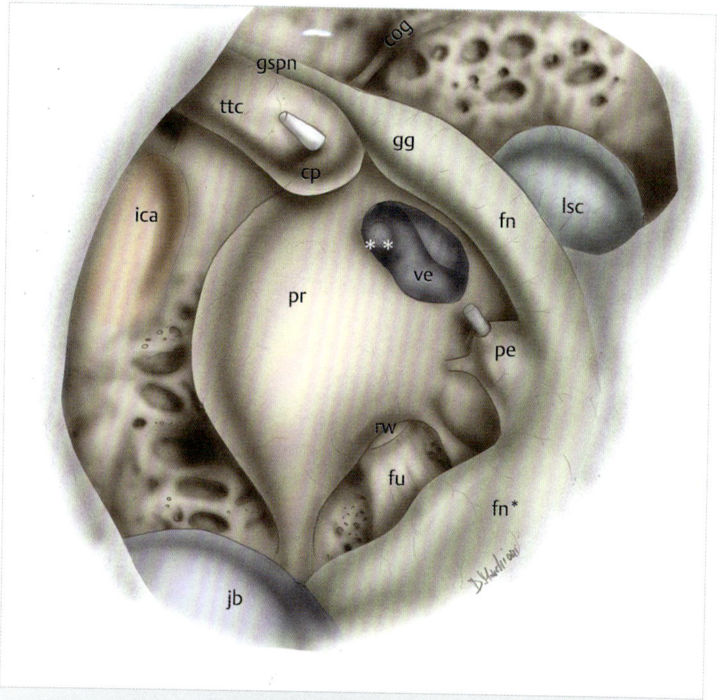

Fig. 11.15 Left side: The internal carotid artery and the jugular bulb are detected in the tympanic cavity, representing the anterior and the inferior limits of the dissection. *cp: cochleariform process; fn: facial nerve; fn*: mastoid portion of facial nerve; fu: fustis; gg: geniculate ganglion; gspn: greater superficial petrosal nerve; ica: internal carotid artery; jb: jugular bulb; lsc: lateral semicircular canal; pe: pyramidal eminence; pr: promontory; rw: round window; ttc: tensor tendon canal; ve: vestibule; **: spherical recess.*

that the finiculus originates just posteriorly to the anterior pillar of the round window and heads toward the bulb of the jugular vein in the hypotympanum. Therefore, we can consider this bony crest as an anatomical landmark to find the jugular bulb, through the drilling of the finiculus and the hypotympanic cellularity, until the blue color of the venous vessel in the hypotympanum is identified. Moreover, in this step, it is recommended to identify the vessel for transparency and not to expose the vessel's wall, like in the next step, during tumor removal, it could be traumatized by the use of the instruments and therefore generate severe bleeding. It is also important to evaluate the preoperative CT scan to understand the jugular bulb height, since a particularly high jugular bulb could make the transcanal surgical procedure particularly difficult to perform. A low jugular bulb requires important drilling of the hypotympanic region until the vessel is identified but allows the surgeon to gain a lot of surgical space, making the next endoscopic maneuvers easier. Once the vascular structures have been identified by drilling with a diamond bur, the bone is gently removed at the level of the third intrapetrous portion of the FN, which represents the posterior limit of the dissection. It is recommended not to uncover the nerve from the bone and to leave a bony layer above the nerve to protect it. During this step, the surgical field must be irrigated with water and a diamond bur can be gently used (see Clinical Case 7). Alternatively, a piezosurgery drill can help to remove the bone above the nerve, avoiding heating that could be dangerous for the nerve itself.

Third Step: Transpromontorial Access to the IAC

Once the anatomical limits of the surgical access have been identified, the opening of the inner ear and the identification of the IAC begin. The access to the vestibule is performed by removing the stapes from the oval window. Afterwards, the opening is enlarged using either a microcurette or a diamond bur or a piezosurgery instrument in order to identify the saccule and the spherical recess. The cribriform area of the spherical recess is found in the anteroinferior portion of the saccule (see ▶ Fig. 11.15 and ▶ Fig. 11.18). Under an endoscopic view, the spherical recess appears as an oval structure of a different color from the remaining medial wall of the vestibule and it can have a whitish or brownish color. This structure represents the termination of the inferior vestibular nerve's fibers and serves as an important landmark indicating the fundus of the IAC (see ▶ Fig. 11.20).

Once the vestibule has been exposed, and the spherical recess has been identified, the promontory is removed leading to the exposure of the cochlear turns, which is necessary for the dissection of the fundus of the IAC (see ▶ Fig. 11.16). The tegmen of the round window is identified and is knocked down by using a diamond bur or a piezoelectric drill, until the membrane of the round window is identified. The further removal of the promontory bone at this level gives access to the cochlea, which is composed of the scala vestibuli and the scala tympani separated by the spiral lamina. The basal turn is therefore anteriorly followed to the junction of the medial turn, removing the promontorial bone (see ▶ Fig. 11.18). Once the basal turn exposure has been performed, the medial and apical turns are identified. In order to find the medial and the apical turns, the medial and anteroinferior portions of the promontory are drilled. The progressive removal of this bone just below the semicanal of the tensor muscle allows for the exposure of the cochlear structures, medial and apical turns up to the helicotrema.

The identification of the apical turn of the cochlea is possible by opening it up where the cochlear bone reaches the bony groove of the tensor tendon muscle canal. The helicotrema is identified. At this point three openings to the labyrinth are present: anteriorly the apical turn of the cochlea with the helicotrema, inferiorly the basal turn of the cochlea, and superiorly the oval window niche indicating the medial part of the vestibule (see ▶ Fig. 11.17, ▶ Fig. 11.18). The bone between these three

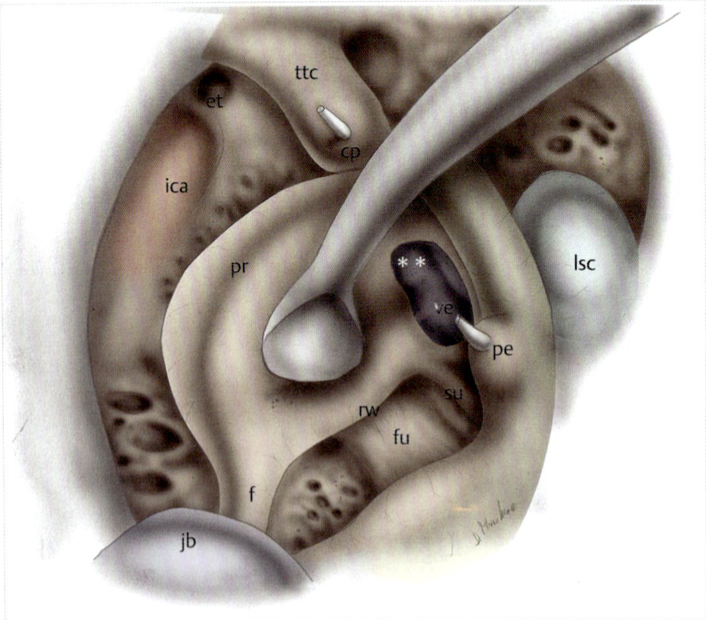

Fig. 11.16 Left side: A piezoelectric device is used to remove the promontory, exposing the cochlear turns. *cp: cochleariform process; et: eustachian tube; f: finiculus; fu: fustis; ica: internal carotid artery; jb: jugular bulb; lsc: lateral semicircular canal; pe: pyramidal eminence; pr: promontory; rw: round window; su: subiculum; ttc: tensor tendon canal; ve: vestibule; **: spherical recess.*

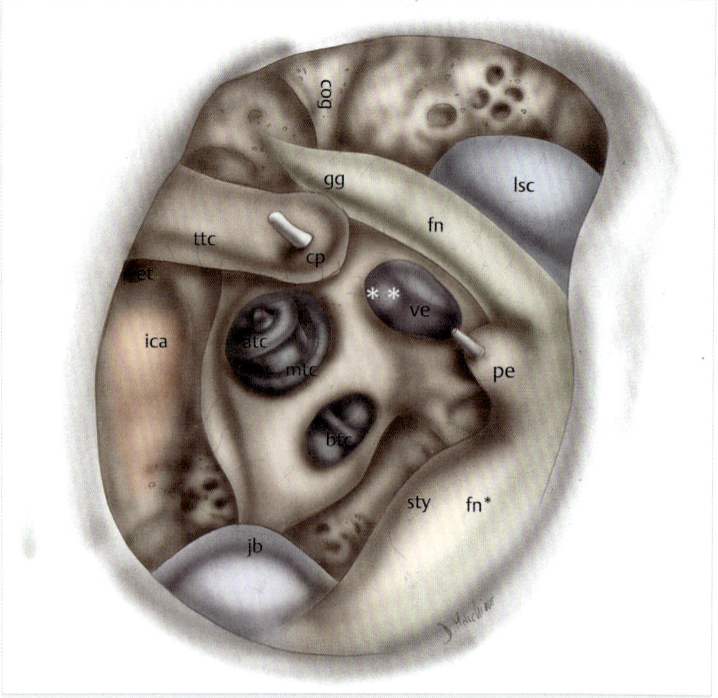

Fig. 11.17 Left side: The promontory has been drilled; the basal, middle, and apical turns of the cochlea are exposed. *atc: apical turn of cochlea; btc: basal turn of cochlea; cp: cochleariform process; et: eustachian tube; fn: facial nerve; fn* mastoid segment of facial nerve; gg: geniculate ganglion; ica: internal carotid artery; jb: jugular bulb; lsc: lateral semicircular canal; mtc: middle turn of cochlea; pe: pyramidal eminence; sty: styloid prominence; ttc: tensor tendon canal; ve: vestibule; **: spherical recess.*

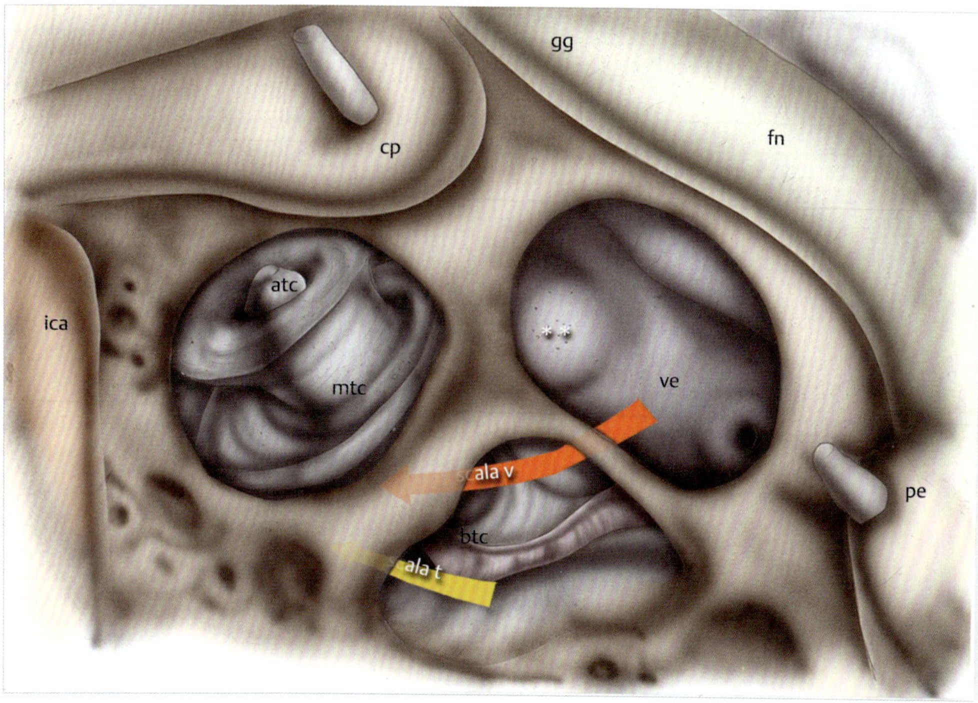

Fig. 11.18 Left side: The anatomical relationship between the basal turn of the cochlea and the vestibule, and the anatomical position of scala vestibuli and the scala tympani are pointed out. The reader can note the connection between the vestibule and scala vestibuli. *atc: apical turn of cochlea; btc: basal turn of cochlea; cp: cochleariform process; fn: facial nerve; gg: geniculate ganglion; ica: internal carotid artery; mtc: middle turn of cochlea; pe: pyramidal eminence; scala t: scala tympani; scala v: scala vestibuli; ve: vestibule; **: spherical recess.*

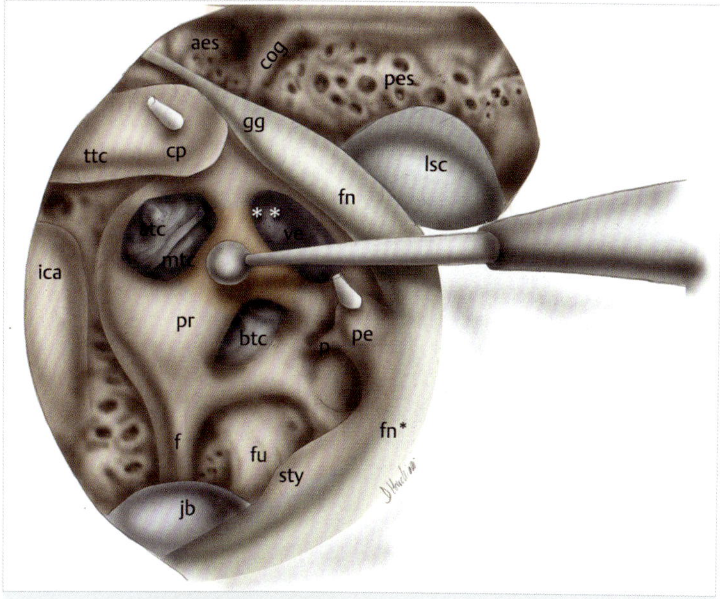

Fig. 11.19 Left side: The cochlear-vestibular bone (orange area) is progressively removed to gain access to the fundus of the internal auditory canal (IAC). *aes: anterior epitympanic space; atc: apical turn of cochlea; btc: basal turn of cochlea; cp: cochleariform process; f: finiculus; fn*: mastoid portion of facial nerve; fn: facial nerve; fu: fustis; gg: geniculate ganglion; ica: internal carotid artery; jb: jugular bulb; lsc: lateral semicircular canal; mtc: middle turn of cochlea; pe: pyramidal eminence; pes: posterior epitympanic space; sty: styloid prominence; ttc: tensor tendon canal; ve: vestibule; **: spherical recess.*

landmarks represents the cochlear-vestibular bone, a thin bone tract of variable shape between the vestibule and the cochlea which gives access to the fundus of the IAC.

Therefore, the cochlear-vestibular bone can be progressively removed by a diamond bur or piezolectric bur (see ▶ Fig. 11.19; see Clinical Case 5). Drilling with extreme care is recommended, since in this surgical route the facial and superior vestibular nerves lie below the cochlear and inferior vestibular nerves. In particular, the removal of this bone allows for the exposure of the cochlear nerve and its insertion to the modiolus, the inferior vestibular nerve, and the spherical recess in a posterior position, while the FN runs anterosuperiorly (see ▶ Fig. 11.20; see Clinical Case 5, ▶ Fig. 11.103).

Once the fundus of IAC has been opened, in case of schwannoma involvement of this area, it is possible to visualize the tumor which completely covers the area of the nerves. The tumor itself can in some cases cause a widening of the IAC, which facilitates the subsequent maneuvers of dissection of the dura of the IAC and also the subsequent maneuvers of dissection of the tumor from the FN. By using a medium-sized diamond bur or a piezosurgery device, the removal of the bone from the fundus of the IAC is performed from a lateral to a medial direction, uncovering the dura of the IAC (see ▶ Fig. 11.21). The anatomical exposure of the IAC is carried out from a lateral to a medial and from an anterior to a posterior direction. The porus is located deeply, about 1 to 1.5 cm from the fundus. By using a diamond drill, the removal of the bone from the surface of the IAC is performed from a lateral to a medial direction, in a horseshoe-like fashion, progressively uncovering the dura of the anterior, inferior, and posterior walls of the IAC (see ▶ Fig. 11.22). The skeletonization of the anterior and posterior limits of the IAC creates a groove between the anterior border and the internal carotid artery anteriorly, and between the posterior wall of the IAC and the third portion of the FN posteriorly (see ▶ Fig. 11.23). Further deeper drilling enables the surgeon to expose the most medial portion of the IAC which corresponds to the porus. The bone removal around the porus allows to expose the dura, until the dural reflection from the IAC meatus to the posterior wall of petrous temporal bone, which corresponds to the deepest limit of the dissection (see ▶ Fig. 11.24). At this level, the dura is characterized by a bluish color and after dural opening, the CPA is seen with the acoustic-facial bundle entering the brainstem. The distance in between the brainstem (entry zone of the acoustic-facial bundle) and the porus is variable, but the enlargement of the opening of the porus may provide a wide surgical view of the acoustic-facial bundle entry zone (see Clinical Case 6).

Fourth Step: Tumor Removal

Once the entire IAC has been skeletonized until the porus and the temporal bone dural reflection in the CPA has been identified, the tumor dissection maneuvers begin. Using a scalpel or

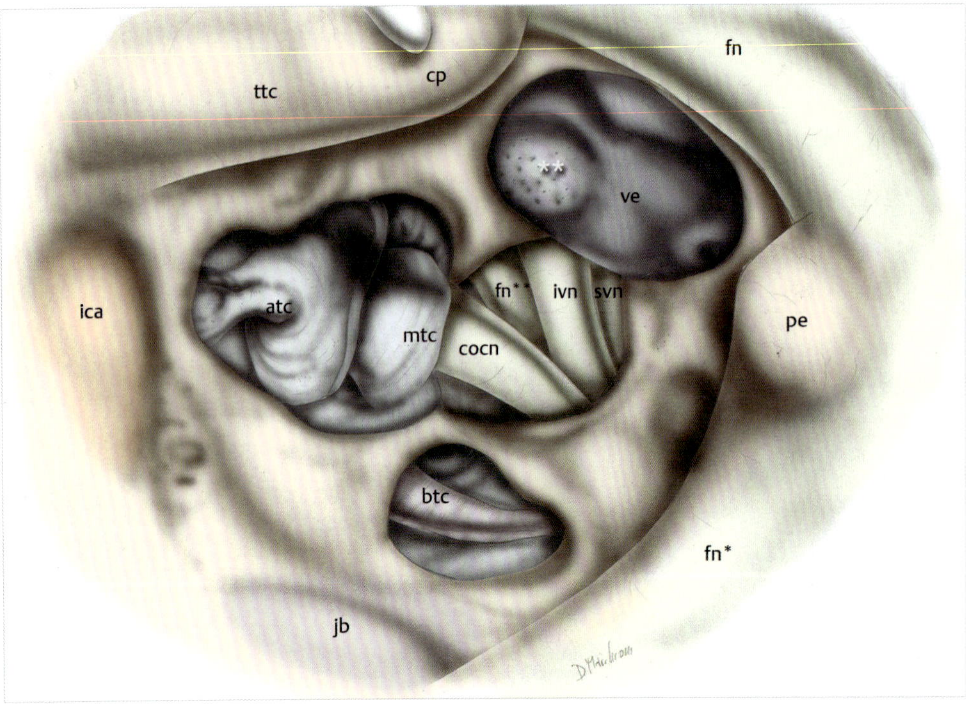

Fig. 11.20 Left side: The cochlear-vestibular bone has been removed; the fundus of the internal auditory canal (IAC) is opened; the anatomical relationship between the nerves at the fundus can be noticed. *atc: apical turn of cochlea; btc: basal turn of cochlea; cocn: cochlear nerve; cp: cochleariform process; fn: facial nerve; fn*: mastoid portion of facial nerve; fn** facial nerve into the IAC; ica: internal carotid artery; ivn: inferior vestibular nerve; jb: jugular bulb; mtc: middle turn of cochlea; pe: pyramidal eminence; svn: superior vestibular nerve; ttc: tensor tendon canal; ve: vestibule; **: spherical recess.*

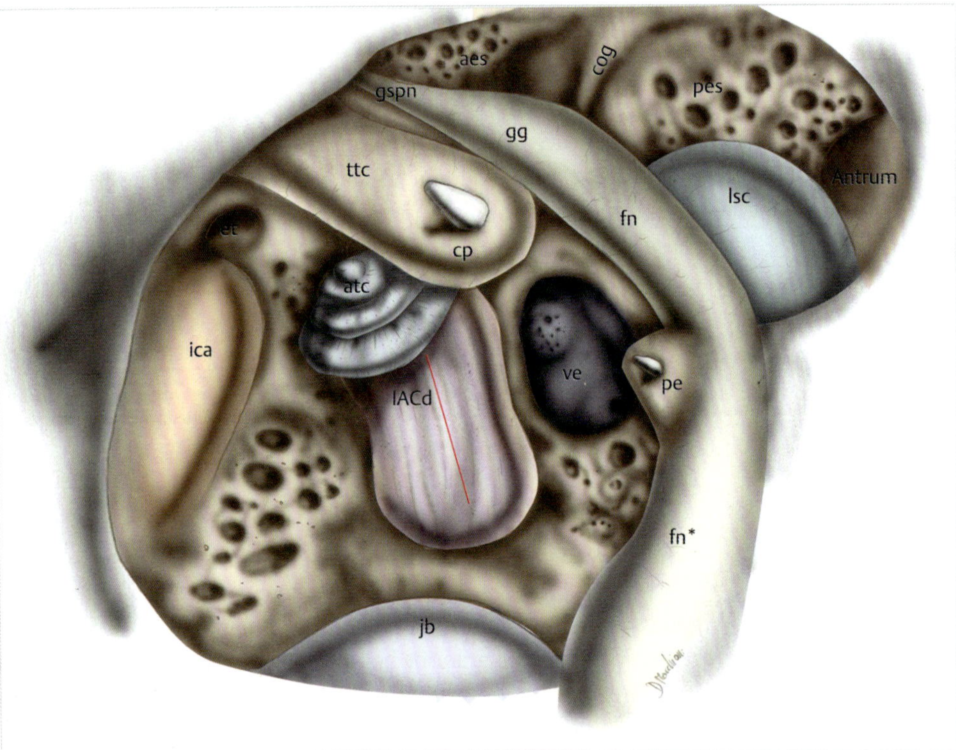

Fig. 11.21 Left side: The dural layer of the internal auditory canal (IAC) is progressively skeletonized using a diamond bur, from the fundus to the porus. The *red line* indicates the major axis and the orientation of the IAC. The same line is the line of incision of the dura of the IAC. *aes: anterior epitympanic space; atc: apical turn of cochlea; cp: cochleariform process; et: eustachian tube; fn*: mastoid portion of facial nerve; fn: facial nerve; gg: geniculate ganglion; gspn: greater superficial petrosal nerve; IACd: dural plane of IAC; ica: internal carotid artery; jb: jugular bulb; lsc: lateral semicircular canal; pe: pyramidal eminence; pes: posterior epitympanic space; ttc: tensor tendon canal; ve: vestibule.*

microscissors, the dura of the IAC is incised parallel to the major axis of the IAC and the tumor is exposed within the IAC. The tumor is identified and the dissection starts strictly following its capsula, delicately removing the arachnoidal adherences and the small vessels that supply the tumor (see Figs. 11.25–11.27). If necessary, an intracapsular debulking of the tumor is performed. Once the most medial part of the lesion has been reached, it is important to allow the cerebrospinal fluid (CSF) to flow, to allow for a better mobilization of the mass and improve the identification of the FN. Since this technique is one-handed, the constant outflow of CSF may hinder a straight-forward dissection. Therefore, a second surgeon may assist holding the suction instrument in order to keep the surgical field clean. After the identification of the FN, the tumor is removed from the nerve and from the IAC until the porus of the IAC is reached (see ▶ Fig. 11.27, ▶ Fig. 11.28, ▶ Fig. 11.29). In this area, we very frequently observe adherences to the FN which are gently released, following the plane of the tumor capsule. At this point, the FN is often flattened and therefore vulnerable. The endoscope allows for a thorough check for any residual disease. The tumor is removed with a piecemeal technique to achieve a radical removal.

Fifth Step: Closure

After the final stimulation of the FN to prove its integrity and an endoscopic exclusion of bleeding, the closure is performed. First, the eustachian tube is sealed using small pieces of muscle. The closure can be carried out with a pedicle flap of tensor tympani muscle. With a microcurette the cochleariform process is opened, and using a dissector the tensor tympani muscle is anteriorly pushed to obtain a pedicle muscular flap with enough length to close the

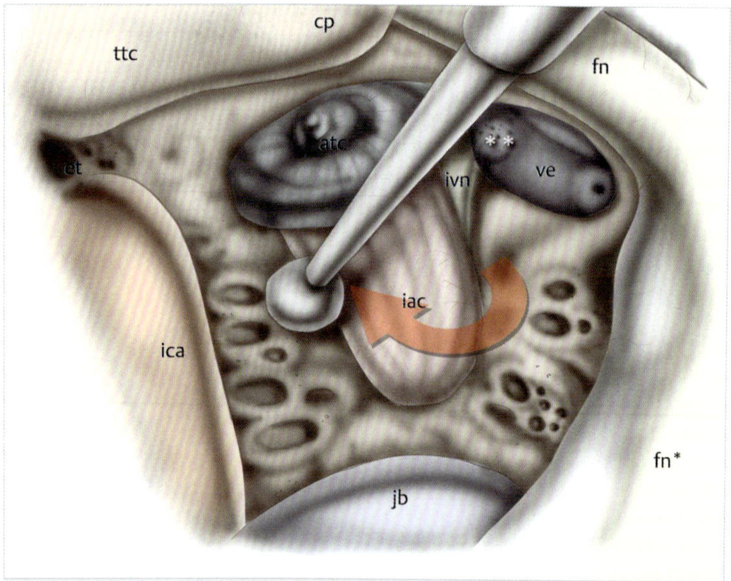

Fig. 11.22 Left side: The bone around the internal auditory canal (IAC) is progressively removed from the surface to the depth using a diamond bur in a horseshoe-like fashion (see *red arrow*), uncovering the dura of the lateral, anterior, and posterior walls of the IAC. *atc: apical turn of cochlea; cp: cochleariform process; et: eustachian tube; fn: facial nerve; fn*: mastoid portion of facial nerve; iac: internal auditory canal; ica: internal carotid artery; ivn: inferior vestibular nerve; jb: jugular bulb; ttc: tensor tendon canal; ve: vestibule; **: spherical recess.*

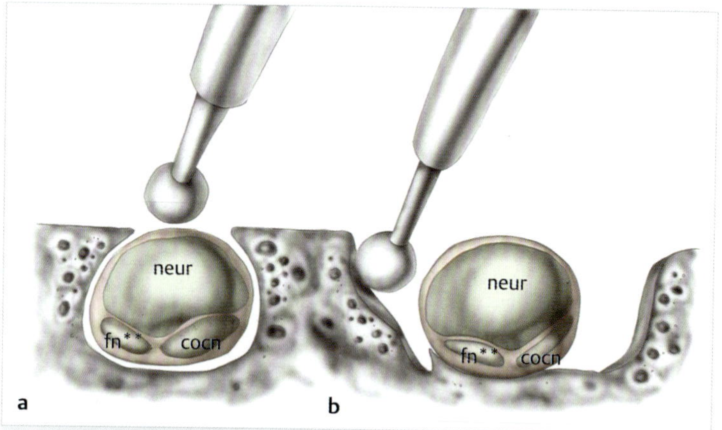

Fig. 11.23 Left side: **(a, b)** The dura of the internal auditory canal (IAC) is progressively uncovered on the lateral, anterior, and posterior walls, creating a deep troughs around the IAC. *cocn: cochlear nerve; fn**: facial nerve into the IAC; neur: acoustic neuroma.*

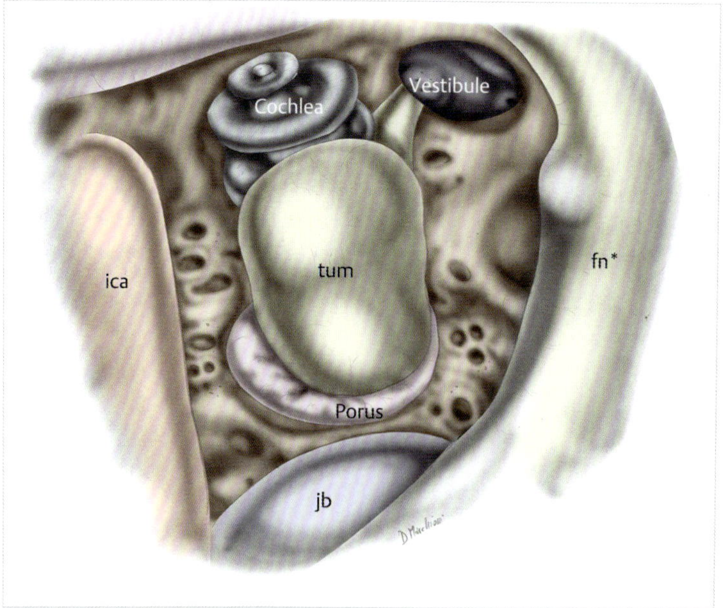

Fig. 11.24 Left side: The dura of the internal auditory canal (IAC) is opened. The tumor in the IAC is exposed from the fundus to the porus. *fn*: mastoid portion of facial nerve; ica: internal carotid artery; jb: jugular bulb; tum: tumor.*

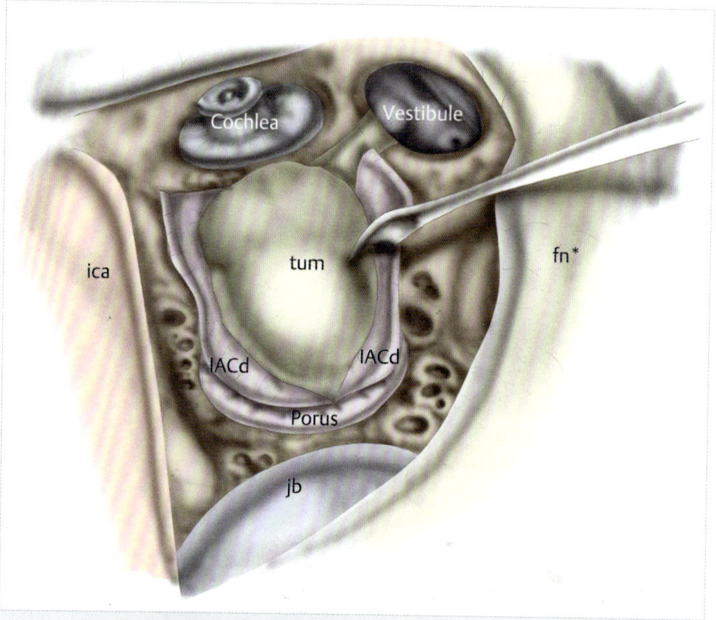

Fig. 11.25 Left side: The dura of the internal auditory canal (IAC) has been opened. The dissection of the tumor is started. *fn*: mastoid portion of facial nerve; IACd: dural plane of the IAC; ica: internal carotid artery; jb: jugular bulb; tum: tumor.*

eustachian tube (▶ Fig. 11.30, ▶ Fig. 11.31). Tabotamp (haemostat absorbable material) is used to push the muscle inside the tube to seal it. Fibrin glue reinforces the closure of the eustachian tube; then, a small piece of fat is added and again hemostatic matrix and fibrin glue are used to seal the site. Through a small abdominal incision, a pad of fat is used to close the defect created between the CPA and the tympanic cavity: the first fat fragment is pushed into the porus area sealing the communication defect between the CPA and the tympanic cavity (see ▶ Fig. 11.32). Fibrin glue is also applied to reinforce the closure. The whole surgical access is then filled with fat and finally the remaining skin of the EAC is sutured.

The skin of the border between the osteocartilaginous portion of the EAC is detached from the cartilage and outwardly pushed (see ▶ Fig. 11.33). Once this has been done, it is sutured with nonabsorbable stitches (i.e., silk) to obtain a blind closure of the skin in a "cul-de-sac" fashion (see ▶ Fig. 11.34).

Then, a dressing is applied.

11.2.7 Hints and Pitfalls

- During the canaloplasty step, it is advisable to extensively drill the EAC to identify its anatomical limits (the temporomandibular joint anteriorly, the third FN portion posteriorly). This allows for a comfortable use of the surgical instruments such as the drills, keeping the noble structures under control at the same time. Moreover, this enlargement allows for the use of the hand of a second surgeon to help the dissection of the IAC tumor lesion by holding a suction instrument.
- A piezosurgery device is recommended during the skeletonization of the inner ear, as it allows for an ultrasonic dissection

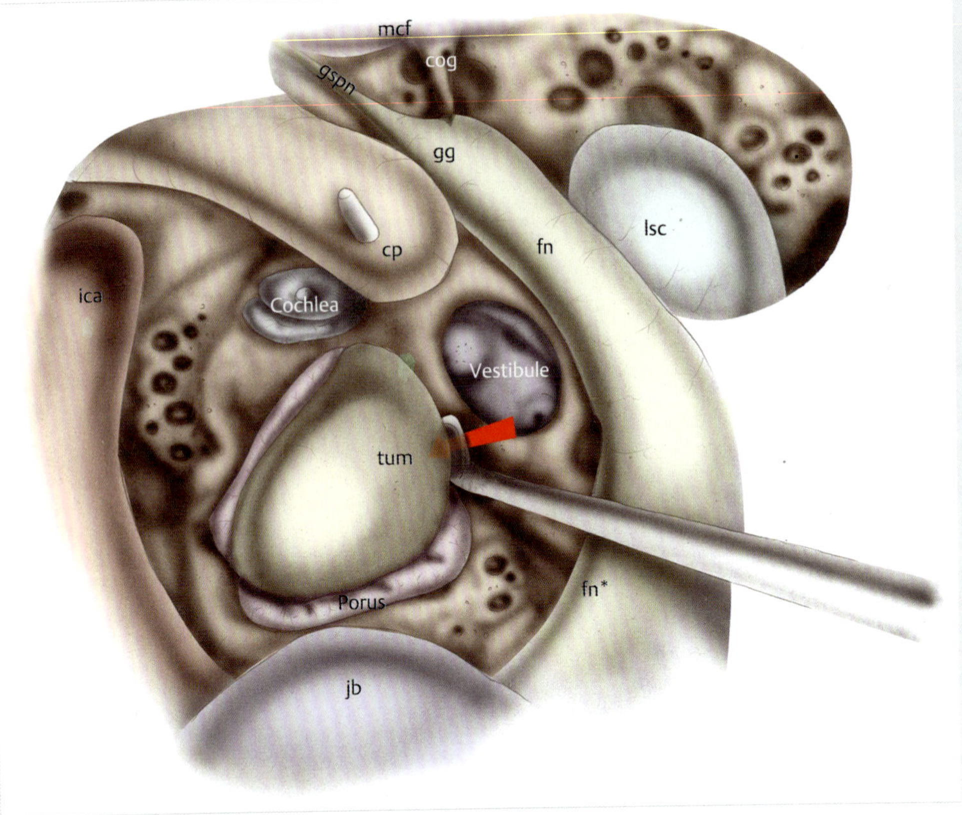

Fig. 11.26 Left side: The tumor is gently dissected and removed, detaching the adherences around the internal auditory canal (IAC), detecting the facial nerve (FN) under the tumor mass. *cp: cochleariform process; fn: facial nerve; fn*: mastoid portion of facial nerve; gg: geniculate ganglion; gspn: greater superficial petrosal nerve; ica: internal carotid artery; jb: jugular bulb; lsc: lateral semicircular canal; mcf: middle cranial fossa; tum: tumor.*

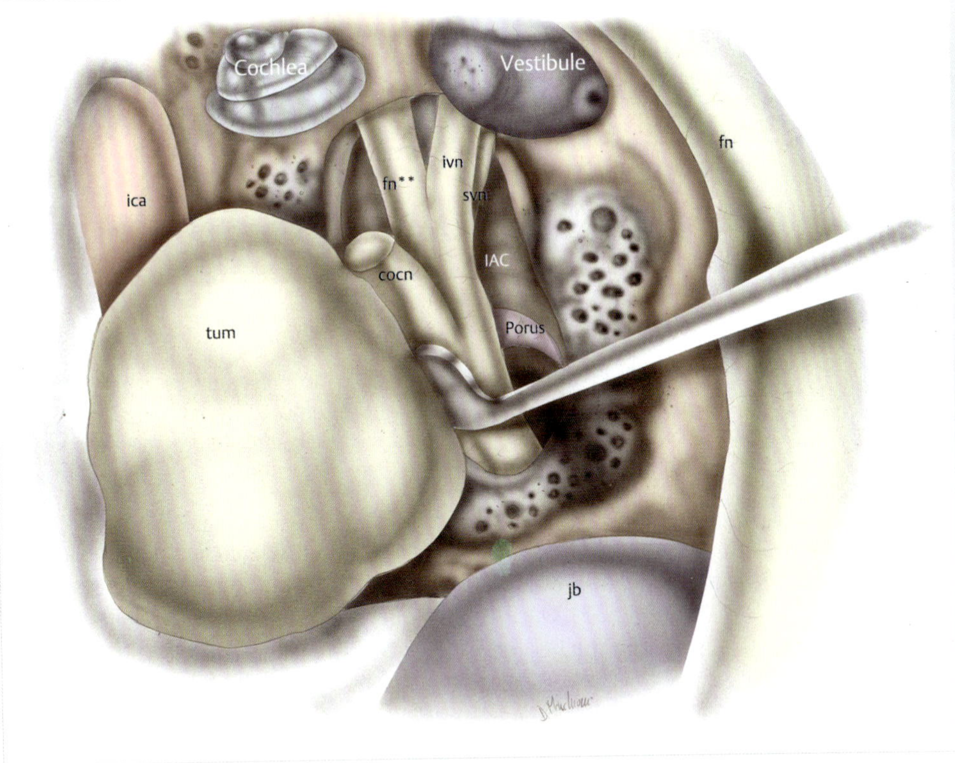

Fig. 11.27 Left side: The facial nerve (FN) is identified in the internal auditory canal (IAC), and the tumor is gently removed, detaching the mass from the arachnoid plane and nerves. *cocn: cochlear nerve; fn**: facial nerve into the IAC; fn: facial nerve; IAC: internal auditory canal; ica: internal carotid artery; ivn: inferior vestibular nerve; jb: jugular bulb; svn: superior vestibular nerve; tum: tumor.*

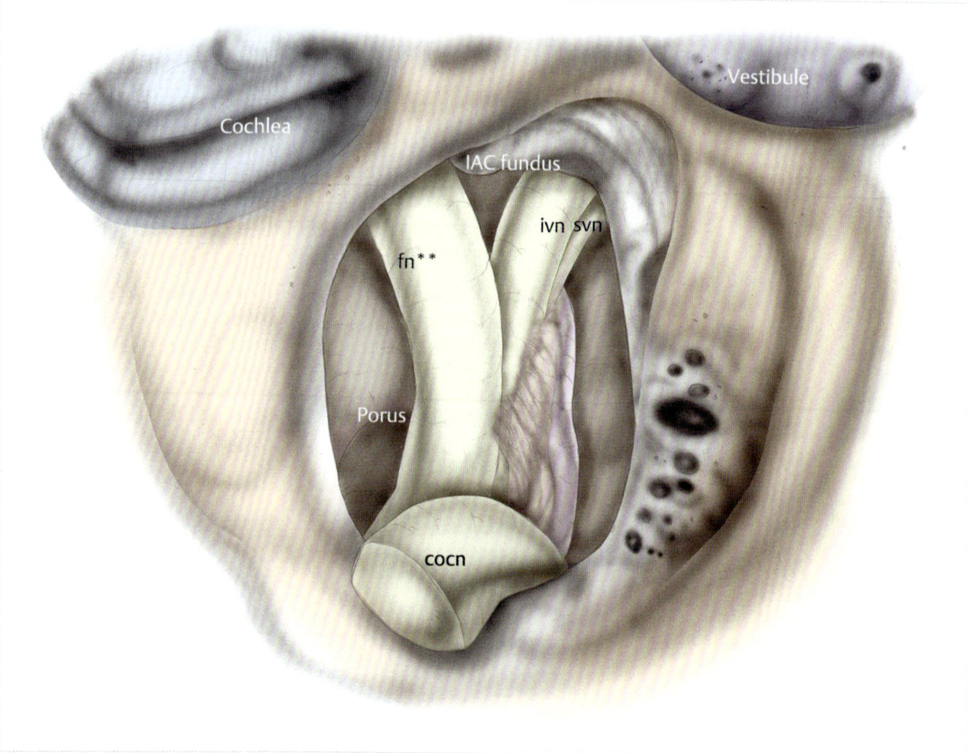

Fig. 11.28 Left side: Endoscopic view of the internal auditory canal (IAC) after tumor removal; the nerves are visible, running into the IAC from the fundus to the porus. *cocn: cochlear nerve; fn**: facial nerve into the IAC; ivn: inferior vestibular nerve; svn: superior vestibular nerve.*

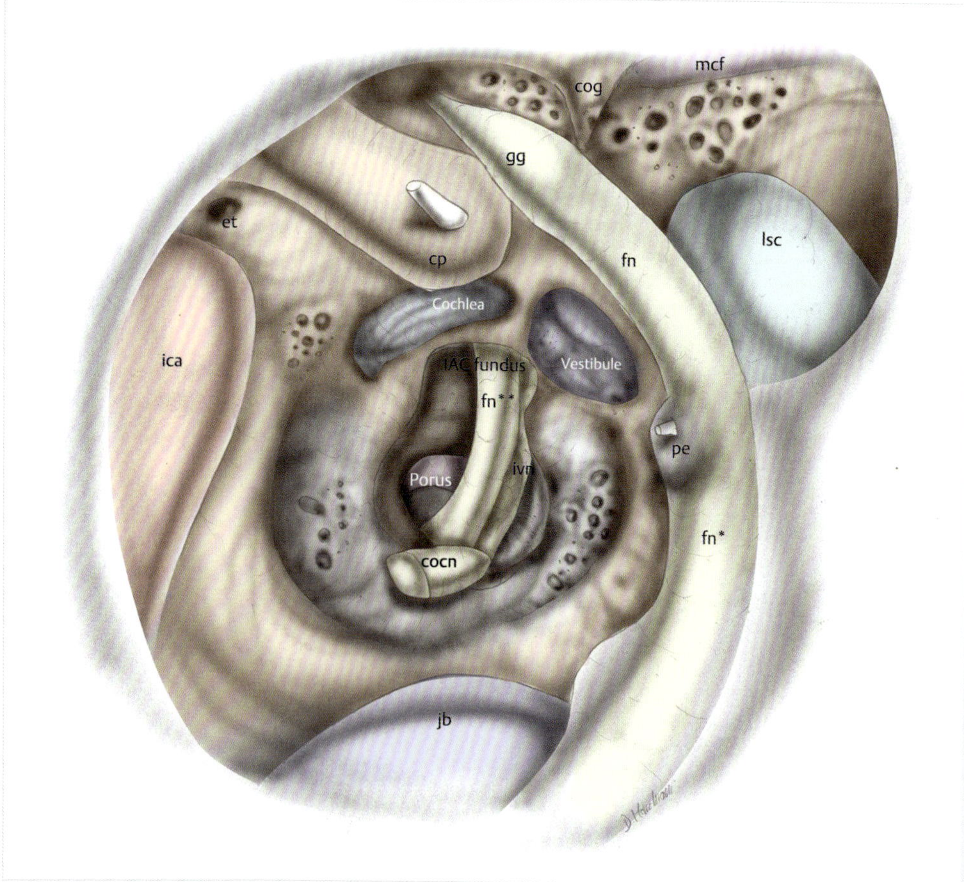

Fig. 11.29 Left side: Final cavity after tumor removal. *cocn: cochlear nerve; cp: cochleariform process; et: eustachian tube; fn: facial nerve; fn*: mastoid portion of facial nerve; fn**: facial nerve into the IAC; gg: geniculate ganglion; ica: internal carotid artery; ivn: inferior vestibular nerve; jb: jugular bulb; lsc: lateral semicircular canal; mcf: middle cranial fossa; pe: pyramidal eminence.*

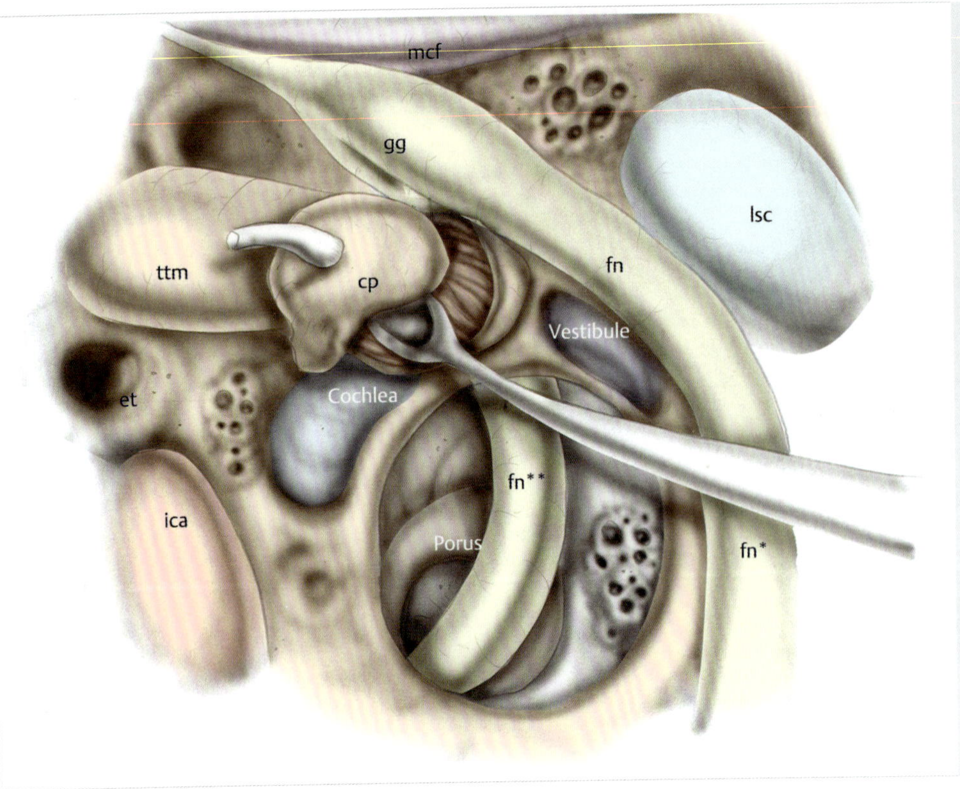

Fig. 11.30 Left side: The cochleariform process is removed through a microcurette, and the tensor tendon muscle is anteriorly pushed. During this maneuver, the surgeon should pay attention to the most superior and anterior portion of the muscle, since this muscle lies in the proximity of the geniculate ganglion, mantaining a strong anatomical relationship. *cp: cochleariform process; et: eustachian tube; fn: facial nerve; fn*: mastoid portion of facial nerve; fn**: facial nerve into the IAC; gg: geniculate ganglion; ica: internal carotid artery; lsc: lateral semicircular canal; mcf: middle cranial fossa; ttm: tensor tendon muscle.*

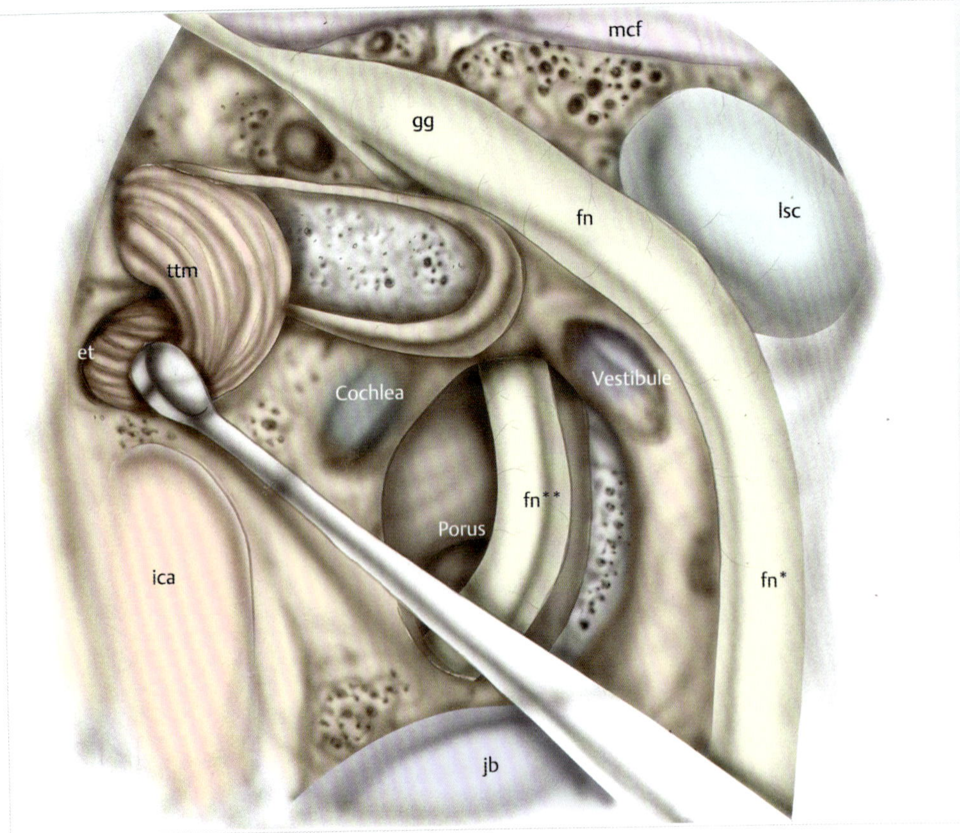

Fig. 11.31 Left side: The tensor tendon muscle is pushed into the eustachian tube, to obliterate the tubaric orifice. Surgicel may be used to deeply push the muscle into the eustachian tube. *et: eustachian tube; fn: facial nerve; fn*: mastoid portion of facial nerve; fn**: facial nerve into the IAC; gg: geniculate ganglion; ica: internal carotid artery; jb: jugular bulb; lsc: lateral semicircular canal; mcf: middle cranial fossa; ttm: tensor tendon muscle.*

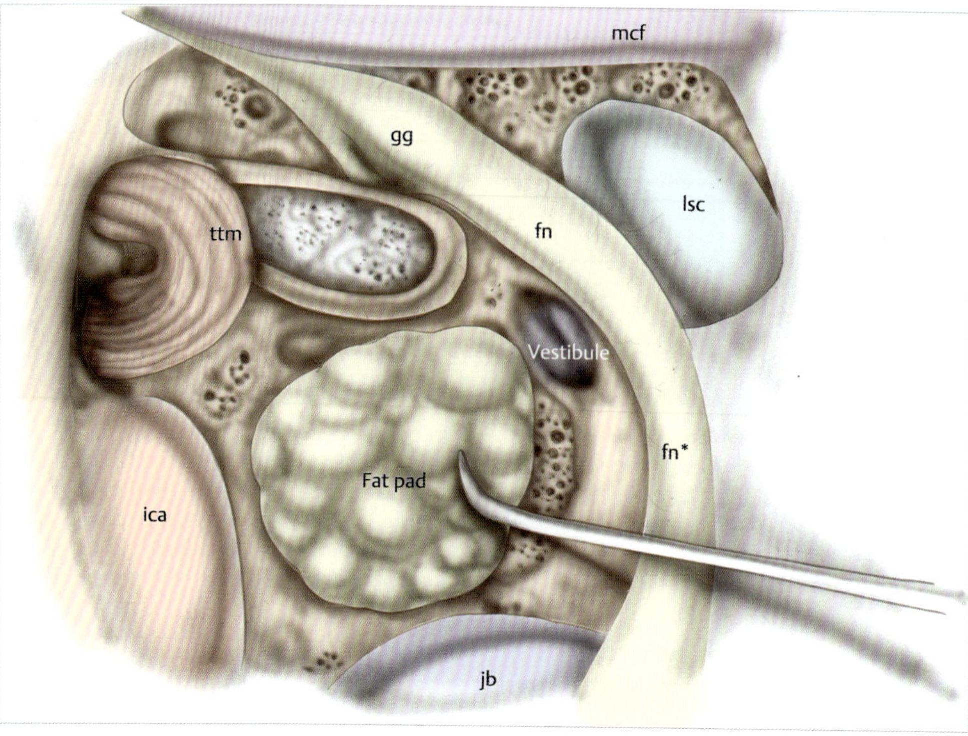

Fig. 11.32 Left side: An abdominal fat pad is used to close the defect between the tympanic cavity and the cerebellopontine angle (CPA). A single piece of fat is pushed through the internal auditory canal (IAC), passing the porus in order to obliterate the defect. *fn: facial nerve; fn*: mastoid portion of facial nerve; gg: geniculate ganglion; ica: internal carotid artery; lsc: lateral semicircular canal; mcf: middle cranial fossa; ttm: tensor tendon muscle.*

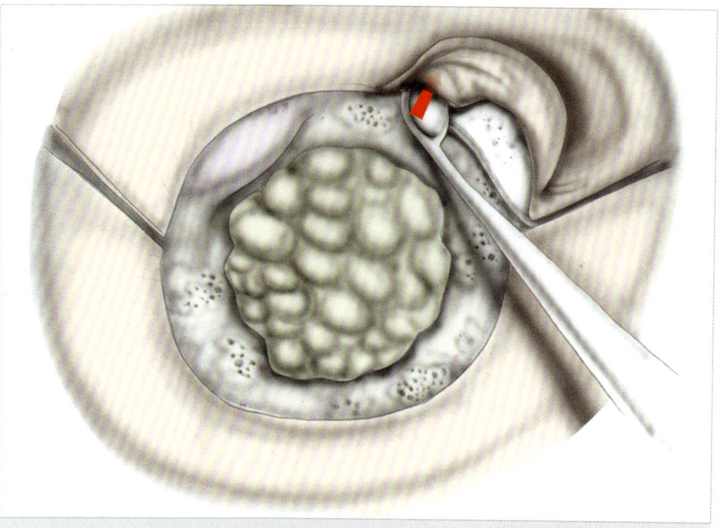

Fig. 11.33 Left side: Abdominal fat is used to close the surgical cavity, and the skin around the cartilage of the external auditory canal (EAC) is detached and everted (see the *red arrow*).

under constant irrigation preserving the nervous structures. Piezosurgery is useful, especially while opening the fundus of the IAC and the cochlea because during these steps the use of the drill can cause heat damage to the intralabyrinthine tract of the FN (see Clinical Case 1, ▸ Fig. 11.46, ▸ Fig. 11.47).

- Wet cottonoids can be useful during the dissection of the tumor from the FN. The dissection should be carried out on the tumor mass and not on the nerve, to avoid its stretching with subsequent palsy.
- Small dural vessels may bleed during the dissection of the IAC. In most cases the use of cottonoids placed on the bleeding area can solve this problem which must be controlled, especially

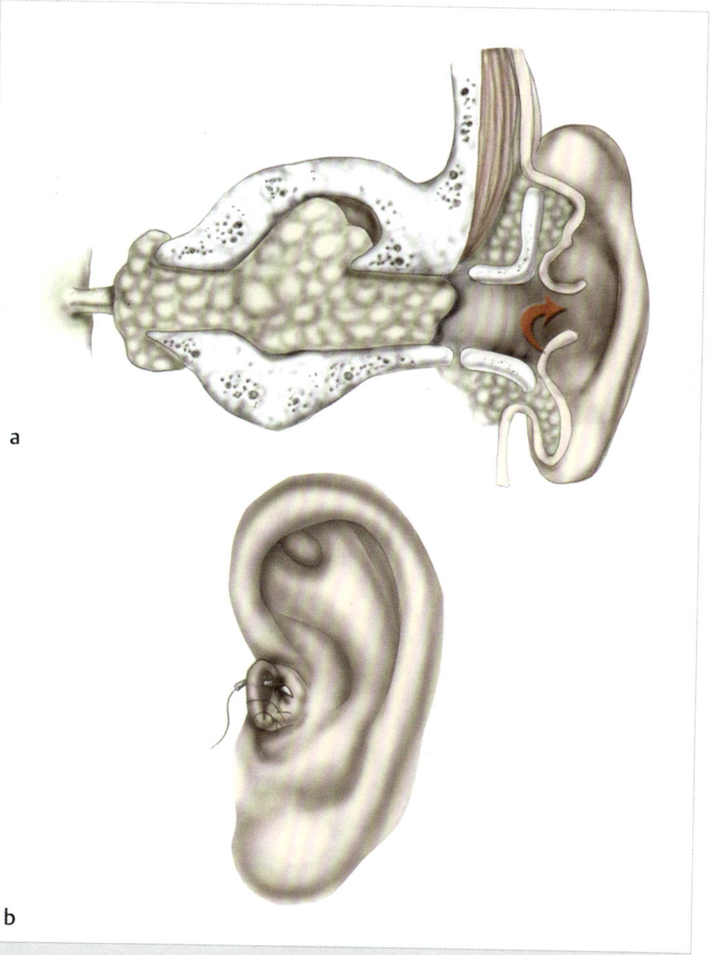

Fig. 11.34 **(a, b)** Left side: After the obliteration of the cavity with abdominal fat, the everted skin of the external auditory canal (EAC) is sutured.

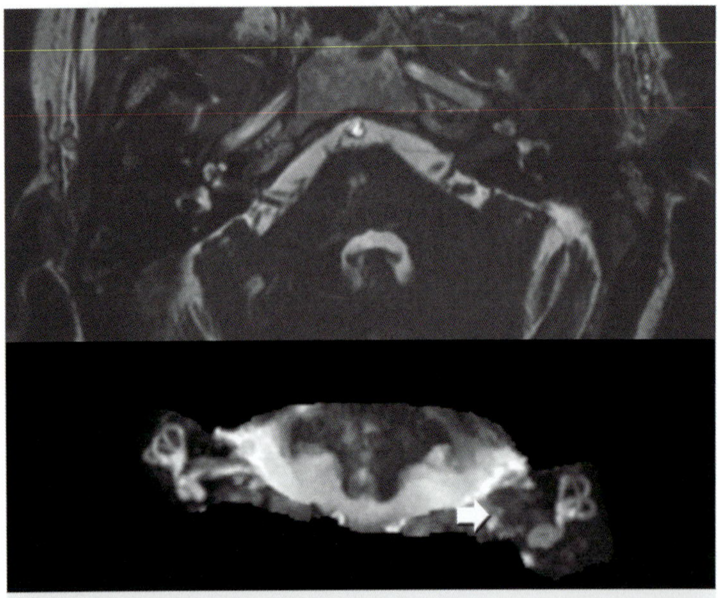

Fig. 11.35 Clinical Case 1: Patient suffering from an intractable vertigo with a profound receptive hearing loss on the left side. The magnetic resonance imaging (MRI) shows an acoustic neuroma involving the whole internal auditory canal (IAC) in the left side.

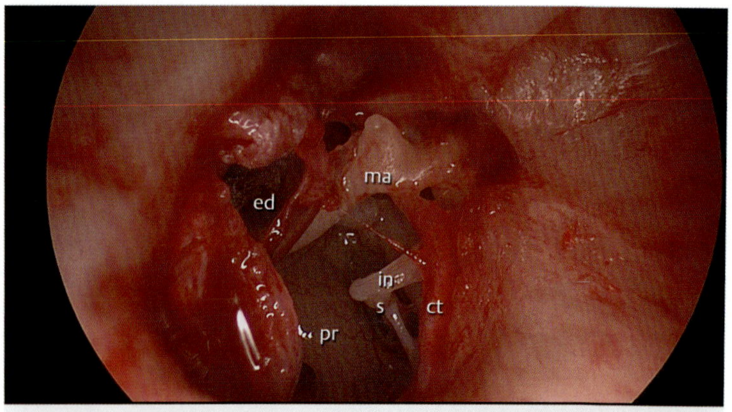

Fig. 11.36 Left side: View through a 0- degree, 4 mm diameter, 15 cm length endoscope. A circumferential incision is performed using a monopolar cautery tool and the skin is elevated until the annulus is reached. The skin of the external auditory canal (EAC) and tympanic membrane are removed en bloc to access the tympanic cavity. *ct: chorda tympani; ed: eardrum; in: incus; ma: malleus; pr: promontory; s: stapes.*

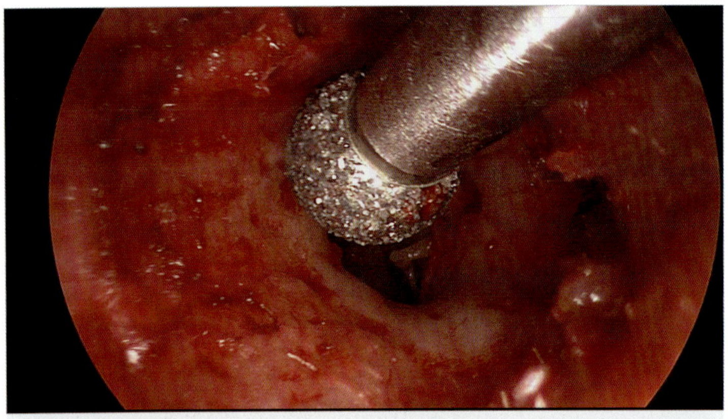

Fig. 11.37 Left side: A medium (4 mm diameter) diamond bur is used to perform a wide circumferencial drilling of the external auditory canal (EAC) in order to allow for a better view of the surgical cavity and a better management of the instruments.

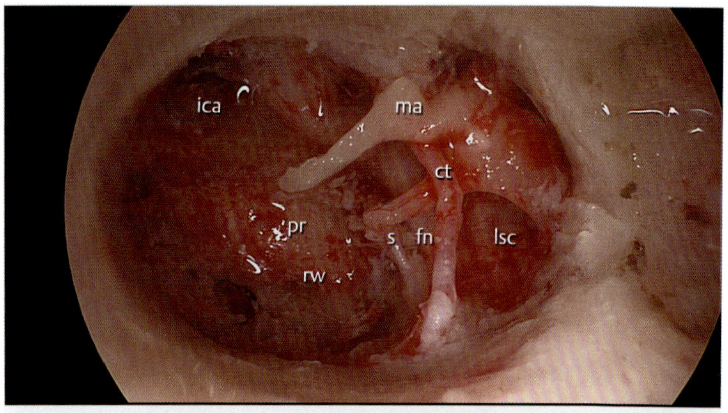

Fig. 11.38 Left side: View of the surgical cavity after drilling the bony portion of the external auditory canal (EAC): a large atticotomy is performed and the bony anulus is drilled to have a good exposure of the epitympanic, retrotympanic, hypotympanic, and protympanic regions. *ct: chorda tympani; fn: facial nerve; ica: internal carotid artery; lsc: lateral semicircular canal; ma: malleus; pr: promontory; rw: round window; s: stapes.*

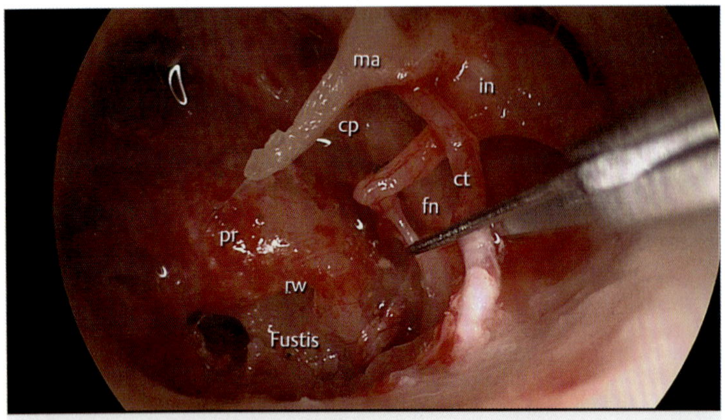

Fig. 11.39 Left side: The chorda tympani is dissected. *cp: cochleariform process; ct: chorda tympani; fn: facial nerve; in: incus; ma: malleus; pr: promontory; rw: round window.*

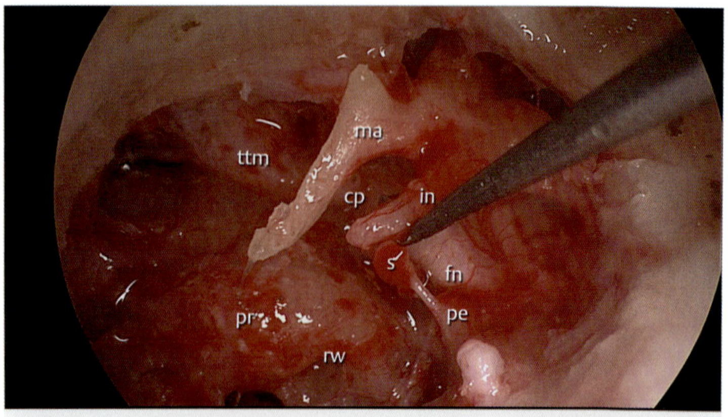

Fig. 11.40 Left side: The incus is disarticulated from the stapes and removed. *cp: cochleariform process; fn: facial nerve; in: incus; ma: malleus; pe: pyramidal eminence; pr: promontory; rw: round window; s: stapes; ttm: tensor tympani muscle.*

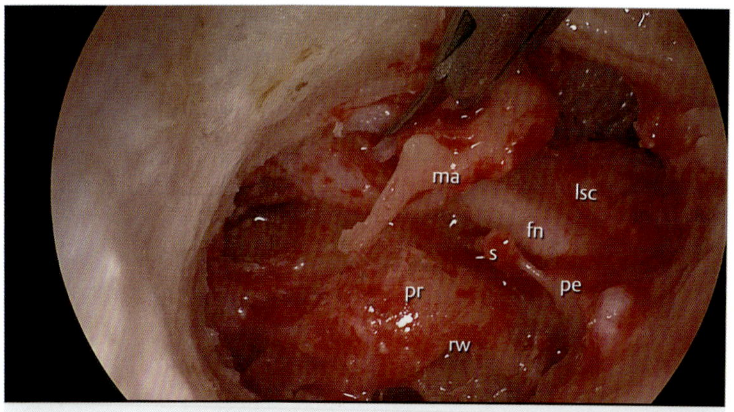

Fig. 11.41 Left side: The anterior malleolar ligamental fold and the tensor tympani tendon are dissected. Afterwards, the malleus is removed. *fn: facial nerve; lsc: lateral semicircular canal; ma: malleus; pe: pyramidal eminence; pr: promontory; rw: round window; s: stapes.*

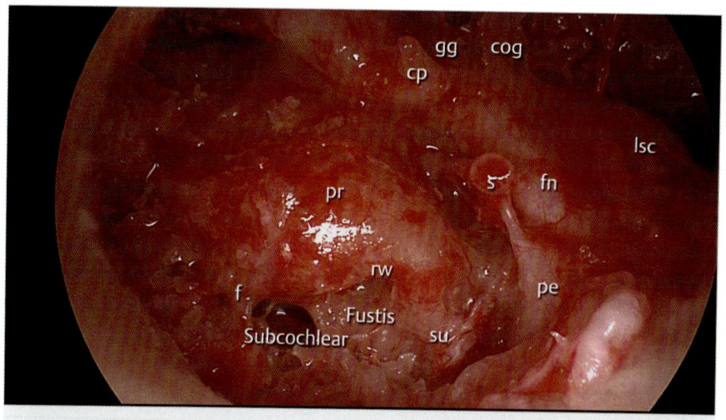

Fig. 11.42 Left side: After incus and malleus removal, the tympanic portion of the facial nerve (FN) is exposed. *cp: cochleariform process; f: fniculus; fn: facial nerve; gg: geniculate ganglion; lsc: lateral semicircular canal; pe: pyramidal eminence; pr: promontory; rw: round window; s: stapes; subcochlear: subcochlear canaliculus.*

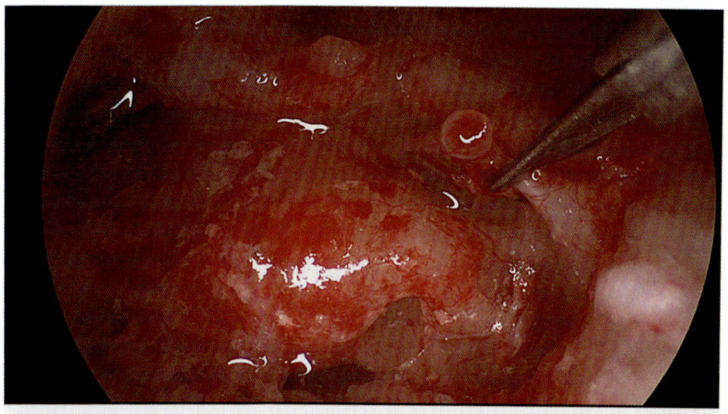

Fig. 11.43 Left side: The stapedial tendon is dissected using Bellucci microscissors.

because it is a one-hand surgical technique. In case of persistent bleeding a microbipolar forceps can be used during the irrigation to coagulate vessels.

- Particular attention must be paid to the management of the tumor in the area between the porus and the CPA for the possible presence of small vessels arising from the AICA. In this case, the use of a microbipolar instrument allows the surgeon to coagulate the vascular adhesions of the tumor and the hand of the second operator could help hold a suction instrument to clean the surgical field.
- A loop of the AICA located within the IAC or in the porus could be dangerous for this technique because an injury to this vessel with a retraction in the CPA requires the conversion of the endoscopic approach to an enlarged microscopic transcanal (see following section) or even a retrosigmoid approach to control the bleeding in the CPA. Therefore, we recommend a detailed preoperative radiological study of the AICA course through MRI. A large circumferential drilling until the porus could be useful to make the surgical window wider and to allow for an adequate management of the vessels in this region, as well as the use of a microbipolar instrument in order to coagulate the vascular adherences to the tumor.
- During the final closure step, the adipose tissue must be gently pushed into the defect area between the CPA and the porus. The push must be constant but gentle to avoid stretching the FN that runs within this anatomical area. A surgicel (hemostat absorbable material) segment is used on the fat pad to allow for an adequate thrust of fat, in an hourglass way, to obliterate and seal the area, in order to avoid any CSF leakage.
- The eversion of the EAC skin and the cul-de-sac closure must be particularly accurate, obtaining a separation between the cartilage and the skin. No skin residues must be left inside the surgical cavity to avoid a secondary cholesteatoma.

11.2.8 Postoperative Care

If the patient has no relevant comorbidities, immediate postoperative extubation and monitoring in the anesthetic recovery room is regularly performed.

No compression dressing is required; a dressing will be placed on the EAC to cover the blind sac suture. Stitches are removed in the outpatient clinic 10 days after surgery.

A CT scan is performed to rule out any hemorrhagic complications on the surgery day, 6 hours after the end of surgery (see ▸ Fig. 11.152).

To allow for the repair of the defect reconstruction, the patient is kept in a supine position for 2 days. On the third day, the patient is mobilized and according to the physical conditions he/she can be discharged 4 or 5 days after surgery.

Medications for pain or dizziness are administered on demand. A pre- and perioperative intravenous antibiotic prophylactic (cephazoline) treatment is administered. The radiological follow-up consists of an MRI scan with gadolinium contrast 1 year after the operation.

Complications

Intraoperative Complications

- Bleeding complications are the most dangerous ones and must be addressed immediately. Among the others, we can list the following complications:
  - Lesions of the AICA loop. In this case, we suggest converting surgery to a microscopic enlarged transpromontorial approach through a retroauricular skin incision, thus widening the surgical window to the CPA and coagulating the vessel.

- Lacerations of the bulb of the internal jugular vein. These events led to copious venous bleeding. Tabotamp is used to perform the packing of the vessel until the bleeding stops. The assistant surgeon can use suction during the venous bleeding and help the first operator in the plugging of the vessel; large tabotamp fragments are pushed between the vessel wall and the hypotympanic bone, extraluminally, to stop the bleeding. A cottonoid can be used to push the tabotamp onto the vessel and kept in place for about 10 minutes.
- Internal carotid artery ruptures are the most fearsome complication. It is a traumatic event which stems from an incorrect surgical technique due to the denudation of the carotid vessel wall during the identification and the subsequent damage of the artery. This event leads to violent and copious bleeding that requires immediate constant pressure on the vessels to reduce it, in order to avoid hypovolemic shock. A surgical pressure bandage has to be placed on the vessel and once the bleeding has been stopped, the surgical procedure must be completed and an immediate neuroradiological angiography performed.

• Lesions of the FN. We distinguish two types of lesions:
  - FN stretching injury. This lesion is caused during tumor dissection maneuvers. The most delicate and fragile tracts of the FN are the tract that passes through the porus from the IAC to the CPA, and the intralabyrinthine tract. These two segments of the nerve are extremely delicate and maneuvers on the nerve should be gentle.
  - Direct lesions of the FN with a section or laceration of the nerve. In these cases, the two ends of the nerve are approached in the IAC and a little fibrin glue is used to connect the nerve. When a direct connection of the two severed portions of the nerve is impossible, a nerve graft is used and fixed to the FN by fibrin glue. The most frequently used graft is the great superficial auricular nerve (see Chapter 14).

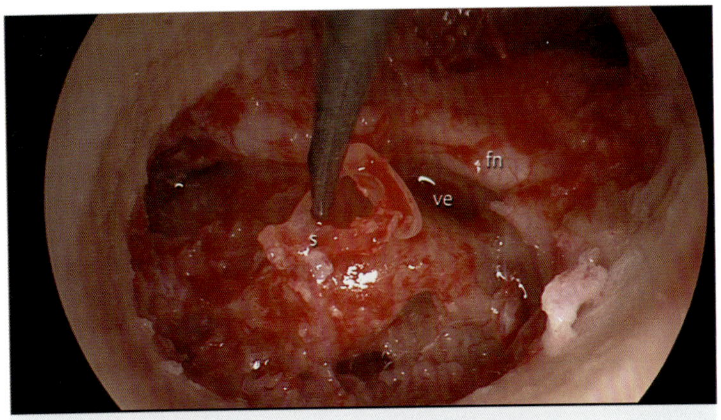

Fig. 11.44 Left side: The stapes is removed from the oval window, inserting a hook between the crura. In this way, the vestibule is opened. *fn: facial nerve; s: stapes; ve: vestibule.*

Postoperative Complications

• Postoperative bleeding from vascular vessels in the posterior cranial fossa is an extremely rare complication due to the type of approach and the features of the schwannomas that are often involved in this type of surgery. In any case, it must always be ruled out by performing a CT scan 6 hours after surgery and by performing a neurological examination of the patient.

In most of the cases, no revision surgery is required. In the rare case of active bleeding, with or without impairment of the neurological status, an immediate surgical revision through a retrosigmoid approach must be performed.

• Dehiscence of the blind sac closure of the EAC can happen even a week after surgery. In case of revision of the cutaneous wound, it is necessary to perform a retroauricular incision and a direct suture of the skin with further skin eversion.
• CSF leakage from the EAC can also arise after 1 to 4 weeks. It is a sign of a direct connection between the CPA and the tympanic cavity. Therefore, the CSF can fill the space within the fat placed in the promontory defect. In case of CSF leakage, the patient must lie down in a supine position to favor a spontaneous resolution. In case the CSF leakage does not stop, an external ventricular drainage is taken into account to allow for the healing of the wound. In the rare cases of persistent liquorrhea after these conservative procedures, a surgical revision is required to place more fat padding in the porus.

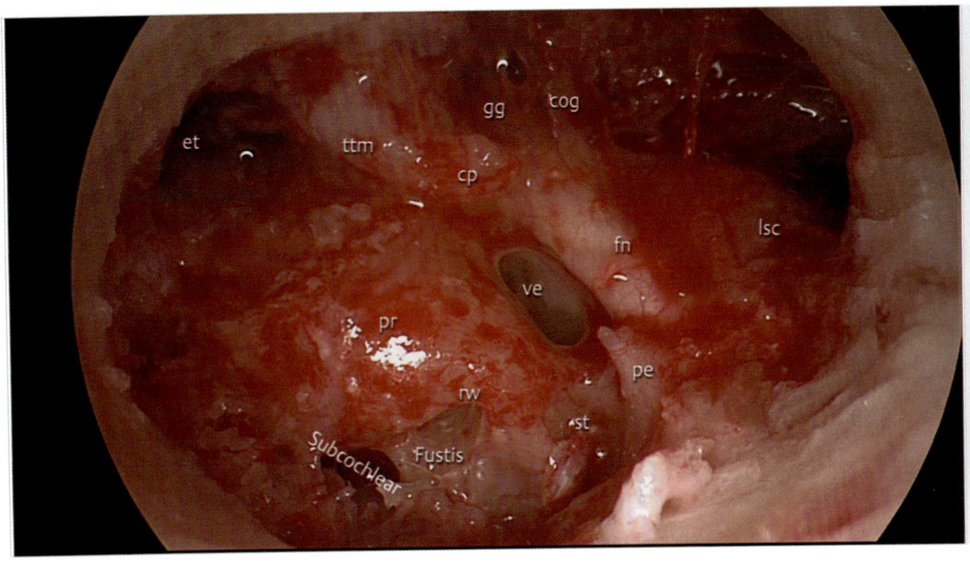

Fig. 11.45 Left side: The saccule in the vestibule is endoscopically exposed. The spherical recess is anteroinferiorly detected, on the medial wall of the vestibule. It represents an important landmark indicating, the fundus of internal auditory canal (IAC). *cp: cochleariform process; et: eustachian tube; fn: facial nerve; gg: geniculate ganglion; lsc: lateral semicircular canal; pe: pyramidal eminence; pr: promontory; rw: round window; st: sinus tympani; subcochlear: subcochlear canaliculus; ttm: tensor tympani muscle; ve: vestibule.*

11.3 Enlarged Transcanal Transpromontorial Approach (ExpTTA)

This surgical technique represents an evolution of the exclusive transpromontoral endoscopic technique, as it allows to expand the surgical window inside the CPA. It enables the surgeon to remove lesions that also affect the CPA with a straight-line extension into the IAC up to the entry zone (Koos II–III). The previous surgical approach was characterized by being exclusively endoscopic. The disadvantages of the one-hand technique are overcome by the new microscopic, endoscopic assisted surgical technique. Thus, the two-hand management typical of the microscope allows for the dissection maneuvers of the tumour component beyond the porus and at the level of the CPA.

11.3.1 Indications

This approach leads to the creation of a surgical window on the CPA with the exposure of the brainstem and of the entry zone of the acoustic-facial boundle. Therefore, it is indicated for tumors with involvement of the CPA with a straight-line extension.

This approach is indicated for:

- Growing masses in serial MRI examinations;
- Vestibular schwannomas: Koos grade I or II tumors: masses located in the IAC with involvement of the porus and extension toward the CPA;
- Schwannomas with a straight-line extension to the CPA with the involvement of the entry zone (Koos III) (see Clinical Case 10, ▶ Fig. 11.262);
- Lesions and/or schwannomas with CPA and petrous apex extension below the vertical and horizontal tracts of the internal carotid artery (see Clinical Case 12, ▶ Fig. 11.291);
- Class D hearing status (severe to profound hearing loss).

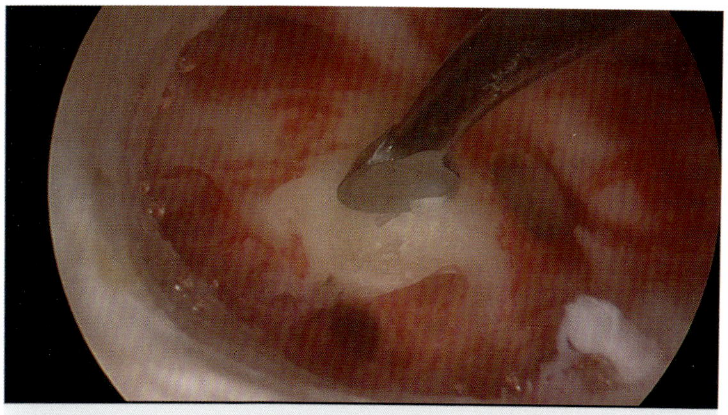

Fig. 11.46 Left side: A piezosurgery device is used to remove the promontorial bone and expose the basal, medial, and apical turns of the cochlea. The promontorial bone is removed inferiorly and anteriorly to the vestibule.

11.3.2 Contraindications

Absolute contraindications are tumours that have a downward extension involving the mixed nerves or an upward extension with the involvement of the trigeminal nerve. A high riding jugular bulb is a relative contraindication.

11.3.3 Advantages

- Very limited external incision (Shambaugh or retroauricular incision), no craniotomy;
- The additional space allows for a bimanual dissection of the tumor;
- Magnification and excellent visualization of the noble structures, especially the FN and the entry zone;
- No need of brainstem or dural traction, the dissection maneuvers are performed on the tumor and there is no retraction of the cerebral structures;
- Easy postoperative care, no intensive care unit (ICU);
- Short operating time, short hospital stay, low morbidity rate.

11.3.4 Disadvantages

- Limited indications in terms of tumor size and location
- Difficult management in case of unexpected bleeding
- Complete hearing loss

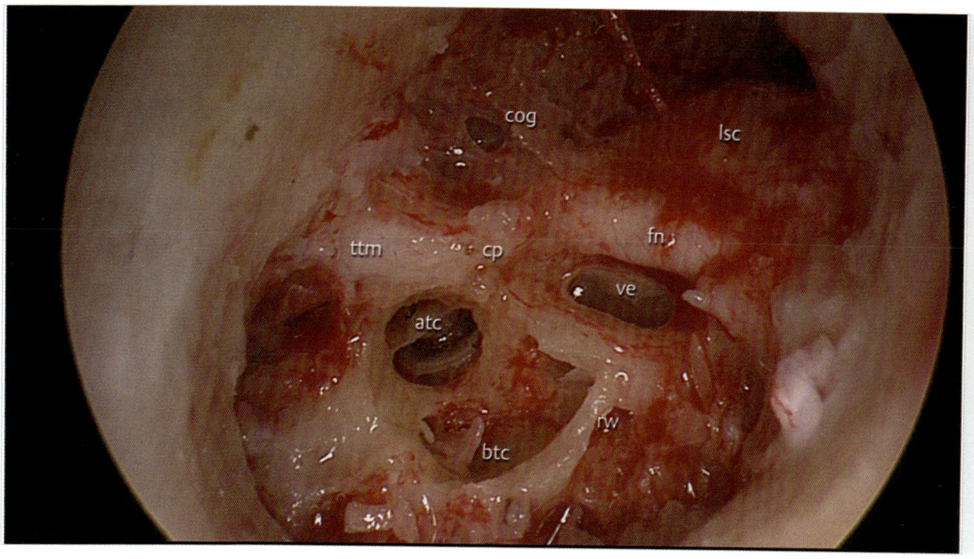

Fig. 11.47 Left side: Once the cochlea has been completely identified, the opening of the fundus of the internal auditory canal (IAC) begins. The drilling starts carefully removing the promontorial bone between the medial turn of the cochlea (anterosuperiorly) and the vestibule (posterosuperiorly). *atc: apical turn of the cochlea; btc: basal turn of the cochlea; cp: cochleariform process; fn: facial nerve; lsc: lateral semicircular canal; rw: round window; ttm: tensor tympani muscle; ve: vestibule.*

11.3.5 Preoperative Assessment

- CT and MRI with gadolinium, angiography in selected cases
- Audiometry: pure tone audiogram and speech audiogram
- Otoneurological examination

The enlarged transpromontorial approach is performed using the microscope. The endoscope assists the procedure during the final phases of the operation to perform the cavity scan and remove any tumor residues; therefore, this is considered an endoscopic assisted approach. Due to the enlarged working space as described below, a bimanual dissection under a microscopic view is allowed from the EAC to the IAC. This is especially useful after opening the dura to manage CSF leakage during tumor removal and to control bleeding during the dissection of intracranial vessels. The approach to the IAC is direct and straight from the EAC to the IAC, offering a good microscopic view. If a panoramic, high-magnification, or angled view is required to detect any residual disease or identify the anatomical landmarks, the endoscope may serve as an appropriate tool. Although derived from the exclusive endoscopic transcanal transpromontorial approach, the extended approach is essentially based on a microscopic technique. The patient's position is the same as the one for the endoscopic transpromontorial approach (see ▶ Fig. 11.4). The patient lies supine, with the head slightly extended and rotated to the contralateral side. Intraoperative FN monitoring is mandatory.

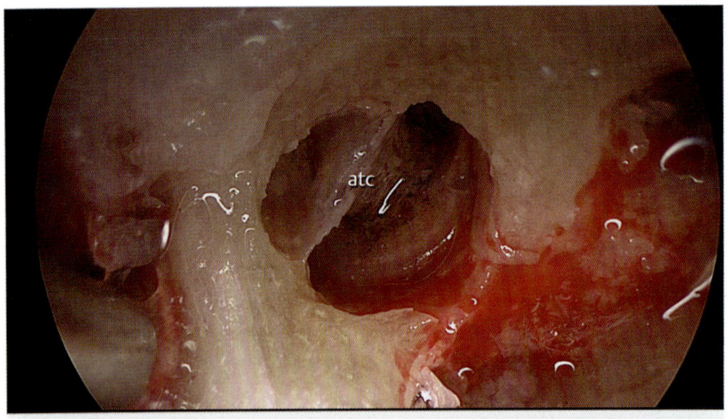

Fig. 11.48 Left side: The medial and basal turns of the cochlea are shown in detail, through endoscopic magnification. *atc: apical turn of the cochlea.*

11.3.6 First Step: Exposition of EAC Bone

The cutaneous incision can be performed in two ways:

- Shambaugh incision
- Retroauricolar incision

Both methods are valid and allow for the exposure of the bony part of the EAC with optimal access to the medial wall of the tympanic cavity. To simplify the execution, we recommend the adoption of a retroauricular skin incision that allows for an easy blind sac closure similar to the one of the transotic pathways which are already codified and well known.

11.3.7 Shambaugh Skin Incision (see Clinical Case 8)

A circular incision of the external ear canal skin, approximately at the level of the osteocartilaginuos junction, is performed. The external skin extension is superiorly performed between the tragus and the helix (Shambaugh incision) and inferiorly until the root of the auricular lobule (see ▶ Fig. 11.153). The upper portion of the incision is continued until the temporal muscle fascia is found; the latter represents the dissection plane to create two flaps, an anterior and a posterior one, to unveil the temporal muscle fascia. These two flaps are joined to the circumferential incision of the EAC to create two continuous skin flaps. The anterior skin and cartilage flap is created by detaching the cartilage from the underlying parotid tissue, and it is then anteriorly everted and pushed forward. The posterior flap is created by detaching the skin from the underlying fibroperiosteal tissue and posteriorly moved. A retractor is positioned to maintain the thus created cutaneous flaps and expose the EAC in its circumference. The temporal muscle is incised at full thickness above the EAC. The incision is continued below to circumnavigate the posterior margin of the EAC (see ▶ Fig. 11.154), thus creating two muscoloperiosteal flaps, one anterior and one posterior. Using a dissector,

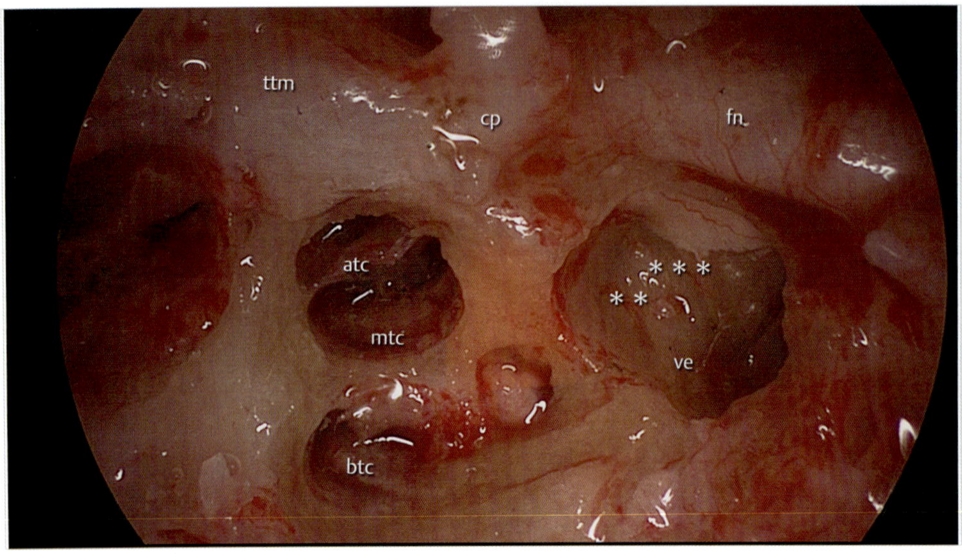

Fig. 11.49 Left side: The promontorial bone between the medial turn of the cochlea and the vestibule (cochlear-vestibular bone) is removed, in this way opening, the fundus of internal auditory canal (IAC). The tumor is exposed in the IAC. *atc: apical turn of the cochlea; btc; basal turn of the cochlea; cp: cochleariform process; fn: facial nerve; mtc: middle turn of the cochlea; ttm: tensor tympani muscle; ve: vestibule; **: spherical recess; ***: elliptical recess.*

the posterior flap is detached from the mastoid bone, and positioned beneath the retractor. This maneuver allows for the exposure of the mastoid bone wall. The anterior flap is pushed under the retractor to uncover the zygomatic bone region above the EAC. At the end of this procedure, the skin of the EAC with the eardrum is removed, and the EAC bone is completely exposed and the calibration procedure can be started (see ▶ Fig. 11.155). A temporal muscle segment is collected and placed in an antibiotic solution. It will be used to close the eustachian tube during the final steps. Particular attention must be paid to the creation of the cutaneous flaps of the EAC, since the final closure of the external meatus will depend on them. The cartilage adhering to the anterior skin flap will be partially removed and detached to allow for the blind sac suture.

11.3.8 Retroauricolar Incision (see Clinical Case 9)

A simple and safe procedure to access the EAC is represented by the retroauricular incision, shaped on the retrauricular groove. The incision is performed up to the level of the temporal muscle fascia that represents the dissection plane. The flap is anteriorly continued following the dissection plane to detach the preauricular soft tissues by dissecting the posterior auricular muscle near the posterior wall of the EAC. The incision is circumferentially continued in the skin of the EAC, at the level of its osteocartilaginous junction, and the flap is anteriorly continued over the parotid gland capsule. The skin of the outer portion of the EAC is detached from the cartilaginous component and outwardly everted to prepare for the blind sac closure (▶ Fig. 11.156). A full-thickness incision of the temporal muscle is performed above the EAC and continued around the posterior wall, at the mastoid level, like in the previously described surgical technique. Periosteal muscle flaps are detached from the mastoid and zygomatic bone and positioned below the retractors to completely expose the external meatus. The skin of the EAC is dissected until the anulus of the tympanic membrane and removed altogether. As for the endoscopic technique, particular care must be taken during this phase to avoid leaving epidermal residues that could give rise to iatrogenic cholesteatoma; therefore, it is recommended to carefully remove the skin along with the tympanic membrane.

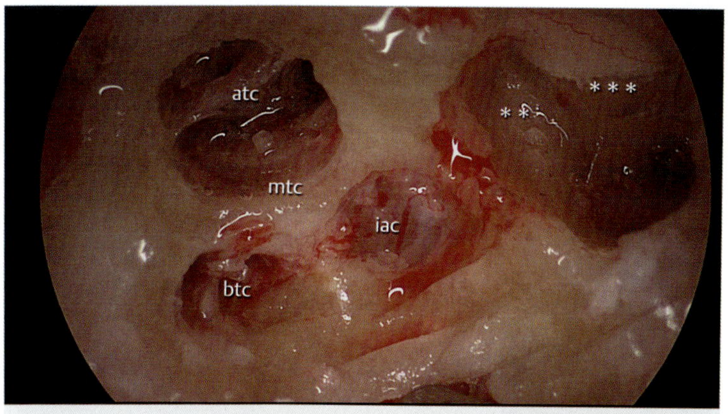

Fig. 11.50 Left side: Further drilling is performed to remove the promontorial bone between the vestibule and the cochlea, in order to expose the tumor and the internal auditory canal (IAC). *atc: apical turn of the cochlea; btc; basal turn of the cochlea; iac: internal auditory canal; mtc: middle turn of the cochlea; **: spherical recess; ***: elliptical recess.*

11.3.9 Second Step: Calibration of the Promontorial Access

A large diamond bur is used to calibrate the EAC beginning on the postero-superior side; Henle spine is removed (see ▶ Fig. 11.157). The calibration must be extended enough to allow for a confortable management of the tumor in the IAC and CPA, if necessary. Therefore, drilling, if necessary, is also extended to the mastoideal cellularity to lead to a better view of the surgical field. The temporomandibular joint is detected by removing the bone of the anterior portion of the EAC. Superiorly extensive drilling is performed, to expose the epitympanum; the dura of the MCF is identified and followed only in case of a "low" riding dural plane; otherwise it is not necessary to identify it. After the calibration of the EAC, the bone annulus is extensively enlarged uncovering the epitympanum, the protympanum, the retrotympanum, and the hypotympanum (see ▶ Fig. 11.158). Posteriorly, the opening of the tympanic antrum allows for the identification of the LSC. In the epitympanum the incudomalleolar joint and the tegmen tympani can be noticed. The anterior limit of the skeletonization

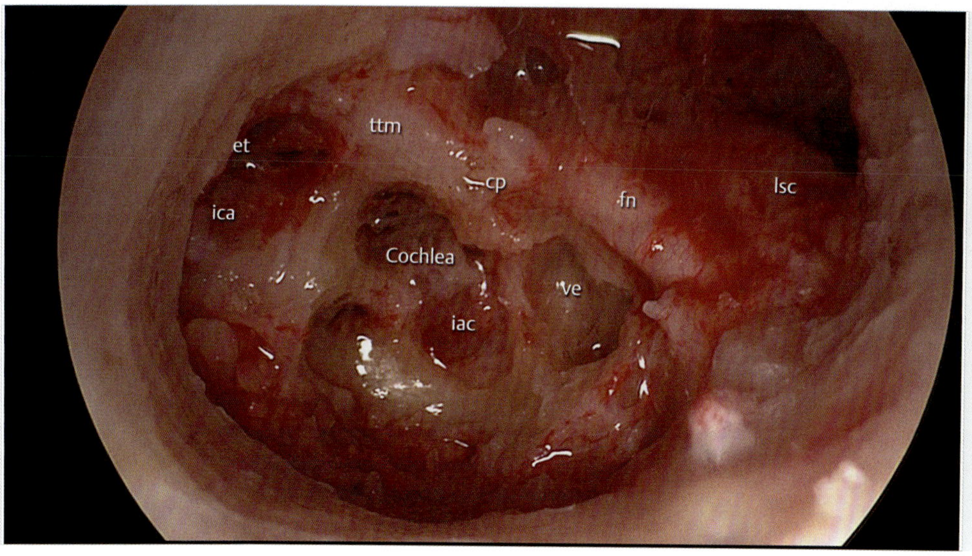

Fig. 11.51 Left side: The internal auditory canal (IAC) is carefully scheletonized from the fundus to the porus. The drilling is carried out in a lateral to medial and superior to inferior direction, circumnavigating the anterior, posterior, and inferior portions of IAC. *cp: cochleariform process; et: eustachian tube; fn: facial nerve; iac: internal auditory canal; ica: internal carotid artery; lsc: lateral semicircular canal; ttm: tensor tympani muscle; ve: vestibule.*

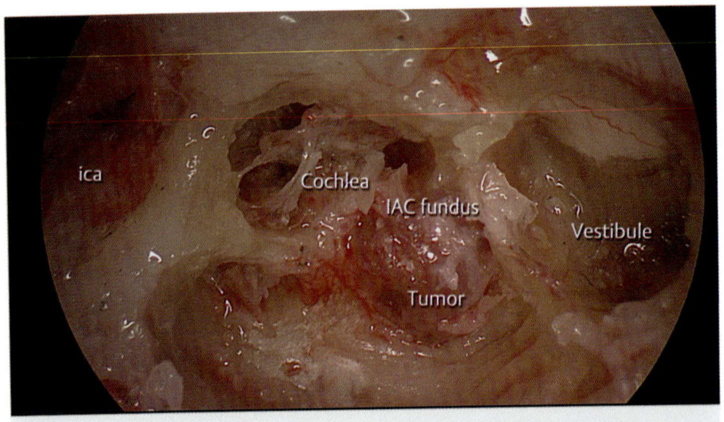

Fig. 11.52 Left side: The tumor is clearly detected between the cochlea and the vestibule. *ica: internal carotid artery.*

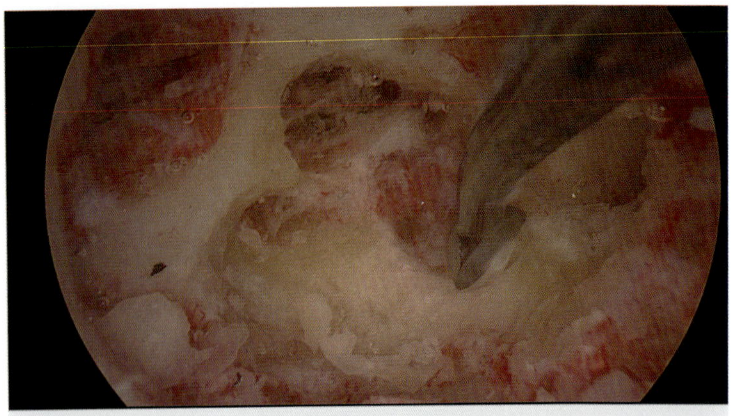

Fig. 11.53 Left side: A piezosurgery device is used to carefully scheletonize the dura of the internal auditory canal (IAC).

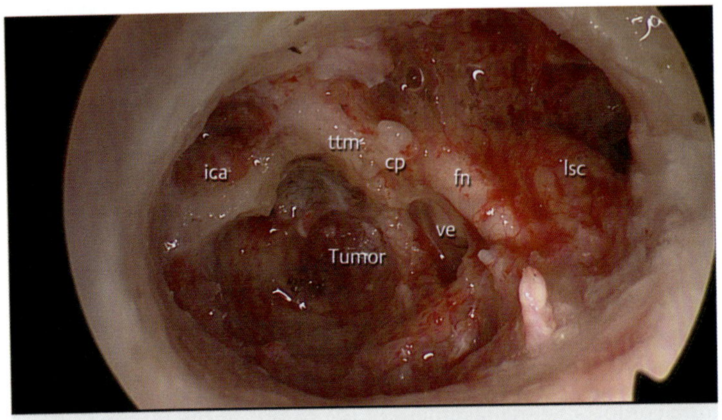

Fig. 11.54 Left side: The internal auditory canal (IAC) is exposed and the tumor is fully identified, and gently removed, preserving the facial nerve (FN). *cp: cochleariform process; fn: facial nerve; ica: internal carotid artery; lsc: lateral semicircular canal; ttm: tensor tympani muscle; ve: vestibule.*

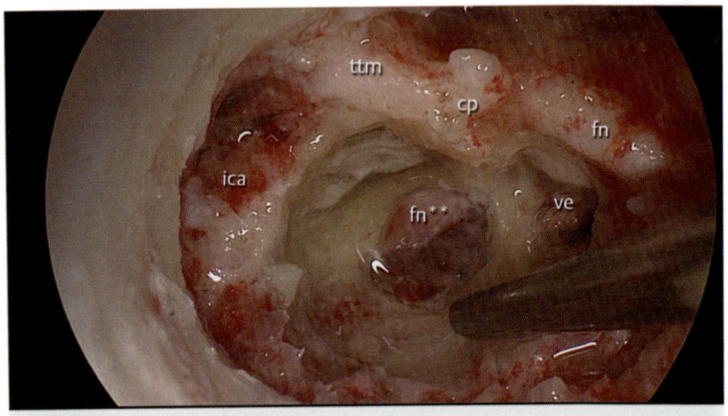

Fig. 11.55 Left side: The facial nerve (FN) is identified in the internal auditory canal (IAC) and the tumor is dissected from the the FN and from the IAC. *cp: cochleariform process; fn: tympanic portion of the facial nerve; fn**: facial nerve into the IAC; ica: internal carotid artery; ttm: tensor tympani muscle; ve: vestibule.*

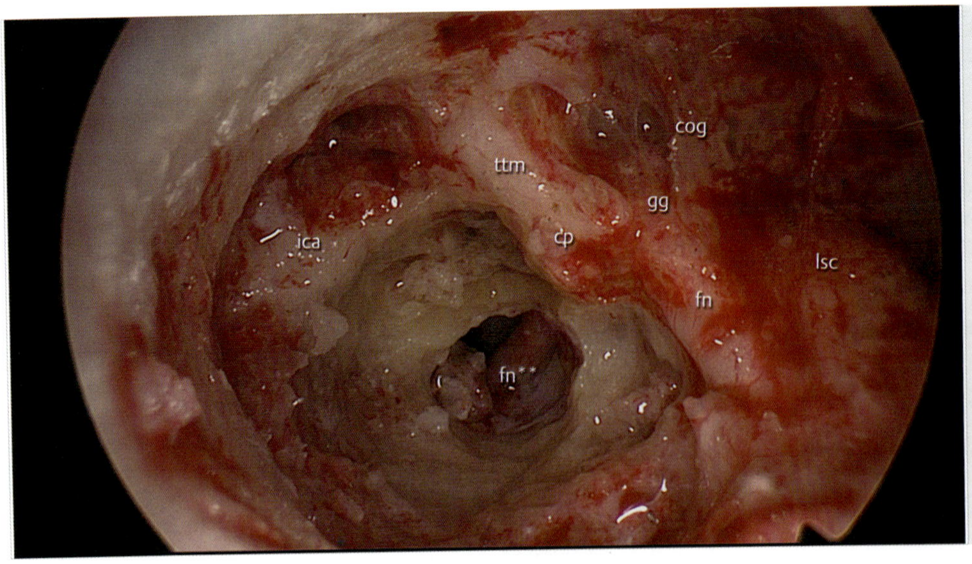

Fig. 11.56 Left side: View of the surgical cavity after tumor removal: the whole internal auditory canal (IAC) is exposed. *cp: cochleariform process; fn**: facial nerve into the IAC; fn: tympanic portion of the facial nerve; gg: geniculate ganglion; ica: internal carotid artery; lsc: lateral semicircular canal; ttm: tensor tympani muscle.*

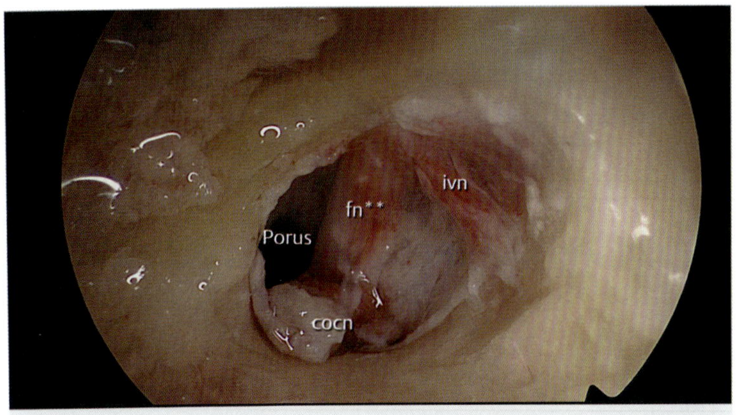

Fig. 11.57 Left side: The facial nerve (FN) is identified in the internal auditory canal (IAC) from the fundus to the porus. It is possible to see the severed cochlear nerve and the vestibular nerves. *cocn: cochlear nerve; fn**: facial nerve into the IAC; ivn: inferior vestibular nerve.*

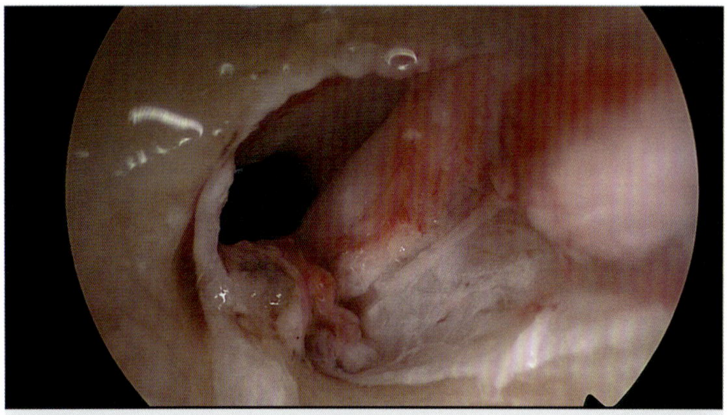

Fig. 11.58 Left side: Magnified endoscopic view of the porus.

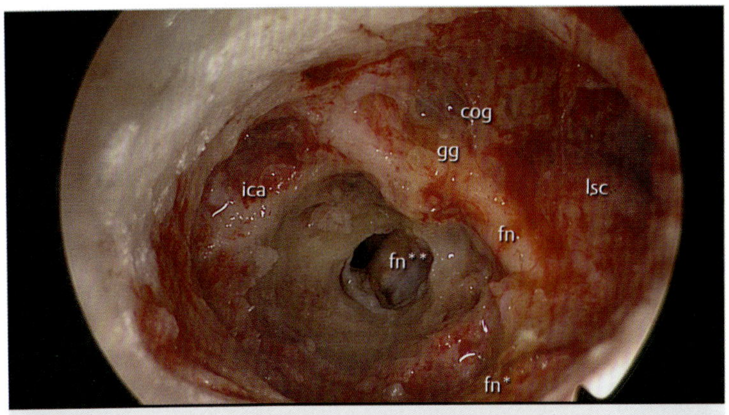

Fig. 11.59 Left side: Final surgical cavity showing the surgical defect that represents a connection between the cerebellopontine angle (CPA) and the tympanic cavity. *ica: internal carotid artery; gg: geniculate ganglion; fn: tympanic portion of facial nerve; fn*: mastoid portion of the facial nerve; fn**: facial nerve into the IAC; lsc: lateral semicircular canal.*

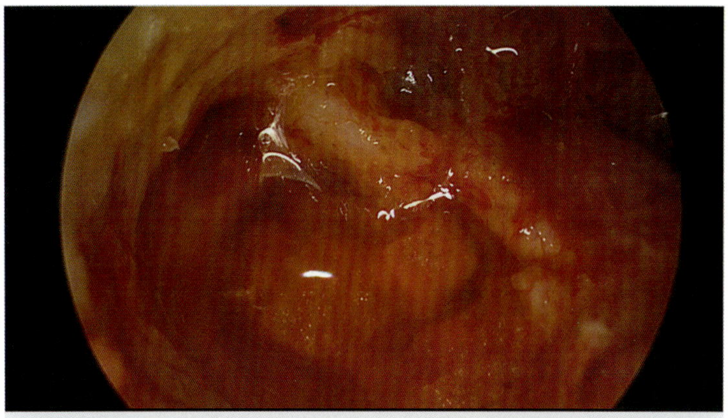

Fig. 11.60 Left side: An abdominal fat pad is harvested and placed into the promontorial defect. The fat pad is pulled into the porus to hermetically seal the defect.

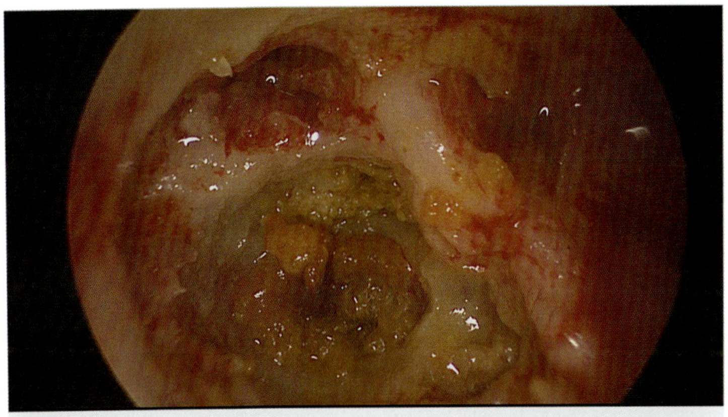

Fig. 11.61 Left side: Surgicel (absorbable hemostat matrix) is placed with the fat tissue into the surgical cavity. The Eustachian tube is obliterated using a small piece of temporal muscle and then a small piece of fat. Afterwards the eustachian tube is sealed using a hemostatic matrix and fibrin glue. The remaining cavity is filled with fat and then the skin of the external auditory canal (EAC) is sutured with a cul-de-sac closure.

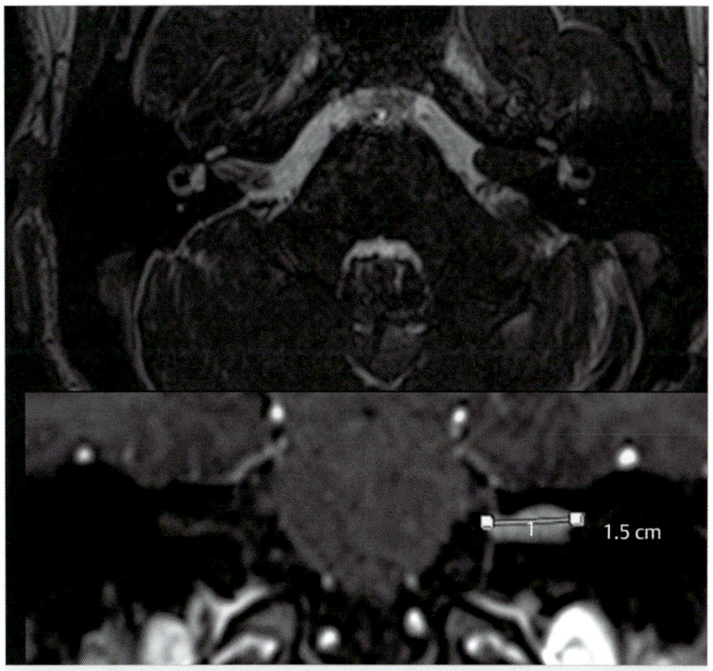

Fig. 11.62 Clinical Case 2, Left side: Magnetic resonance imaging (MRI) scan showing the growth of an acoustic neuroma during the wait and scan policy, occupying the whole internal auditory canal (IAC), protruding into the cerebellopontine angle (CPA), in a patient with a left profound sensorineural hearing loss.

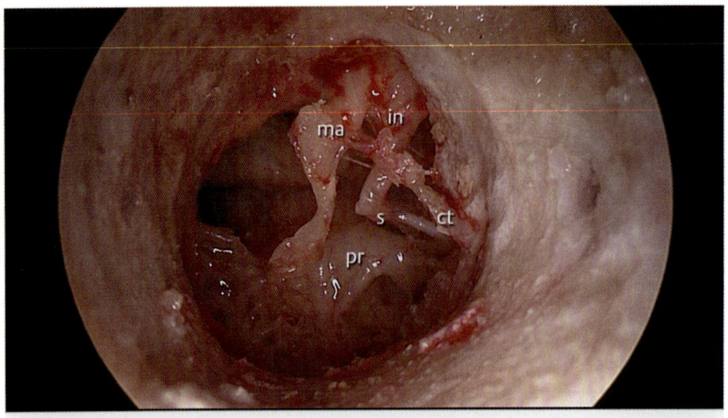

Fig. 11.63 Left side: View through a 0-degree, 4 mm diameter, 15 cm length endoscope. The tympanic cavity is exposed after a canalplasty and a scutotomy. The ossicular chain is shown. *ct: chorda tympani; in: incus; ma: malleus; pr: promontory; s: stapes.*

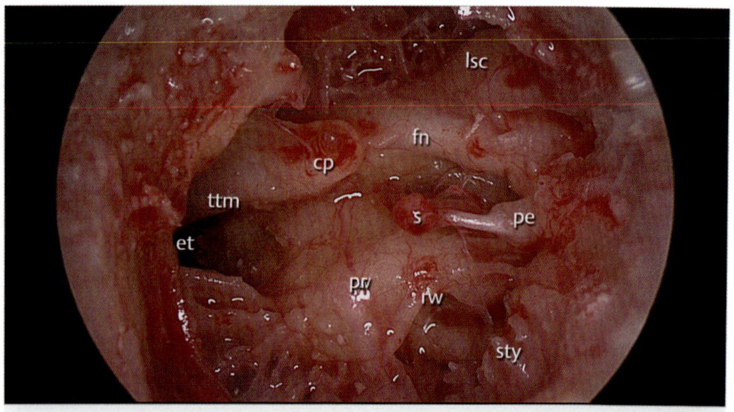

Fig. 11.64 Left side: Removal of the malleus and incus, in order to expose the whole medial wall of the tympanic cavity. *cp: cochleariform process; et: eustachian tube; fn: facial nerve; lsc: lateral semicircular canal; pe: pyramidal eminence; pr: promontory; rw: round window; s: stapes; sty: styloid eminence; ttm: tensor tympani muscle semicanal.*

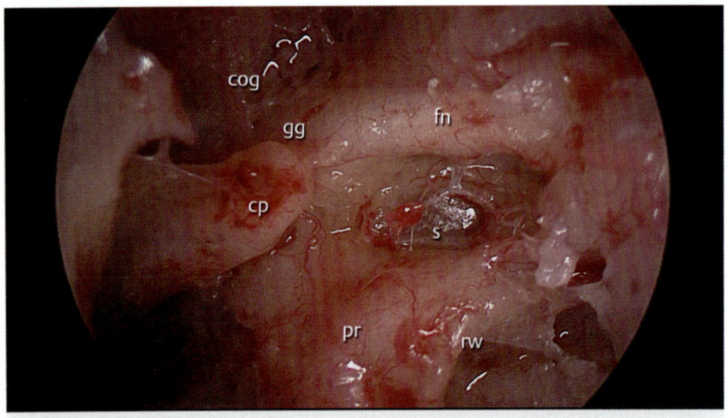

Fig. 11.65 Left side: The stapes superstructure is removed. The geniculate ganglion is detected over the cochleariform process. *cp: cochleariform process; fn: facial nerve; gg: geniculate ganglion; pr: promontory; rw: round window; s: stapes (footplate).*

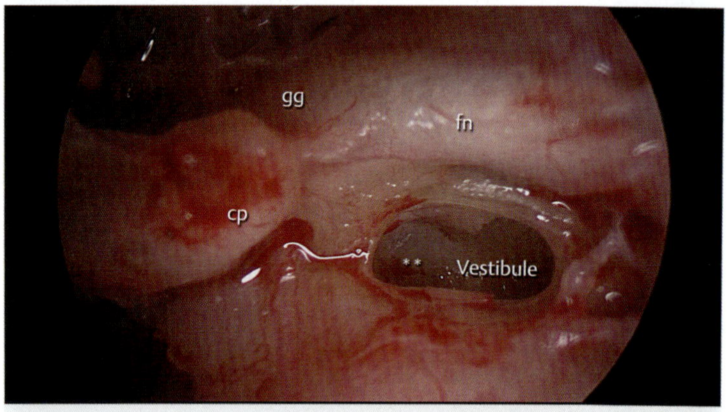

Fig. 11.66 Left side: The footplate is removed exposing the spherical recess in the saccule. The spherical recess is situated in the anteroinferior portion of the vestibule and indicates where the fundus of the internal auditory canal (IAC) is located. *cp: cochleariform process; fn: facial nerve; gg: geniculate ganglion; **: spherical recess.*

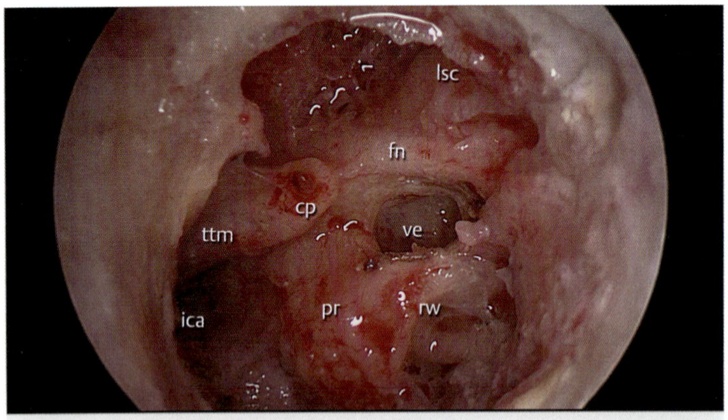

Fig. 11.67 Left side: The bone around the oval window is removed, in order to obtain a wider access to the vestibule and a direct view of the spherical recess. *cp: cochleariform process; fn: facial nerve; ica: internal carotid artery; lsc: lateral semicircular canal; pr: promontory; ttm: tensor tympani muscle semicanal; ve: vestibule.*

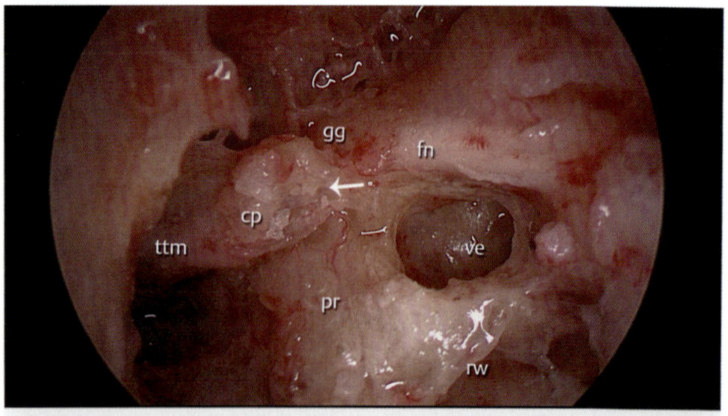

Fig. 11.68 Left side: The cochleariform process is identified following the tensor tympani muscle bony canal. The cochleariform process is opened. The eustachian tube is obliterated using a tensor tympani muscular flap. Here, particular attention must be paid to the facial nerve (see the *arrow*), as in this region, the nerve fibers are in direct contact with the tensor tympani muscle. *cp: cochleariform process; fn: facial nerve; gg: geniculate ganglion; pr: promontory; rw: round window; ttm: tensor tympani muscle semicanal; ve: vestibule.*

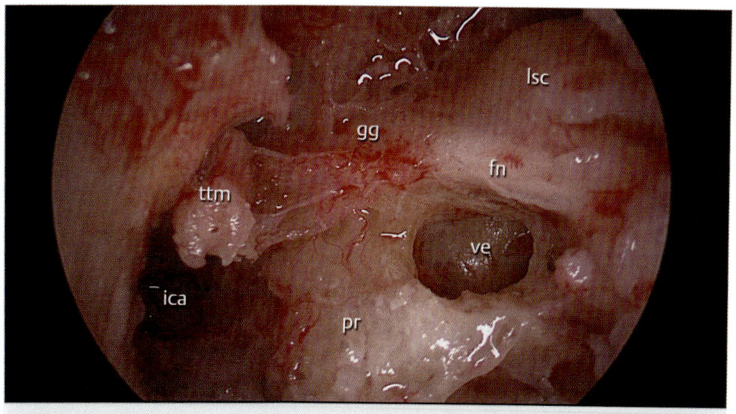

Fig. 11.69 Left side: The tensor tympani muscle is gently pushed forward keeping it pedunculated. For this step, it is recommended to use a small curette or a small round knife. Notice how the closest contact between the facial nerve (FN) and the tensor tympani canal is at the level of the postero-superior portion of the cochleariform process. *fn: facial nerve; gg: geniculate ganglion; ica: internal carotid artery; lsc: lateral semicircular canal; pr: promontory; ttm: tensor tympani muscle semicanal; ve: vestibule.*

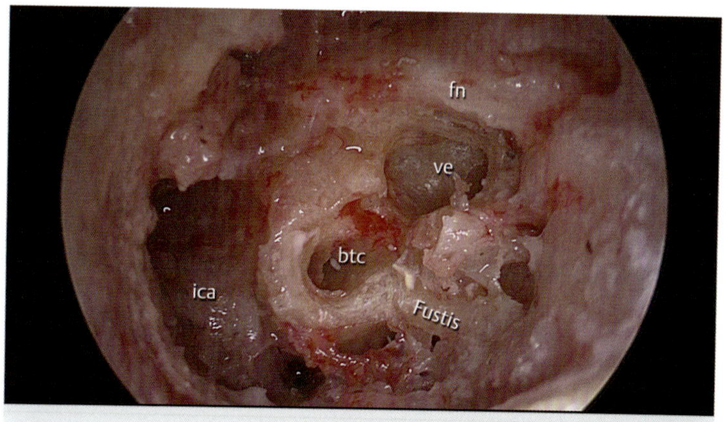

Fig. 11.70 Left side: The basal turn of the cochlea is identified. *btc: basal turn of the cochlea; fn: facial nerve; ica: internal carotid artery; ve: vestibule.*

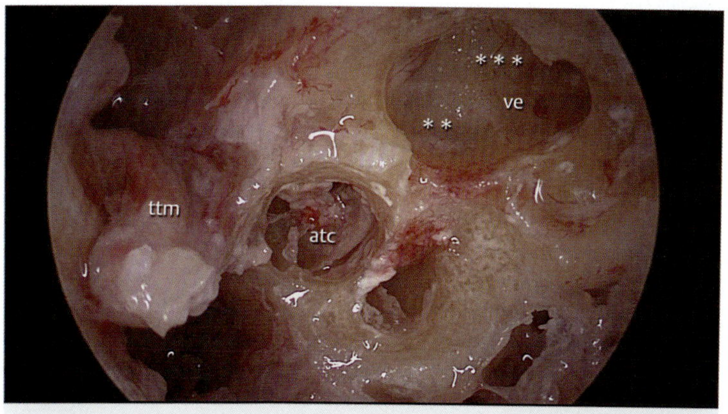

Fig. 11.71 Left side: After the dura of the internal auditory canal (IAC) is skeletonized, the medial and apical turns of the cochlea are identified. *atc: apical turn of the cochlea; ttm: tensor tympani muscle semicanal; ve: vestibule; **: spherical recess; ***: elliptical recess.*

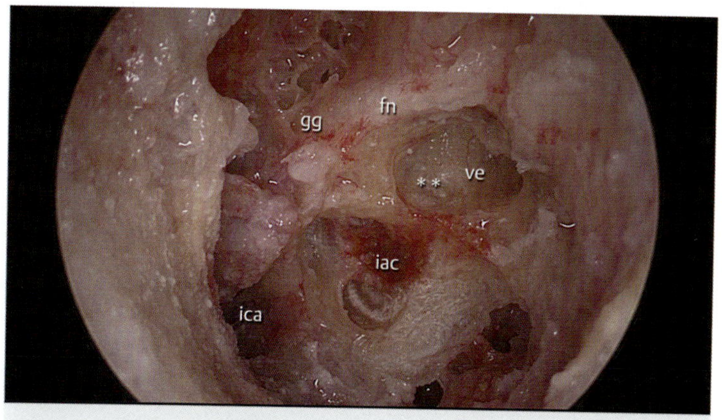

Fig. 11.72 Left side: The dura of the internal auditory canal (IAC) is skeletonized, first by removing the cochlear-vestibular bone. *fn: facial nerve; gg: geniculate ganglion; iac: internal auditory canal; ica: internal carotid artery; ve: vestibule; **: spherical recess.*

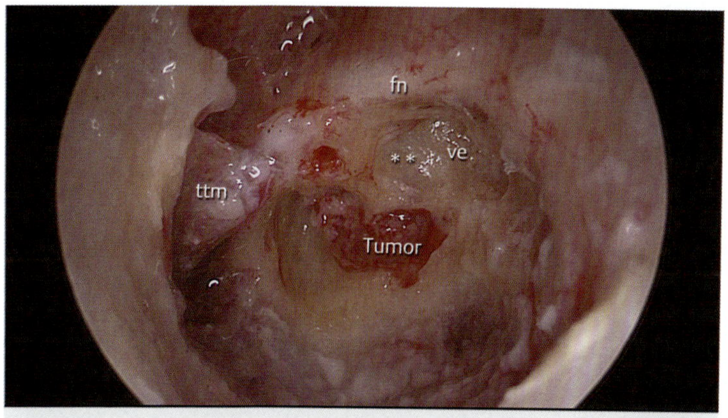

Fig. 11.73 Left side: The tensor tympani muscle is pushed inside the eustachian tube. The tumor is identified in the internal auditory canal (IAC). *fn: facial nerve; ttm: tensor tympani muscle semicanal; ve: vestibule; **: spherical recess.*

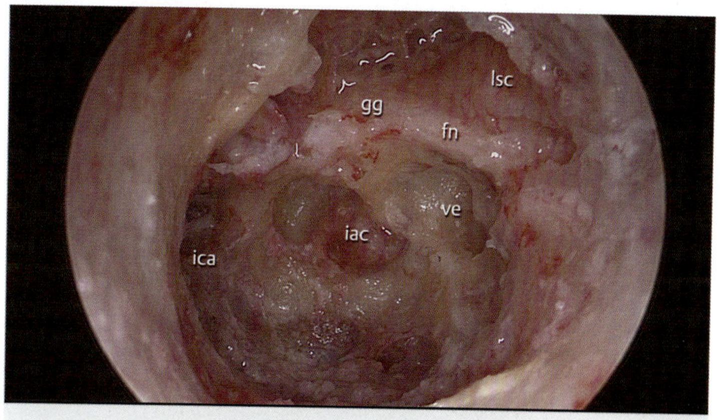

Fig. 11.74 Left side: The internal auditory canal (IAC) is skeletonized by drilling the bone around the anterior, inferior, and posterior portions of the IAC dura. *fn: facial nerve; gg: geniculate ganglion; iac: internal auditory canal; ica: internal carotid artery; lsc: lateral semicircular canal; ve: vestibule.*

is the temporomandibular joint, the superoposterior limit is the tympanic antrum, and the posterior limit is represented by the mastoid tract of the FN. The FN must also be identified in the facial recess, thus detecting its second knee and the pyramidal eminence which are important landmarks to understand the depth of the FN third tract (see ▶ Fig. 11.159). The corda tympani can be followed until its insertion into the mastoid tract of the FN. The nerve is skeletonized and followed in its entire length from the second knee to the stylomastoid foramen. It is important to identify it without uncovering the nerve, but leaving a layer of bone for protection. During this phase, it is crucial to use a medium-sized diamond bur and constant irrigation that avoids heat damage to the nerve itself (see Clinical Case 9, ▶ Fig. 11.238). At this point the superficial anatomical landmarks serving as boundaries of the dissection are:

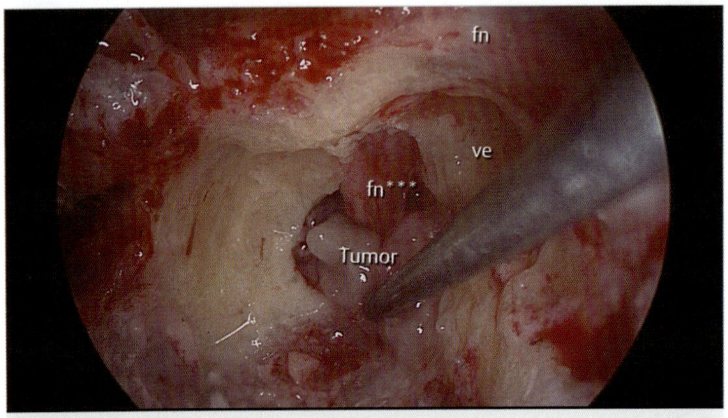

Fig. 11.75 Left side: The facial nerve (FN) is identified and then the tumor is removed paying attention not to damage the nerve. During tumor removal, it is better to use mild suction and work on the tumor and not on nervous structures. It is also possible to perform a three-handed technique; the surgeon's assistant holds the suction and the surgeon holds the endoscope in one hand, and the dissector in the other hand. This technique allows for tumor removal, avoiding to stretch or damage the nervous structures underneath. *fn: facial nerve; fn***: facial nerve into the IAC; ve: vestibule.*

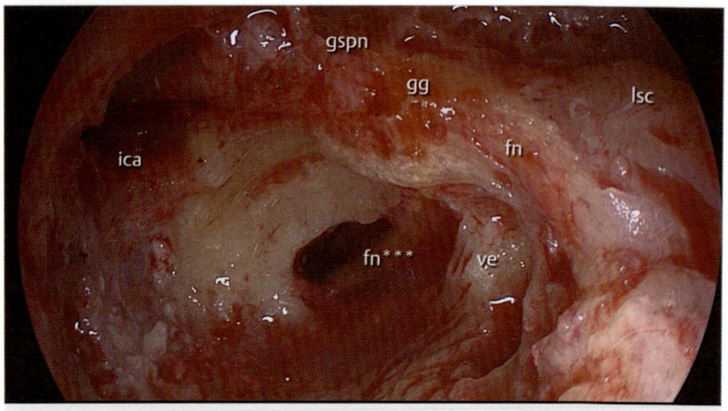

Fig. 11.76 Left side: The tumor is removed. *fn: facial nerve; fn***: facial nerve into the IAC; gg: geniculate ganglion; gspn: greater superficial petrosal nerve; ica: internal carotid artery; lsc: lateral semicircular canal; ve: vestibule.*

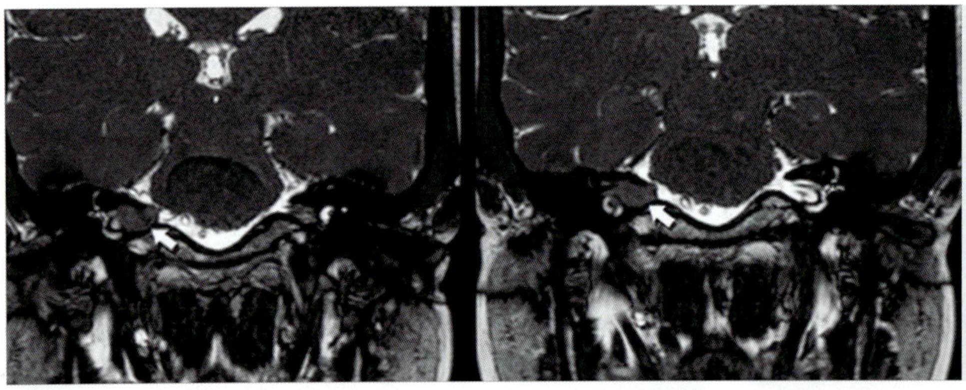

Fig. 11.77 Clinical Case 3: Magnetic resonance imaging (MRI) scan. Acoustic neuroma on the right side, occupying and enlarging the internal auditory canal (IAC), entering the cochlea, without cerebellopontine angle (CPA) extension (the *white arrow* is indicating the porus).

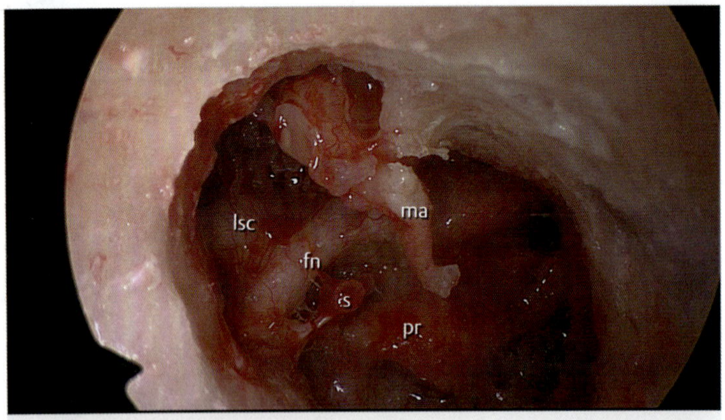

Fig. 11.78 Right side: View through a 0-degree, 4 mm diameter and 15 cm length endoscope. The skin of the external auditory canal (EAC) and the tympanic membrane is removed. The bone of the EAC is circumferentially drilled; the incus is removed, exposing the medial wall of the tympanic cavity. *fn: facial nerve; lsc: lateral semicircular canal; ma: malleus; pr: promontory; s: stapes.*

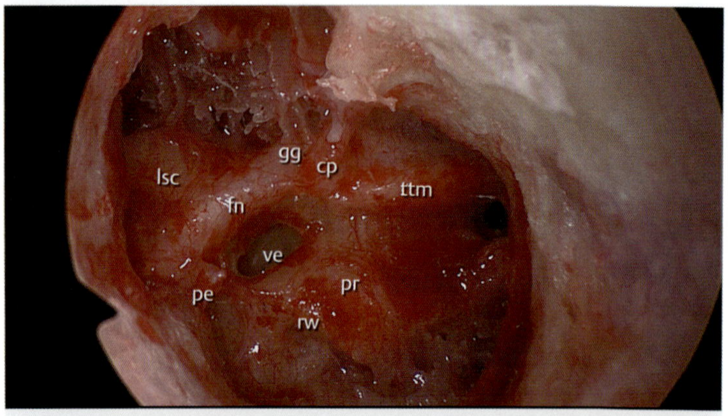

Fig. 11.79 Right side: The incus and the stapes are removed in order to identifiy the vestibule and the spherical recess. *cp: cochleariform process; fn: facial nerve; gg: geniculate ganglion; lsc: lateral semicircular canal; pe: pyramidal eminence; pr: promontory; rw: round window; ttm: tensor tympani muscle semicanal; ve: vestibule.*

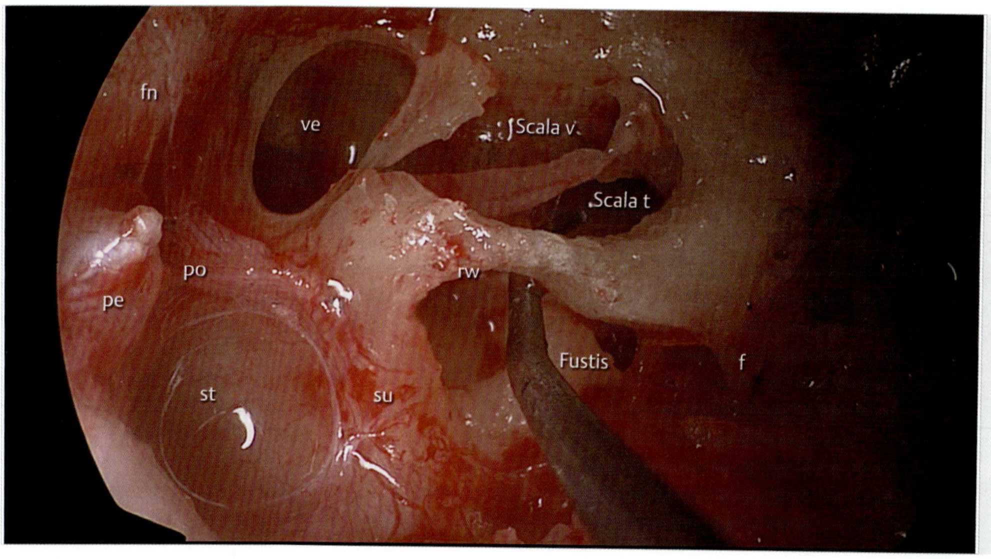

Fig. 11.80 Right side: The basal turn of the cochlea is opened, preserving the tegmen of the round window. It is possible to detect the fustis anatomy, which is a landmark to identify the scala tymani (see Chapter 12 on endoscopic surgery of the cochlea). *fn: facial nerve; pe: pyramidal eminence; po: ponticulus; rw: round window; scala t: scala tympani; scala v: scala vestibuli; st: sinus tympani; su: subiculum; ve: vestibule.*

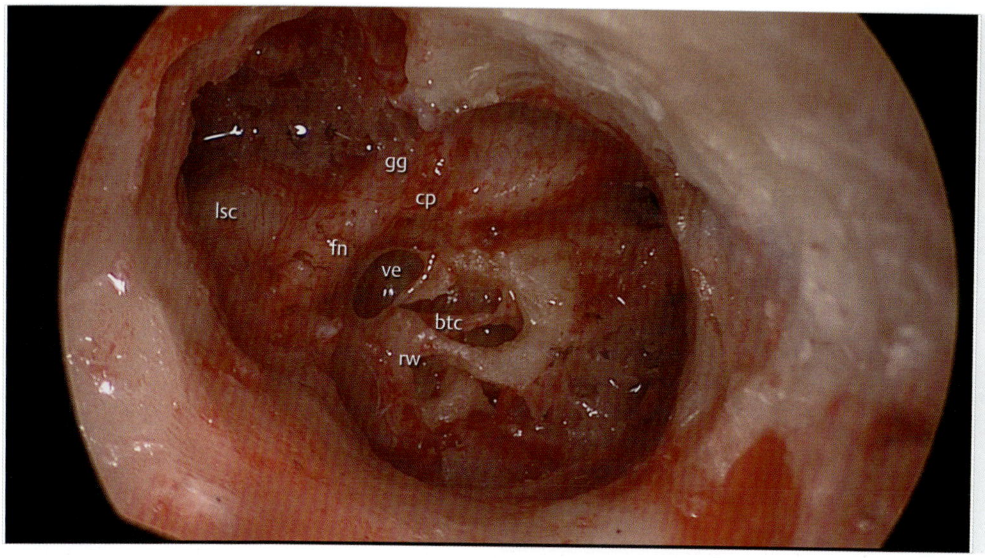

Fig. 11.81 Right side: Tympanic cavity after the partial removal of the basal turn of the cochlea. *btc: basal turn of the cochlea; cp: cochleariform process; fn: facial nerve; gg: geniculate ganglion; lsc: lateral semicircular canal; rw: round window; ve: vestibule.*

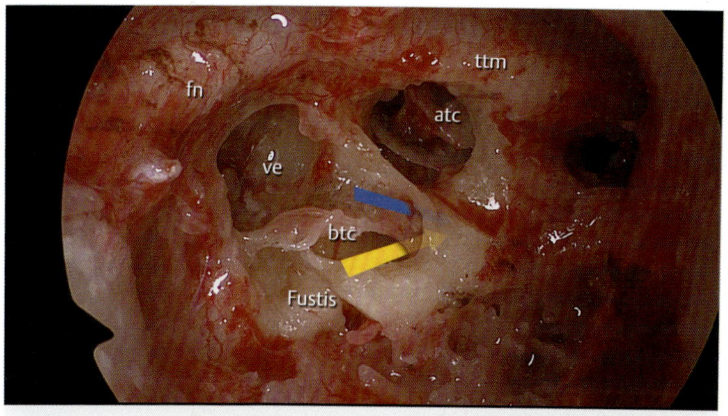

Fig. 11.82 Right side: After removing the promontorial bone using a piezoelectric bur, the medial and apical turns of the cochlea are identified as anterior to the vestibule. *atc: apical turn of the cochlea; btc: basal turn of the cochlea; fn: facial nerve; ttm: tensor tympani muscle semicanal; ve: vestibule; blue arrow: scala vestibuli; yellow arrow: scala tympani.*

- Anterior limit: the capsule of the temporomandibular joint
- Superior: the antrum and the tegmen tympani
- Posterior: the third tract of the FN
- Inferior: the hypotympanic cells

The corda timpani is then sectioned.

11.3.10 Third Step: Middle Ear Dissection

Once the tympanic cavity has been externalized, the exposure of the anatomical landmarks is started, which will serve to delineate the surgical window in relation to the CPA and the IAC. After the removal of the ossicular chain, the FN is exposed in its tympanic tract, from the second knee up to the geniculate ganglion, localized between the cochleariform process and the COG (see ▶ Fig. 11.160). The stapes entering the vestibule is removed and a diamond bur is used to identify the anatomical boundaries of the internal carotid artery and the jugular bulb. Then the surgeon must proceed to the identification of the deep anatomical limits of the dissection and the vascular structures, like in the previous technique. The carotid artery is identified below the eustachian tube in its vertical course by drilling the protympanic region using a medium-sized diamond bur. The exposure of the vessel is progressively obtained avoiding the exposure of the vessel's wall, maintaining a bone layer above it. The exposure of the jugular vein, like in the endoscopic technique, is reached by drilling the hypotympanum beneath the finiculus, exposing the gulf of the jugular vein, maintaining a thin bone layer above the vessel (see ▶ Fig. 11.161). The carotid artery and the jugular bulb,

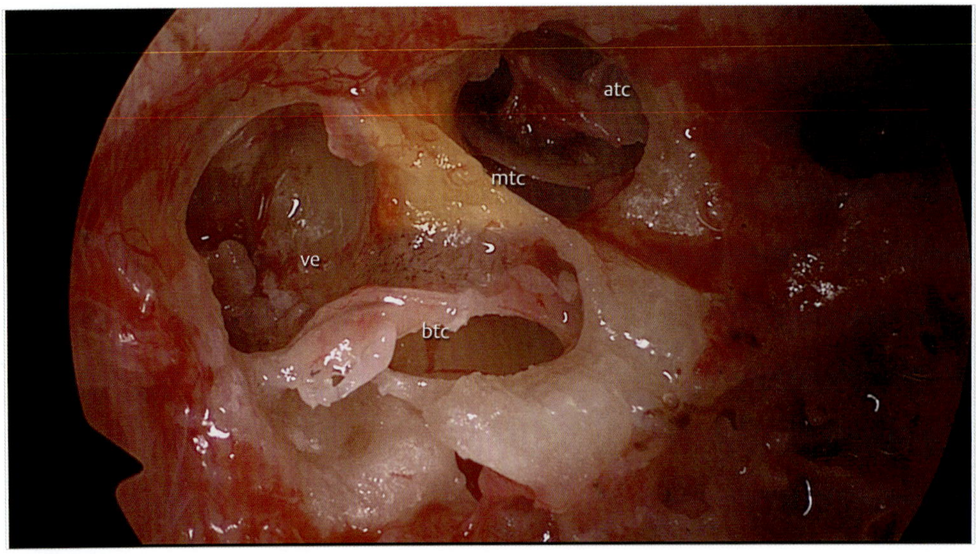

Fig. 11.83 Right side: The fundus of the internal auditory canal (IAC) is opened by removing the bony area between medial and basal turns of the cochlea and the vestibule. This bony area is the cochlear-vestibular bone, which is a thin bony crest that divides the tympanic cavity from the IAC. *atc: apical turn of the cochlea; btc: basal turn of the cochlea; mtc: middle turn of the cochlea; ve: vestibule.*

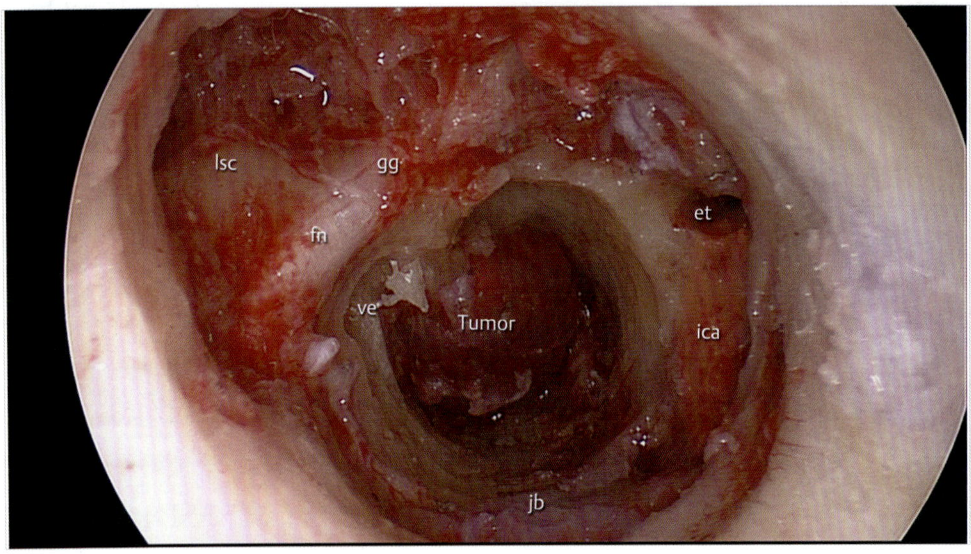

Fig. 11.84 Right side: The internal auditory canal (IAC) is skeletonized from the fundus to the porus, exposing the acoustic neuroma, first identifying anteriorly, the vertical tract of the internal carotid artery and inferiorly the bulb of jugular vein. The IAC should be skeletonized for at least 180 degrees, in a lateral to medial direction. Particular attention must be paid to the drilling of anterior portion of IAC because the anterior limit of the dissection is the vertical tract of the internal carotid artery. *et: eustachian tube; fn: facial nerve; gg: geniculate ganglion; ica: internal carotid artery; jb: jugular bulb; lsc: lateral semicircular canal; ve: vestibule.*

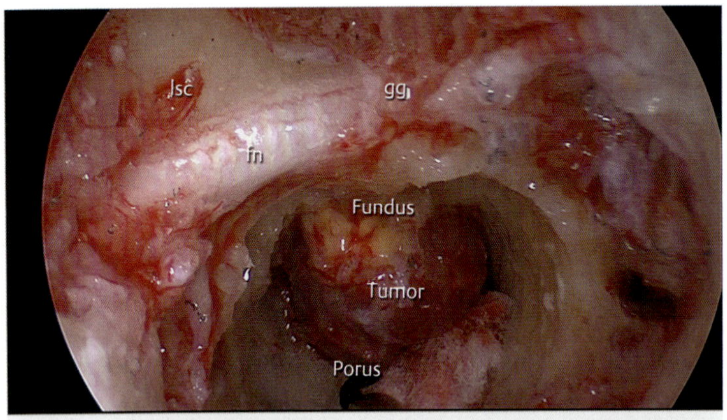

Fig. 11.85 Right side: A cottonoid is used to control the bleeding from the dura, in proximity to the porus. *fn: facial nerve; gg: geniculate ganglion; lsc: lateral semicircular canal.*

respectively, represent the anterior and the inferior anatomical limits. Once the vascular structures have been identified, the removal of the promontory and the identification of the inner ear structures can begin, generally starting by removing the round window tegmen entering the basal turn of the cochlea (see ▶ Fig. 11.162). In the expanded approach, the cochleariform process and the tensor tympani muscle must be removed to allow for an adequate exposure of the cochlea that would otherwise remain hidden from microscopic view, below the semichannel of the tensor tympani. Before removing the cochleariform process, a microbipolar tool is used to coagulate the Jacobson plexus that runs on the promontory. This allows the surgeon to minimize the annoying bleeding at this level. A courette is used to anteriorly fracture the cochleariform process; the tensor timpani muscle is identified and detached from its canal, paying attention to the posterosuperior portion of the muscle, near the cochleariform process that is closely related to the FN. The muscle is then sectioned and excised, allowing for the exposure of the promontory bone (see ▶ Fig. 11.163).

11.3.11 Fourth Step: Transpromontorial Approach to the IAC

As previously described, the stapedial tendon is sectioned and the stapes removed from the oval window. The removal of the stapes allows for the identification of the vestibule and its contents, the saccule. On the medial wall of the vestibule in the anteroinferior portion, the spherical recess appears in a different brownish/whitish color. The terminal nerve fibers of the inferior vestibular nerve are present in this region and are composed by a thin bone layer representing also a landmark for the IAC. Once the vestibule has been uncovered, exposing its medial wall, the surgeon must begin opening the cochlea, removing the tegmen of the round window and identifying the round window membrane. Entering the round window gives access to the basal turn of the cochlea with the tympanic and vestibular scale (see ▶ Fig. 11.163). When the basal turn is completely exposed, the skeletonization of the medial and apical turns of the cochlea starts by drilling the anteroinferior portion of the promontory, identifying the apical turn of the cochlea by opening it up where the cochlear bone reaches the bony groove of the tensor timpani muscle (see ▶ Fig. 11.164). The helicotrema is also identified. At this point, three openings are present: anteriorly the apical turn of the cochlea with the heilcotrema, inferiorly the basal turn of the cochlea, and superiorly the oval window niche indicating the medial part of the vestibule. The bone bridge between these structures represents the cochleovestibular bone, a very thin bone that separates the promontory from the bottom of the IAC. The removal of this bone component allows the surgeon to enter the bottom of the IAC near the cochlear nerve (see ▶ Fig. 11.165; see also Clinical Case 11). The cochlear nerve, at this level, is anteroinferiorly positioned while the inferior vestibular nerve is more superficial and in a posterior position until it adheres to the spherical recess in the saccular fossa. The labyrinthine tract of the FN follows an imaginary line passing from the geniculate ganglion to the spherical recess turning around the apical turn of the cochlea (see Clinical Case 11, ▶ Fig. 11.284). The IAC runs almost parallel to the EAC but with a slight oblique movement from anterior to posterior from the surface to the depth in a lateromedial direction (see ▶ Fig. 11.165). After the identification of the fundus at the level of the medial vestibule, the IAC dura is progressively exposed. Drilling of the promontory and the tympanic cavity will proceed on the whole perimeter, delimited anteriorly by the carotid artery, inferiorly by the jugular bulb, posteriorly by the third tract of the FN, and superiorly by the tympanic tract. The bone is progressively removed by exposing the dura of the IAC, from the surface to the depth reaching the petrous apex and the porus region (see ▶ Fig. 11.166; see also Clinical Case 11).

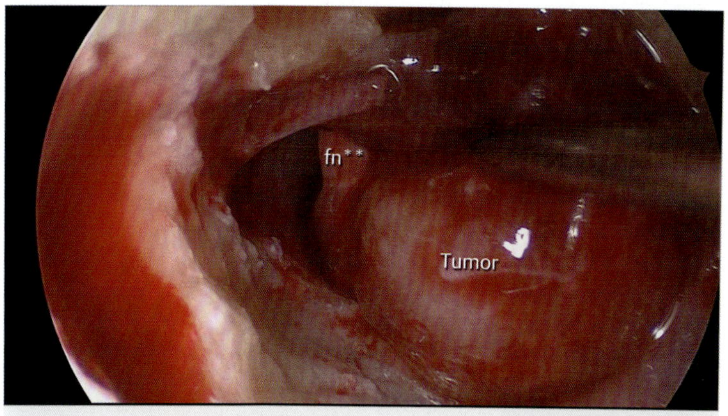

Fig. 11.86 Right side: The tumor is gently dissected, keeping the facial nerve (FN) in the internal auditory canal (IAC) under constant observation. *fn**: facial nerve into the IAC.*

In this phase, we recommend a medium-sized diamond bur. The IAC will be progressively skeletonized and its lateral, anterior, and posterior walls fully exposed in the tympanic cavity. Once the porus has been identified, the dural reflection of the medial surface of the temporal bone is uncovered (dura of the posterior fossa). The exposure of this area is crucial to determine the surgical window on the CPA and to access the intracysternal tumor component (see ▶ Fig. 11.167). The inferior limit of the approach should not be in the projection area of the junction between the jugular bulb and the internal carotid artery as this anatomical area represents the projection area of the mixed nerves. Once the IAC and dura of the temporal bone have been skeletonized, an incision of the dura under the porus is performed by accessing the CPA far from the IAC. With this maneuver, when the tumor does not have considerable dimensions, it is possible to deliquor the cistern that will allow the subsequent maneuvers to mobilize the tumor (see ▶ Fig. 11.168). The exposure of the CPA is obtained with the identification of the tumor. The entry zone of the acoustic-facial bundle in cases of good exposure usually lies in front of the operator.

11.3.12 Fifth Step: Tumor Dissection

The dura is medially incised along the IAC from the bottom to the porus, and it is elevated by exposing the tumor capsule from the IAC to the CPA. The tumor is identified and the dissection is started strictly following its capsula, delicately removing the arachnoidal adherences and the small vessels supplying the tumor (see ▶ Fig. 11.169). As soon as the most medial pole of the neoplasm is reached, a remarkable outflow of CSF is observed. In this porus area, we frequently observe adherences to the FN, which are gently released following the plane of the tumor capsula. The FN at this point is often flattened and therefore

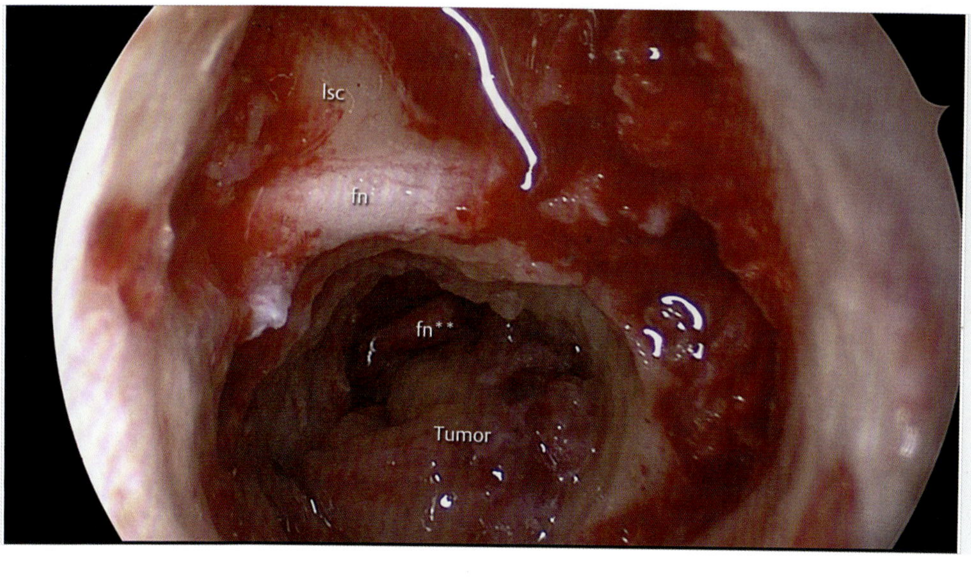

Fig. 11.87 Right side: The tumor is removed en bloc. Notice the facial nerve (FN) course through a transcanal endoscopic view: the tympanic and the intracanalicular tracts of the nerve till the porus. *fn: tympanic portion of the facial nerve; fn**: facial nerve into the IAC; lsc: lateral semicircular canal.*

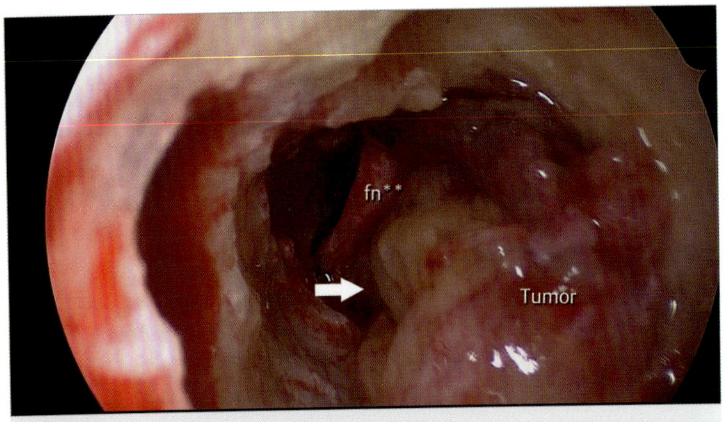

Fig. 11.88 Right side: Endoscopic magnification of the facial nerve (FN) in the internal auditory canal (IAC). *fn**: facial nerve into the IAC.*

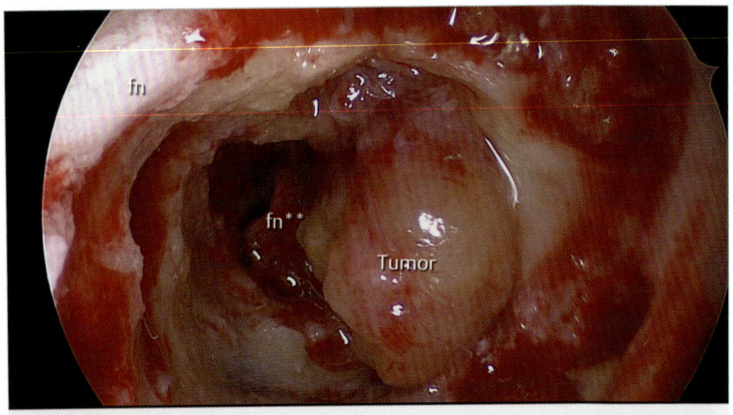

Fig. 11.89 Right side: The tumor is dissected from the inferior vestibular nerve. *fn: tympanic portion of the facial nerve; fn**: facial nerve into the IAC.*

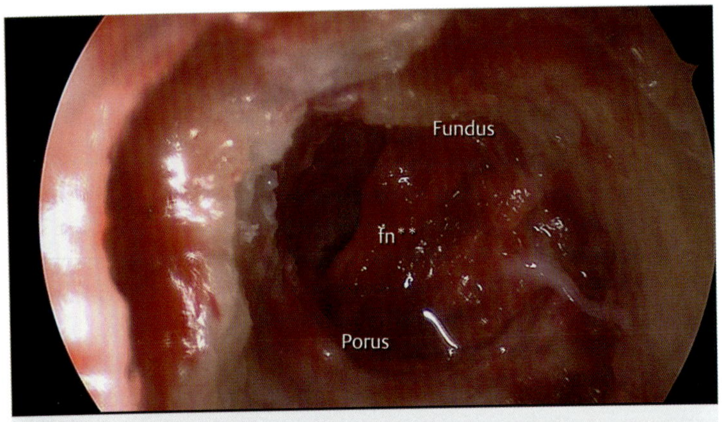

Fig. 11.90 Right side: Endoscopic magnification of the facial nerves (FN) and vestibular nerves in the internal auditory canal (IAC). *fn**: facial nerve into the IAC.*

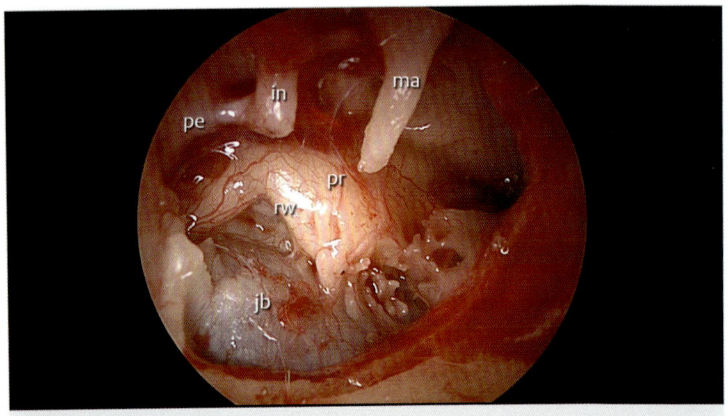

Fig. 11.91 Clinical case 4: Right intracanalicular acoustic neuroma. Right side. Endoscopic view with a 0-degree endoscope of 4 mm diameter and 15 cm length. The skin of the external auditory canal (EAC) and the tympanic membrane is removed. The EAC is drilled and the tympanic cavity is exposed. Notice the jugular bulb inferiorly, which represents the inferior limit of the dissection. *in: incus; jb: jugular bulb; ma: malleus; pe: pyramidal eminence; pr: promontory; rw: round window.*

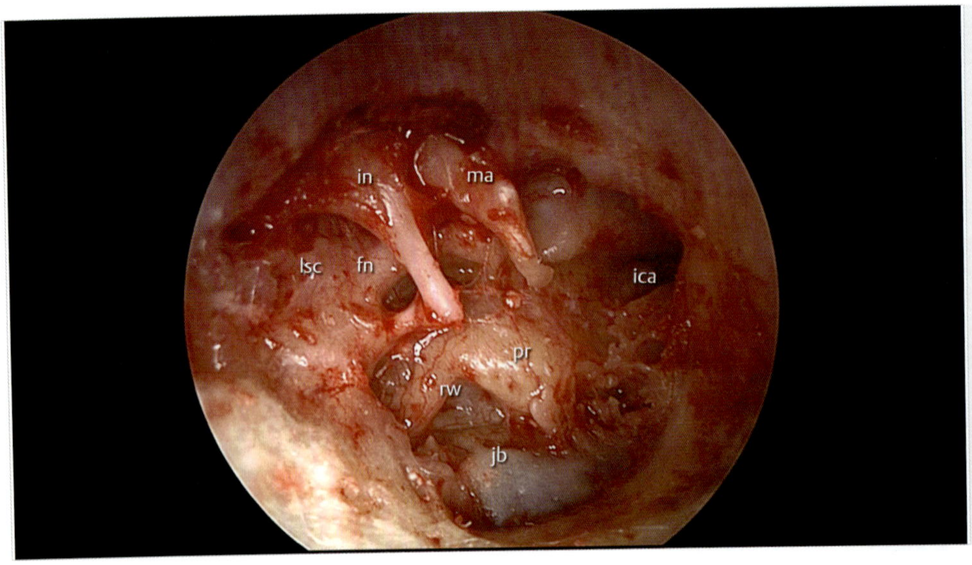

Fig. 11.92 Right side: Endoscopic view of the medial wall of the tympanic cavity. *fn: tympanic portion of the facial nerve; ica: internal carotid artery; in: incus; jb: jugular bulb; lsc: lateral semicircular canal; ma: malleus; pr: promontory; rw: round window.*

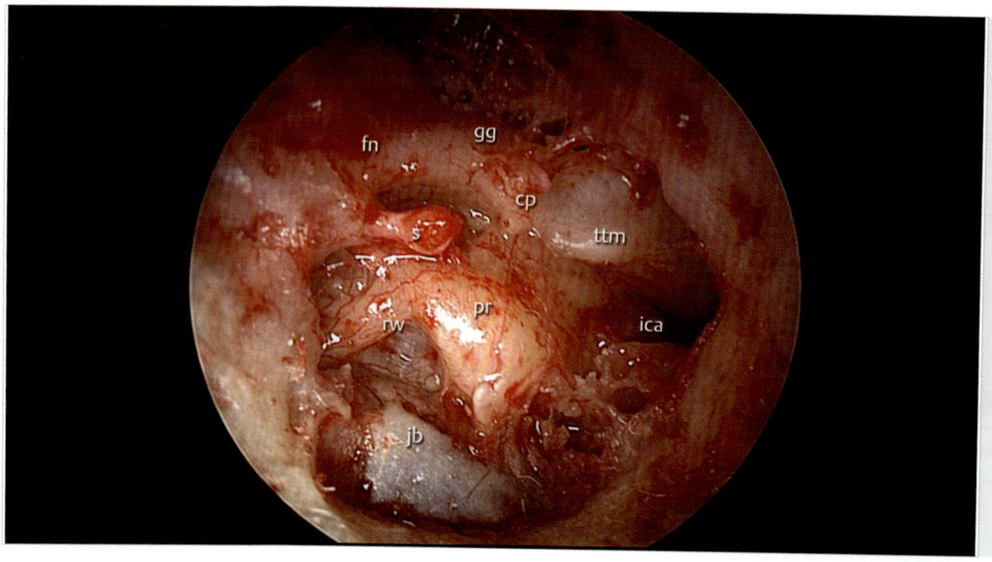

Fig. 11.93 Right side: Limits of the dissection: superiorly the tympanic portion of the facial nerve (FN), anteriorly the vertical segment of the petrous internal carotid artery, inferiorly the jugular bulb, and posteriorly the mastoid portion of the FN. *cp: cochleariform process; fn: tympanic portion of the facial nerve; gg: geniculate ganglion; ica: internal carotid artery; jb: jugular bulb; pr: promontory; rw: round window; s: stapes; ttm: tensor tympani muscle semicanal.*

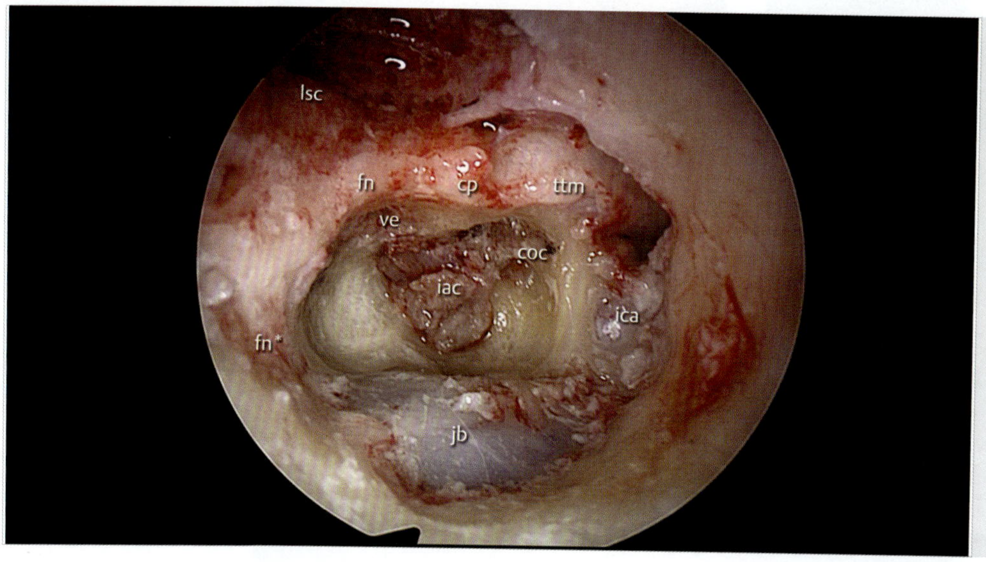

Fig. 11.94 Right side: The internal auditory canal (IAC) is identified and skeletonized through the landmarks already shown in the previous clinical cases. *coc: cochlea; cp: cochleariform process; fn: tympanic portion of the facial nerve; fn*: mastoid portion of the facial nerve; iac: internal auditory canal; ica: internal carotid artery; jb: jugular bulb; lsc: lateral semicircular canal; ttm: tensor tympani muscle semicanal; ve: vestibule.*

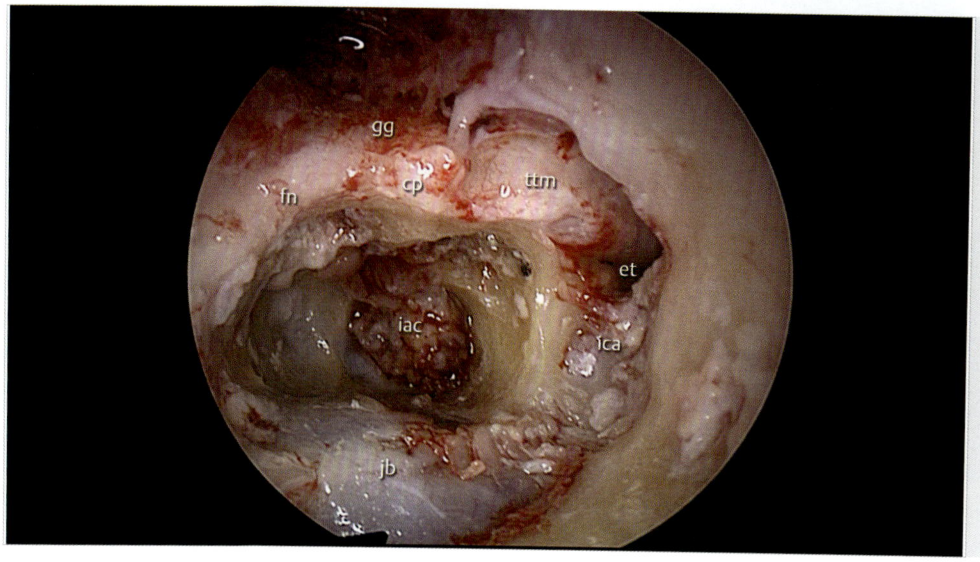

Fig. 11.95 Right side: The internal auditory canal (IAC) dura is skeletonized till the reflection of the dura from the IAC to the posterior surface of the temporal bone is identified. The dural reflection represents the end of the IAC and beyond this dura, we can find the cerebellopontine angle (CPA). *cp: cochleariform process; et: eustachian tube; fn: tympanic portion of the facial nerve; gg: geniculate ganglion; iac: internal auditory canal; ica: internal carotid artery; jb: jugular bulb; ttm: tensor tympani muscle semicanal.*

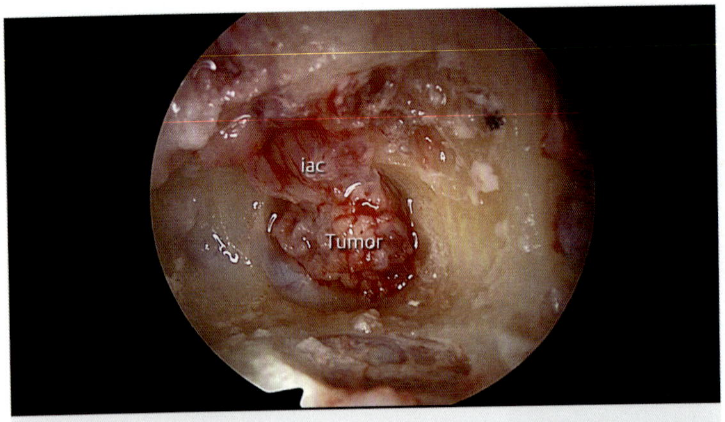

Fig. 11.96 Right side: Endoscopic detail of the blue line of the dura covering the medial surface of the temporal bone. *iac: internal auditory canal.*

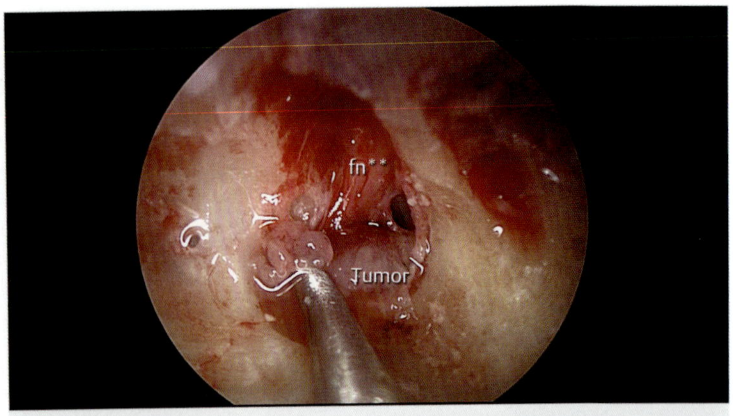

Fig. 11.97 Right side: The tumor is removed from the porus, preserving the facial nerve (FN). *fn**: facial nerve into the IAC.*

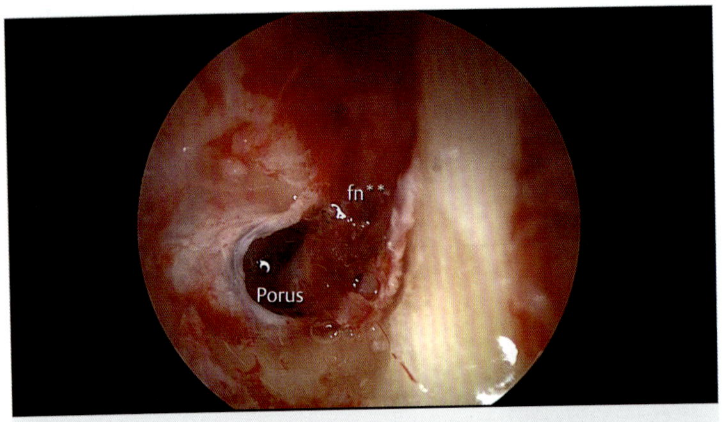

Fig. 11.98 Right side: Endoscopic view of the internal auditory canal (IAC) after tumor removal. *fn**: facial nerve into the IAC.*

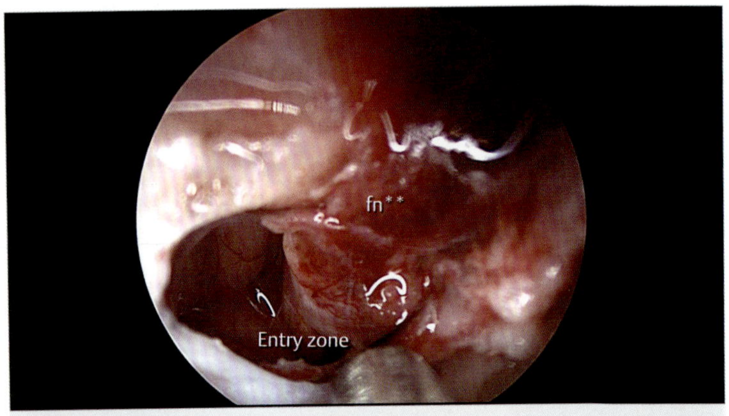

Fig. 11.99 Right side: Facial nerve's root entry zone in the brainstem. *fn**: facial nerve into the IAC.*

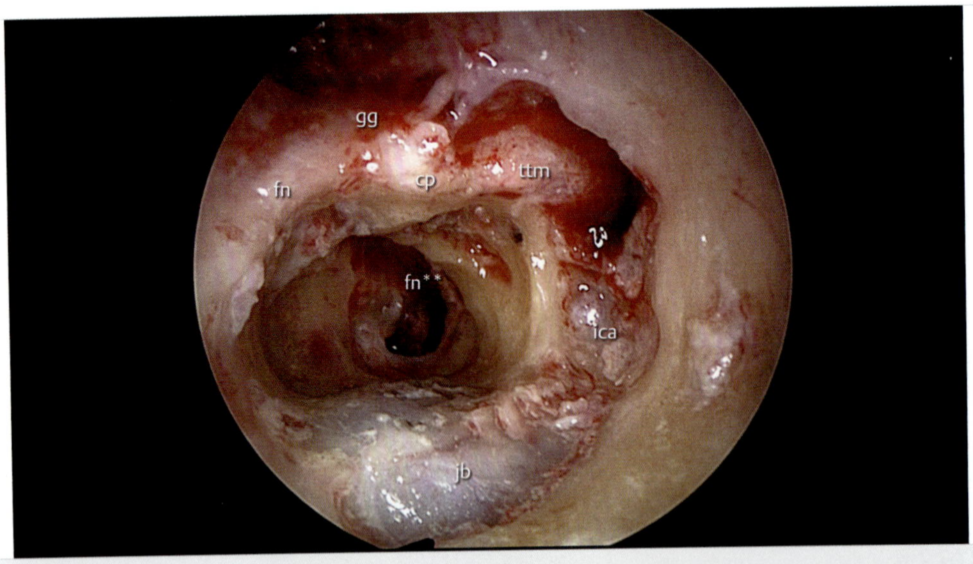

Fig. 11.100 Right side: Final surgical cavity after tumor removal. The opening of the fundus of the IAC should be always started with cochlear-vestibular bone removal. This is a thin bony crest located between the medial turn, the basal turn of the cochlea, and the vestibule. The cochlear-vestibular bone divides the promontory from the fundus, where the cochlear, facial, and vestibular nerve attachments are located. Once the cochlear-vestibular bone has been removed, the cochlear nerve is visible while entering the cochlea and the superior and inferior vestibular nerves are detected in the fundus, respectively, before the attachment to the spherical and elliptical recesses. The facial nerve (FN) runs into the IAC, between the cochlear nerve and the inferior vestibular nerve. The FN becomes intralabynthine just over the cochlea. *cp: cochleariform process; fn: tympanic portion of the facial nerve; fn**: facial nerve into the IAC; gg: geniculate ganglion; ica: internal carotid artery; jb: jugular bulb; ttm: tensor tympani muscle semicanal.*

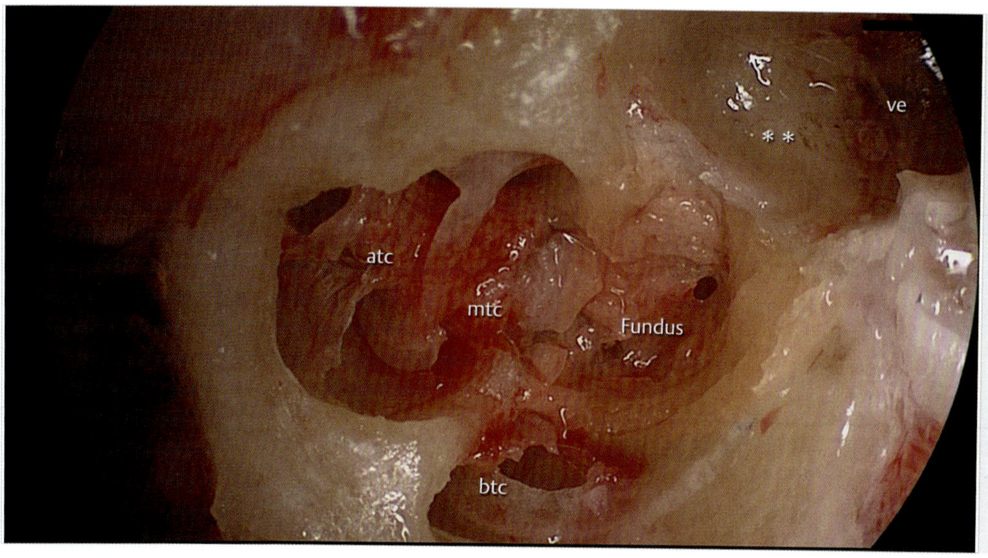

Fig. 11.101 Clinical Case 5, Left side: Fundus of internal auditory canal (IAC) opening: after the identification of the basal, medial, and apical turns of the cochlea, the medial portion of the vestibule, and the spherical recess, the fundus of the IAC can be opened by removing the cochlear-vestibular bone (orange area) with a piezoelectric bur. *atc: apical turn of the cochlea; btc: basal turn of the cochlea; mtc: middle turn of the cochlea; ve: vestibule; **: spherical recess.*

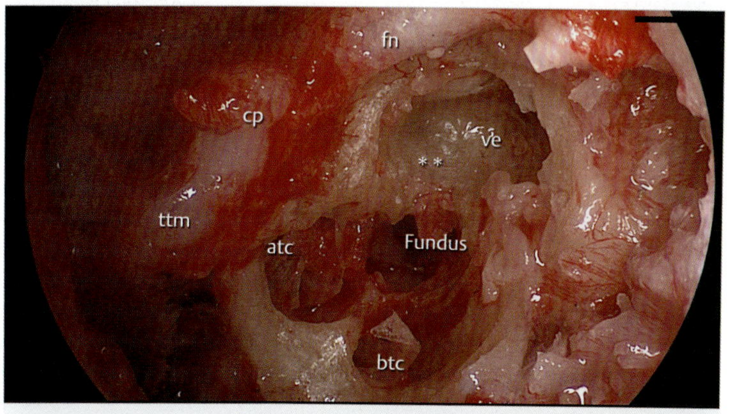

Fig. 11.102 Left side: The cochlear-vestibular bone is removed. The fundus of the internal auditory canal (IAC) is opened. *atc: apical turn of the cochlea; btc: basal turn of the cochlea; cp: cochleariform process; fn: tympanic portion of the facial nerve; ttm: tensor tympani muscle semicanal; ve: vestibule; **: spherical recess.*

vulnerable. The most posterior and medial part of the tumor is progressively released and thereafter removed. When the lesion occupies the CPA near the porus, a central debulking of the tumor is performed, emptying the central component of the neurinoma; so the mobilization maneuvers as well as the dissection of the vasal components, such as the AICA, and also the identification of the FN up to its entry zone become easier (see ▶ Fig. 11.170, ▶ Fig. 11.171). Once the tumor has been removed, an inspection of the cavity of the IAC and the CPA is performed using a 0-degree, 4-mm endoscope, inserted through the promontory defect in search of any tumor residues. In case of tumor remnants, an endoscopic removal technique will be adopted in the above-mentioned way (see Clinical Case 10). The introduction of the optics allows for a direct and magnified vision of the entry zone, of the trigeminal nerve, and of the abducent nerve in depth. Moreover, in patients with lesions extending in the petrous apex, below the internal carotid artery, in its vertical and horizontal tracts, disease residues can be exposed with straight or curved optics (0 or 45 degrees) and removed with angled instruments with extreme precision (see Clinical Case 12). The final microscopic inspection through the porus offers a direct view of the acustic-facial bundle that runs toward the CPA; superiorly the trigeminal nerve and more medially the AICA are identified (see ▶ Fig. 11.171).

11.3.13 Sixth Step: Closure

After a final stimulation of the FN to prove its integrity and the exclusion of bleeding, we proceed with the closure of the approach. First, the eustachian tube is closed using a piece of muscle (harvested from the temporal muscle) followed by a small piece of fat and sealed using a hemostatic matrix and fibrin glue (see ▶ Fig. 11.172). Then a pad of abdominal fat is placed into the created defect, which immediately stops the liquorrhea (see ▶ Fig. 11.173). The graft is further sealed using a hemostatic matrix and fibrin glue. The whole access is then filled with fat, and finally the remaining skin at the level of the meatus of the EAC and the skin incisions are closed in layers.

In case of a Shambaugh incision, the temporalis muscle is sutured, and the periosteum layer replaced and sutured to cover the surgical cavity (see ▶ Fig. 11.174). The skin is tightly sutured in layers, and the EAC skin everted and sutured (see ▶ Fig. 11.175).

11.3.14 Hints and Pitfalls

- Performing this technique with a retroauricular incision facilitates the blind sac closure; therefore, this choice is to be preferred to the anterior incision.
- In case of lesions of 2 cm or more, an extensive mastoid exposure is recommended. If necessary, the transcanal technique can be converted into a transotic approach to expose the whole CPA.
- The carotid and the jugular bulb must be covered by a thin bone to protect the vascular structures.
- The drilling toward the medial surface of the temporal bone must be particularly accurate to broadly expose the temporal reflection of the posterior fossa. Around the porus, the wider the dural exposure the greater the surgical window in the CPA will be.
- Never uncover the mastoid tract of the FN as it could result in a traumatic damage during deep tumor removal maneuvers. A protective bone wall must therefore always be maintained.
- During the dissection of the tumor, we suggest to surround the tumor in the APC with cottonoids soaked in water. This procedure allows the surgeon to protect the brainstem and to avoid traumatic damage to the vascular structures. The surgical

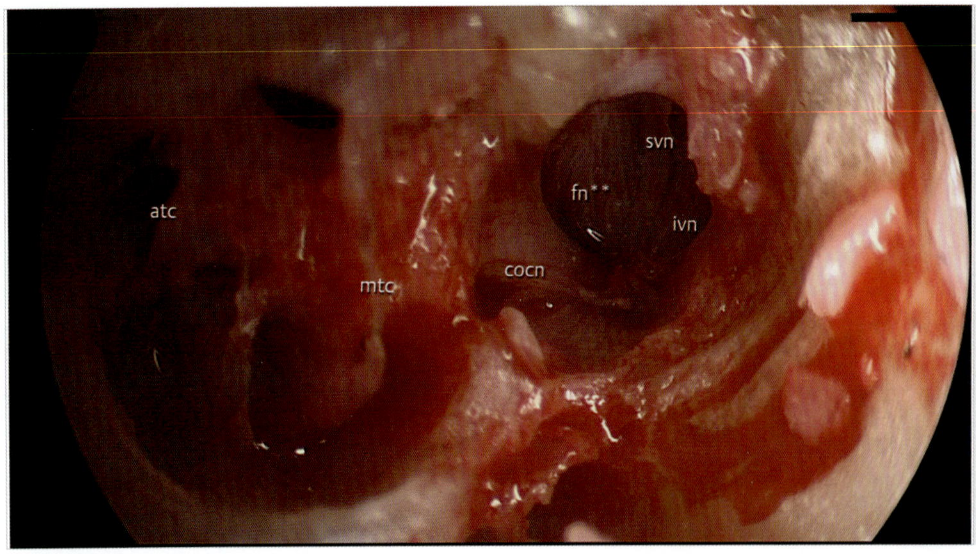

Fig. 11.103 Left side: The removal of cochlearvestibular bone enables the surgeon to expose the nervous structures of the acoustic-facial bundle. It is possible to see the terminal portion of the cochlear nerve attached to the posteroinferior portion of the cochlea and the terminal portion of inferior vestibular nerve more deeply if compared to the cochlear nerve. *atc: apical turn of the cochlea; cocn: cochlear nerve; fn**: facial nerve into the IAC; ivn: inferior vestibular nerve; mtc: medial turn of the cochlea; svn: superior vestibular nerve.*

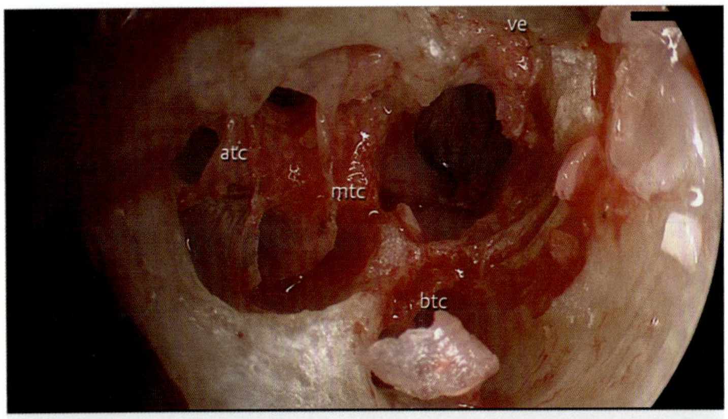

Fig. 11.104 Left side: The dissection proceeds deeply following the dura a lateral to medial direction, from the fundus of the internal auditory canal (IAC) to the porus. *atc: apical turn of the cochlea; btc: basal turn of the cochlea; mtc: medial turn of the cochlea; ve: vestibule.*

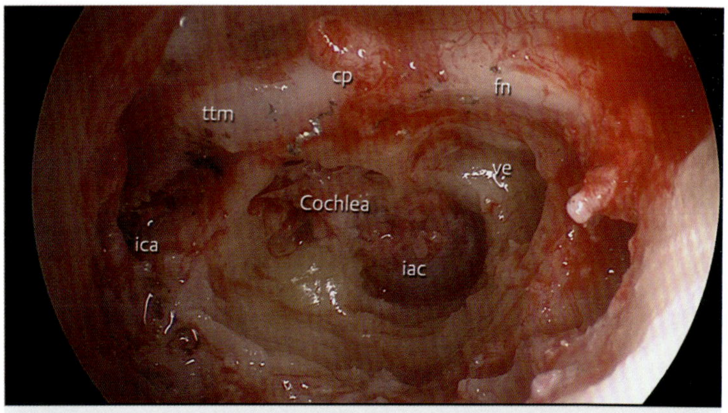

Fig. 11.105 Left side: Drilling is performed in a horseshoe manner around the dura of inferior, posterior, and anterior portions of the internal auditory canal (IAC), in a lateral to medial direction until the porus is identified. *cp: cochleariform process; fn: tympanic portion of the facial nerve; iac: internal auditory canal; ica: internal carotid artery; ttm: tensor tympani muscle semicanal; ve: vestibule.*

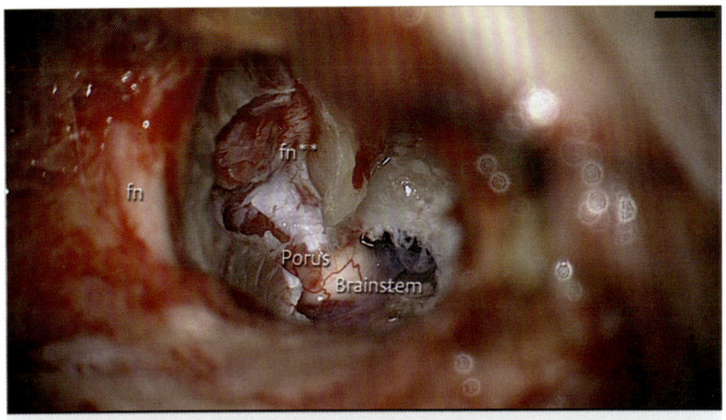

Fig. 11.106 Clinical Case 6, Right side: Microscopic view of the internal auditory canal (IAC) during a transcanal transpromontorial expanded approach; it is possible to observe the drilling below the porus and the access to the cerebellopontine angle (CPA). Notice how close the brainstem is. *fn: tympanic portion of the facial nerve; fn**: facial nerve into the IAC.*

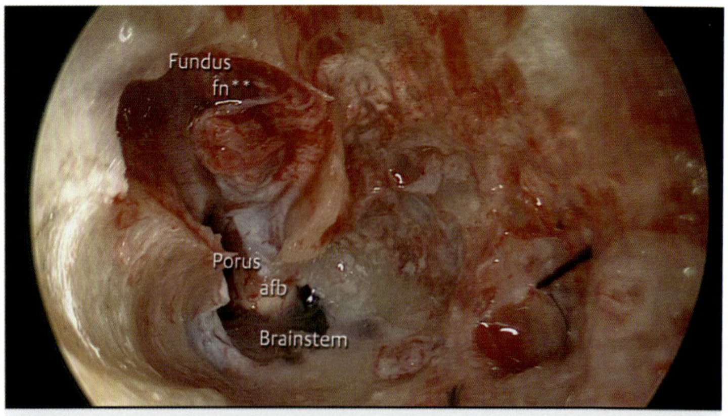

Fig. 11.107 Right side: Endoscopic view with 0-degree endoscope. Internal auditory canal (IAC) is skeletonized and the inferior section of the porus is drilled to obtain a wide access to the cerebellopontine angle (CPA). Notice the root entry zone of the acoustic-facial bundle in the brainstem. *afb: acoustic-facial bundle; fn**: facial nerve into the IAC.*

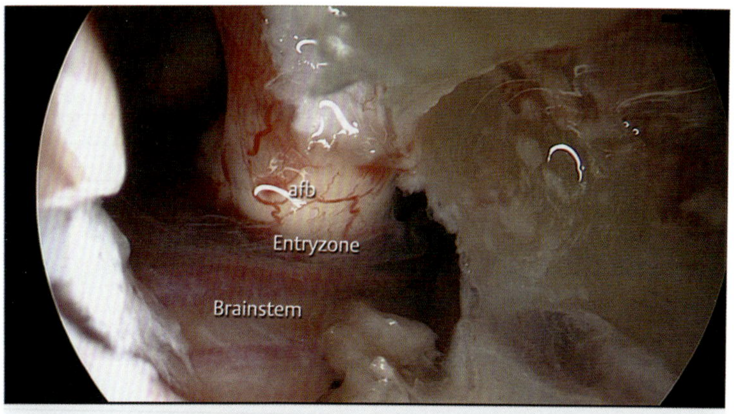

Fig. 11.108 Right side: An endoscopic detail of the root exit zone during a transcanal transpromontorial approach. Notice the narrow space between the posterior portion of the petrous bone around the porus and the brainstem. *fn**: facial nerve into the IAC.*

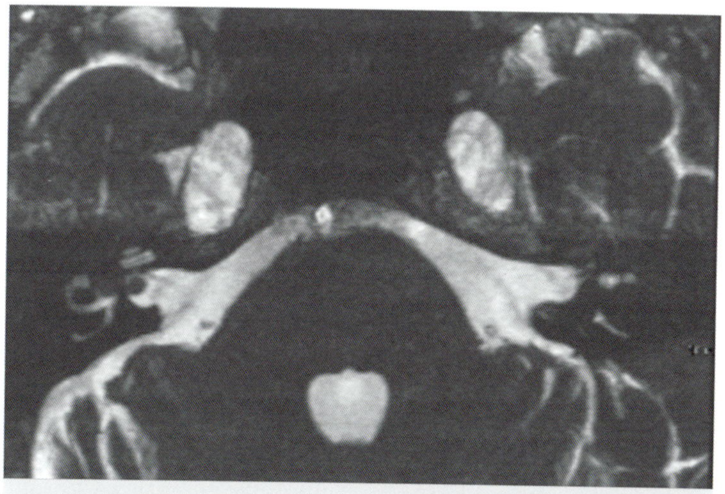

Fig. 11.109 Clinica Case 7: Patient with intractable vertigo associated with profound hearing loss on the right side; on the magnetic resonance imaging (MRI) an intralabyrinthine schwannoma occupying the vestibule and the fundus of the internal auditory canal is seen (IAC).

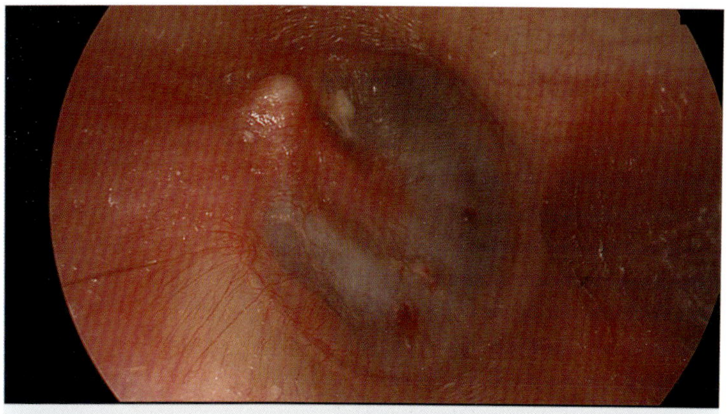

Fig. 11.110 Right side: Endoscopic view of the tympanic membrane, with a 0-degree endoscope of 4 mm diameter and 15 cm length.

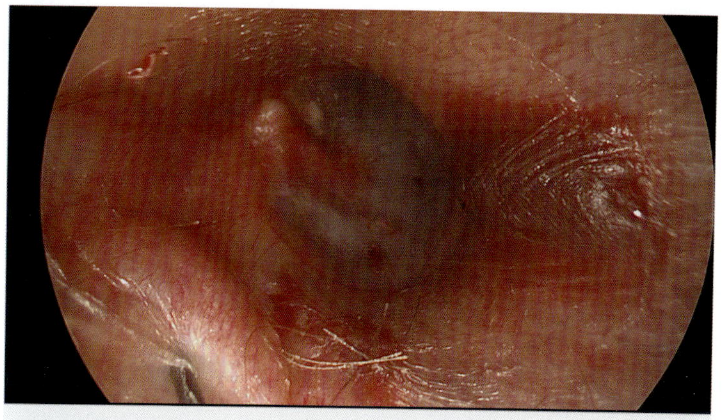

Fig. 11.111 Right side: Posterior skin infiltration with local anesthetic and vasoconstrictor solutions.

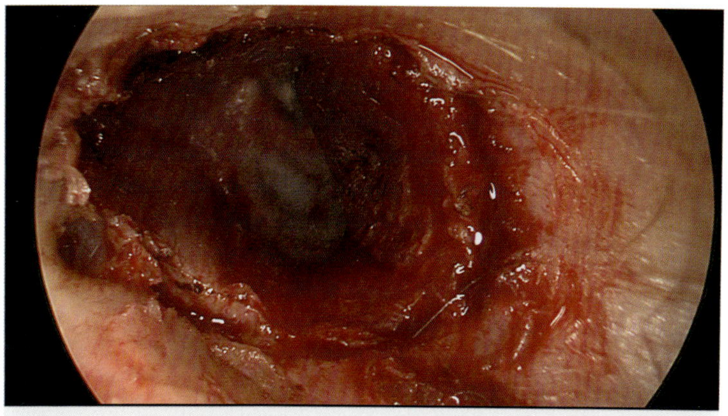

Fig. 11.112 Right side: Circumferential incision of the skin of the external auditory canal (EAC) at the cartilage-bone junction.

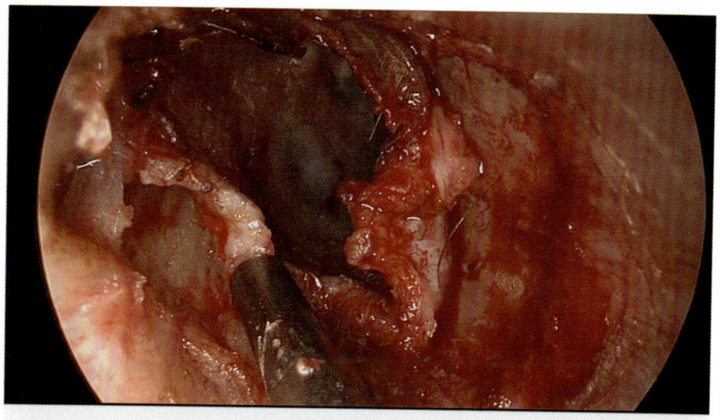

Fig. 11.113 Right side: A suction tube or a round knife is used to circumferentially lift the skin of external auditory canal (EAC).

maneuvers will be carried out around the tumor and not on the brain. In tumors larger than 2 cm, a central debulking of the mass will grant a reduction in the size of the tumor with greater maneuverability during the subsequent phases of removal and preservation of the FN.

- During the closure phase, if the breach is very large, it is better to close the defect with abdominal fat, by stratifying it to tightly seal the defect.

11.3.15 Postoperative Care

Postoperative care is similar to the one of the exclusive endoscopic technique. The patient must be kept in a supine position for 48 hours and then mobilized on the 3rd day. Discharge is scheduled from the 5th day after surgery. If the patient has no relevant comorbidities, immediate postoperative extubation and monitoring in the recovery room is the normal procedure. A CT

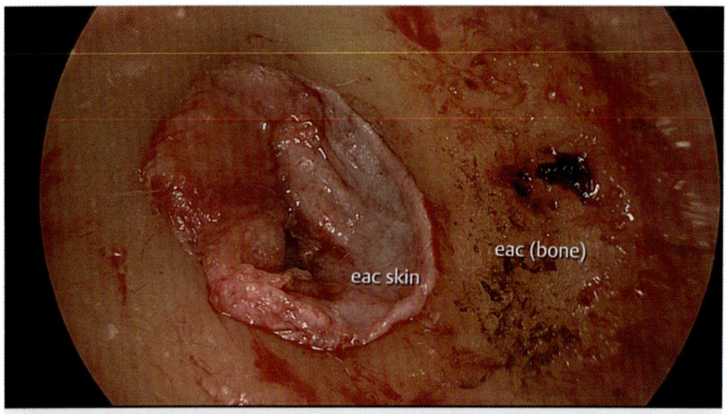

Fig. 11.114 Right side: The skin of the canal is elevated over the tympanic membrane. The dissection and the removal of the tympanic membrane is carried out en bloc with the skin of the canal. *eac (bone): bone of external auditory canal; eac skin: skin of external auditory canal.*

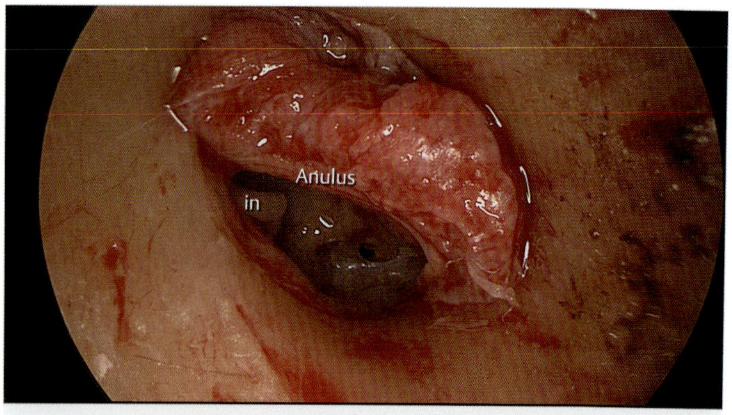

Fig. 11.115 Right side: The annulus is reached and detached from the bony annulus. Afterwards it is lifted forward with the tympanic membrane and the skin. *in: incus.*

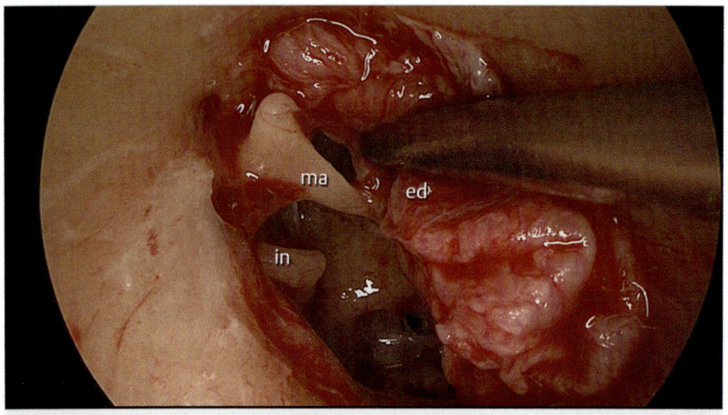

Fig. 11.116 Right side: The tympanic membrane is detached from the handle of the malleus and the fibrous layer of the umbus is dissected. *ed: eardrum; in: incus; ma: malleus.*

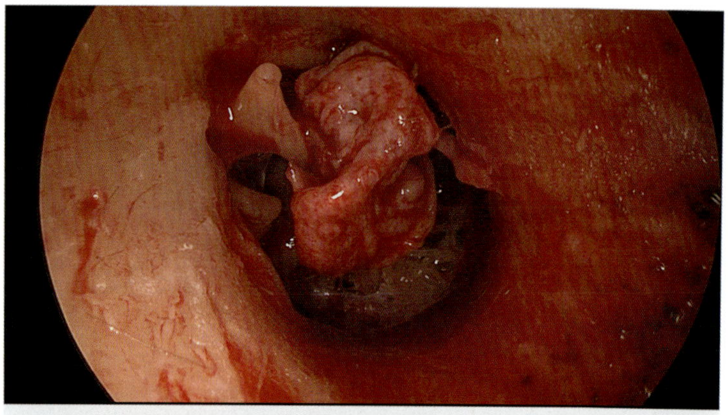

Fig. 11.117 Right side: The skin of the external auditory canal (EAC) and the tympanic membrane are removed en bloc.

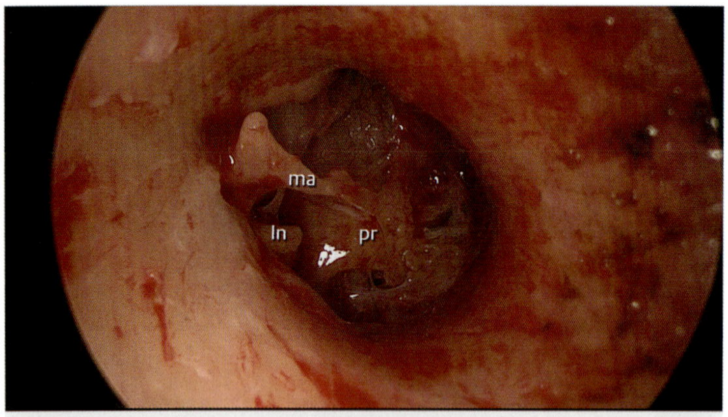

Fig. 11.118 Right side: Endoscopic view of the tympanic cavity after the removal of the tympanic membrane and skin of the canal. *in: incus; ma: malleus; pr: promontory.*

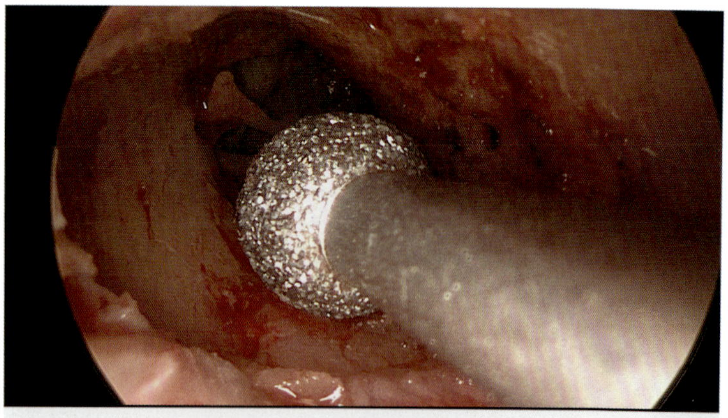

Fig. 11.119 Right side: A diamond bur (3 or 4 mm of diameter) is used to circumferentially drill the external auditory canal (EAC).

scan to rule out hemorrhagic complications is performed on the day of the surgery after 6 hours. Then the patient is sent to the ward. Subjective medications for pain or dizziness are administered on demand. No postoperative antibiotic treatment is required. The follow-up consists mainly of an MRI scan with gadolinium 1 year after the operation. Perioperative and postoperative complications do not differ from those previously listed for the exclusive endoscopic technique and also mirror the ones of the transtemporal techniques.

- Damage to the vascular structures (jugular vein and carotid artery)
- Intraoperative hemorrhage from the AICA vessel or from the venous plexuses of Dandy
- Postoperative hemorrhage and APC hematoma represent the most fearsome complications that must be promptly treated through revision surgery

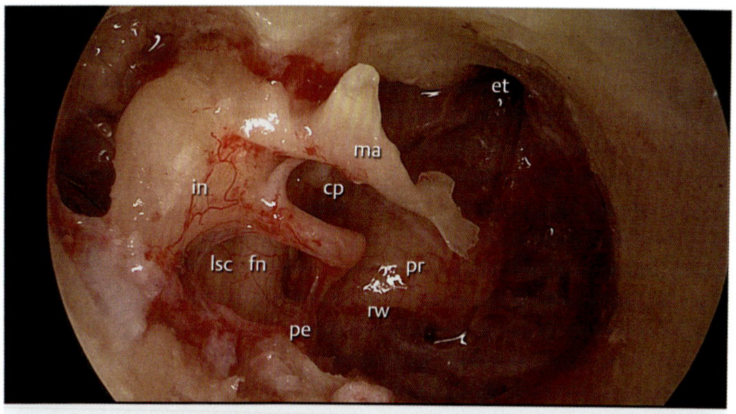

Fig. 11.120 Right side: The scutum is removed and drilling of the bony canal is performed till the hypotympanic and protympanic areas are completely exposed. Drilling of the posterior portion of bony anulus has to be performed carefully, until the mastoid portion of the facial nerve (FN) is identified, without uncovering it. *et: eustachian tube; fn: tympanic portion of the facial nerve; in: incus; lsc: lateral semicircular canal; ma: malleus; pr: promontory; rw: round window.*

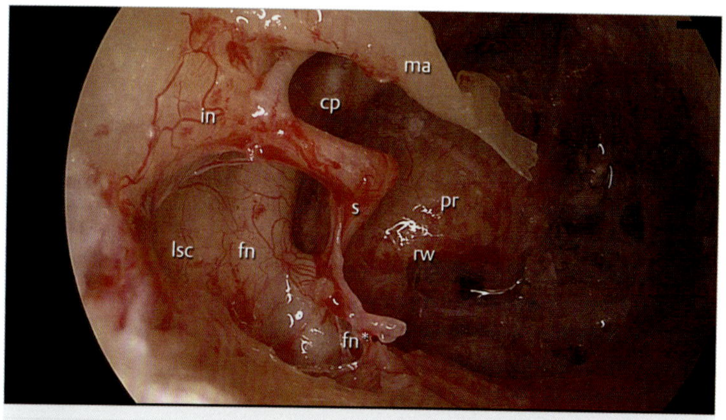

Fig. 11.121 Right side: The facial nerve (FN) and the pyramidal eminence are clearly visible. The pyramidal eminence represents a landmark to identify the depth and the direction of the mastoid portion of the FN. *cp: cochleariform process; fn: tympanic portion of the facial nerve; fn*: mastoid portion of the facial nerve; in: incus; lsc: lateral semicircular canal; ma: malleus; pr: promontory; rw: round window.*

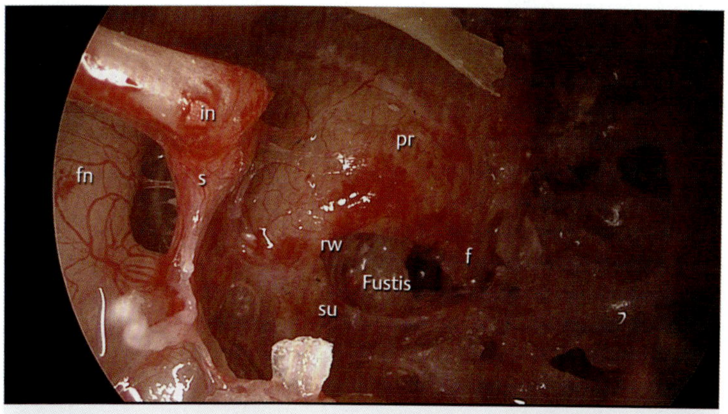

Fig. 11.122 Right side: The retrotympanic and promontorial regions are widely exposed. *f: finiculus; fn: tympanic portion of the facial nerve; in: incus; pr: promontory; rw: round window; s: stapes; su: subiculum.*

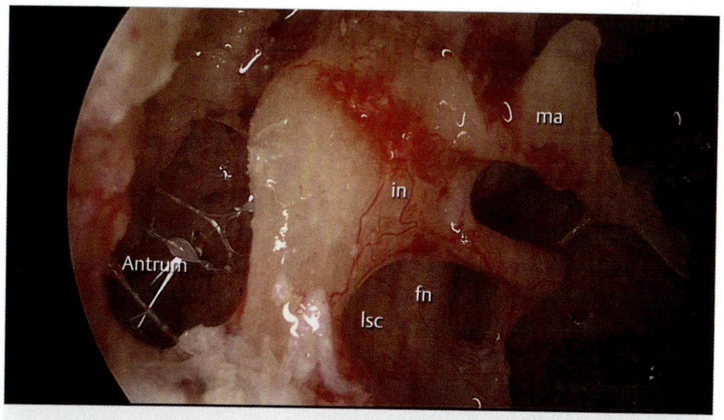

Fig. 11.123 Right side: The epitympanic space and the antrum are well exposed. *fn: tympanic portion of the facial nerve; in: incus; lsc: lateral semicircular canal; ma: malleus.*

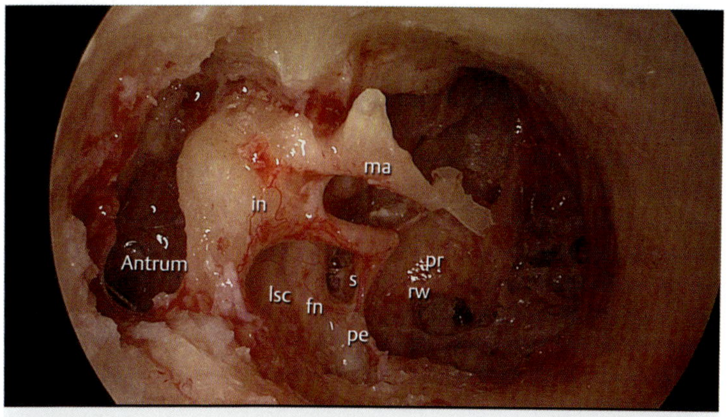

Fig. 11.124 Right side: The ossicular chain is shown. The hypotympanum, the protympanum, and retrotympanum are exposed and the antrum is opened into the external auditory canal (EAC). *fn: tympanic portion of the facial nerve; in: incus; ma: malleus; lsc: lateral semicircular canal; pe: pyramidal eminence; pr: promontory; rw: round window; s: stapes.*

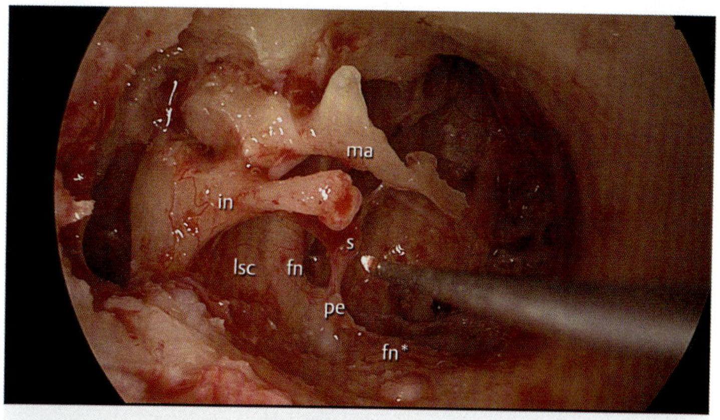

Fig. 11.125 Right side: The incus is removed. *fn: tympanic portion of the facial nerve; fn*: mastoid portion of the facial nerve; in: incus; lsc: lateral semicircular canal; ma: malleus; pe: pyramidal eminence; s: stapes.*

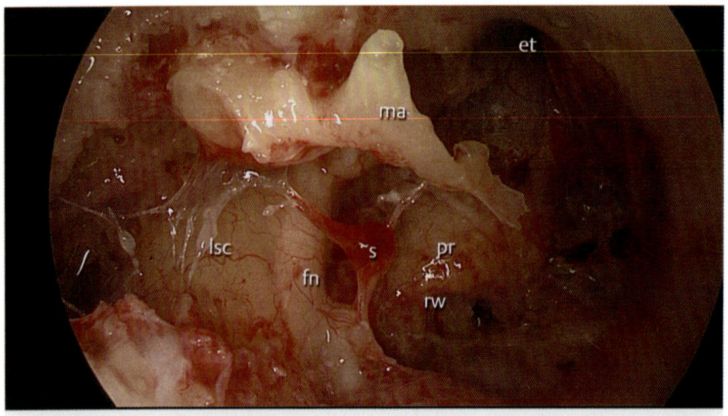

Fig. 11.126 Right side: After the incus removal, the tympanic portion of the facial nerve (FN) is exposed. *et: eustachian tube; fn: tympanic portion of the facial nerve; lsc: lateral semicircular canal; ma: malleus; pr: promontory; rw: round window; s: stapes.*

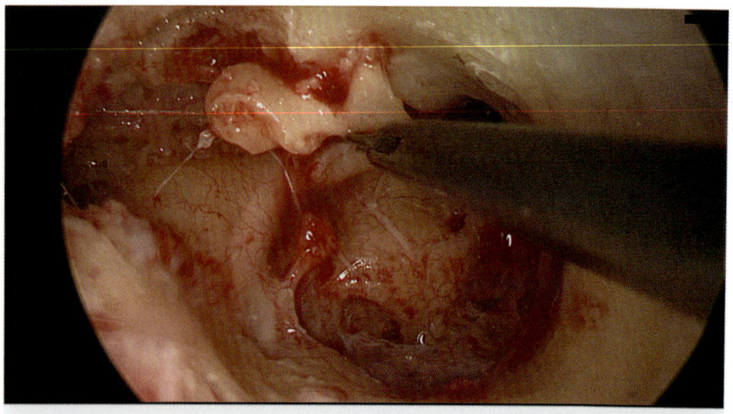

Fig. 11.127 Right side: The tensor tympani tendon is cut and the malleus is removed.

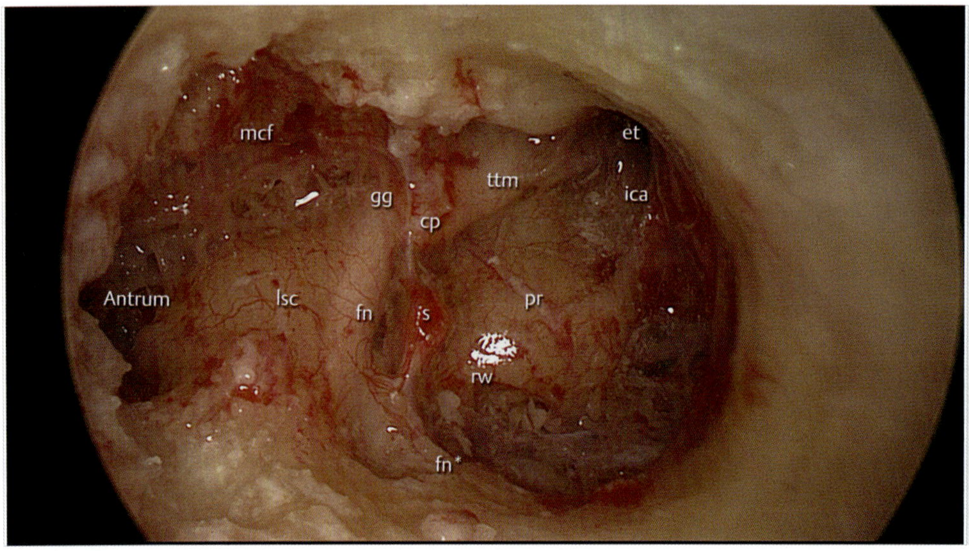

Fig. 11.128 Right side: The medial wall of tympanic cavity and the antrum with the lateral semicircular canal (LSC) posteriorly are shown. The tympanic portion of the facial nerve (FN) is visible from the geniculate ganglion to the second genu. The mastoid portion of the FN is identified but not exposed. *cp: cochleariform process; et: eustachian tube; fn: tympanic portion of the facial nerve; fn*: mastoid portion of the facial nerve; gg: geniculate ganglion; ica: internal carotid artery; lsc: lateral semicircular canal; mcf: middle cranial fossa; pr: promontory; rw: round window; s: stapes; ttm: tensor tympani muscle semicanal.*

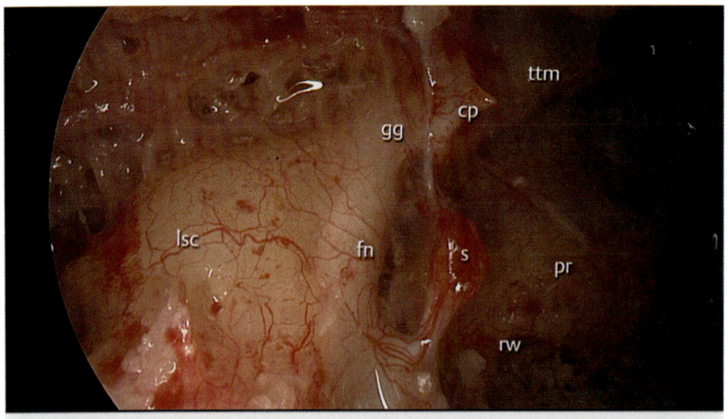

Fig. 11.129 Right side: Notice the anatomical relationship between the lateral semicircular canal (LSC) and the tympanic tract of the facial nerve (FN). *cp: cochleariform process; fn: tympanic portion of the facial nerve; gg: geniculate ganglion; lsc: lateral semicircular canal; pr: promontory; rw: round window; s: stapes; ttm: tensor tympani muscle semicanal.*

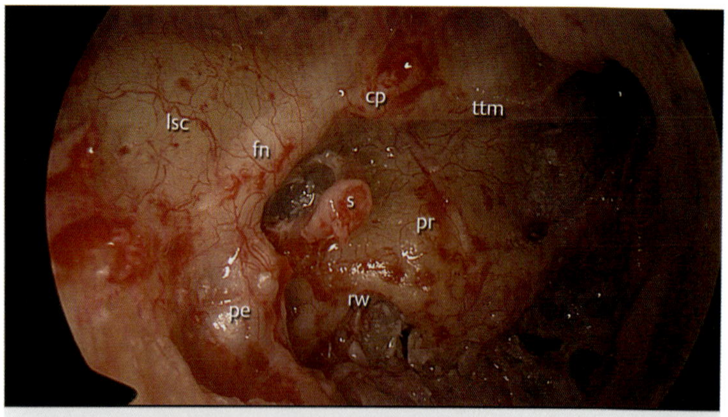

Fig. 11.130 Right side: The stapedial tendon is dissected. *cp: cochleariform process; fn: tympanic portion of the facial nerve; lsc: lateral semicircular canal; pe: pyramidal eminence; pr: promontory; rw: round window; s: stapes; ttm: tensor tympani muscle semicanal.*

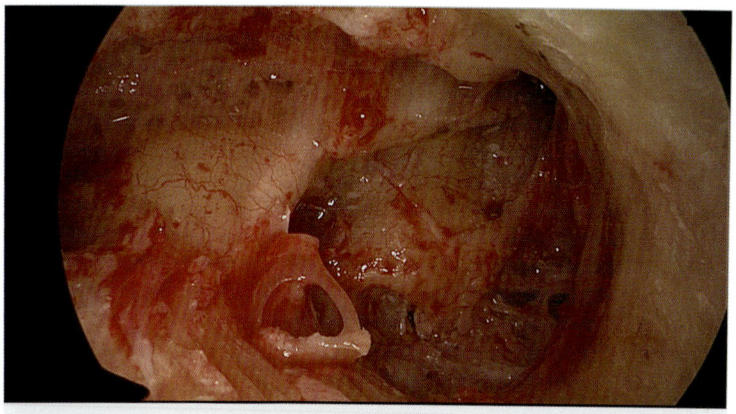

Fig. 11.131 Right side: The stapes is removed to gain access to the vestibule.

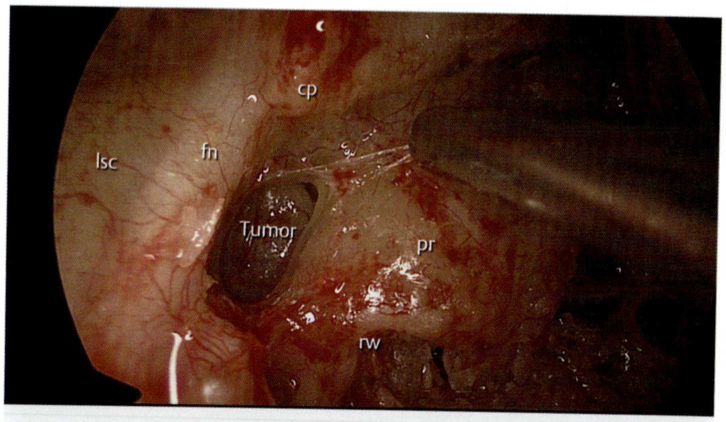

Fig. 11.132 Right side: The tumor is visible inside the vestibule. *cp: cochleariform process; fn: tympanic portion of the facial nerve; lsc: lateral semicircular canal; pr: promontory; rw: round window.*

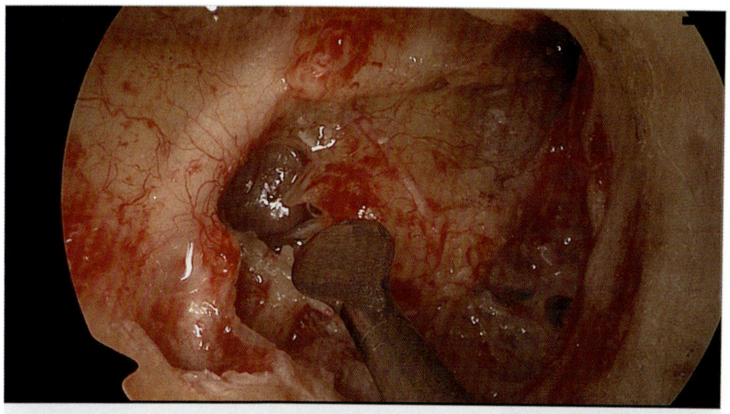

Fig. 11.133 Right side: A piezoelectric bur is used to enlarge the access to the vestibule and open the basal turn of the cochlea.

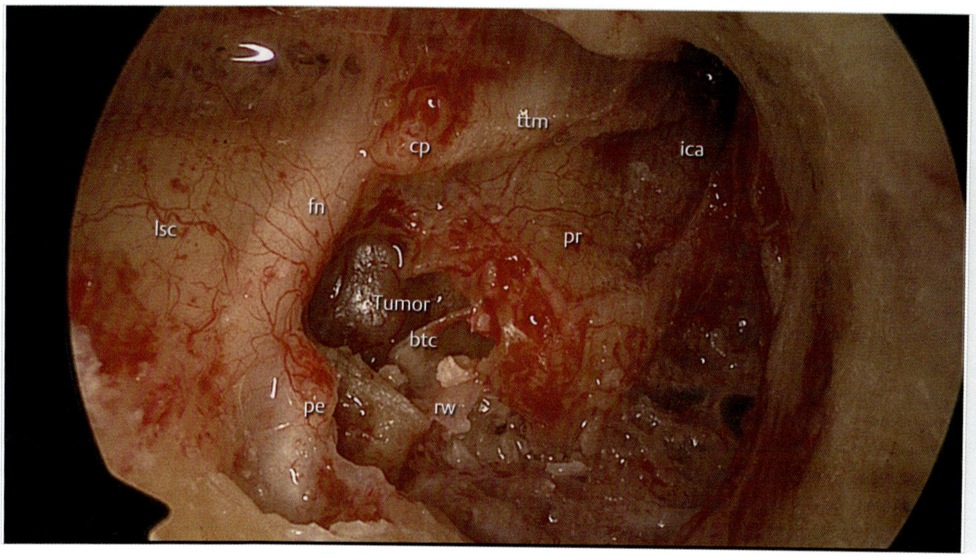

Fig. 11.134 Right side: Endoscopic view of the surgical cavity after vestibule and basal turn opening. *btc: basal turn of the cochlea; cp: cochleariform process; fn: tympanic portion of the facial nerve; ica: internal carotid artery; lsc: lateral semicircular canal; pe: pyramidal eminence; pr: promontory; rw: round window; ttm: tensor tympani muscle semicanal.*

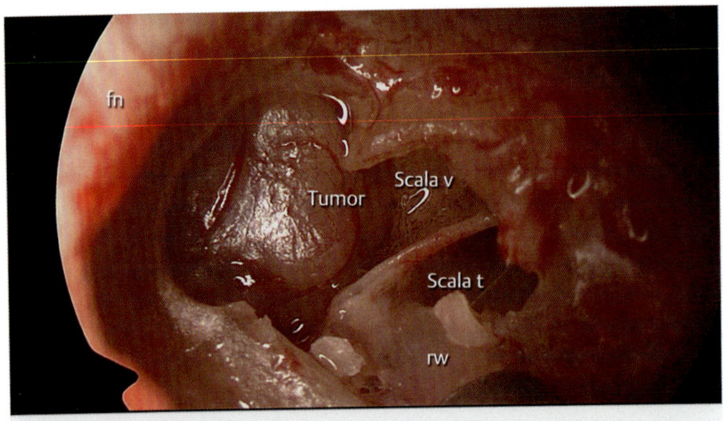

Fig. 11.135 Right side: The tympanic scala and the vestibular scala are exposed. The inferior portion of the schwannoma is located in the vestibular scala extending superiorly into the vestibule and medially to the tympanic segment of the facial nerve (FN). *fn: tympanic portion of the facial nerve; rw: round window; scala t: scala tymani; scala v: scala vestibuli.*

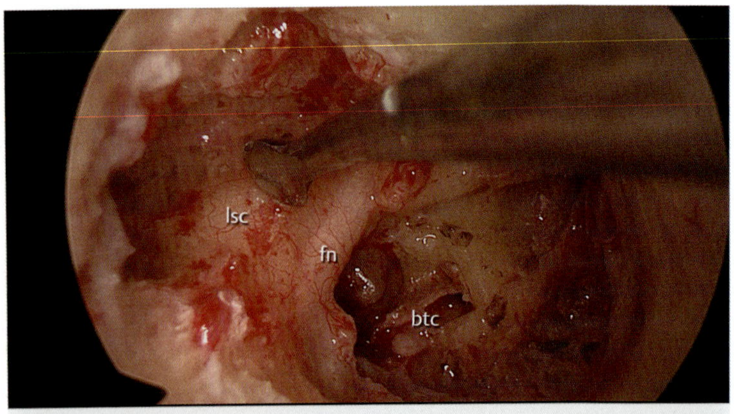

Fig. 11.136 Right side: The lateral semicircular canal (LSC) is opened using a piezoelectric bur. The facial nerve (FN) is kept under endoscopic view allowing for an easy control and preservation of the nerve. *btc: basal turn of the cochlea; fn: tympanic portion of the facial nerve; lsc: lateral semicircular canal.*

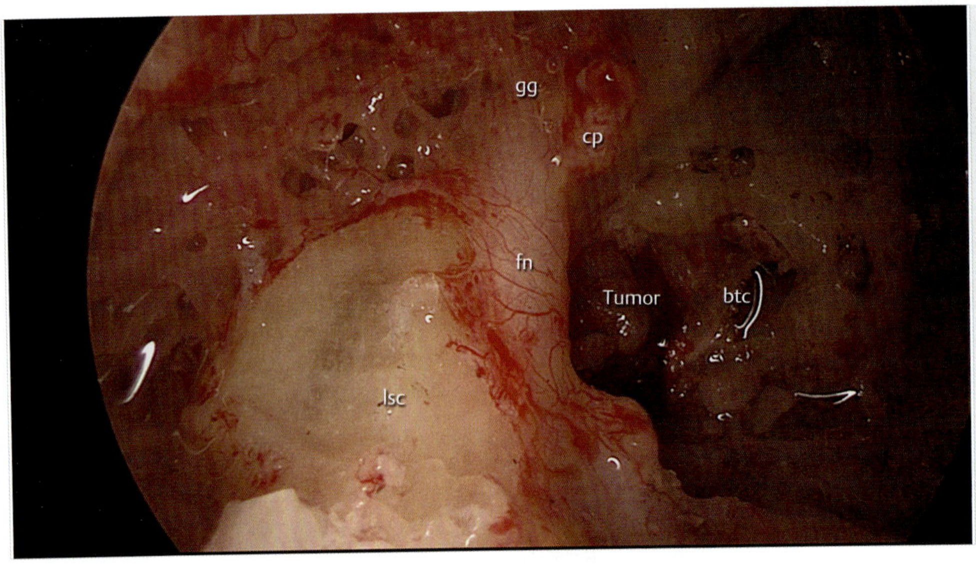

Fig. 11.137 Right side: Notice the blue line of the lateral semicircular canal (LSC). The access through the LSC is indicated in this case to control the upper portion of the tumor, keeping the facial nerve (FN) in its bony canal. *btc: basal turn of the cochlea; cp: cochleariform process; fn: tympanic portion of the facial nerve; gg: geniculate ganglion; lsc: lateral semicircular canal.*

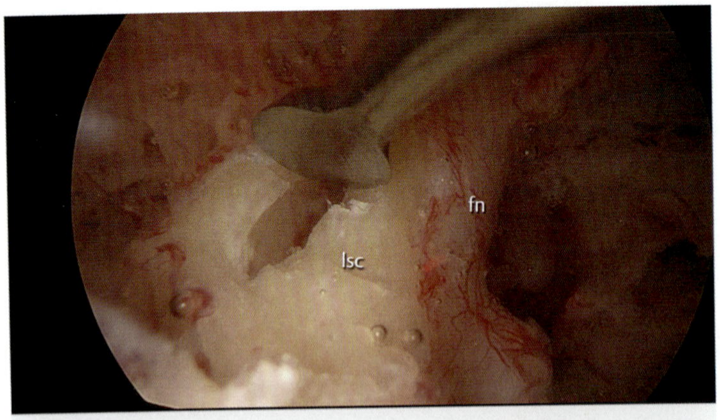

Fig. 11.138 Right side: While drilling the lateral semicircular canal (LSC), it is important to work continuously under water to avoid a thermal damage to the facial nerve (FN), which is very close to the working area. The LSC is drilled behind the tympanic tract of the FN. *fn: tympanic portion of the facial nerve; lsc: lateral semicircular canal.*

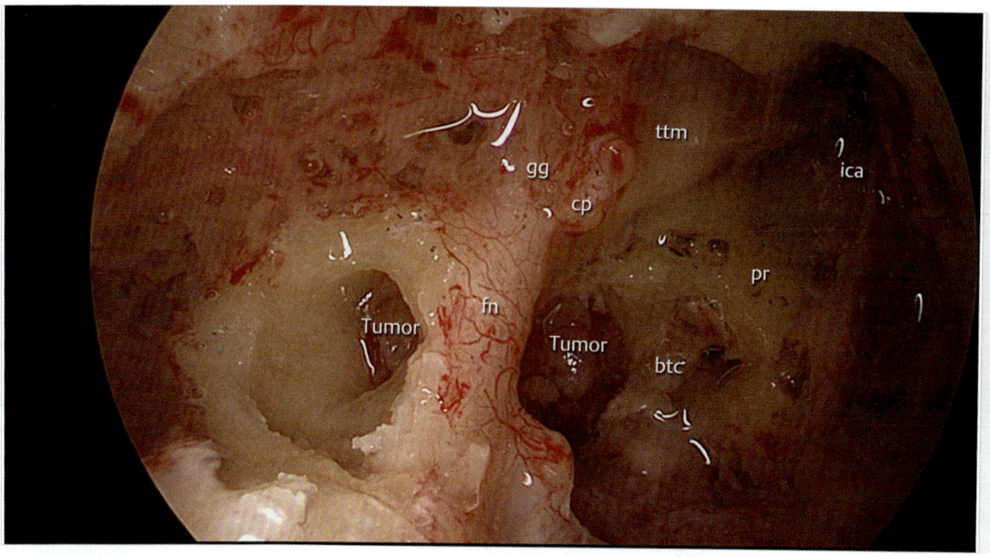

Fig. 11.139 Right side: The upper portion of the vestibule is now visible and it is possible to have a good surgical control of the superior extension of the tumor. *btc: basal turn of the cochlea; cp: cochleariform process; fn: tympanic portion of the facial nerve; gg: geniculate ganglion; ica: internal carotid artery; pr: promontory; ttm: tensor tympani muscle semicanal.*

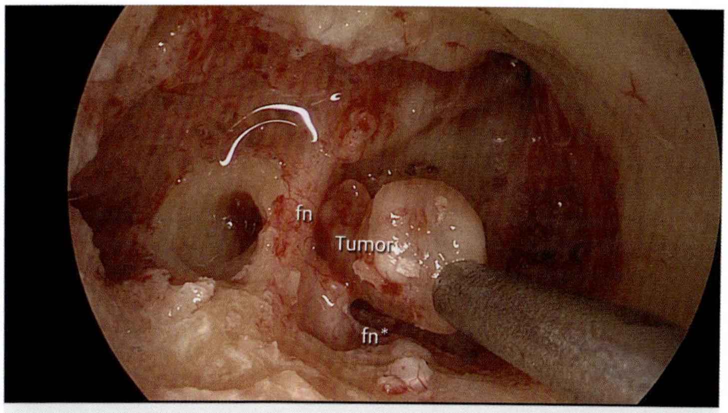

Fig. 11.140 Right side: The tumor is gently detached from the surfaces of the vestibule and removed en bloc using a small suction tube. *fn: tympanic portion of the facial nerve; fn*: mastoid portion of the facial nerve.*

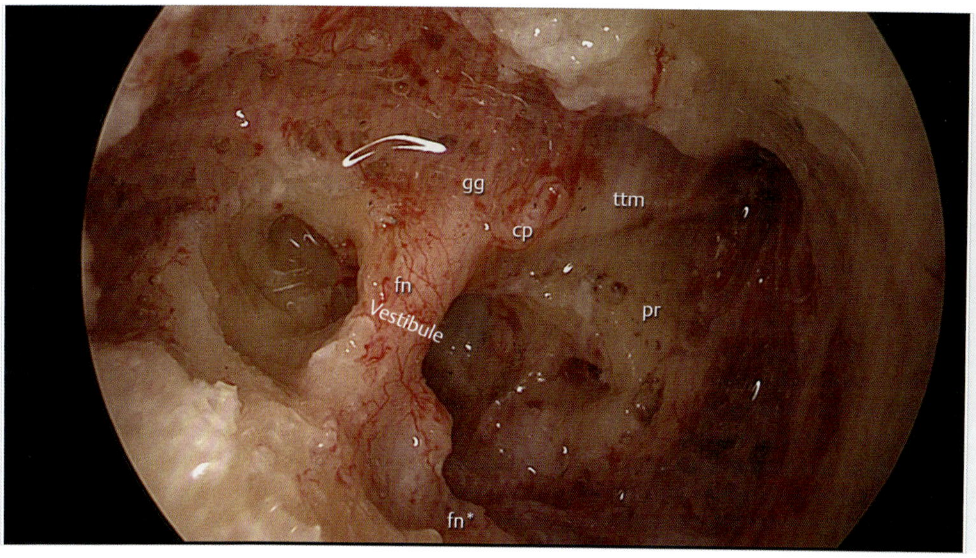

Fig. 11.141 Right side: The vestibule is clear, without evidence of tumor remains. *cp: cochleariform process; fn: tympanic portion of the facial nerve; fn*: mastoid portion of the facial nerve; gg: geniculate ganglion; pr: promontory; ttm: tensor tympani muscle semicanal.*

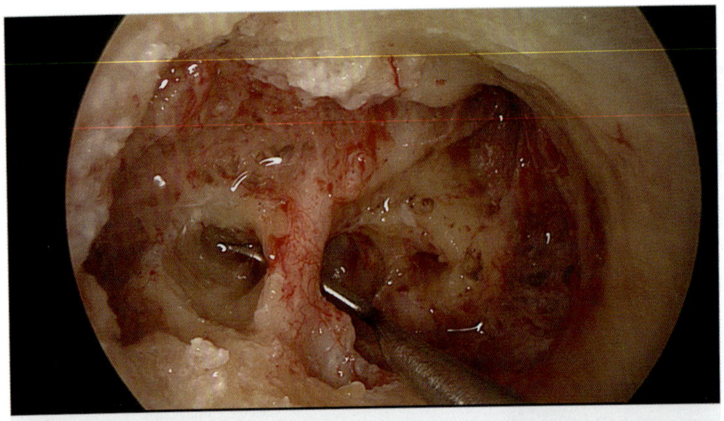

Fig. 11.142 Right side: A curved dissector is introduced into the vestibule underneath the fallopian canal.

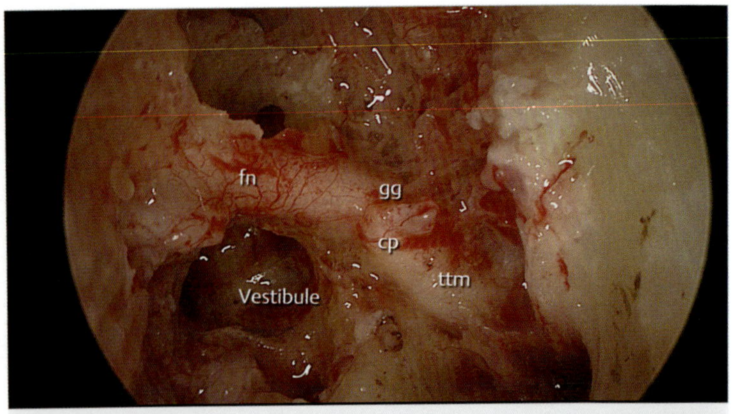

Fig. 11.143 Right side: Endoscopic view with 45-degrees endoscope of 4 mm diameter and 15 cm length. An angled endoscope is used to check the vestibular region under the fallopian canal to detect any residual disease. *cp: cochleariform process; fn: tympanic portion of the facial nerve; gg: geniculate ganglion; ttm: tensor tympani muscle semicanal.*

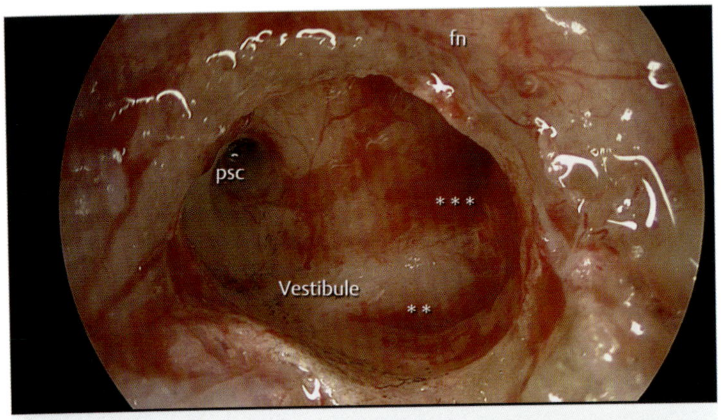

Fig. 11.144 Right side: The vestibule under the fallopian canal is magnified. *fn: tympanic portion of the facial nerve; psc: ampulla of posterior semicircular canal; **: spherical recess; ***: elliptical recess.*

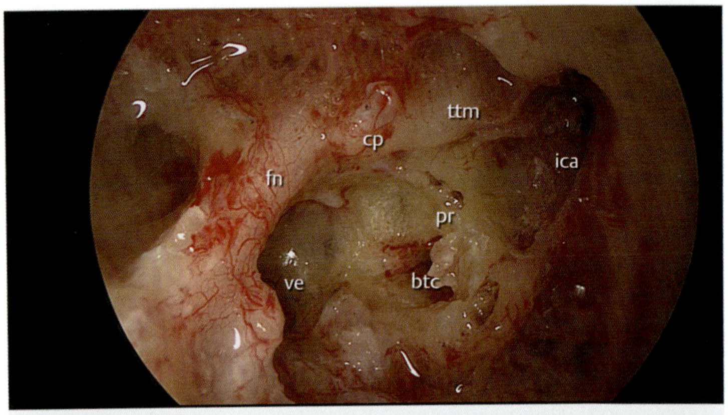

Fig. 11.145 Right side: Further drilling anteriorly and inferiorly to the spherical recess allows to identify the fundus of the internal auditory canal (IAC). *btc: basal turn of the cochlea; cp: cochleariform process; fn: tympanic portion of the facial nerve; ica: internal carotid artery; pr: promontory; ttm: tensor tympani muscle semicanal; ve: vestibule.*

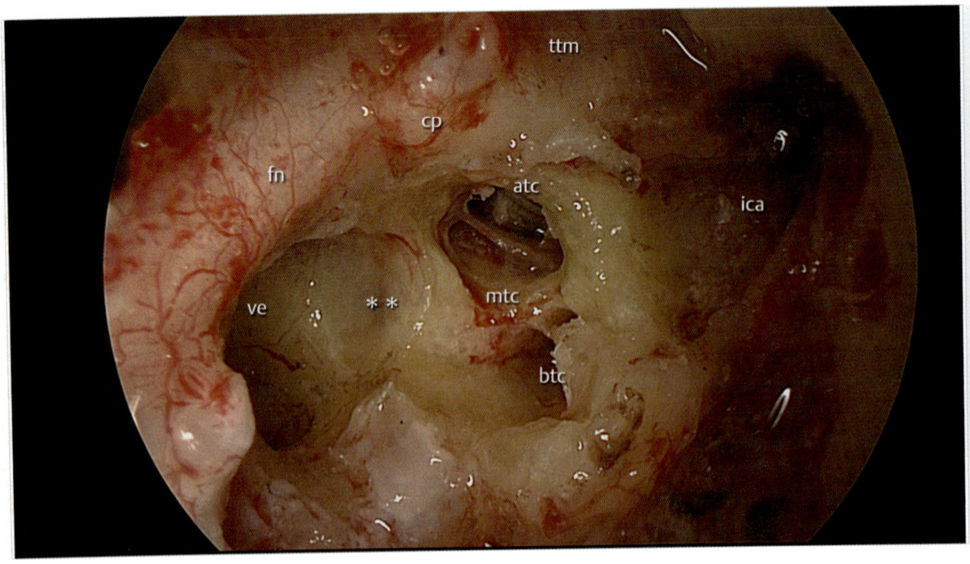

Fig. 11.146 Right side: The medial and apical turns of the cochlea are exposed. *atc: apical turn of the cochlea; btc: basal turn of the cochlea; cp: cochleariform process; fn: tympanic portion of the facial nerve; ica: internal carotid artery; mtc: middle turn of the cochlea; ttm: tensor tympani muscle semicanal; ve: vestibule; **: spherical recess.*

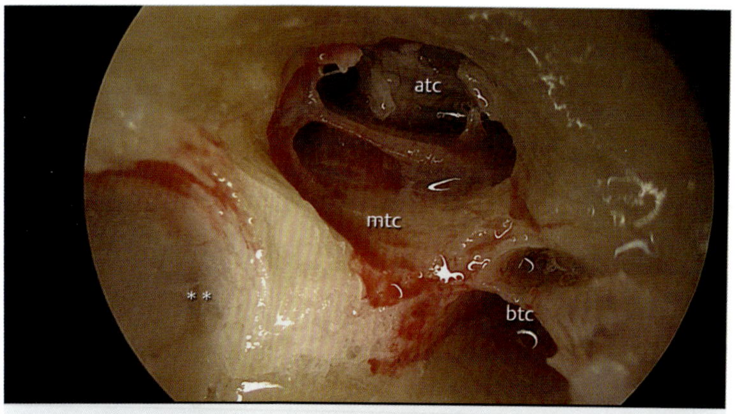

Fig. 11.147 Right side: The basal, middle, and apical turns of the cochlea are exposed. The spherical recess is located in the vestibule, anterosuperiorly, and it represents the landmark for the fundus of internal auditory canal (IAC). *atc: apical turn of the cochlea; btc: basal turn of the cochlea; mtc: medial turn of the cochlea; **: spherical recess.*

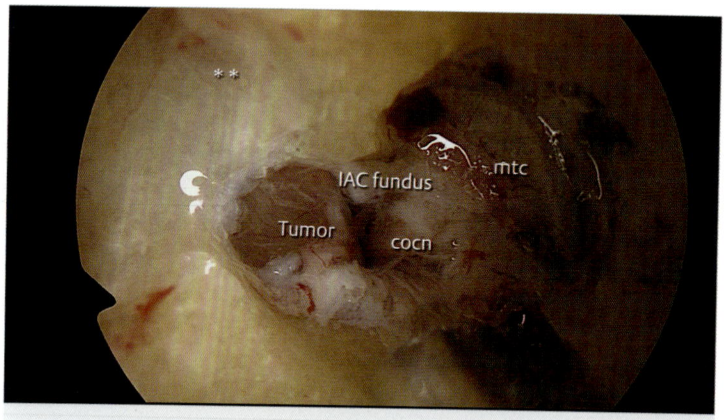

Fig. 11.148 Right side: The fundus of internal auditory canal (IAC) is opened, allowing for the identification of the residual tumor located in this area. The tumor arises from the inferior vestibular nerve, in its attachment to the spherical recess. *cocn: cochlear nerve; iac fundus: fundus of internal auditory canal; mtc: middle turn of the cochlea; **: spherical recess.*

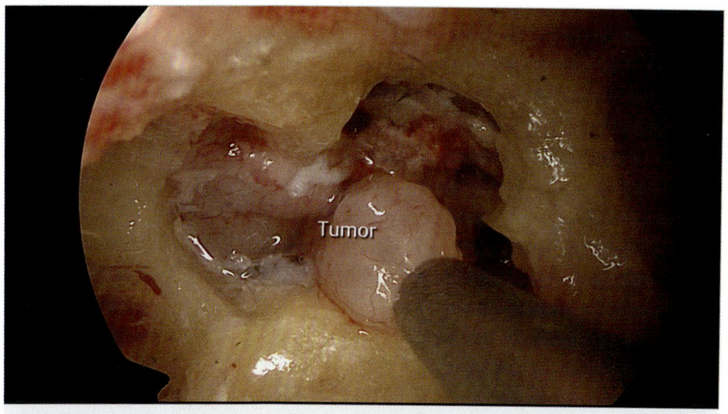

Fig. 11.149 Right side: The tumor is gently removed, preserving the facial nerve (FN).

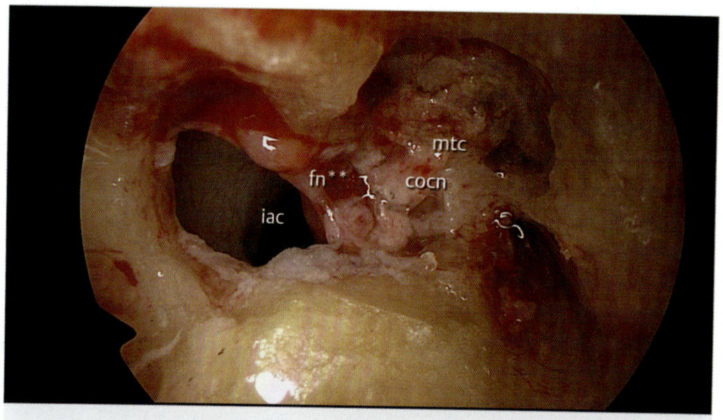

Fig. 11.150 Right side: Last portion of the tumor is removed and the intracanalicular portion of the facial nerve (FN) is exposed till the porus. *cocn: cochlear nerve; fn**: facial nerve into the internal auditory canal; iac: internal auditory canal; mtc: medial turn of the cochlea.*

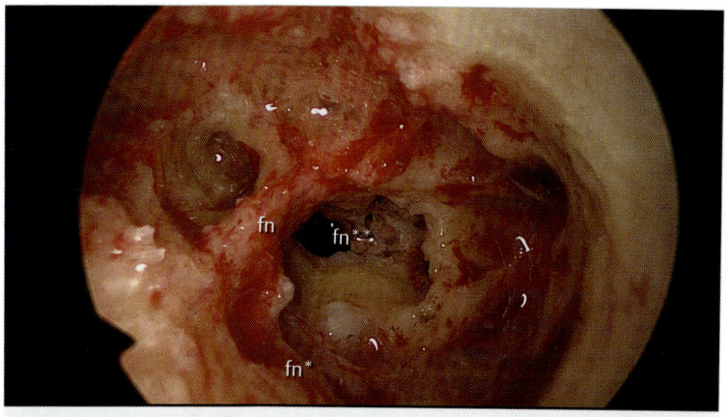

Fig. 11.151 Right side: The promontorial defect is obliterated using abdominal fat. The eustachian tube is obliterated with muscle. A cul-de-sac closure of the skin of the external auditory canal (EAC) is performed. The course of the facial nerve (FN) is shown in the picture. *fn: tympanic portion of the facial nerve; fn*: mastoid portion of the facial nerve; fn**: facial nerve into the internal auditory canal.*

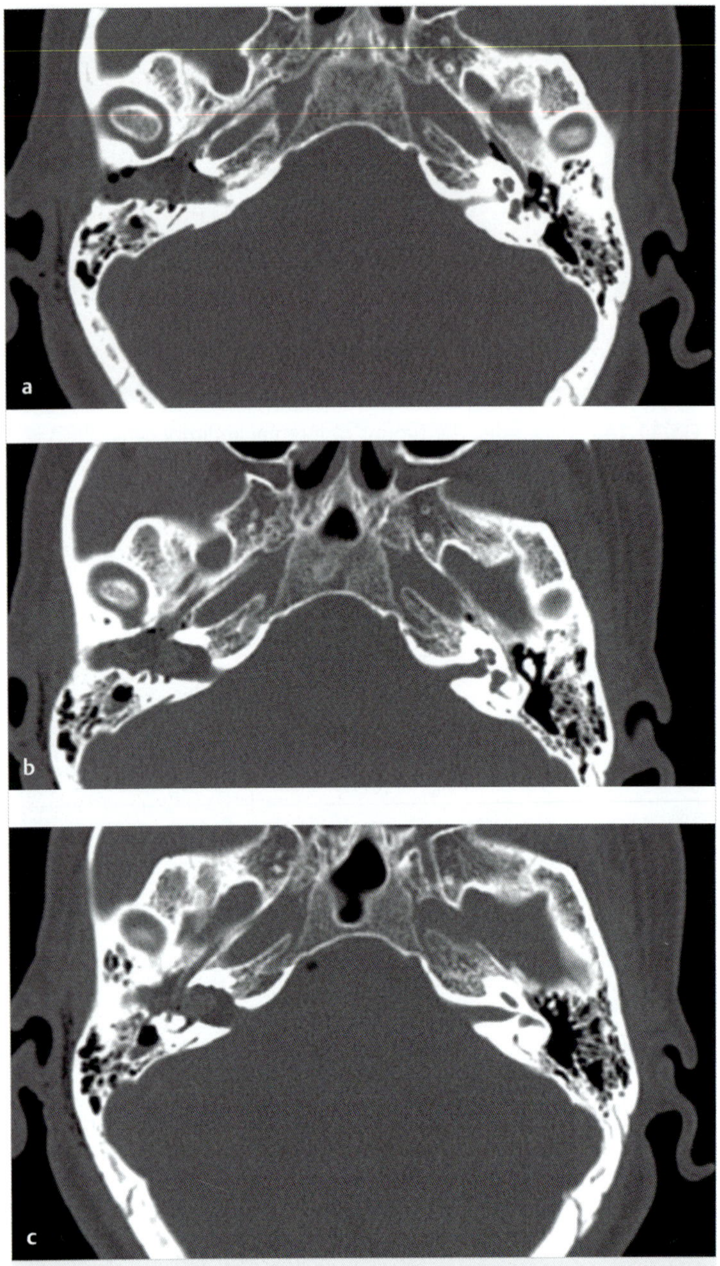

Fig. 11.152 (a–c) Computed tomography (CT) scan of the temporal bone 6 hours after the surgery. We can notice the surgical route from the external auditory canal (EAC) to the internal auditory canal (IAC) which is typical of the transcanal transpromontorial approach.

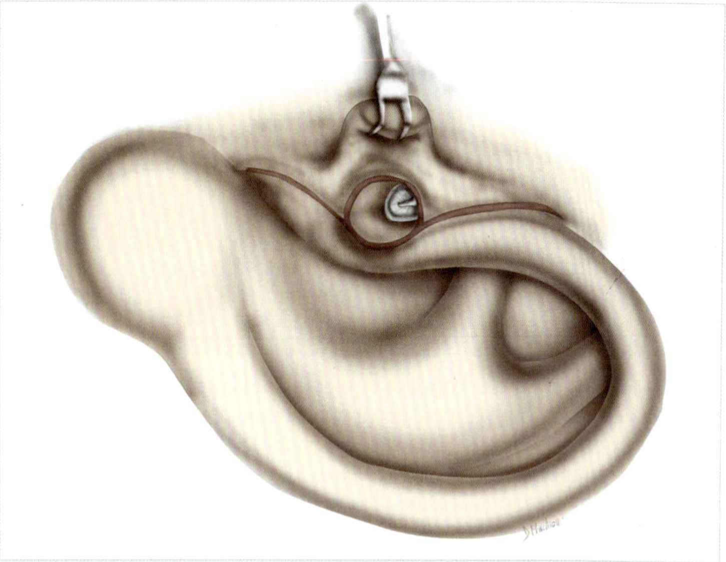

Fig. 11.153 Left side: A circular incision at the osteocartilagineous junction of the external ear canal skin is made, extending superiorly between the tragus and the helix, and inferiorly until the root of the auricular lobule.

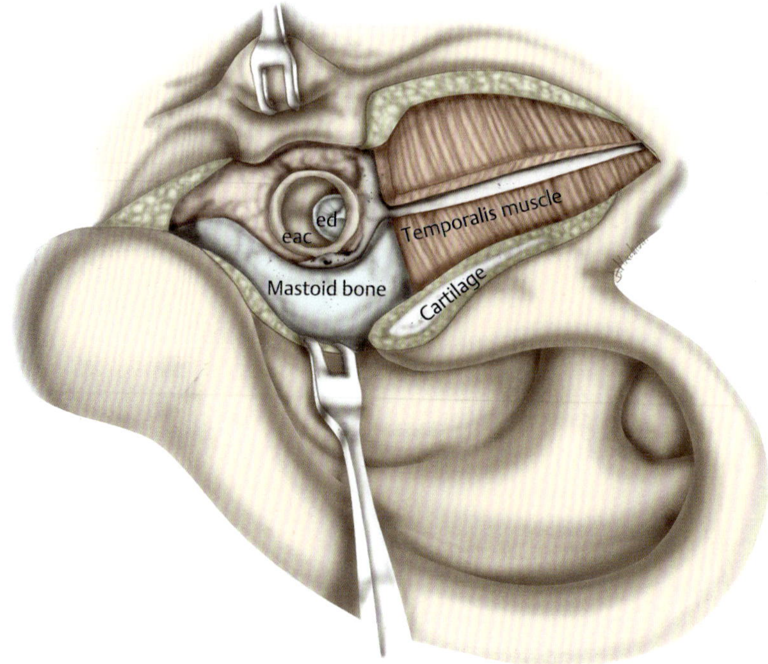

Fig. 11.154 Left side: The two skin flaps are created uncovering the temporal fascia. A deep line of incision is then performed untill the bony plane, dividing the temporalis muscle just above the external auditory canal (EAC), continuing below the fibroperiosteal layer over the mastoid bone, to circumnavigate the posterior margin of the EAC. *Eac: external auditory canal; ed: eardrum.*

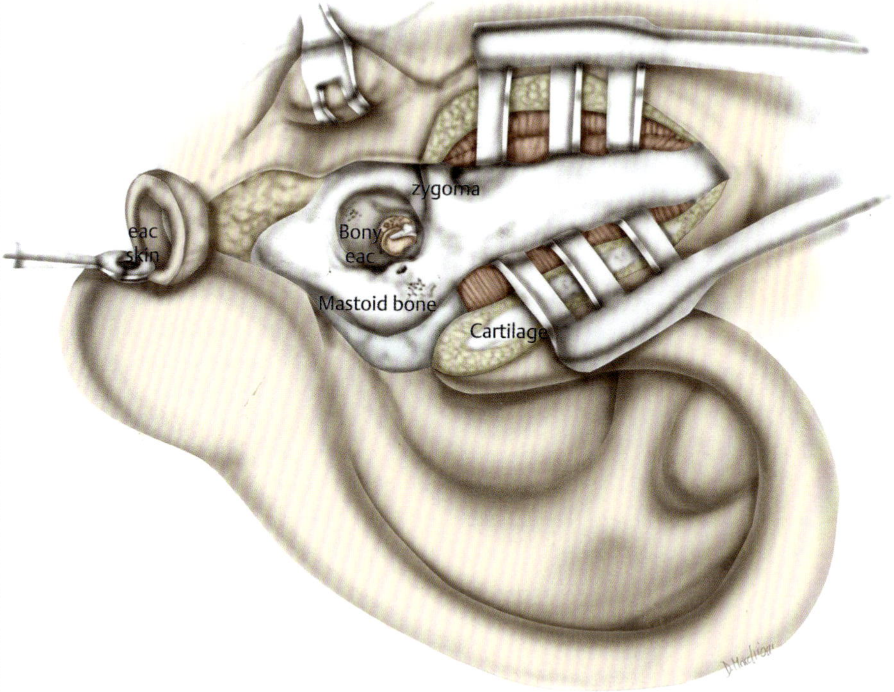

Fig. 11.155 Left side: A retractor is placed over the fibroperiosteal and temporalis muscle flaps, exposing the mastoid bone wall. The external auditory canal (EAC) skin toghether with the eardrum are removed exposing the bony wall of the EAC.

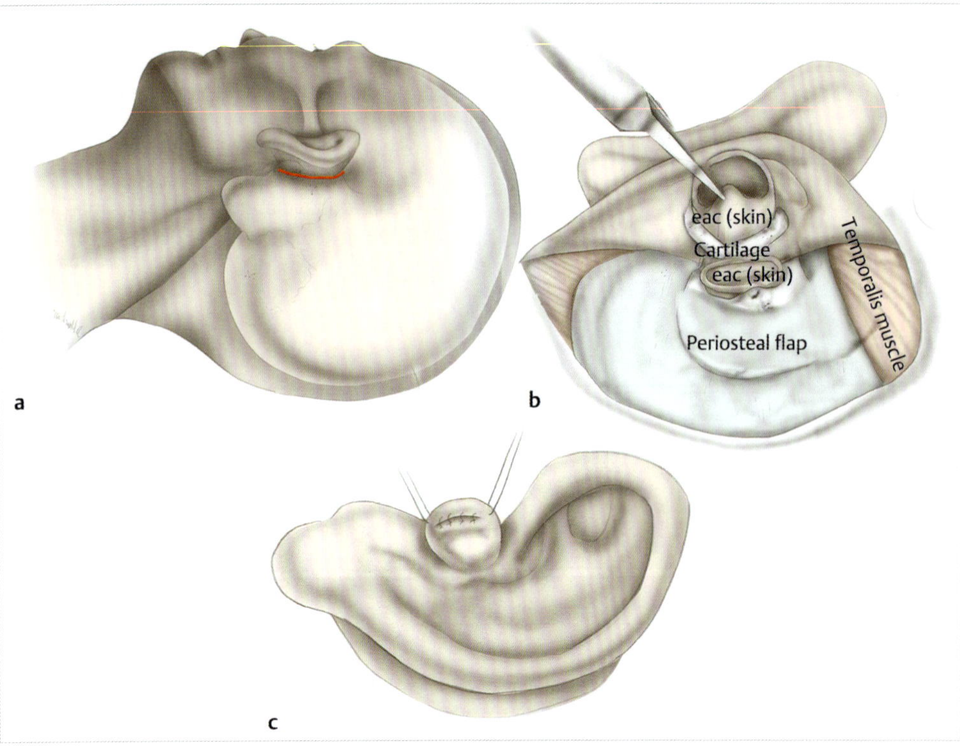

Fig. 11.156 Left side: The incision is performed in the retroauricular sulcus **(a)**. A periosteal muscle flap with a superior based pedicle is performed to uncover the mastoid bone. The skin of the outer portion of the external auditory canal (EAC) is detached from the cartilaginous component and everted to prepare for the blind sac closure **(b)**. An eversion of the EAC skin with a blind sac closure is performed. *eac: external auditory canal.*

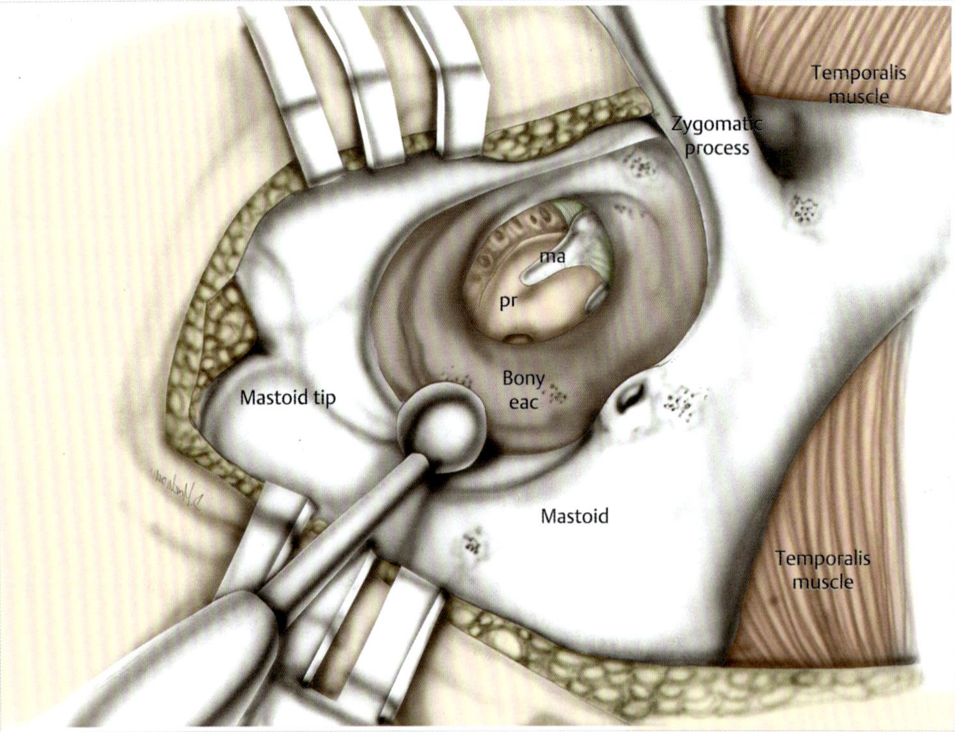

Fig. 11.157 Left side: A calibrage of the bony external auditory canal (EAC) is performed, using a large diamond bar. *ma: malleus; pr: promontory.*

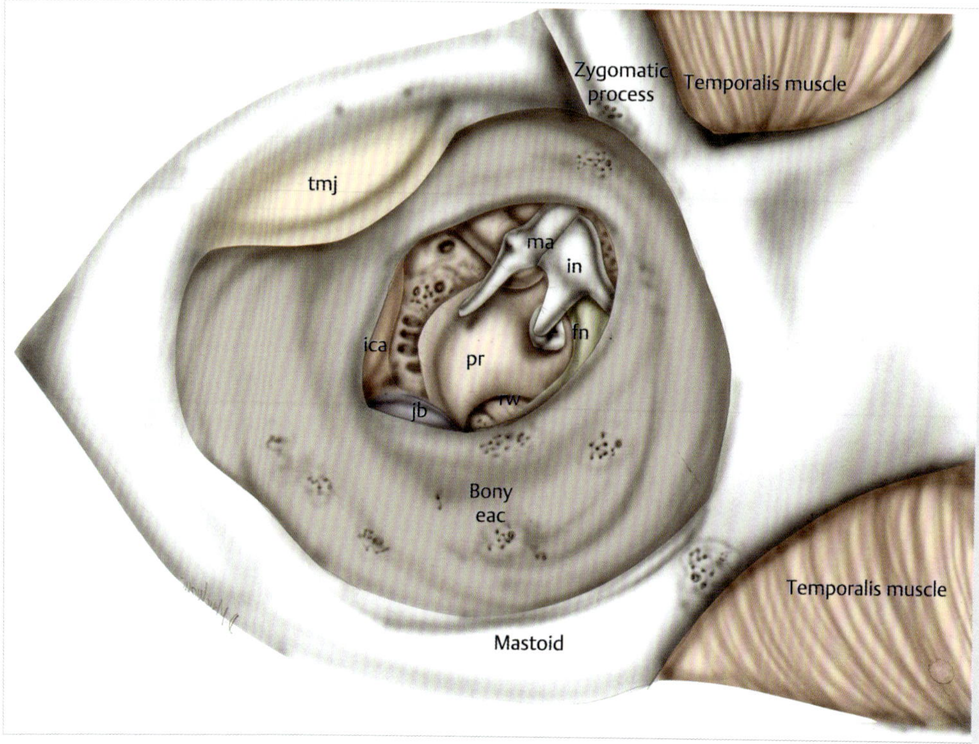

Fig. 11.158 Left side: Microscopic view after external auditory canal (EAC) calibration. The temporomandibular joint is detected in the anterior portion of the EAC. The ossicular chain is visible in the epitympanum; the protympanum, the retrotympanum, and the hypotympanum are progressively exposed, and the major vascular structues lying in the tympanic cavity are noted. *fn: facial nerve; ica: internal carotid artery; in: incus; jb: jugular bulb; ma: malleus; pr: promontory; rw: round window; Tmj: temporomandibular joint.*

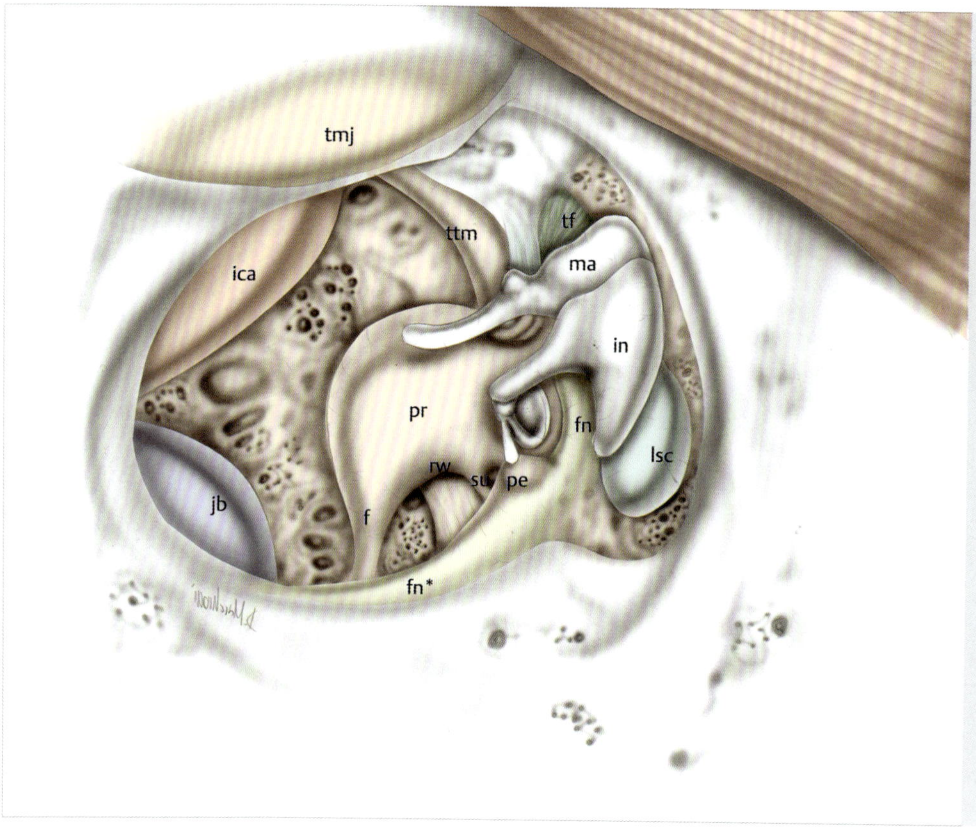

Fig. 11.159 Left side: The tympanic cavity is exposed; the temporomandibular joint represents the anterior limit of the dissection; the supero-posterior limit is the tympanic antrum; the posterior limit is represented by the mastoid tract of the facial nerve (FN). *f: finiculus; fn: facial nerve; fn*: mastoid segment of facial nerve; ica: internal carotid artery; in: incus; jb: jugular bulb; lsc: lateral semicircular canal; ma: malleus; pe: pyramidal eminence; pr: promontory; rw: round window; su: subiculum; tf: tensor fold; Tmj: temporomandibular joint; ttm: tensor tendon muscle.*

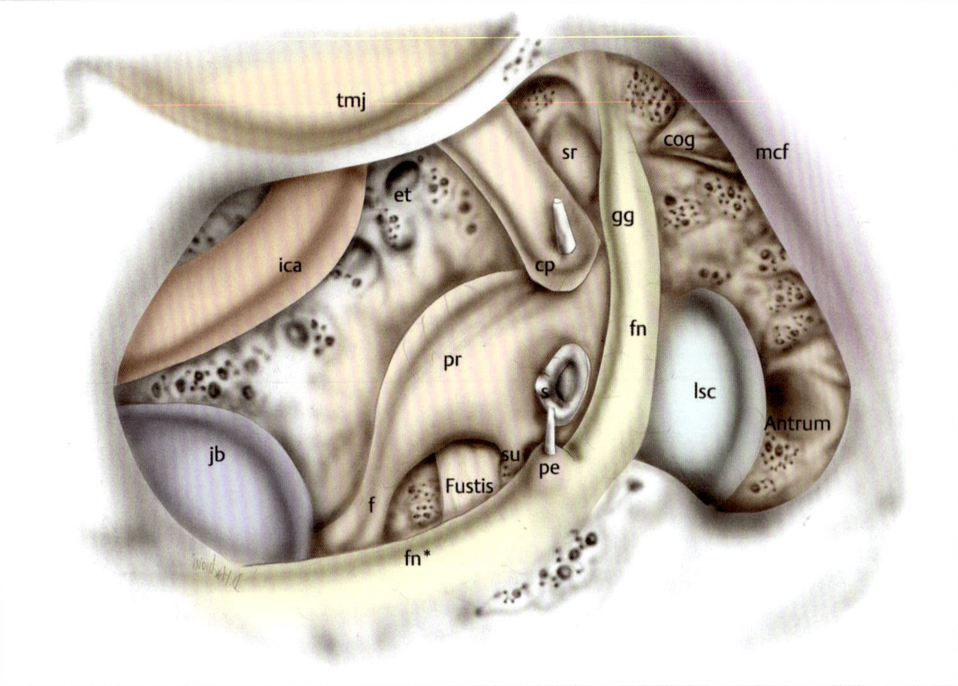

Fig. 11.160 Left side: The ossicular chain has been removed allowing for the detection of the facial nerve (FN) inside the tympanic cavity from the geniculate ganglion to the mastoid portion. *et: eustachian tube; f: finiculus; fn: facial nerve; fn* mastoid segment of facial nerve; gg: geniculate ganglion; ica: internal carotid artery; jb: jugular bulb; lsc: lateral semicircular canal; mcf: middle cranial fossa; pe: pyramidal eminence; pr: promontory; s: stapes; sr: supratubal recess; su: subiculum; Tmj: temporomandibular joint.*

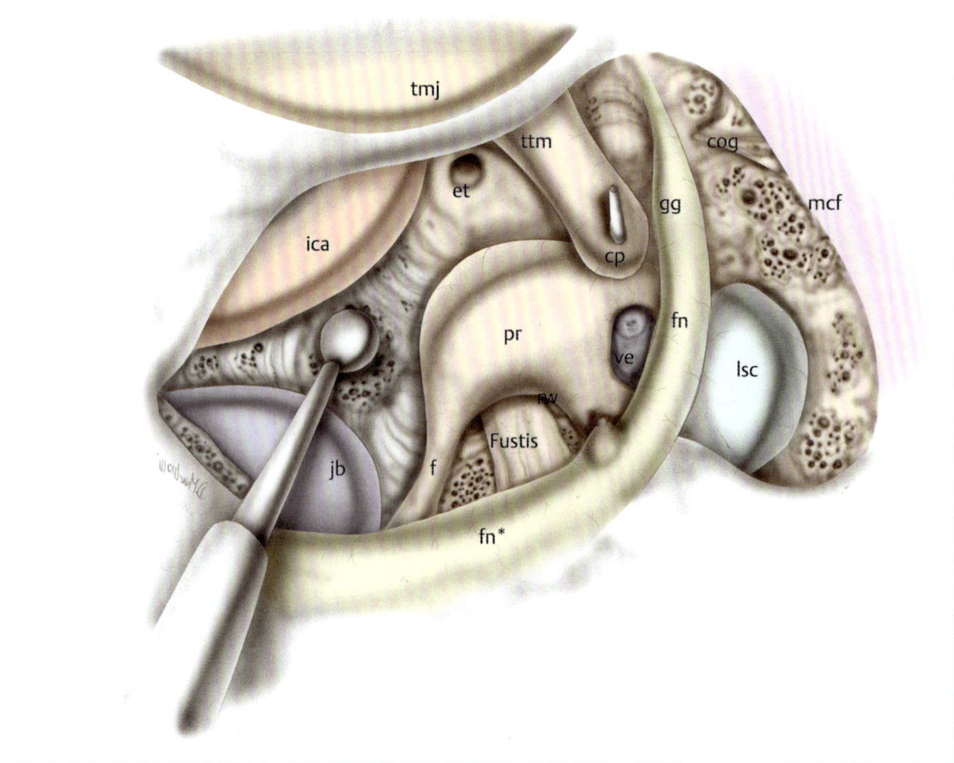

Fig. 11.161 Left side: After stapes removal, a diamond bur is used to detect the internal carotid artery and the jugular bulb. *et: eustachian tube; f: finiculus; fn: facial nerve; fn* mastoid segment of facial nerve; gg: geniculate ganglion; ica: internal carotid artery; jb: jugular bulb; lsc: lateral semicircular canal; mcf: middle cranial fossa; pr: promontory; rw: round window; Tmj: temporomandibular joint; ttm: tensor tendon muscle canal.*

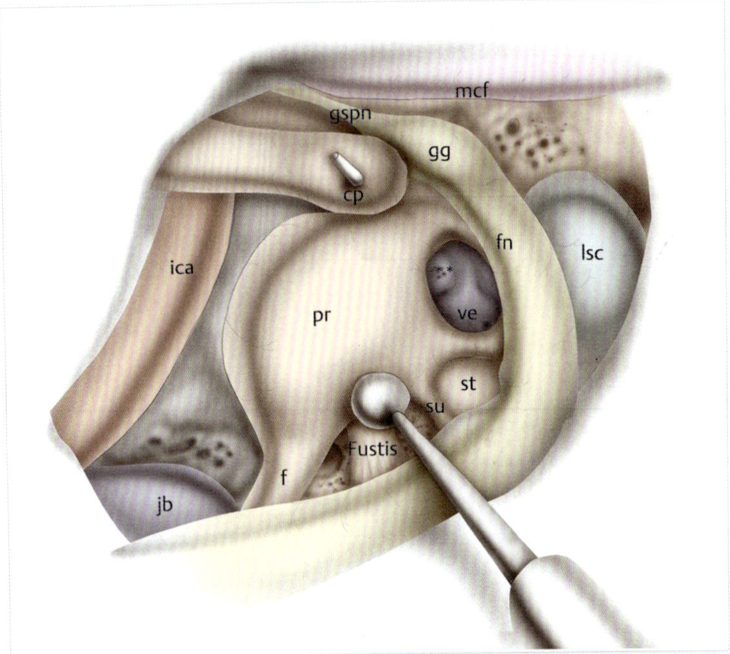

Fig. 11.162 Left side: The round window tegmen is removed using a diamond bur, exposing the round window membrane, entering the basal turn of the cochlea. *f: finiculus; fn: facial nerve; gg: geniculate ganglion; gspn: greater superficial petrosal nerve; ica: internal carotid artery; jb: jugular bulb; lsc: lateral semicircular canal; mcf: middle cranial fossa; pr: promontory; st: sinus tympani; su: subiculum; ve: vestibule.*

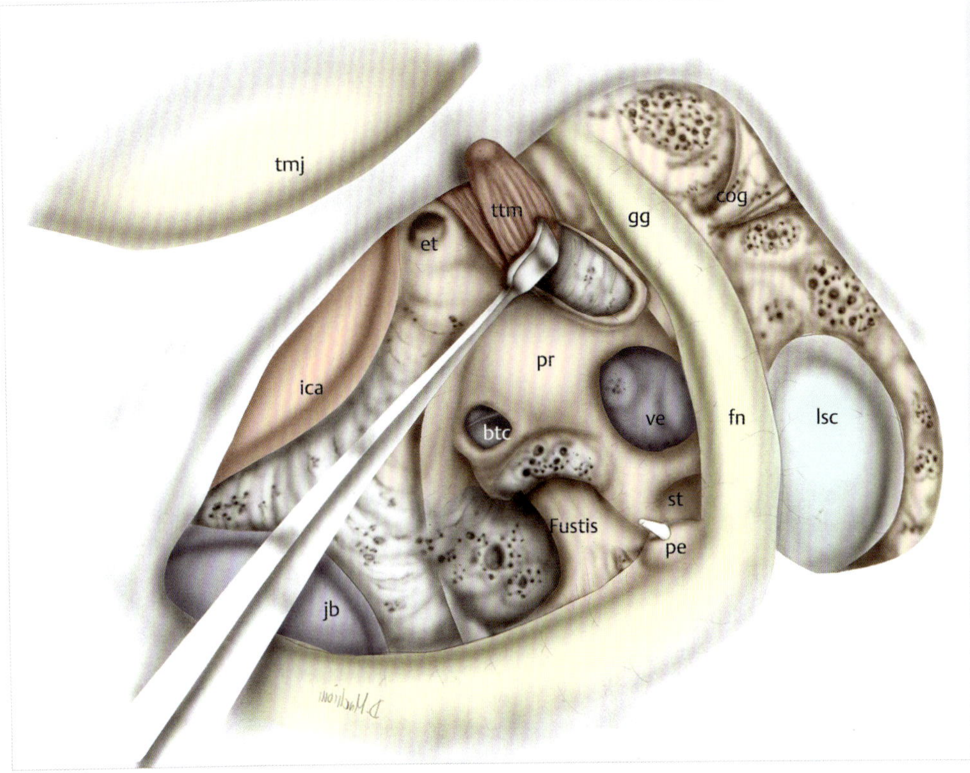

Fig. 11.163 Left side: The basal turn of the cochlea has been opened. The cochleariform process is removed and the tensor tympani muscle is detached from its canal, and pushed anteriorly. *btc: basal turn of the cochlea; et: eustachian tube; fn: facial nerve; gg: geniculate ganglion; ica: internal carotid artery; jb: jugular bulb; lsc: lateral semicircular canal; pe: pyramidal eminence; pr: promontory; st: sinus tympani; tmj: temporal mandibular joint; ttm: tensor timpani muscle; ve: vestibule.*

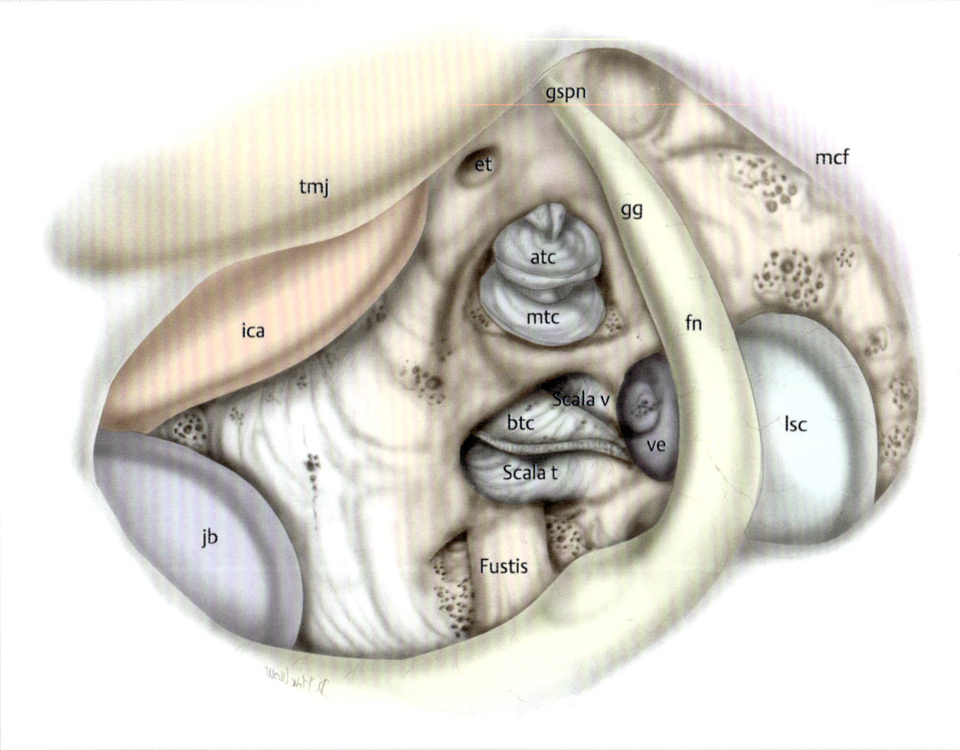

Fig. 11.164 Left side: The promontory is removed and the cochlear turns are exposed, from the basal to the apical turns. *atc: apical turn of cochlea; btc: basal turn of the cochlea; et: eustachian tube; fn: facial nerve; gg: geniculate ganglion; gspn: greater superficial petrosal nerve; ica: internal carotid artery; jb: jugular bulb; lsc: lateral semicircular canal; mcf: middle cranial fossa; mtc: middle turn of the cochlea; scala t: scala tympani; scala v: scala vestibuli; tmj: temporal mandibular joint; ve: vestibule.*

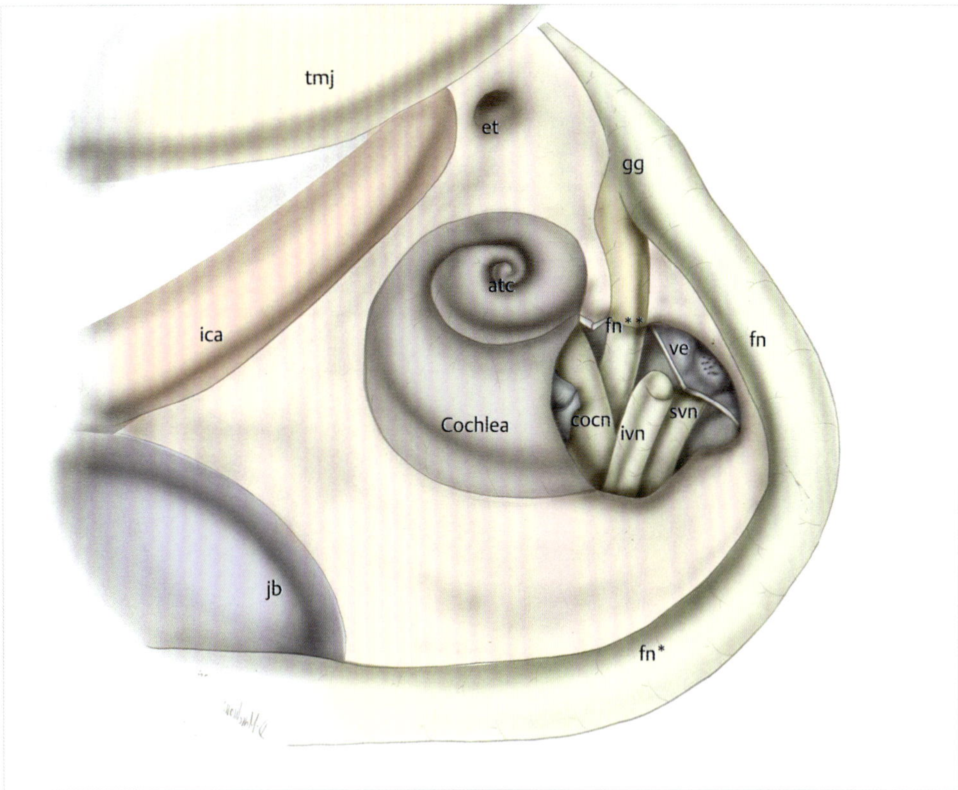

Fig. 11.165 Left side: Schematic drawing representing the anatomy of the fundus of the internal auditory canal (IAC) after cochleovestibular bone removal; the anatomical orientation of the nerves are visible. *atc: apical turn of the cochlea; cocn: cochlear nerve; et: eustachian tube; fn: facial nerve; fn*: mastoid segment of facial nerve; fn**: facial nerve into the IAC; gg: geniculate ganglion; ica: internal carotid artery; ivn: inferior vestibular nerve; jb: jugular bulb; svn: superior vestibular nerve; tmj: temporal mandibular joint; ve: vestibule.*

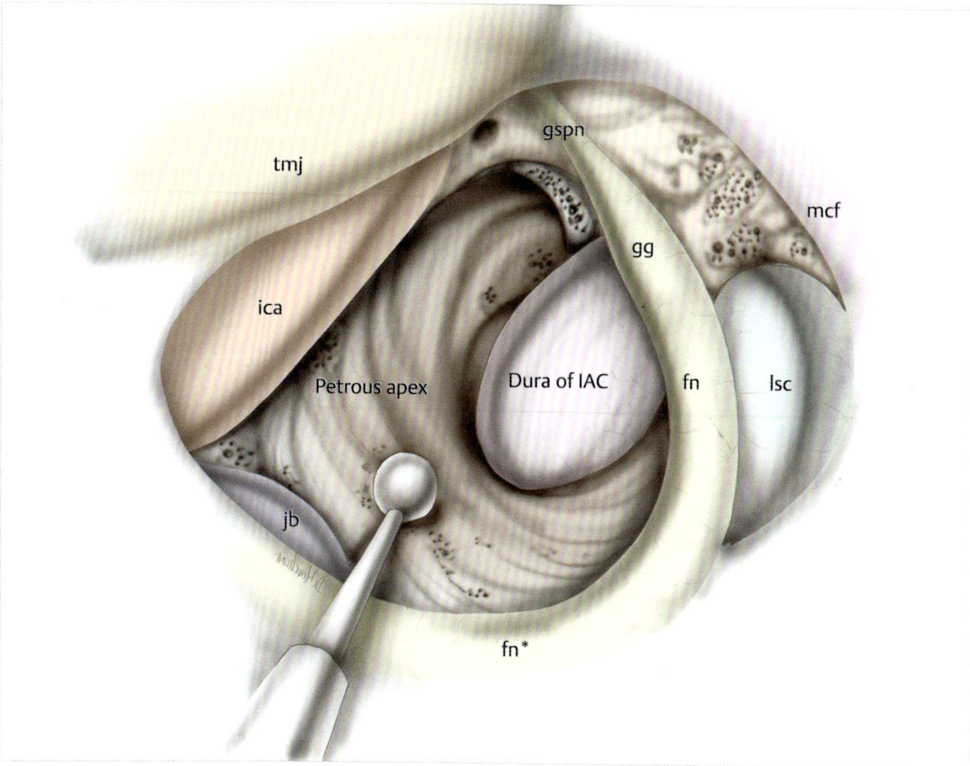

Fig. 11.166 Left side: The dural layer of the internal auditory canal (IAC) is progressively skeletonized, drilling around the vascular structures and the facial nerve (FN) with a diamond bur. *fn: facial nerve; fn*: mastoid segment of facial nerve; gg: geniculate ganglion; gpsn: greater superficial petrosal nerve; ica: internal carotid artery; jb: jugular bulb; lsc: lateral semicircular canal; mcf: middle cranial fossa; tmj: temporal mandibular joint.*

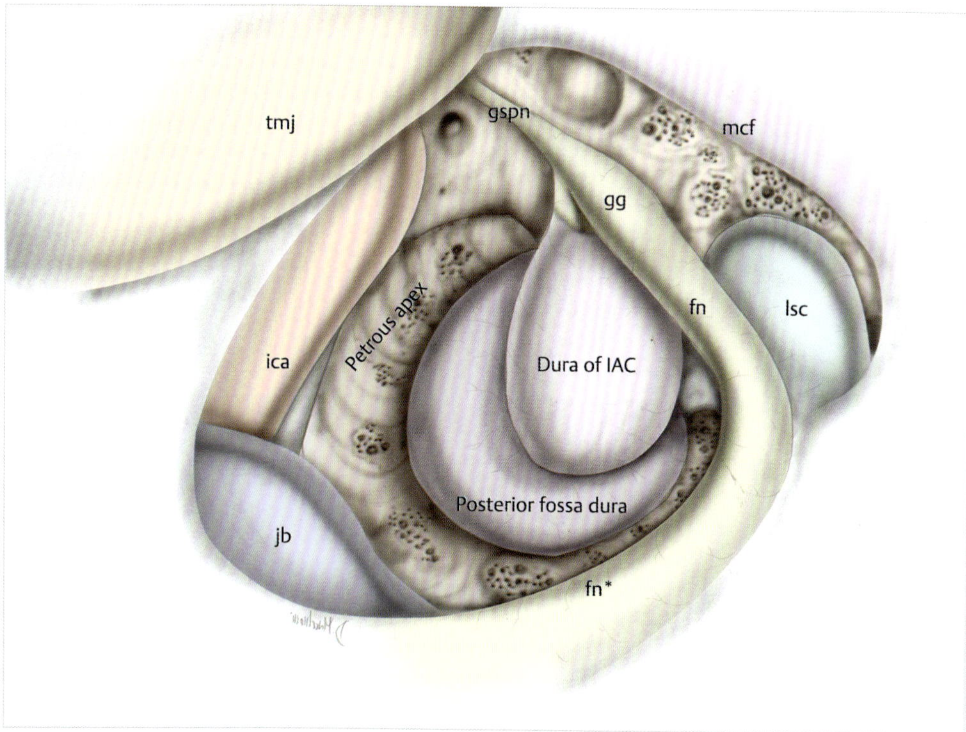

Fig. 11.167 Left side: The internal auditory canal (IAC) is skeletonized from the fundus to the porus. The dural layer of the posterior fossa around the porus is widely exposed to gain access to the cerebellopontine angle (CPA). *fn: facial nerve; fn*: mastoid segment of facial nerve; gg: geniculate ganglion; gspn: greater superficial petrosal nerve; ica: internal carotid artery; jb: jugular bulb; lsc: lateral semicircular canal; mcf: middle cranial fossa; tmj: temporal mandibular joint.*

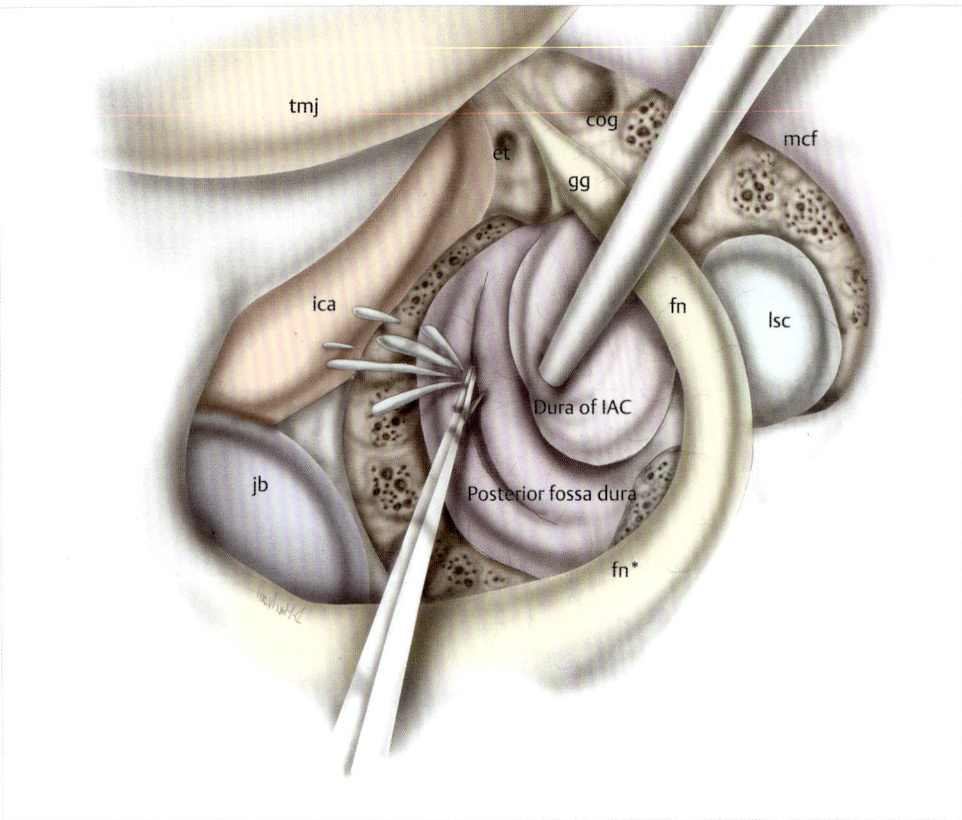

Fig. 11.168 Left side: An incision of the posterior fossa dura is performed; during this procedure, a CSF leak is expected. *et: eustachian tube; fn: facial nerve; fn*: mastoid segment of facial nerve; gg: geniculate ganglion; ica: internal carotid artery; jb: jugular bulb; lsc: lateral semicircular canal; mcf: middle cranial fossa; tmj: temporal mandibular joint.*

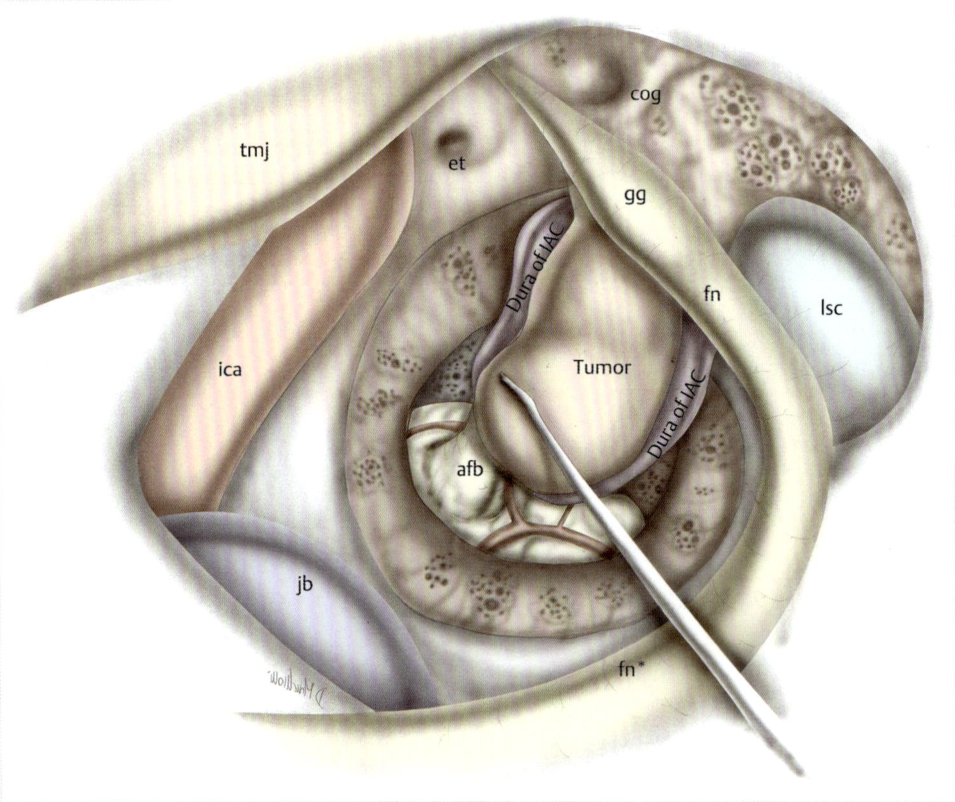

Fig. 11.169 Left side: The dura of the internal auditory canal (IAC) is incised, exposing the tumor in the IAC and cerebellopontine angle (CPA). The tumor dissection is started. *afb: acoustic-facial bundle; et: eustachian tube; fn: facial nerve; fn*: mastoid segment of facial nerve; gg: geniculate ganglion; ica: internal carotid artery; jb: jugular bulb; lsc: lateral semicircular canal; tmj: temporal mandibular joint.*

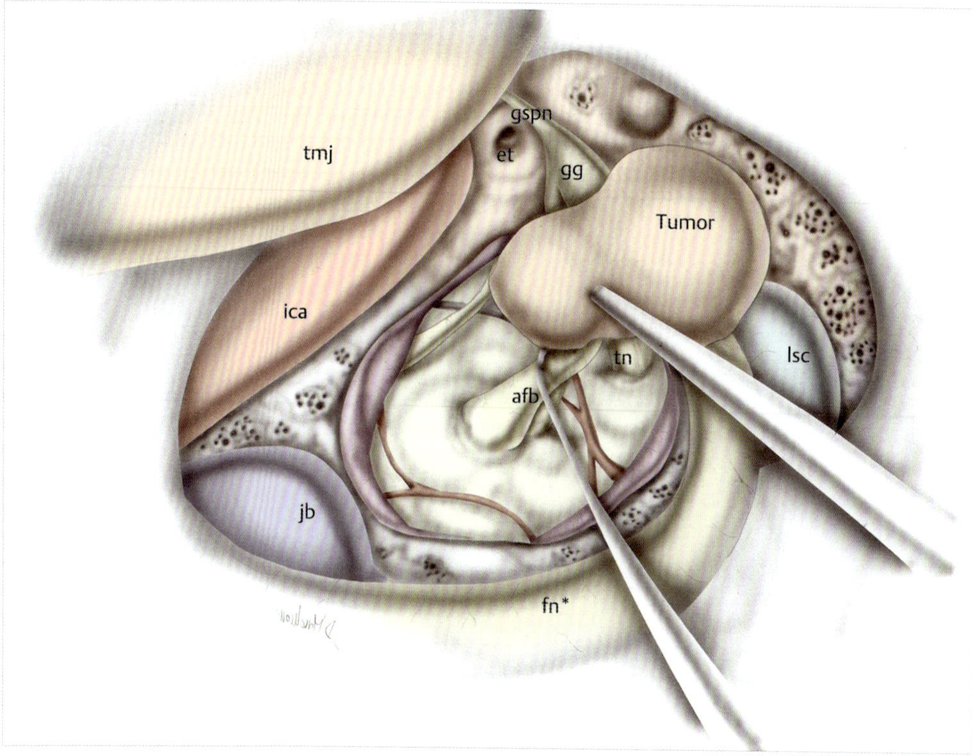

Fig. 11.170 Left side: The tumor is gently dissected from the facial nerve (FN). *afb: acoustic-facial bundle; et: eustachian tube; fn*: mastoid segment of facial nerve; gg: geniculate ganglion; gspn: greater superficial petrosal nerve; ica: internal carotid artery; jb: jugular bulb; lsc: lateral semicircular canal; tmj: temporal mandibular joint; tn: trigeminal nerve.*

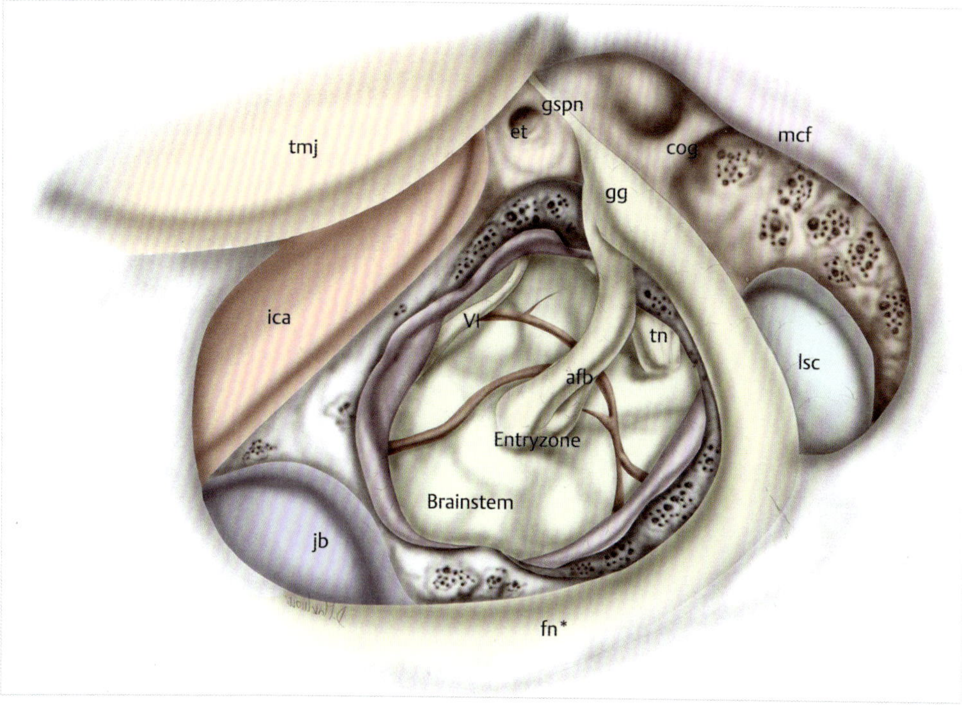

Fig. 11.171 Left side: Final surgical cavity after tumor removal. *afb: acoustic-facial bundle; et: eustachian tube; fn*: mastoid segment of facial nerve; gg: geniculate ganglion; gspn: greater superficial petrosal nerve; ica: internal carotid artery; jb: jugular bulb; lsc: lateral semicircular canal; mcf: middle cranial fossa; tmj: temporal mandibular joint; tn: trigeminal nerve.*

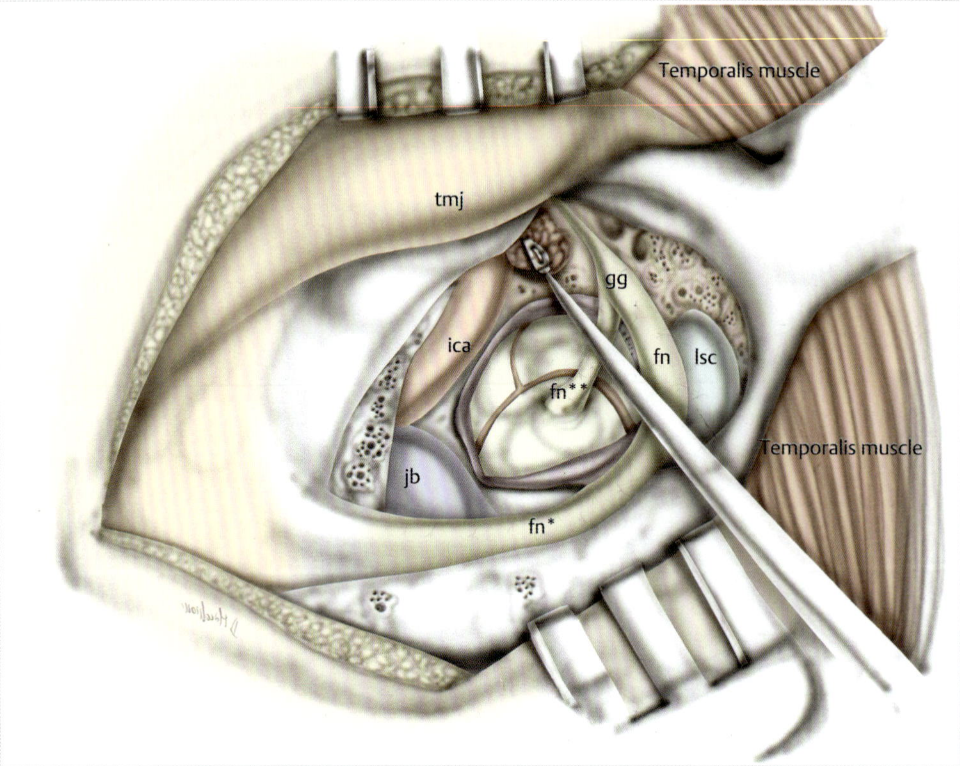

Fig. 11.172 Left side: A fragment of the temporalis muscle is used to close the eustachian tube orifice, pushing it into the lumen. *fn: facial nerve; fn*: mastoid segment of facial nerve; fn** facial nerve into the CPA; gg: geniculate ganglion; ica: internal carotid artery; jb: jugular bulb; lsc: lateral semicircular canal; tmj: temporal mandibular joint.*

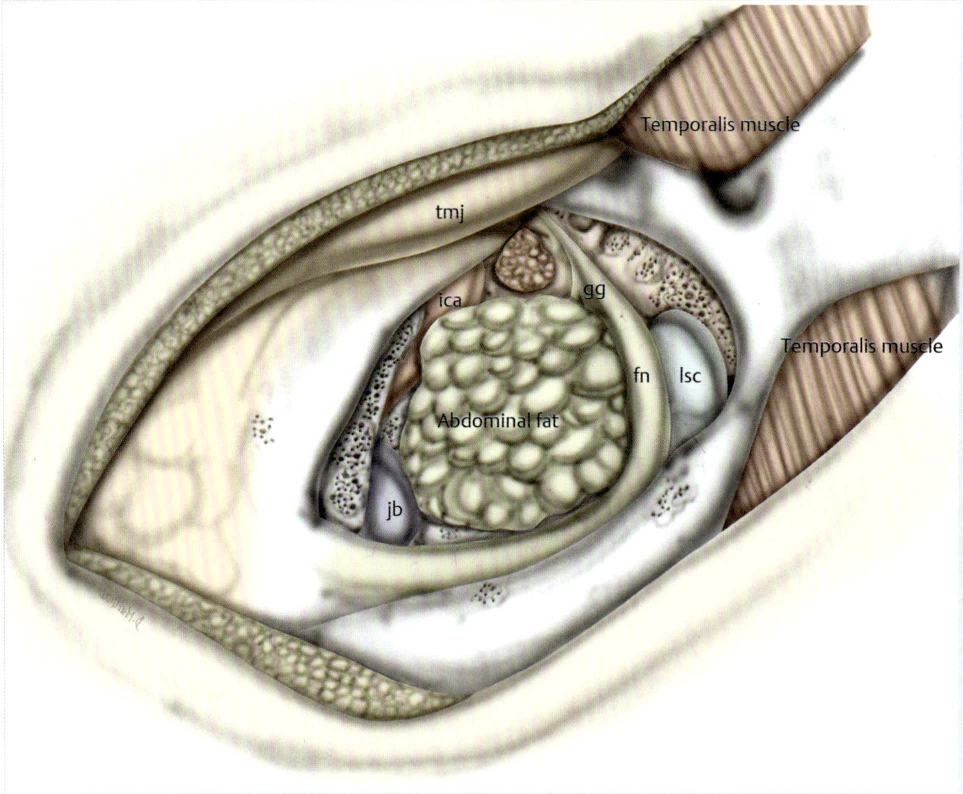

Fig. 11.173 Left side: Abdominal fat is used to fill the surgical cavity, to close the defect between the cerebellopontine angle (CPA) and the tympanic cavity. *fn: facial nerve; gg: geniculate ganglion; ica: internal carotid artery; jb: jugular bulb; lsc: lateral semicircular canal; tmj: temporal mandibular joint.*

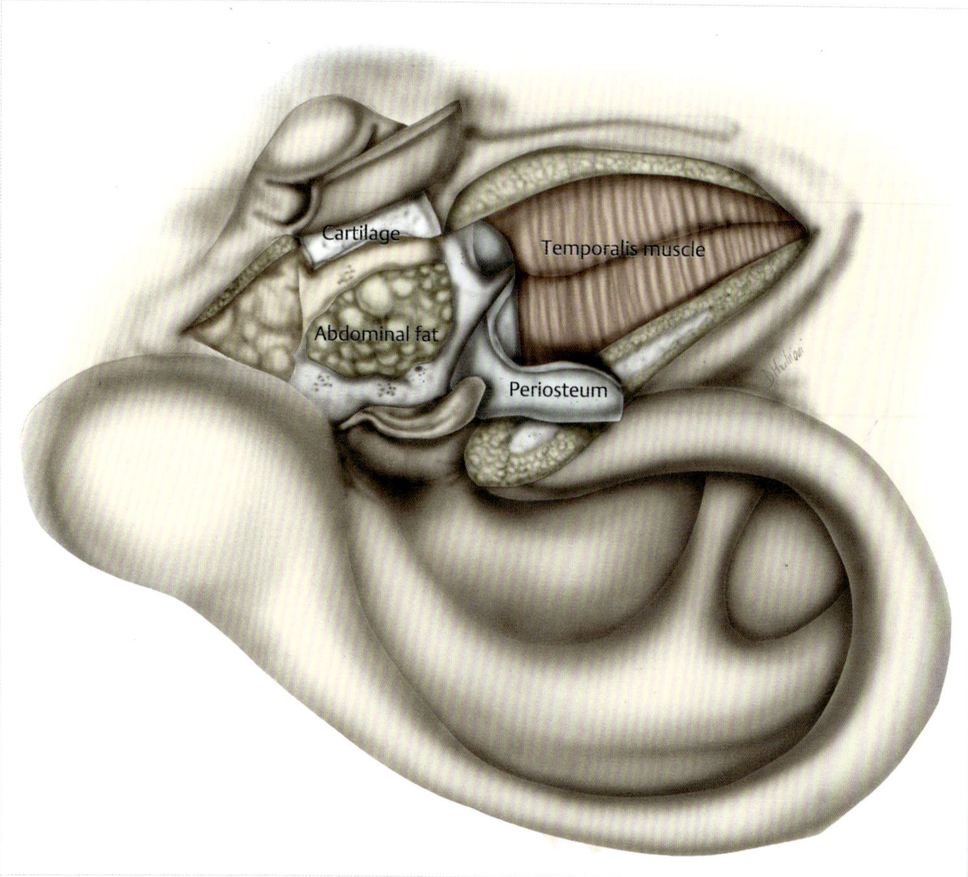

Fig. 11.174 Left side: The temporalis muscle is sutured, and the periosteum layer replaced and sutured to cover the surgical cavity.

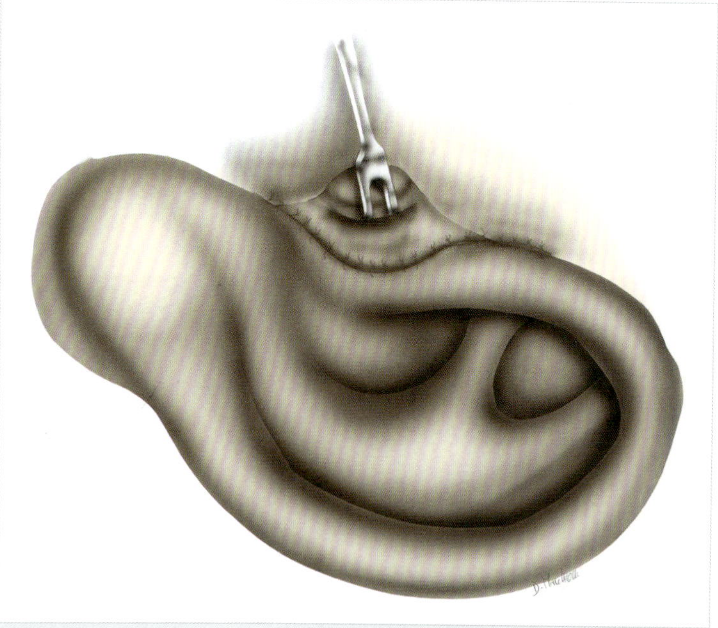

Fig. 11.175 Left side: The skin of the external auditory canal (EAC) is everted and sutured; the skin of the incision is accurately sutured.

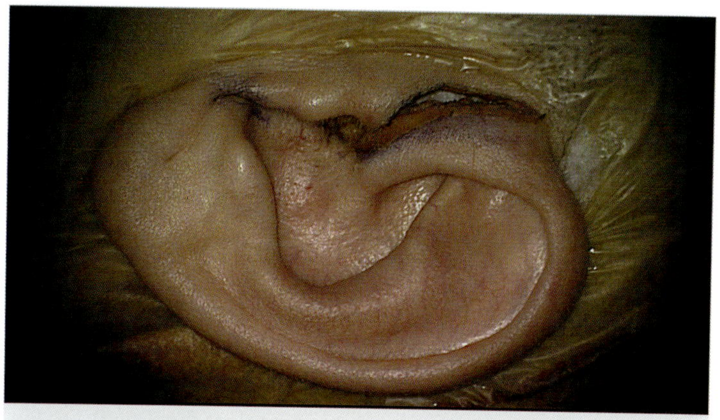

Fig. 11.176 Left side: A preauricolar incision (Shambaugh incision) is performed between the tragus and the helix and inferiorly continued in the external auditory canal (EAC) in an anular shape.

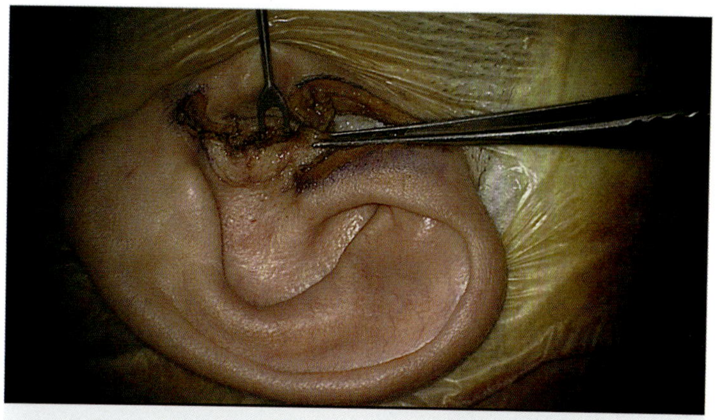

Fig. 11.177 Left side: The skin of the anterior portion of the external auditory canal (EAC) is detached and anteriorly dislocated along with the tragal cartilage.

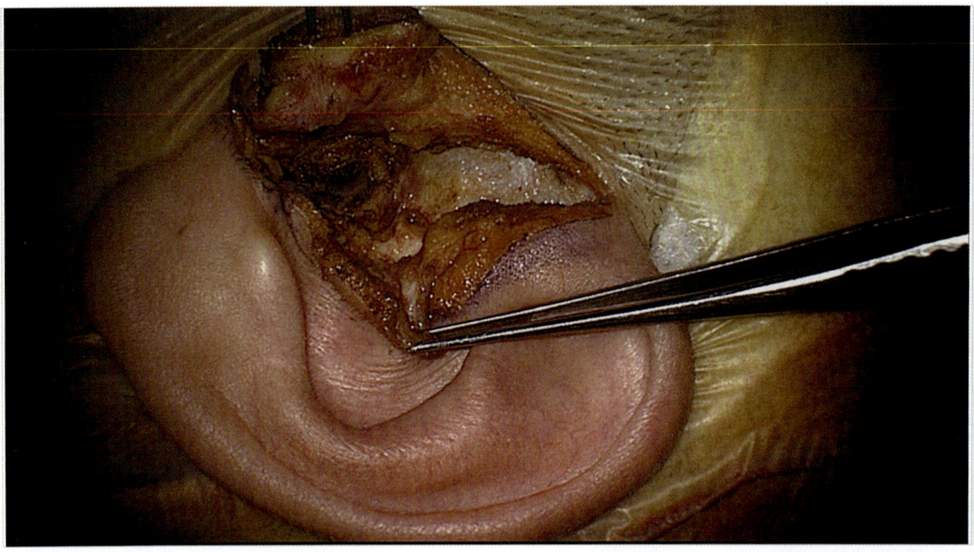

Fig. 11.178 Left side: The anterior and the posterior flaps are detached from the plane of the temporalis muscle fascia. A circular incision is then made in the skin of the external auditory canal (EAC) at its osteocartilaginous junction.

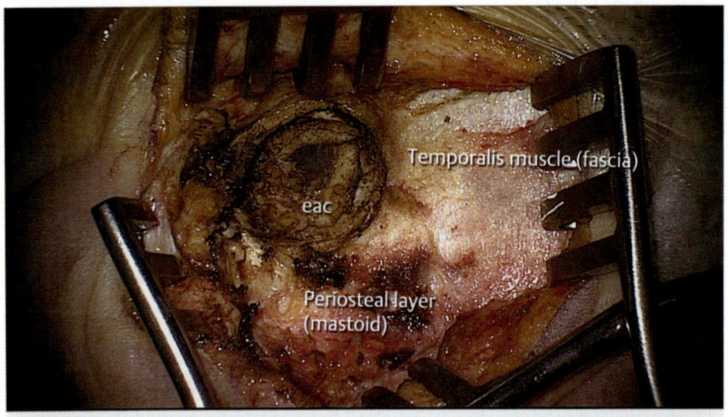

Fig. 11.179 Left side: Two autostatic retractors are placed to expose the distal part of the external auditory canal (EAC). *eac: external auditory canal.*

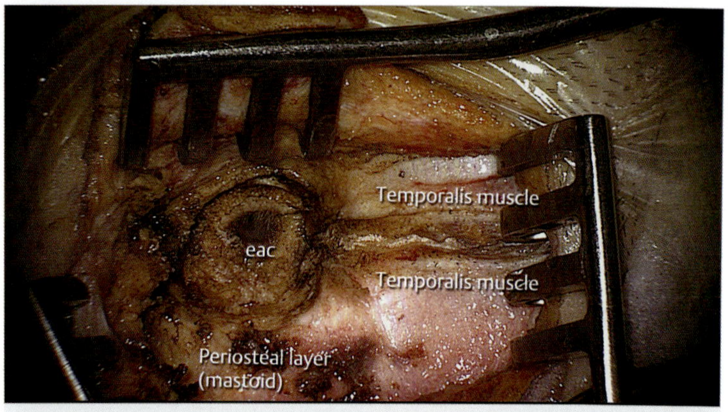

Fig. 11.180 A vertical incision in the temporalis muscle is made from the superior part of the external auditory canal (EAC). The incision must reach the bone to create a muscle-periosteal flap. An anterior and a posterior flap, are sculpted to uncover the mastoid and zygomatic bone. *eac: external auditory canal.*

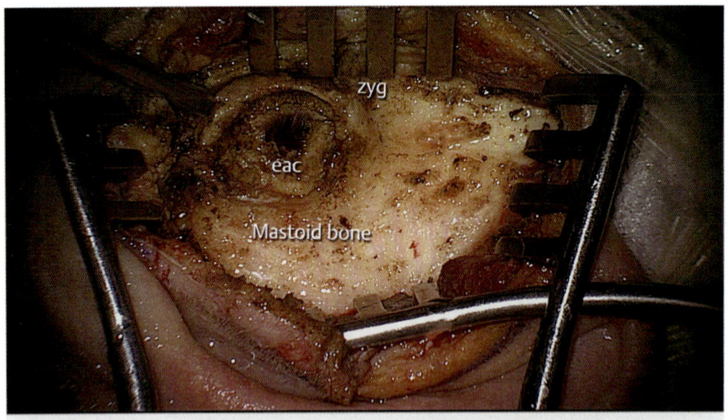

Fig. 11.181 To expose the mastoid bone, posteriorly, and the zygomatic bone, anteriorly, the retractors are placed under the muscle-periosteal flaps. *eac: external auditory canal, zyg: zygomatic bone.*

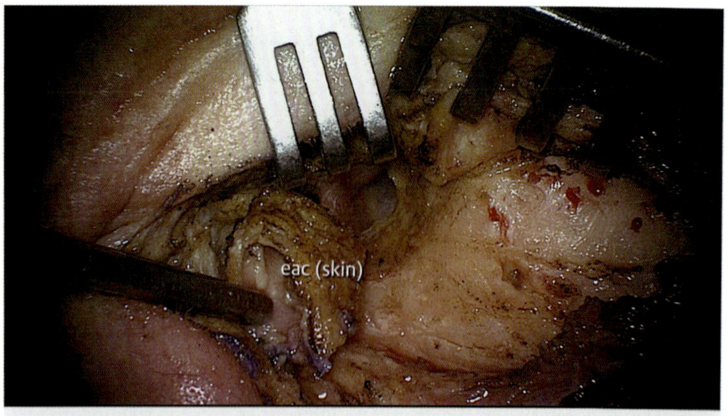

Fig. 11.182 The skin of the lateral portion of the external ear canal is removed. *eac: external auditory canal.*

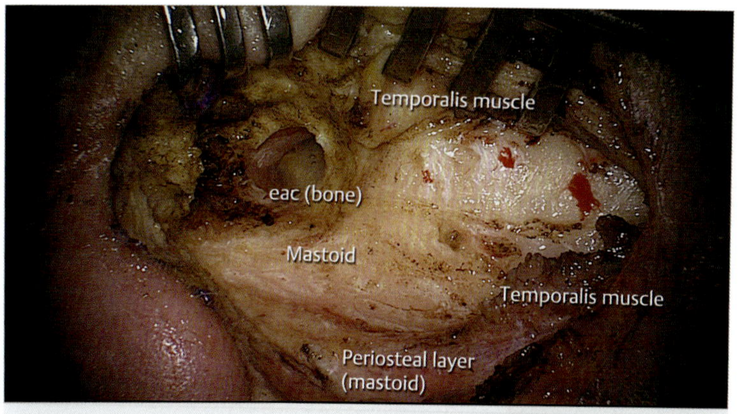

Fig. 11.183 The eardrum, at this point, is completely exposed. *eac: external auditory canal.*

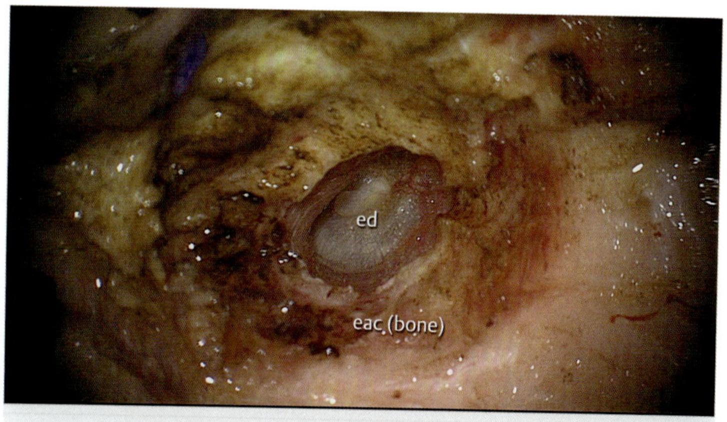

Fig. 11.184 The medial portion of the external auditory canal (EAC) and the eardrum can now be closely visualized. *eac: external auditory canal, ed: eardrum.*

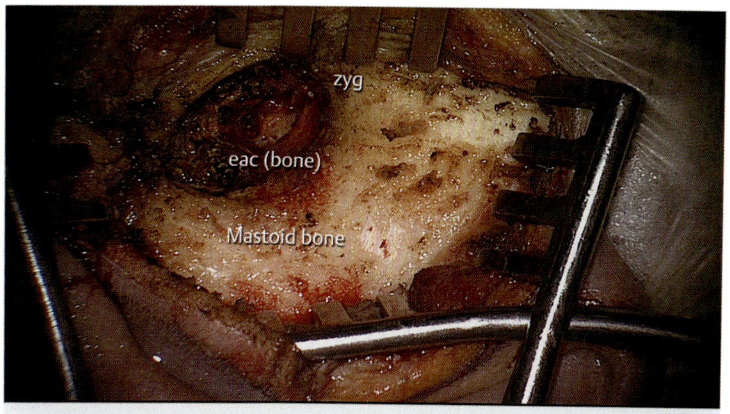

Fig. 11.185 The skin of the medial portion of the external auditory canal (EAC) is removed en bloc with the eardrum, paying attention not to leave any residual skin in the tympanic cavity. *eac: external auditory canal, zyg: zygomatic bone.*

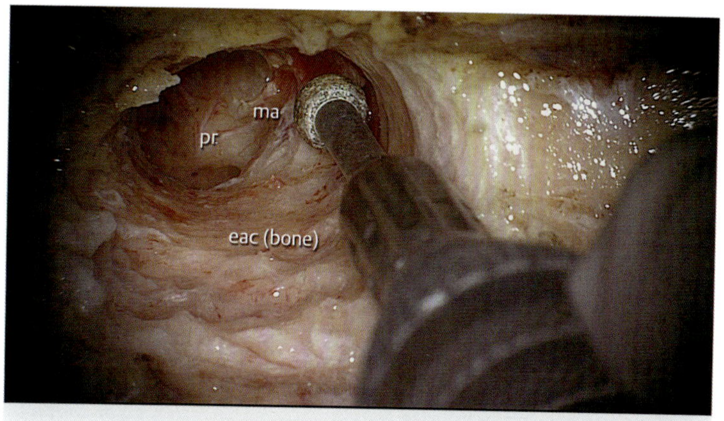

Fig. 11.186 A medium-sized diamond bur is used to circumferentially drill and enlarge the bony segment of the external auditory canal (EAC). *eac: external auditory canal; ma: malleus; pr: promontory.*

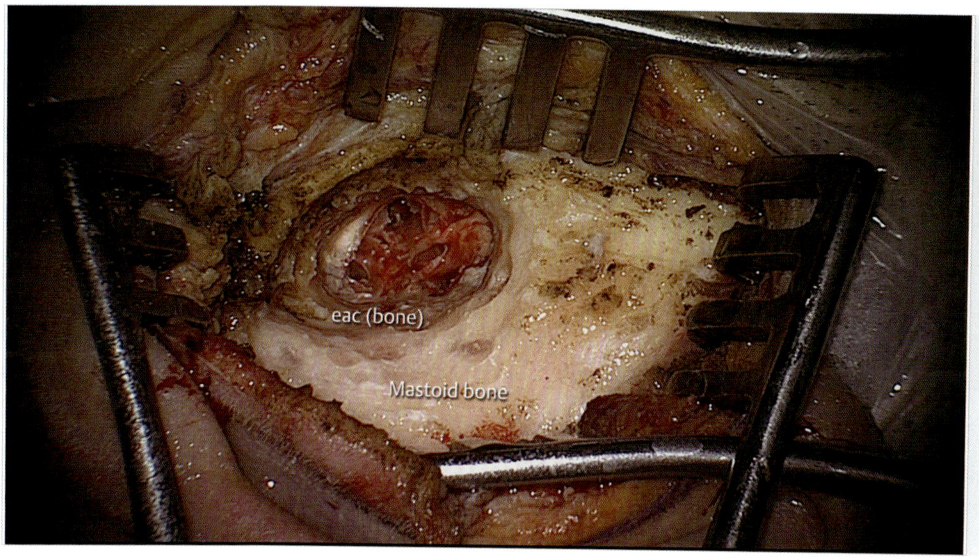

Fig. 11.187 The temporomandibular joint represents the anterior limit. Superiorly a wide atticotomy is made to remove the scutum and uncover the incudomalleolar joint. Posteriorly the bone must be carefully drilled to detect the third part of the facial nerve (FN). The jugular bulb, inferiorly, represents the limit of the dissection. *eac: external auditory canal.*

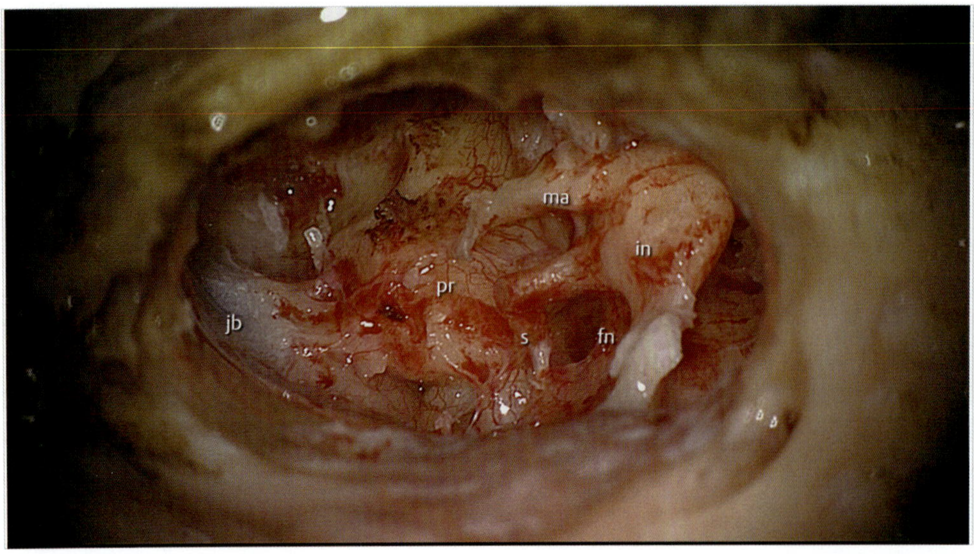

Fig. 11.188 Microscopic view of the tympanic cavity after the enlargement of the external auditory canal (EAC) and the atticotomy; the jugular bulb is inferiorly visible. *fn: facial nerve; in: incus; jb: jugular bulb; ma: malleus; pr: promontory; s: stapes.*

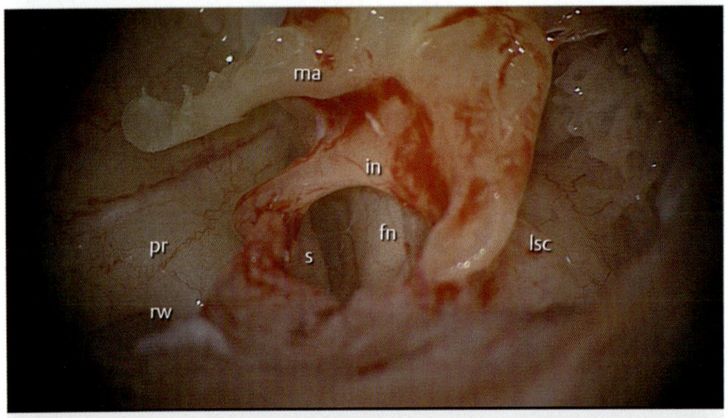

Fig. 11.189 The tympanic tract of the facial nerve (FN) is visible under the incus, till its second genu. *fn: facial nerve; in: incus; lsc: lateral semicircular canal; ma: malleus; pr: promontory; rw: round window; s: stapes.*

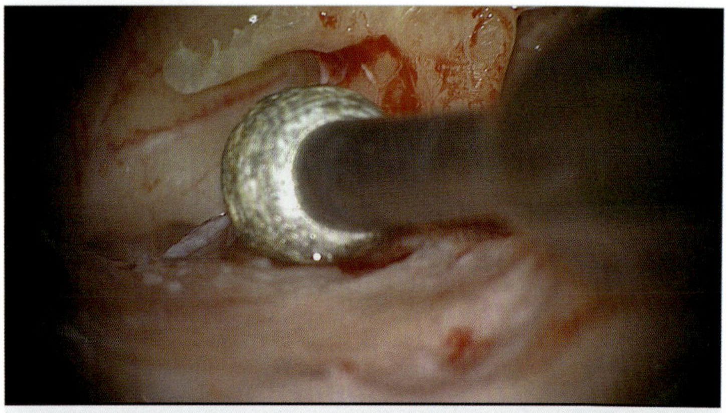

Fig. 11.190 The posterior portion of the external auditory canal (EAC) is carefully drilled to expose the retrotympanum, paying attention to the III segment of the facial nerve (FN) (mastoid portion).

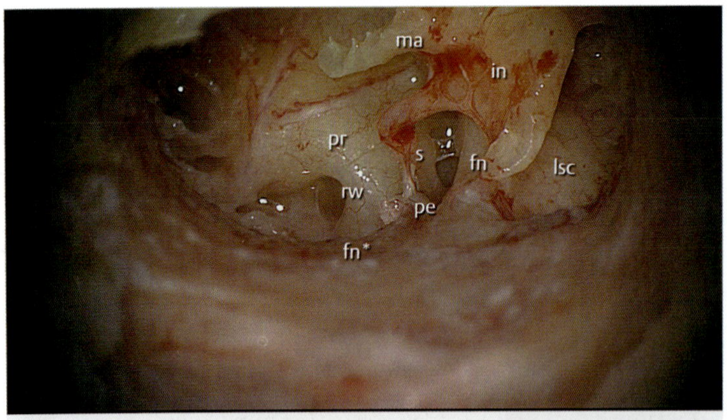

Fig. 11.191 The retrotympanum, the round window area, and the hypotympanum are now clearly visible. *fn: facial nerve; fn*: mastoid segment of the facial nerve; in: incus; lsc: lateral semicircular canal; ma: malleus; pr: promontory; rw: round window; rw: round window; s: stapes.*

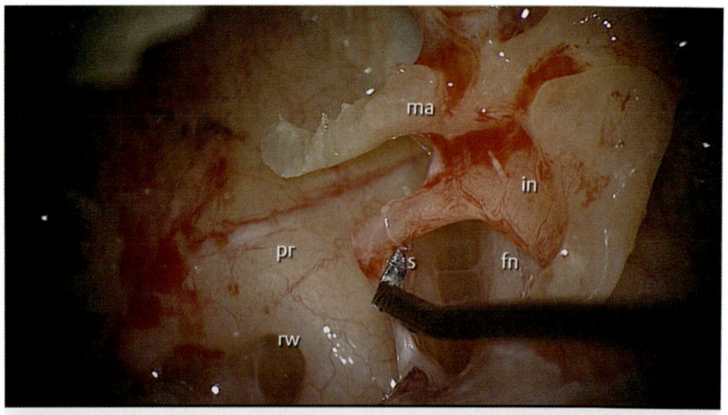

Fig. 11.192 The incus and the malleus are removed. *fn: facial nerve; in: incus; ma: malleus; pr: promontory; rw: round window; s: stapes.*

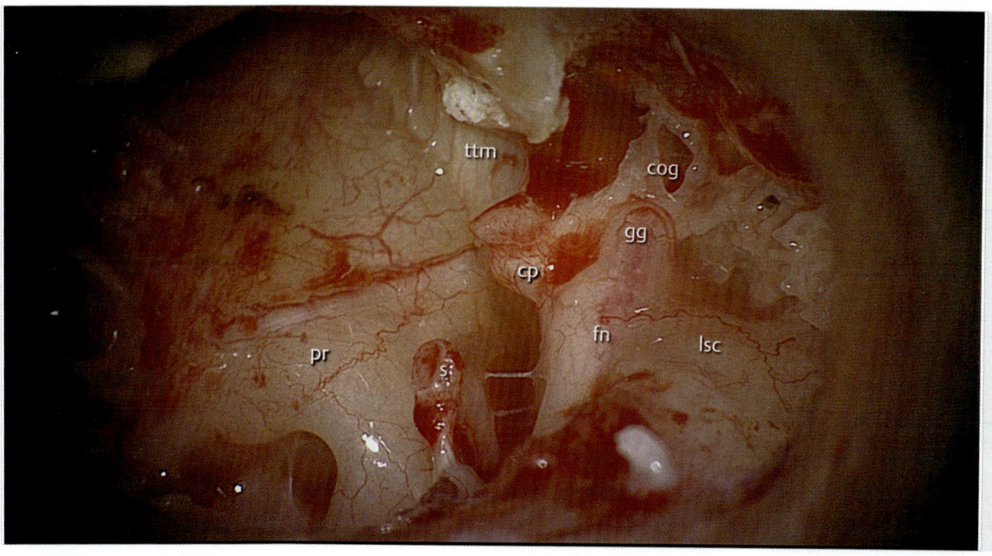

Fig. 11.193 The facial nerve (FN) is exposed till the second genu. *cog: cog; cp: cochleariform process; fn: facial nerve; gg: geniculate ganglion; lsc: lateral semicircular canal; pr: promontory; s: stapes; ttm: tensor tendon muscle.*

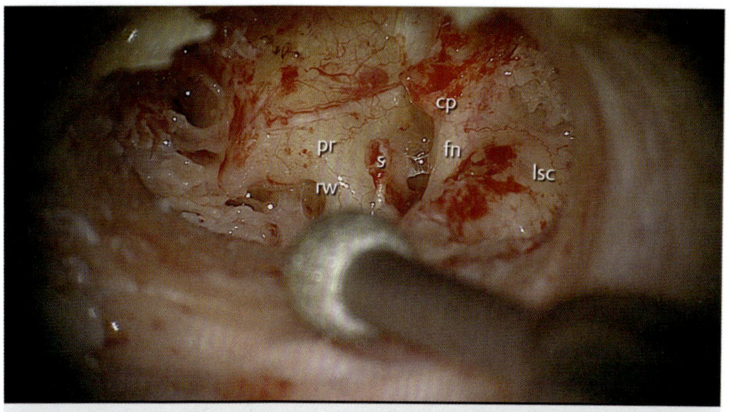

Fig. 11.194 A diamond bur is used to remove the bone over the III portion of the facial nerve (FN). This step grants a better exposition of the internal acoustic canal (IAC) and cerebellopontine angle (CPA). *cp: cochleariform process; fn: facial nerve; lsc: lateral semicircular canal; pr: promontory; rw: round window; s: stapes.*

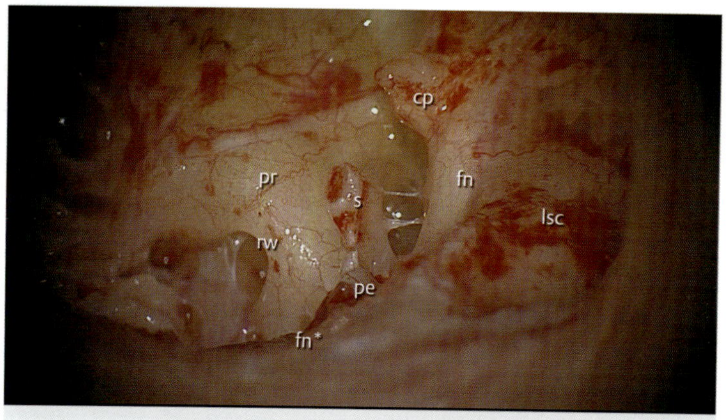

Fig. 11.195 Drilling the external auditory canal (EAC) helps uncover the round window area. This area represents the external projection of the internal auditory canal (IAC). *cp: cochleariform process; fn: facial nerve; fn*: mastoid segment of the facial nerve; lsc: lateral semicircular canal; pr: promontory; rw: round window; s: stapes.*

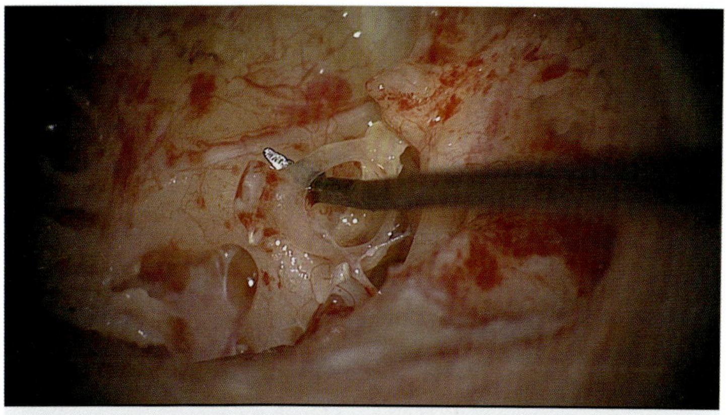

Fig. 11.196 The stapes is removed uncovering the vestibule.

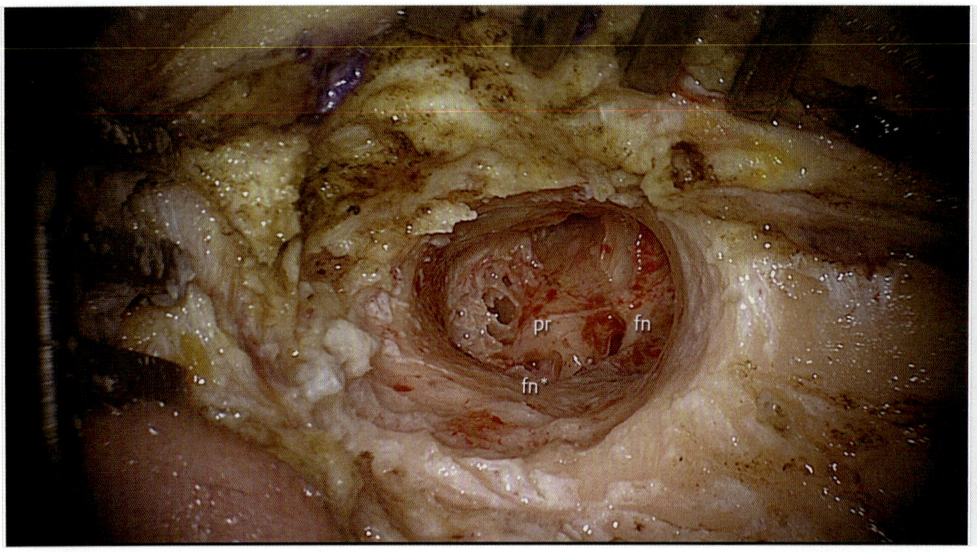

Fig. 11.197 Operative field after drilling the external auditory canal (EAC). *fn: facial nerve; fn*: mastoid segment of the facial nerve; pr: promontory.*

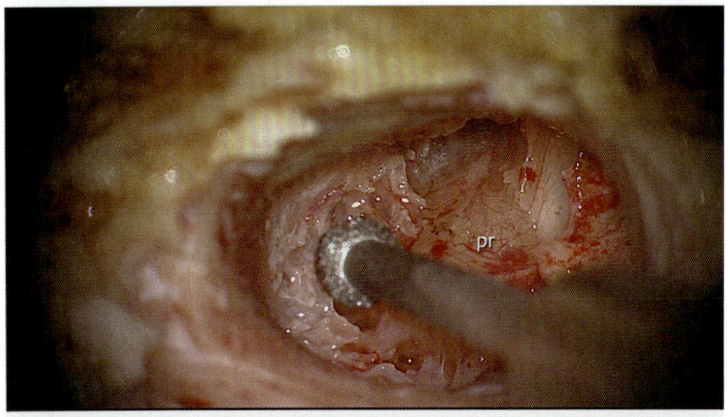

Fig. 11.198 A medium-sized diamond bur is used to remove the protympanic cell and uncover the vertical tract of the internal carotid artery, which is the anterior limit of the dissection. *pr: promontory.*

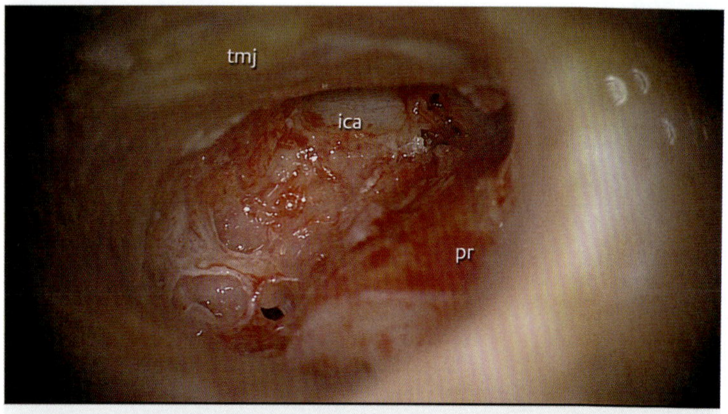

Fig. 11.199 The vertical tract of the internal carotid artery is identified. The bone covering the vascular structure is maintained to avoid possible damages during tumor removal. *ica: internal carotid artery; pr: promontory; tmj: temporomandibular joint.*

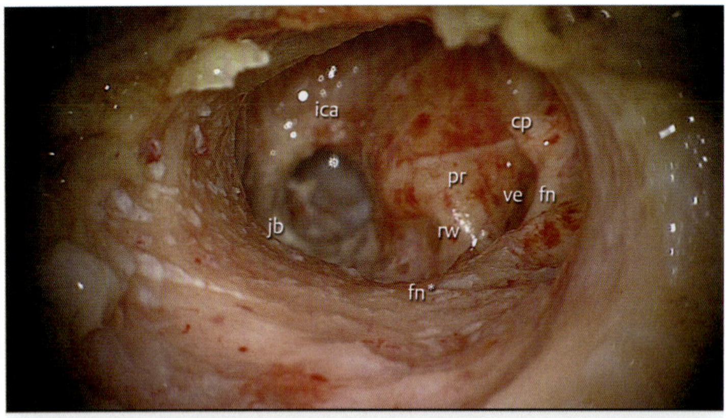

Fig. 11.200 The jugular bulb is inferiorly exposed. *cp: cochleariform process; fn: facial nerve; fn*: mastoid segment of the facial nerve; ica: internal carotid artery; jb: jugular bulb; pr: promontory; rw: round window; ve: vestibule.*

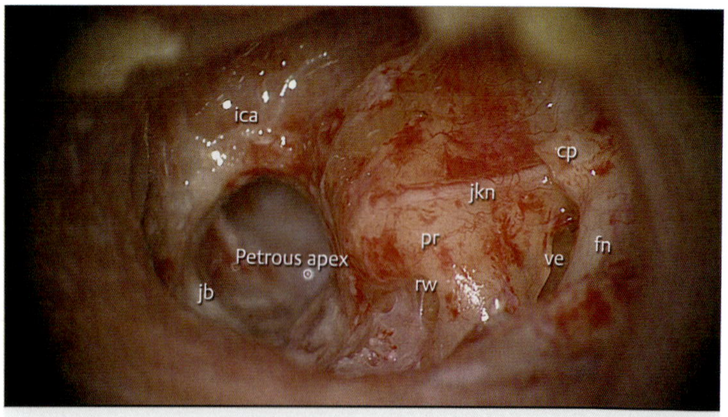

Fig. 11.201 The landmarks of the dissection are identified. The limits are the internal carotid artery anteriorly, the jugular bulb inferiorly, the III segment of the facial nerve (FN) posteriorly, and the tympanic segment of the FN superiorly. *cp: cochleariform process; fn: facial nerve; ica: internal carotid artery; jb: jugular bulb; jkn: Jacobson's nerve; pr: promontory; rw: round window; ve: vestibule.*

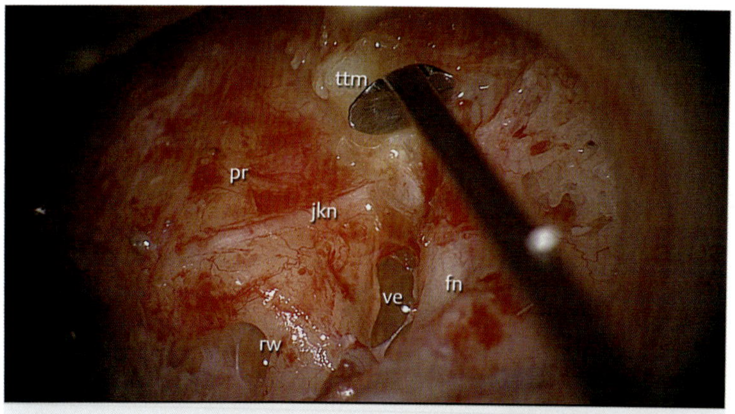

Fig. 11.202 The cochleariform process is removed and the tensor tympani muscle is dissected anteriorly, exposing the geniculate ganglion. In this way we can identify the apical turn of the cochlea which is otherwise hidden. *fn: facial nerve; jkn: Jacobson's nerve; pr: promontory; rw: round window; ttm: tensor tendon muscle; ve: vestibule.*

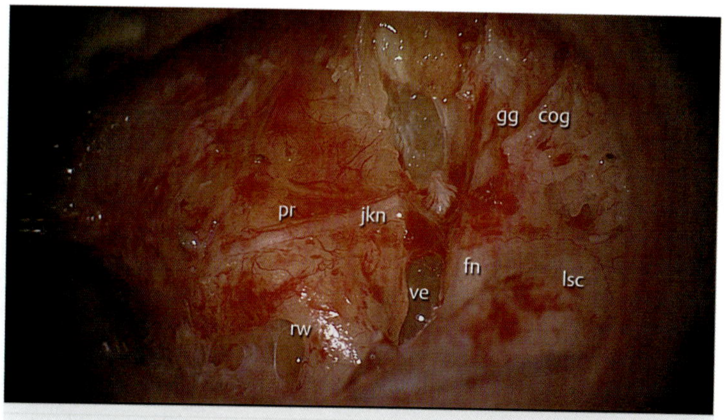

Fig. 11.203 The tensor tympani muscle is pushed anteriorly, and detached from its bony canal. *fn: facial nerve; gg: geniculate ganglion; jkn: Jacobson's nerve; lsc: lateral semicircular canal; pr: promontory; rw: round window; ve: vestibule.*

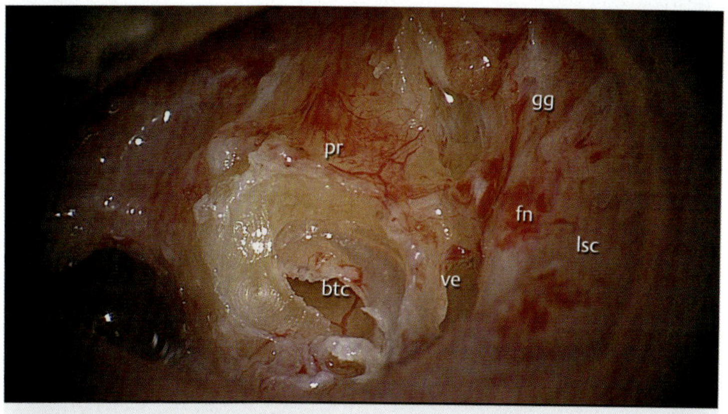

Fig. 11.204 The bone of the promontory is removed, starting from the round window, identifying the basal turn of the cochlea. *btc: basal turn of the cochlea; fn: facial nerve; gg: geniculate ganglion; lsc: lateral semicircular canal; pr: promontory; ve: vestibule.*

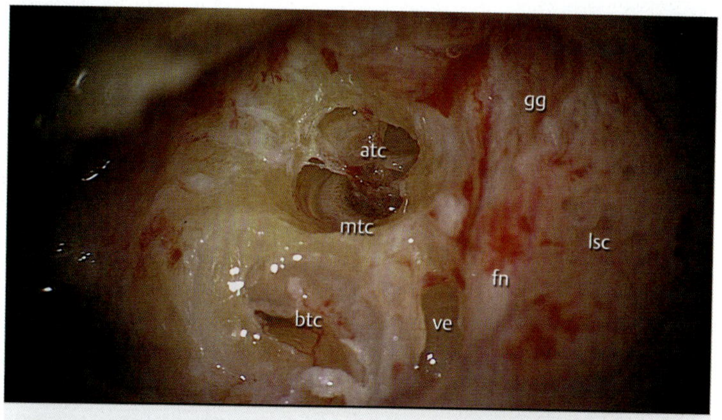

Fig. 11.205 The medial and apical turns of the cochlea are identified superiorly. Now it is clear how important the removal of the tensor tympani muscle is to uncover the apical turn of the cochlea. *atc: apical turn of the cochlea; btc: basal turn of the cochlea; fn: facial nerve; gg: geniculate ganglion; lsc: lateral semicircular canal; mtc: middle turn of the cochlea; ve: vestibule.*

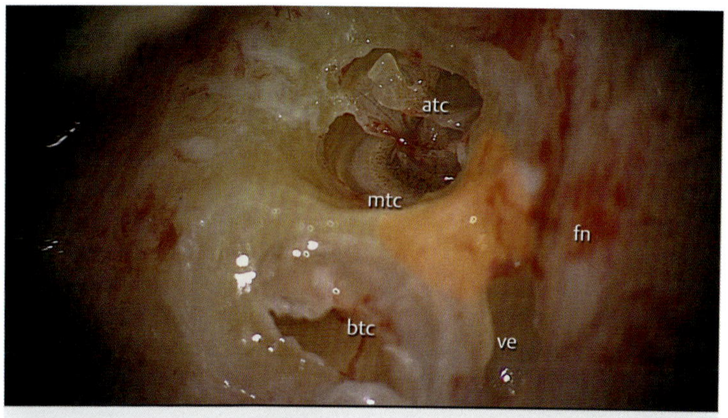

Fig. 11.206 The promontorial bone (cochlear-vestibular bone), a bone bridge between the vestibule and the cochlea, represents the ideal projection of the fundus of the internal auditory canal (IAC). *atc: apical turn of the cochlea; btc: basal turn of the cochlea; fn: facial nerve; mtc: middle turn of the cochlea; ve: vestibule.*

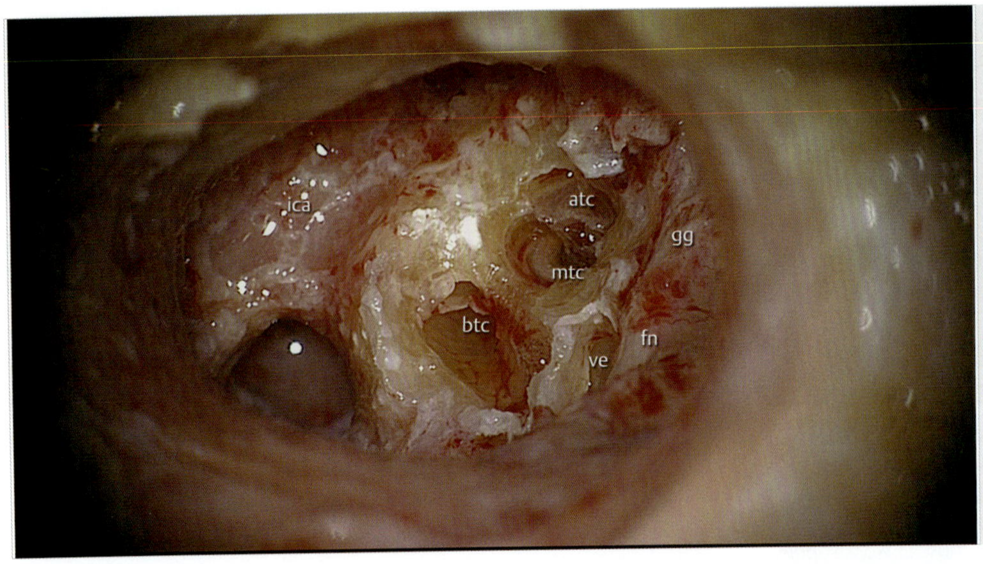

Fig. 11.207 All the landmarks are visible. The identification of the fundus can start. *atc: apical turn of the cochlea; btc: basal turn of the cochlea; fn: facial nerve; gg: geniculate ganglion; mtc: middle turn of the cochlea; ve: vestibule.*

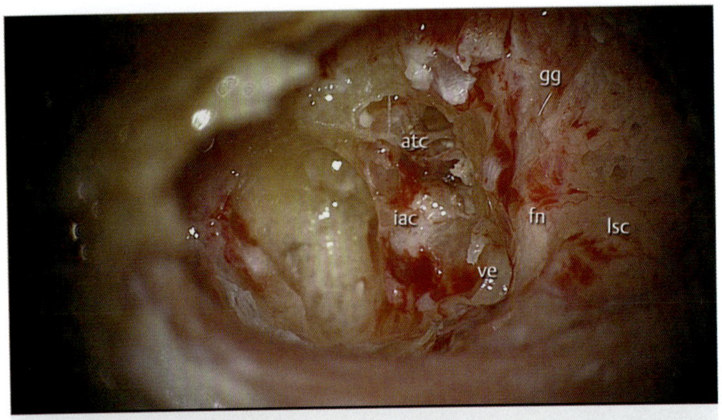

Fig. 11.208 The internal auditory canal (IAC) is skeletonized circumferentially removing the bone. In this picture, the orientation of the IAC is clear, starting from the cochlear modiolus and going posteriorly and under the vestibule. *atc: apical turn of the cochlea; fn: facial nerve; gg: geniculate ganglion; iac: internal auditory canal; lsc: lateral semicircular canal; ve: vestibule.*

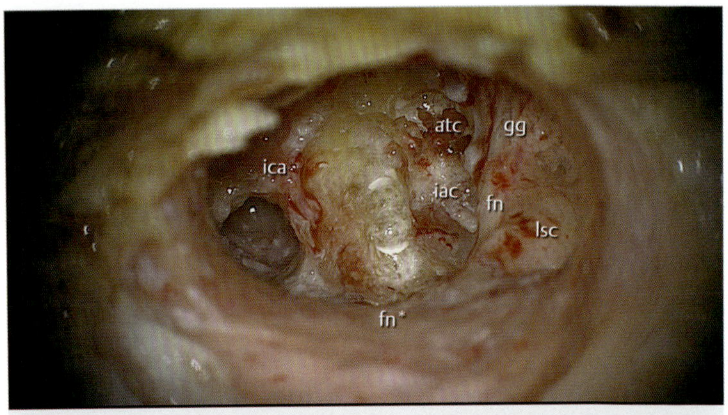

Fig. 11.209 The skeletonization of the internal auditory canal (IAC) continues, drilling the promontorial bone under the IAC. *atc: apical turn of the cochlea; fn: facial nerve; gg: geniculate ganglion; iac: internal auditory canal; ica: internal carotid artery; lsc: lateral semicircular canal.*

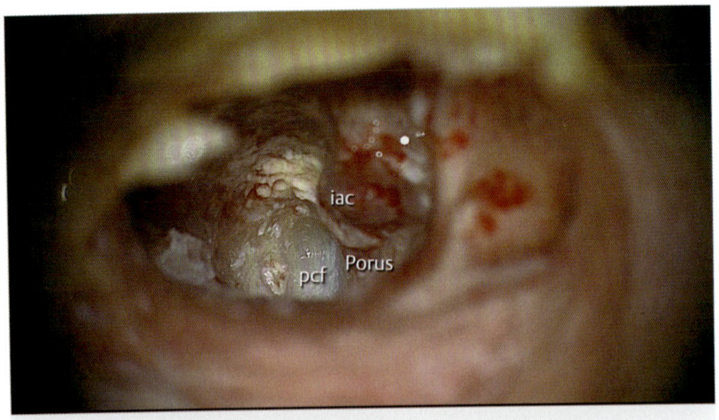

Fig. 11.210 The reflection of the dura on the medial surface of petrous bone represents the deepest limit of the dissection. The blue color of the dural lining is a landmark for the porus acousticus. *iac: internal auditory canal; pcf: posterior cranial fossa.*

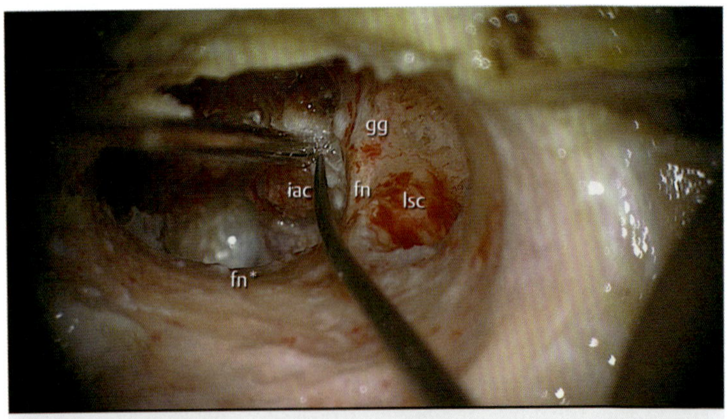

Fig. 11.211 The dura of the internal auditory canal (IAC) is longitudinally opened to expose the neuroma. With this approach the removal of the vestibular schwannoma can be made using the microscope and a two-handed technique. *fn: facial nerve; fn*: mastoid segment of facial nerve; gg: geniculate ganglion; iac: internal auditory canal; lsc: lateral semicircular canal.*

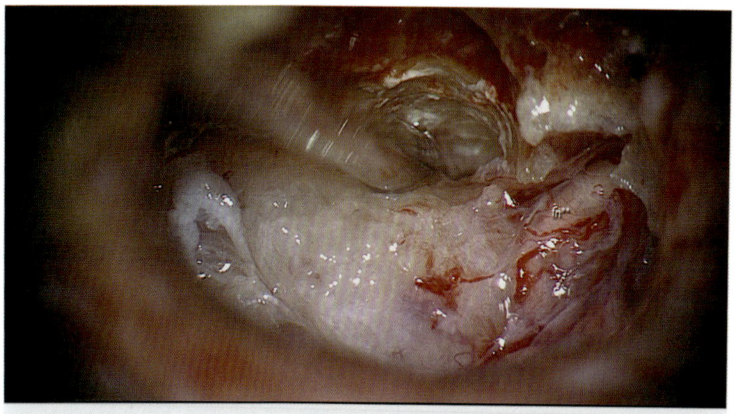

Fig. 11.212 The vestibular schwannoma (VS) is removed and the facial nerve is identified and preserved. In this case the VS involves the internal auditory canal (IAC), till the porus.

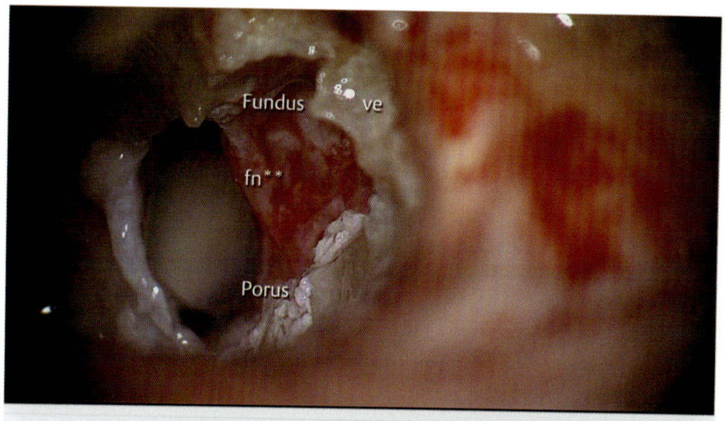

Fig. 11.213 Microscopic view of the porus after the vestibular schwannoma removal. The facial nerve (FN) is identified and visualized. *fn**: facial nerve into the IAC; ve: vestibule.*

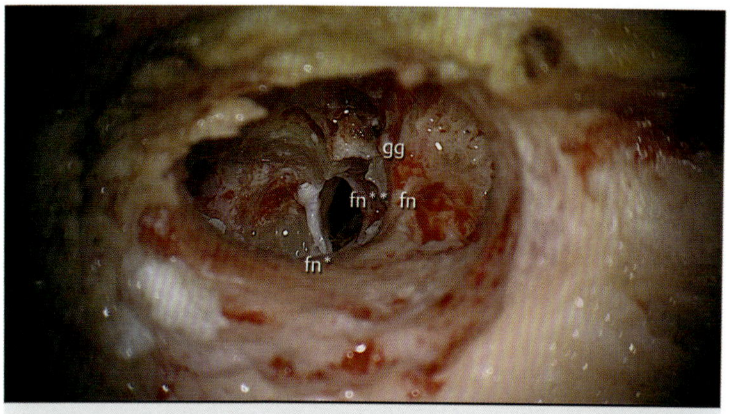

Fig. 11.214 The operative field after the removal of the vestibular schwannoma. The promontorial defect is clearly visible after the dissection. *fn: facial nerve; fn*: mastoid segment of facial nerve; fn**: facial nerve into the IAC; gg: geniculate ganglion.*

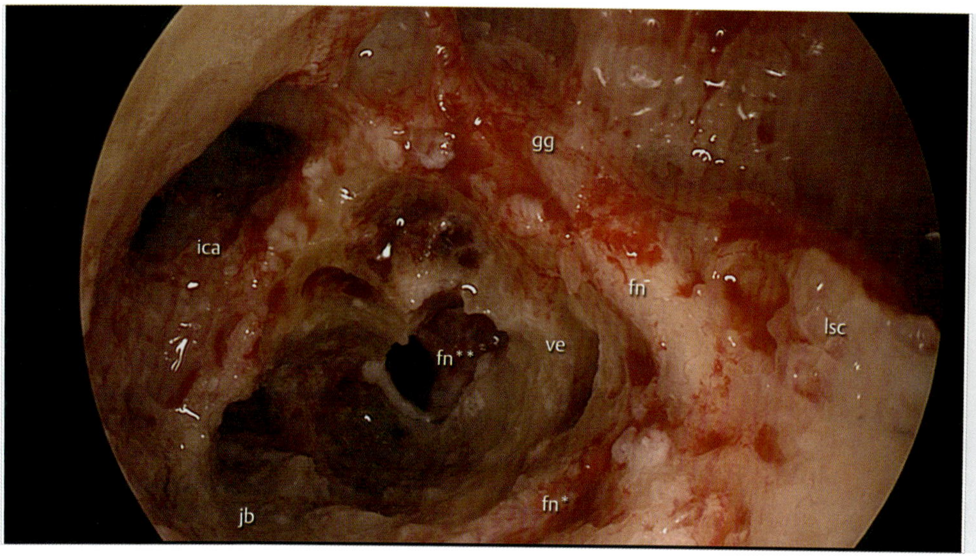

Fig. 11.215 View through a 0-degree, 15 cm long, 4 mm diameter endoscope. *fn: facial nerve; fn*: mastoid segment of facial nerve; fn**: facial nerve into the IAC; gg: geniculate ganglion; ica: internal carotid artery; jb: jugular bulb; lsc: lateral semicircular canal; ve: vestibule.*

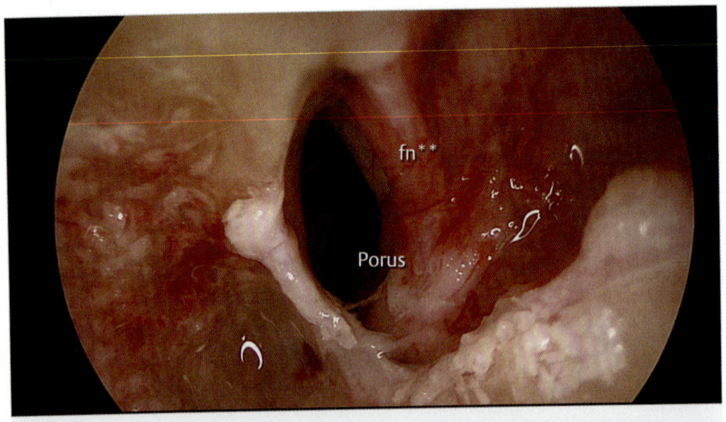

Fig. 11.216 The power of magnification of the endoscope permits to identify any residual fragment of the lesion. *fn**: facial nerve into the internal auditory canal (IAC).*

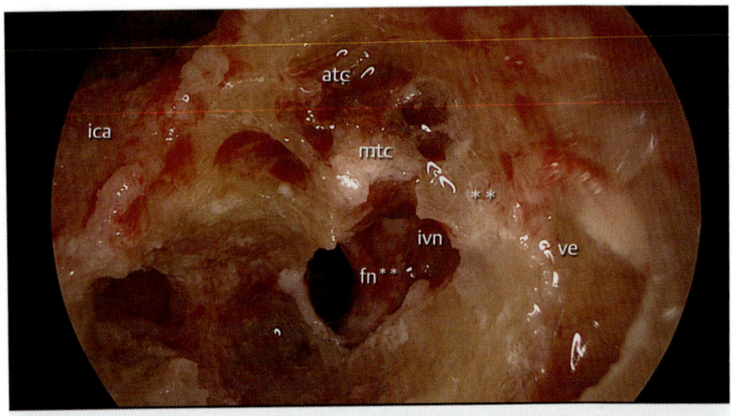

Fig. 11.217 The bone defect is clearly visible under the middle and apical turns of the cochlea and the medial wall of the vestibule; the facial nerve (FN) is visible in all its segments till the fundus of the internal auditory canal (IAC). *atc: apical turn of the cochlea; fn**: facial nerve into the IAC; ica: internal carotid artery; ivn: inferior vestibular nerve; mtc: middle turn of the cochlea; ve: vestibule; **: spherical recess.*

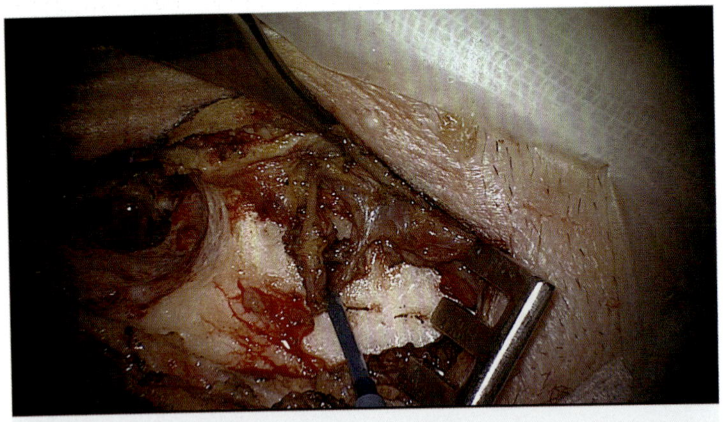

Fig. 11.218 A fragment of muscle is harvested from the temporalis muscle.

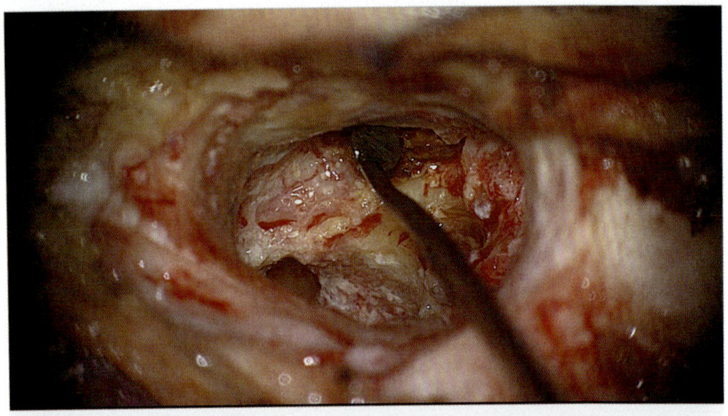

Fig. 11.219 The muscle fragment is used to close the eustachian tube.

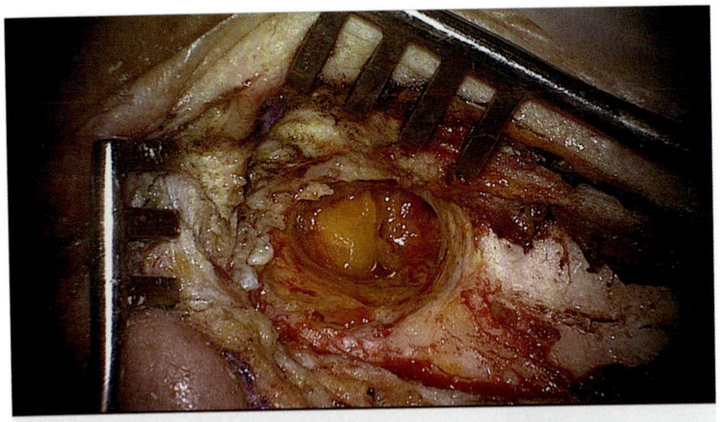

Fig. 11.220 Fat, harvested in the abdomen, is placed in the promontorial defect to fill the tympanic cavity, blocking any cerebrospinal fluid (CSF) leaks. Fibrin glue is then used to seal.

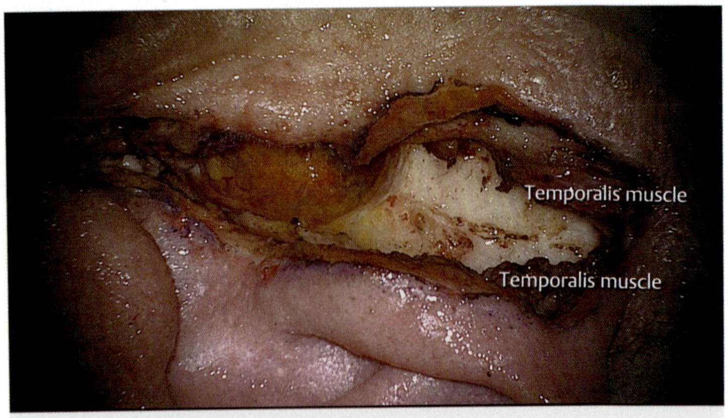

Fig. 11.221 The retractors are removed.

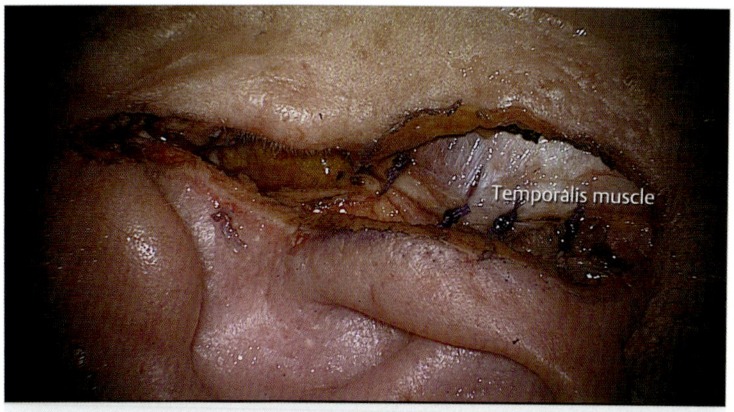

Fig. 11.222 The temporalis muscle is sutured.

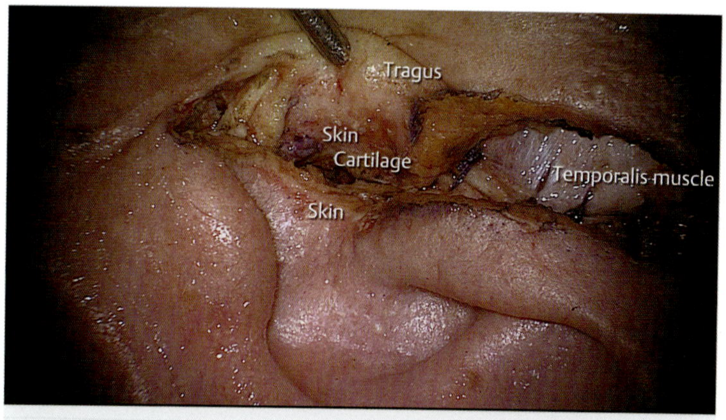

Fig. 11.223 The cutaneous flaps of the external ear canal are sutured.

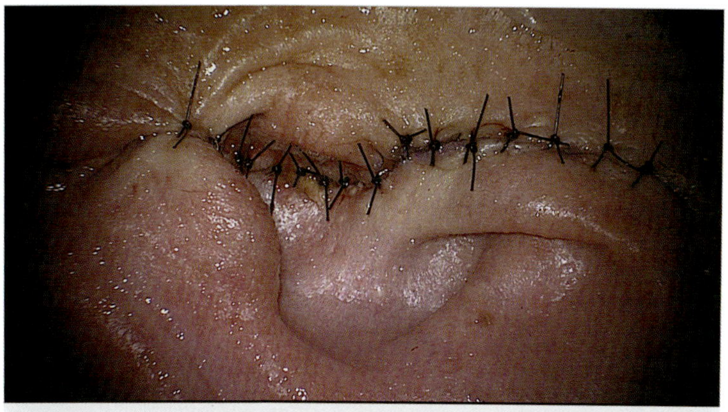

Fig. 11.224 The skin flaps are sutured. There is no need for a compressive wound dressing; an adhesive dressing is placed over the wound.

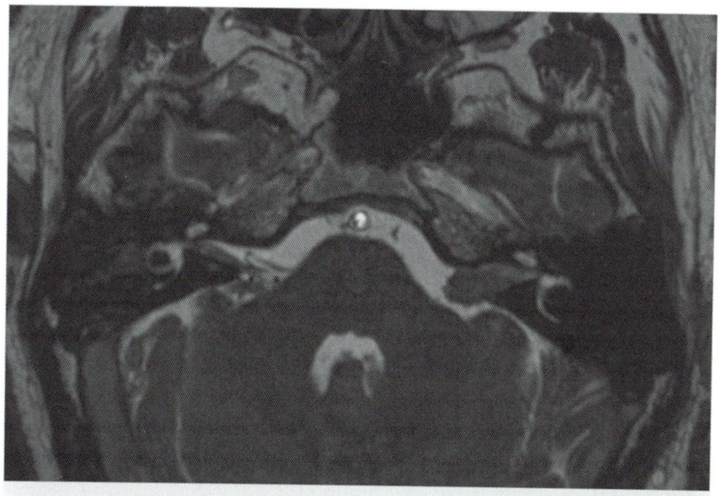

Fig. 11.225 Left side: Axial magnetic resonance imaging (MRI). Acoustic neuroma (Koos II) involving the internal auditory canal (IAC) till the fundus.

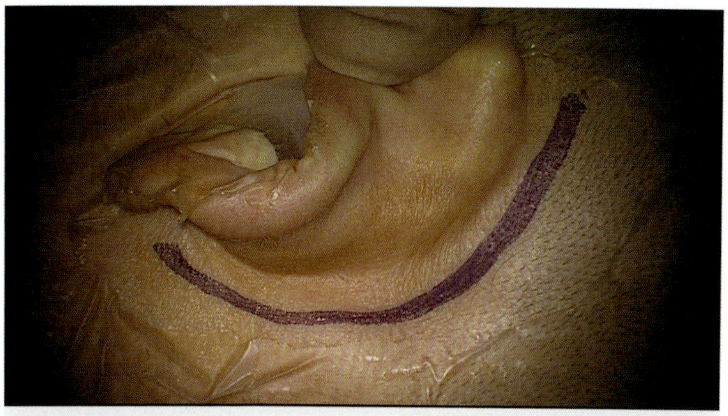

Fig. 11.226 Left side: A skin incision is made following the retroauricolar sulcus.

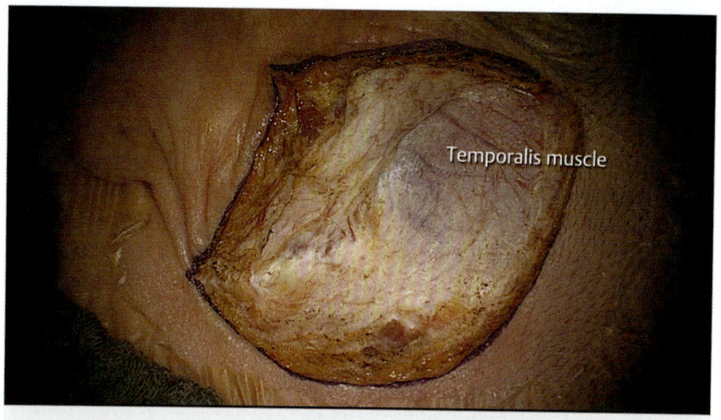

Fig. 11.227 The skin flap is raised over the temporalis muscle fascia; the posterior edge of the external auditory canal (EAC) must be identified.

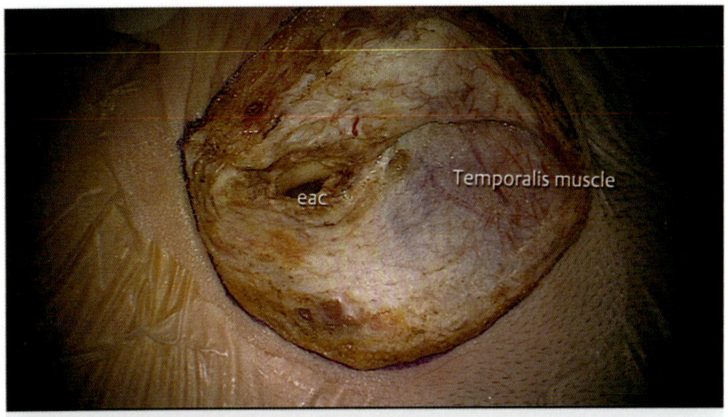

Fig. 11.228 The skin of the external auditory canal (EAC) is circumferentially cut at the ostecartilaginous junction; then the flap is raised anteriorly. *eac: external auditory canal.*

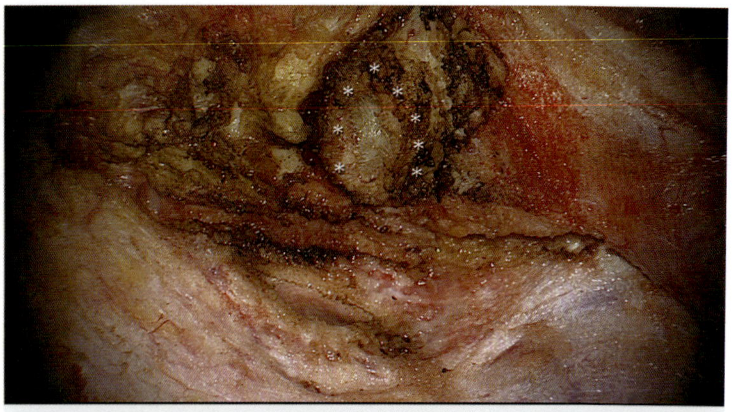

Fig. 11.229 The skin of the external auditory canal (EAC) is detached from the cartilaginous portion of the EAC.

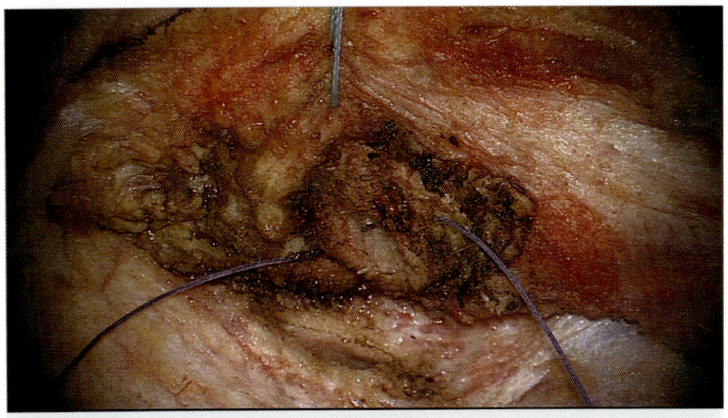

Fig. 11.230 A suture is passed through the internal margins of the skin of the external auditory canal (EAC).

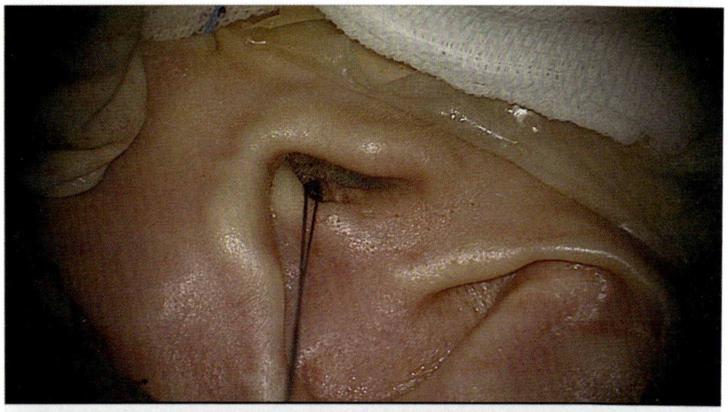

Fig. 11.231 The suture is outwardly pulled through the external auditory canal (EAC) to evert the EAC skin flaps.

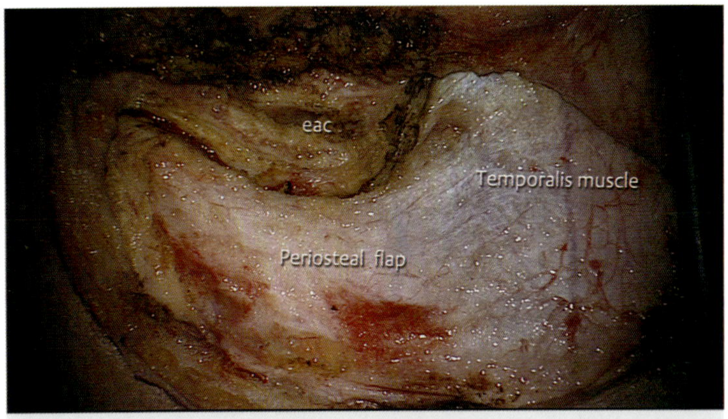

Fig. 11.232 The incision is then made through the temporalis muscle and the periosteal layer, following the posterior border of the external auditory canal (EAC), to uncover the mastoid bone. *eac: external auditory canal.*

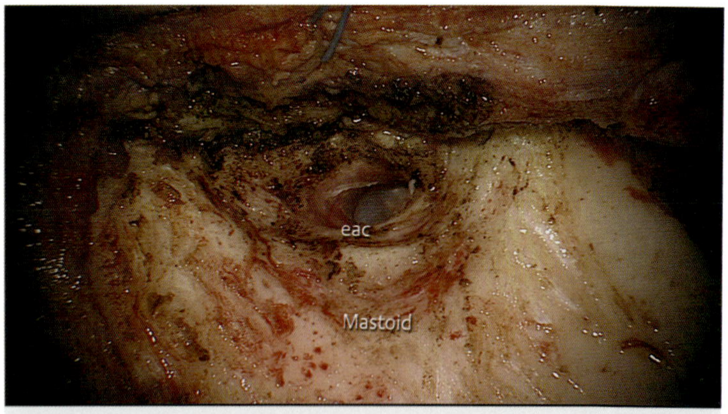

Fig. 11.233 The muscle-periosteal flap is superiorly elevated uncovering the mastoid bone and the skin is detached from the lateral portion of the external auditory canal (EAC) and removed. *eac: external auditory canal.*

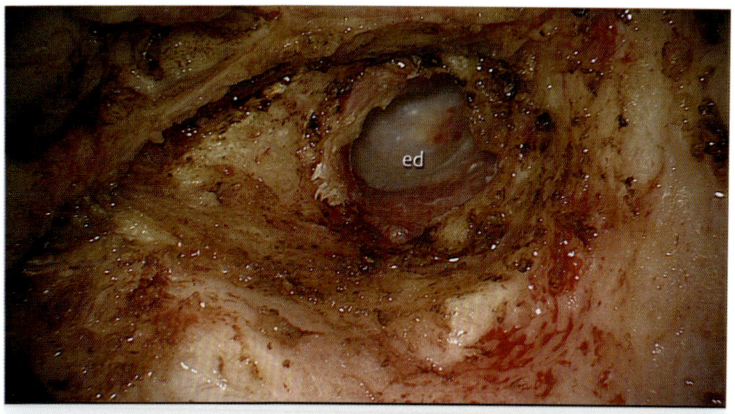

Fig. 11.234 The eardrum is then visualized. *ed: eardrum.*

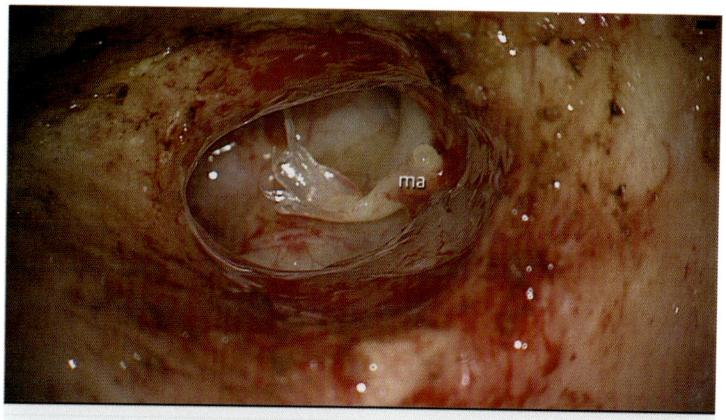

Fig. 11.235 The skin of the medial portion of the external auditory canal (EAC) and the eardrum are removed en bloc. *Ma: malleus.*

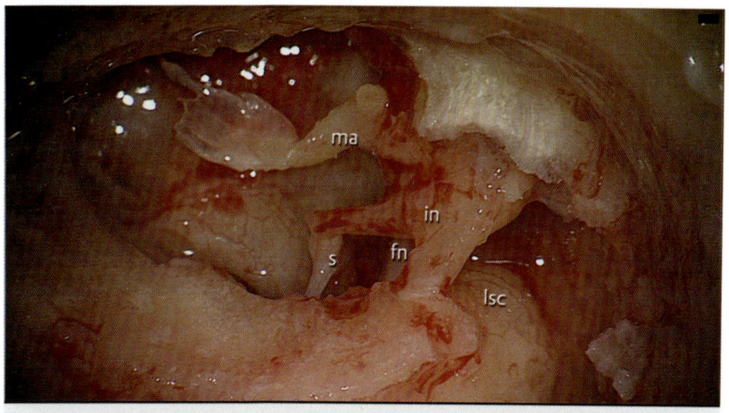

Fig. 11.236 The external ear canal is circumferentially drilled to expose the tympanic cavity. *fn: facial nerve; in: incus; lsc: lateral semicircular canal; ma: malleus; s: stapes.*

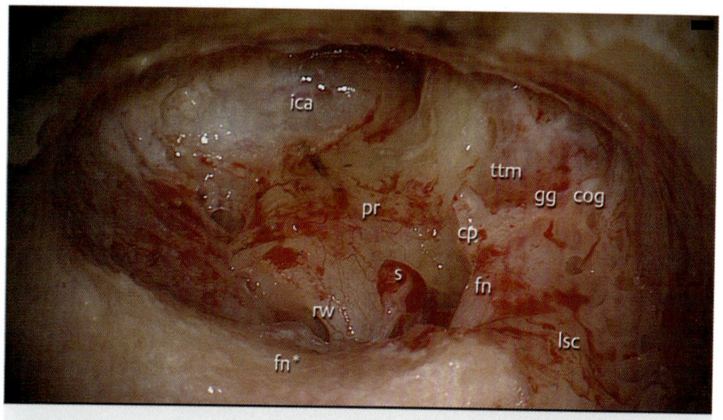

Fig. 11.237 The incus and the malleus are removed. The promontory, the tympanic tract of the facial nerve, the area of the geniculate ganglion, and the internal carotid are visible. *cog: cog; cp: cochleariform process; fn: facial nerve; fn*: mastoid segment of facial nerve; gg: geniculate ganglion; ica: internal carotid artery; lsc: lateral semicircular canal; pr: promontory; rw: round window; s: stapes; ttm: tensor tendon muscle.*

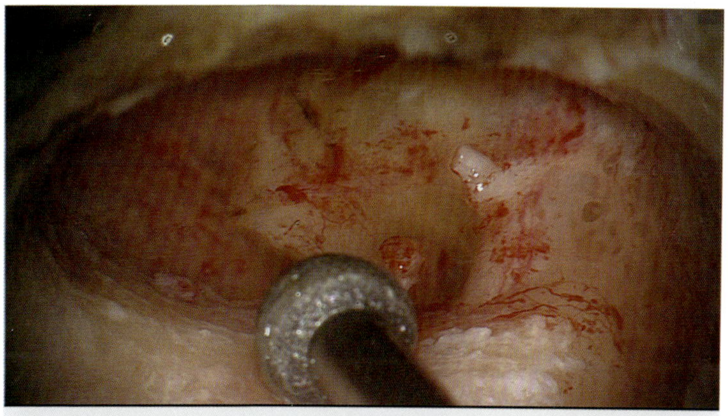

Fig. 11.238 The facial wall is drilled and lowered; during this step the surgical field must be irrigated to prevent thermal damage to the nerve.

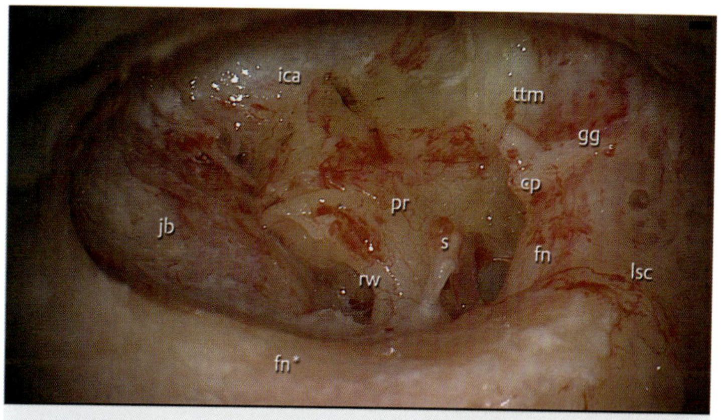

Fig. 11.239 The III tract of the facial nerve (FN) is identified. The jugular bulb represents the inferior limit of the dissection. This case is an example of high riding jugular bulb. An high riding jugular bulb can be an exclusion criterion for this type of approach because it limits the operative space to get to the porus. *cp: cochleariform process; fn: facial nerve; fn*: mastoid segment of facial nerve; gg: geniculate ganglion; ica: internal carotid artery; jb: jugular bulb; lsc: lateral semicircular canal; pr: promontory; rw: round window; s: stapes; ttm: tensor tendon muscle.*

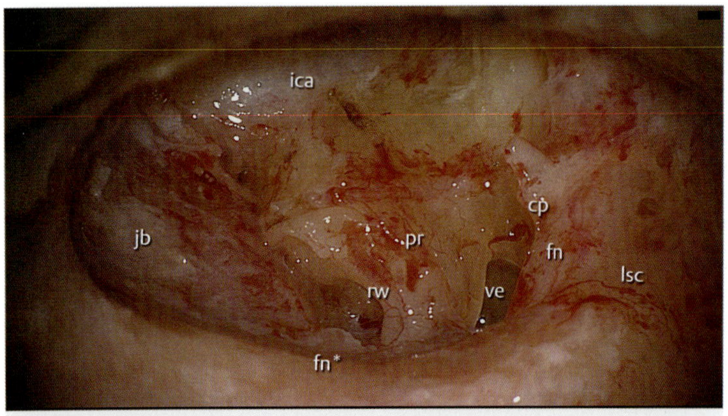

Fig. 11.240 The stapes is removed and the vestibule uncovered. *cp: cochleariform process; fn: facial nerve; fn*: mastoid segment of facial nerve; ica: internal carotid artery; jb: jugular bulb; lsc: lateral semicircular canal; pr: promontory; rw: round window; ve: vestibule.*

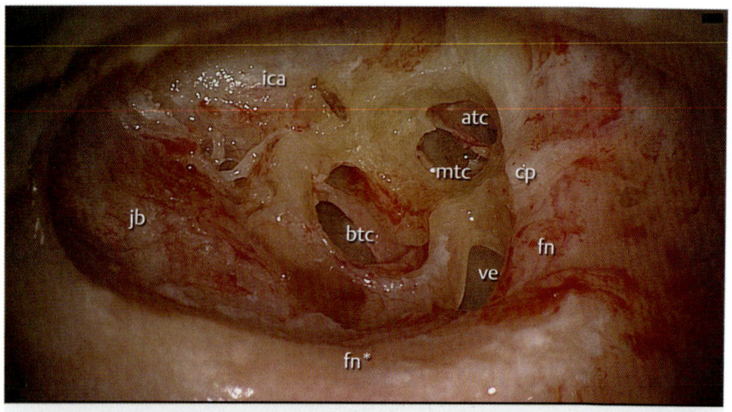

Fig. 11.241 The cochlea is opened and the basal, middle, and apical turns exposed. *atc: apical turn of the cochlea; btc: basal turn of the cochlea; cp: cochleariform process; fn: facial nerve; fn*: mastoid segment of facial nerve; ica: internal carotid artery; jb: jugular bulb; mtc: middle turn of the cochlea; ve: vestibule.*

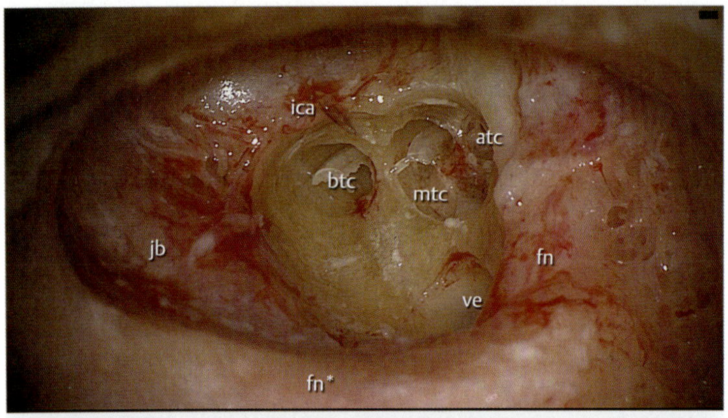

Fig. 11.242 The cochleovestibular bone is a landmark for the internal auditory canal (IAC). *atc: apical turn of the cochlea; btc: basal turn of the cochlea; fn: facial nerve; fn*: mastoid segment of facial nerve; ica: internal carotid artery; jb: jugular bulb; mtc: middle turn of the cochlea; ve: vestibule.*

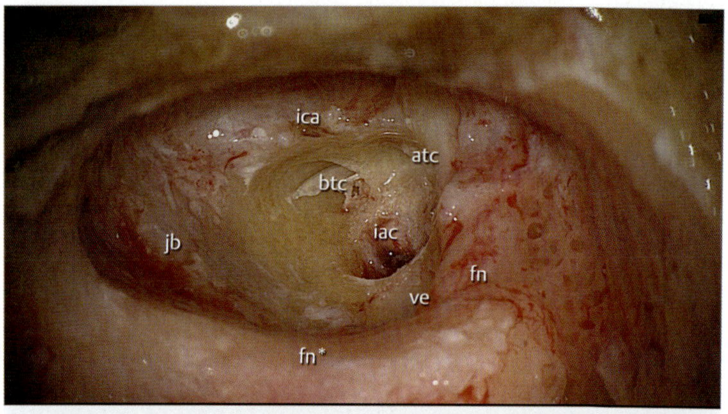

Fig. 11.243 The cochleovestibular bone is removed to gain access to the fundus of the internal auditory canal (IAC). It is important to notice the borders of the dissection: the jugular bulb inferiorly, the internal carotid artery anteriorly, and the facial nerve (FN) posteriorly (mastoid segment) and superiorly (tympanic segment). *atc: apical turn of the cochlea; btc: basal turn of the cochlea; fn: facial nerve; fn*: mastoid segment of facial nerve; iac: internal auditory canal; ica: internal carotid artery; jb: jugular bulb; ve: vestibule.*

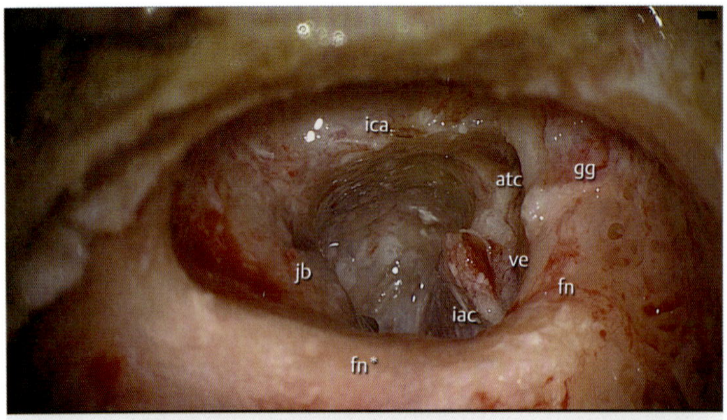

Fig. 11.244 The internal auditory canal (IAC) is skeletonized, drilling the bone inferiorly in a horseshoe shape till the porus. *atc: apical turn of the cochlea; fn: facial nerve; fn*: mastoid segment of facial nerve; gg: geniculate ganglion; iac: internal auditory canal; ica: internal carotid artery; jb: jugular bulb; ve: vestibule.*

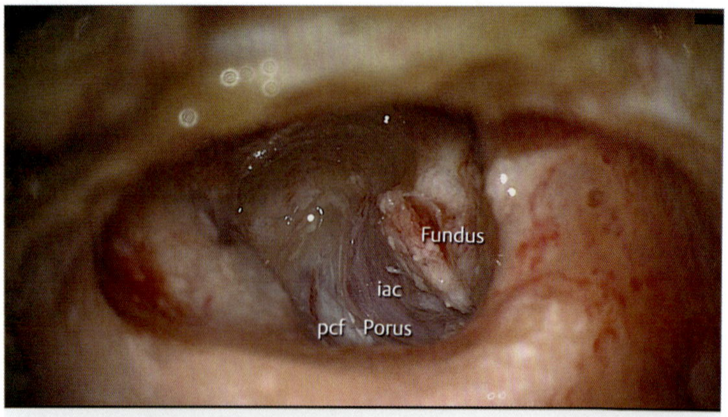

Fig. 11.245 Drilling has to be carried out from the internal carotid artery to the anterior portion of the internal auditory canal (IAC), from the juguar bulb to the inferior edge of the IAC, from the III tract of the facial nerve (FN) to the posterior edge of the FN. The skeletonization is performed till the porus; the blue lining of the dura reflecting on the petrous bone represents the in-depth limit of the dissection. *iac: internal auditory canal; pcf: posterior cranial fossa.*

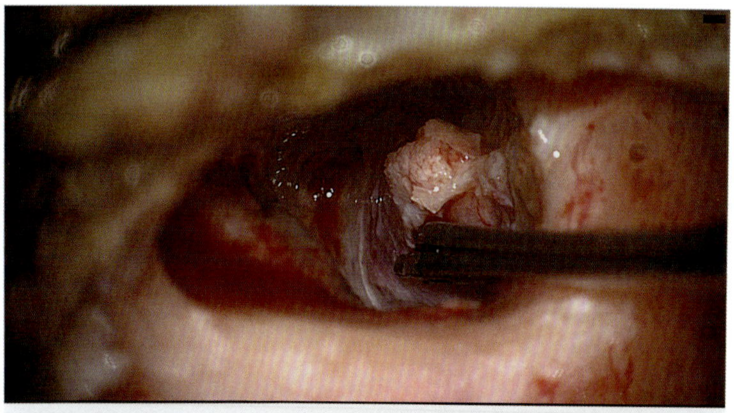

Fig. 11.246 The dura is longitudinally cut using microscissors.

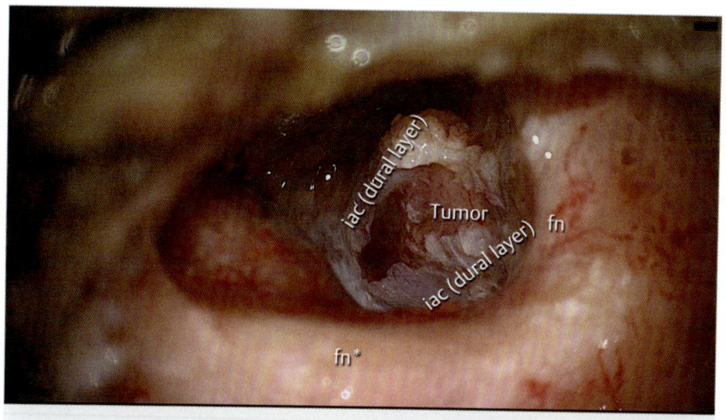

Fig. 11.247 The neuroma is exposed under the dural lining. *fn: facial nerve; fn*: mastoid segment of facial nerve; iac: internal auditory canal.*

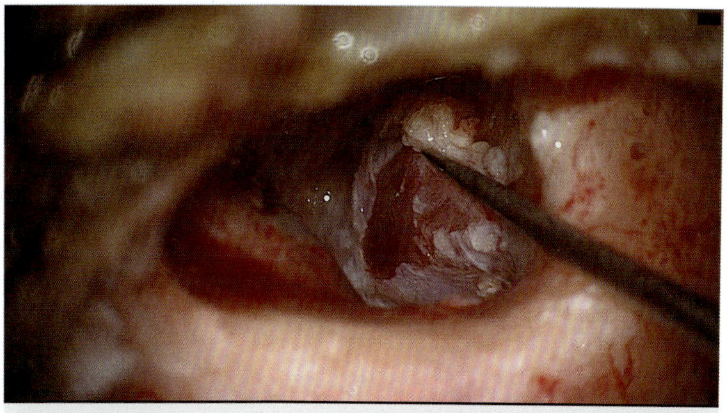

Fig. 11.248 The dural flaps are detached from the underlying neuroma, to expose the whole lesion in the internal auditory canal (IAC).

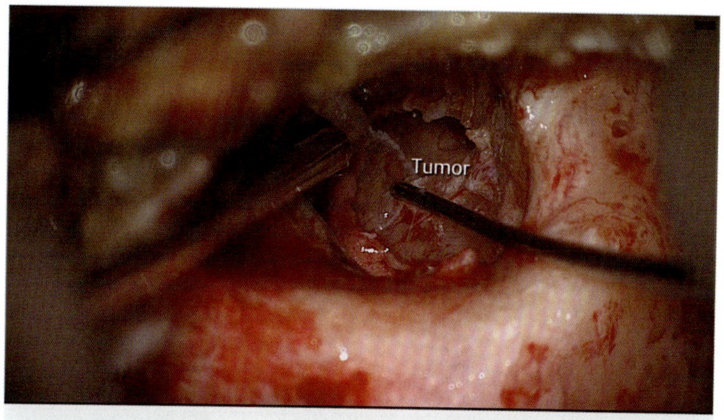

Fig. 11.249 The vestibular schwannoma is dissected keeping its capsule intact, using a two-handed microscopic technique.

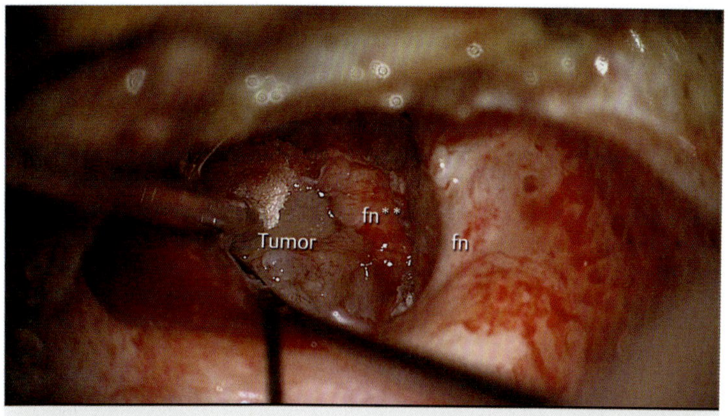

Fig. 11.250 The vestibular schwannoma is very gently detached from the nervous structures. *fn: facial nerve; fn**: facial nerve into the IAC.*

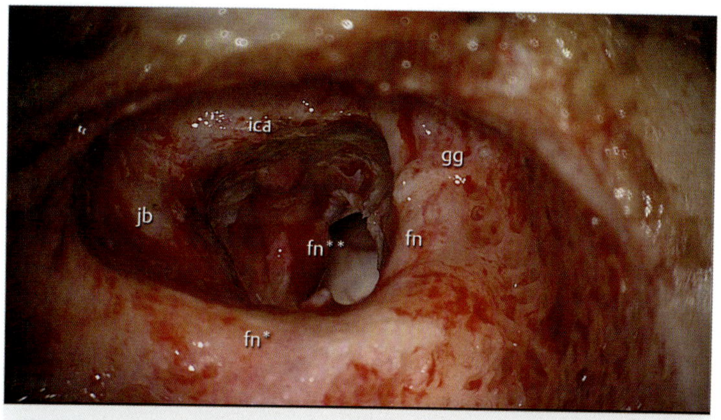

Fig. 11.251 The vestibular schwannoma has been entirely removed. The porus is visible through the promotorial defect. *fn: facial nerve; fn*: mastoid segment of facial nerve; fn**: facial nerve into the IAC; gg: geniculate ganglion; ica: internal carotid artery; jb: jugular bulb.*

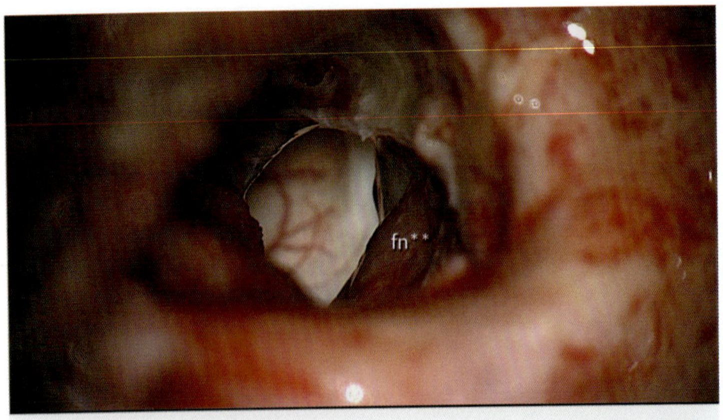

Fig. 11.252 Closer microscopic look at the facial nerve (FN) inside the cerebellopontine angle. *fn**: facial nerve into the cerebellopontine angle (CPA).*

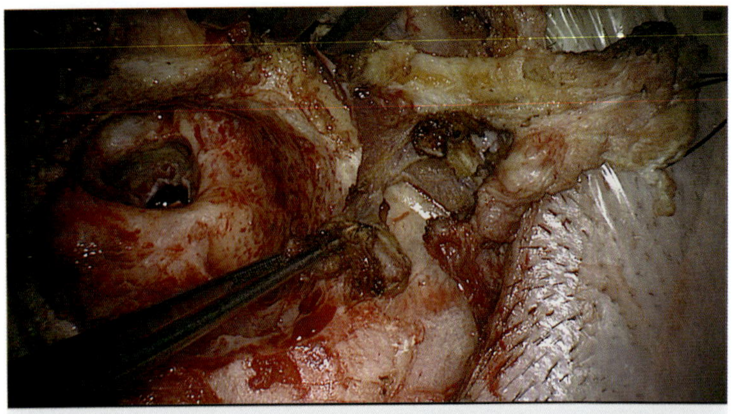

Fig. 11.253 A muscle fragment is harvested from the temporalis muscle.

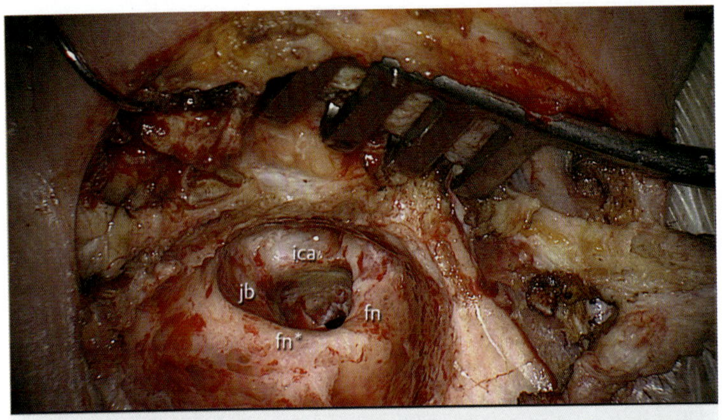

Fig. 11.254 The surgical field is checked and washed with an antibiotic solution. *fn: facial nerve; fn*: mastoid segment of facial nerve; ica: internal carotid artery; jb: jugular bulb.*

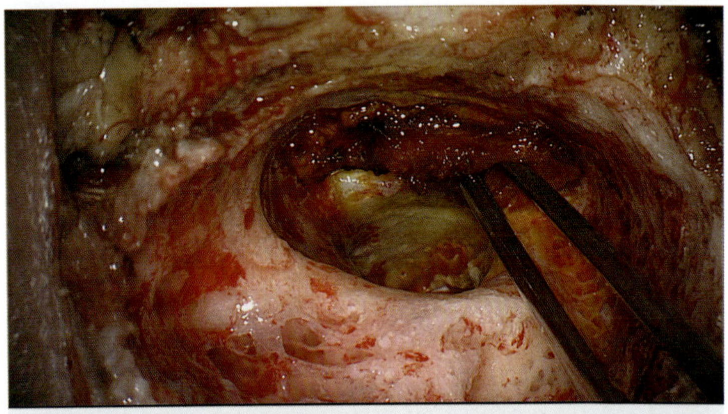

Fig. 11.255 The muscle fragment is pushed inside the eustachian tube to close it.

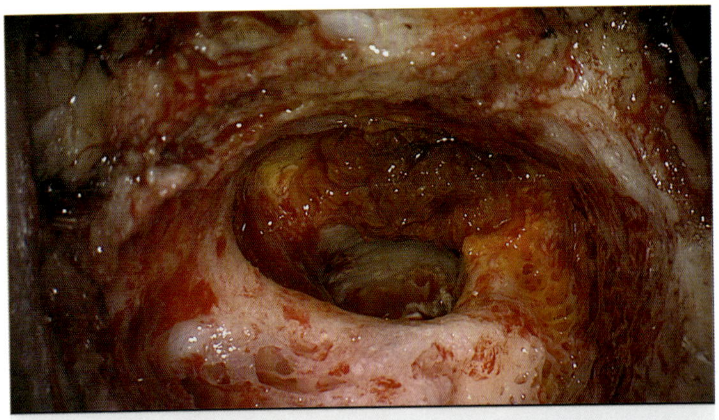

Fig. 11.256 Tabotamp and fibrin glue are used to reinforce the closure of the eustachian tube.

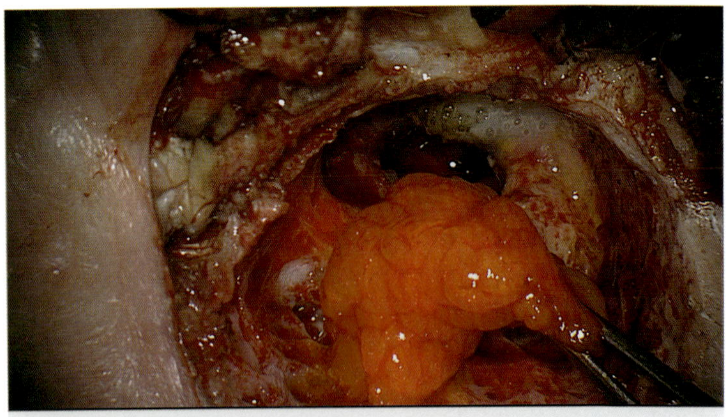

Fig. 11.257 Fat, harvested from the abdomen, is placed in the promontorial defect, to seal the cavity and separate the cerebellopontine angle (CPA) from the timpanic cavity.

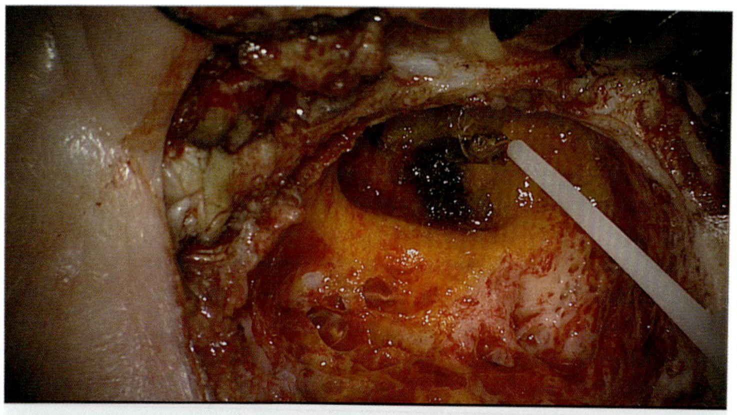

Fig. 11.258 Tabotamp is used to push the fat inside the promonotrial defect and then fibrin glue is poured over to stabilize the seal.

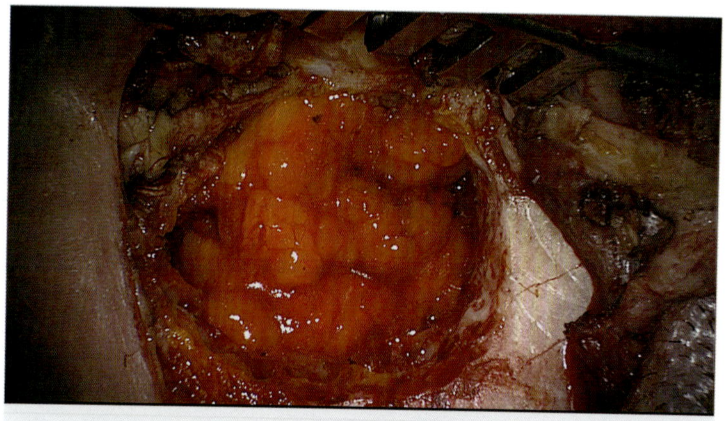

Fig. 11.259 The surgical cavity is filled with fat.

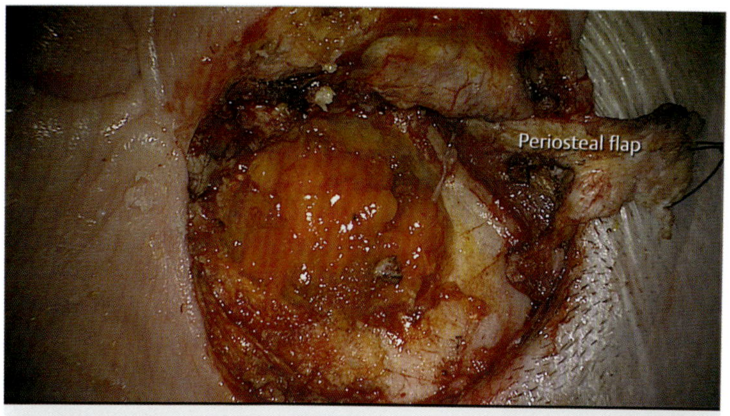

Fig. 11.260 The temporalis muscle flap is repositioned and sutured.

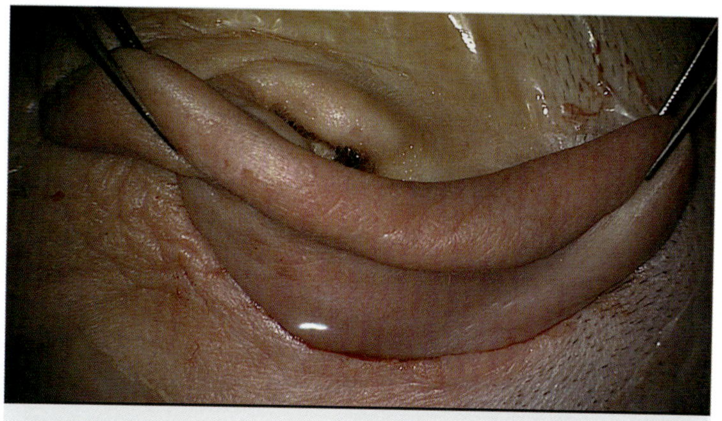

Fig. 11.261 The skin is sutured using intradermal stiches.

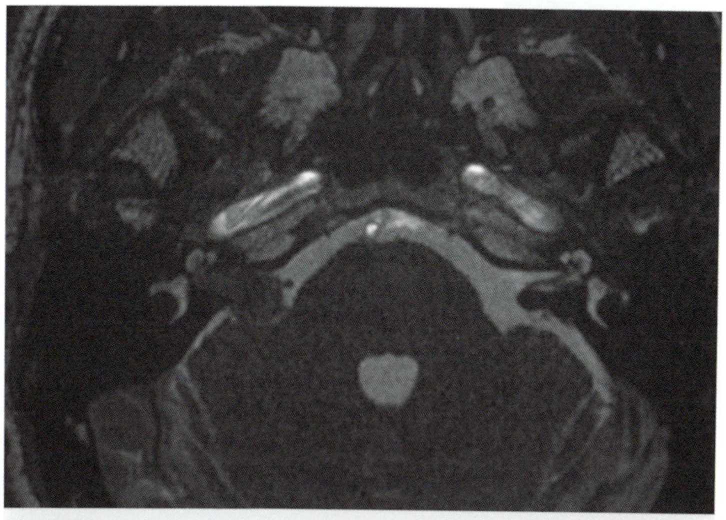

Fig. 11.262 Right side: Axial magnetic resonance imaging (MRI). Acoustic neuroma (Koos III) involving the internal auditory canal (IAC) till the fundus and with a straight-line extension into the cerebello-pontine angle (CPA) with involvement of the entry zone.

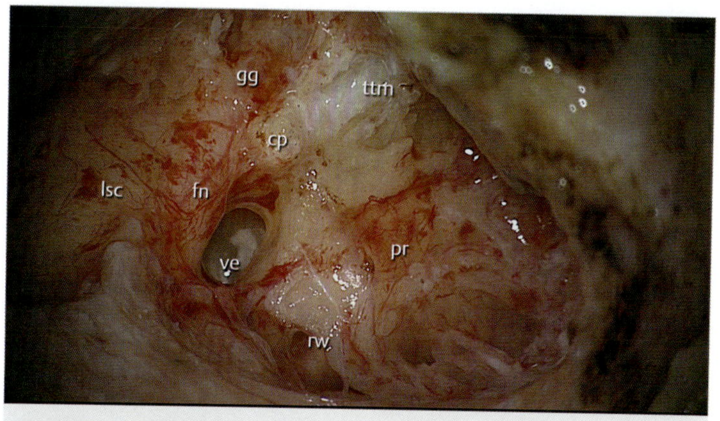

Fig. 11.263 Right side: The ossicular chain has been removed uncovering the vestibule. The spherical recess is visible in its depth. *cp: cochleariform process; fn: facial nerve; gg: geniculate ganglion; lsc: lateral semicircular canal; pr: promontory; rw: round window; ttm: tensor tendon muscle; ve: vestibule.*

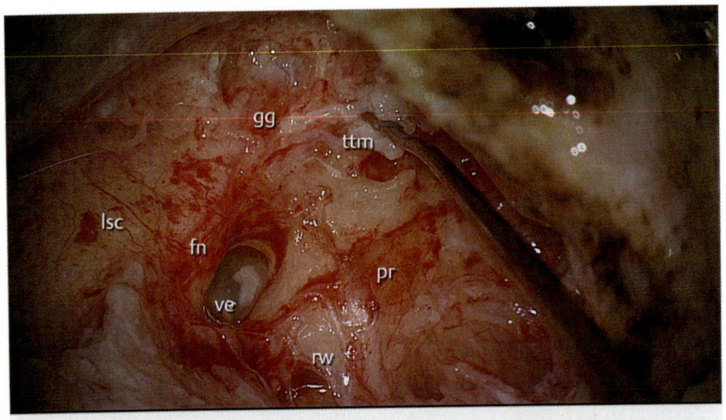

Fig. 11.264 The tensor tympani muscle is removed to enlarge the operative field. *fn: facial nerve; gg: geniculate ganglion; lsc: lateral semicircular canal; pr: promontory; rw: round window; ttm: tensor tendon muscle; ve: vestibule.*

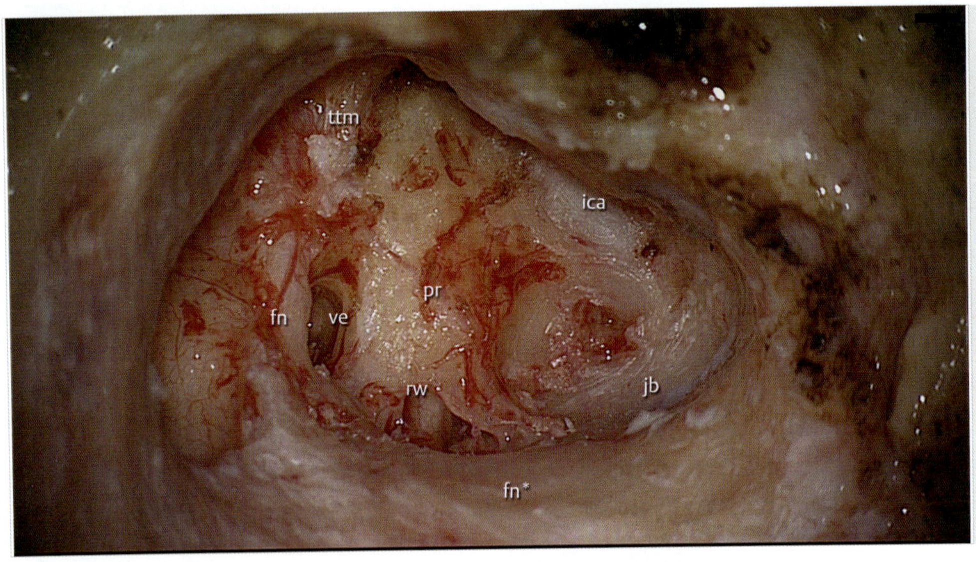

Fig. 11.265 The jugular bulb and the carotid artery are identified; they represent our surgical boundaries. *fn: facial nerve; fn*: mastoid segment of facial nerve; ica: internal carotid artery; jb: jugular bulb; pr: promontory; rw: round window; ttm: tensor tendon muscle; ve: vestibule.*

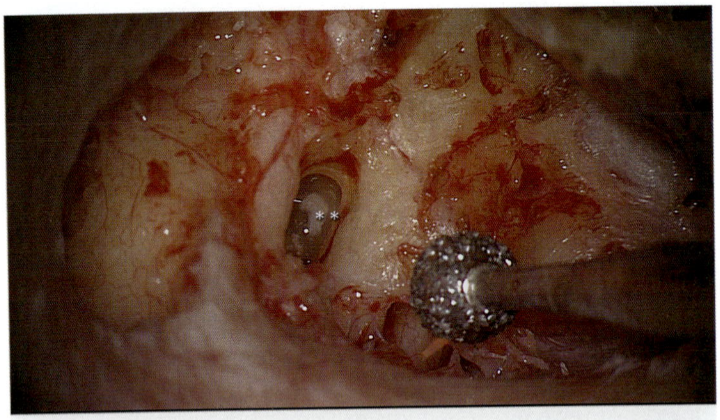

Fig. 11.266 The promontory is drilled and the cochlea uncovered. **: *spherical recess.*

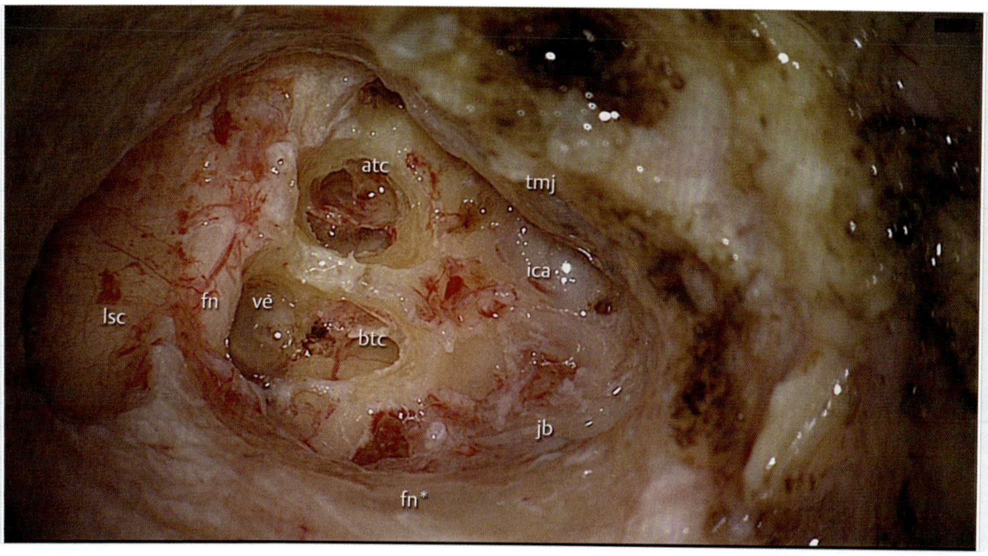

Fig. 11.267 The basal and apical turns of the cochlea are unroofed. All the landmarks of the dissection are now visible. *atc: apical turn of the cochlea; btc: basal turn of the cochlea; fn: facial nerve; fn*: mastoid segment of facial nerve; ica: internal carotid artery; jb: jugular bulb; lsc: lateral semicircular canal; tmj: temporomandibular joint; ve: vestibule.*

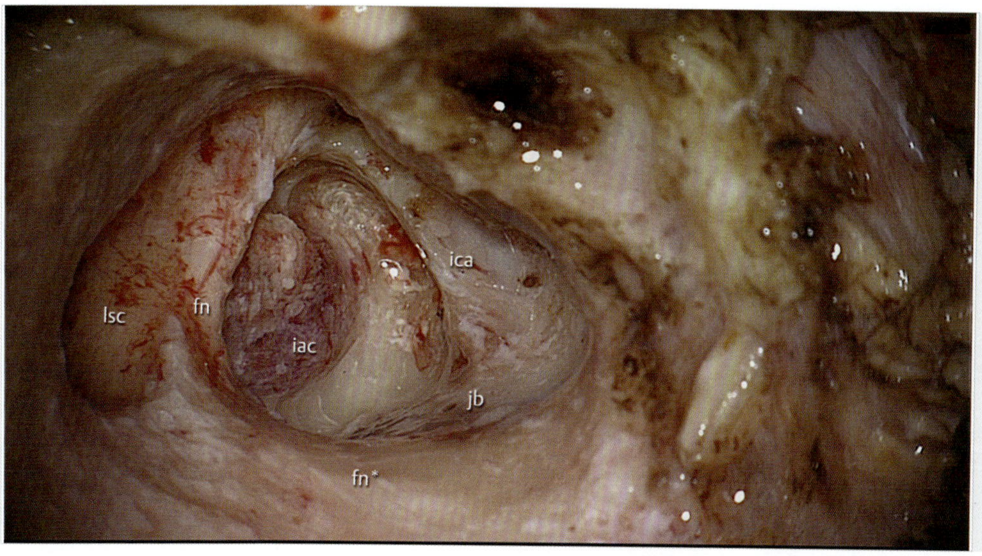

Fig. 11.268 The bone between the facial nerve (FN), the internal carotid artery, and the jugular bulb is removed and the dura of the internal auditory canal (IAC) exposed till the porus. *fn: facial nerve; fn*: mastoid segment of facial nerve; iac: internal auditory canal; ica: internal carotid artery; jb: jugular bulb; lsc: lateral semicircular canal.*

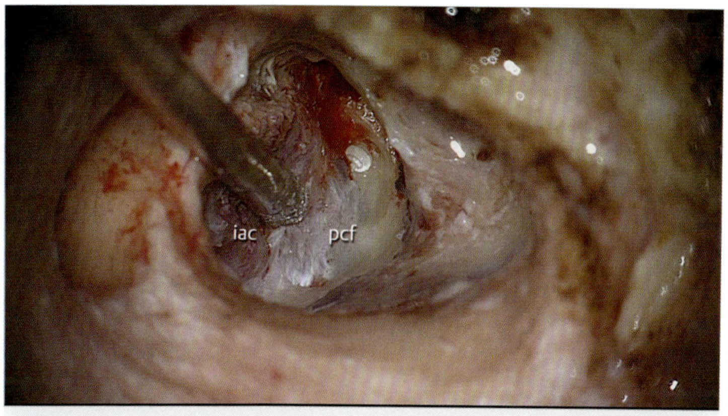

Fig. 11.269 In this image, the internal auditory canal (IAC) is anterosuperiorly gently pushed with the aspirator to expose the bone between the vascular structures that must be removed to completely skeletonize the IAC and to reach the blue lining of the dura of the medial surface of the petrous bone. *iac: internal auditory canal; pcf: posterior cranial fossa.*

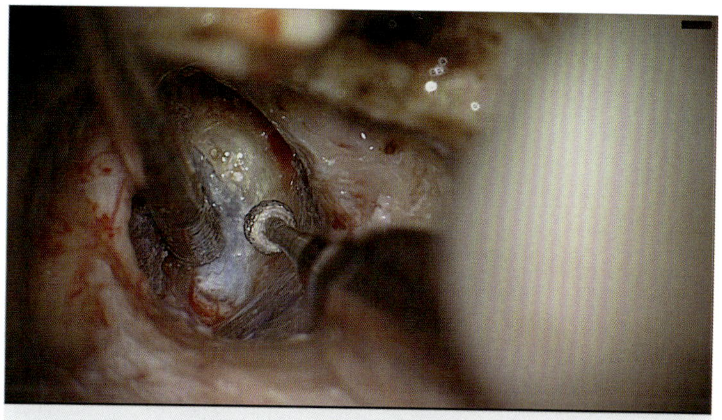

Fig. 11.270 A diamond bur is used to drill the last layer of bone; the blue color of the dura is clearly visible in the depth of the operative field. This meningeal sheet must be cut to enter the cerebellopontine angle (CPA).

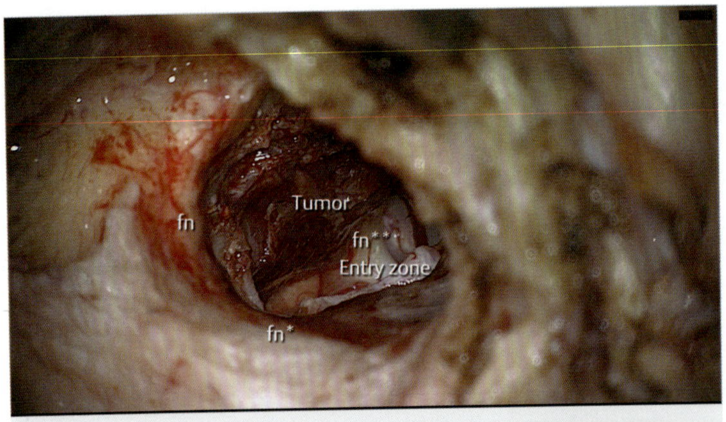

Fig. 11.271 The dura of the posterior cranial fossa is incised. The incision is carried out below the porus, the projection area of the entry zone. *fn: facial nerve; fn*: mastoid segment of facial nerve; fn**: facial nerve into the cerebellopontine angle (CPA).*

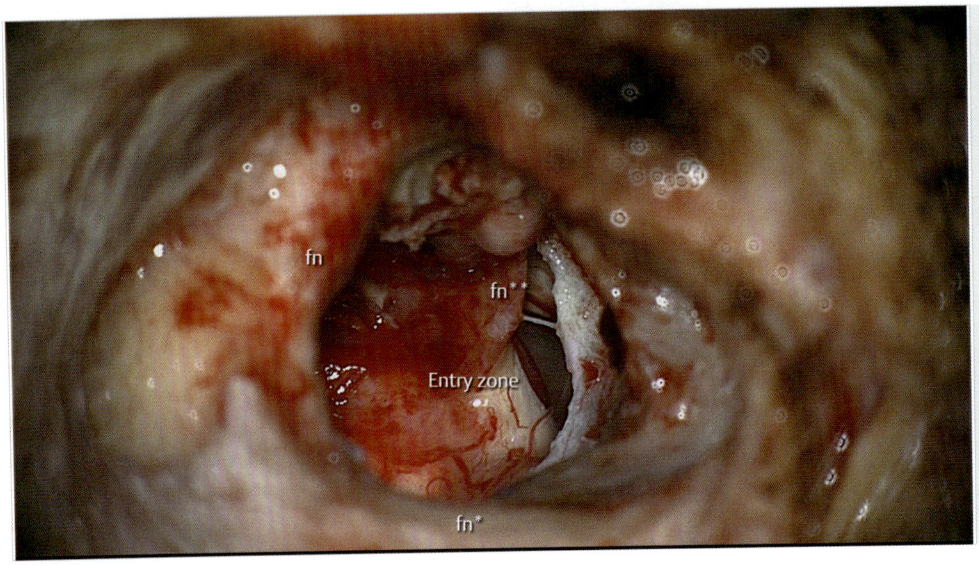

Fig. 11.272 The vestibular schwannoma is removed starting from the entry zone to the fundus of the internal auditory canal (IAC). *fn: facial nerve; fn*: mastoid segment of facial nerve; fn**: facial nerve into the cerebellopontine angle (CPA).*

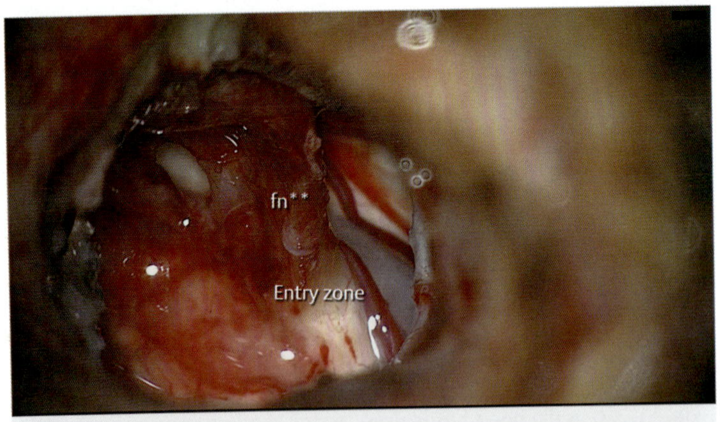

Fig. 11.273 Microscopic magnification of the entry zone area. Notice how the surgeon is just in front of this region after performing the transcanal enlarged approach. *fn**: facial nerve into the cerebellopontine angle (CPA).*

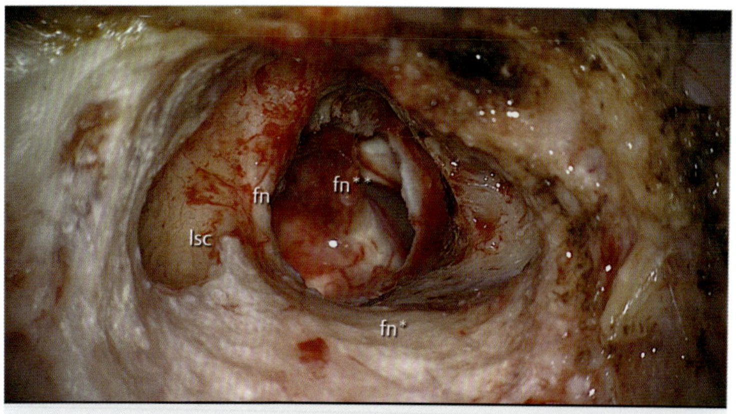

Fig. 11.274 Microscopic view of the CPA after vestibular schwannoma removal. *fn: facial nerve; fn*: mastoid segment of facial nerve; fn**: facial nerve into the cerebellopontine angle (CPA); lsc: lateral semicircular canal.*

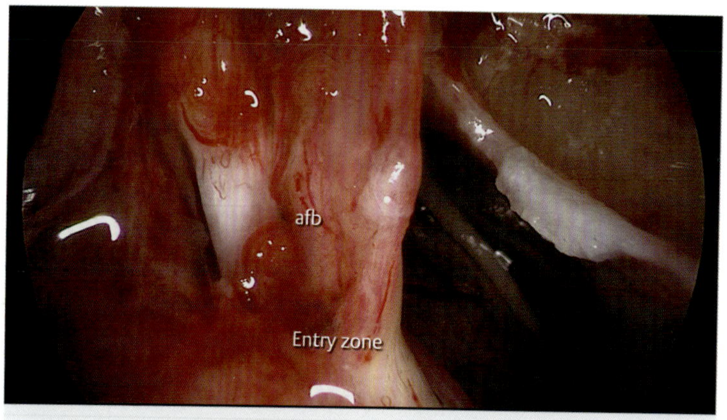

Fig. 11.275 Endoscopic view of the cerebellopontine angle (CPA) (0 degree, 15 cm length, 4 mm diameter). The endoscope is inserted to check the radicality of the excision. The entry zone area is just in front of the surgeon. *afb: acoustic-facial bundle.*

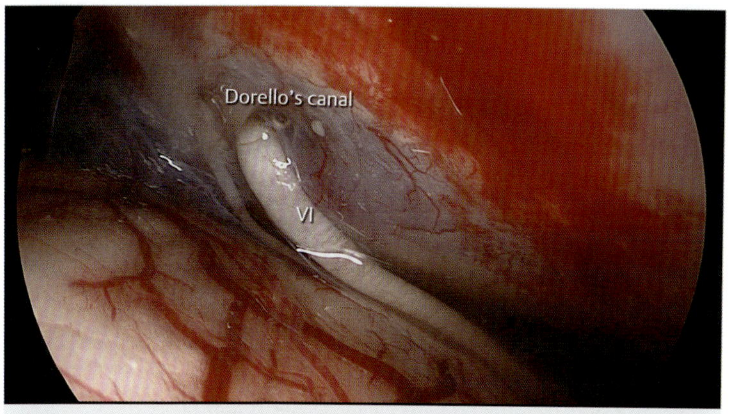

Fig. 11.276 The VI cranial nerve can be pointed out through this approach, till its entry in the Dorello's canal.

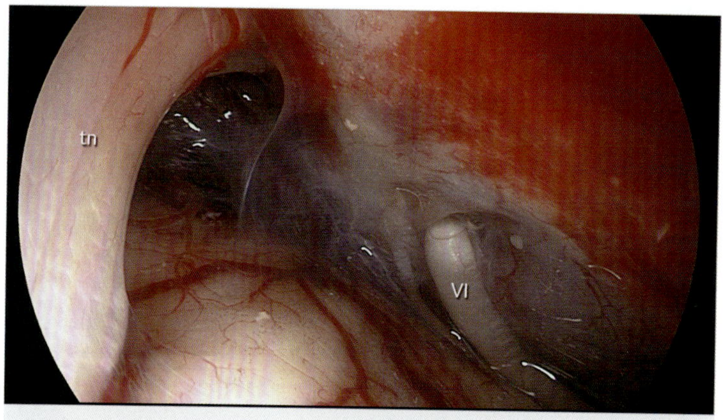

Fig. 11.277 Endoscopic view of the trigeminal nerve arising from the brainstem. *tn: trigeminal nerve.*

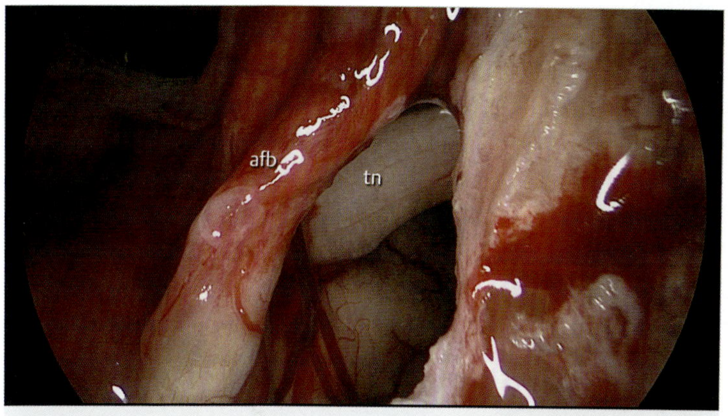

Fig. 11.278 Endoscopic view of the VIII cranial nerve and its relations with the trigeminal nerve. *afb: acoustic-facial bundle; tn: trigeminal nerve.*

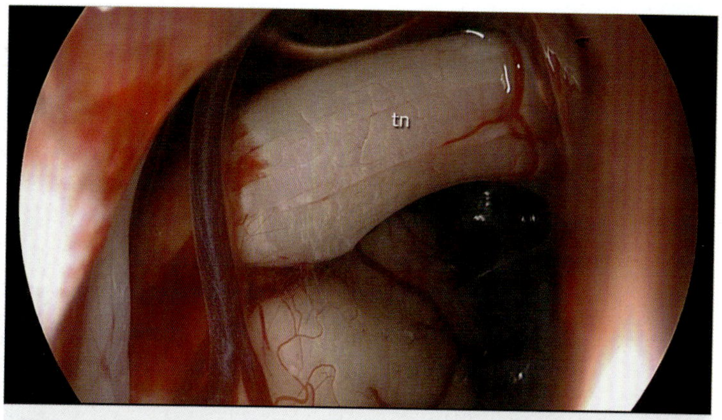

Fig. 11.279 Trigeminal nerve, endoscopic magnification. *tn: trigeminal nerve.*

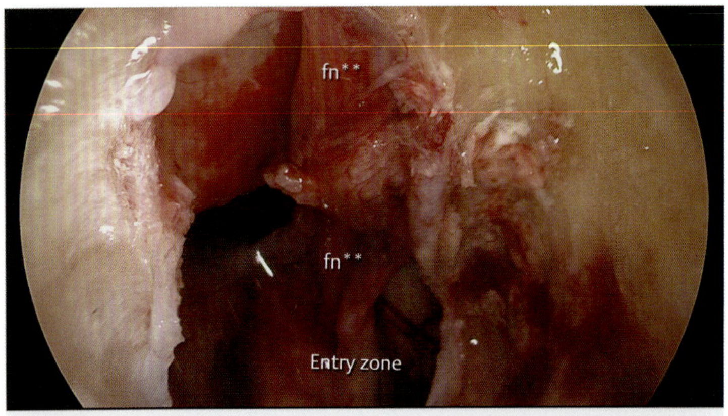

Fig. 11.280 Endoscopic check of the surgical field after the surgical excision. *fn**: facial nerve into the cerebellopontine angle (CPA).*

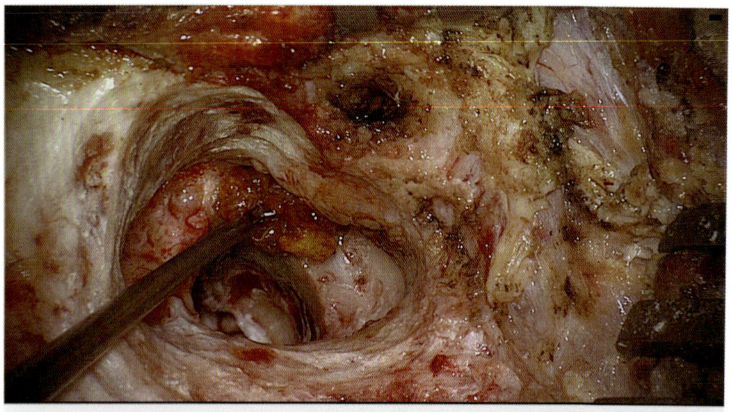

Fig. 11.281 The tube is sealed with a fragment of temporalis muscle.

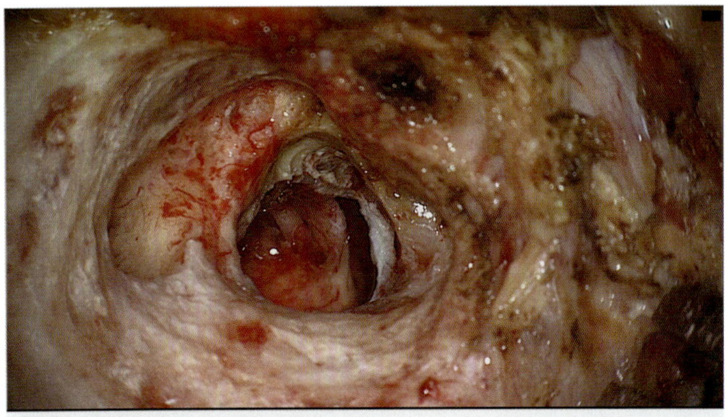

Fig. 11.282 The promontorial defect is microscopically checked.

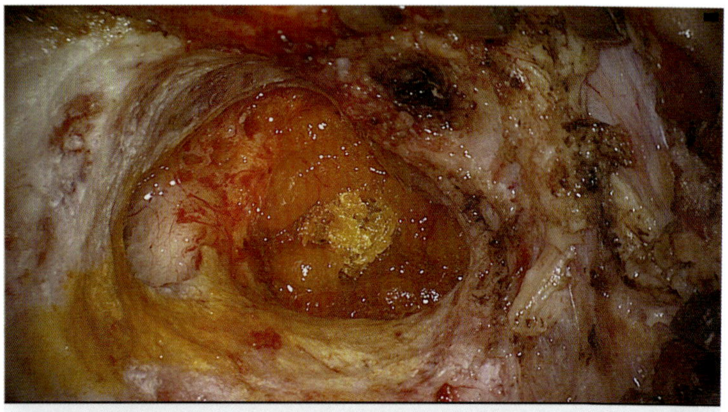

Fig. 11.283 Fat, harvested from the abdomen, is used to fill the surgical cavity, reinforced with cellulose mesh and fibrin glue.

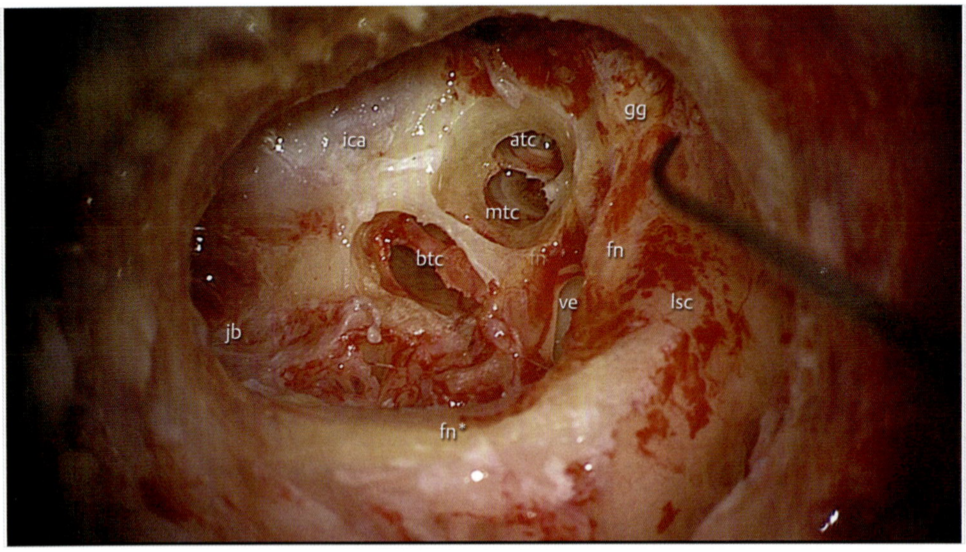

Fig. 11.284 Clinical Case 11, Left side: The promontory has been removed, uncovering the cochlear turns; the vestibule is opened. The tympanic segment, the mastoid segment, and the labyrinthine portions of the facial nerve (FN) are pointed out. *atc: apical turn of the cochlea; btc: basal turn of the cochlea; fn: facial nerve; fn*: mastoid segment of facial nerve; fn**: labyrinthine portion of facial nerve; gg: geniculate ganglion; ica: internal carotid artery; jb: jugular bulb; lsc: lateral semicircular canal; mtc: middle turn of the cochlea; ve: vestibule.*

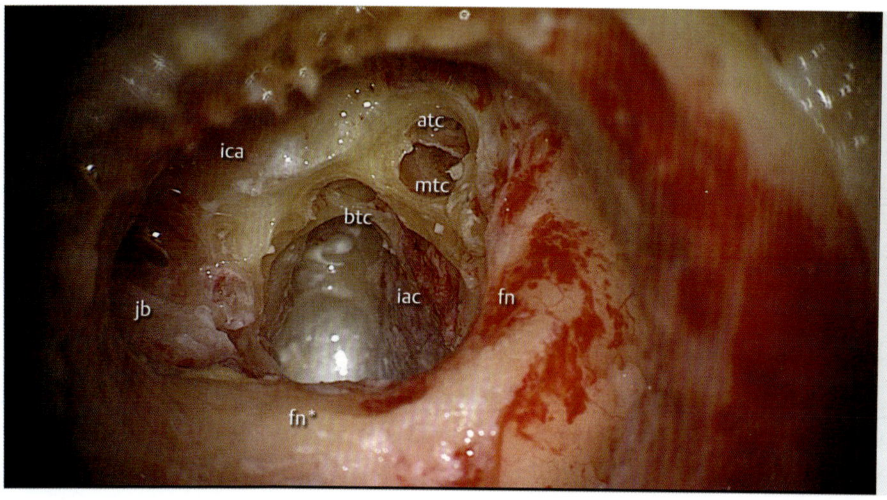

Fig. 11.285 Left side: The dural layer of the internal auditory canal (IAC) is exposed, by drilling the bone between the vestibule and the basal turn of the cochlea; the anatomical orientation of the IAC in relation to the basal, middle, and apical turns of the cochlea is visible. *atc: apical turn of the cochlea; btc: basal turn of the cochlea; fn: facial nerve; fn*: mastoid segment of facial nerve; ica: internal auditory canal; iac: internal carotid artery; jb: jugular bulb; mtc: middle turn of the cochlea.*

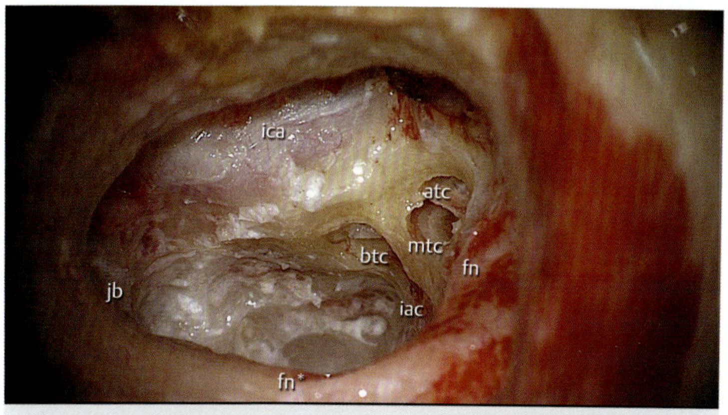

Fig. 11.286 Left side: The vertical portion of the internal carotid artery is exposed. The reader can note the anatomical relationship between the artery and the cochlear turns. *atc: apical turn of the cochlea; btc: basal turn of the cochlea; fn: facial nerve; fn*: mastoid segment of facial nerve; iac: internal auditory canal; ica: internal carotid artery; jb: jugular bulb; mtc: middle turn of the cochlea.*

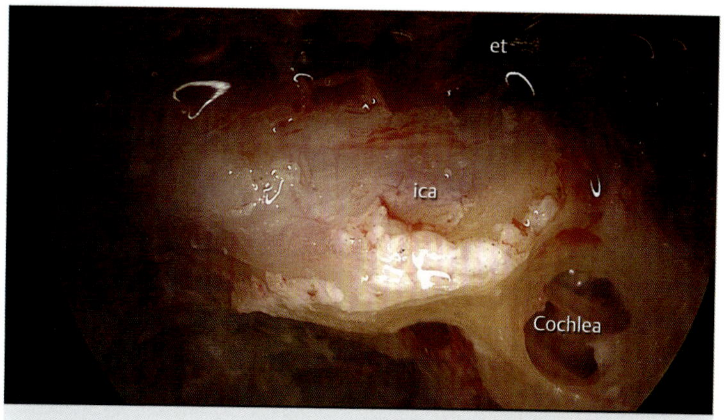

Fig. 11.287 Left side: Endoscopic magnification of the vertical portion of the internal carotid artery. *et: eustachian tube; ica: internal carotid artery.*

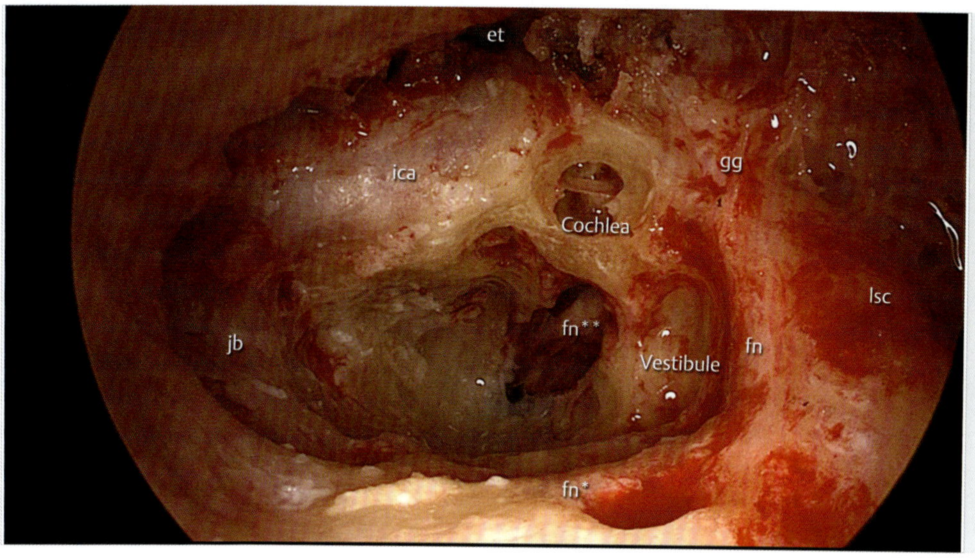

Fig. 11.288 Left side: Endoscopic view after tumor removal from the internal auditory canal (IAC). The facial nerve (FN) inside the IAC can be noticed; the anatomical relationship between the vestibule, cochlea, and IAC is also clearly visible. *et: eustachian tube; fn: facial nerve; fn*: mastoid segment of facial nerve; fn**: facial nerve into the IAC; gg: geniculate ganglion; ica: internal carotid artery; jb: jugular bulb; lsc: lateral semi-circular canal.*

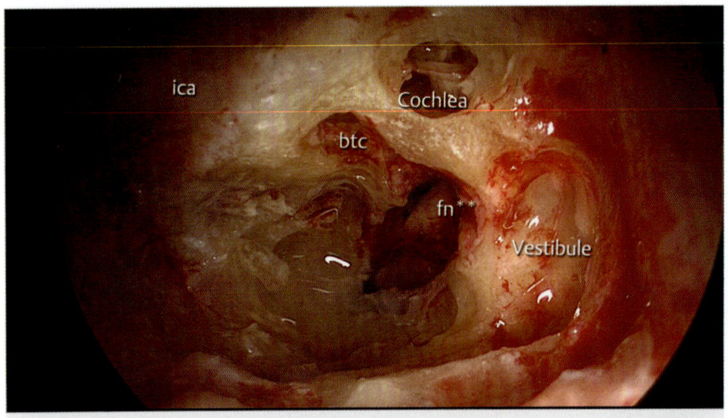

Fig. 11.289 Left side:. Endoscopic view of the fundus of the internal auditory canal (IAC). *btc: basal turn of the cochlea; fn**: facial nerve into the IAC; ica: internal carotid artery.*

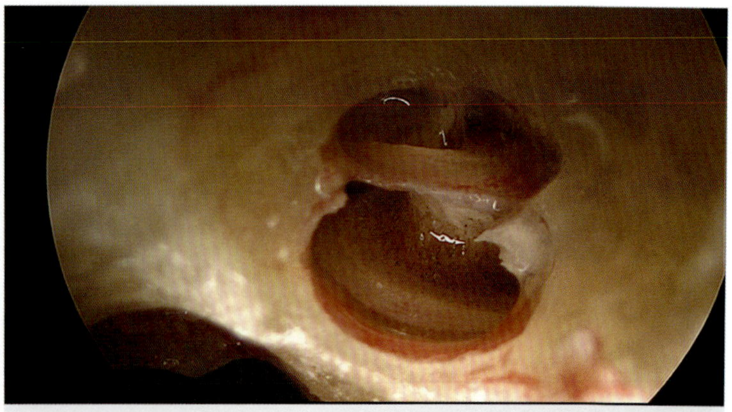

Fig. 11.290 Left side: Endoscopic magnification of the middle and apical turns of the cochlea.

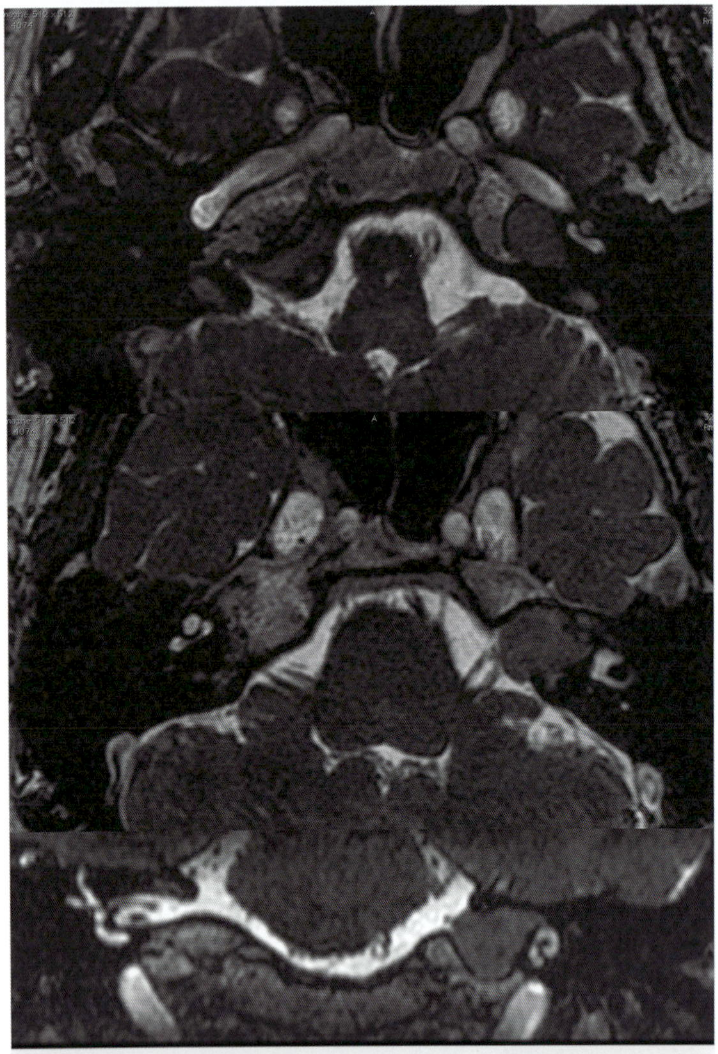

Fig. 11.291 Left side: Axial magnetic resonance imaging (MRI). Acoustic neuroma with atypical extension to the petrous apex extending below the horizontal segment of the internal carotid artery.

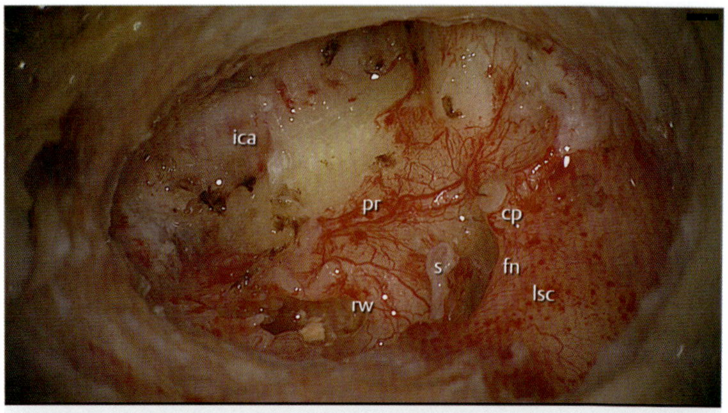

Fig. 11.292 Left side: Microscopic view of the middle ear. The eardrum and the ossicuar chain have been removed. *cp: cochleariform process; fn: facial nerve; ica: internal carotid artery; lsc: lateral semicircular canal; pr: promontory; rw: round window; s: stapes.*

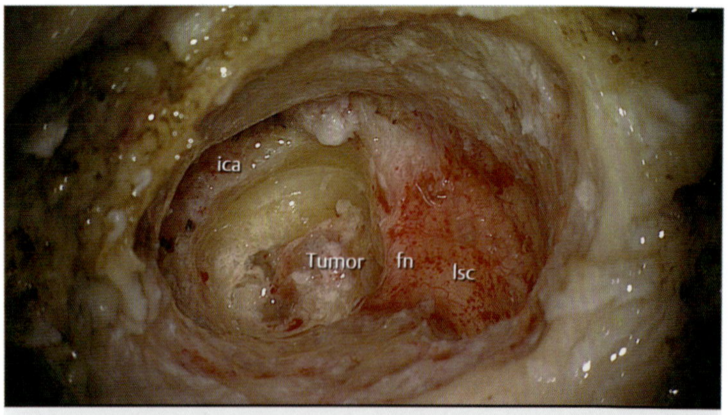

Fig. 11.293 Left side: The internal auditory canal (IAC) is carefully skeletonized till the porus. The area is drilled in a lateral to medial direction and from superiorly to inferiorly, circumnavigating the anterior, posterior, and inferior portions of the IAC. *fn: facial nerve; ica: internal carotid artery; lsc: lateral semicircular canal; tum: tumor.*

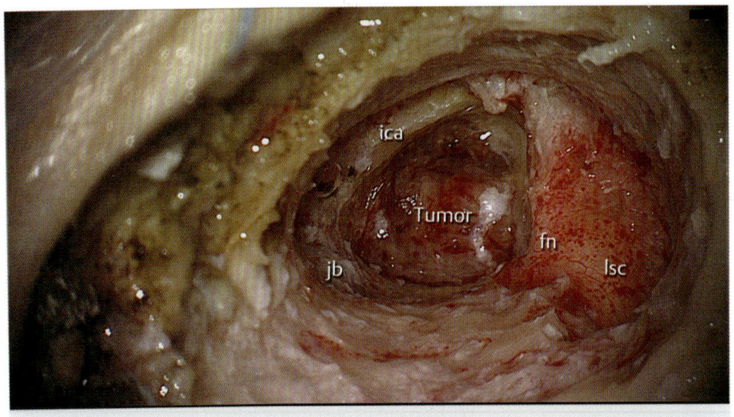

Fig. 11.294 Left side: The dura is longitudinally opened exposing the tumor. *fn: facial nerve; ica: internal carotid artery; jb: jugular bulb; lsc: lateral semicircular canal; tum: tumor.*

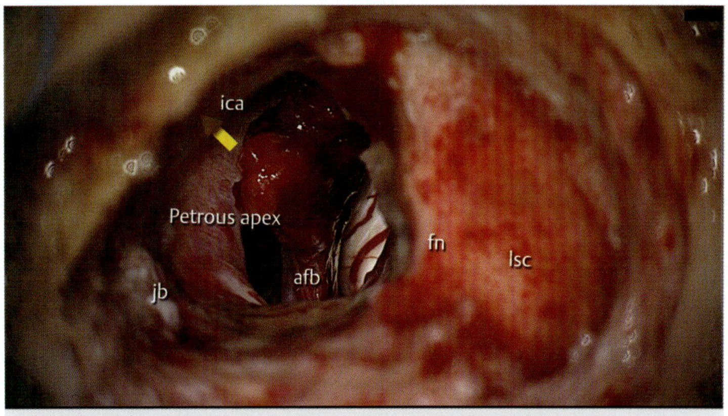

Fig. 11.295 Left side: The lesion extends in the petrous apex, below the vertical and horizontal tracts of the internal carotid artery. *afb: acoustic-facial bundle; fn: facial nerve; ica: internal carotid artery; jb: jugular bulb; lsc: lateral semicircular canal; tum: tumor.*

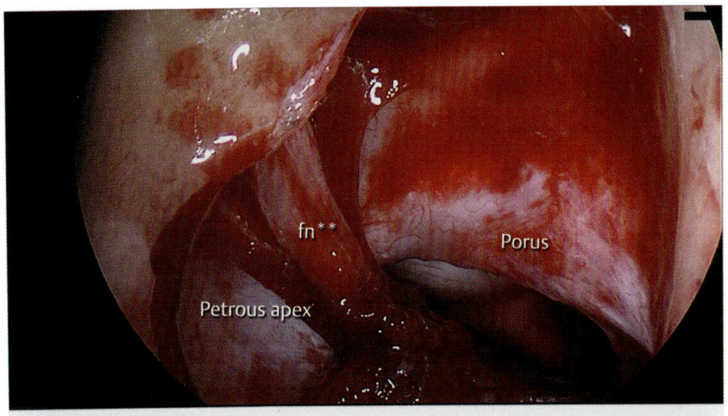

Fig. 11.296 Left side: Endoscopic view of the petrous apex and IAC below the vertical and horizontal tracts of the carotid artery. The residual desease can be removed with curved instruments. *fn**: facial nerve into the IAC.*

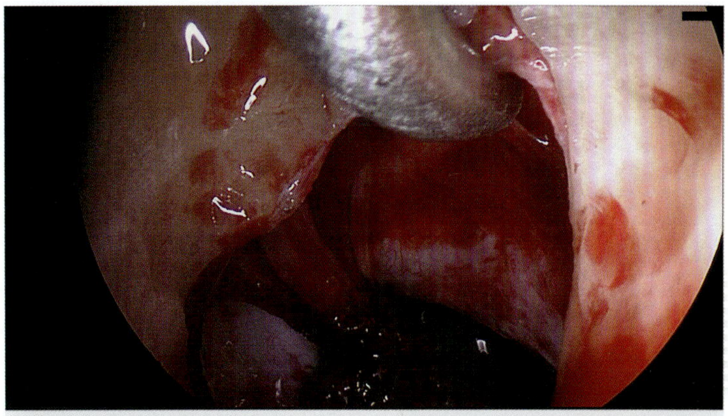

Fig. 11.297 Left side: Endoscopic view of the petrous apex and IAC. The residual desease can be removed with curved instruments.

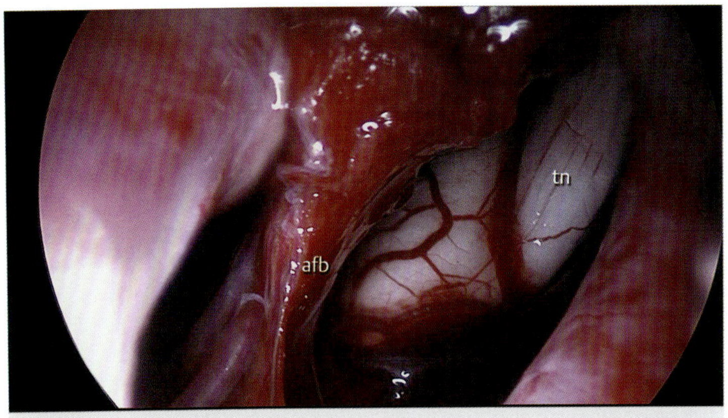

Fig. 11.298 Left side: Endoscopic view of the cerebellopontine angle (CPA); endoscopic check of the surgical cavity. *afb: acoustic-facial bundle; tn: trigeminal nerve.*

Suggested Readings

Alicandri-Ciufelli M, Piccinini A, Grammatica A, et al. A step backward: the "rough" facial nerve grading system. J Craniomaxillofac Surg. 2013; 41(7):e175–e179

Ansari SF, Terry C, Cohen-Gadol AA. Surgery for vestibular schwannomas: a systematic review of complications by approach. Neurosurg Focus. 2012; 33(3):E14

Bennett M, Haynes DS. Surgical approaches and complications in the removal of vestibular schwannomas. Otolaryngol Clin North Am. 2007; 40(3):589–609, ix–x

Jacob JT, Pollock BE, Carlson ML, Driscoll CL, Link MJ. Stereotactic radiosurgery in the management of vestibular schwannoma and glomus jugulare: indications, techniques, and results. Otolaryngol Clin North Am. 2015; 48(3):515–526

Magnan J, Chays A, Lepetre C, Pencroffi E, Locatelli P. Surgical perspectives of endoscopy of the cerebellopontine angle. Am J Otol. 1994; 15(3):366–370

Marchioni D, Alicandri-Ciufelli M, Mattioli F, et al. From external to internal auditory canal: surgical anatomy by an exclusive endoscopic approach. Eur Arch Otorhinolaryngol. 2013; 270(4):1267–1275

Marchioni D, Alicandri-Ciufelli M, Molteni G, Genovese E, Presutti L. Endoscopic tympanoplasty in patients with attic retraction pockets. Laryngoscope. 2010; 120 (9):1847–1855

Marchioni D, Alicandri-Ciufelli M, Rubini A, Masotto B, Pavesi G, Presutti L. Exclusive endoscopic transcanal transpromontorial approach: a new perspective for internal auditory canal vestibular schwannoma treatment. J Neurosurg. 2017; 126(1):98

Marchioni D, Alicandri-Ciufelli M, Rubini A, Presutti L. Endoscopic transcanal corridors to the lateral skull base: initial experiences. Laryngoscope. 2015; 125 Suppl 5:S1–S13

Patnaik U, Prasad SC, Tutar H, Giannuzzi AL, Russo A, Sanna M. The long-term outcomes of wait-and-scan and the role of radiotherapy in the management of vestibular schwannomas. Otol Neurotol. 2015; 36(4):638–646

Presutti L, Alicandri-Ciufelli M, Cigarini E, Marchioni D. Cochlear schwannoma removed through the external auditory canal by a transcanal exclusive endoscopic technique. Laryngoscope. 2013; 123(11):2862–2867

Presutti L, Marchioni D, Mattioli F, Villari D, Alicandri-Ciufelli M. Endoscopic management of acquired cholesteatoma: our experience. J Otolaryngol Head Neck Surg. 2008; 37(4):481–487

Presutti L, Nogueira JF, Alicandri-Ciufelli M, Marchioni D. Beyond the middle ear: endoscopic surgical anatomy and approaches to inner ear and lateral skull base. Otolaryngol Clin North Am. 2013; 46(2):189–200

Tarabichi M. Endoscopic management of limited attic cholesteatoma. Laryngoscope. 2004; 114(7):1157–1162

Thakur JD, Banerjee AD, Khan IS, et al. An update on unilateral sporadic small vestibular schwannoma. Neurosurg Focus. 2012; 33(3):E1

Thomassin JM, Korchia D, Doris JM. Endoscopic-guided otosurgery in the prevention of residual cholesteatomas. Laryngoscope. 1993; 103(8):939–943

Chapter 12

Endoscopic Assisted and Transcanal Procedures in Cochlear Implant

12

12 Endoscopic Assisted and Transcanal Procedures in Cochlear Implant

Daniele Marchioni, Davide Soloperto, Luca Bianconi, Joao Flavio Nogueira, Domenico Villari and Marco Carner

Abstract

The traditional microscopic technique for cochlear implant (CI) surgery is a standardized, safe, and easy procedure due to a well-known technical approach which is well codified, with extremely rare complications, and a highly successful treatment rate. The microscope does not allow for a complete exploration of the round window (RW) area, while through the endoscope the landmarks of the RW area can be easily identified to grant a safe surgery also in difficult situations. The endoscope can be used to increase the success rate in specific conditions such as unfavorable anatomy, malformed ears, or advanced otosclerosis, using the traditional or the trans-attic technique. The trans-attic endoscopic assisted technique allows the surgeon to overcome some surgical problems such facial nerve anomalies, inner ear anomalies, RW or scala tympani obliteration, a high jugular bulb, or a sclerotic mastoid. The infrapromontorial approach is a variation of the transcanal tranpromontorial approach with the preservation of the most anterior portion of the cochlea with the middle and apical turns giving the surgeon the opportunity to preserve and restore hearing during vestibular schwannoma surgery.

Keywords: endoscopic cochlear implant, round window anatomy, CHARGE syndrome, trans-attic endoscopic assisted cochlear implant, cochlear implant in vestibular schwannoma, infrapromontorial approach

12.1 Introduction

Although the use of the endoscopic transcanal route is becoming more and more widespread among otologists, the cochlear implant (CI) procedure remains a microscopic transmastoid based procedure.

As the endoscope magnifies the anatomical structures, it should be used especially for complicated cases or in case of difficult orientation due to an unfavorable anatomy.

The endoscope can also help during microscopic based procedures for CI, especially in malformed ears. The trans-attic endoscopic assisted procedure was codified to help the surgeon especially in complicated cases.

Another instance concerns the possibility to use the transcanal route for acoustic neuroma removal with simultaneous CI placement. A variation of the transcanal transpromontorial technique may be useful for the removal of the acoustic neuroma limited to the internal auditory canal (IAC) preserving the cochlea and the cochlear nerve, allowing for the insertion of a simultaneous CI to restore the hearing function.

In this chapter, we will focus our attention especially on two procedures:

- The trans-attic endoscopic assisted procedure for CI placement
- The transcanal infrapromontorial approach with simultaneous CI placement

12.2 Trans-attic Endoscopic Assisted Cochlear Implantation

12.2.1 Endoscopic Anatomy of the Round Window

The round window (RW) chamber has been described as an area lying between the subiculum posteriorly and slightly superiorly and the finiculus anteriorly and slightly inferiorly. The round window niche is formed in a triangular shape by the posterior pillar, the anterior pillar, and the tegmen, and the apex of this triangular shape is the round window membrane (see ▶ Fig. 12.1). The subiculum (from Latin, “support”) extends from the posterior pillar toward the styloid eminence, inferiorly limiting the sinus tympani.

The finiculus (from Latin, “borderline”) is a ridge of bone connecting the anterior pillar of the round window niche to the

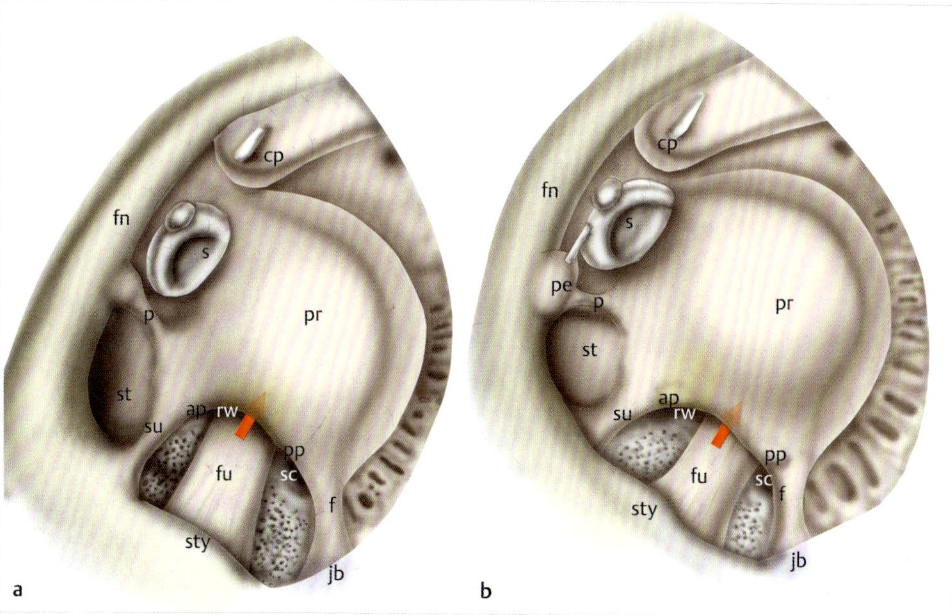

Fig. 12.1 Right ear. The anatomy of the round window (RW) is shown. The variation of the fustis is represented in the drawing. **(a)** The fustis has an oblique orientation from the styloid eminence to the RW. This structure points to the RW membrane and scala tympani (*yellow line*). **(b)** The fustis has an oblique orientation from the styloid eminence to the RW, running just below the RW, forming the floor of the scala tympani (*yellow line*). *ap: anterior pillar; cp: cochleariform process; f: finiculus; fn: facial nerve; fu: fustis; jb: jugular bulb; p: ponticulus; pp: posterior pillar; pe: pyramidal eminence; pr: promontory; rw: round window; s: stapes; sc: subcochlear caniluculus; st: sinus tympani; sty: styloid eminence; su: subiculum; red arrow: direction of fustis bone.*

jugular wall of the tympanum, first called the sustentaculum promontorii, because of its orientation to sustain the inferior tympanic artery, enveloping it during the development of the middle ear. The finiculus extends from the anterior pillar toward the jugular dome, separating the retrotympanum from the hypotympanum (▶ Fig. 12.1).

The fustis is a smooth bony structure, which forms the floor of the RW chamber and seems to indicate the entrance to the RW niche. The structure links the styloid eminence to the basal turn of the cochlea.

The fustis crosses the RW chamber in an oblique direction from the styloid eminence posteriorly and inferiorly to the RW niche anteriorly and superiorly, pointing at the RW membrane. This smooth bone represents a constant anatomical landmark to find the right orientation of the scala tympani since this anatomical structure forms the floor of the scala tympani (see ▶ Fig. 12.1).

Between the fustis and the finiculus, a subcochlear canaliculus which is a tunnel connecting the RW chamber to the petrous apex via a series of pneumatized cells, is often seen.

Three different types of subcochlear canaliculus have been described (see Chapter 13):

- Type A: The subcochlear canaliculus is a large endoscopically detectable tunnel leading to the petrous apex.
- Type B: The subcochlear canaliculus is a small tunnel whose connection to the petrous apex is not endoscopically detectable.
- Type C: The subcochlear canaliculus provides no connection between the RW chamber and the petrous apex.

12.2.2 General Considerations on Cochlear Implants

Cochlear implant surgery is a standardized, safe, and easy procedure due to well-known technical approaches. Nowadays, the most commonly used technique is the posterior tympanotomy with mastoidectomy and with the aid of a microscope. In the authors' opinion, the use of an endoscopic technique during CI surgery in patients with normal anatomy of the ear is not recommended. The traditional approaches are well codified, with extremely rare complications and a highly successful rate of treatment. In this case, the transcanal endoscopic cochlear implantation should be avoided, due to the risks of this surgical procedure, such as iatrogenic cholesteatoma and the possible extrusion of the array.

Although the microscope provides a multiplanar visualization of the anatomical spaces, it does not allow the RW niche to be fully visualized in all conditions, and especially in unfavorable anatomical conditions (like in malformed ears and in children), this area can sometimes be difficult to explore. The maneuver for electrode positioning in these conditions can be very difficult, causing additional possible damage to the facial nerve (FN), the ossicular chain, or the tympanic membrane.

In children, even without congenital anatomical malformations, the RW membrane is less accessible than in adults, due to a more obtuse angle between the cochlear basal axis and the mid-sagittal plane of the temporal bone. Moreover, in pediatric patients, the subcochlear canaliculus is wider, and it may easily be confused with the RW niche, resulting in a misplaced location of the electrodes in the cochlea or a damage of the cochlear turns.

In patients with malformed ears audiological outcomes after surgery are worse for several reasons, not only related to the condition of the cochlear nerve, but also related to the difficult insertion of the array in relation to the grade of malformations of the middle ear and cochlear structures. In these cases, the correct exposure of the anatomical landmarks is crucial to perform a safe and successful surgery avoiding FN injury and showing the correct location of the cochleostomy for array insertion. In order to overcome these difficulties, many more surgical approaches have been proposed. Despite their advantages many complex and controversial issues have been reported in literature, sometimes obliging the surgeon to abandon such attempts.

Especially in patients with congenital anomalies of the FN (see ▶ Fig. 12.2), the traditional transmastoid approach with posterior tympanotomy may be difficult due to the position of the nerve and the high risk of nerve injury. The introduction of the endoscopic approach in recent years has allowed for the development of a trans-attic endoscopic assisted technique trying to identify the correct position of the implant in the presence of unfavorable anatomical conditions.

12.2.3 Indications

The trans-attic endoscopic assisted technique allows the surgeon to overcome some problems:

- FN anatomical malformations (as in CHARGE syndrome) (see Clinical Case 1)
- CHARGE syndrome with inner ear anomalies (see Clinical Case 2)
- RW and scala tympani obliteration (see ▶ Fig. 12.82)
- High jugular bulb preventing posterior tympanotomy (see ▶ Fig. 12.30)
- Sclerotic mastoid

12.2.4 Cochlear Implant in Otosclerosis

The obliteration of the RW and the ossification of the cochlea have been reported in cases of cochlear otosclerosis (see ▶ Fig. 12.82). Histopathological studies have demonstrated that the most common region of cochlear ossification, regardless of the etiology, is the basal turn of the scala tympani. A complete obliteration of the RW may occur, particularly in advanced otosclerosis, with intracochlear foci of ossification extending to the basal turn and leading to a complete remodeling of the labyrinth. Cochlear implantation in patients suffering from otosclerosis, however, is mainly characterized by two risks: the difficulty in electrode placement, linked to the degree of cochlear ossification, and the stimulation of the FN. The possibility of a labyrinthine fistula with liquorrea is also described. The most commonly used technique for managing a partially ossified cochlea is tunneling through the ossified portion of the lower basal turn toward the scala tympani. This procedure could be difficult due to the complex anatomy of the RW, which is altered by the otospongiotic process; so in some cases, it could be hard to identify the correct anatomical orientation and thus identify the scala tympani.

In these unfavorable anatomical conditions, the use of the endoscopic technique enables the surgeon to determine the morphology of the RW membrane and to visualize the fustis, the area concamerata, and the subcochlear canaliculus, and to clearly identify the orientation of the scala tympani of the basal turn. It provides useful information about the spatial orientation of the modiolus and ensures the correct placement and advancement of

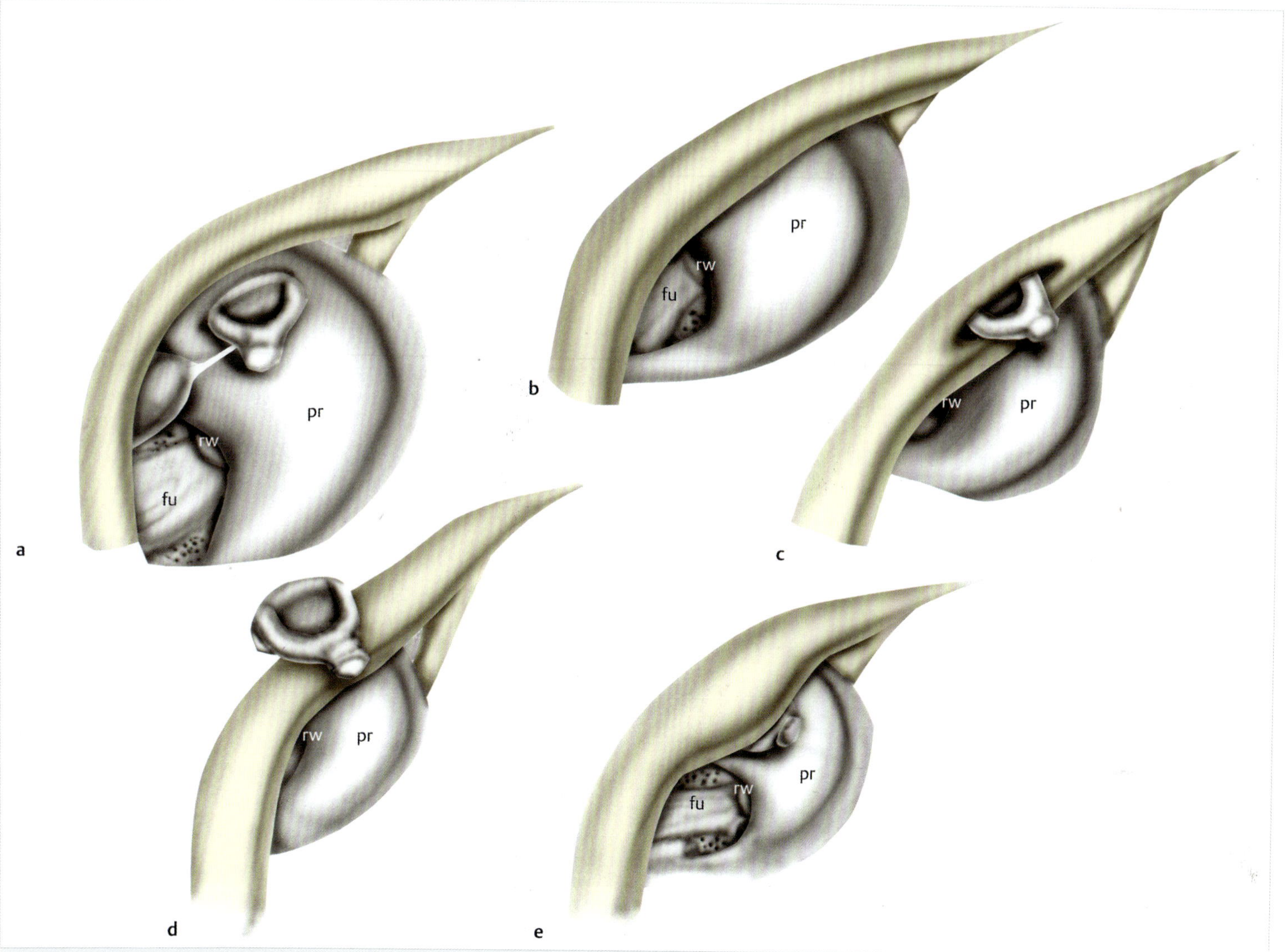

Fig. 12.2 Patterns of facial nerve (FN) displacement (dystopia) in a patient with congenital middle ear malformations. **(a)** Normal anatomy of the tympanic segment of the FN. **(b)** Dehiscence of the FN over the oval window. **(c)** Duplication of the tympanic segment of the FN. **(d)** The FN runs below the oval window covering the round window (RW). **(e)** FN dehiscence over the stapes. *fu: fustis; pr: promontory; rw: round window; s: stapes.*

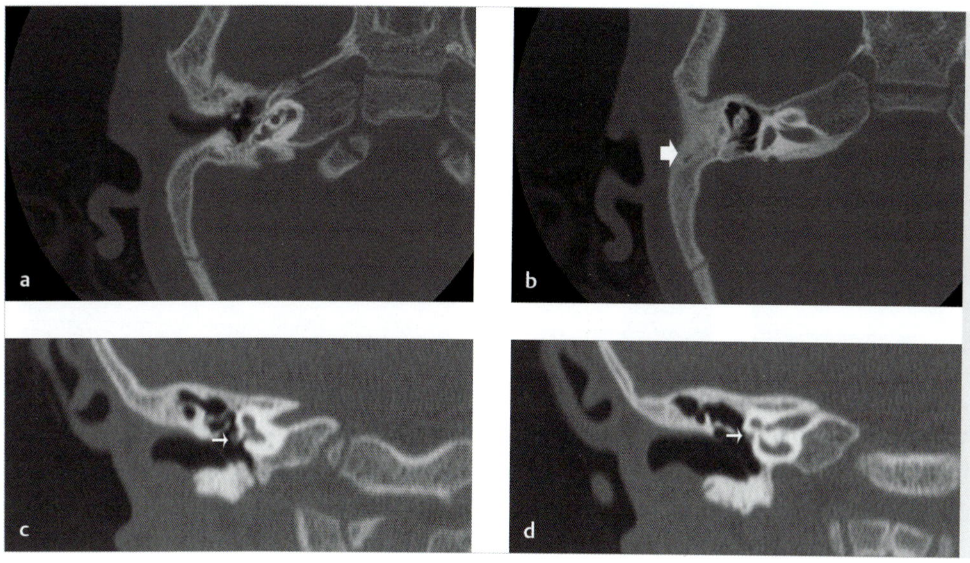

Fig. 12.3 Clinical Case 1: Preoperative computed tomography (CT) scan a patient suffering from CHARGE syndrome. **(a, b)** CT scan in axial view. In **(a)** the anomalous displacement of the facial nerve (FN) is seen on the promontory, in **(b)**, a sclerotic mastoid is seen (*large white arrow*). **(c–d)** CT scan in coronal view. In these scans, an abnormal displacement of the FN over the promontory, obscuring the round window (RW), is noted (*small white arrow*).

the electrodes in the cochlea, by means of the best vector of insertion, coaxial to the centerline of the scala tympani.

The advantage of RW endoscopic magnification is the direct visualization of the structures of the round window and labyrinth affected by the disease, allowing the recently formed bone to be removed for the detection of the scala tympani. In particular, the magnification of the RW and the perifenestral area helps us to better understand the anatomical relationships existing between the RW and its niche.

We have to consider some anatomical landmarks in order to have the right orientation during CI placement in cochlear ossification (see ▶ Fig. 12.31):

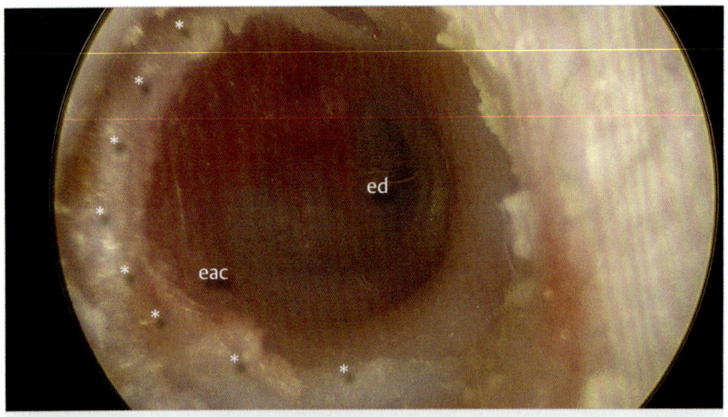

Fig. 12.4 Clinical Case 1, Right ear: Patient suffering from CHARGE syndrome. The endoscopic time starts with the incision (***) of the external auditory canal (EAC), to create the tympanomeatal flap. A 0-degree endoscope, of 15 cm length and 3 mm diameter, is used. *eac: external auditory canal; ed: eardrum.*

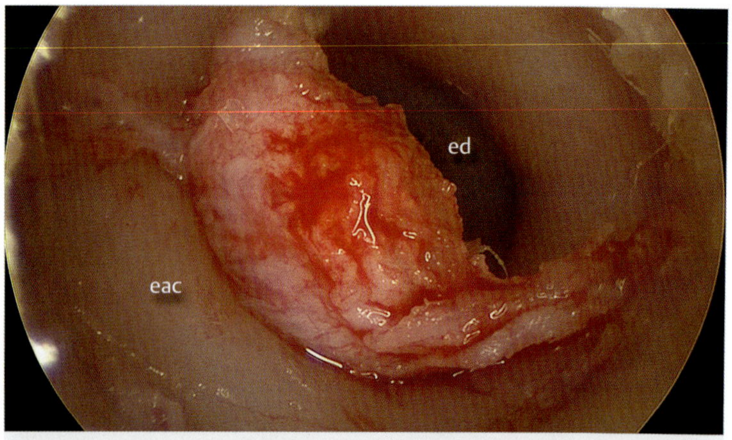

Fig. 12.5 Clinical Case 1, Right ear: Patient suffering from CHARGE syndrome. The tympanomeatal flap is progressively endoscopically elevated. *eac: external auditory canal; ed: eardrum.*

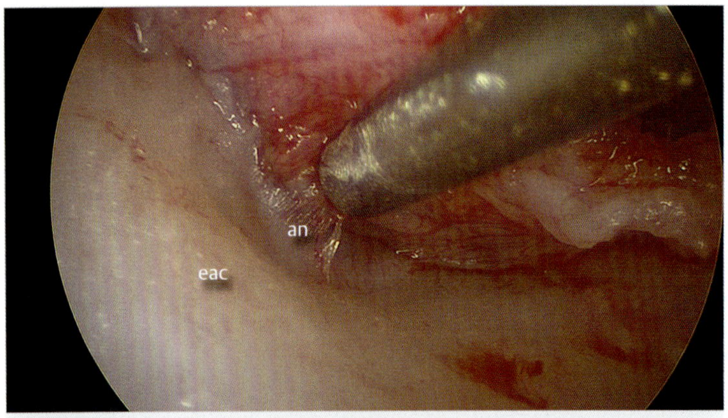

Fig. 12.6 Clinical Case 1, Right ear: Patient suffering from CHARGE syndrome. The fibrous anulus is endoscopically detected and progressively detached from the bony anulus. *an: fibrous anulus, eac: external auditory canal.*

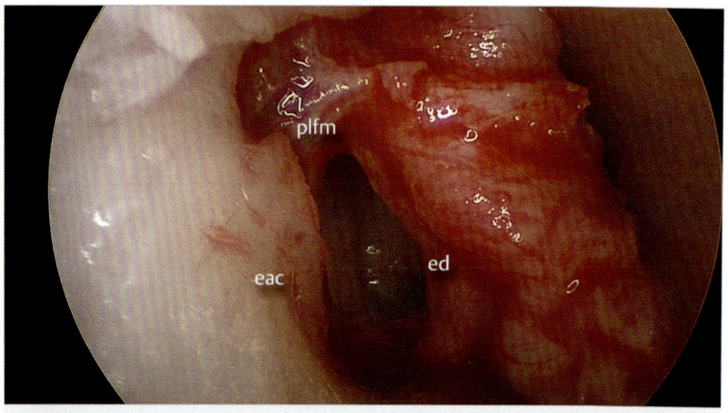

Fig. 12.7 Clinical Case 1, Right ear: Patient suffering from CHARGE syndrome. The tympanomeatal flap is anteriorly elevated until the handle of the malleus, entering the tympanic cavity. *eac: external auditory canal; ed: eardrum; plfm: posterior ligamental fold of the malleus.*

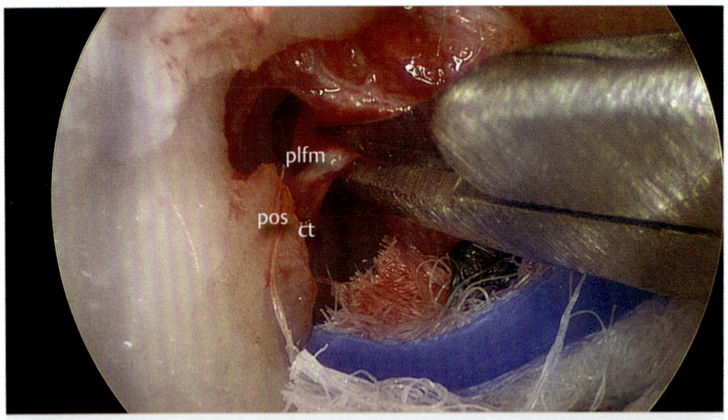

Fig. 12.8 Clinical Case 1, Right ear: Patient suffering from CHARGE syndrome. The posterior ligamental fold of the malleus is endoscopically cut. This surgical maneuver allows the complete elevation of the flap over the malleus. During this step, the surgeon should be careful to avoid damage of the chorda tympani, since this nerve runs just medial to the posterior ligamental fold of the malleus. *ct: chorda tympani; plfm: posterior ligamental fold of the malleus; pos: posterior spine.*

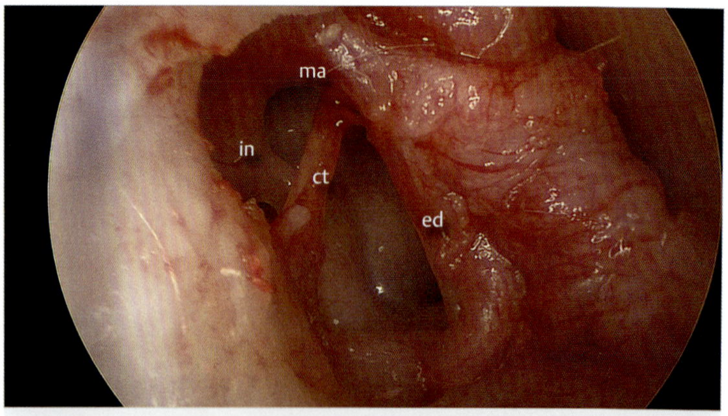

Fig. 12.9 Clinical Case 1, Right ear: Patient suffering from CHARGE syndrome. The flap is anteriorly transposed over the malleus. *ct: chorda tympani; ed: eardrum; in: incus: ma: malleus.*

The fustis bone is located in the pars media of the area concamerata (Proctor's fustis) of the RW chamber. It is a smooth bony structure forming the floor of the RW niche. The fustis may be easily endoscopically identified. This bony structure is the main landmark to find the scala tympani, since the fustis represents the floor of the scala tympani itself (see ▶ Fig. 12.1 and ▶ Fig. 12.31).

In fact, in case of obliteration of the RW and the scala tympani, the use of the fustis bone as a landmark is crucial. The fustis is a bony structure which has a smooth evolution from a posterior to an anterior direction and from an inferior to a superior one. Its anterior limit is the RW membrane and it forms the floor of the

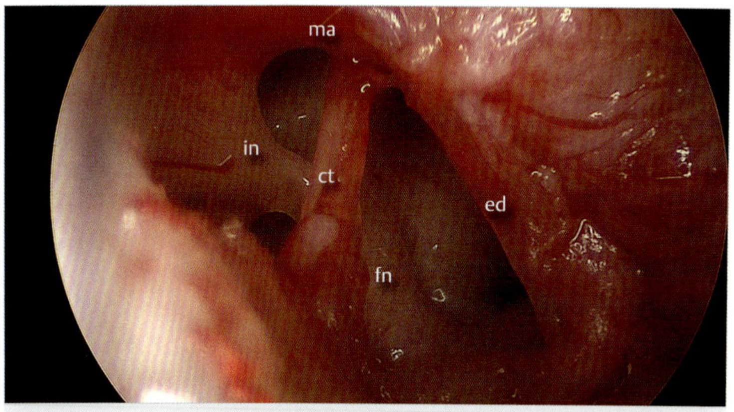

Fig. 12.10 Clinical Case 1, Right ear: Patient suffering from CHARGE syndrome. Endoscopic exploration of the tympanic cavity. A dystopic facial nerve (FN) located under the stapes and over the promontory is detected. *ct: chorda tympani; ed: eardrum; fn: facial nerve; in: incus: ma: malleus.*

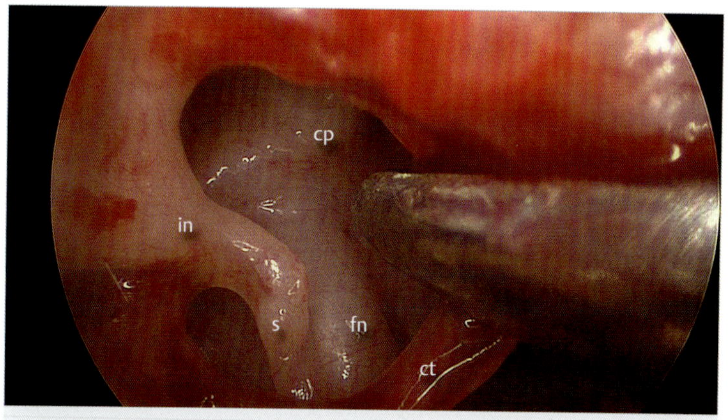

Fig. 12.11 Clinical Case 1, Right ear: Patient suffering from CHARGE syndrome. Endoscopic magnification of the anomalous position of the facial nerve (FN) below the stapes. *cp: cochleariform process; ct: chorda tympani; fn: facial nerve; in: incus; s: stapes.*

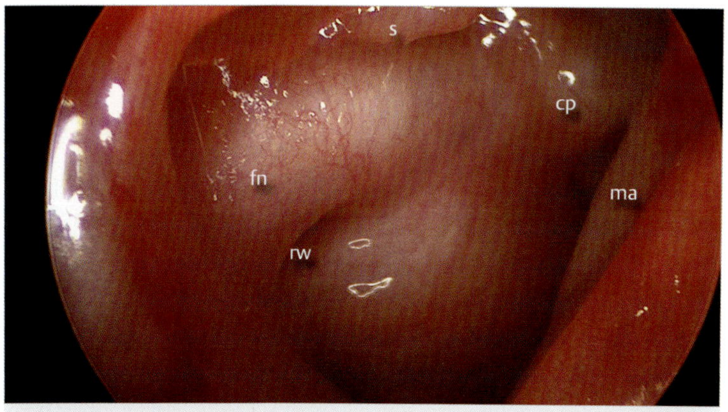

Fig. 12.12 Clinical Case 1, Right ear: Patient suffering from CHARGE syndrome. The dystopic facial nerve (FN) runs over the promontory obscuring the round window (RW) niche; in this case a cochleostomy through the RW is not recommendable. *cp: cochleariform process; fn: facial nerve; ma: malleus; rw: round window, s: stapes.*

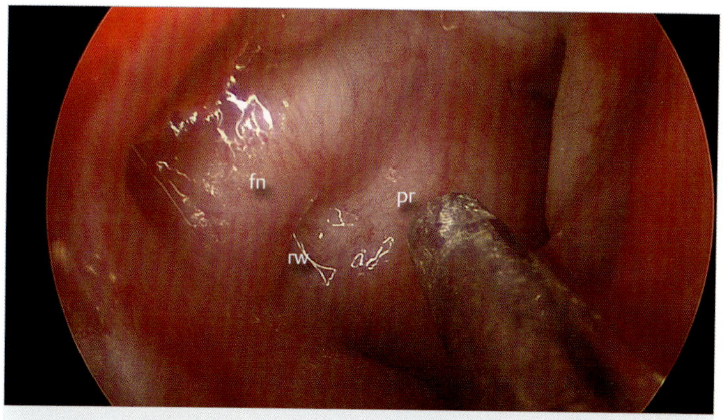

Fig. 12.13 Clinical Case 1, Right ear: Patient suffering from CHARGE syndrome. In the light of the computed tomography (CT) scan, an anterior inferior cochleostomy is planned; the suction instrument indicates the right place to endoscopically start the cochleostomy. *fn: facial nerve; pr: romontory; rw: round window.*

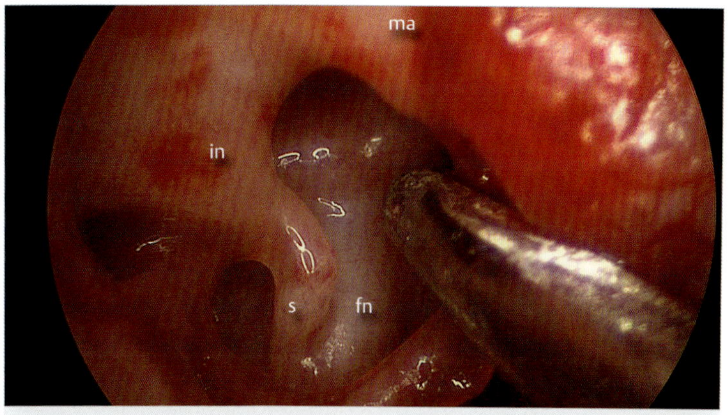

Fig. 12.14 Clinical Case 1, Right ear: Patient suffering from CHARGE syndrome. Before starting the drilling time, the whole tympanic segment of the facial nerve (FN) is endoscopically detected in order to know the right position of the nerve, avoiding possible trauma. *fn: facial nerve; in: incus; ma: malleus; s: stapes.*

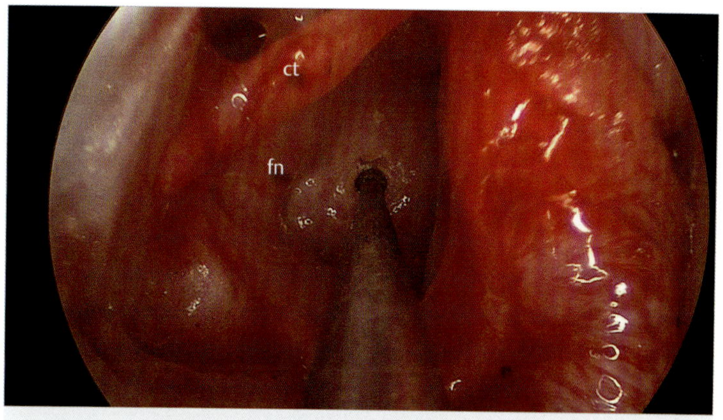

Fig. 12.15 Clinical Case 1, Right ear: Patient suffering from CHARGE syndrome. Maintaining the facial nerve (FN) under endoscopic view, a small diamond bur is used over the promontory to create a cochleostomy located anteroinferiorly to the position of the round window (RW). *ct: chorda tympani; fn: facial nerve.*

scala tympani. Therefore, it represents an important landmark to find the correct position of the RW membrane. We can have two different types of fustis in relation to the anatomy of the RW membrane (see ▶ Fig. 12.1):

- Type A: The fustis has an oblique orientation from a posterior to an anterior direction pointing at the RW membrane.
- Type B: The fustis has an oblique orientation from a posterior to an anterior direction, running just below the RW membrane.

The fustis bone should be endoscopically detected and using a diamond bur on the ossification, and following from the fustis bone in a posterior to anterior direction, the opening of the scala tympani will be detected (see ▶ Fig. 12.32, ▶ Fig. 12.33, ▶ Fig. 12.34).

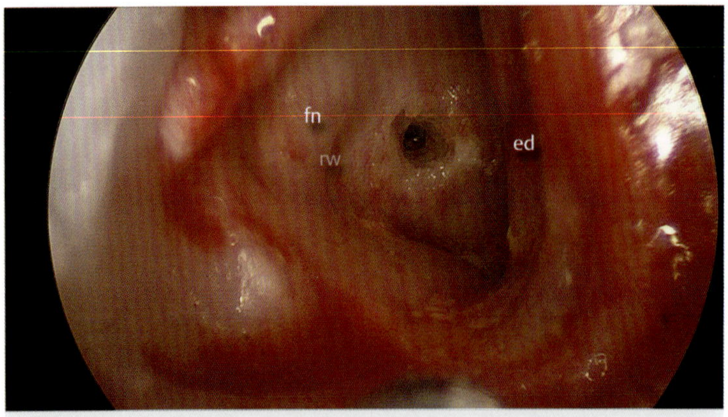

Fig. 12.16 Clinical Case 1, Right ear: Patient suffering from CHARGE syndrome. The promontorial cochleostomy is endoscopically performed. *ed: eardrum; fn: facial nerve; rw: round window.*

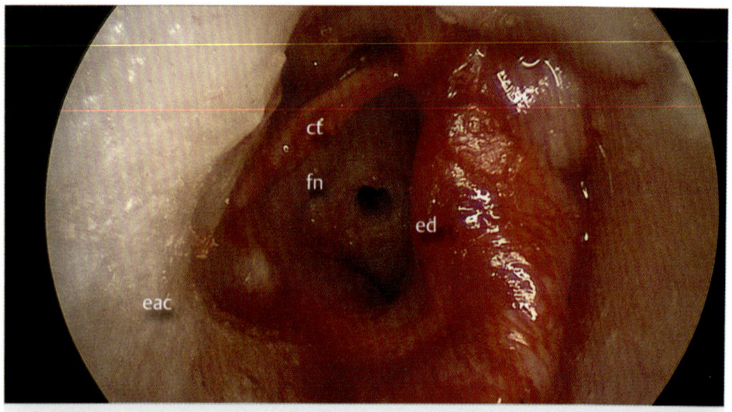

Fig. 12.17 Clinical Case 1, Right ear: Patient suffering from CHARGE syndrome. View of the tympanic cavity at the end of endoscopic time. *ct: chorda tympani; eac: external auditory canal; ed: eardrum; fn: facial nerve.*

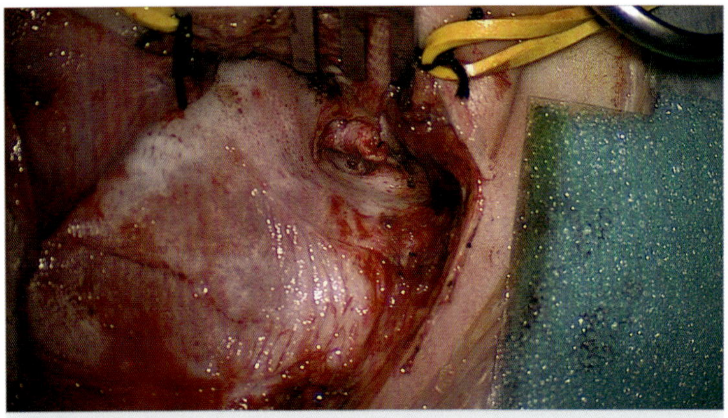

Fig. 12.18 Clinical Case 1, Right ear: Patient suffering from CHARGE syndrome. The microscopic time is started. A retrouricular incision is made; a fibromastoid flap is superiorly elevated to uncover the mastoid bone; and the skin of the posterior portion of the external auditory canal (EAC) is elevated to expose the tympanic cavity.

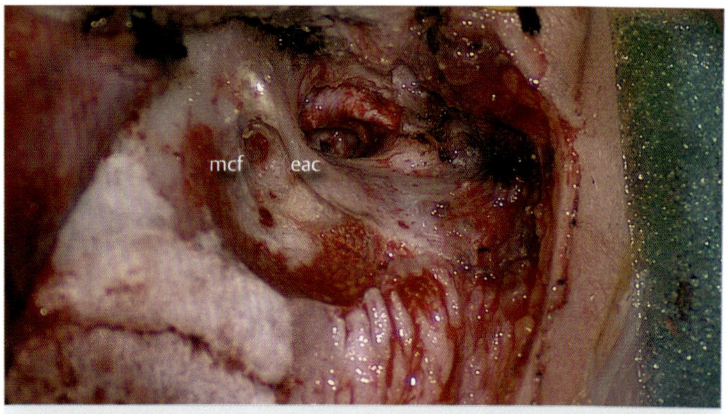

Fig. 12.19 Clinical Case 1, Right ear: Patient suffering from CHARGE syndrome. A microscopic mastoidectomy is performed in a sclerotic mastoid detecting the plane of the middle cranial fossa and preserving the posterior wall of the external auditory canal (EAC). *eac: external auditory canal; mcf: middle cranial fossa dura.*

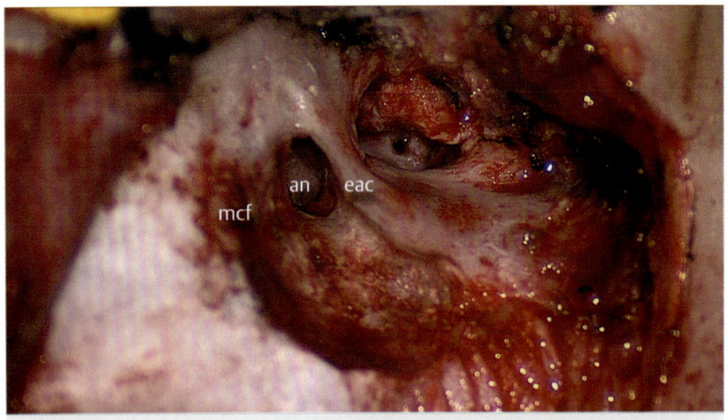

Fig. 12.20 Clinical Case 1, Right ear: Patient suffering from CHARGE syndrome. The aditus ad antrum is exposed through the mastoidectomy. *an: antrum; eac: external auditory canal; mcf: middle cranial fossa dura.*

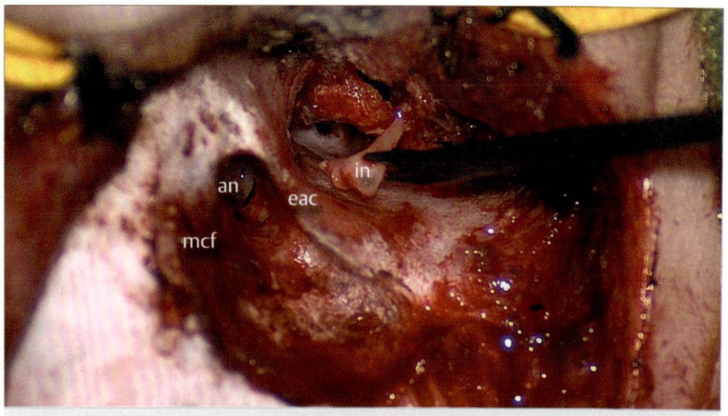

Fig. 12.21 Clinical Case 1, Right ear: Patient suffering from CHARGE syndrome. The incus is removed, creating a wide connection between the antrum, the attic, and the mesotympanic spaces. *an: antrum; eac: external auditory canal; in: incus; mcf: middle cranial fossa dura.*

12.2.5 Cochlear Implantation in CHARGE Syndrome

The trans-attic endoscopic assisted CI placement should be considered when a variation of the course of the FN is detected in a congenitally malformed ear. A great variety of FN arrangements is present within the temporal bone. Especially in congenitally malformed ears two anatomical conditions are common: the displacement of the nerve (dystopia) and the absence of the bony canal covering the nerve (see ▶ Fig. 12.2).

In these cases, the FN may transit at the level of the oval window, it may press against the suprastructure of the stapes, or it may run below the oval window covering the RW (see Clinical Case 1, ▶ Fig. 12.3).

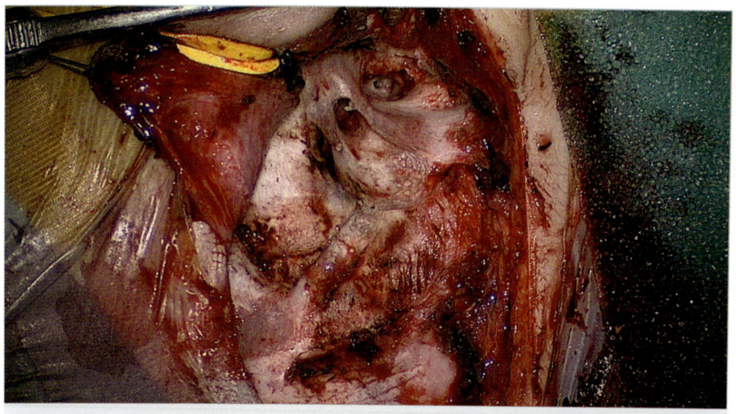

Fig. 12.22 Clinical Case 1, Right ear: Patient suffering from CHARGE syndrome. A placement for the receiver–stimulator is created under the temporalis muscle.

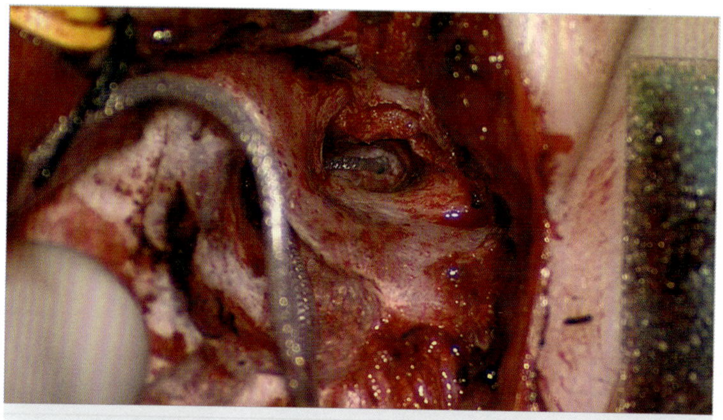

Fig. 12.23 Clinical Case 1, Right ear: Patient suffering from CHARGE syndrome. The array of the cochlear implant (CI) is gently pushed through the mastoidectomy, from the antrum to the tympanic cavity into the cochleostomy.

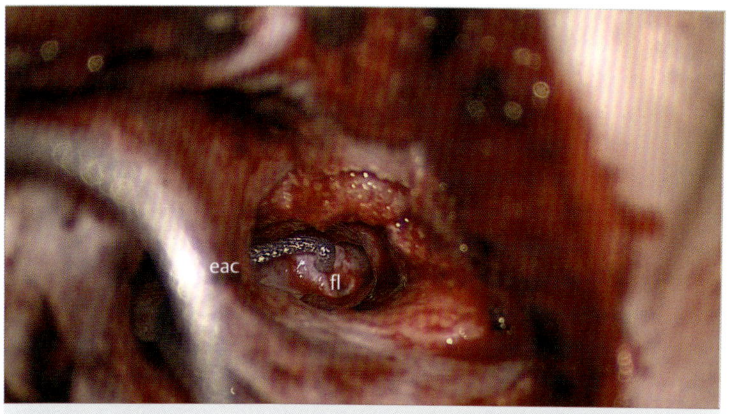

Fig. 12.24 Clinical Case 1, Right ear: Patient suffering from CHARGE syndrome. Once the insertion of the array has been completed, a piece of temporalis fascia layer is placed around the cochleostomy, to cover the promontory. *eac: external auditory canal; fl: temporalis fascia layer.*

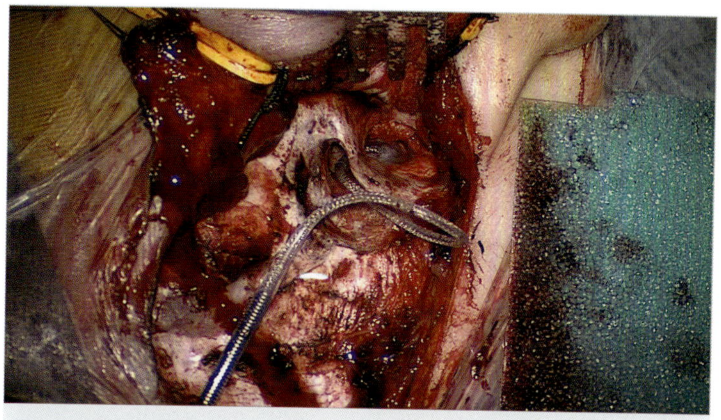

Fig. 12.25 Clinical Case 1, Right ear: Patient suffering from CHARGE syndrome. Final view of the surgical cavity after cochlear implant (CI) positioning.

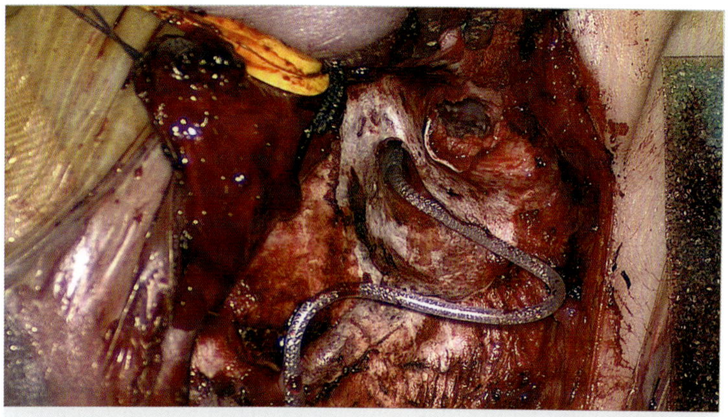

Fig. 12.26 Clinical Case 1, Right ear: Patient suffering from CHARGE syndrome. The tympanomeatal flap is replaced; a temporalis fascia is used to reinforce the eardrum.

Since the displacement of FN is frequently noticed, special care should be taken during cochlear implantation when dealing with patients suffering from CHARGE syndrome.

CHARGE syndrome has a prevalence of approximately 1/8,500 newborns/year. Children suffering from CHARGE syndrome usually show an abnormal cup shaped pinna, hearing loss (conductive, sensorineural, or mixed), abnormal ossicles, cochlear hypoplasia, absent semicircular canals (particularly lateral), choanal atresia, and cranial nerve deficiencies (vestibular, cochlear, facial, and olfactory nerves). Cochlear nerve aplasia and hypoplasia can occur *de novo* and are particularly associated with CHARGE syndrome. Only a small proportion of children with CHARGE syndrome requires a CI. However, CHARGE syndrome is one of the most common syndromes seen in CI programs. Ear abnormalities and hearing loss are common in children with CHARGE syndrome. Both conductive hearing loss, due to chronic otitis media, cholesteatoma, or ossicular chain abnormalities, and sensorineural hearing loss, due to inner ear abnormalities, can be found. CHARGE syndrome is also associated with cranial nerve abnormalities, particularly involving the olfactory, facial, vestibular, and cochlear nerves. A small number of these children have a profound hearing loss and are eligible for CI. However, children with CHARGE syndrome have worse audiological outcomes after surgery for several reasons, especially related to the difficulty in array insertion in the malformed site and to the degree of cochlear malformation. In this case, a correct exposure of the anatomical landmarks is crucial to perform safe and successful surgery avoiding FN injury and showing the correct location of the cochleostomy for the array insertion. Furthermore, the high risk of gusher in these patients and the condition of the cochlear nerve in the IAC must be considered before surgery. Several risks related to CI surgery in these patients should be taken into account. Parental counseling regarding risks and benefits of this surgical procedure is mandatory, due to our inability to predict the audiological results. First of all, the risk of FN injury during

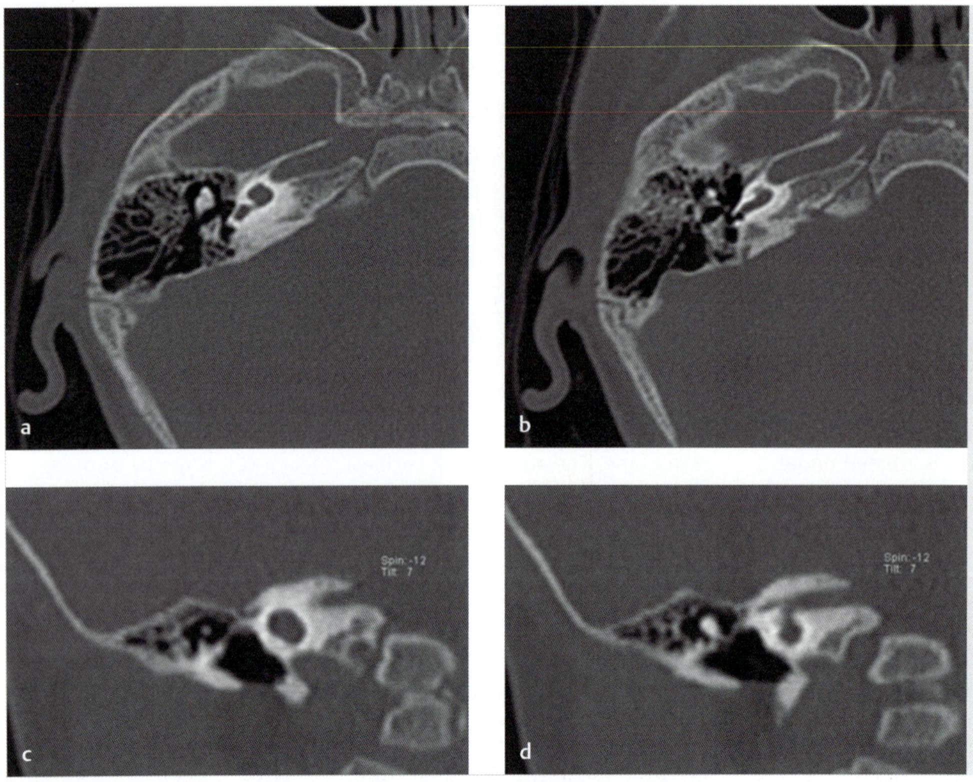

Fig. 12.27 (a–d) Clinical Case 2: Computed tomography (CT) scan in axial and coronal view. An anomalous inner ear with a labyrinthine and vestibule aplasia with a cystic cochlea is noted.

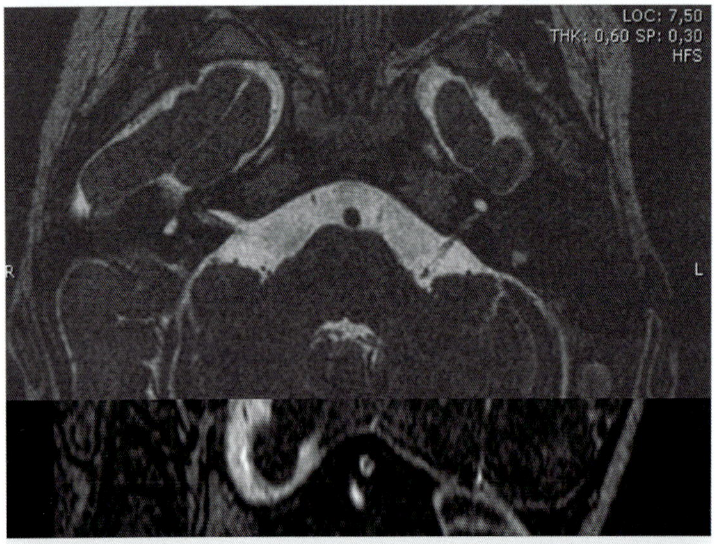

Fig. 12.28 Clinical Case 2: In the magnetic resonance imaging (MRI) in axial view a bilateral cochlear nerve hypoplasia is shown.

surgery is considerable, because an anomalous position of the FN in the tympanic cavity has been reported in 43% of patients with a malformed cochlea, in association to a sclerotic mastoid. Another important anatomical detail is related to the RW access; in some cases, the FN is located over the RW niche, obscuring it. In literature the percentage of totally hidden or absent RW niches varies from 4 to 14% in children with malformed ears. In these conditions, the identification of the RW region and the control of the FN course could be very difficult with the traditional microscopic CI surgery. Some authors have suggested the use of a subtotal petrosectomy, others a suprameatal approach in order to perform a safe CI procedure and to reduce the incidence of FN injury in these patients (see Clinical Case 3). However, from the previous experiences, the selection of a specific surgical technique does not seem to influence the audiological outcome. Also, the inner ear distorted anatomy may represent a high risk during surgery. The trans-attic endoscopic assisted CI approach should be considered in the preoperative planning of these patients, in order to detect the anatomical landmarks' safety in the tympanic cavity during surgery, such as the position of the FN, the RW membrane, and the scala tympani, to perform a "safe" cochleostomy. The endoscopic assistance also enables the surgeon to perform a transmastoid/transattic microscopic step more safely even in patients with a sclerotic mastoid, since the surgeon knows the exact location of the anatomical structures inside the tympanic cavity, especially the course of the FN. Finally, this procedure allows the surgeon to preserve the integrity of the posterior canal wall and to have a direct exposure of the tympanic cavity anatomy, avoiding a complex subtotal petrosectomy or an open approach as some authors have suggested for the treatment of malformed ears.

Although the trans-attic endoscopic assisted cochlear implantation is a safe procedure and represents the main surgical choice in these cases, in the authors' opinion, a subtotal petrosectomy should be considered in case of CHARGE syndrome in association with an extensive cholesteatoma or in case of an uncontrollable gusher during surgery.

12.2.6 Surgical Steps

The trans-attic endoscopic assisted CI placement procedure is performed in two sequential steps: a transcanal endoscopic and a transmastoid trans-attic microscopic time. The endoscopic magnification enables the surgeon to recognize the anatomical conformation of the tympanic cavity and to perform the cochleostomy. The array is then inserted, under a microscopic view, through the attic into the mesotympanum, into the previously endoscopically created cochleostomy (see Clinical Case 3). The details of these steps are given below.

12.2.7 Endoscopic Step

A 0-degree 3 mm diameter and 15 cm length endoscope, is inserted through the external auditory canal (EAC) and used to

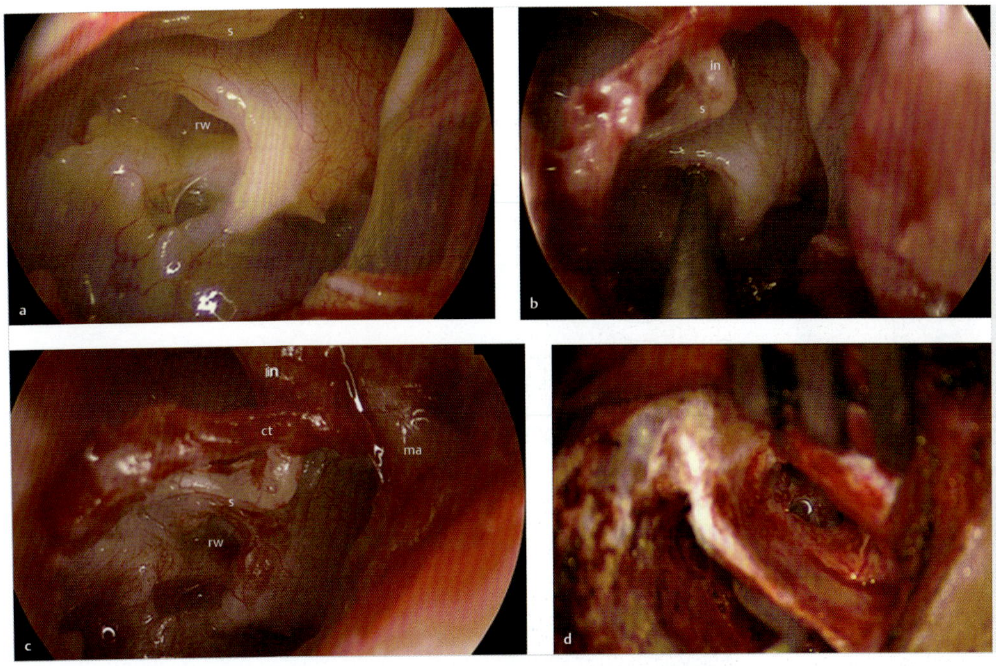

Fig. 12.29 Clinical Case 2, Right ear: Patient with inner ear malformation. **(a)** The round window (RW) niche is endoscopically detected. **(b)** A diamond bur is used to remove the tegmen of the RW, uncovering the membrane of the window. **(c)** The RW membrane can be seen in an anomalous position just below the oval window. **(d)** A microscopic transattic approach is performed and the insertion of the array is noted. *ct: chorda tympani; in: incus; ma: malleus; rw: round window; s: stapes.*

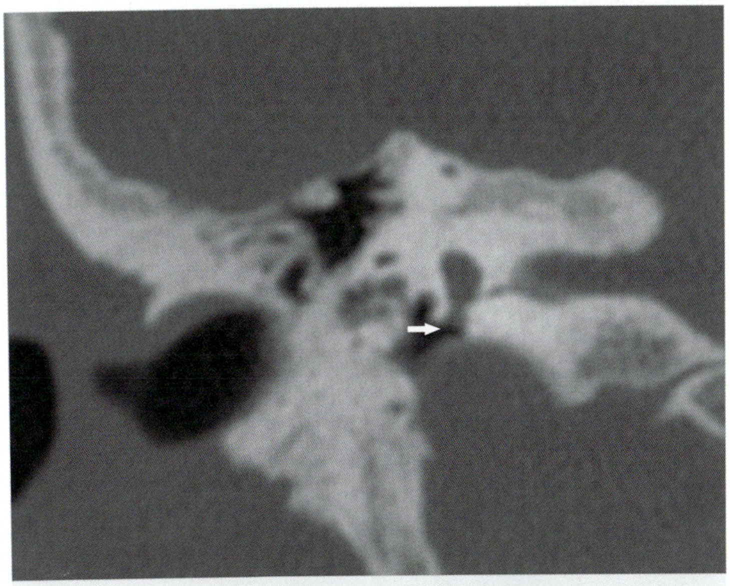

Fig. 12.30 Computed tomography (CT) scan in coronal view showing a high jugular bulb reaching the round window (RW) niche (*white arrow*).

create a tympanomeatal flap that is then anteriorly pulled, until the posterior border of the malleus is identifiable (see ▶ Fig. 12.35 and ▶ Fig. 12.36). A curette is used to remove the bone in the posterior portion of the EAC to enlarge the tympanic cavity view (see ▶ Fig. 12.37). During this step, the surgeon should try to avoid damage to the chorda tympani. A dissector may be used to inferiorly pull the chorda tympani (see ▶ Fig. 12.38). The anatomical structures in the tympanic cavity are supervised, inspecting the relationship between the course of the FN, the ossicular chain structures, the RW niche, and the promontory.

In case of RW obliteration due to otosclerosis, the RW niche is identified, valuating its accessibility; the tegmen, the finiculus, and the subiculum are evaluated; and especially the fustis bone is detected inside the RW chamber where the obliterative bone is present. To obtain a better exposure of the RW membrane, a diamond bur is used under endoscopic view to drill the obliterative bone in the RW chamber, following the fustis, until the tegmen of the RW is visible. Further drilling may be necessary to expose the RW membrane. A micro-hook is then used to open the membrane, to access to the scala tympani and to observe the orientation of the basal turn and of the modiolus. A piece of Gelfoam is placed on the cochleostomy site. In case of scala tympani obliteration, the fustis is again used as a landmark. A diamond bur should be used on the obliterative bone in the scala tympani creating a tunnel. The tunnel should be created following the orientation of the fustis, until the opening of the scala is found (see ▶ Fig. 12.32, ▶ Fig. 12.33, ▶ Fig. 12.34). Once the opening of the scala tympani has been detected, irrigation with corticosteroid may be performed to clean the scala from the bony dust. A piece of absorbable gelatin sponge (i.e., Gelfoam) is placed on the cochleostomy site.

In case of anomalous anatomy of the middle ear like in the CHARGE syndrome, when the RW is inaccessible, due to the anomalous course of the FN, hiding the RW niche, or due to the absence of the RW, an endoscopic promontorial cochleostomy must be performed (see ▶ Fig. 12.39, ▶ Fig. 12.40). In this case, it is mandatory to maintain the FN and the RW niche under endoscopic control, to avoid any surgical injury or misplacement of the electrode into the subcochlear canaliculus. A diamond bur is used to perform the cochleostomy just anteriorly and inferiorly to the position of the RW, based on the CT scan anatomy. During this step, the facial nerve (FN) is maintained under an endoscopic view and the fustis is detected in order to have the right orientation to find the scala tympani. A piece of absorbable gelatin sponge is then placed on the cochleostomy site.

12.2.8 Microscopic Step

Once the cochleostomy has been performed, the endoscopic step is over. A retroauricular skin incision is made, identifying the plane of the temporal muscle fascia; a superior based fibromuscular-periosteal flap is created and elevated, uncovering the mastoid bone (see ▶ Fig. 12.41). The skin of the posterior portion of the EAC is elevated and the tympanic cavity is exposed under a microscopic view (see ▶ Fig. 12.42). A mastoidectomy is

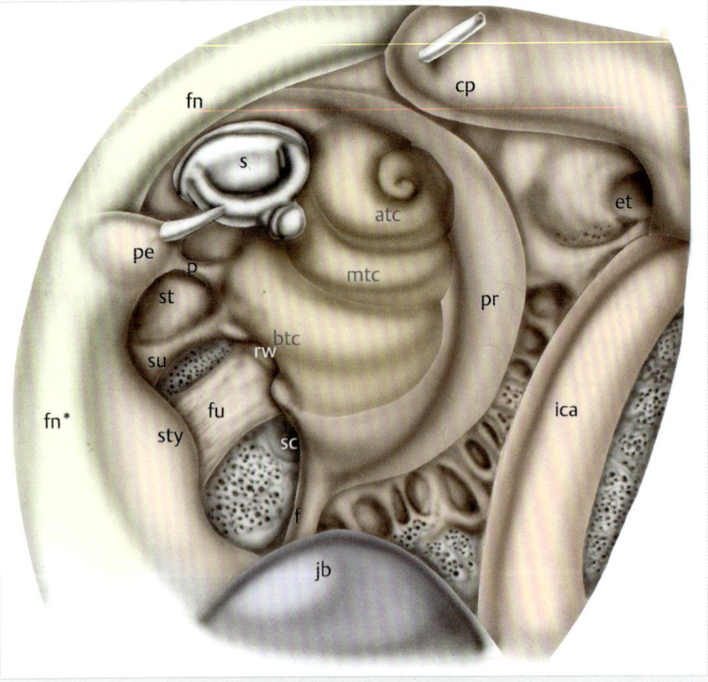

Fig. 12.31 Right side: Schematic drawing representing the anatomical relationship between the cochlea, the internal carotid artery, and the facial nerve (FN). The round window (RW) chamber showing the relationship between the fustis bone and the RW membrane is seen. *atc: apical turn of cochlea; btc: basal turn of cochlea; cp: cochleariform process; et: eustachian tube; f: finiculus; fn: tympanic segment of facial nerve; fn*: mastoid portion of facial nerve; fu: fustis; ica: internal carotid artery; jb: jugular bulb; mtc: middle turn of cochlea; p: ponticulus; pe: pyramidal eminence; pr: promontory; rw: round window; s: stapes; sc: subcochlear canaliculus; st: sinus tympani; sty: styloid eminence; su: subiculum.*

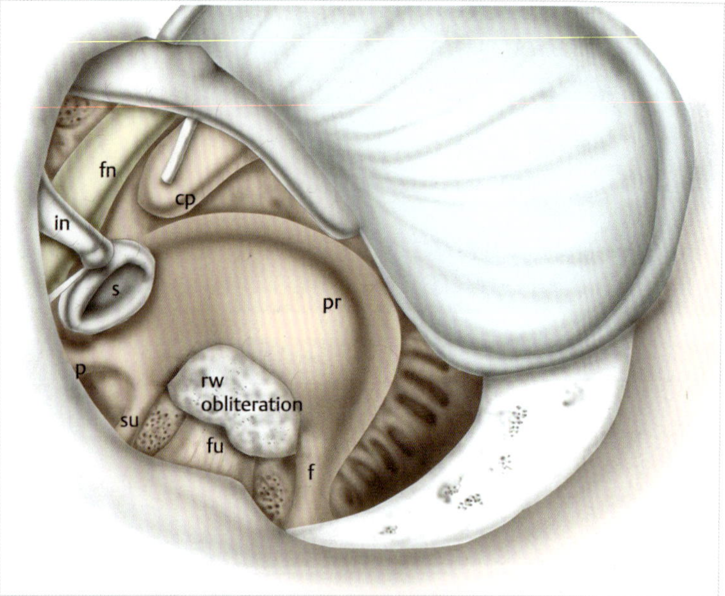

Fig. 12.32 Right side: The tympanomeatal flap is endoscopically elevated; an obliteration of the round window (RW) is noted. *cp: cochleariform process; f: finiculus; fn: tympanic segment of facial nerve; fu: fustis; in: incus; p: ponticulus; pr: promontory; rw: round window; s: stapes; su: subiculum.*

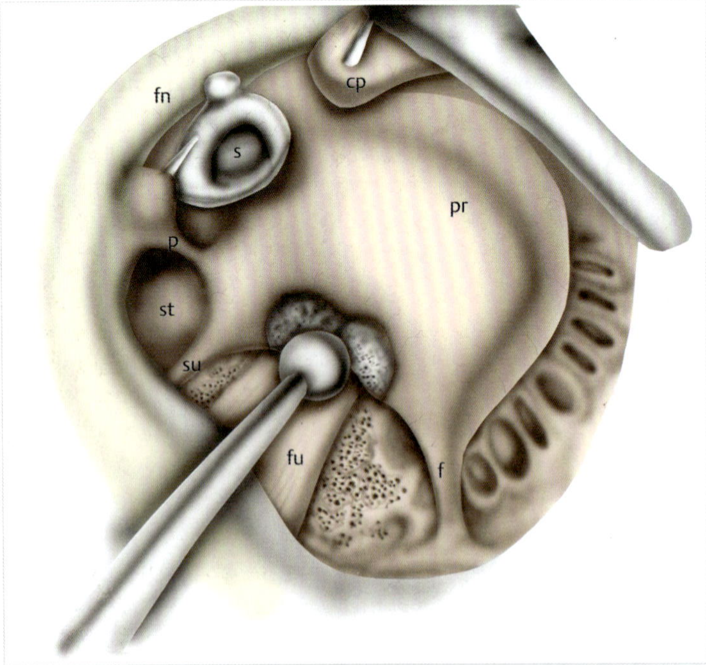

Fig. 12.33 Right side: A diamond bur is used in the endoscopic transcanal approach. The obliterated bone over the round window (RW) is removed following the fustis bone as an anatomical landmark to find the scala tympani. *cp: cochleariform process; f: finiculus; fn: tympanic segment of facial nerve; fu: fustis; p: ponticulus; pr: promontory; s: stapes; st: sinus tympani; su: subiculum.*

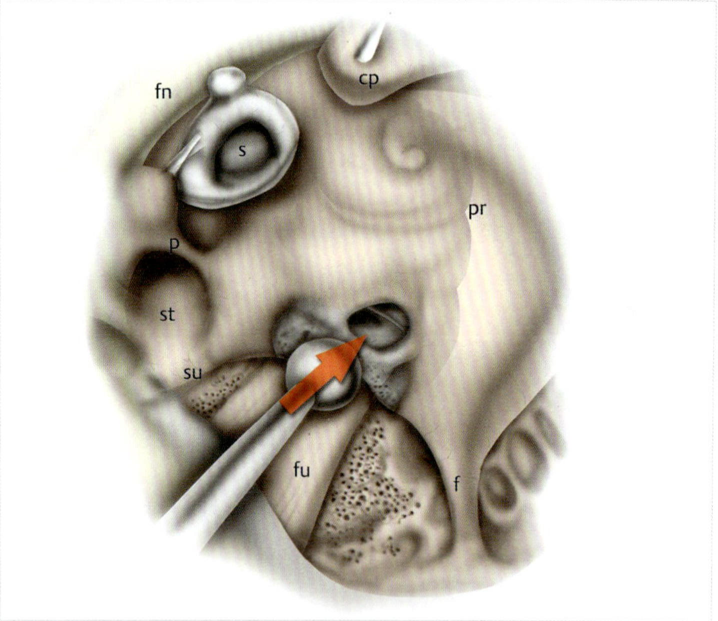

Fig. 12.34 Right side: The scala tympani is endoscopically detected following the orientation of the fustis bone (see *the red arrow*). *cp: cochleariform process; f: finiculus; fn: tympanic segment of facial nerve; fu: fustis; p: ponticulus; pr: promontory; s: stapes; st: sinus tympani; su: subiculum.*

carried out until the antrum is exposed; an anterior atticotomy is then performed uncovering the incudomalleolar joint (see ▶ Fig. 12.43). When mastoid air cells are absent and the space through the suprameatal route is insufficient, the incus is removed, creating a wide connection between the posterior epitympanum and the mesotympanic spaces (▶ Fig. 12.44). In cases in which the mastoid air cells are well represented, a limited posterior tympanotomy is performed, to enlarge the surgical

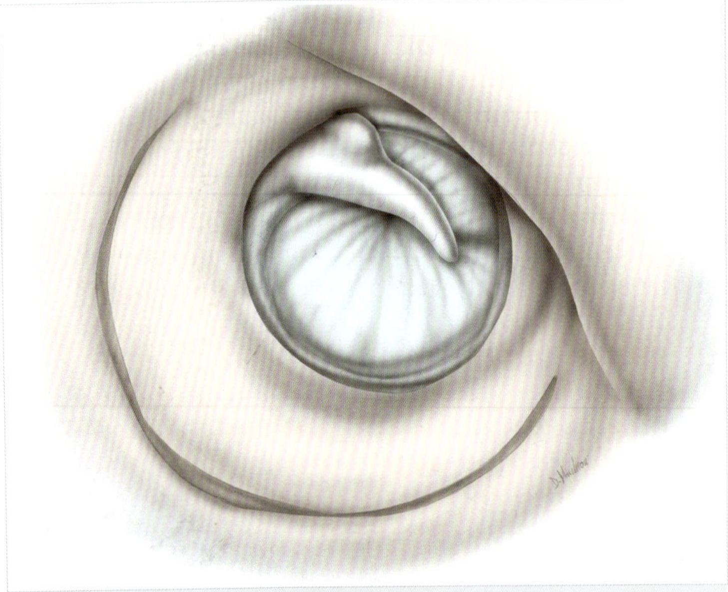

Fig. 12.35 Right side: Endoscopic time. An incision is made in the posterior portion of the external auditory canal (EAC).

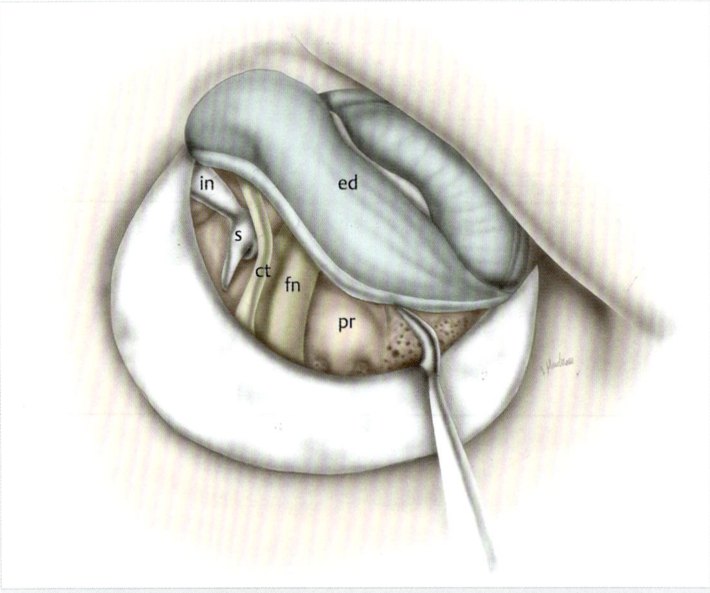

Fig. 12.36 Right side: Endoscopic time. The tympanomeatal flap is elevated, entering the tympanic cavity. *ct: chorda tympani; ed: eardrum; fn: tympanic segment of facial nerve; in: incus; pr: promontory; s: stapes.*

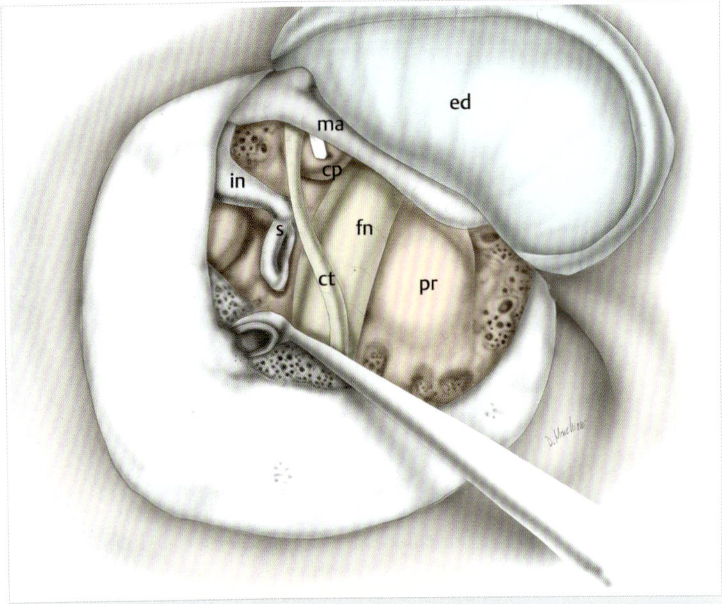

Fig. 12.37 Right side: Endoscopic time. A curette is used to remove the superoposterior portion of the bony anulus to gain some surgical space inside the tympanic cavity. *cp: cochleariform process; ct: chorda tympani; ed: eardrum; fn: facial nerve; in: incus; ma: malleus; pr: promontory; s: stapes.*

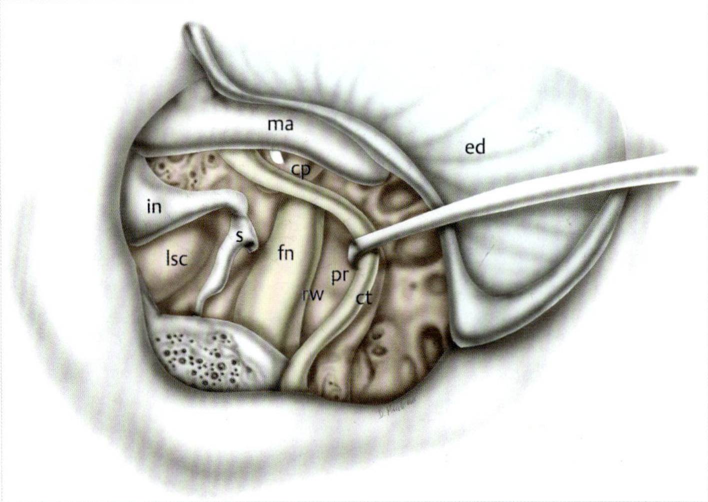

Fig. 12.38 Right side: Endoscopic time. The chorda tympani is gently inferiorly pulled, and an endoscopic magnification of the tympanic cavity is possible. In this case a CHARGE syndrome malformed middle ear is shown; the ossicular chain is abnormal and the facial nerve (FN) runs under the stapes on the promontory, covering the round window (RW) niche. *cp: cochleariform process; ct: chorda tympani; ed: eardrum; fn: facial nerve; in: incus; lsc: lateral semicircular canal; ma: malleus; pr: promontory; rw: round window; s: stapes.*

space for the array introduction and maintain the integrity of the ossicles. The receiver–stimulator of the implant is fixed and covered under the temporalis muscle. The array is gently microscopically pushed through the previously created passage, from the epitympanum into the mesotympanum (transattic route) and inserted into the cochleostomy, through the EAC (see ▶ Fig. 12.45). In malformed ears, an endoscopic check of the array insertion may be useful, especially to push the final portion of the array, to be sure of the correct positioning of the implant (see ▶ Fig. 12.46).

Since some electrodes are particularly flexible and springy, while some others may require removal of the stylet with one hand and insertion with the other, it is an unnecessary challenge to try to insert the electrode while one hand is holding the endoscope. Therefore, we do not recommend to routinely insert the electrode under an endoscopic view. The technique hereby described is recommended as an auxiliary approach to dominate the abnormal anatomical conditions of malformed middle and inner ears in children, and to perform a safe and effective cochleostomy. The endoscopic step through a transcanal corridor is to be favored since, as it is well known, it offers the best frontal direct view of the RW area.

Once the electrode has been inserted, a small piece of temporalis fascia or muscle is used with fibrin glue to seal the cochleostomy (see ▶ Fig. 12.47). The tympanomeatal flap is finally replaced and the EAC packed with Gelfoam (see ▶ Fig. 12.48). The subperiosteal flap is used to cover the receiver-stimulator and the retroauricular skin incision is sutured.

12.3 Transcanal Infrapromontorial Approach with Simultaneous Coclear Implant

The transcanal infrapromontorial approach is a variation of the transcanal transpromontorial approach (see Chapter 13). This approach includes the same steps as the ones of the transpromontorial approach; the difference is the preservation of the most anterior portion of the basal turn of the cochlea with the middle and apical turns. The IAC must be skeletonized from the fundus to the porus, identifying the fundus through the cochlear-vestibular bone and preserving the cochlea. This approach allows for the removal of an acoustic neuroma located in the IAC, allowing for the insertion of the CI through the remnant cochlea to restore the hearing function, whenever possible (see Clinical Case 4).

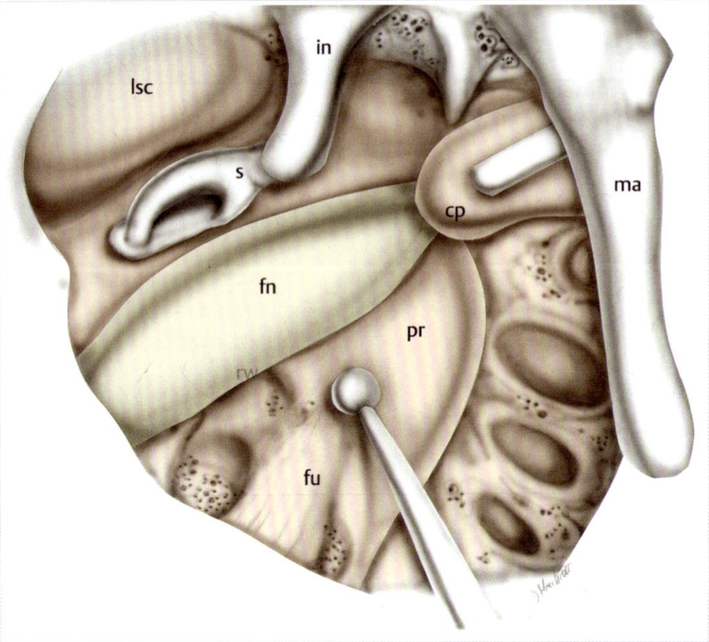

Fig. 12.39 Right side: Endoscopic time. A diamond bur is used to perform the cochleostomy just anteriorly and inferiorly to the position of the round window (RW). During this step, the facial nerve (FN) is maintained under endoscopic view. The fustis helps to have the right orientation to find the scala tympani. *cp: cochleariform process; fn: facial nerve; fu: fustis; in: incus; lsc: lateral semicircular canal; ma: malleus; pr: promontory; rw: round window, s: stapes.*

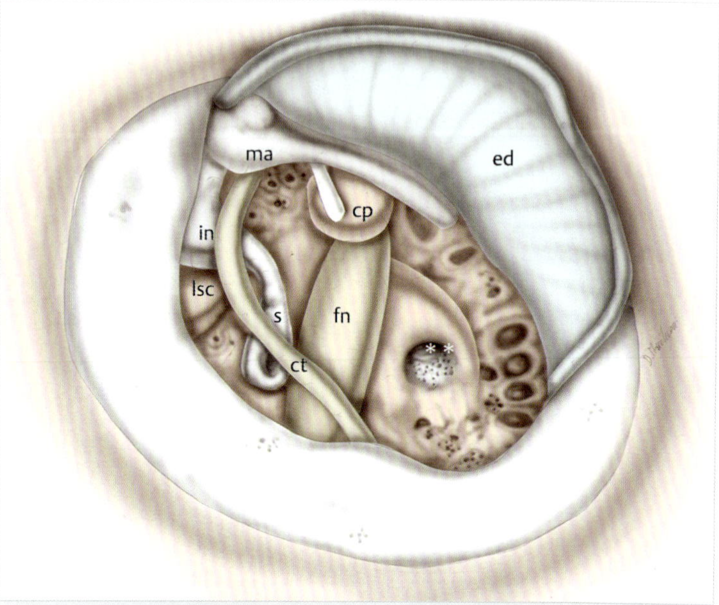

Fig. 12.40 Right side: Endoscopic time. The cochleostomy is endoscopically performed on the promontory (see **). *cp: cochleariform process; ct: chorda tympani; ed: eardrum; fn: facial nerve; in: incus; lsc: lateral semicircular canal; ma: malleus; s: stapes.*

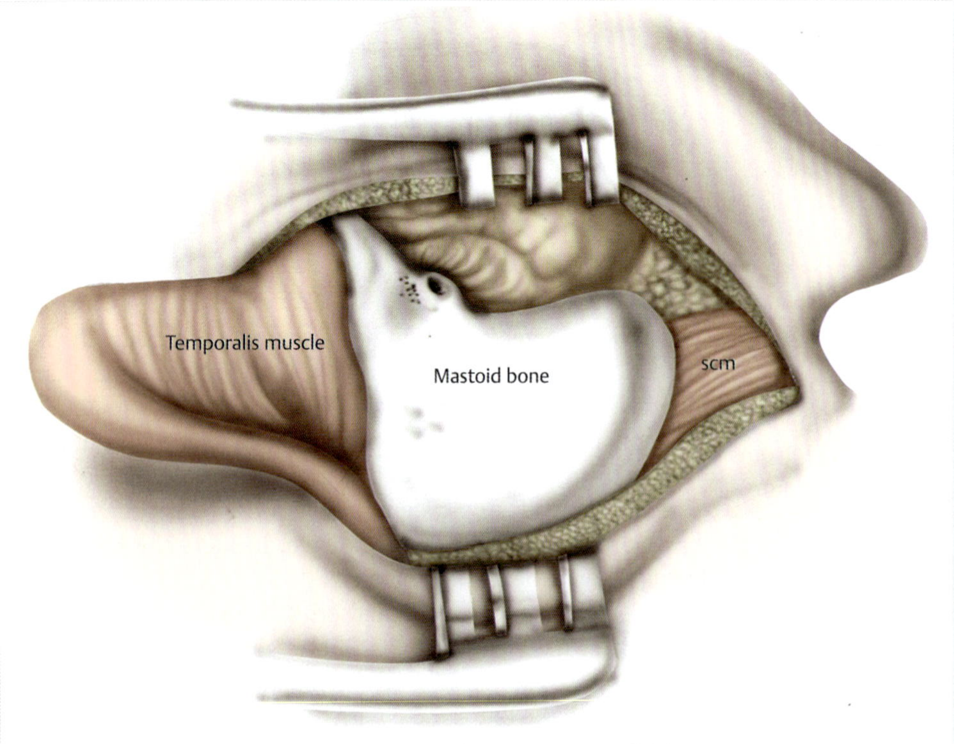

Fig. 12.41 Right side: Microscopic time. A retroauricular incision is made and a superior pedicle based fibro-muscular-periosteal flap is created. The mastoid bone is exposed. *scm: sternocleidomastoid muscle.*

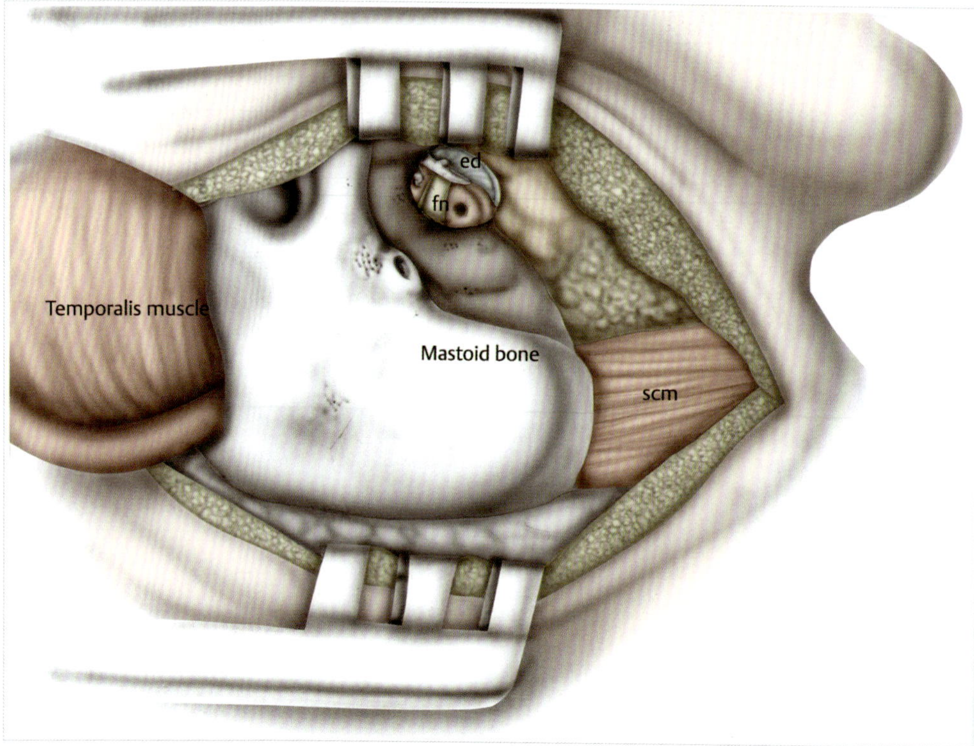

Fig. 12.42 Right side: Microscopic time. The skin of the posterior portion of the external auditory canal (EAC) is elevated in order to allow the microscopic view of the tympanic cavity; a self-retractor is placed to maintain the skin of the EAC elevated. *ed: eardrum; fn: facial nerve; scm: sternocleidomastoid muscle.*

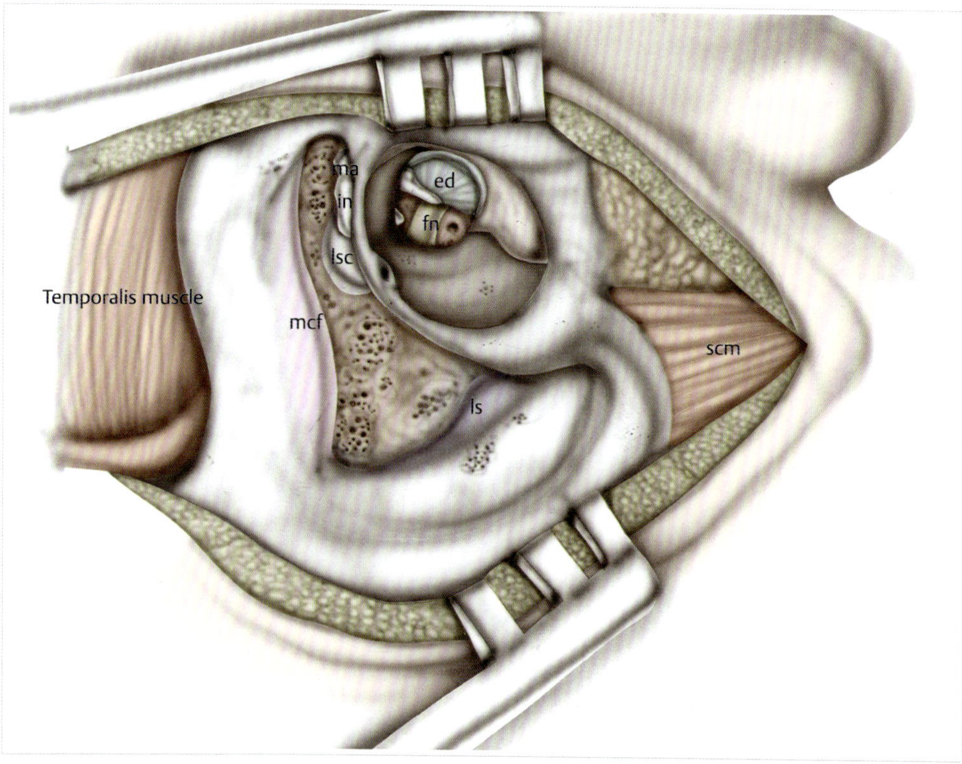

Fig. 12.43 Right side: Microscopic time. A mastoidectomy with an anterior tympanotomy is performed, exposing the antrum and the epitympanum with the incudomalleolar joint. *ed: eardrum; fn: facial nerve; in: incus; lsc: lateral semicircular canal; ma: malleus; mcf: middle cranial fossa; scm: sternocleidomastoid muscle; ss: sigmoid sinus.*

12.3.1 Indications

Relative indications for simultaneous CI surgery should include small tumors (with a high likelihood of cochlear nerve preservation) in poor hearing ears where sensory (rather than neural) loss is suspected. To distinguish sensory (cochlear) loss from neural (cochlear nerve) hearing loss, promontory stimulation should be considered before surgery.

Relative Indications (see ▶ Fig. 12.88)

- Acoustic neuromas limited to the IAC requiring surgery in patients with unserviceable hearing function with compromised contralateral hearing function (presbycusis, chronic otitis media, and unstable hearing function)
- NF2 tumors limited to the IAC in patients with unserviceable hearing function where surgery is required

Another consideration should be made for hearing rehabilitation in acoustic neuroma surgery. In patients undergoing labyrinthectomy during a translabyrinthine approach, postsurgical cochlear ossification was observed, which can preclude CI. Imaging studies to examine cochlear patency after labyrinthectomy have demonstrated that about one-third of patients develop some degree of cochlear ossification after surgery. This condition after a translabyrinthine approach

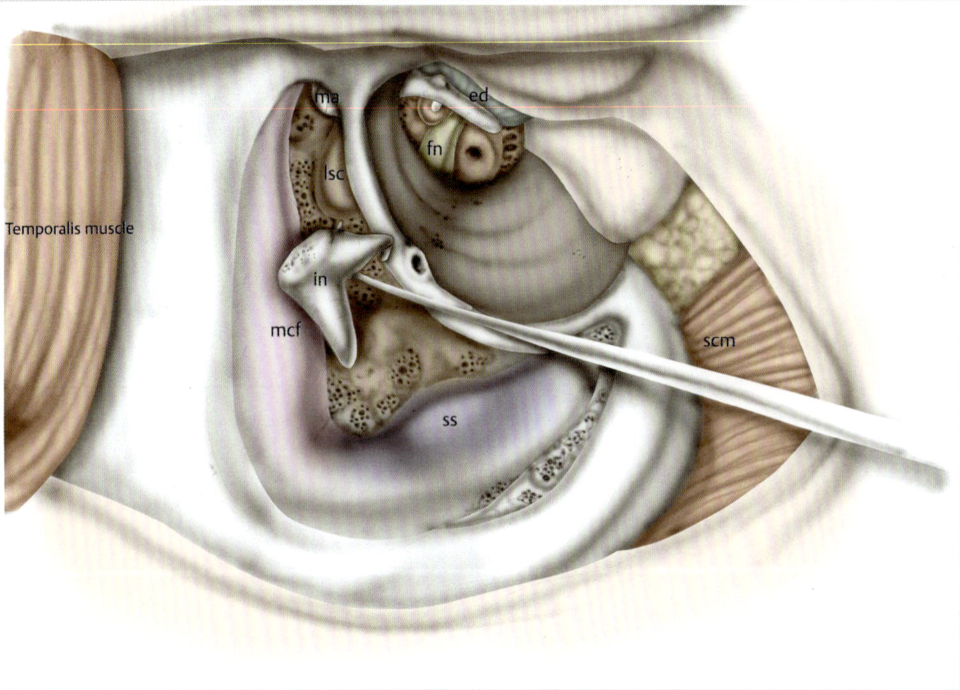

Fig. 12.44 Right side: Microscopic time. The incus is removed, creating a connection between the antrum, the epitympanum and the mesotympanum. *ed: eardrum; fn: facial nerve; in: incus; lsc: lateral semicircular canal; ma: malleus; mcf: middle cranial fossa; scm: sternocleidomastoid muscle; ss: sigmoid sinus.*

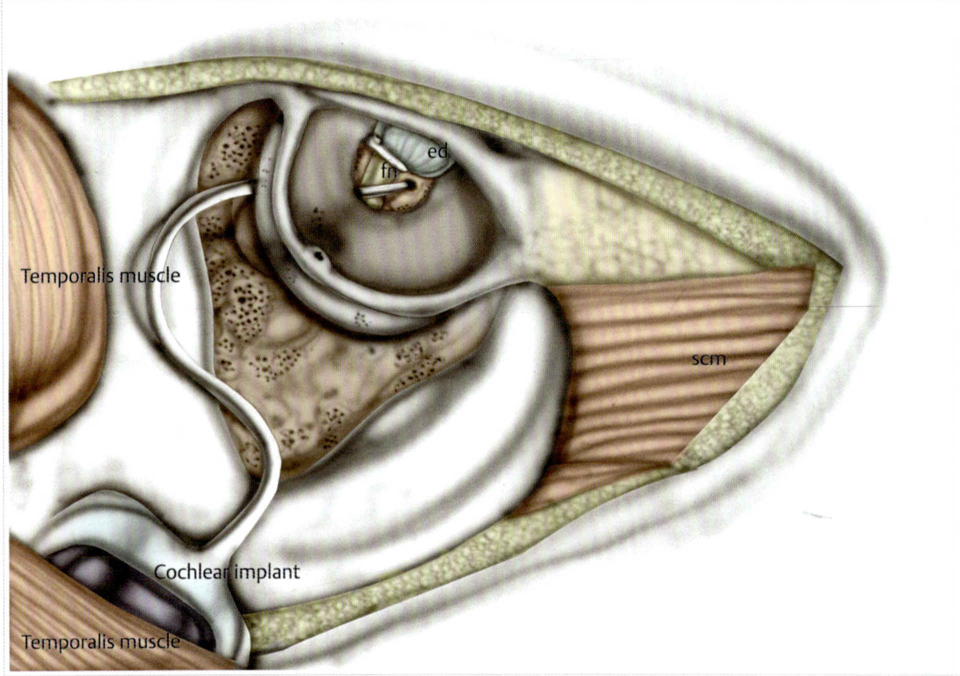

Fig. 12.45 Right side: Microscopic time. The receiver–stimulator is placed and fixed under the temporalis muscle. The array is gently inserted through the mastoidectomy and pushed from the attic to the mesotympanum inside the cochleostomy. *ed: eardrum; fn: facial nerve; scm: sternocleidomastoid muscle.*

could provoke a cochlear ossification during the postoperative time which is associated with a poorer hearing outcome after implantation as reported in literature (Wang and Zhang, 2014). In the transcanal infrapromontorial approach, the semicircular canals and the cochlea are preserved, thus avoiding cochlear ossification in the postoperative time probably yielding better hearing results.

12.3.2 Limitations

Even though the cochlea and the cochlear nerve are preserved during this approach, the transcanal infrapromontorial route may present some limitations that should be underlined to enable the surgeon to make the right choice:

- The preservation of the cochlea during the transcanal infrapromontorial approach is possible, but the sacrifice of the most posterior portion of the basal turn is required; at the end of the procedure, in fact the array is inserted from the most anterior portion of the basal turn to the apical turn of the cochlea.
- The association of the infrapromontorial route with a CI is indicated only for acoustic neuromas limited to the IAC (Koos I); if the acoustic neuroma is growing inside the cerebellopontine angle (CPA), a translabyrinthine approach with CI is suggested, since the preservation of the cochlea may be difficult and the visibility of the tumor in the CPA may be limited, forcing the surgeon to perform a blind dissection of the tumor in this anatomical area.

12.3.3 Surgical Steps

The initial surgical steps are the same as the ones described for the transcanal transpromontorial approaches to the IAC and in the CPA chapter (for more surgical details, see Chapter 11).

Summary of the surgical technique: Under a microscopic view, a postauricular incision is performed and the auricle is moved

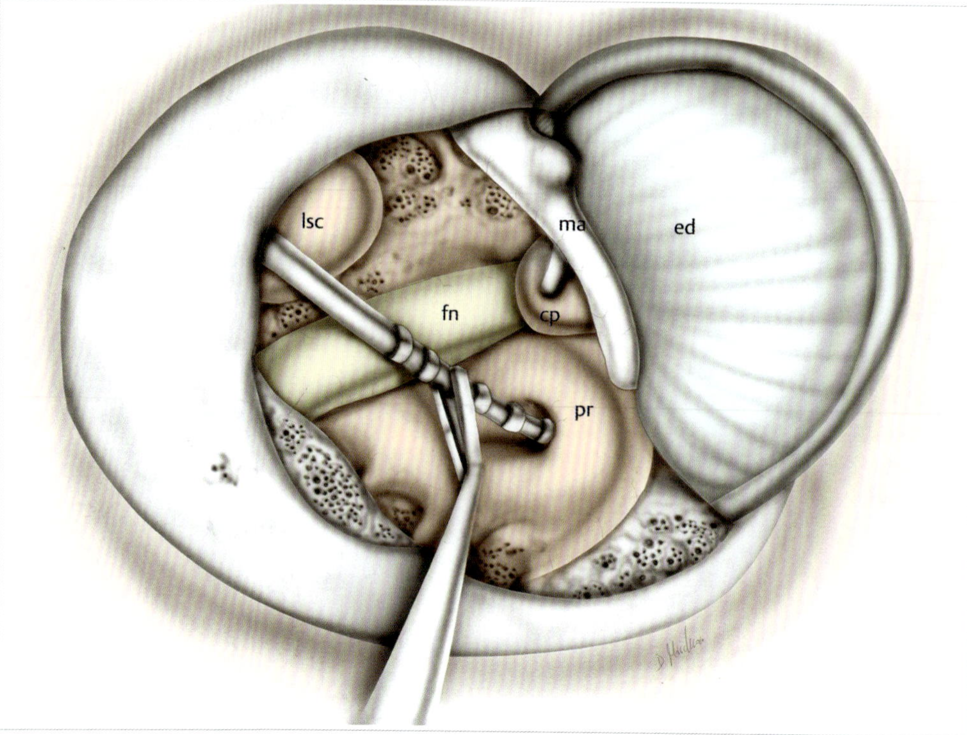

Fig. 12.46 Right side: The endoscopic magnification of the tympanic cavity may favor the correct insertion of the array through the cochleostomy. *cp: cochleariform process; ed: eardrum; fn: facial nerve; lsc: lateral semicircular canal; ma: malleus; pr: promontory.*

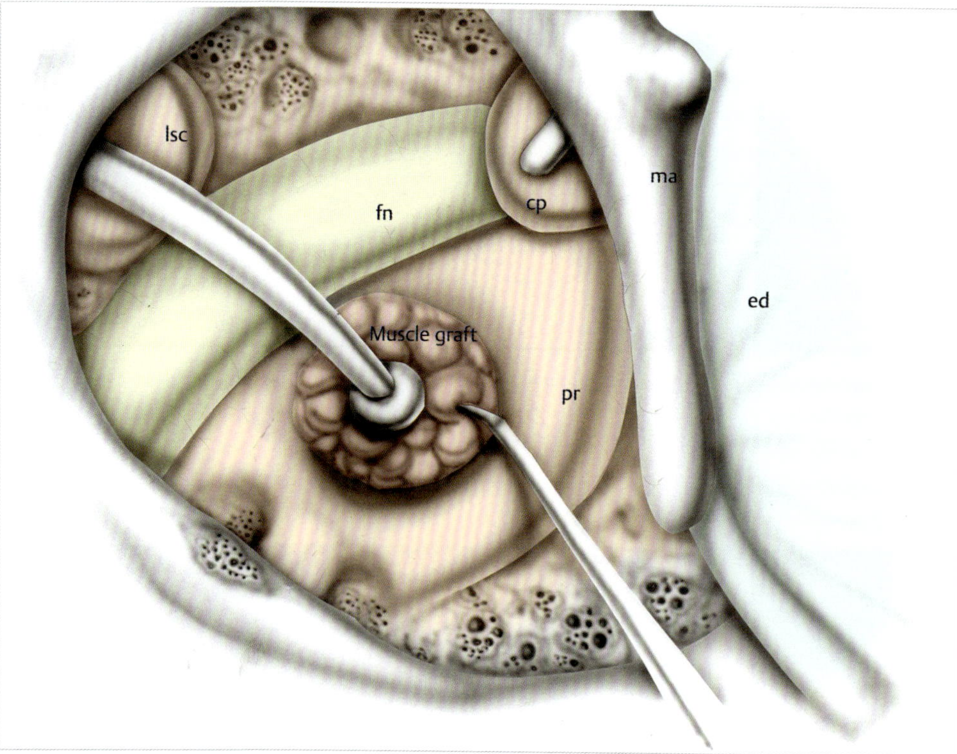

Fig. 12.47 Right side: A piece of muscle is placed to cover the cochleostomy. *cp: cochleariform process; ed: eardrum; fn: facial nerve; lsc: lateral semicircular canal; ma: malleus; pr: promontory.*

forward. The skin of the EAC is circumferentially incised and a blind sac closure of the EAC is performed. The skin of the EAC is completely dissected in an orthogonal way and removed along with the tympanic membrane en bloc. Then, a wide canalplasty is performed. During this step, the temporomandibular joint is anteriorly skeletonized and a wide atticotomy is performed. The tympanic and the mastoid portions of the FN are identified and skeletonized. The incus and the malleus are removed, to better expose the medial wall of the tympanic cavity and the tympanic portion of the FN. The microscopic dissection proceeds, using a diamond bur, to identify the main landmarks of the dissection: posteriorly, the mastoid portion of the FN; inferiorly, the jugular bulb; and anteriorly, the internal carotid artery. Once the working area has been created, the stapes is removed entering the vestibule, and the identification of the IAC preserving the cochlea should start.

12.3.4 Preservation of the Cochlea and the Cochlear Nerve

Once the medial wall of the vestibule with the spherical recess has been detected, the anatomy of the RW niche and the RW chamber, especially the tegmen, the finiculus, the subiculum, and the fustis with the subcochlear canaliculus, should be observed. In order to get a microscopic view of these anatomical observed, the mastoid segment of the FN should be skeletonized in a proper way, maintaining just a thin bony layer over the nerve to protect the FN during the dissection of the tumor.

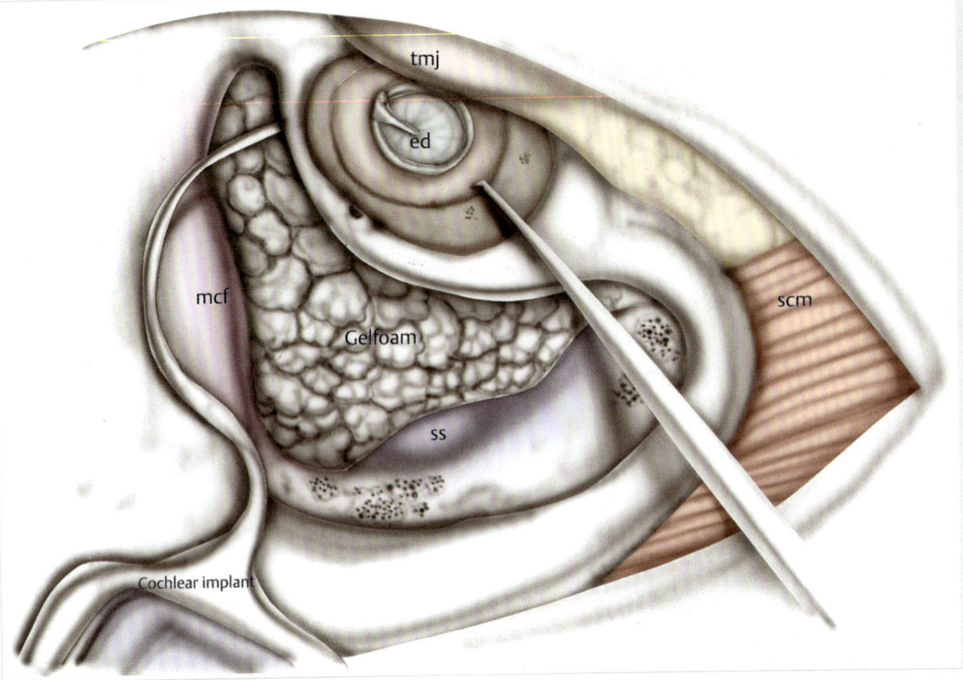

Fig. 12.48 Right side: The mastoid is filled with absorbable gelatin sponge. The tympanomeatal flap is replaced. *ed: eardrum; mcf: middle cranial fossa; scm: sternocleidomastoid muscle; tmj: temporomandibular joint; ss: sigmoid sinus.*

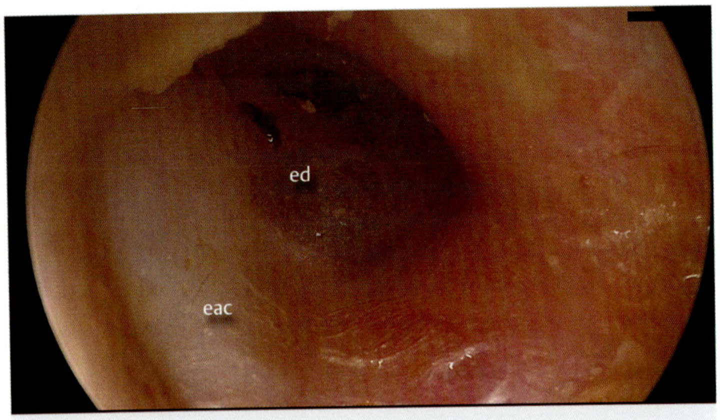

Fig. 12.49 Clinical Case 3, Right side: CHARGE syndrome. Endoscopic time. The external auditory canal (EAC) is injected with a diluted anesthetic/adrenaline solution. *eac: external auditory canal; ed: eardrum.*

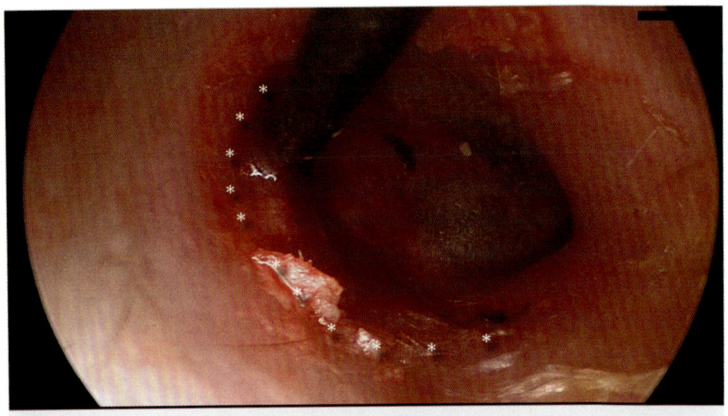

Fig. 12.50 Clinical Case 3, Right side: CHARGE syndrome. Endoscopic time. An external auditory canal (EAC) incision is endoscopically performed (****).

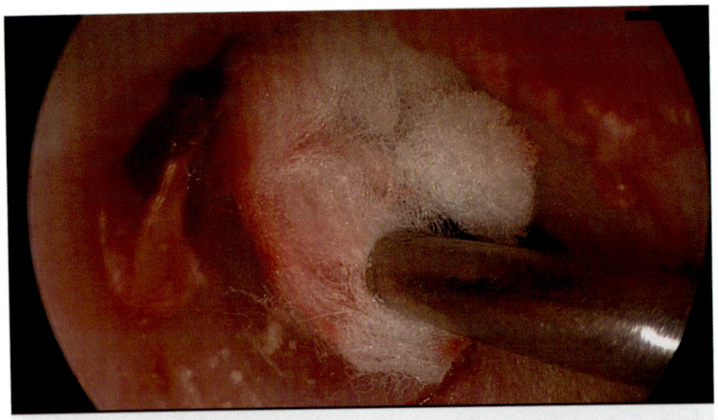

Fig. 12.51 Clinical Case 3, Right side: CHARGE syndrome. Endoscopic time. A cottonoid is used to pull the tympanomeatal flap, and to maintain the surgical field clean.

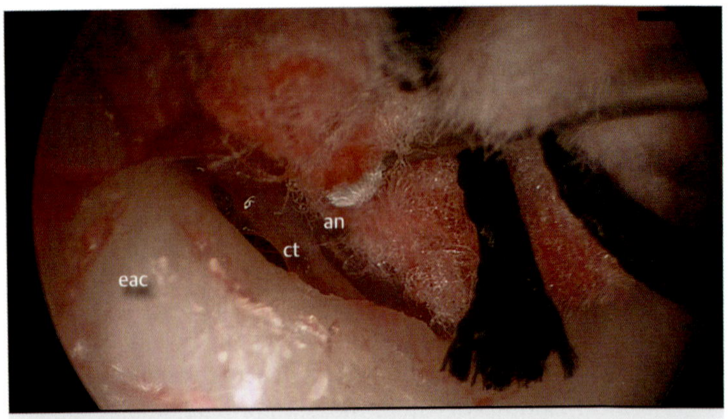

Fig. 12.52 Clinical Case 3, Right side: CHARGE syndrome. Endoscopic time. The tympanomeatal flap is elevated with the anulus entering the tympanic cavity. *an: fibrous anulus; ct: chorda tympani; eac: external auditory canal.*

A diamond bur is used on the tegmen of the RW to open the basal turn of the cochlea. Once the basal turn of the cochlea has been carefully opened, preserving the modiolar structure, the scala tympani and the scala vestibuli are detected (see ▶ Fig. 12.89, ▶ Fig. 12.90). A diamond bur is used to progressively remove the most posterior portion of the basal turn, creating a good visualization of the space between the cochlea, the vestibule, and the fundus of the IAC, uncovering the cochlear-vestibular bone (see ▶ Fig. 12.91, ▶ Fig. 12.92). After this step, careful

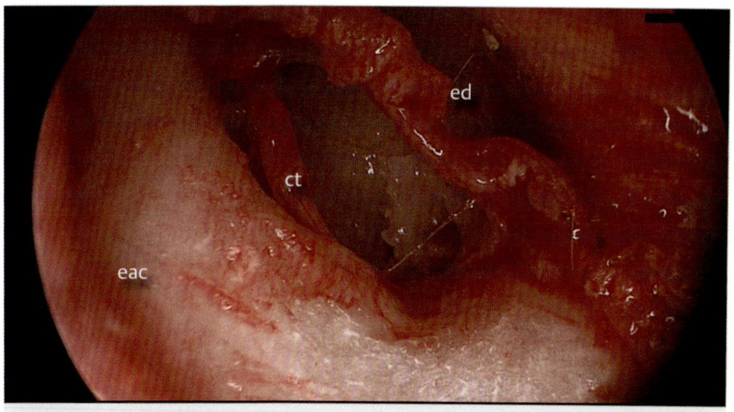

Fig. 12.53 Clinical Case 3, Right side: CHARGE syndrome. Endoscopic time. The tympanic cavity is endoscopically exposed. *ct: chorda tympani; eac: external auditory canal; ed: eardrum.*

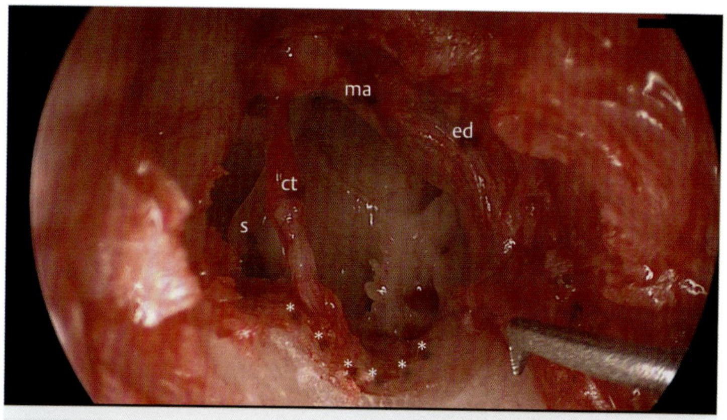

Fig. 12.54 Clinical Case 3, Right side: CHARGE syndrome. Endoscopic time. A curette is used to partially remove the posterior portion of the bony anulus (see ****) to gain an endoscopic view of the promontory. A malformed stapes is present. *ct: chorda tympani; ed: eardrum; ma: malleus; s: stapes.*

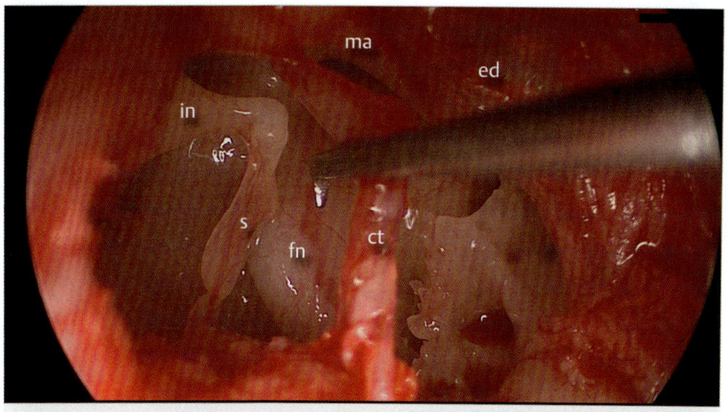

Fig. 12.55 Clinical Case 3, Right side: CHARGE syndrome. Endoscopic time. The chorda tympani is gently inferiorly pulled. A dystopic facial nerve (FN), located below the stapes, is shown running over the promontory. *ct: chorda tympani; ed: eardrum; fn: facial nerve; in: incus; ma: malleus; s: stapes.*

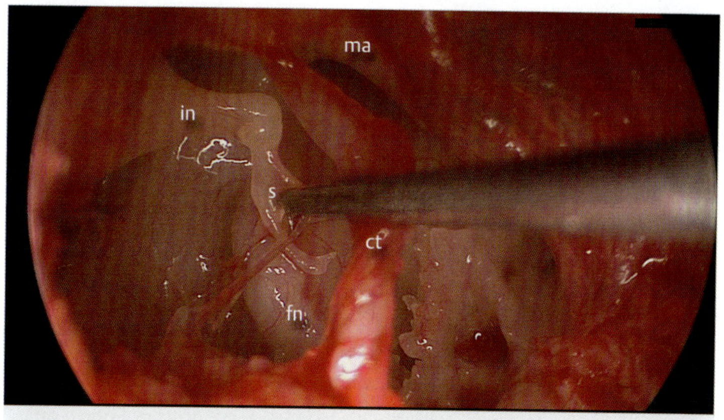

Fig. 12.56 Clinical Case 3, Right side: CHARGE syndrome. Endoscopic time. The stapes is disjointed from the incus. *ct: chorda tympani; fn: facial nerve; in: incus; ma: malleus, s: stapes.*

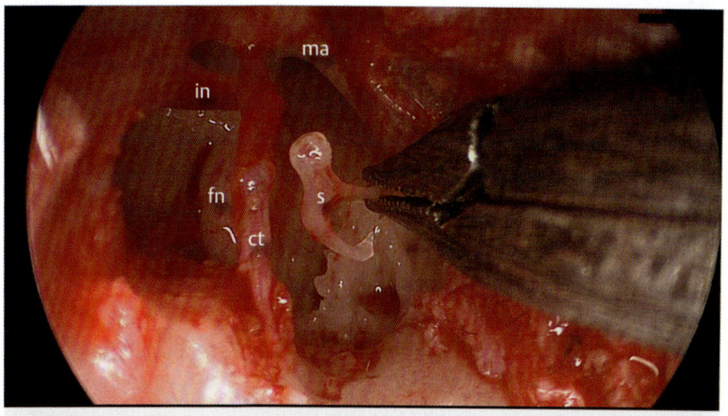

Fig. 12.57 Clinical Case 3, Right side: CHARGE syndrome. Endoscopic time. The stapes is removed. *ct: chorda tympani; fn: facial nerve; in: incus; ma: malleus; s: stapes.*

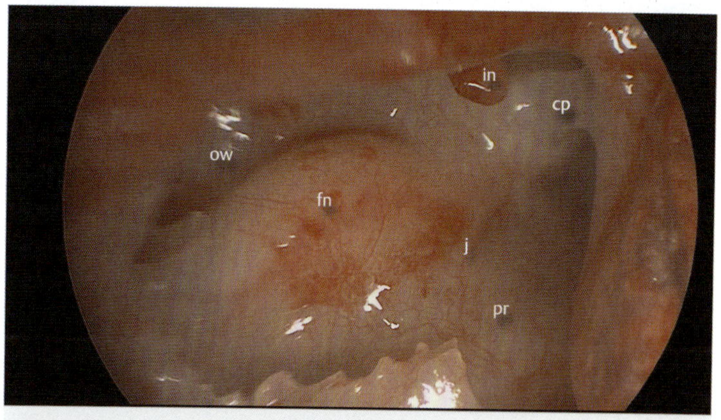

Fig. 12.58 Clinical Case 3, Right side: CHARGE syndrome. Endoscopic time. Endoscopic magnification of the anomalous facial nerve (FN); the nerve runs over the promontory, obscuring the round window (RW). *cp: cochleariform process; in: incus; j: Jacobson's nerve; ow: oval window; pr: promontory.*

drilling of the cochlear vestibular bone should be carried out until the skeletonization of the fundus of the IAC trying to preserve the medial and the apical turns of the cochlea (see ▶ Fig. 12.92, ▶ Fig. 12.93). The bony wall of the promontory should be preserved in order to protect the medial, the apical, and the most anterior portion of the basal turns of the cochlea. The fundus of the IAC is opened just between the vestibule and the posterior portion of the basal turn of the cochlea, uncovering the dura of the IAC. A diamond bur is used to remove the hypotympanic, retrotympanic, and protympanic bone; the IAC in the petrous apex area is progressively skeletonized from the fundus to the porus. Once the porus has been detected, the dura of the

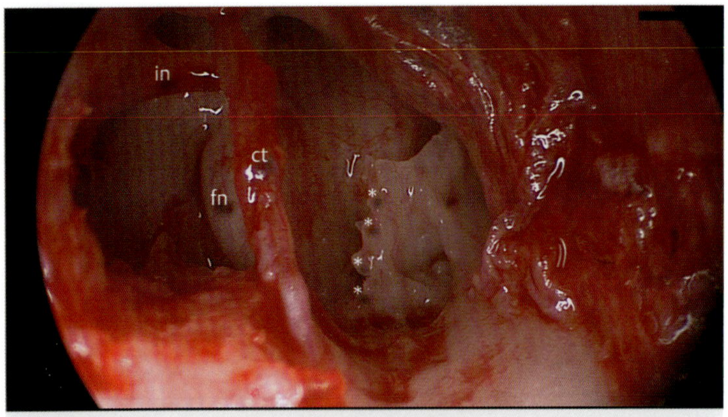

Fig. 12.59 Clinical Case 3, Right side: CHARGE syndrome. Endoscopic time. The round window (RW) chamber with the fustis is endoscopically detected (*****). *ct: chorda tympani; fn: facial nerve; in: incus.*

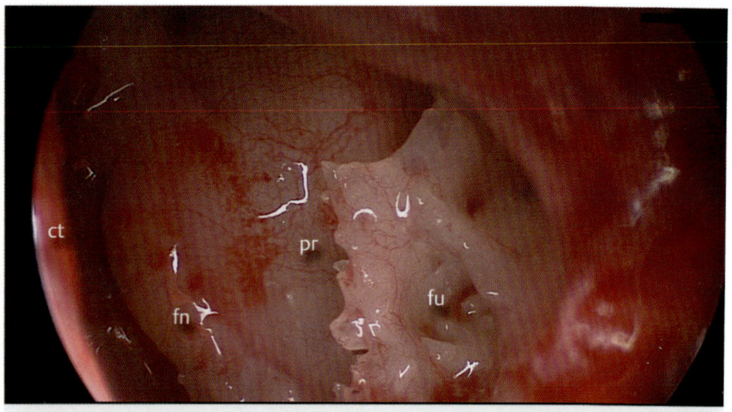

Fig. 12.60 Clinical Case 3, Right side: CHARGE syndrome. Endoscopic time. The fustis bone is endoscopically magnified and used as a landmark to find the cochlea. *ct: chorda tympani; fn: facial nerve; fu: fustis; pr: promontory.*

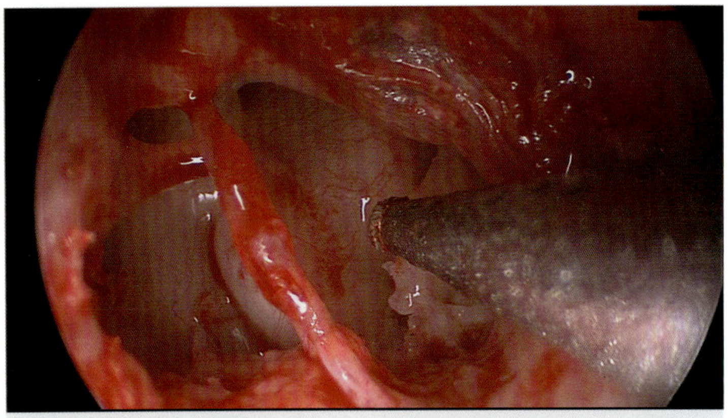

Fig. 12.61 Clinical Case 3, Right side: CHARGE syndrome. Endoscopic time. A diamond bur is used following the fustis' orientation to perform the cochleostomy.

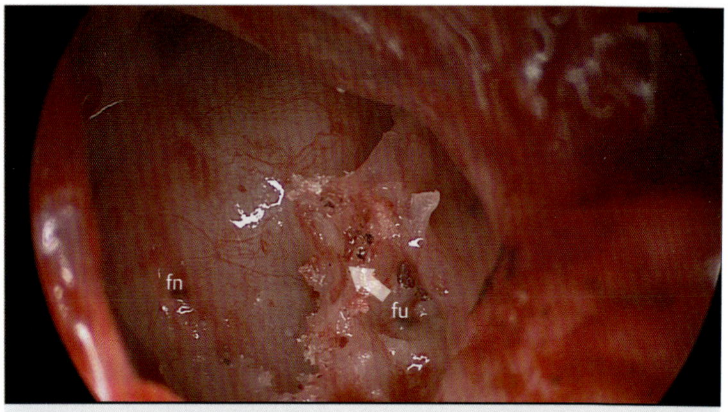

Fig. 12.62 Clinical Case 3, Right side: CHARGE syndrome. Endoscopic time. The *white arrow* shows the direction of the fustis. *fn: facial nerve; fu: fustis.*

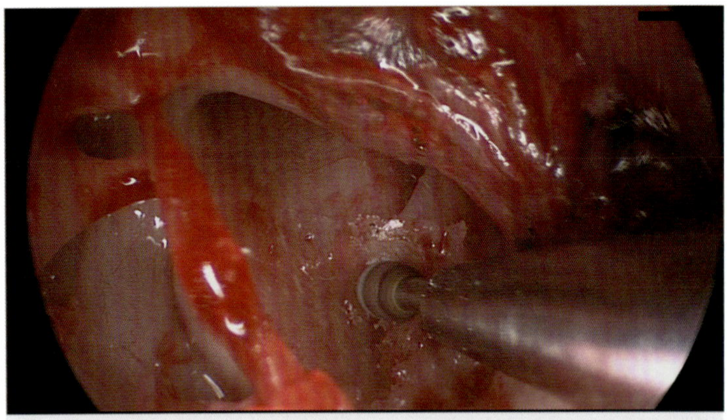

Fig. 12.63 Clinical Case 3, Right side: CHARGE syndrome. Endoscopic time. The drilling time is started.

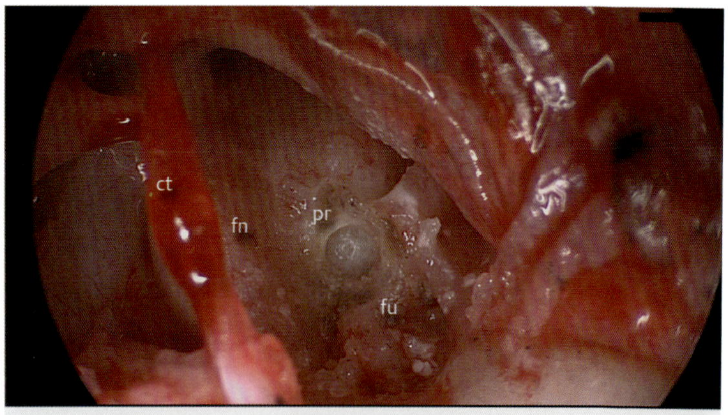

Fig. 12.64 Clinical Case 3, Right side: CHARGE Ssndrome. Endoscopic time. The cochleostomy is performed in the promontory following the fustis' orientation. *ct: chorda tympani; fn: facial nerve; fu: fustis; pr: promontory.*

posterior fossa is gently exposed around the porus. The folding of the dura on the medial surface of the petrous bone represents the deepest limit of the dissection. The IAC dura is opened exposing the acoustic neuroma. A gentle dissection is performed over the tumor. During this step, a careful preservation of the cochlear nerve is mandatory. The cochlear nerve is identified at its entrance to the modiolus, in the spiral ganglion, and the nerve should be preserved during the excision of the acoustic neuroma (see ▶ Fig. 12.94 and Clinical Case 5).

In case of a difficult orientation during surgery, the lateral wall of the promontory may be carefully drilled to just expose the medial and apical turns of the cochlea. This procedure is performed in order to provide an anatomical view of the cochlear structures and to get the right orientation, exposing the anatomical relationship between the cochlea and the surrounding anatomical structures (see ▶ Fig. 12.95, ▶ Fig. 12.96, ▶ Fig. 12.97 and see Clinical Case 7). Once the microscopic acoustic neuroma removal has been performed, a 0-degree 4 mm diameter endoscope is introduced into the surgical cavity to detect the status of the cochlear nerve and of the FN, looking for any residual disease

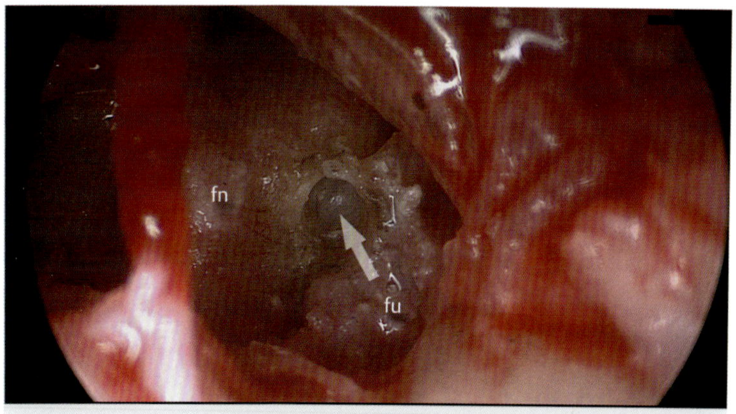

Fig. 12.65 Clinical Case 3, Right side: CHARGE syndrome. Endoscopic time. The *white arrow* shows the fustis' orientation in relation to the cochleostomy site. *fn: facial nerve; fu: fustis.*

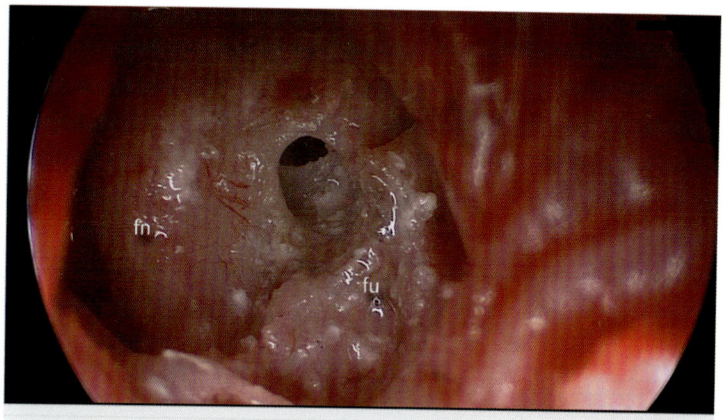

Fig. 12.66 Clinical Case 3, Right side: CHARGE syndrome. Endoscopic time. The cochleostomy is performed. *fn: facial nerve; fu: fustis.*

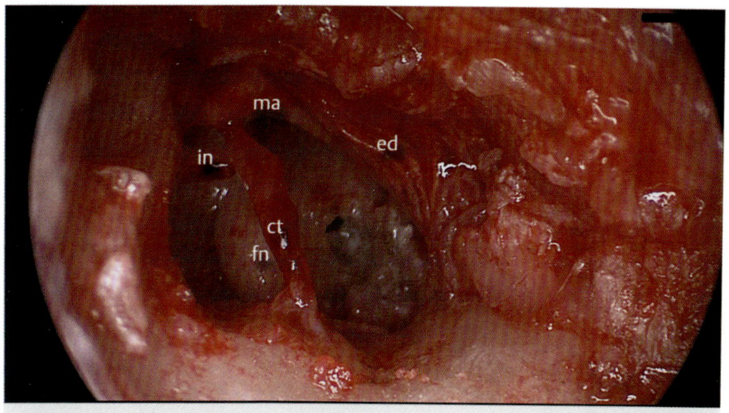

Fig. 12.67 Clinical Case 3, Right side: CHARGE syndrome. Endoscopic time. Final endoscopic view of the tympanic cavity. *ct: chorda tympani; ed: eardrum; fn: facial nerve; in: incus; ma: malleus.*

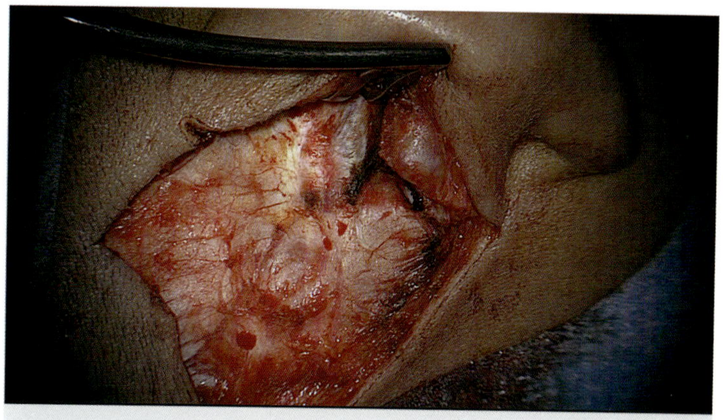

Fig. 12.68 Clinical Case 3, Right side: CHARGE syndrome. Microscopic time. A retroauricular incision is made; the fascia of the temporalis muscle and the posterior portion of the external auditory canal (EAC) are exposed.

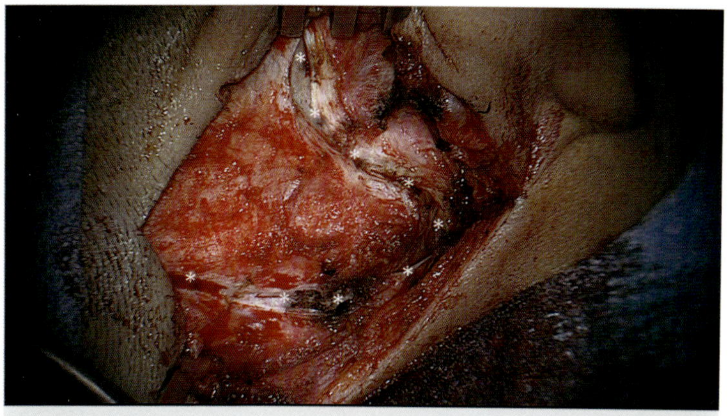

Fig. 12.69 Clinical Case 3, Right side: CHARGE syndrome. Microscopic time. A superior based pedicle fibro-muscular-periosteal flap is created (****** = line of incision).

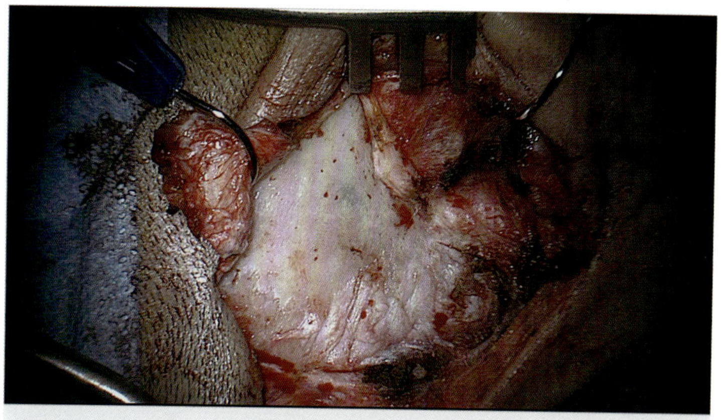

Fig. 12.70 Clinical Case 3, Right side: CHARGE syndrome. Microscopic time. The mastoid bone is exposed.

(see Clinical Case 6). In case of a residual disease, an endoscopic dissection of the remnants should be carefully performed in order to avoid damage to the insertion of the cochlear nerve into the cochlea. In some cases, a 45-degree endoscope may be useful to remove the remnant disease located in the fundus.

Once the acoustic neuroma has been removed, electrophysiological tests are performed in order to have a map of the status of the cochlear nerve before the placement of the CI.

The receiver–stimulator of the implant is fixed and covered under the temporalis muscle. The array is gently microscopically pushed through the previously created cochleostomy in the basal turn of the cochlea (see ▶ Fig. 12.94b). When the drilling of the lateral wall of the promontory is necessary, the insertion of the array should be carefully performed in order to control the most apical portion of the cochlea, where the array could be misplaced (see ▶ Fig. 12.98). In this case, a piece of muscle may be used to cover the promontory defect, and to help the insertion of the array, protecting the cochlea (see ▶ Fig. 12.99).

A muscle fragment is placed in the eustachian tube and fibrin glue is used to secure the closure.

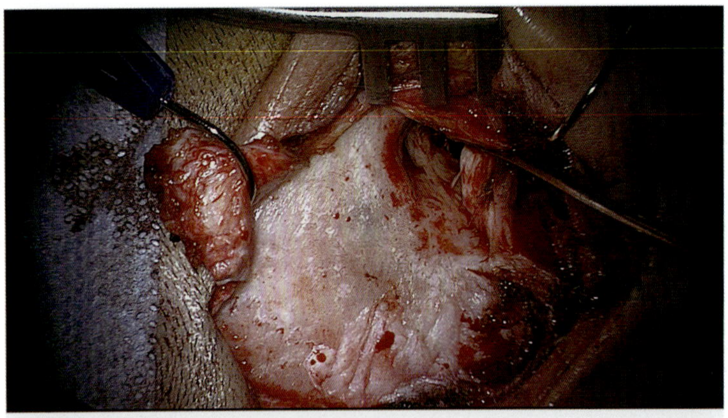

Fig. 12.71 Clinical Case 3, Right side: CHARGE syndrome. Microscopic time. The skin of the posterior portion of the external auditory canal (EAC) is gently detached from the bony canal. This maneuver allows to expose the tympanic cavity through the EAC.

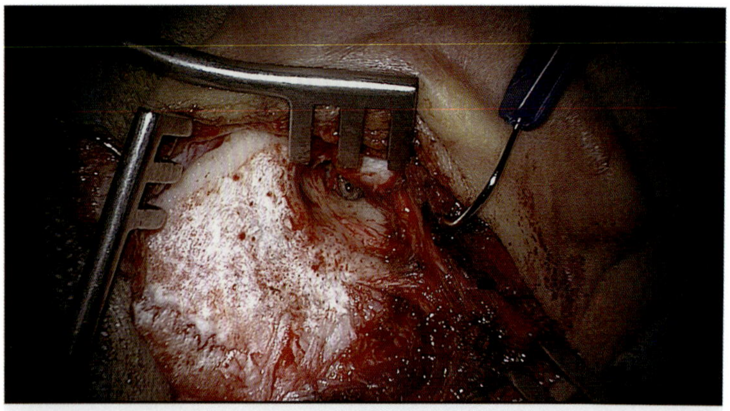

Fig. 12.72 Clinical Case 3, Right side: CHARGE syndrome. Microscopic time. A retractor is placed to maintain the opening through the external canal, optimizing the microscopic view of the tympanic cavity.

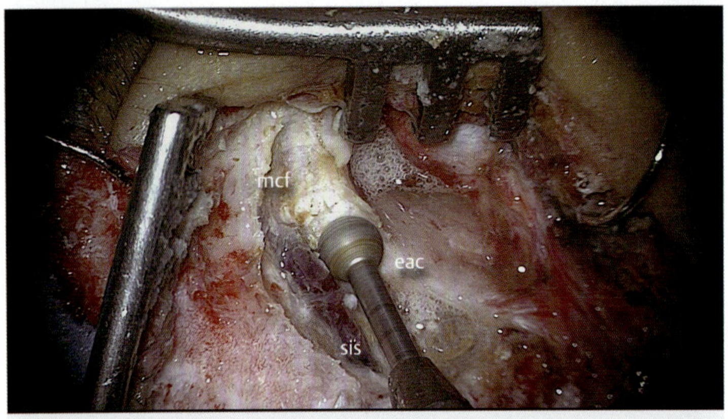

Fig. 12.73 Clinical Case 3, Right side: CHARGE syndrome. Microscopic time. A mastoidectomy is performed; in this case a sclerotic contracted mastoid is found. *eac: external auditory canal; mcf: middle cranial fossa; sis: sigmoid sinus.*

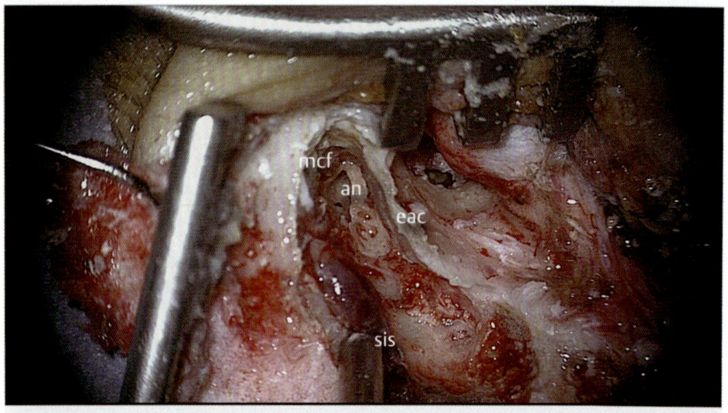

Fig. 12.74 Clinical Case 3, Right side: CHARGE syndrome. Microscopic time. The mastoidectomy is carried out reaching the antrum. *an: antrum; eac: external auditory canal; mcf: middle cranial fossa; sis: sigmoid sinus.*

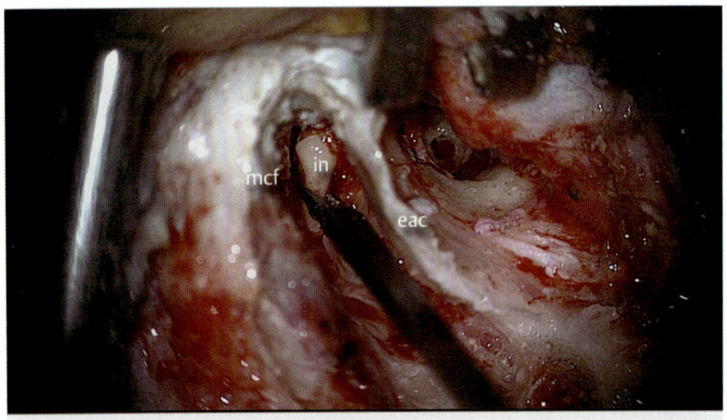

Fig. 12.75 Clinical Case 3, Right side: CHARGE syndrome. Microscopic time. The incus is removed. *eac: external auditory canal; in: incus; mcf: middle cranial fossa.*

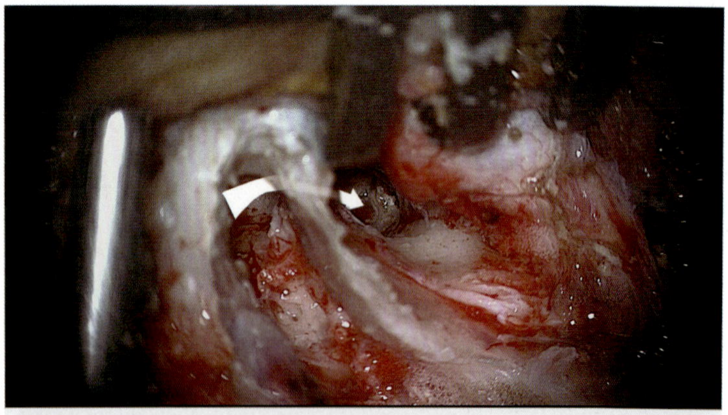

Fig. 12.76 Clinical Case 3, Right side: CHARGE syndrome. Microscopic time. After incus is removed, a connection between the attic and the mesotympanum is created (see the *white arrow*).

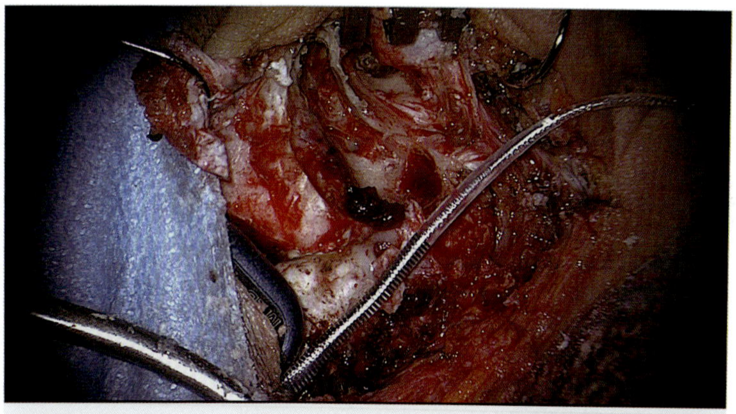

Fig. 12.77 Clinical Case 3, Right side: CHARGE syndrome. Microscopic time. The receiver–stimulator is placed and fixed under the temporalis muscle.

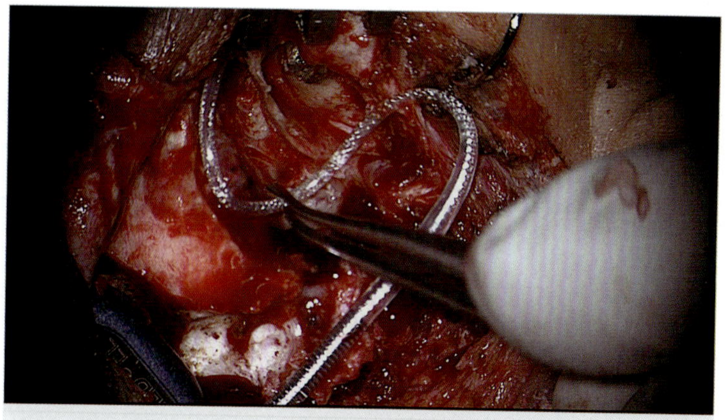

Fig. 12.78 Clinical Case 3, Right side: CHARGE syndrome. Microscopic time. The array is gently inserted through the mastoidectomy from the attic to the mesotympanum.

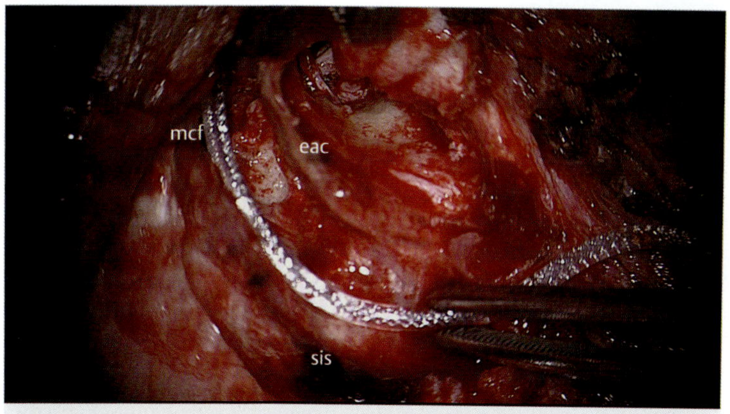

Fig. 12.79 Clinical Case 3, Right side: CHARGE syndrome. Microscopic time. The array is pushed inside the previously created cochleostomy. *eac: external auditory canal; mcf: middle cranial fossa; sis: sigmoid sinus.*

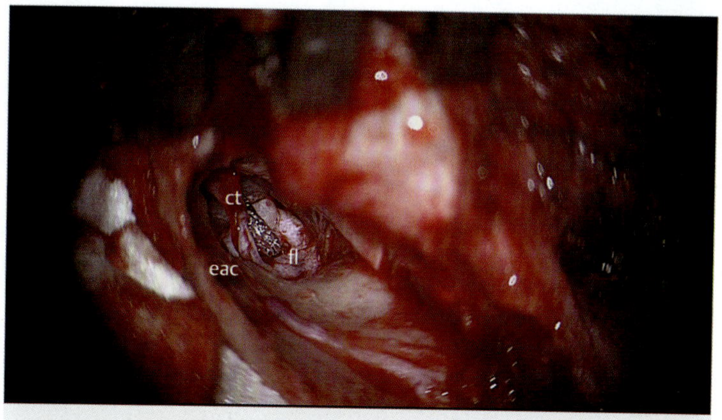

Fig. 12.80 Clinical Case 3, Right side: CHARGE syndrome. Microscopic time. A piece of temporalis fascia is used to cover the cochleostomy and protect the array. *ct: chorda tympani; eac: external auditory canal; fl: fascia layer.*

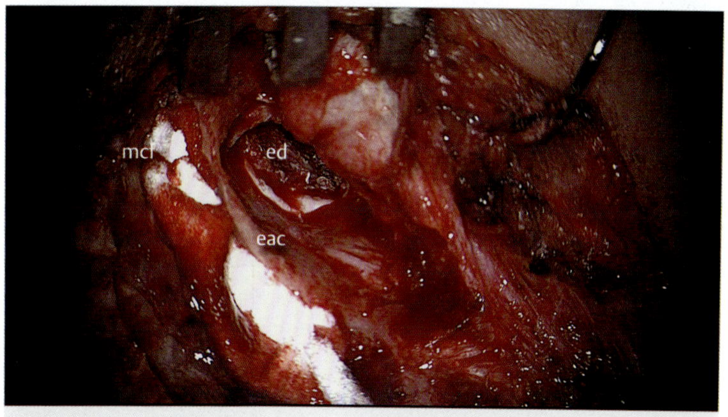

Fig. 12.81 Clinical Case 3, Right side: CHARGE syndrome. Microscopic time. The eardrum is replaced; an absorbable gelatin sponge is placed into the mastoid cavity. *eac: external auditory canal; ed: eardrum; mcf: middle cranial fossa.*

The surgical cavity is then obliterated using a fat pad harvested from the abdomen to occlude the inner ear defect and the middle ear.

12.3.5 Postoperative Care

The transcanal infrapromontorial approach follows the same principles as the transcanal transpromontorial approach (see Chapter 11).

The CI is activated 1 month after surgery and a rehabilitation protocol is followed in order to evaluate the final hearing result.

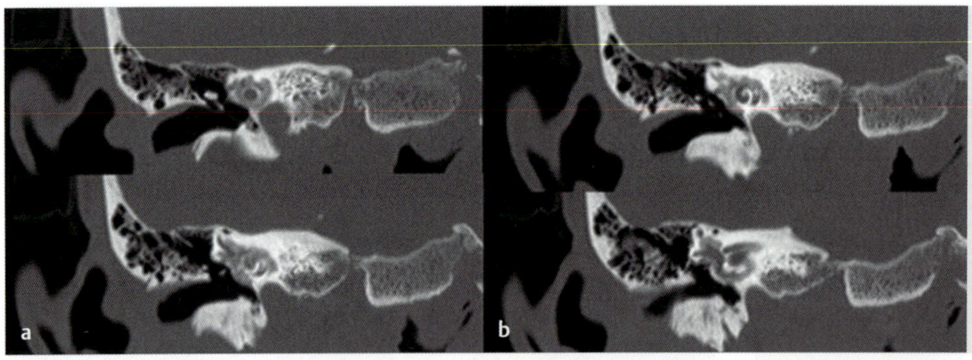

Fig. 12.82 (a, b) Computed tomography (CT) scan in coronal view of a patient with cochlear otosclerosis; an obliterative round window (RW) is noted.

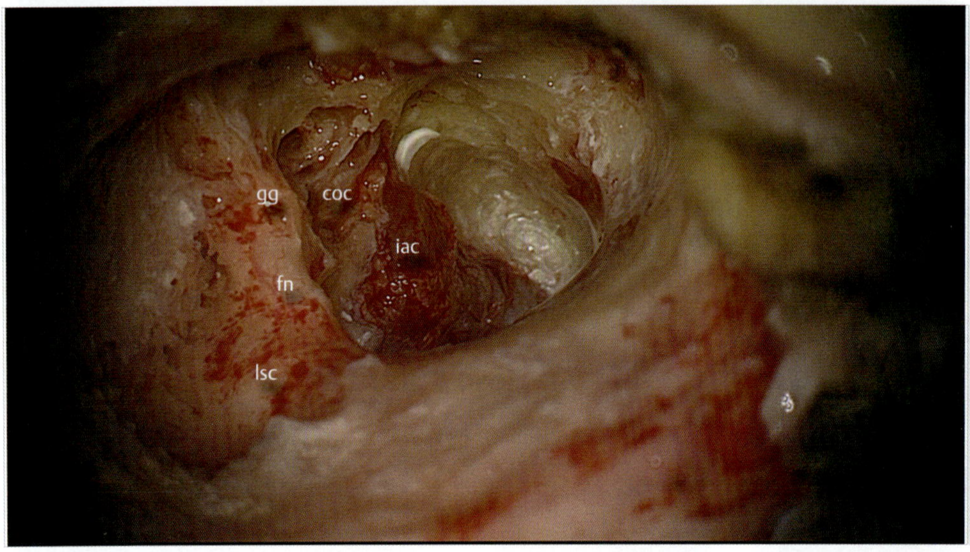

Fig. 12.83 Clinical Case 4, Right side: Transcanal infrapromontorial approach. Microscopic view. The ossicular chain is removed, the vestibule is exposed, and the facial nerve (FN) is skeletonized from the tympanic to the mastoid segment. The promontory is partially removed and the cochlear turns are exposed; the internal auditory canal (IAC) is skeletonized just below the cochlea from the fundus to the porus. The anatomical relationship between the cochlea and the IAC is well visible. *coc: cochlea; fn: facial nerve; gg: geniculate ganglion; iac: internal auditory canal; lsc: lateral semicircular canal.*

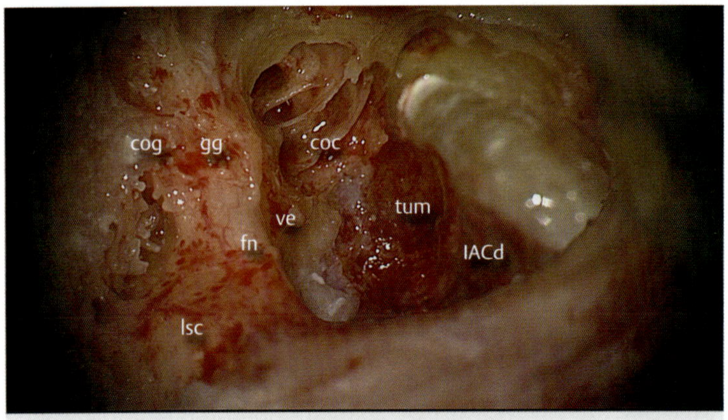

Fig. 12.84 Clinical Case 4, Right side: Transcanal infrapromontorial approach, Microscopic view. The dura of the internal auditory canal is opened exposing the acoustic neuroma. *coc: cochlea; fn: facial nerve; gg: geniculate ganglion; IACd: dura layer of internal auditory canal; lsc: lateral semicircular canal; tum: tumor; ve: vestibule.*

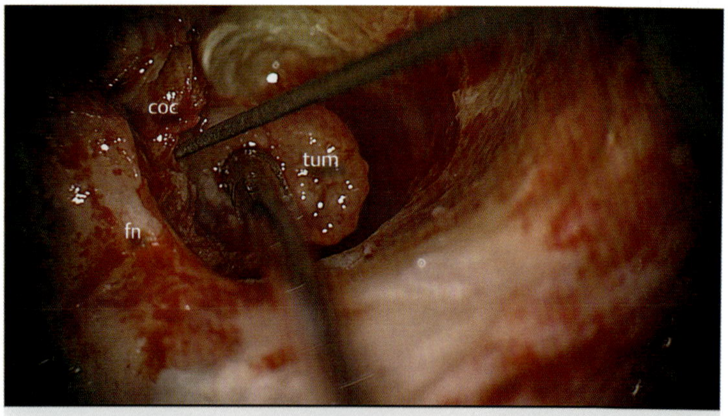

Fig. 12.85 Clinical Case 4, Right side: Transcanal infrapromontorial approach. The tumor is microscopically removed. *coc: cochlea, fn: facial nerve; tum: tumor.*

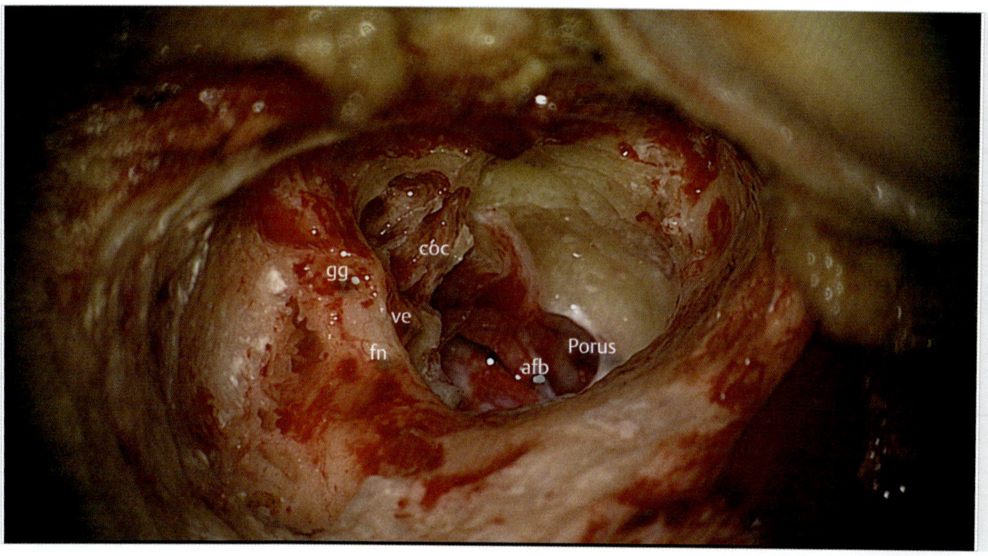

Fig. 12.86 Clinical Case 4, Right side: Transcanal infrapromontorial approach. Microscopic view. The tumor is removed; the acoustic-facial bundle is preserved. The anatomy of the internal auditory canal is visible from the fundus to the porus. *afb: acoustic-facial bundle; coc: cochlea; fn: facial nerve; gg: geniculate ganglion; ve: vestibule.*

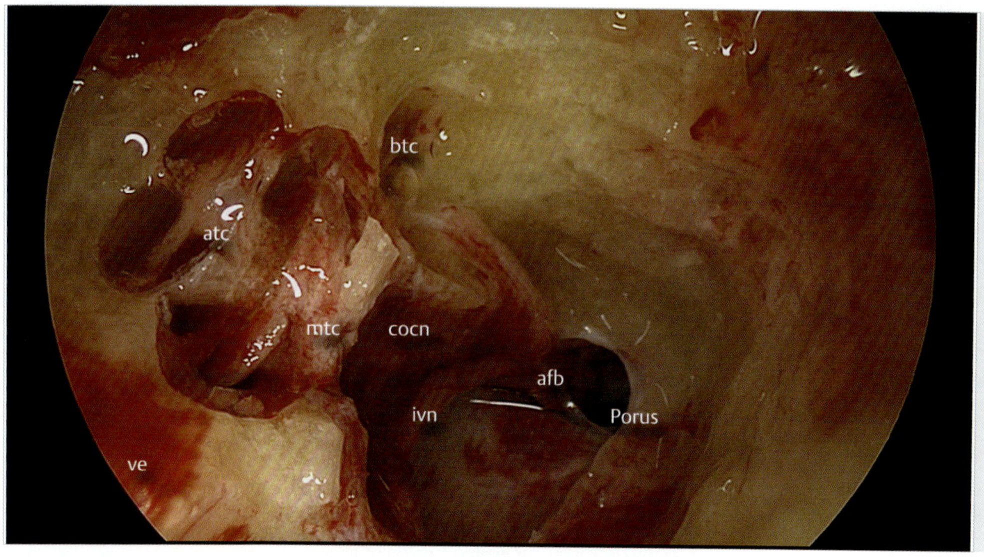

Fig. 12.87 Clinical Case 4, Right side: Transcanal infrapromontorial approach. Endoscopic view. A 0-degree endoscope is inserted into the surgical cavity to check the presence of any residual disease and to see the status of the cochlear nerve. The most anterior portion of the basal turn is noted. *afb: acoustic-facial bundle; atc: apical turn of the cochlea; btc: basal turn of the cochlea; cocn: cochlear nerve; ivn: inferior vestibular nerve; mtc: middle turn of the cochlea; ve: vestibule.*

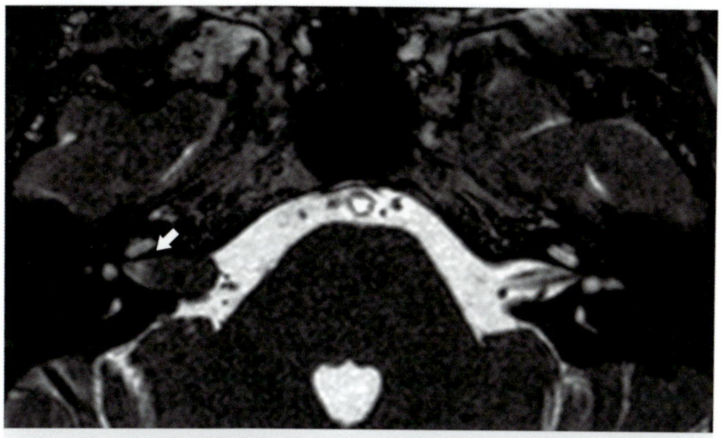

Fig. 12.88 Magnetic resonance imaging (MRI) in axial view. Typical indication for a transcanal infrapromontorial approach. The acoustic neuroma is limited to the internal auditory canal (IAC) with a minimal extension to the cerebellopontine angle cistern. The fundus of the IAC is not completely occupied by the tumor, and the insertion of the cochlear nerve in the modiolus is visible (see the *white arrow*). In this case a preservation of the cochlear nerve with simultaneous cochlear implant (CI) is feasible.

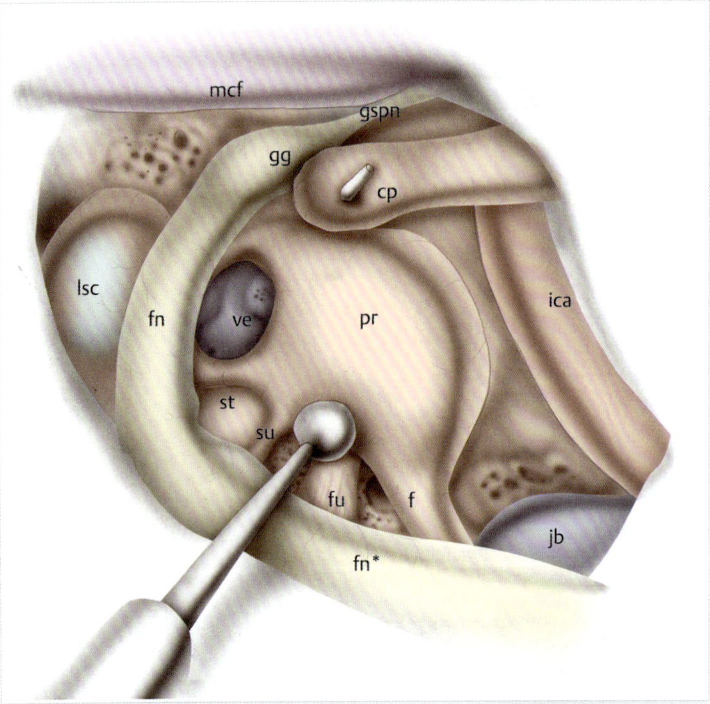

Fig. 12.89 Right side: Transcanal infrapromontorial approach. The ossicular chain is removed; the vestibule and the medial wall of the tympanic cavity are exposed. A diamond bur is used on the round window (RW) to open the basal turn of the cochlea following the basal turn until the most anterior portion. *cp: cochleariform process; f: finiculus; fn: tympanic segment of facial nerve; fn*: mastoid portion of facial nerve; fu: fustis; gg: geniculate ganglion; gspn: greater superficial petrosal nerve; ica: internal carotid artery; jb: jugular bulb; lsc: lateral semicircular canal; mcf: middle cranial fossa; pr: promontory; st: sinus timpani; su: subiculum; ve: vestibule.*

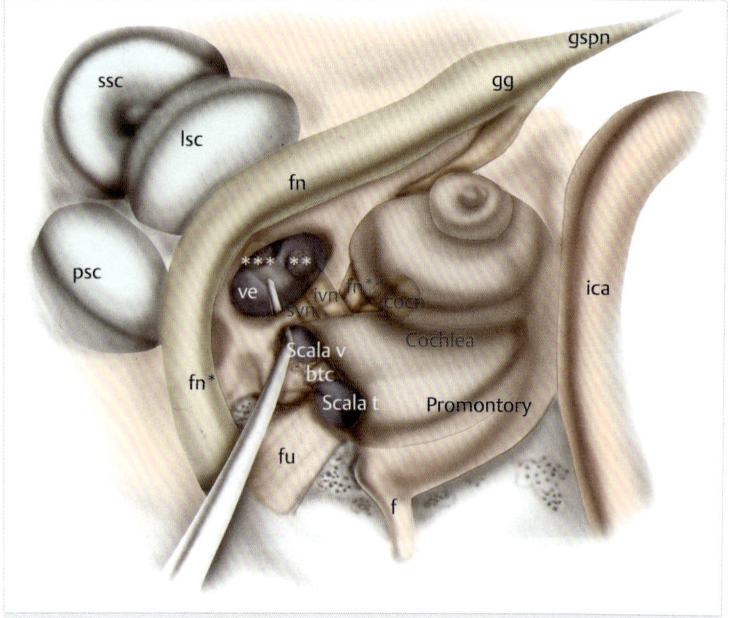

Fig. 12.90 Right side: Transcanal infrapromontorial approach. The basal turn of the cochlea is opened; the scala tympani and the scala vestibuli are identified; the cochlear turns and the fundus of the internal auditory canal with the nerves are represented in transparency. *bct: basal turn of the cochlea; cocn: cochlear nerve; f: finiculus; fn: tympanic segment of facial nerve; fn*: mastoid portion of facial nerve; fn**: labyrinthine portion of facial nerve; fu: fustis; gg: geniculate ganglion; gspn: greater superficial petrosal nerve; ica: internal carotid artery; ivn: inferior vestibular nerve; lsc: lateral semicircular canal; psc: posterior semicircular canal; scala t: scala tympani; scala v: scala vestibuli; ssc: superior semicircular canal; svn: superior vestibular nerve; ve: vestibule; **: spherical recess; ***: elliptical recess.*

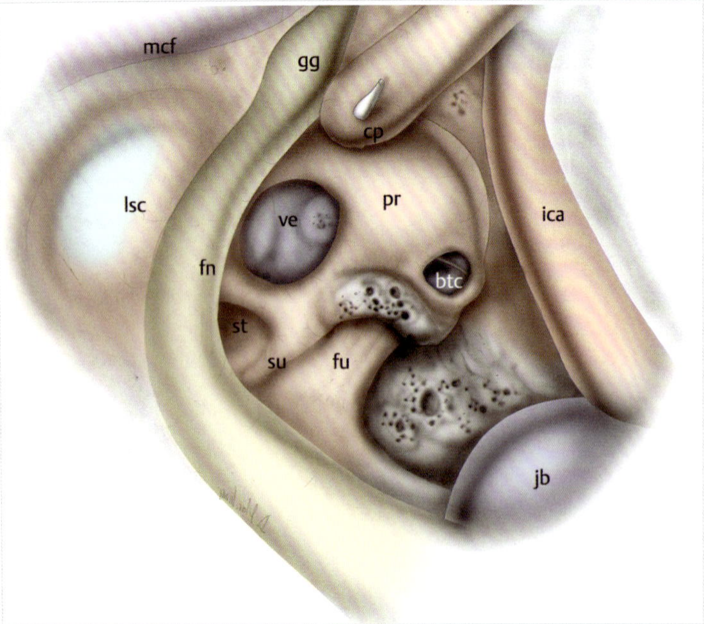

Fig. 12.91 Right side: Transcanal infrapromontorial approach. A diamond bur is used to open the basal turn of the cochlea; the surgeon stops drilling when the most anterior portion of the basal turn is reached. *btc: basal turn of the cochlea; cp: cochleariform process; fn: tympanic segment of facial nerve; fu: fustis; gg: geniculate ganglion; ica: internal carotid artery; jb: jugular bulb; lsc: lateral semicircular canal; mcf: middle cranial fossa; pr: promontory; st: sinus timpani; su: subiculum; ve: vestibule.*

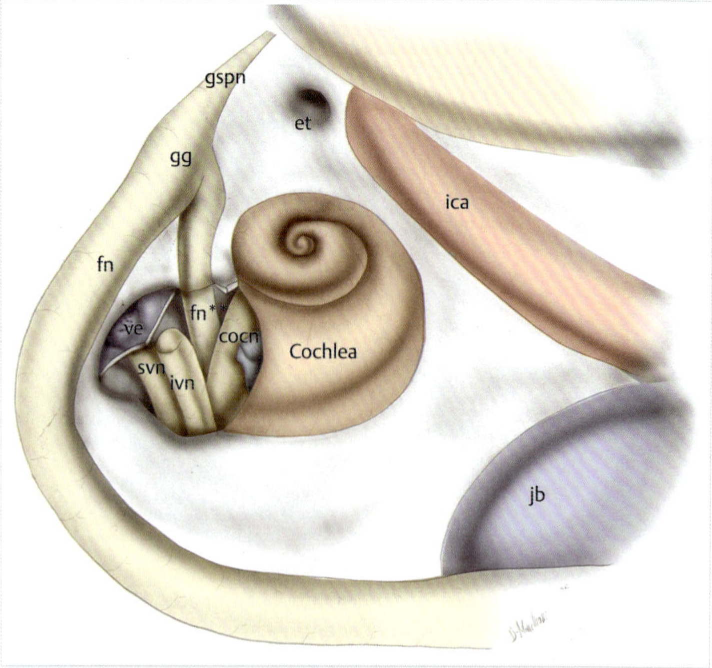

Fig. 12.92 Right side: Transcanal infrapromontorial approach. Schematic drawing showing the anatomical position of the nerves inside the fundus of the internal auditory canal after cochlear-vestibular bone removal through a transcanal infrapromontorial approach. *cocn: cochlear nerve; et: eustachian tube; fn: tympanic segment of facial nerve; fn**: facial nerve into the IAC; gg: geniculate ganglion; gspn: greater superficial petrosal nerve; ica: internal carotid artery; ivn: inferior vestibular nerve; jb: jugular bulb; svn: superior vestibular nerve; ve: vestibule.*

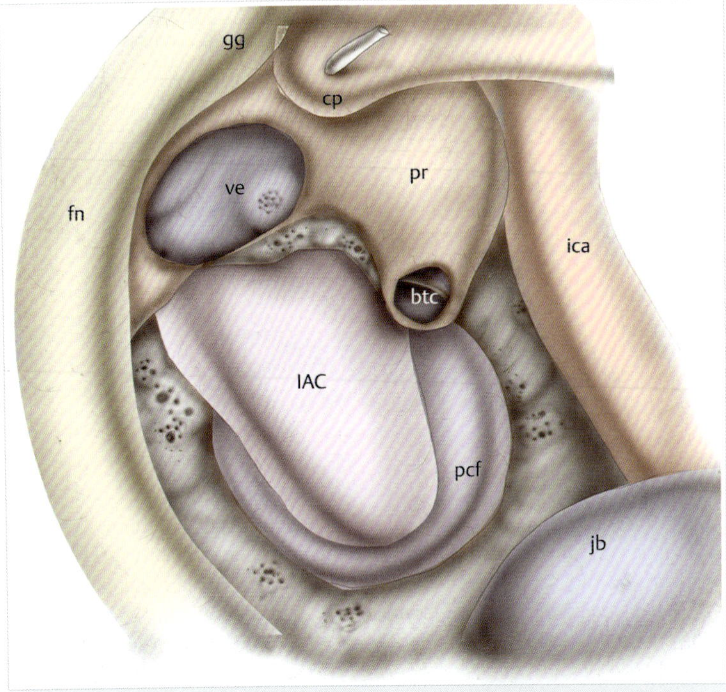

Fig. 12.93 Right side: Transcanal infrapromontorial approach. The cochlear-vestibular bone is removed and the internal auditory canal skeletonized from the fundus to the porus, preserving both the promontory and the cochlea. *btc: basal turn of the cochlea; cp: cochleariform process; fn: tympanic segment of facial nerve; gg: geniculate ganglion; IAC: internal auditory canal; ica: internal carotid artery; jb: jugular bulb; pcf: posterior fossa dura; pr: promontory; ve: vestibule.*

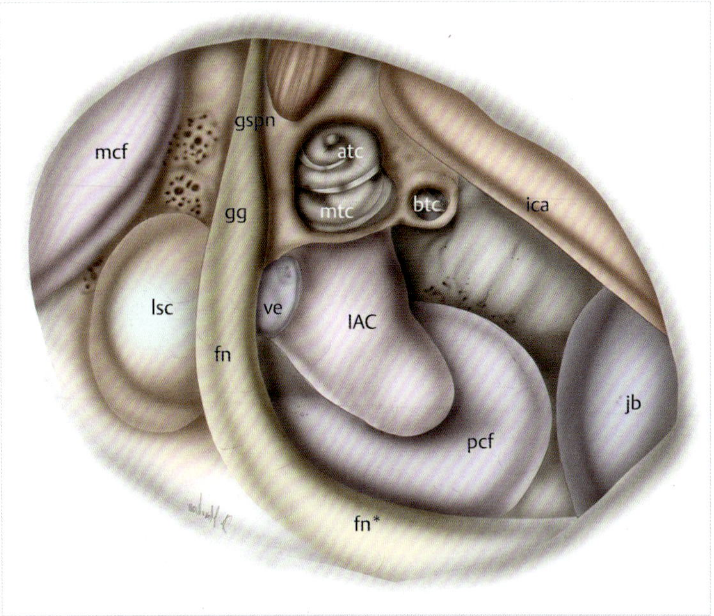

Fig. 12.95 Right side: Transcanal infrapromontorial approach. In this case, the promontory is partially removed just to uncover the cochlear turns; this surgical maneuver is suggested in case of difficult orientation during surgery. The internal auditory canal is skeletonized from the fundus to the porus keeping the cochlear turns under surgical view. *atc: apical turn of cochlea; btc: basal turn of the cochlea; fn: tympanic segment of facial nerve; fn*: mastoid segment of facial nerve; gg: geniculate ganglion; gspn: greater superficial petrosal nerve; IAC: internal auditory canal; ica: internal carotid artery; jb: jugular bulb; lsc: lateral semicircular canal; mcf: middle cranial fossa; mtc: middle turn of cochlea; pcf: posterior cranial fossa dura; ve: vestibule.*

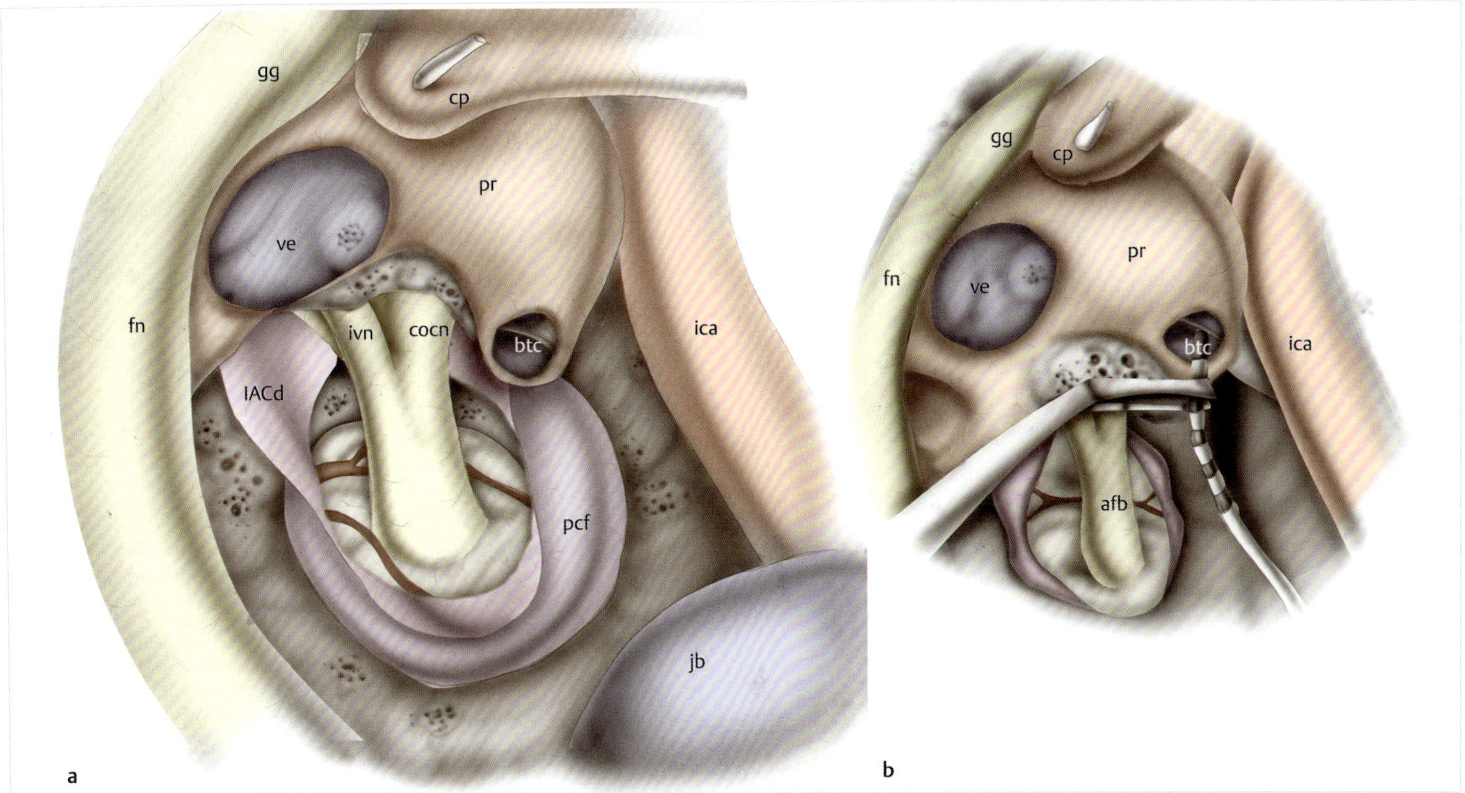

Fig. 12.94 Right side: Transcanal infrapromontorial approach: **(a)** The dura of the internal auditory canal (IAC) is opened and the tumor is removed. The content of the IAC is seen; the nerves are preserved, especially the cochlear nerve and the cochlea are preserved in order to permit a simultaneous cochlear implant (CI). **(b)** The array of the CI is gently inserted through the cochleostomy on the basal turn of the cochlea. *afb: acoustic facial bundle; btc: basal turn of the cochlea; cocn: cochlear nerve; cp: cochleariform process; fn: tympanic segment of facial nerve; gg: geniculate ganglion; IACd: dural layer of the IAC; ica: internal carotid artery; ivn: inferior vestibular nerve; jb: jugular bulb; pcf: posterior fossa dura; pr: promontory; ve: vestibule.*

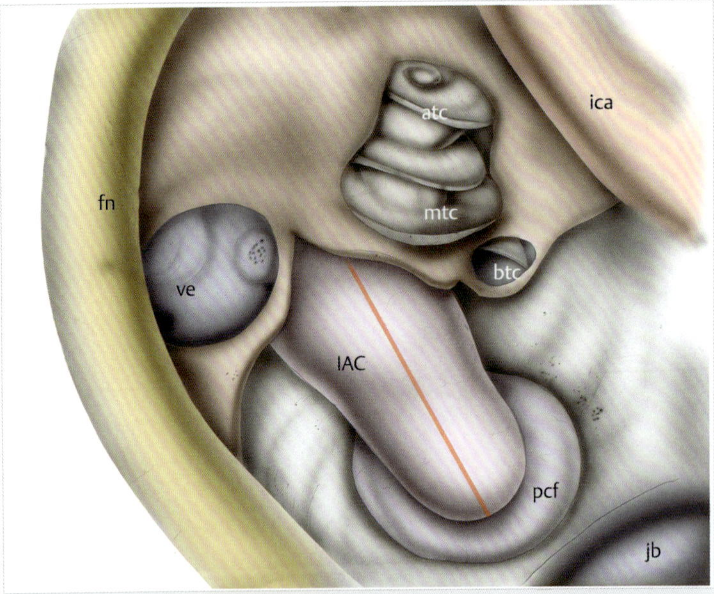

Fig. 12.96 Right side: Transcanal infrapromontorial approach. The dura of the internal auditory canal is opened through an incision performed along the axis of the IAC. *atc: apical turn of cochlea; btc: basal turn of cochlea; fn: tympanic segment of facial nerve; IAC: internal auditory canal; ica: internal carotid artery; jb: jugular bulb; mtc: middle turn of cochlea; pcf: posterior fossa dura; ve: vestibule.*

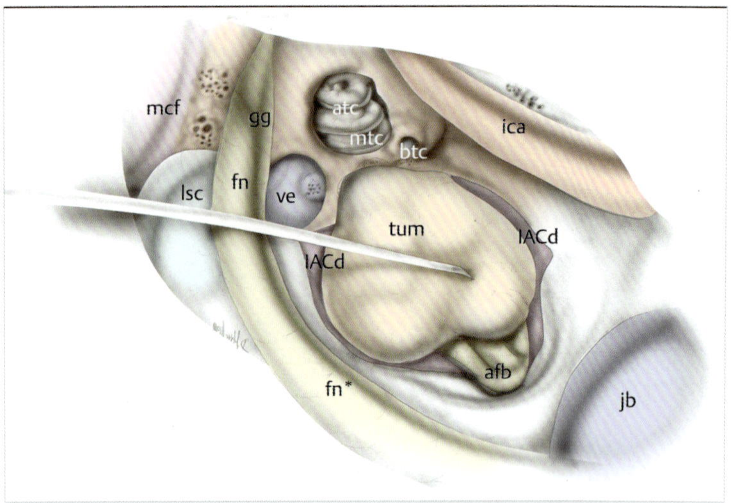

Fig. 12.97 Right side: Transcanal infrapromontorial approach. The acoustic neuroma is carefully removed from the internal auditory canal preserving the integrity of the facial nerve (FN) and the cochlear nerve. *afb: acoustic facial bundle; atc: apical turn of cochlea; btc: basal turn of the cochlea; fn: tympanic segment of facial nerve; fn*: mastoid portion of facial nerve; gg: geniculate ganglion; IACd: dura of internal auditory canal; ica: internal carotid artery; jb: jugular bulb; lsc: lateral semicircular canal; mcf: middle cranial fossa; mtc: middle turn of cochlea; tum: tumor; ve: vestibule.*

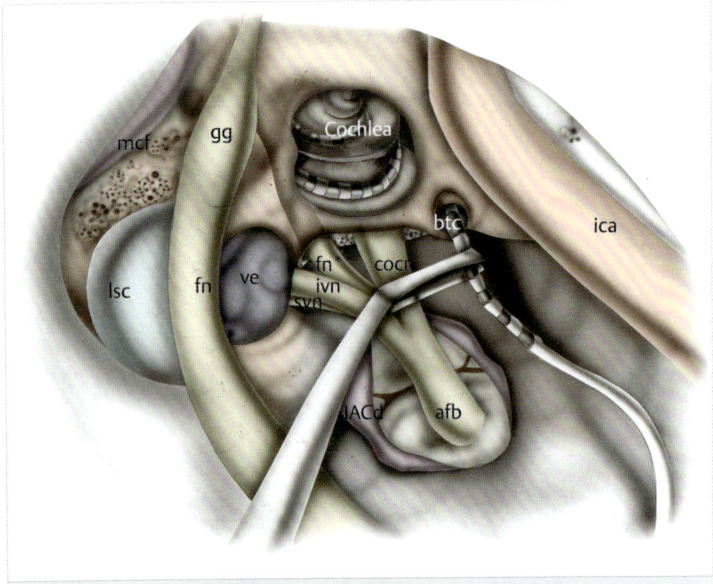

Fig. 12.98 Right side: Transcanal infrapromontorial approach. The array of the cochlear implant (CI) is gently inserted through the basal turn of the cochlea. Since the lateral wall of the promontory is opened during this step, the surgeon should pay attention to check the progression of the electrode array insertion in the middle and apical turns of the cochlea to avoid a misplacement. *afb: acoustic facial bundle; btc: basal turn of the cochlea; cocn: cochlear nerve; fn: tympanic segment of facial nerve; fn**: facial nerve into the IAC; gg: geniculate ganglion; IACd: dura of internal auditory canal; ica: internal carotid artery; ivn: inferior vestibular nerve; lsc: lateral semicircular canal; mcf: middle cranial fossa; svn: superior vestibular nerve; ve: vestibule.*

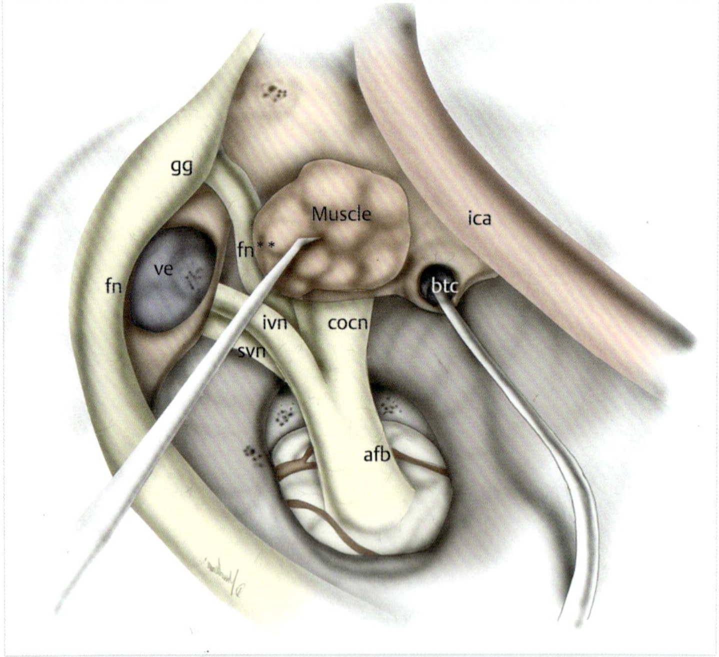

Fig. 12.99 Right side: Transcanal infrapromontorial approach. A piece of muscle is placed over the cochlea to protect the electrode array and cover the cochlear turns. *afb: acoustic facial bundle; btc: basal turn of the cochlea; cocn: cochlear nerve; fn**: facial nerve into the IAC; fn: tympanic segment of facial nerve; gg: geniculate ganglion; ica: internal carotid artery; ivn: inferior vestibular nerve; svn: superior vestibular nerve; ve: vestibule.*

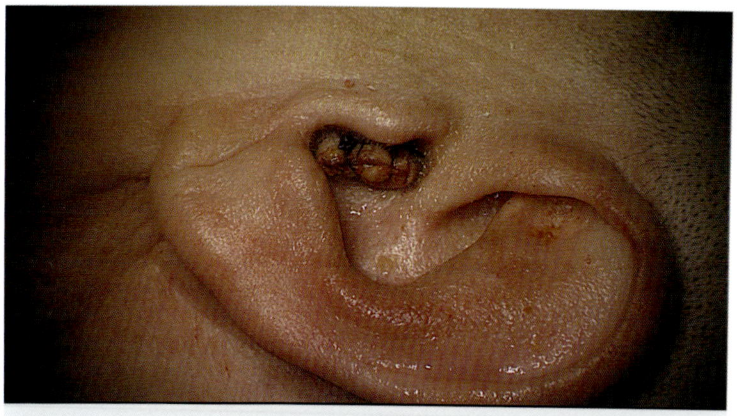

Fig. 12.100 Clinical Case 5, Left side: Transcanal infrapromontorial approach. The skin of external auditory canal (EAC) is everted and sutured in a blind sac closure fashion.

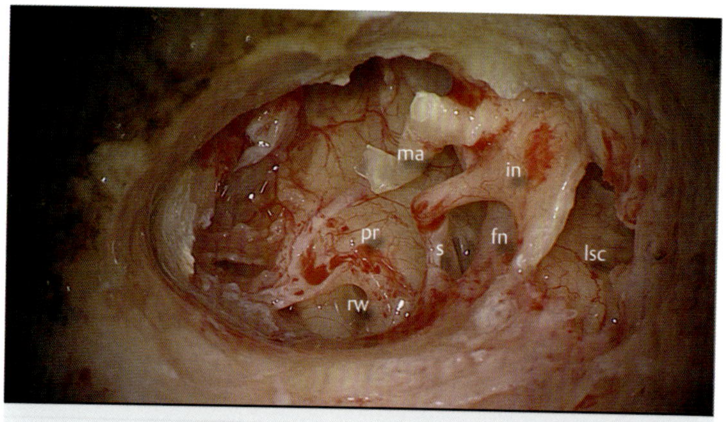

Fig. 12.101 Clinical Case 5, Left side: Transcanal infrapromontorial approach. An enlarged transcanal approach is performed, drilling the external canal bony walls. The medial wall of the tympanic cavity with the ossicular chain is exposed. *fn: facial nerve; in: incus; lsc: lateral semicircular canal; ma: malleus; pr: promontory; rw: round window; s: stapes.*

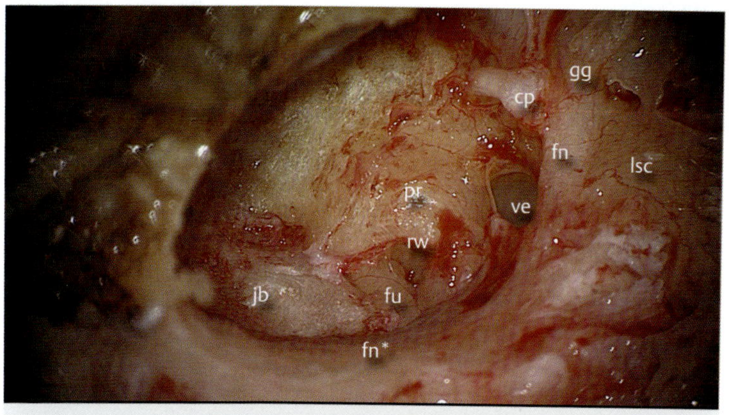

Fig. 12.102 Clinical Case 5, Left side: Transcanal infrapromontorial approach. The ossicular chain is removed and the vestibule exposed. *cp: cochleariform process; fn: facial nerve; fn*: mastoid segment of facial nerve; fu: fustis; gg: geniculate ganglion; jb: jugular bulb; lsc: lateral semicircular canal; pr: promontory; rw: round window; ve: vestibule.*

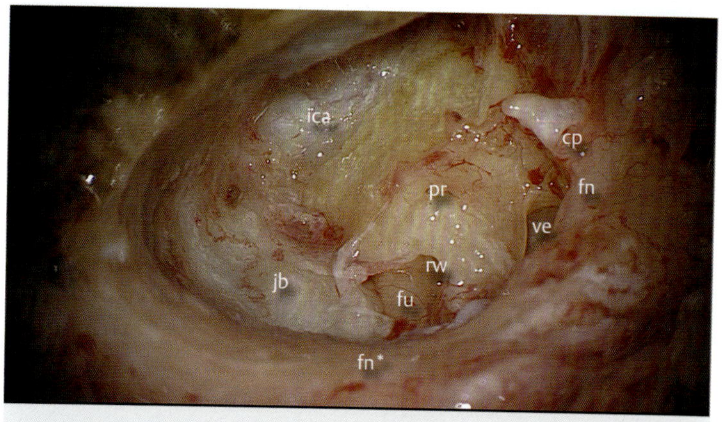

Fig. 12.103 Clinical Case 5, Left side: Transcanal infrapromontorial approach. The internal carotid artery and the jugular bulb are detected. *cp: cochleariform process; fn: facial nerve; fn*: mastoid segment of facial nerve; fu: fustis; ica: internal carotid artery; jb: jugular bulb; pr: promontory; rw: round window; ve: vestibule.*

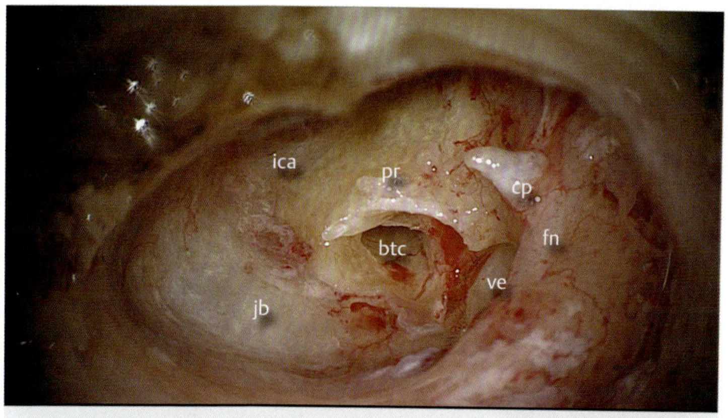

Fig. 12.104 Clinical Case 5, Left side: Transcanal infrapromontorial approach. A diamond bur is used to open the round window (RW), exposing the basal turn of the cochlea. *btc: basal turn of the cochlea; cp: cochleariform process; fn: facial nerve; ica: internal carotid artery; jb: jugular bulb; pr: promontory; ve: vestibule.*

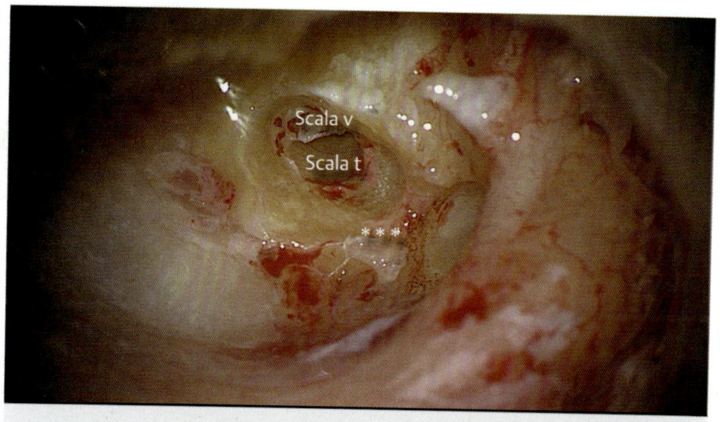

Fig. 12.105 Clinical Case 5, Left side: Transcanal infrapromontorial approach. The basal turn of the cochlea is drilled until the most anterior portion of the basal turn of the cochlea. This surgical maneuver allows for the exposure of the cochlear-vestibular bone (see the ***). This anatomical structure is a thin bone anterior to the vestibule, separating the fundus of the internal auditory canal from the surgical cavity. *scala t: scala tympani; scala v: scala vestibuli.*

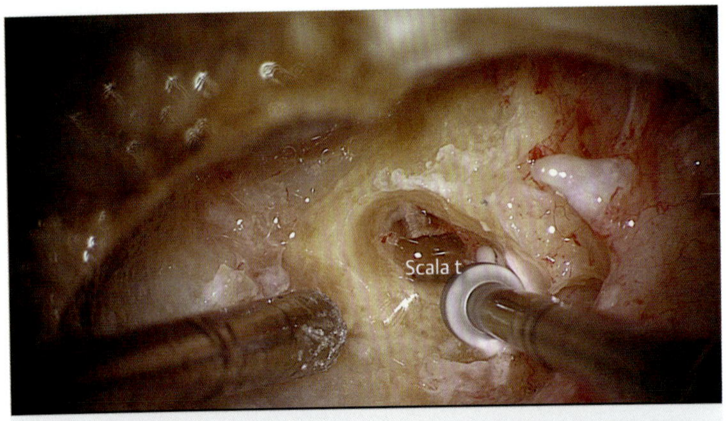

Fig. 12.106 Clinical Case 5, Left side: Transcanal infrapromontorial approach. A small diamond bur is used to remove the cochlear-vestibular bone between the vestibule and the most anterior portion of the basal turn of the cochlea, opening the fundus of the internal auditory canal. *scala t: scala tympani.*

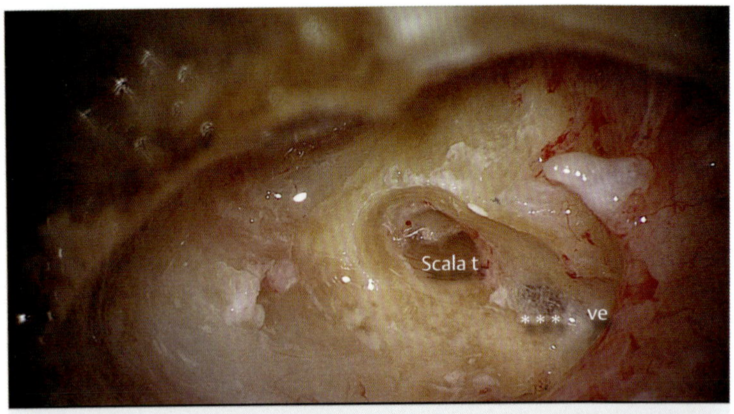

Fig. 12.107 Clinical Case 5, Left side: Transcanal infrapromontorial approach. An opening in the fundus of the internal auditory canal between the vestibule and the cochlea is seen (***). *scala t: scala tympani; ve: vestibule.*

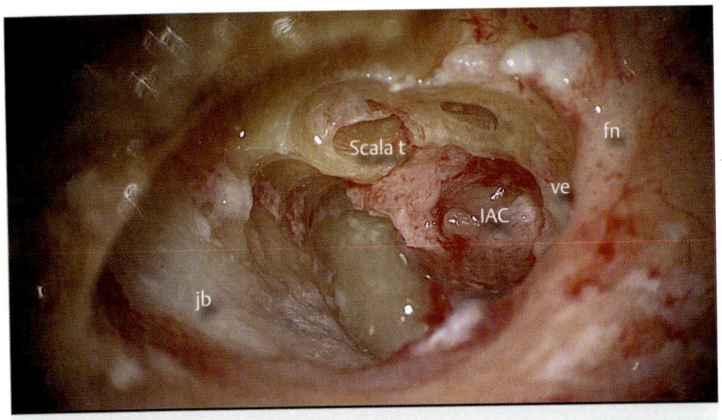

Fig. 12.108 Clinical Case 5, Left side: Transcanal infrapromontorial approach. The internal auditory canal is exposed and opened; the tumor is noticed inside the internal auditory canal. *fn: facial nerve; IAC: internal auditory canal; jb: jugular bulb; scala t: scala tympani; ve: vestibule.*

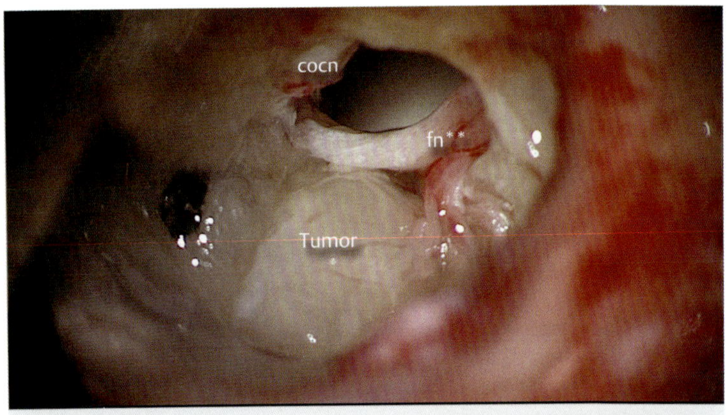

Fig. 12.110 Clinical Case 5, Left side: Transcanal infrapromontorial approach. The tumor is dissected from the nerves and removed. *cocn: cochlear nerve; fn**: facial nerve into the internal auditory canal.*

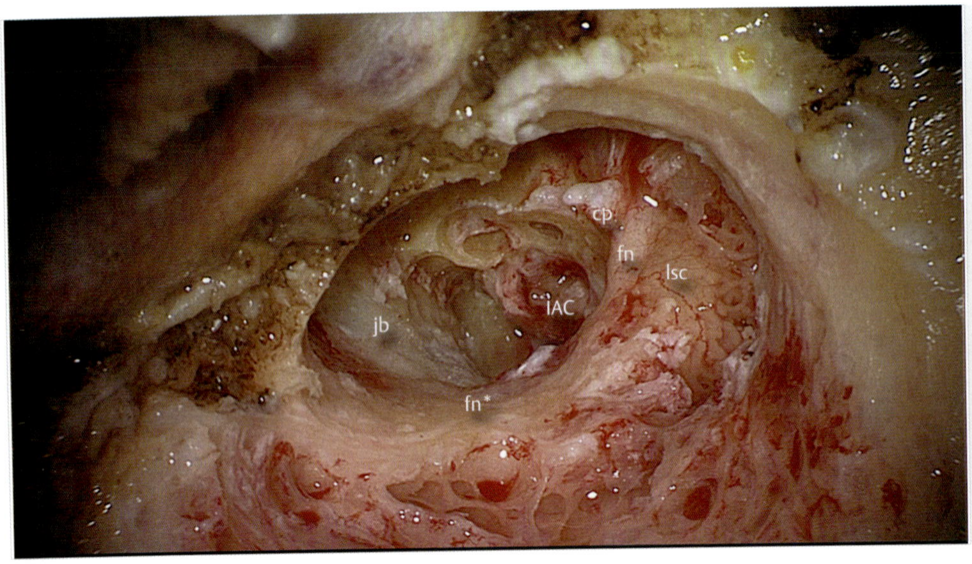

Fig. 12.109 Clinical Case 5, Left side: Transcanal infrapromontorial approach. Microscopic view of the surgical cavity after the detection of the tumor in the internal auditory canal (IAC). *cp: cochleariform process; fn: tympanic segment of facial nerve; fn*: mastoid segment of facial nerve; IAC: internal auditory canal; jb: jugular bulb; lsc: lateral semicircular canal.*

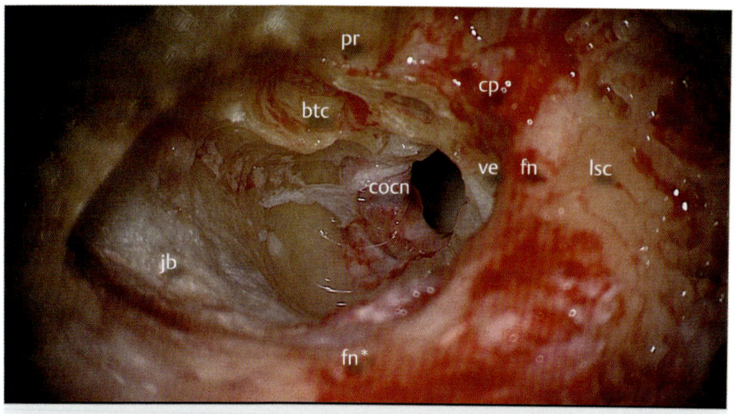

Fig. 12.111 Clinical Case 5, Left side: Transcanal infrapromontorial approach. The tumor is removed and the cochlear nerve is preserved. *btc: basal turn of the cochlea; cocn: cochlear nerve; cp: cochleariform process; fn*: mastoid segment of facial nerve; fn: tympanic segment of facial nerve; jb: jugular bulb; lsc: lateral semicircular canal; pr: promontory; ve: vestibule.*

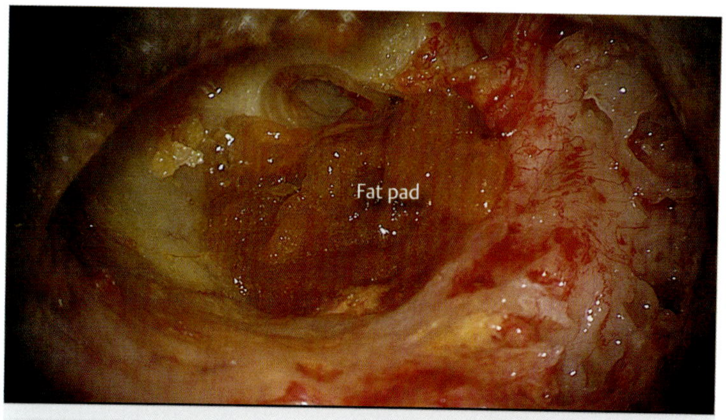

Fig. 12.112 Clinical Case 5, Left side: Transcanal infrapromontorial approach. A fat pad is placed through the defect between the internal auditory canal and the tympanic cavity.

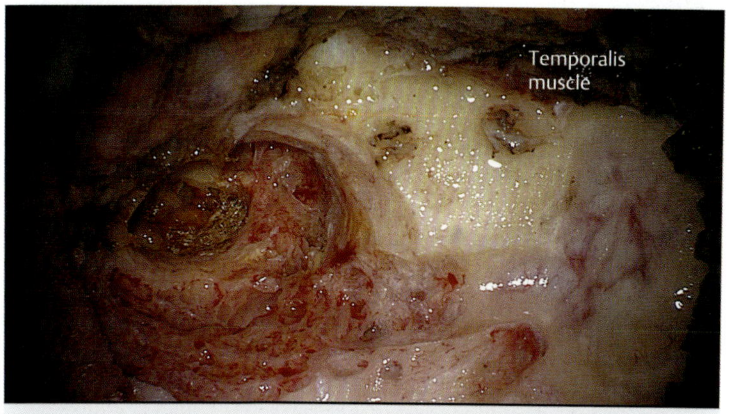

Fig. 12.113 Clinical Case 5, Left side: Transcanal infrapromontorial approach. Some room for the receiver-stimulator is created under the temporalis muscle.

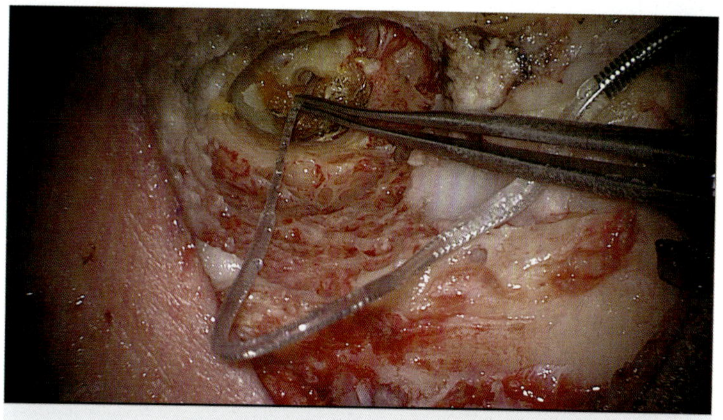

Fig. 12.114 Clinical Case 5, Left side: Transcanal infrapromontorial approach. The array of the cochlear implant (CI) is gently inserted through the basal turn of the cochlea.

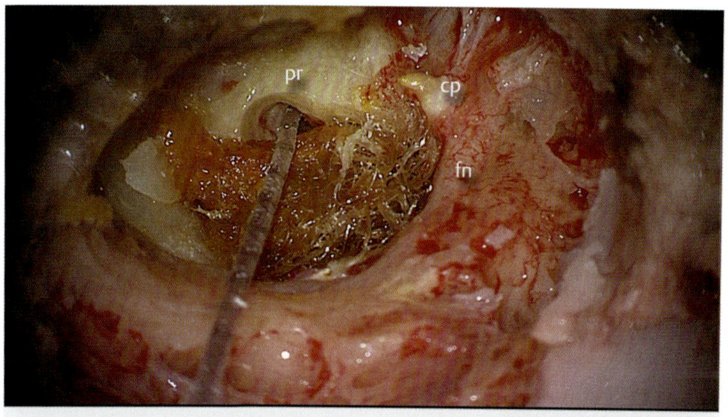

Fig. 12.115 Clinical Case 5, Left side: Transcanal infrapromontorial approach. The array is progressively pushed into the scala tympani. *cp: cochleariform process; fn: facial nerve; pr: promontory.*

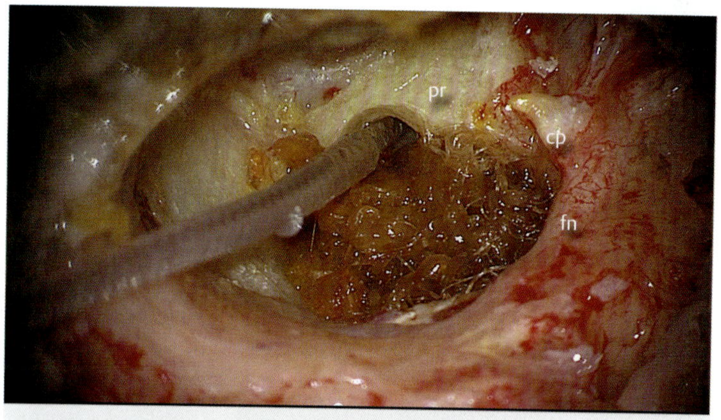

Fig. 12.116 Clinical Case 5, Left side: Transcanal infrapromontorial approach. The array is completely inserted into the cochlea until the final marker. *cp: cochleariform process; fn: facial nerve; pr: promontory.*

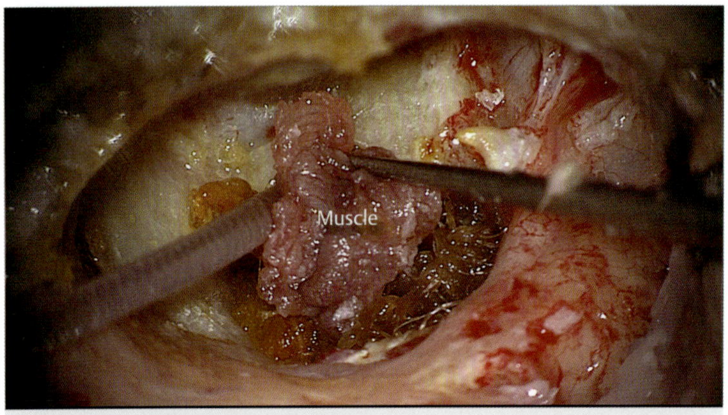

Fig. 12.117 Clinical Case 5, Left side: Transcanal infrapromontorial approach. A fragment of muscle is placed to protect the cochleostomy.

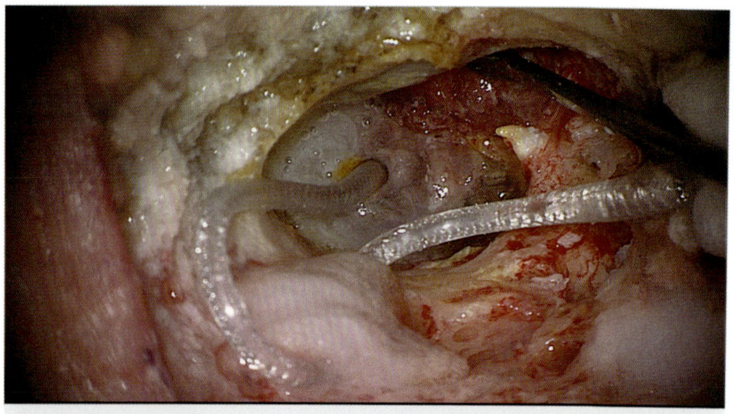

Fig. 12.118 Clinical Case 5, Left side: Transcanal infrapromontorial approach. Some fibrin glue is used to fix the muscle on the cochleostomy; a piece of muscle is also used to obliterate the eustachian tube lumen.

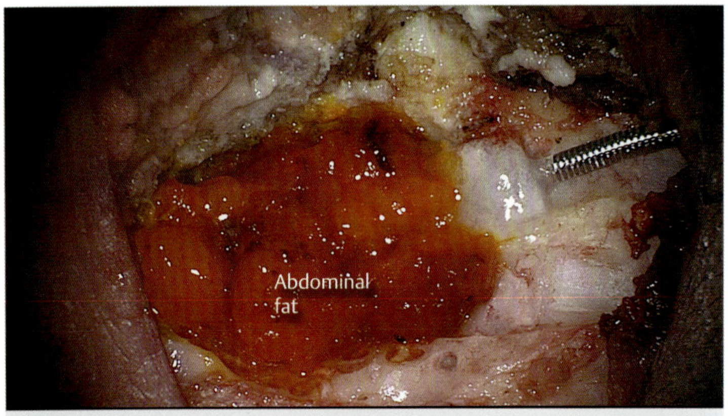

Fig. 12.119 Clinical Case 5, Left side: Transcanal infrapromontorial approach. The surgical cavity is filled with abdominal fat.

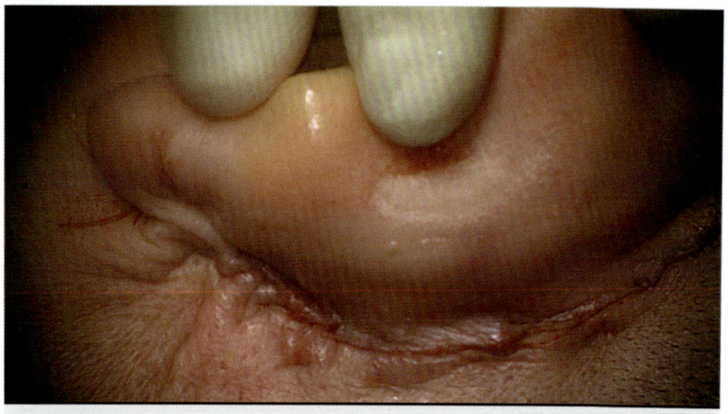

Fig. 12.120 Clinical Case 5, Left side: Transcanal infrapromontorial approach. An accurate layer by layer suture is performed; the skin layer is sutured with absorbable materials.

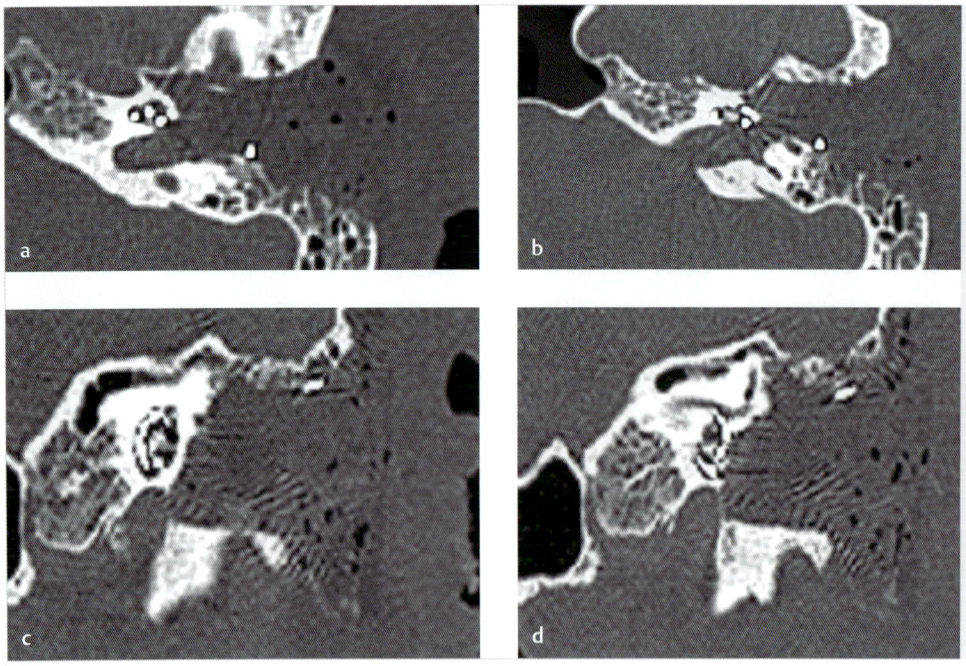

Fig. 12.121 (a–d) Clinical Case 5, Left side: Transcanal infrapromontorial approach. The computed tomography (CT) scan carried out immediately after surgery shows the right positioning of the electrode array inside the cochlea, and the bony work of the infrapromontorial approach to the internal auditory canal (IAC) with cochlear preservation.

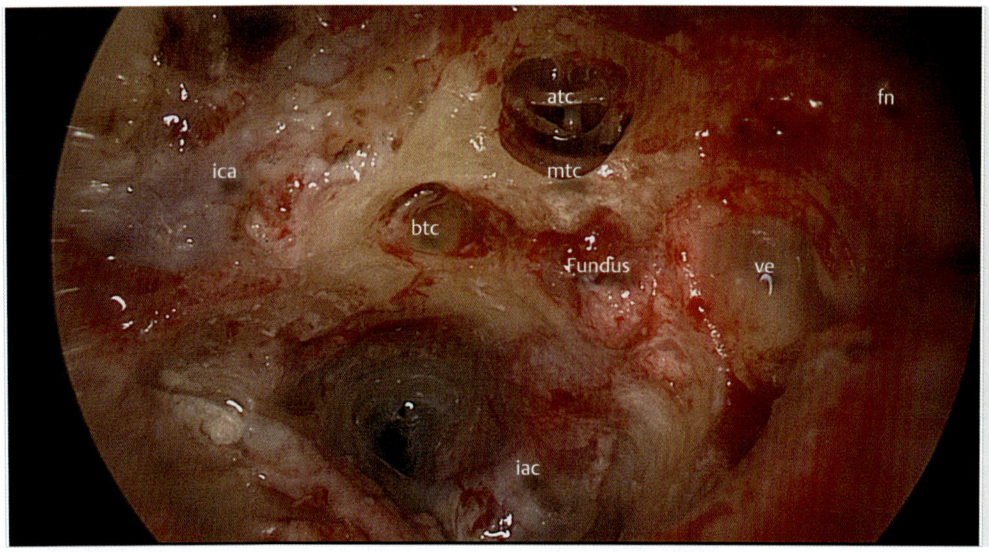

Fig. 12.122 Clinical Case 6, Left side: Transcanal infrapromontorial approach. Endoscopic view: In this case, the cochlear turns are exposed, and the internal auditory canal (IAC) is skeletonized from the fundus to the porus. The location of the fundus of the IAC is noted between the cochlea and the vestibule. *atc: apical turn of cochlea; btc: basal turn of the cochlea; fn: tympanic segment of facial nerve; ica: internal carotid artery; mtc: middle turn of cochlea; ve: vestibule.*

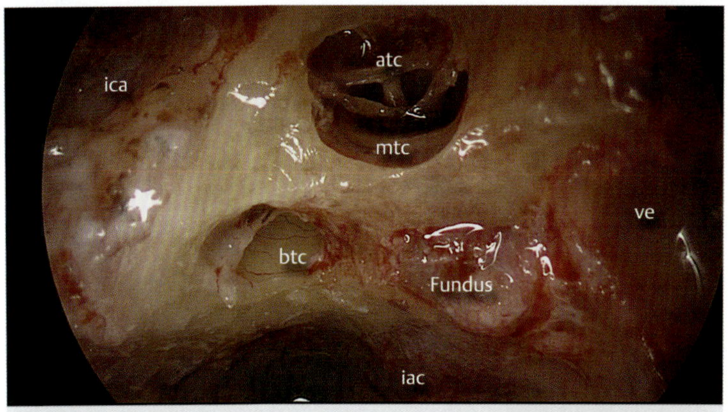

Fig. 12.123 Clinical Case 6, Left side: Transcanal infrapromontorial approach. Endoscopic magnification of the fundus. The anatomical relationship between the vestibule the cochlea and the fundus is visible. *atc: apical turn of cochlea; btc: basal turn of the cochlea; iac: internal auditory canal; ica: internal carotid artery; mtc: middle turn of cochlea; ve: vestibule.*

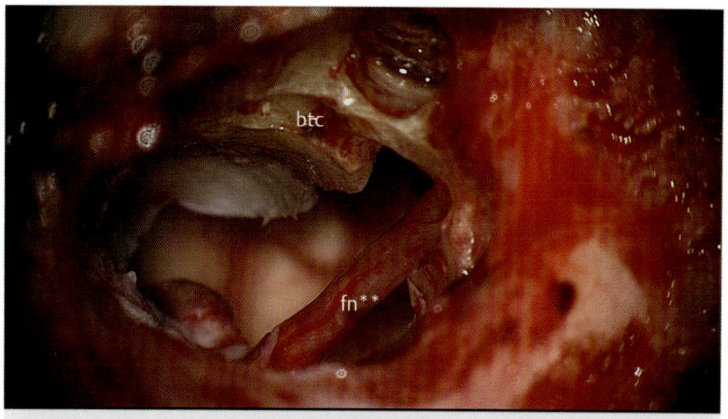

Fig. 12.125 Clinical Case 6, Left side: Transcanal infrapromontorial approach. Microscopic magnification of the facial nerve (FN) in the internal auditory canal. *btc: basal turn of the cochlea; fn**: facial nerve into the IAC.*

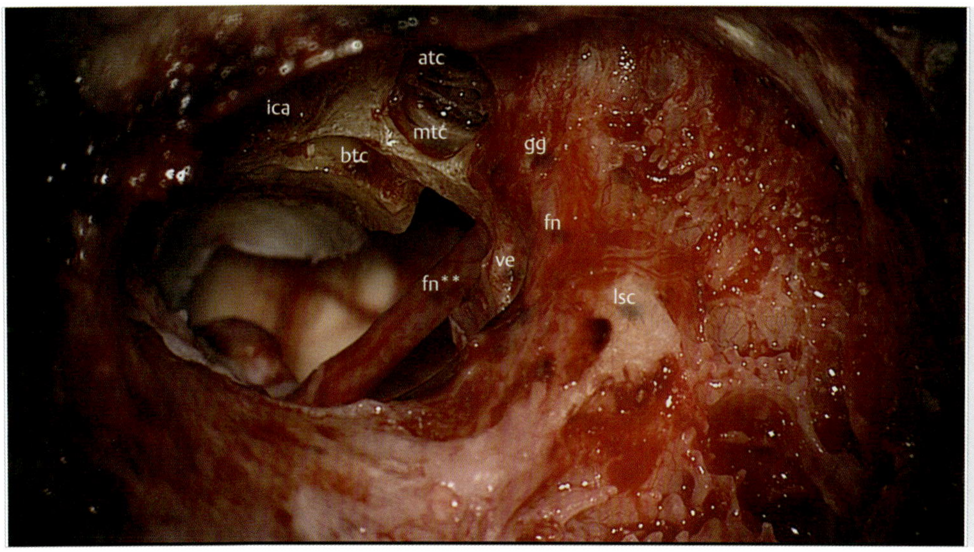

Fig. 12.124 Clinical Case 6, Left side: Transcanal infrapromontorial approach. In this case, despite the preservation of the cochlear turns, the cochlear nerve is sacrificed, since a large window on the cerebellopontine angle (CPA) is created to allow for tumor removal. The facial nerve (FN) can be seen in the internal auditory canal. *atc: apical turn of cochlea; btc: basal turn of the cochlea; fn: tympanic segment of facial nerve; fn**: facial nerve into the IAC; gg: geniculate ganglion; ica: internal carotid artery; lsc: lateral semicircular canal; mtc: middle turn of cochlea; ve: vestibule.*

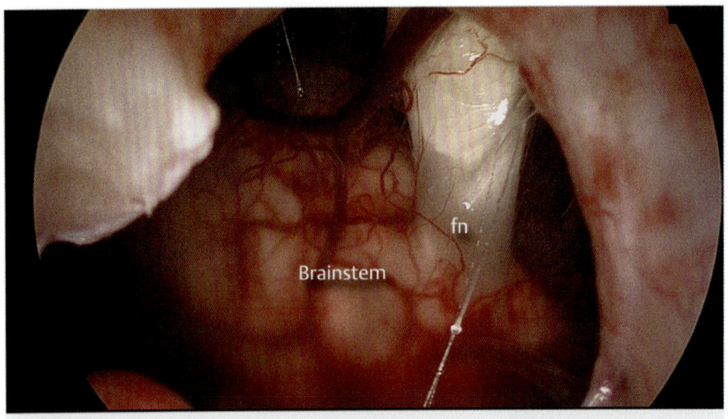

Fig. 12.126 Clinical Case 6, Left side: Transcanal infrapromontorial approach. Endoscopic magnification of the cerebellopontine angle (CPA) through the tympanic cavity defect. *fn: trigeminal nerve.*

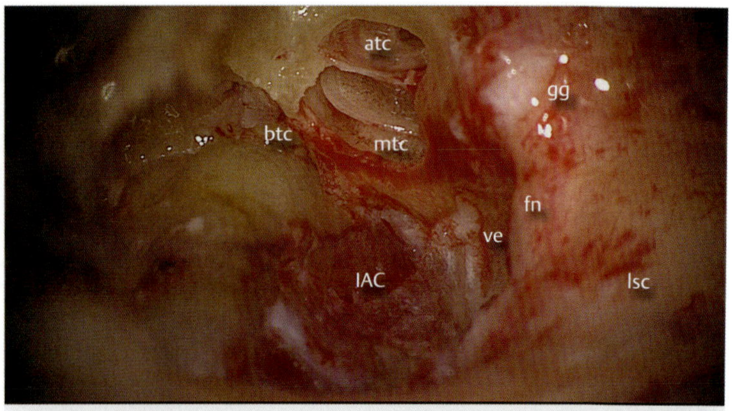

Fig. 12.128 Clinical Case 7, Left side: Transcanal infrapromontorial approach. The dura of the internal auditory canal is gently opened, progressively exposing the tumor. *atc: apical turn of cochlea; btc: basal turn of the cochlea; fn: tympanic segment of facial nerve; gg: geniculate ganglion; IAC: internal auditory canal; lsc: lateral semicircular canal; mtc: middle turn of cochlea; ve: vestibule.*

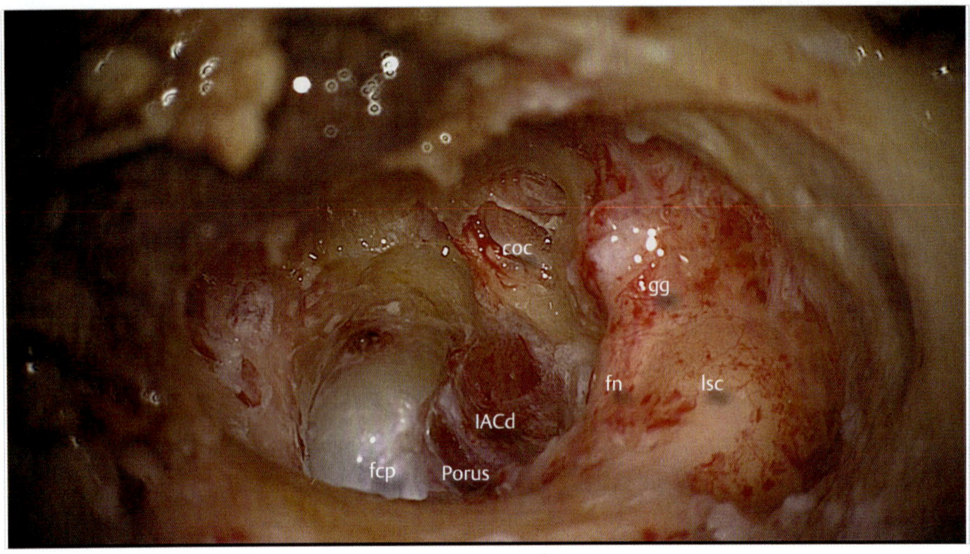

Fig. 12.127 Clinical Case 7, Left side: Transcanal infrapromontorial approach. The cochlear turns are exposed; the internal auditory canal is skeletonized from the fundus to the porus. *coc: cochlea; fcp: posterior cranial fossa dura; fn: tympanic segment of facial nerve; gg: geniculate ganglion; IACd: dura of internal auditory canal; lsc: lateral semicircular canal.*

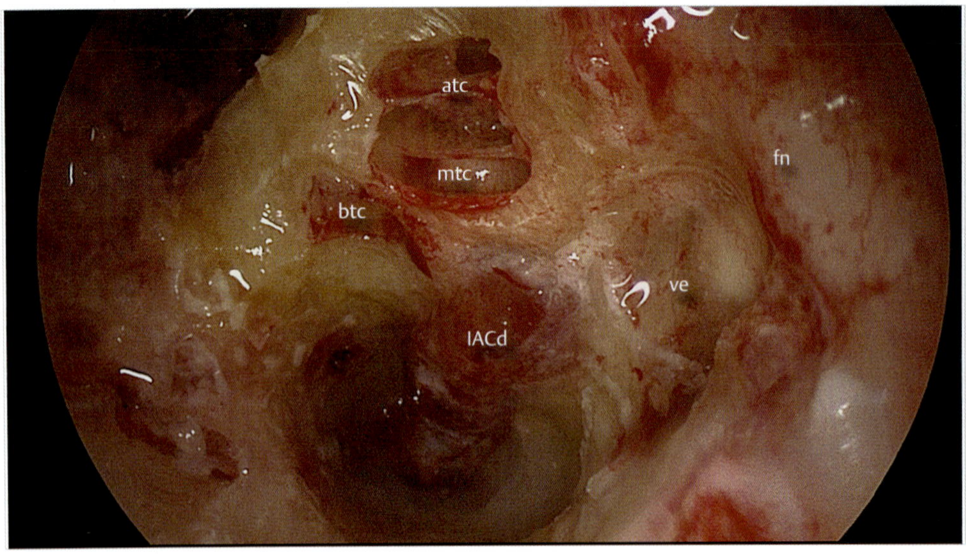

Fig. 12.129 Clinical Case 7, Left side: Transcanal infrapromontorial approach. Endoscopic view of the tympanic cavity after the skeletonization of the internal auditory canal. *atc: apical turn of cochlea; btc: basal turn of the cochlea; fn: tympanic segment of facial nerve; IACd: dura of internal auditory canal; mtc: middle turn of cochlea; ve: vestibule.*

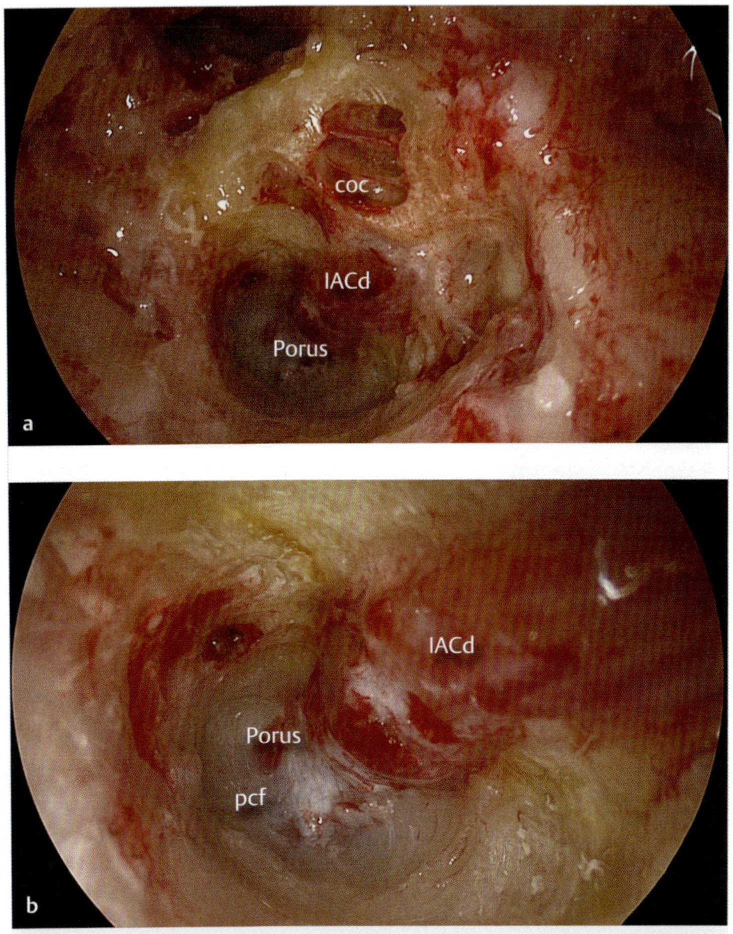

Fig. 12.130 Clinical Case 7, Left side: Transcanal infrapromontorial approach: **(a, b)** The internal auditory canal is exposed from the fundus to the porus, exposing the posterior fossa dura around the porus. *coc: cochlea; IACd: dura of internal auditory canal; pcf: posterior cranial fossa dura.*

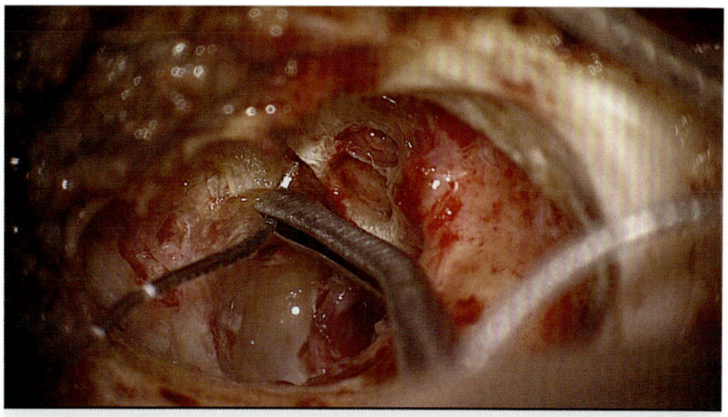

Fig. 12.132 Clinical Case 7, Left side: Transcanal infrapromontorial approach. The array of the cochlear implant (CI) is inserted through the basal turn of the cochlea.

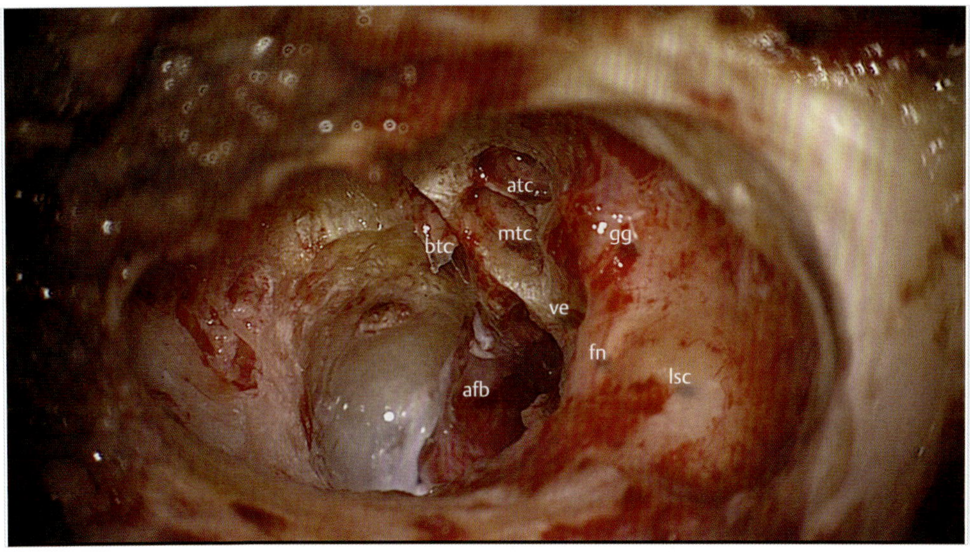

Fig. 12.131 Clinical Case 7, Left side: Transcanal infrapromontorial approach. The tumor is removed, preserving the facial and cochlear nerves. *afb: acoustic-facial bundle; atc: apical turn of cochlea; btc: basal turn of the cochlea; fn: tympanic segment of facial nerve; gg: geniculate ganglion; lsc: lateral semicircular canal; mtc: middle turn of cochlea; ve: vestibule.*

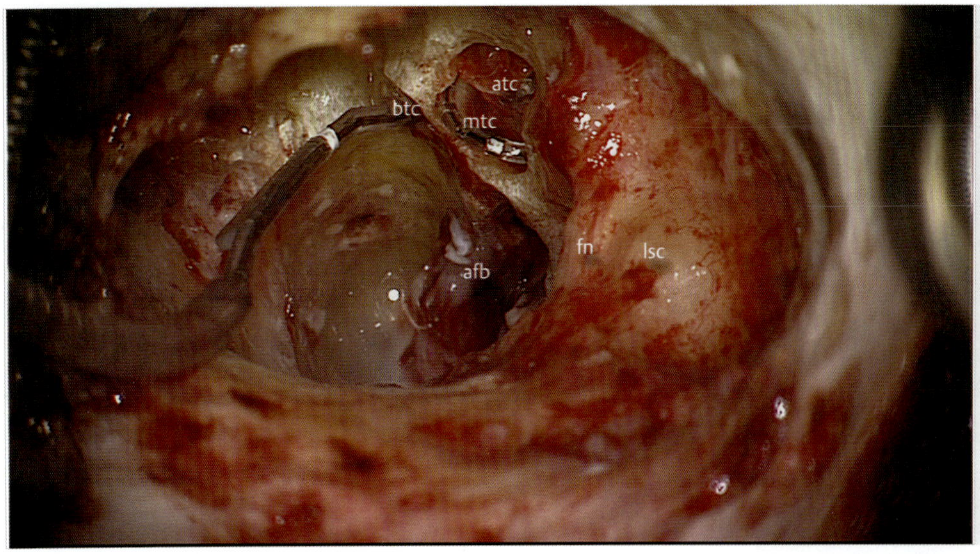

Fig. 12.133 Clinical Case 7, Left side: Transcanal infrapromontorial approach. The placement of the array inside the cochlea is seen. *afb: acoustic-facial bundle; atc: apical turn of cochlea; btc: basal turn of the cochlea; fn: tympanic segment of facial nerve; lsc: lateral semicircular canal; mtc: middle turn of cochlea.*

Suggested Readings

Ahsan S, Telischi F, Hodges A, Balkany T. Cochlear implantation concurrent with translabyrinthine acoustic neuroma resection. Laryngoscope. 2003; 113(3):472–474

Arístegui M, Denia A. Simultaneous cochlear implantation and translabyrinthine removal of vestibular schwannoma in an only hearing ear: report of two cases (neurofibromatosis type 2 and unilateral vestibular schwannoma). Otol Neurotol. 2005; 26(2):205–210

Bajaj Y, Gibbins N, Fawkes K, et al. Surgical aspects of cochlear implantation in syndromic children. Cochlear Implants Int. 2012; 13(3):163–167

Birman CS, Brew JA, Gibson WP, Elliott EJ. CHARGE syndrome and cochlear implantation: difficulties and outcomes in the paediatric population. Int J Pediatr Otorhinolaryngol. 2015; 79(4):487–492

Bruijnzeel H, Ziylan F, Cattani G, Grolman W, Topsakal V. Retrospective complication rate comparison between surgical techniques in paediatric cochlear implantation. Clin Otolaryngol. 2016; 41(6):666–672

Carlson ML, Breen JT, Driscoll CL, et al. Cochlear implantation in patients with neurofibromatosis type 2: variables affecting auditory performance. Otol Neurotol. 2012; 33(5):853–862

Charlett SD, Biggs N. The prevalence of cochlear obliteration after labyrinthectomy using magnetic resonance imaging and the implications for cochlear implantation. Otol Neurotol. 2015; 36(8):1328–1330

Chen YH, Liu TC, Yang TH, Lin KN, Wu CC, Hsu CJ. Using endoscopy to locate the round window membrane during cochlear implantation: our experience with 25 patients. Clin Otolaryngol. 2018; 43(1):357–362

Cruz OL, Vellutini EA. Cochlear implant in type 2 neurofibromatosis: an option for better hearing rehabilitation. Rev Bras Otorrinolaringol (Engl Ed). 2011; 77 (4):538

Güneri EA, Olgun Y. Endoscope-assisted cochlear implantation. Clin Exp Otorhinolaryngol. 2018; 11(2):89–95

Leong AC, Jiang D, Agger A, Fitzgerald-O'Connor A. Evaluation of round window accessibility to cochlear implant insertion. Eur Arch Otorhinolaryngol. 2013; 270 (4):1237–1242

Lloyd SK, Glynn FJ, Rutherford SA, et al. Ipsilateral cochlear implantation after cochlear nerve preserving vestibular schwannoma surgery in patients with neurofibromatosis type 2. Otol Neurotol. 2014; 35(1):43–51

Lloyd SK, Kasbekar AV, Kenway B, et al. Developmental changes in cochlear orientation—implications for cochlear implantation. Otol Neurotol. 2010; 31(6):902–907

Marchioni D, Alicandri-Ciufelli M, Pothier DD, Rubini A, Presutti L. The round window region and contiguous areas: endoscopic anatomy and surgical implications. Eur Arch Otorhinolaryngol. 2015; 272(5):1103–1112

Marchioni D, Carner M, Soloperto D, et al. Endoscopic-assisted cochlear implant procedure in CHARGE syndrome: preliminary report. Acta Oto-Laryngologica Case Reports. 2017; 2(1):52–58

Marchioni D, Carner M, Soloperto D, et al. Expanded transcanal transpromontorial approach: a novel surgical technique for cerebellopontine angle vestibular schwannoma removal. Otolaryngol Head Neck Surg. 2018; 158(4):710–715

Marchioni D, Carner M, Soloperto D, et al. The kaleidoscope of the operative solutions for hearing restoration in Charge syndrome: a critical review. Otolaryngol (Sunnyvale). 2017; 7(3):309–313

Marchioni D, Grammatica A, Alicandri-Ciufelli M, Genovese E, Presutti L. Endoscopic cochlear implant procedure. Eur Arch Otorhinolaryngol. 2014; 271(5):959–966

Marchioni D, Soloperto D, Guarnaccia MC, Genovese E, Alicandri-Ciufelli M, Presutti L. Endoscopic assisted cochlear implants in ear malformations. Eur Arch Otorhinolaryngol. 2015; 272(10):2643–2652

Marchioni D, Soloperto D, Masotto B, et al. Transcanal transpromontorial acoustic neuroma surgery: results and facial nerve outcomes. Otol Neurotol. 2018; 39 (2):242–249

Marchioni D, Veronese S, Carner M, et al. Hearing restoration during vestibular schwannoma surgery with transcanal approach: anatomical and functional preliminary report. Otol Neurotol. 2018; 39(10):1304–1310

McRackan TR, Reda FA, Rivas A, et al. Comparison of cochlear implant relevant anatomy in children versus adults. Otol Neurotol. 2012; 33(3):328–334

Meshik X, Holden TA, Chole RA, Hullar TE. Optimal cochlear implant insertion vectors. Otol Neurotol. 2010; 31(1):58–63

Morimoto AK, Wiggins RH, III, Hudgins PA, et al. Absent semicircular canals in CHARGE syndrome: radiologic spectrum of findings. AJNR Am J Neuroradiol. 2006; 27(8):1663–1671

Neff BA, Wiet RM, Lasak JM, et al. Cochlear implantation in the neurofibromatosis type 2 patient: long-term follow-up. Laryngoscope. 2007; 117(6):1069–1072

Orhan KS, Polat B, Çelik M, Çomoğlu Ş, Güldiken Y. Endoscopic-assisted cochlear implantation: a case series. J Int Adv Otol. 2016; 12(3):337–340

Roland PS, Wright CG, Isaacson B. Cochlear implant electrode insertion: the round window revisited. Laryngoscope. 2007; 117(8):1397–1402

Tran Ba Huy P, Kania R, Frachet B, Poncet C, Legac MS. Auditory rehabilitation with cochlear implantation in patients with neurofibromatosis type 2. Acta Otolaryngol. 2009; 129(9):971–975

Vesseur AC, Verbist BM, Westerlaan HE, et al. CT findings of the temporal bone in CHARGE syndrome: aspects of importance in cochlear implant surgery. Eur Arch Otorhinolaryngol. 2016; 273(12):4225–4240

Zanetti D, Campovecchi CB, Pasini S, Nassif N. Simultaneous translabyrinthine removal of acoustic neuroma and cochlear implantation. Auris Nasus Larynx. 2008; 35(4):562–568

Zheng Y, Schachern PA, Djalilian HR, Paparella MM. Temporal bone histopathology related to cochlear implantation in congenital malformation of the bony cochlea. Otol Neurotol. 2002; 23(2):181–186

Chapter 13

Endoscopic Transcanal Infracochlear Approach

13 Endoscopic Transcanal Infracochlear Approach

Seiji Kakeatha, Daniele Marchioni, and Brandon Isaacson

Abstract

The endoscopic transcanal infracochlear approach provides a direct corridor to the petrous apex running just below the cochlea and the internal auditory canal (IAC), thus preserving the hearing function. A detailed knowledge of the endoscopic anatomy of the middle ear is mandatory to correctly create the surgical corridor, using a deep tunnel, called "subcochlear canaliculus," as a guide to reach the petrous apex cells lying under the IAC. The subcochlear canaliculus is bordered superiorly by the promontory, posteriorly by the fustis, anteriorly by the finiculus, and inferiorly by the jugular bulb. By removing the finiculus and using the vertical portion of the carotid artery as the anterior limit of the dissection, it is possible to create an infracochlear corridor to the petrous apex. The major advantages of this technique concern the possibility to have better anatomical magnifications of the round window chamber and vascular structures, which are to preserve the cochlea and the cochlear function, avoiding at the same time a retroauricular incision. The indications include: (1) petrous apex cholesterol granulomas; (2) tympanic cavity cholesteatomas with subcochlear canaliculus extension; (3) biopsy of petrous apex lesions when malignant or metastatic tumors are suspected; and (4) rare middle ear benign tumors with limited extension into the tympanic cavity with protympanic and hypotympanic adhesions, like middle ear adenoma, schwannoma, or carcinoid tumor. Conversely, this approach cannot be used for large petrous apex cholesteatomas. Unfavorable anatomical condition, like a high jugular bulb, represents a contraindication to this surgical approach.

Keywords: endoscopic infracochlear approach, subcochlear canaliculus, petrous apex cholesteatoma, petrous apex cholesterol granuloma, hypotympanic anatomy

13.1 Introduction

The infracochlear approach is a well-known surgical approach among otologists, used for the drainage of petrous apex cholesterol granulomas, especially during a microscopic approach.

Recently, the introduction of the endoscopic approach for middle ear lesion removal has progressively increased the anatomical knowledge of the tympanic cavity, mostly about the round window region and surrounding areas. This knowledge enables the surgeon to use the infracochlear approach not only for the evacuation of cholesterol granulomas of the petrous apex, but also for the treatment of some tumors adherent to the hypotympanic and protympanic areas, and for cholesteatomas with subcochlear extension.

13.2 Rationale

This surgical approach consists of creating a transcanal infracochlear surgical corridor to reach lesions in the petrous apex, with inferior extension to the internal auditory canal (IAC). The approach preserves the ossicular chain and the hearing function, in keeping with the preoperative ossicular chain and hearing function situation (▶ Fig. 13.1).

13.3 Advantages

Although the infracochlear microscopic approach is a well-established technique, some advantages of the endoscopic infracochlear approach should be emphasized:

- The retroauricular incision is not required.
- A better anatomical magnification of the round window chamber and the vascular structures is necessary to preserve the cochlea and the cochlear function, by reaching the lesion inside the petrous apex.
- In case of cholesterol granuloma, the endoscopic magnification of the cyst content inside the petrous apex allows for a more radical surgery. Visualizing what is inside the cyst allows for the lysis of any additional intracystic loculations.
- It is possible to create an infracochlear corridor also in case of a tympanic cavity cholesteatoma invading the petrous apex through the subcochlear canaliculus, or in case of benign tumor with hypotympanic cell adhesion, avoiding damage to the cochlea.

13.4 Disadvantages and Limitations

- The endoscopic infracochlear approach is a one-hand dissection technique.
- This technique is suitable just for limited infralabyrinthine petrous apex cholesteatoma, involving the petrous apex through the subcochlear canaliculus, but it is not suitable for petrous apex cholesteatomas (large infralabyrinthine and infralabyrinthine-apical types).

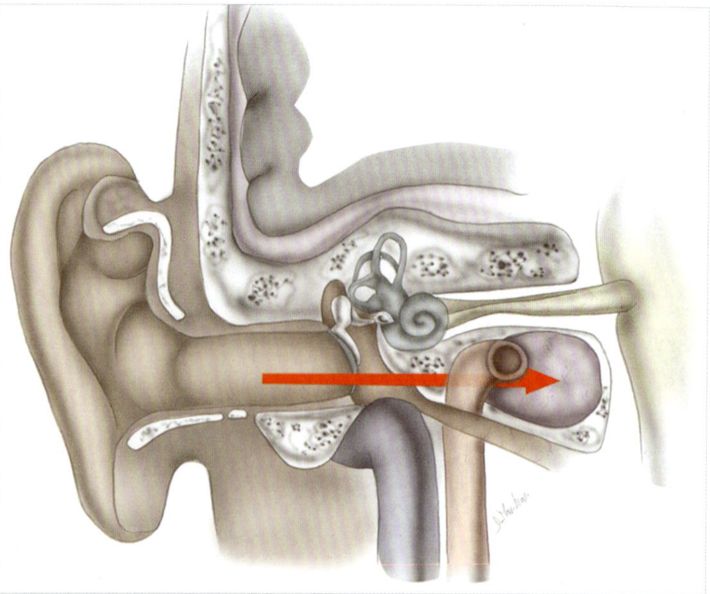

Fig. 13.1 Schematic drawing representing the surgical route of the transcanal endoscopic infracochlear approach: A surgical corridor between the intrapetrous vertical tract of the internal carotid artery (ICA) and the jugular bulb is created, under the cochlea. Through this corridor it is possible to reach the lesion in the petrous apex cells, lying under the internal auditory canal (IAC) (see the *red arrow*).

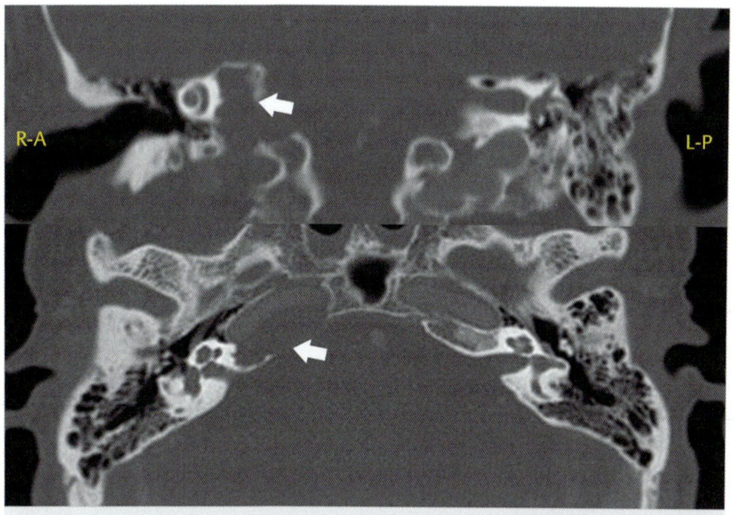

Fig. 13.2 (a,b) Computed tomography (CT) scan of a temporal bone in coronal and axial views: A petrous apex lesion with extension along the course of the intrapetrous horizontal portion of the internal carotid artery (ICA) is detected (see the *white arrow*).

13.5 Indications

- Petrous apex cholesterol granulomas (▶ Fig. 13.2);
- Tympanic cavity cholesteatomas with subcochlear canaliculus extension;
- Biopsy of petrous apex lesions when malignant or metastatic tumors are suspected;
- Rare benign tumors of the middle ear with limited extension to the tympanic cavity with protympanic and hypotympanic adhesions, such as middle ear adenoma, schwannoma, or carcinoid tumor. In these cases when a medial adhesion of the tumor to the ossicular chain is present, ossicular chain removal should be considered, since surgical radicality is mandatory in order to avoid recurrence.

13.6 Contraindications

The radiological study of the anatomical conformation of the jugular bulb with a computed tomography (CT) scan is mandatory in the preoperative patient selection. In fact, an unfavorable anatomical condition, such as a high jugular bulb, represents a contraindication to this surgical approach (see ▶ Fig. 13.43).

13.7 Surgical Considerations about the Round Window Chamber and the Hypotympanum (▶ Fig. 13.3)

To understand the anatomical landmarks used during the endoscopic infracochlear approach, it is crucial to know the anatomy of the round window chamber and the connections between this anatomical area and the petrous apex.

The development of the bony round window niche begins during the 16th fetal week. The anterior, superior, and posterior walls of the round window are the first to appear, while the inferior wall is completely absent at this time. One week later, a bony process grows inside the niche forming its inferior wall but this process will only reach the anterior wall by the 18th week. In the 23-week-old fetus the bony structure forming the inferior wall appears, the so-called fustis. This structure runs in the middle of the inferior wall and points to the crest of the round window. After the 20th prenatal week an intensive growth can be observed in the anterior wall, where the inferior tympanic artery and the tympanic nerve run. During this week, a complete bony canal takes shape around the tympanic nerve and the inferior tympanic artery; this bony structure arises from the anterior pillar and runs inferiorly to the hypotympanic cells, forming the so-called finiculus.

In some patients a deep tunnel between the fustis and the finiculus inside Proctor's area concamerata is formed. This is the "subcochlear canaliculus" connecting directly with the petrous apex cells located inferiorly to the IAC. This tunnel has an anatomical importance, particularly during the infracochlear approach to cholesterol granuloma or during cholesteatoma surgery, because it consists of a deep extension toward the petrous apex cells lying below the cochlea, and medial to the vertical portion of the internal carotid artery (ICA). The subcochlear canaliculus probably arises from a merging defect between the inferior wall (fustis and area concamerata) and the superior wall (anterior pillar and finiculus) of the round window during fetal development. This event could be the basis of the formation of the subcochlear canaliculus with a variable extension to the petrous apex cells lying under the cochlea. On the contrary, when a well-developed area concamerata merges with the finiculus, the subcochlear canaliculus is not present. Considering the anatomy, the endoscopic infracochlear approach uses the subcochlear canaliculus as a guide to reach the petrous apex cells lying under the IAC, removing the finiculus and the bone of the area concamerata located anteriorly to the fustis. The bone removal is performed between the fustis posteriorly, the ICA anteriorly, and jugular bulb inferiorly.

13.8 Surgical Procedure

A 0-degree 3mm diameter and 14 cm length endoscope is used.

A canal incision from 2 to 9 o'clock position along the inferior wall of the external auditory canal (EAC) is performed to create a superiorly based tympanomeatal flap (▶ Fig. 13.4). The flap is progressively elevated, the fibrous anulus is identified, and elevated, entering the tympanic cavity (▶ Fig. 13.5). The fibrous anulus is then followed in its inferior and anterior portions. In this way the flap is superiorly elevated, maintaining the attachment on the malleus and uncovering the hypotympanic and protympanic areas (▶ Fig. 13.6). Once the flap has been elevated a diamond bur is used to enlarge the EAC and to drill the posterior and inferior aspects of the bony anulus in order to have a wide surgical access to the hypotympanic cells (▶ Fig. 13.7, ▶ Fig. 13.8). During this step, particular attention should be paid, since the mastoid segment of the facial nerve runs just posteriorly to the styloid prominence (see ▶ Fig. 13.9).

The round window chamber is endoscopically detected; the tegmen, the posterior pillar and the anterior pillar, and the finiculus bone are recognized. The fustis bone is also detected in the middle of the round window chamber. The endoscopic examination of the round window chamber is necessary to find the subcochlear canaliculus, which represents the connection between the round window chamber and the petrous apex cells, in case of subcochlear canaliculus type A (see ▶ Fig. 13.3). This anatomical connection is used as a landmark to find the petrous apex cells

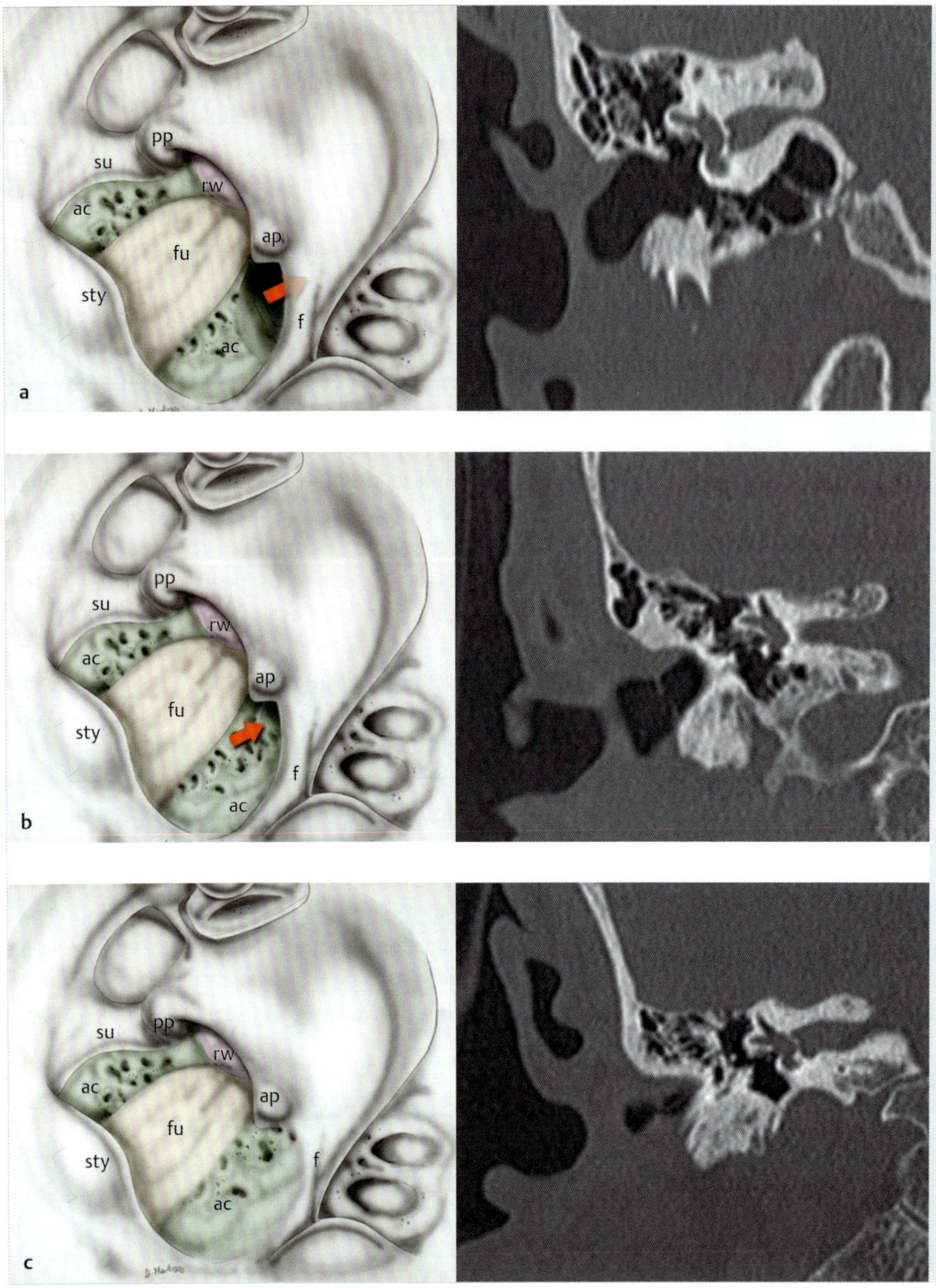

Fig. 13.3 Right side: Here we see three possible conformations of the round window chamber according to the relationship among the fustis, area concamerata, and finiculus bone. **(a, b)** Type A: Between the fustis and the finiculus, a deep hole/tunnel (subcochlear canaliculus) is present with deep extension to the petrous apex cells lying below the cochlea. In these cases, a computed tomography (CT) scan in a sagittal view shows the presence of a well-pneumatized temporal bone at the level of the most inferior and medial portion of the petrous apex, below the internal auditory canal (IAC). **(c, d)** Type B: Between the fustis and the finiculus, a small hole (subcochlear canaliculus) is present. The connection between this hole and the apex is not endoscopically recognizable because of the dimension of this area. In this case, a CT scan in a sagittal view shows the presence of a limited pneumatized bone below the cochlea. **(e, f)** Type C: The fustis and the area concamerata are merged to the finiculus and anterior pillar. There are no connections between the round window chamber and the petrous apex. In these cases, no air cells are present at the level of the most inferior and medial portion of the petrous apex on sagittal view CT scans. *ac: area concamerata; ap: anterior pillar; f: finiculus; fu: fustis; pp: posterior pillar; rw: round window; sty: styloid complex; su: subiculum; su: subiculum; red arrow: tunnel of subcochlear canaliculus.*

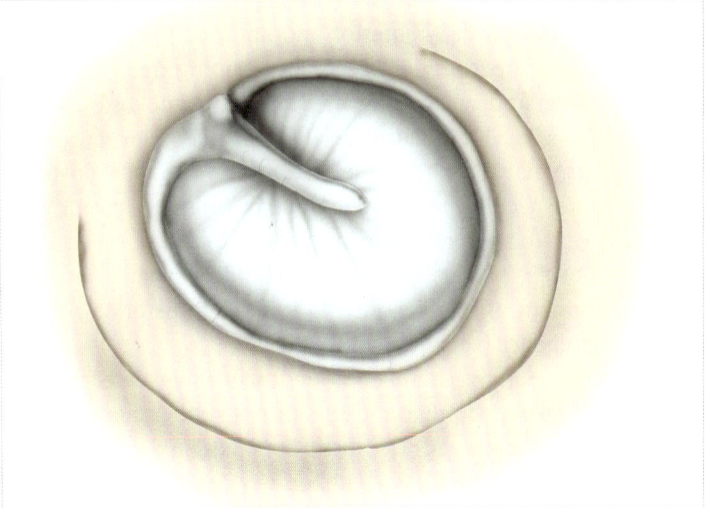

Fig. 13.4 Right side: An incision is endoscopically made to create a superior based tympanomeatal flap.

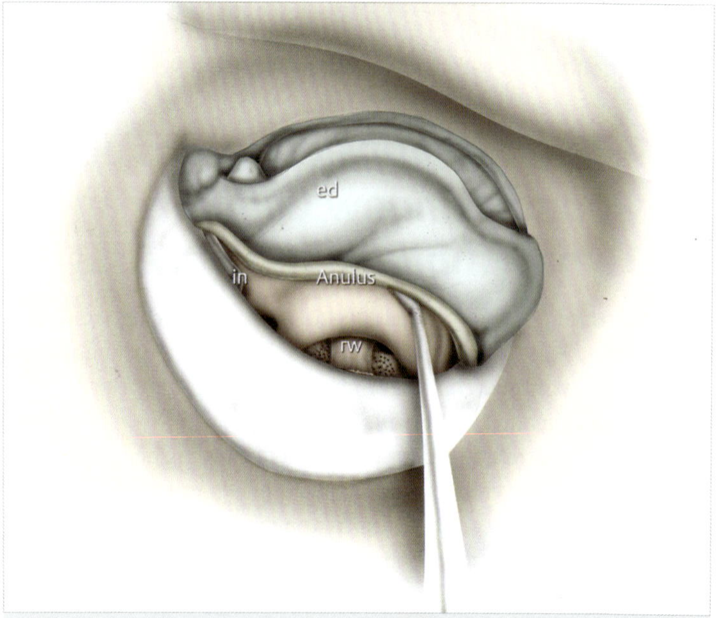

Fig. 13.5 Right side: The annulus is elevated, entering the tympanic cavity. *ed: eardrum; in: incus; rw: round window.*

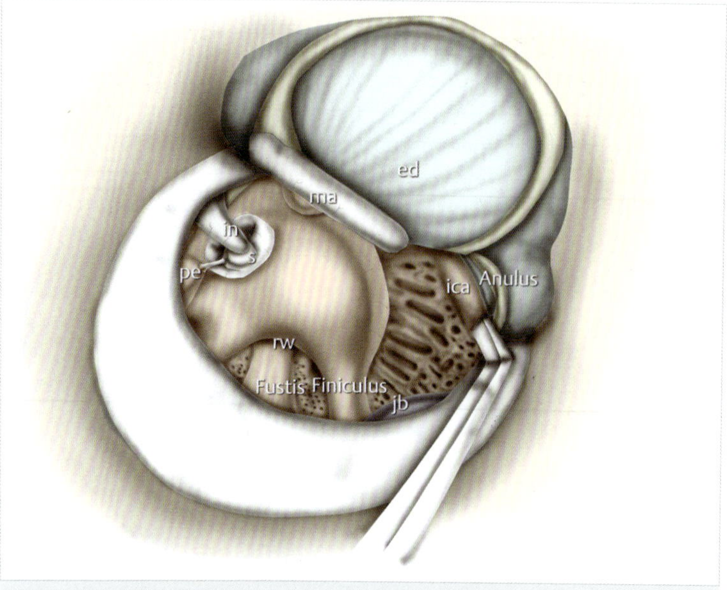

Fig. 13.6 Right side: The anulus is inferiorly and anteriorly followed, elevating the eardrum and exposing the protympanum and the hypotympanum. *ica: internal carotid artery; in: incus; jb: jugular bulb; ma: malleus; pe: pyramidal eminence; rw: round window; s: stapes.*

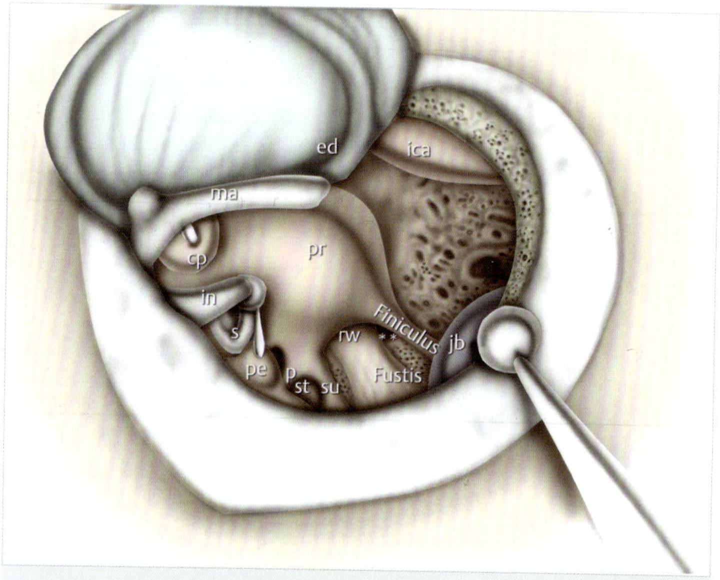

Fig. 13.7 Right side: A diamond bur is used to perform a canaloplasty, removing the bony anulus in the inferior and posterior portions, to get a wide exposure of the vascular structures (jugular bulb and internal carotid artery). *cp: cochleariform process; ed: eardrum; ica: internal carotid artery; in: incus; jb: jugular bulb; ma: malleus; p: ponticulus; pe: pyramidal eminence; pr: promontory; rw: round window; s: stapes; st: sinus tympani; su: subiculum; **: subcochlear canaliculus.*

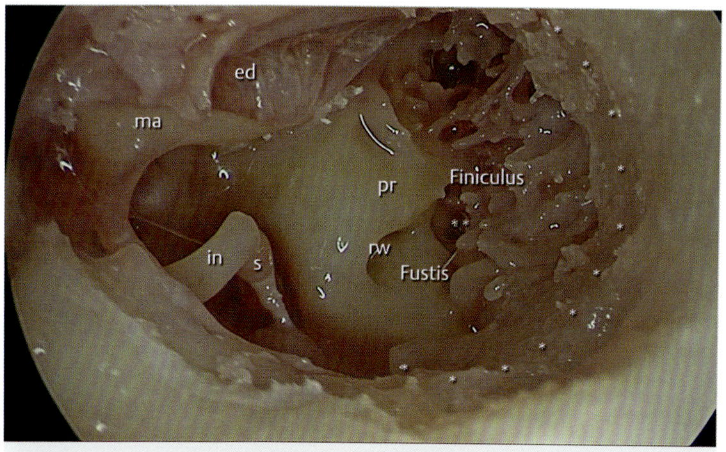

Fig. 13.8 Right side, Dissection: The bony anulus was drilled exposing the hypotympanic and protympanic cells (see the **** line). *ed: eardrum; in: incus; ma: malleus; pr: promontory; rw: round window; s: stapes; **: subcochlear canaliculus.*

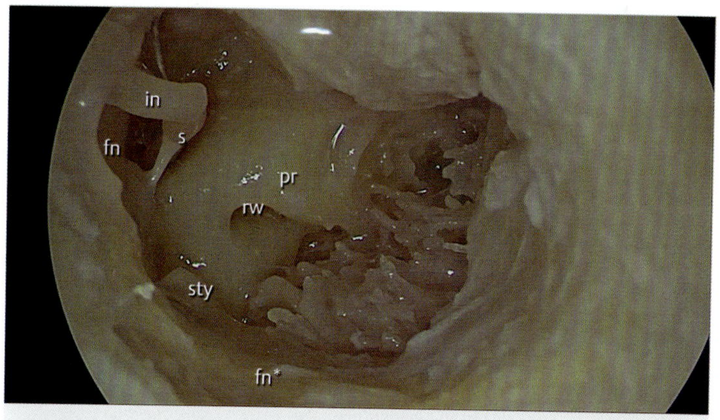

Fig. 13.9 Right side: In this dissection the relationship between the styloid prominence and the mastoid segment of the facial nerve is noted. *fn: tympanic segment of facial nerve; fn*: mastoid segment of facial nerve; in: incus; pr: promontory; rw: round window; s: stapes; sty: styloid prominence.*

under the cochlea (▶ Fig. 13.10, ▶ Fig. 13.11). The fustis represents the posterior limit of the dissection of the infracochlear endoscopic approach, due to the singular nerve lying in depth postero-superior to the fustis canal (canalis singularis). The singular nerve innervates the posterior semicircular canal ampulla.

A diamond bur is used to inferiorly detect the jugular bulb, inferiorly following the finiculus as landmark. Once the jugular bulb has been detected, the vertical portion of the ICA is recognized in the protympanic space; the ICA is detected just under the eustachian tube at the level of its junction between the vertical and the horizontal intrapetrous tracts, where the ICA is more superficial.

After the identification of the major vessels is achieved, the infracochlear cell dissection is started. The finiculus bone is removed using a curette, uncovering the subcochlear canaliculus (▶ Fig. 13.12, ▶ Fig. 13.13). A medium sized diamond bur is used to remove the infracochlear cells between the fustis posteriorly, the vertical portion of carotid artery anteriorly, the jugular bulb inferiorly, and the promontory superiorly, creating an infracochlear corridor to the petrous apex (▶ Fig. 13.14, ▶ Fig. 13.15, ▶ Fig. 13.16). Before drilling is started, some drops of a saline are instilled into the surgical field. The surgeon's assistant can hold a suction instrument to help the surgeon to maintain the surgical field clean during the drilling procedure.

The deeper the dissection to reach the lesion in the petrous apex, the better the anatomical knowledge of the IAC orientation should be, to avoid complications (see ▶ Fig. 13.17, ▶ Fig. 13.18, ▶ Fig. 13.19). The lateral end of the IAC (the fundus) is located just behind the medial wall of the vestibule. The medial end of the IAC is the porus, which is the deepest portion of the IAC, before the access to the cerebellopontine angle. The IAC has an oblique orientation: from anterior to posterior and from lateral to medial.

The extension and the type of surgical procedure depend on the nature of the lesion.

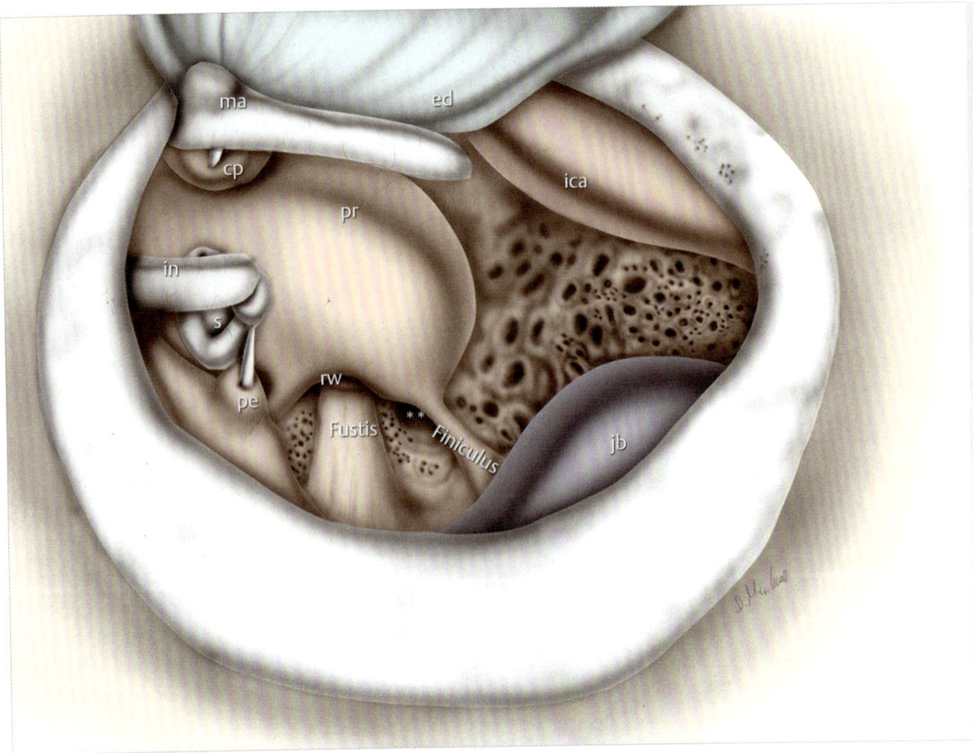

Fig. 13.10 Right side: Endoscopic round window chamber recognition. The round window tegmen, the finiculus bone, and the fustis are well visible. The subcochlear canaliculus (see the **) is located between the fustis and the finiculus, connecting the round window chamber with the petrous apex cells. *cp: cochleariform process; ed: eardrum; ica: internal carotid artery; in: incus; jb: jugular bulb; ma: malleus; pe: pyramidal eminence; pr: promontory; rw: round window; s: stapes; **: subcochlear canaliculus.*

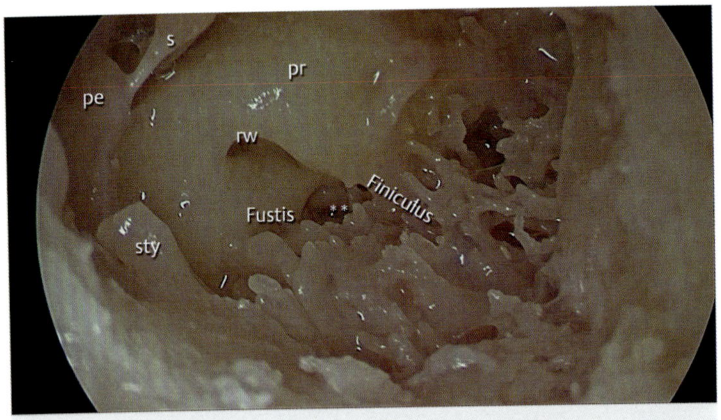

Fig. 13.11 Right side: Endoscopic magnification of the round window chamber and subcochlear canaliculus. *pe: pyramidal eminence; pr: promontory; rw: round window; s: stapes; sty: styloid prominence; **: subcochlear canaliculus.*

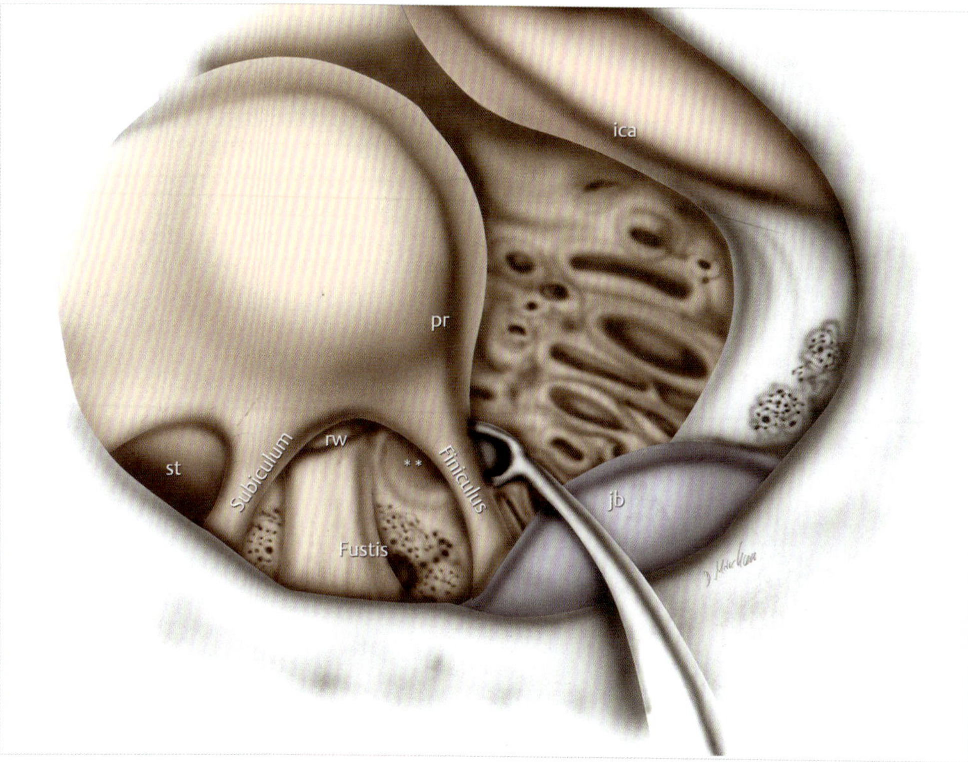

Fig. 13.12 Right side: The internal carotid artery (ICA) and the jugular bulb are detected; the finiculus bone is removed using a curette. *ica: internal carotid artery; jb: jugular bulb; pr: promontory; rw: round window; st: sinus tympani; **: subcochlear canaliculus.*

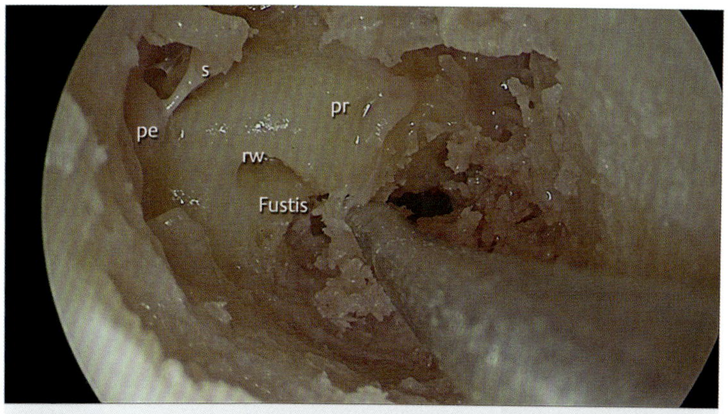

Fig. 13.13 Right side, Dissection: A curette is used to remove the finiculus bone. During this maneuver, bleeding from the Jacobson nerve plexus is expected; a microbipolar may be useful to coagulate the plexus. *pe: pyramidal eminence; pr: promontory; rw: round window; s: stapes.*

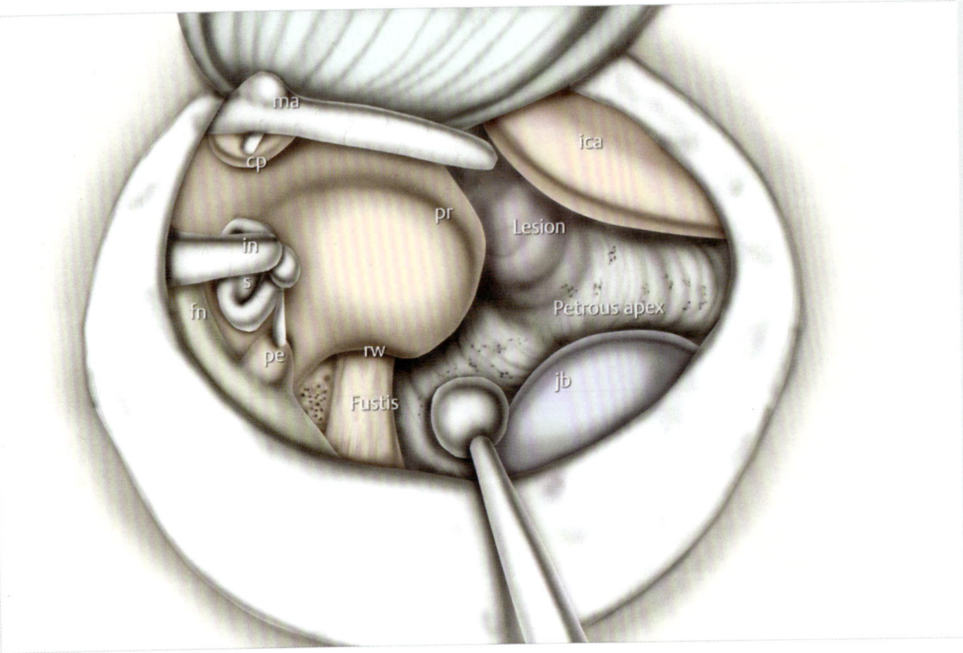

Fig. 13.14 Right side: A diamond bur is used to remove the bone between the cochlea, the internal carotid artery (ICA), and the jugular bulb; the fustis is the posterior limit of the dissection. The lateral wall of the lesion is progressively exposed. *cp: cochleariform process; fn: facial nerve; ica: internal carotid artery; in: incus; jb: jugular bulb; ma: malleus; pe: pyramidal eminence; pr: promontory; rw: round window; s: stapes.*

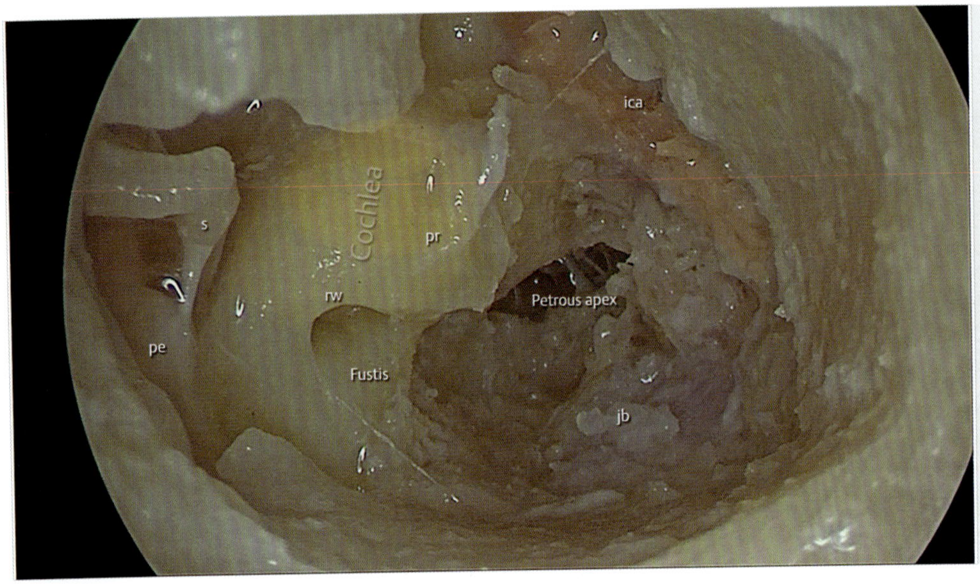

Fig. 13.15 Right side, Dissection: Transcanal infracochlear approach. The anatomical landmarks are emphasized in this anatomical picture. The petrous apex is exposed under the cochlea. *ica: internal carotid artery; jb: jugular bulb; pe: pyramidal eminence; pr: promontory; rw: round window; s: stapes.*

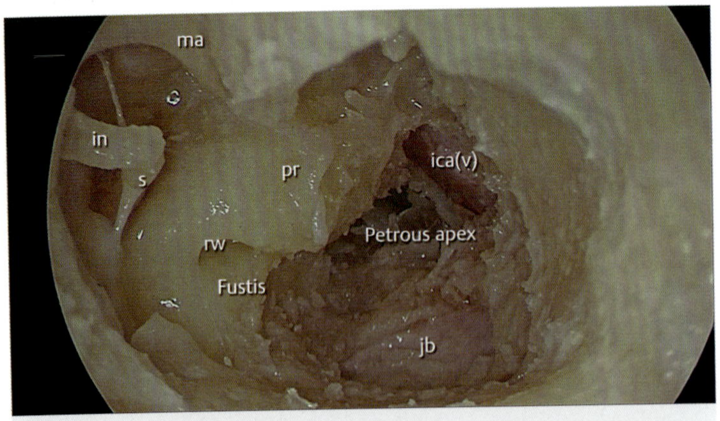

Fig. 13.16 Right side, Dissection: Endoscopic magnification of the petrous apex cells under the cochlea, during the infracochlear approach. *ica: internal carotid artery; in: incus; ma: malleus; jb: jugular bulb; pr: promontory; rw: round window; s: stapes.*

13.8.1 Cholesterol Granuloma (see Clinical Case 1)

In case of cholesterol granuloma, during the infracochlear approach, the lateral wall of the cyst is progressively exposed in the petrous apex. Once the lateral portion of the cyst has been isolated, a fenestration with drainage of the cyst is performed using an otologic knife, opening the lateral wall of the cyst (▶ Fig. 13.20). The cyst cavity is irrigated with antibiotic and saline solutions and then suction is carried out inside the cyst, to remove the granuloma. An adequate fenestration and connection between the petrous apex and the tympanic cavity are created, in order to maintain a correct ventilation of the surgical cavity, avoiding recurrence (▶ Fig. 13.21).

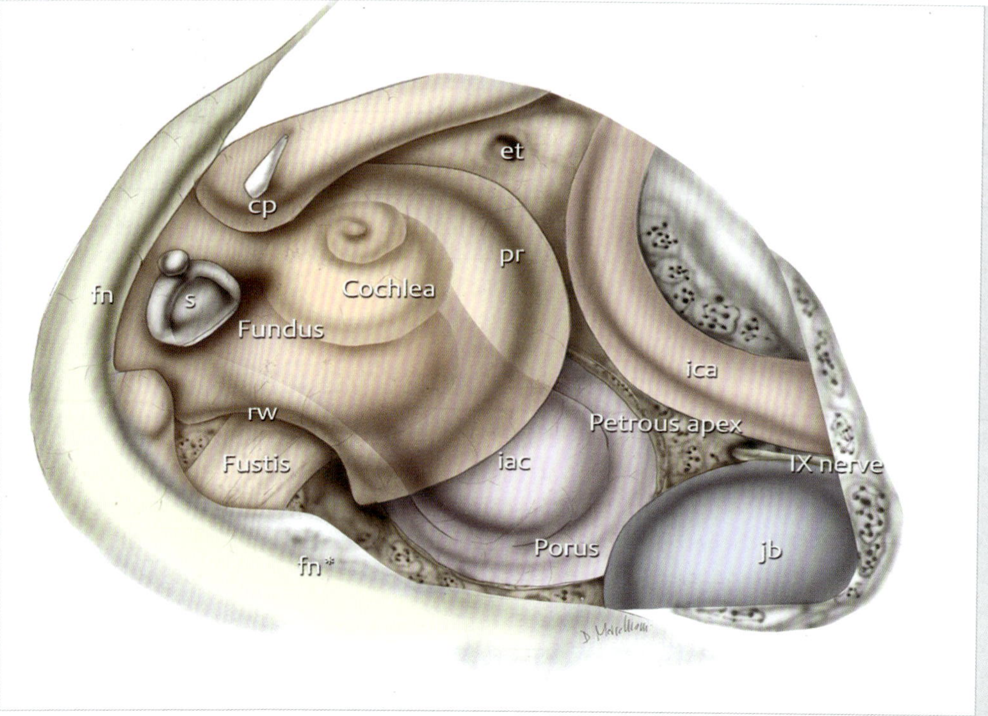

Fig. 13.17 Right side: Schematic drawing showing the anatomical relationship between the cochlea and the internal auditory canal (IAC) related to the infracochlear approach. The oblique orientation of the IAC is seen from the most lateral portion (fundus) to the deepest and most medial portion (porus) in the petrous apex. The glossopharyngeal nerve connection is noted in the deepest and most inferior portion of the petrous apex at the level of the junction between the internal carotid artery (ICA) and the jugular bulb. *cp: cochleariform process; fn: facial nerve; fn* mastoid segment of the facial nerve; ica: internal carotid artery; jb: jugular bulb; pr: promontory; rw: round window; s: stapes.*

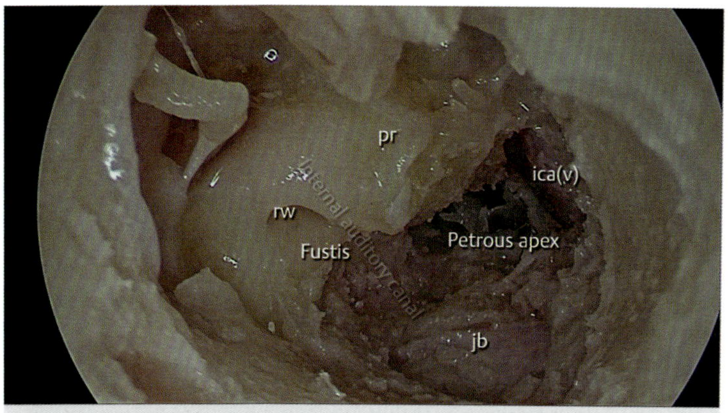

Fig. 13.18 Right side, Dissection: The infracochlear approach is performed. The reader can note the orientation of the internal auditory canal (IAC) in relation to the promontory and the fustis bone. *ica (v): vertical portion of internal carotid artery; jb: jugular bulb; pr: promontory; rw: round window.*

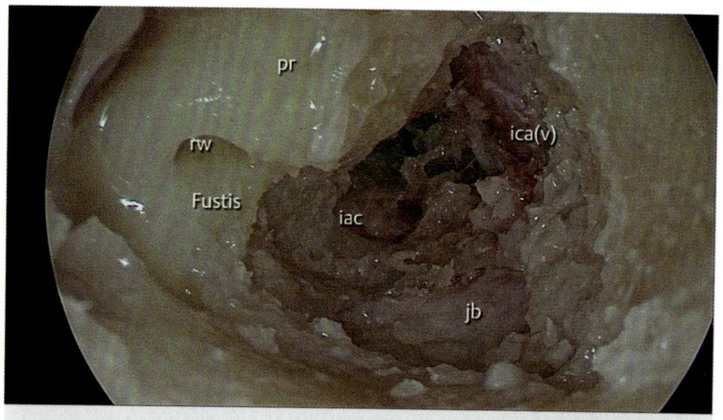

Fig. 13.19 Right side, Dissection: Endoscopic magnification. An infracochlear surgical corridor is created, reaching the petrous apex under the cochlea and under the internal auditory canal (IAC). *IAC: internal auditory canal; ica (v): vertical portion of internal carotid artery; jb: jugular bulb; pr: promontory; rw: round window.*

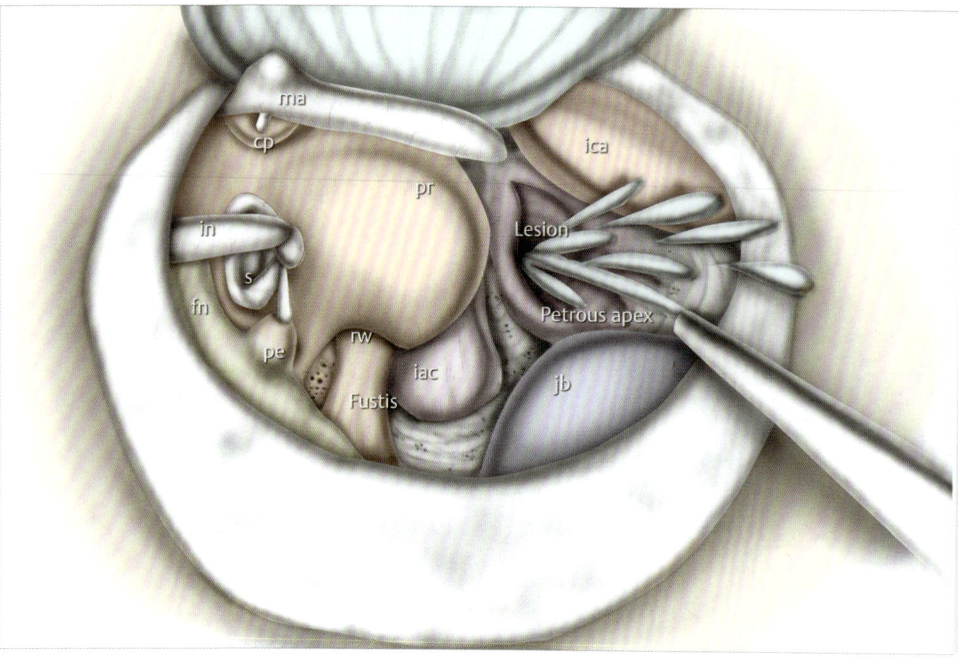

Fig. 13.20 Right side: Once the lateral wall of the cyst has been exposed, an otologic knife is used to cut the wall and a suction instrument is used to drain the content of the cyst. *cp: cochleariform process; fn: facial nerve; IAC: internal auditory canal; ica: internal carotid artery; in: incus; jb: jugular bulb; ma: malleus; pe: pyramidal eminence; pr: promontory; rw: round window; s: stapes.*

13.8.2 Cholesteatoma (see Clinical Case 2)

In case of a tympanic cavity cholesteatoma, with round window chamber extension, an endoscopic recognition of the subcochlear canaliculus should be performed, particularly in case of an infiltrative matrix. This subcochlear canalicus check is important because in case of a subcochlear involvement, a possible spreading into the petrous apex may be found. The subcochlear canaliculus is a tunnel located between the fustis posteriorly and the finiculus anteriorly (see ▶ Fig. 13.3). In case of a cholesteatoma spreading to the petrous apex through the subcochlear canaliculus, an infracochlear endoscopic approach must be considered. The endoscopic infracochlear procedure is similar to the previously described one (▶ Fig. 13.29).

The nerves of Jacobson and the tympanic plexus that run over the finiculus bone are coagulated (▶ Fig. 13.30), and the finiculus is then removed using a microcurette. A diamond bur is used to remove the infracochlear cells under the promontory after jugular bulb and vertical portion of the ICA recognition (▶ Fig. 13.31), reaching the cholesteatoma in its deepest portion. An angulated dissector and suction instruments are used to remove the cholesteatoma matrix from the petrous apex (▶ Fig. 13.32).

In case of bleeding from the jugular bulb, absorbable hemostatic material (e.g., Surgicel) is placed over the vein, and a cottonoid is used to press it against the vascular structure to stop the bleeding (▶ Fig. 13.33).

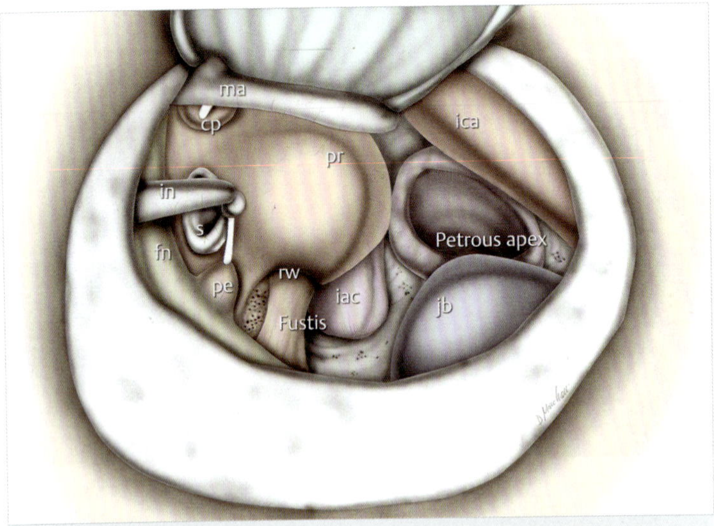

Fig. 13.21 Right side: The lateral wall of the cyst is removed creating a connection between the cyst and the tympanic cavity, to maintain the ventilation into the petrous apex and avoid recurrence. *cp: cochleariform process; fn: facial nerve; IAC: internal auditory canal; ica: internal carotid artery; in: incus; jb: jugular bulb; ma: malleus; pe: pyramidal eminence; pr: promontory; rw: round window; s: stapes.*

13.9 Postoperative Care

The patient is discharged 48 hours after surgery. After 3 months of follow-up, at the end of the healing process, a computed tomography (CT) scan is performed to detect the aeration of the petrous bone. Magnetic resonance imaging (MRI) is also planned 1 year after the surgery to detect the ventilation of the petrous apex.

13.10 Intraoperative Complications

Although this approach is considered safe, possible complications should be considered, before deciding the surgical plan:

- In case of a high jugular bulb, the access to the petrous apex via an infracochlear approach is limited, so a different approach (transphenoid and middle cranial fossa approaches) should be considered (▶ Fig. 13.43).
- Cerebrospinal fluid (CSF) leak from a damage of the dura of the IAC or the posterior cranial fossa or from cochlear duct opening. In this case a fat pad is used to close the defect.
- Vascular injury; rupture of the ICA or jugular bulb lesion.
- Injury of the cochlea causing profound sensorineural hearing loss.

In case of excessive bleeding which is difficult to manage with one hand, a retroauricular incision should be made. A diamond bur is used to calibrate the EAC to join the previously created cavity and a microscopic approach should be considered because of the possibility to use two hands to control the bleeding (see Clinical case 3).

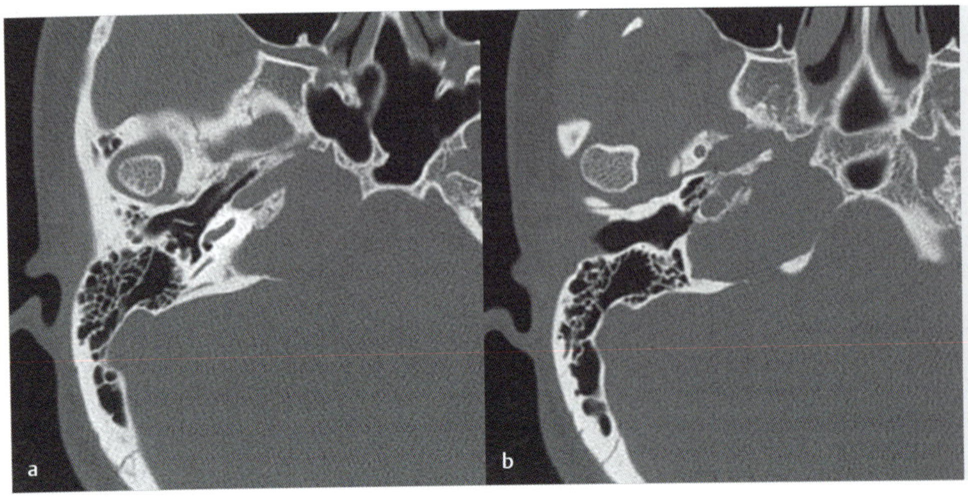

Fig. 13.22 Clinical case 1. **(a, b)** The computed tomography (CT) scan in axial view shows a lesion occupying the petrous apex in a patient with a normal hearing function.

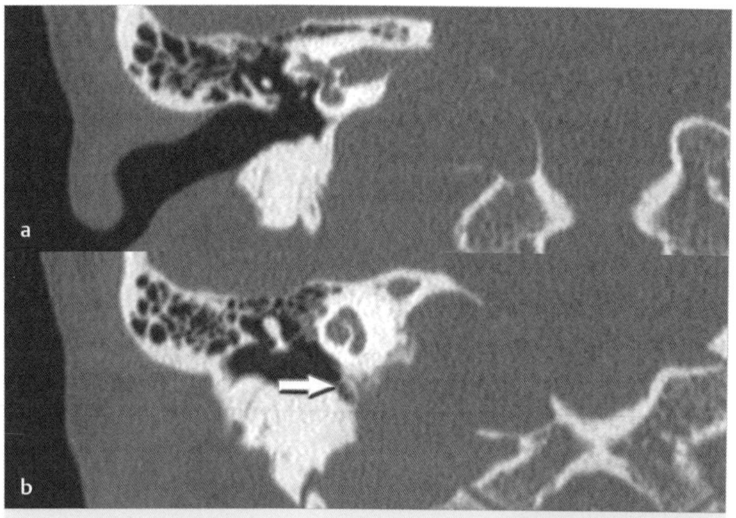

Fig. 13.23 Clinical case 1. **(a, b)** Computed tomography (CT) scan in coronal view. A petrous apex lesion running under the internal auditory canal (IAC) is detected. The reader can note the close relationship between the lesion and the subcochlear canaliculus route (see the *white arrow*).

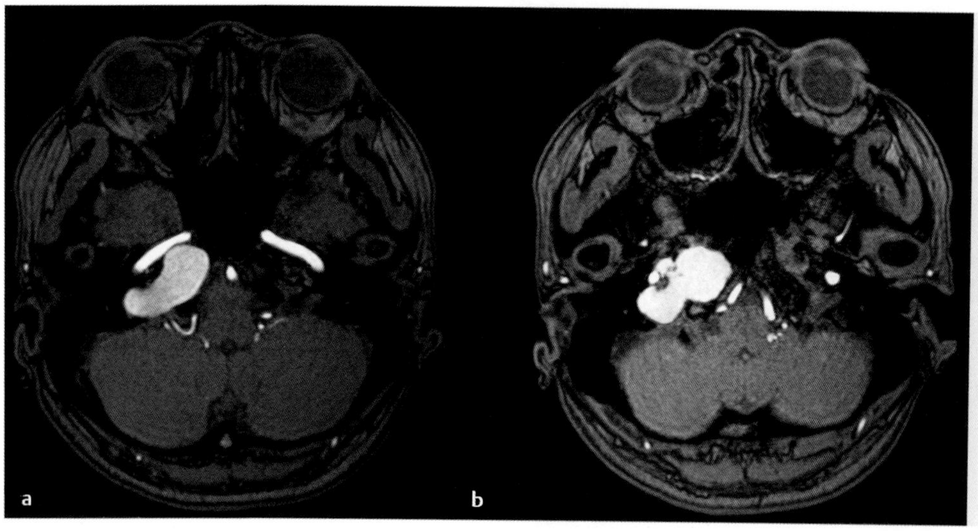

Fig. 13.24 Clinical case 1. **(a, b)** The magnetic resonance imaging (MRI) scan confirms the presence of an hyperintense lesion in the petrous apex, running along the horizontal portion of internal carotid artery (ICA) with the typical features of a cholesterol granuloma.

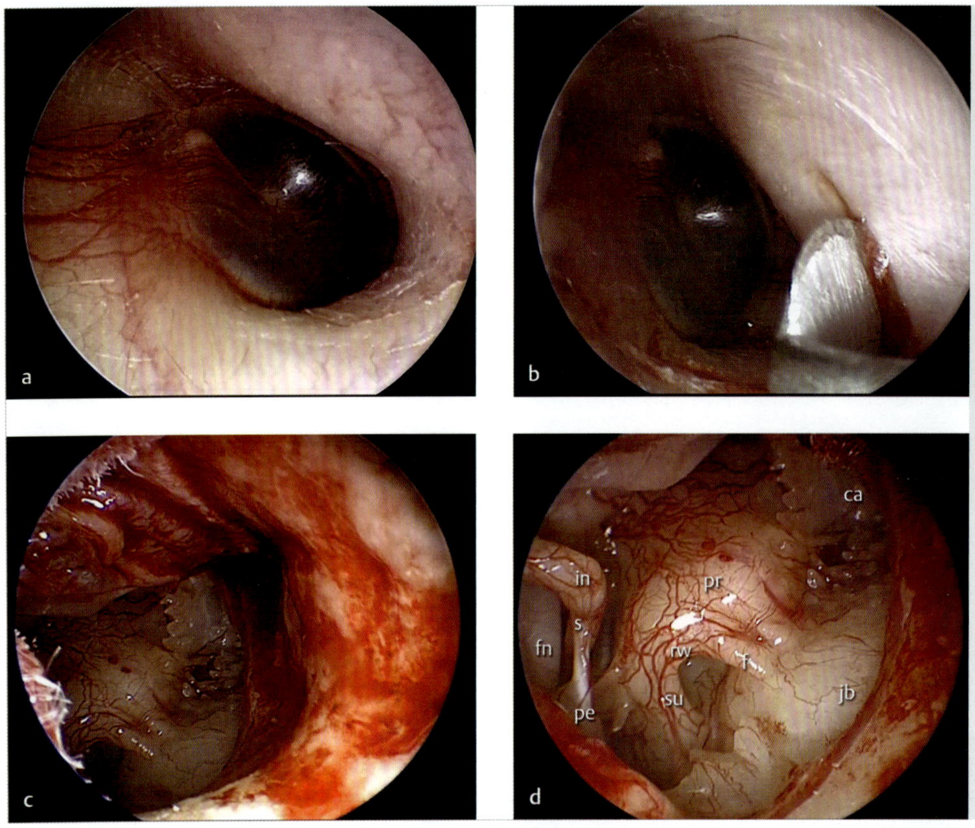

Fig. 13.25 Clinical Case 1, Right side **(a)** The ear drum is endoscopically exposed. **(b)** A tympanomeatal flap is performed and elevated. **(c)** The tympanomeatal flap is elevated in a posterior to an anterior direction and in an inferior to a superior one, maintaining the attachment of the eardrum on the malleus. **(d)** The hypotympanic and protympanic areas are progressively endoscopically exposed. The jugular bulb and the internal carotid artery (ICA) are detected. *f: finiculus; fn: facial nerve; ica: internal carotid artery; in: incus; in: incus; jb: jugular bulb; pe: pyramidal eminence; pr: promontory; rw: round window; s: stapes; su: subiculum.*

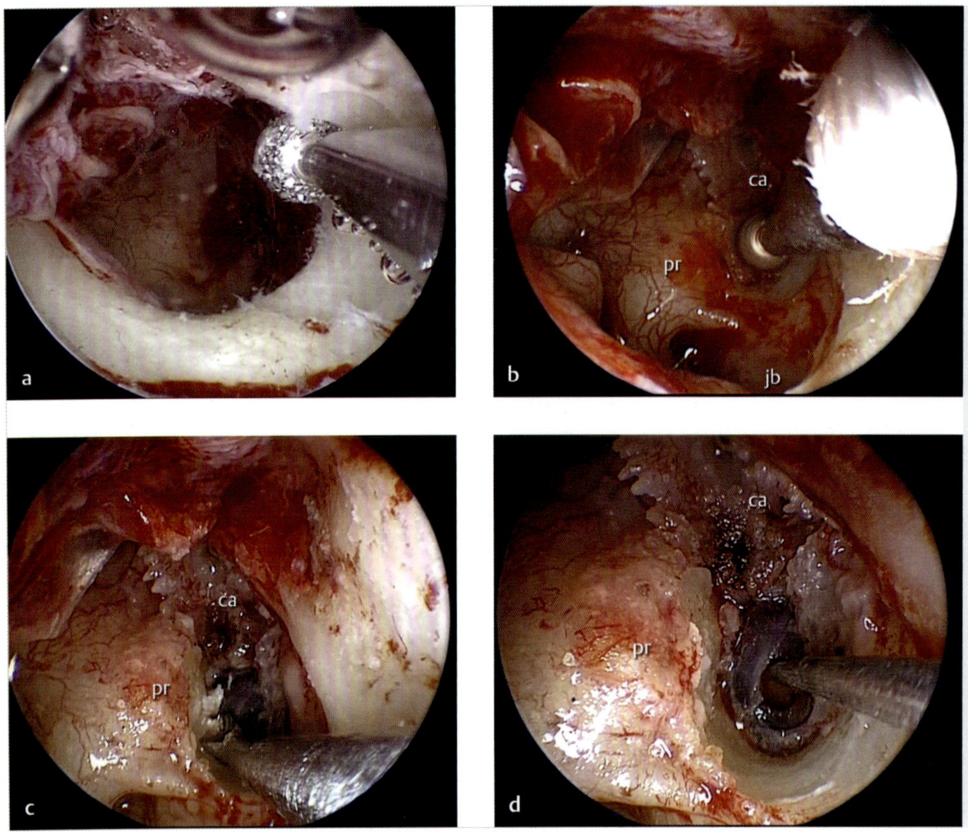

Fig. 13.26 Clinical Case 1, Right side. **(a)** A diamond bur is used to perform a canaloplasty and to remove the inferior portion of the bony anulus, uncovering the hypotympanum. **(b)** A diamond bur is used to remove the bony cells between the internal carotid artery (ICA), the jugular bulb, and the promontory, reaching the lateral wall of the cyst. **(c)** The lateral wall of the cyst is exposed; a curette is used to enlarge the surgical window, opening the wall of the cyst. **(d)** The lateral wall of the cyst is incised; a suction instrument is used to remove the content of the cyst. *ica: internal carotid artery; jb: jugular bulb; pr: promontory.*

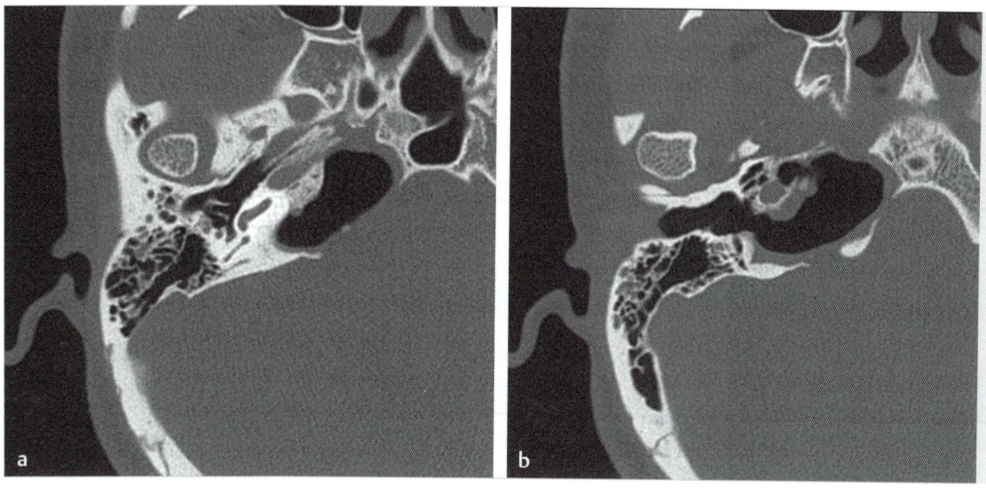

Fig. 13.27 Clinical Case 1. **(a, b)** Computed tomography (CT) scan in axial view. A postoperative check: A well-ventilated petrous apex cavity is seen through the infracochlear route.

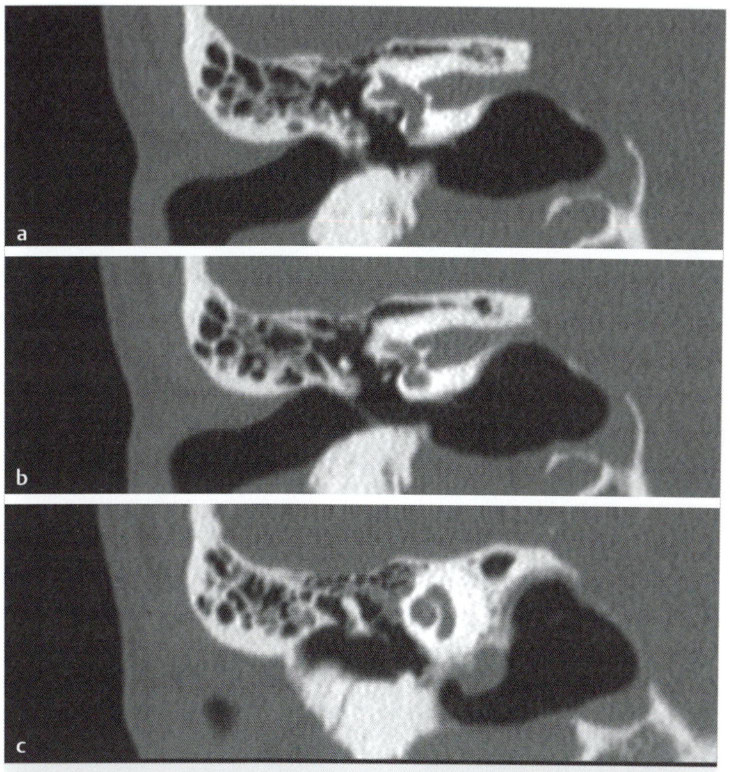

Fig. 13.28 Clinical Case 1. **(a–c)** Computed tomography (CT) scan in coronal view. A postoperative check: The infracochlear surgical route is seen; the connection between the tympanic cavity and the petrous apex is well visible, allowing for the ventilation and the drainage of the petrous apex cells.

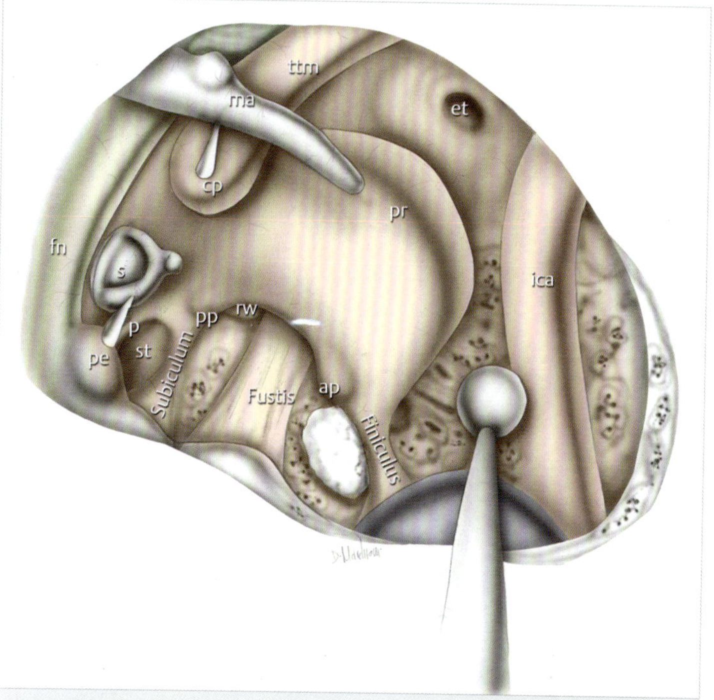

Fig. 13.29 Right side: Once the tympanic cavity cholesteatoma has been removed, a residual disease under the subcochlear canaliculus, spreading into the petrous apex, is found. A diamond bur is used to detect the major vascular structures. *ap: anterior pillar; cp: cochleariform process; et: eustachian tube; fn: facial nerve; ica: internal carotid artery; ma: malleus; p: ponticulus; pe: pyramidal eminence; pp: posterior pillar; pr: promontory; rw: round window; s: stapes; st: sinus tympani; ttm: tensor tendon muscle of the malleus.*

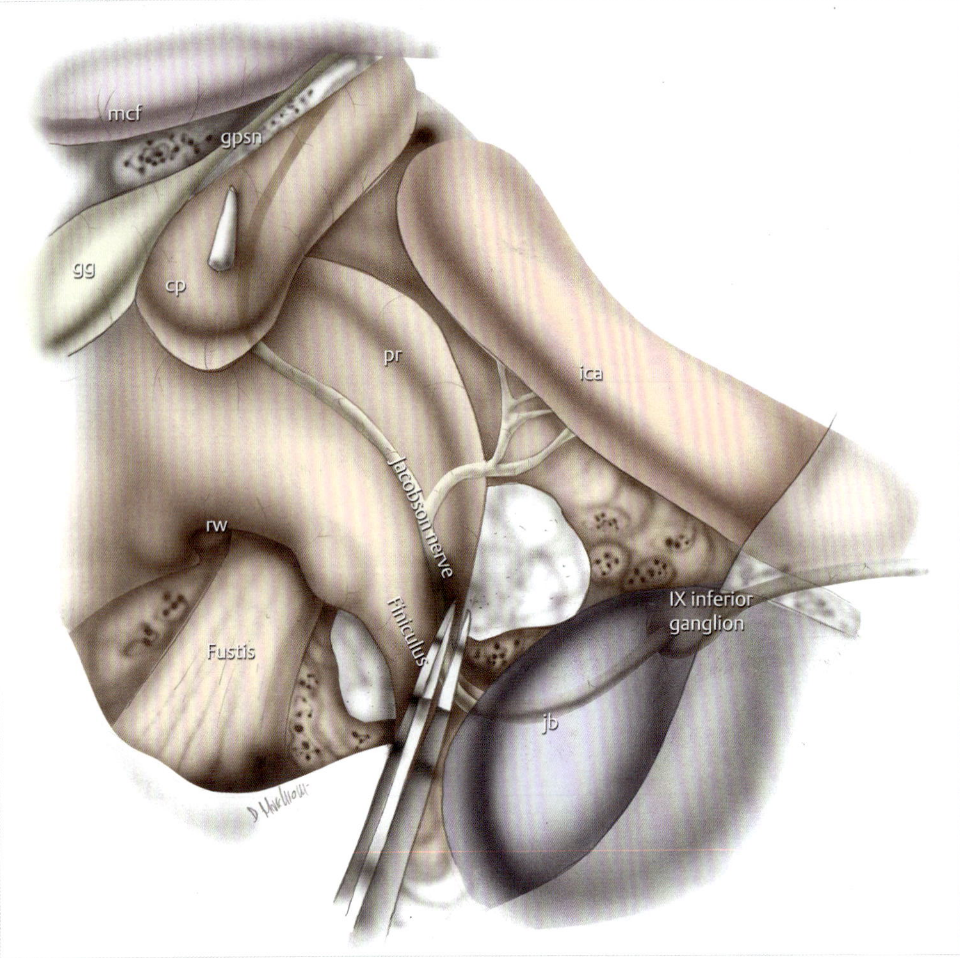

Fig. 13.30 Right side: A microbipolar instrument is used to coagulate the Jacobson plexus before the removal of the finiculus bone, to avoid bleeding. The connection between the Jacobson's nerve and the IX inferior ganglion can be noticed in the schematic drawing. *cp: cochleariform process; gg: geniculate ganglion; gpsn: greater petrosal superficial nerve; ica: internal carotid artery; jb: jugular bulb; mcf: middle cranial fossa; pr: promontory; rw: round window.*

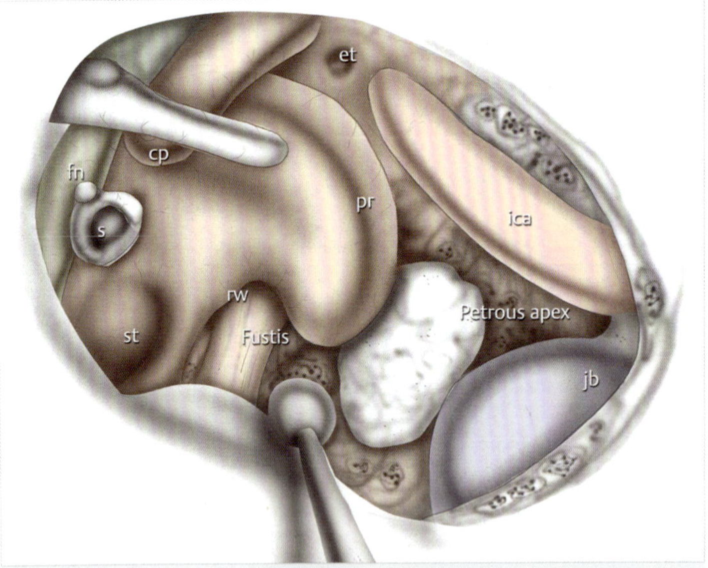

Fig. 13.31 Right side: A diamond bur is used to remove the hypotympanic cells among the internal carotid artery (ICA), the fustis, the jugular bulb, and the cochlea, to reach the cholesteatoma in the petrous apex. *cp: cochleariform process; et: eustachian tube; fn: facial nerve; ica: internal carotid artery; jb: jugular bulb; pr: promontory; rw: round window; s: stapes; st: snus tympani.*

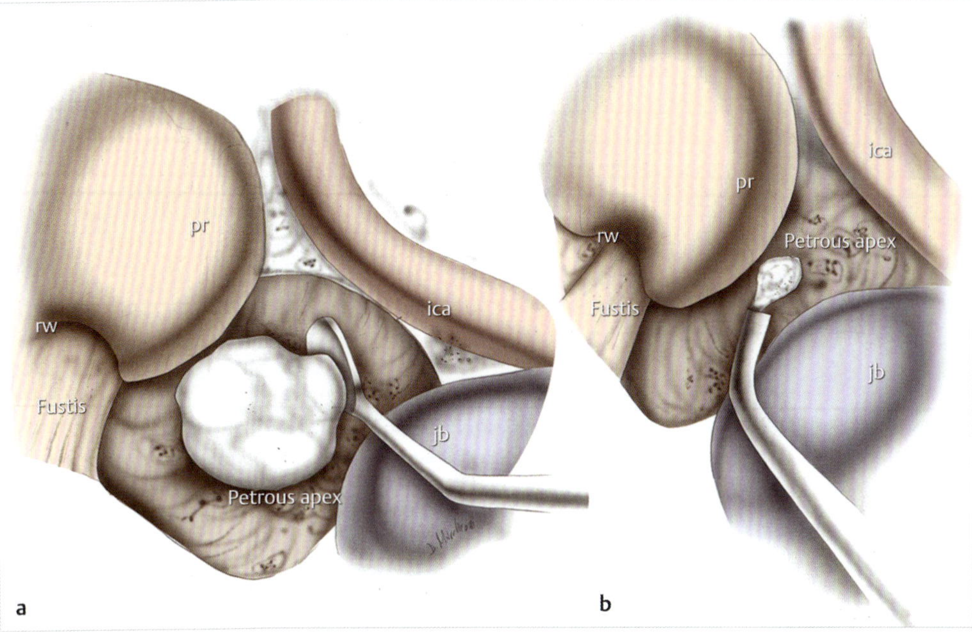

Fig. 13.32 Right side: Once the cholesteatoma has been exposed in the petrous apex, an angulated instrument is used to remove the disease **(a)**; an angulated suction instrument is used to remove remnant disease in the petrous apex **(b)**. *ica: internal carotid artery; jb: jugular bulb; pr: promontory; rw: round window.*

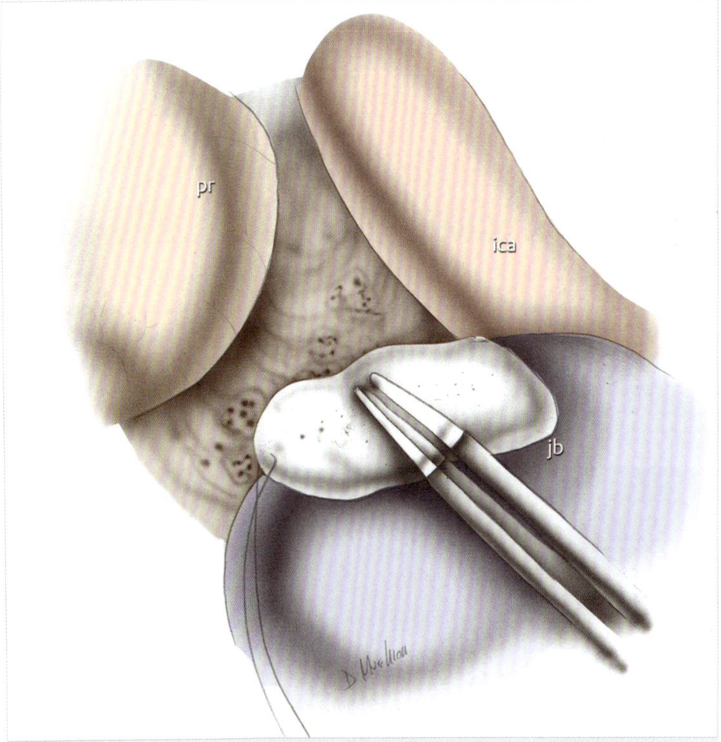

Fig. 13.33 Right side: In case of bleeding from the jugular bulb, a cottonoid is used to pack the vein. *ica: internal carotid artery; jb: jugular bulb; pr: promontory; rw: round window.*

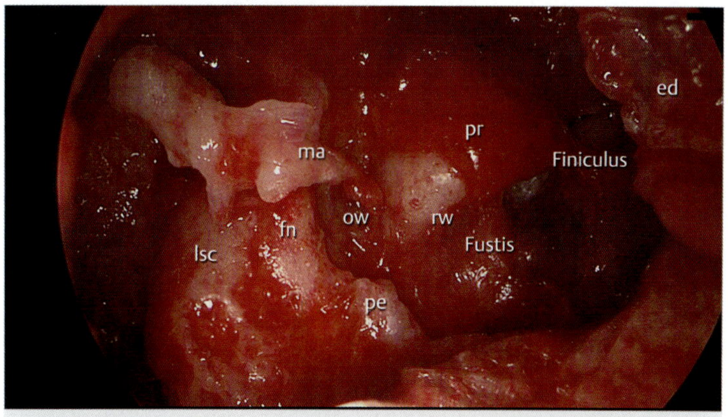

Fig. 13.34 Clinical Case 2, Right side: Tympanic cavity cholesteatoma. The cholesteatoma is removed from the tympanic cavity and a final endoscopic check of the whole cavity is performed (0-degree endoscope, 3 mm diameter). *ed: eardrum; fn: facial nerve; lsc: lateral semicircular canal; ma: malleus; ow: oval window; pe: pyramidal eminence; pr: promontory; rw: round window.*

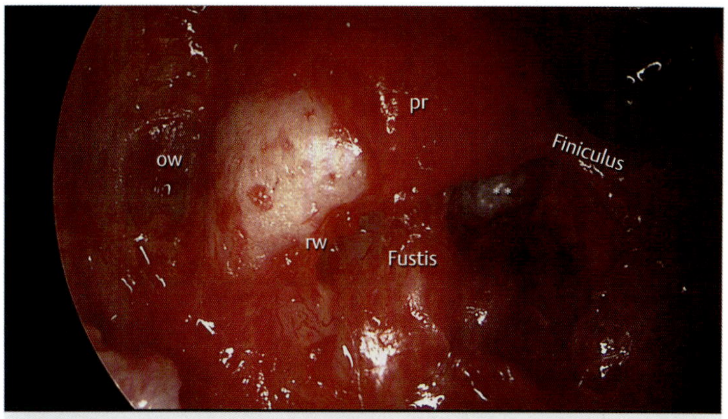

Fig. 13.35 Clinical Case 2, Right side: A remnant disease under the cochlea, is endoscopically found inside the subcochlear canaliculus (the reader can note that the subcochlear canaliculus is located between the fustis and the finiculus bone). *ow: oval window; pr: promontory; rw: round window; **: residual cholesteatoma.*

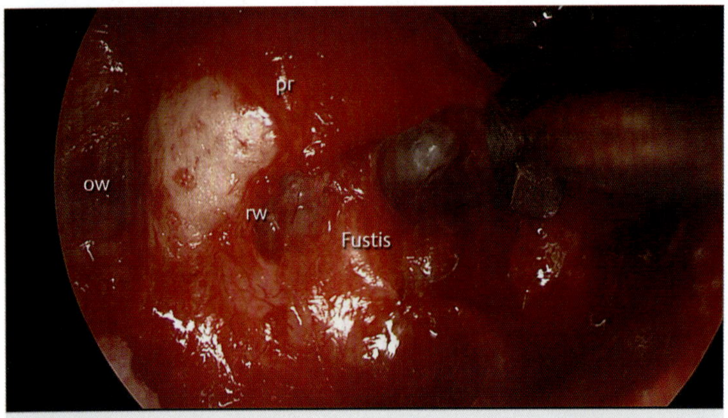

Fig. 13.36 Clinical Case 2, Right side: A piezosurgery device is used to enlarge the subcochlear area. *ow: oval window; pr: promontory; rw: round window.*

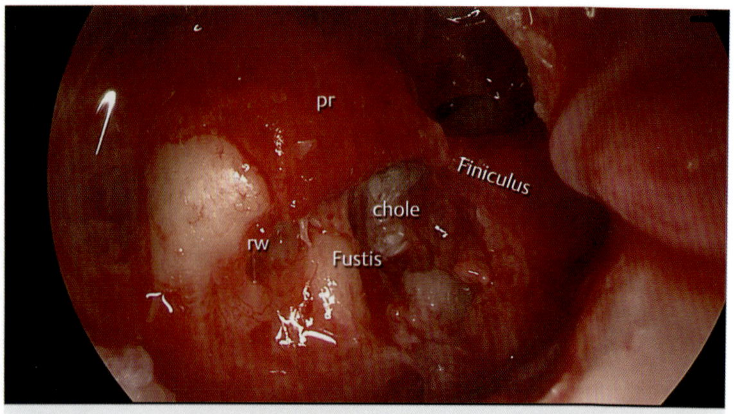

Fig. 13.37 Clinical Case 2, Right side: A residual cholesteatoma, spreading into the petrous apex, through the subcochlear canaliculus can be seen. *chole: cholesteatoma; pr: promontory; rw: round window.*

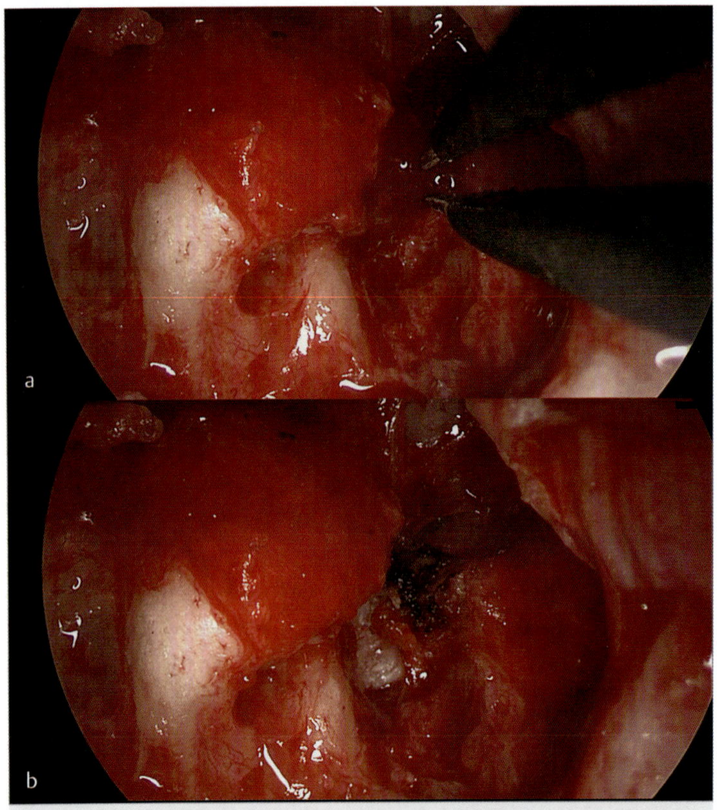

Fig. 13.38 Clinical case 2. **(a, b)** Right side: A bipolar instrument is used to coagulate the Jacobson plexus.

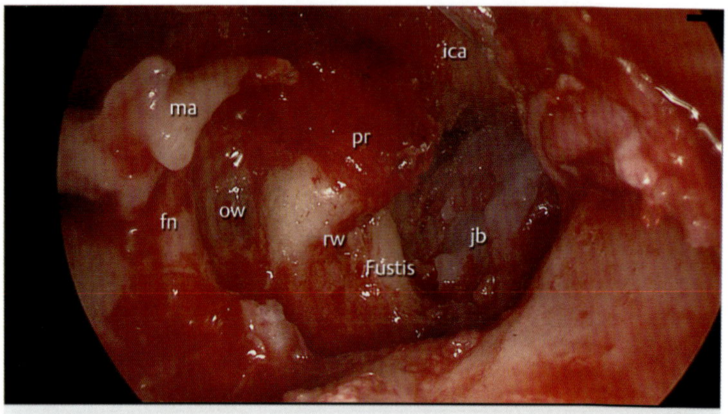

Fig. 13.39 Clinical Case 2, Right side: Once the finiculus has been removed, the Jugular bulb and the internal carotid artery (ICA) are endoscopically detected, and the cholesteatoma is removed from the petrous apex. *fn: facial nerve; ica: internal carotid artery; jb: jugular bulb; ma: malleus; ow: oval window; pr: promontory; rw: round window.*

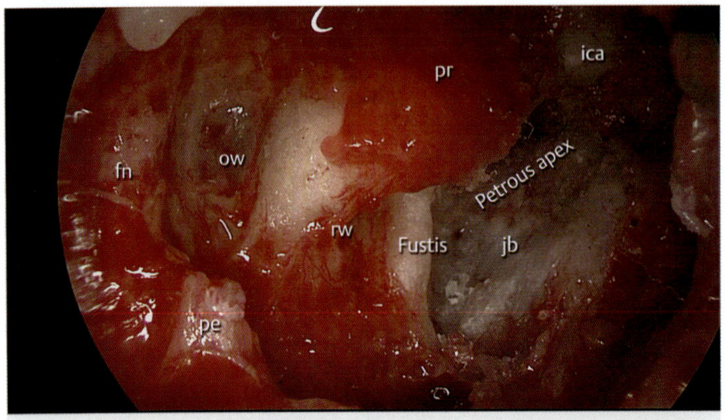

Fig. 13.40 Clinical Case 2, Right side: Final view of the subcochlear surgical route after cholesteatoma removal. *ica: internal carotid artery; jb: jugular bulb; ow: oval window; pr: promontory; rw: round window.*

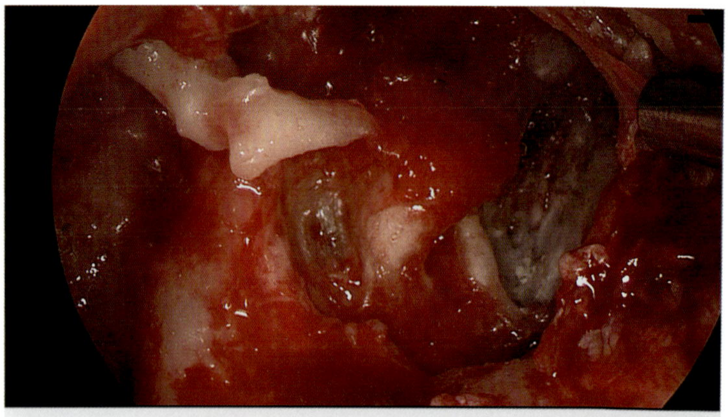

Fig. 13.41 Clinical Case 2, Right side: The malleus is maintained in the tympanic cavity.

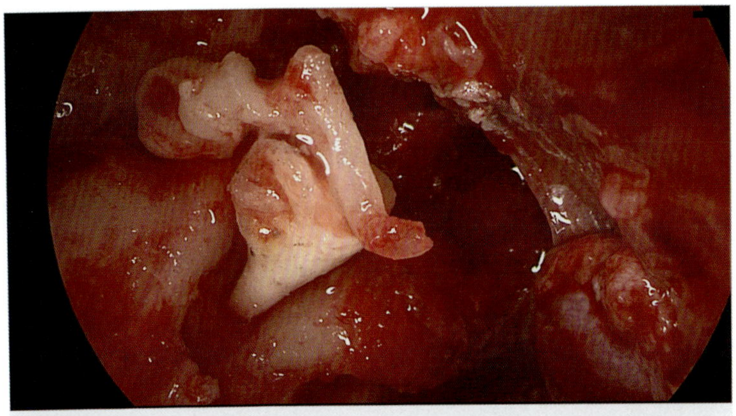

Fig. 13.42 Clinical Case 2, Right side: A remodelled incus is used to reconstruct the ossicular chain as a prosthesis between the oval window and the malleus.

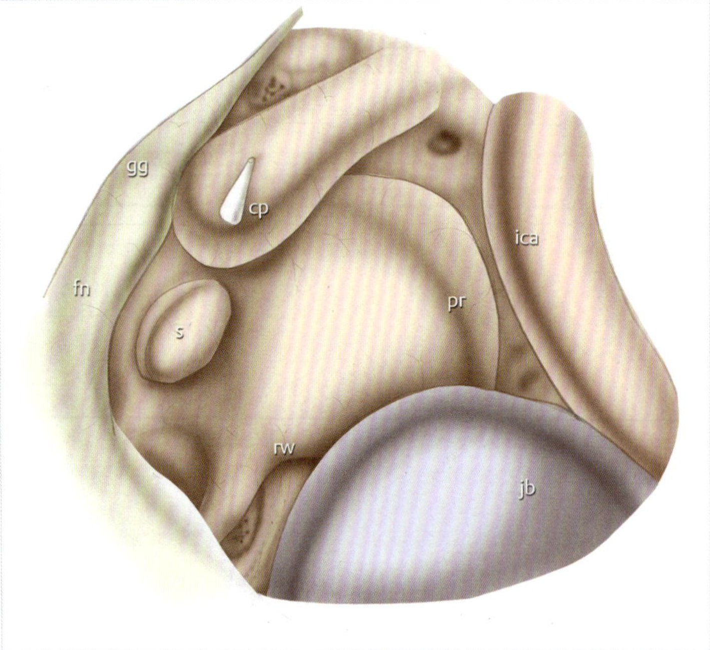

Fig. 13.43 Right side: A high jugular bulb is noted; in this case an infracochlear procedure is contraindicated. *cp: cochleariform process; fn: facial nerve; gg: geniculate ganglion; ica: internal carotid artery; jb: jugular bulb; pr: promontory; rw: round window; s: stapes.*

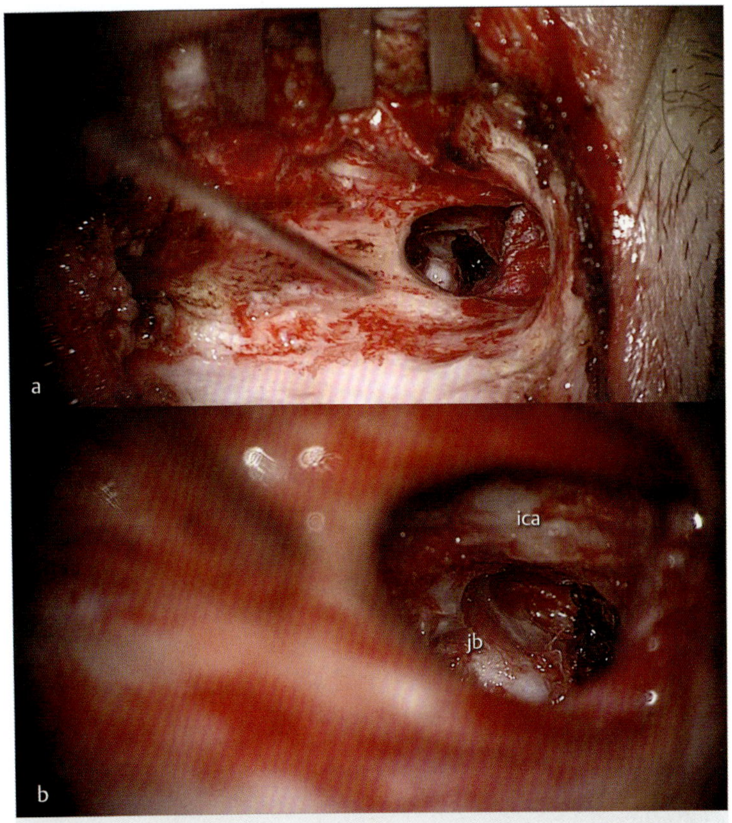

Fig. 13.44 Clinical case 3. **(a, b)** Left side: Microscopic infracochlear approach. A retroauricular incision is performed; the external auditory canal (EAC) is drilled to enlarge the surgical corridor; the inferior bony anulus is removed and the major vascular structures are detected; and the petrous apex cells among the internal carotid artery (ICA), the jugular bulb, and the promontory are removed. *ica: internal carotid artery; jb: jugular bulb.*

Suggested Readings

Brackmann DE, Toh EH. Surgical management of petrous apex cholesterol granulomas. Otol Neurotol. 2002; 23(4):529–533

Ghorayeb BY, Jahrsdoerfer RA. Subcochlear approach for cholesterol granulomas of the inferior petrous apex. Otolaryngol Head Neck Surg. 1990; 103(1):60–65

Giddings NA, Brackmann DE, Kwartler JA. Transcanal infracochlear approach to the petrous apex. Otolaryngol Head Neck Surg. 1991; 104(1):29–36

Kempfle JS, Fiorillo B, Kanumuri VV, et al. Quantitative imaging analysis of transcanal endoscopic Infracochlear approach to the internal auditory canal. Am J Otolaryngol. 2017; 38(5):518–520

Leung R, Samy RN, Leach JL, Murugappan S, Stredney D, Wiet G. Radiographic anatomy of the infracochlear approach to the petrous apex for computer-assisted surgery. Otol Neurotol. 2010; 31(3):419–423

Marchioni D, Alicandri-Ciufelli M, Pothier DD, Rubini A, Presutti L. The round window region and contiguous areas: endoscopic anatomy and surgical implications. Eur Arch Otorhinolaryngol. 2015; 272(5):1103–1112

Marchioni D, Alicandri-Ciufelli M, Rubini A, Presutti L. Endoscopic transcanal corridors to the lateral skull base: Initial experiences. Laryngoscope. 2015; 125 Suppl 5:S1–S13

Marchioni D, Soloperto D, Colleselli E, Tatti MF, Patel N, Jufas N. Round window chamber and fustis: endoscopic anatomy and surgical implications. Surg Radiol Anat. 2016; 38(9):1013–1019

Mattox DE. Endoscopy-assisted surgery of the petrous apex. Otolaryngol Head Neck Surg. 2004; 130(2):229–241

Mosnier I, Cyna-Gorse F, Grayeli AB, et al. Management of cholesterol granulomas of the petrous apex based on clinical and radiologic evaluation. Otol Neurotol. 2002; 23(4):522–528

Presutti L, Nogueira JF, Alicandri-Ciufelli M, Marchioni D. Beyond the middle ear: endoscopic surgical anatomy and approaches to inner ear and lateral skull base. Otolaryngol Clin North Am. 2013; 46(2):189–200

Rhoton ALJ, Jr. The temporal bone and transtemporal approaches. Neurosurgery. 2000; 47(3) Suppl:S211–S265

Scopel TF, Fernandez-Miranda JC, Pinheiro-Neto CD, et al. Petrous apex cholesterol granulomas: endonasal versus infracochlear approach. Laryngoscope. 2012; 122 (4):751–761

Wick CC, Hansen AR, Kutz JW, Jr, Isaacson B. Endoscopic infracochlear approach for drainage of petrous apex cholesterol granulomas: a case series. Otol Neurotol. 2017; 38(6):876–881

Chapter 14

Complications and Management in Lateral Skull Base Surgery

14 Complications and Management in Lateral Skull Base Surgery

Daniele Marchioni, Andrea Martone, and Matteo Alicandri Ciufelli

Abstract

Open approaches to lateral skull base are technically challenging due to the complex anatomy of this area, and various types of complications can occur. Lower cranial nerves deficit, typically related to glossopharyngeal and vagus injuries, may result in significant swallowing dysfunction and vocal cord paralysis with weak voice and requires a swallowing rehabilitation with a speech therapist in the postoperative period. Facial nerve paralysis causes a significant functional and aesthetic impair and has to be treated as quickly as possible. Among the various techniques described, the end-to-end anastomosis remains the procedure of choice if the residual nerve is long enough so that no dislocation of the facial nerve is needed, while cable nerve grafting is usually the best option if a direct graft is not feasible. CSF leak, resulting from a communication between the subarachnoid spaces and the extracranial spaces, poses a great infectious risk for the patient. Up to 80% of CSF leaks due to lateral skull base surgery can be treated conservatively. Recurrent leaks must be treated surgically and the technique is driven by the location and cause of the fistula. Intraoperative bleeding is generally caused by an accidental injury of the jugular bulb, sigmoid sinus, or emissary veins. In contrast, the ICA hemorrhage is uncommon but represents a surgical emergency. Postoperative intracranial bleeding can result in a life-threatening situation due to the space-occupying effect on brain tissue. Therefore, control CT scans are usually recommended after lateral skull base surgery. Surgical decompression of the hematoma is mandatory in these cases and the technique is driven by the type of surgical approach previously performed.

Keywords: lateral skull base complications, facial nerve paralysis, ICA bleeding, CSF leak, cranial nerves deficit, facial nerve rehabilitation

14.1 Cranial Nerves Deficit

Lower cranial nerve deficits are perhaps the most significant causes of morbidity in lateral skull base surgery. Glossopharyngeal and vagus nerve injuries may result in significant swallowing dysfunction and vocal cord paralysis with weak voice. This disability requires a swallowing rehabilitation with a speech therapist in the postoperative time. When significant aspiration and dysphonia are present, thyroplasty and gastrostomy are considered.

Especially in case of repeated bouts of aspiration pneumonia, a tracheostomy should be considered in the postoperative time to avoid lung infections.

A swallowing rehabilitation in this phase is crucial to have the gradual resolution of the aspiration, since the contralateral vocal cord compensation is the most effective treatment for this condition. In case of inadequate compensation of the vocal cord, a type A thyroplasty should be considered in order to medialize the paretic vocal cord surgically. This surgical procedure should improve glottic closure and decrease aspiration risk.

14.1.1 Facial Nerve Reparation

Facial nerve paralysis causes a significant functional and aesthetic impair. Axonotmesis and neurotmesis lead to sensory and motor deficits, muscular atrophy, Wallerian degeneration distal to the injured tract, and scar tissue formation.

A severely damaged or sectioned facial nerve must be surgically repaired if return of function is to be achieved. Surgery is indicated in those cases where a spontaneous recovery is not likely. Testing of the residual nerve function can be useful to assess if spontaneous recovery is probable, especially if there is facial nerve palsy but anatomical continuity was maintained. Electromyography (EMG) and electroneurography (ENoG) are the most widely used procedures for this purpose. If facial palsy occurs immediately after mastoid surgery and doubt of having anatomically damaged the nerve arises, urgent re-exploration of the facial nerve with decompression of several millimeters on either side of the injured segment is indicated. If the surgeon is absolutely sure that there was no disruption of the nerve, observation of the patient and high dosage corticosteroid therapy may be indicated. There are several procedures for the repair of facial nerve injuries, such as: direct end-to-end suture, cable nerve grafting, and nerve crossover. The mechanism of injury, amount of time between nerve damage to treatment, and patient's age are the most important factors determining which approach is most likely to obtain a desirable outcome and the location of the hematoma. As a general principle, the sooner the nerve is repaired, the better the long-term results can be expected. Regardless of the technique chosen, synkinesis is expected and the best achievable result is House-Brackmann grade III.

14.1.2 Primary Nerve Grafting

The direct grafting of the two nervous stumps (end-to-end anastomosis) is the procedure of choice if the residual nerve is long enough so that no dislocation of the facial nerve is needed and it can be achieved without undue tension. Better functional outcomes with this technique can be explained since by performing only one anastomosis, there is a smaller percentage of new fiber dispersion. In order to have a successful graft, some functional motor units must remain to receive reinnervation and there shouldn't be excessive muscular atrophy or motor endplate fibrosis. The key to a successful graft is the reapproximation of the two stumps atraumatically and without tension, keeping in mind that the terminal ends should match as precisely as possible to each other (see ▶ Fig. 14.1 and Clinical Case 1, ▶ Fig. 14.2). Epineurial microsutures, wherever possible, or a fibrin glue with temporalis fascia should be used to realize the anastomosis.

14.1.3 Cable Nerve Grafting

Cable nerve grafting is usually the best option if a direct graft is not feasible. Inserted nerve segments provide endoneurial tubes for axonal regeneration. The most commonly used nerves are the great auricular nerve and the sural nerve since both are sensory

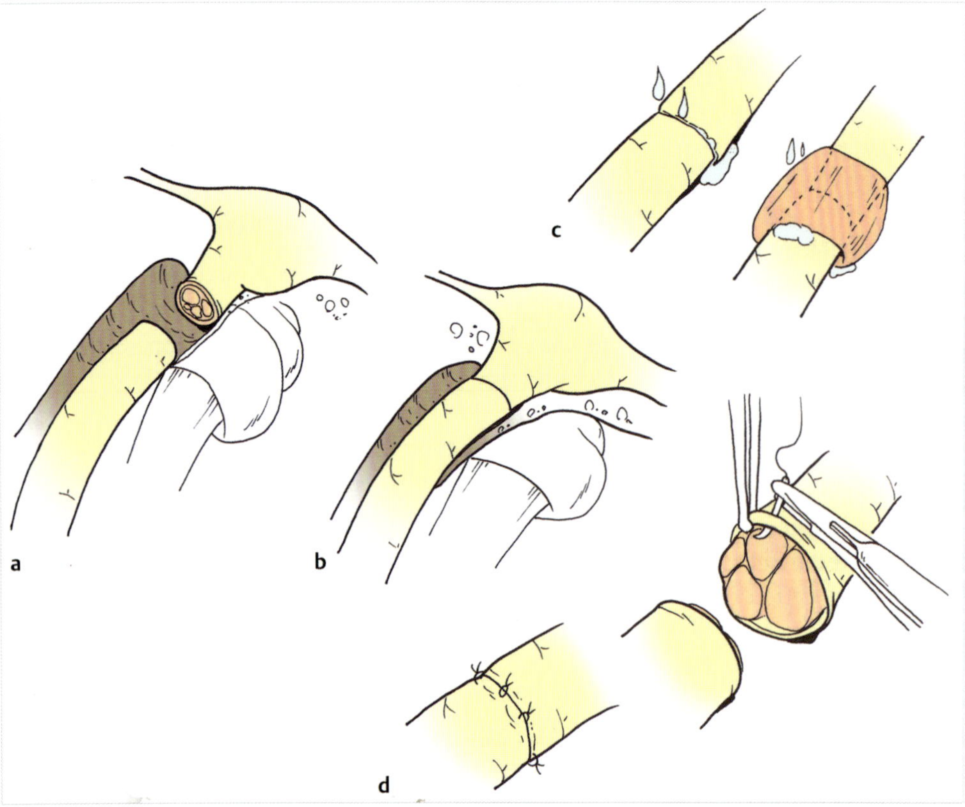

Fig. 14.1 Schematic drawing of left temporal bone during middle fossa approach: **(a)** A nerve interruption between the labyrinthine segment of the facial nerve and geniculate ganglion is noticed. **(b)** An end-to-end anastomosis is performed. For the end-to-end procedure to be successful, there must be enough length on both the proximal and distal stumps of the facial nerve to allow approximation of the two ends in such a way that the endoneural surfaces lie in contact and are completely tension free. Two options are available to create the nerve anastomosis: **(c)** A fibrin glue should be used to fix the anastomosis; a temporalis fascia placed around the anastomosis and fixed with fibrin glue may be used to reinforce the nerve reparation. **(d)** The other option in order to create the end-to-end anastomosis is the epineurial microsutures.

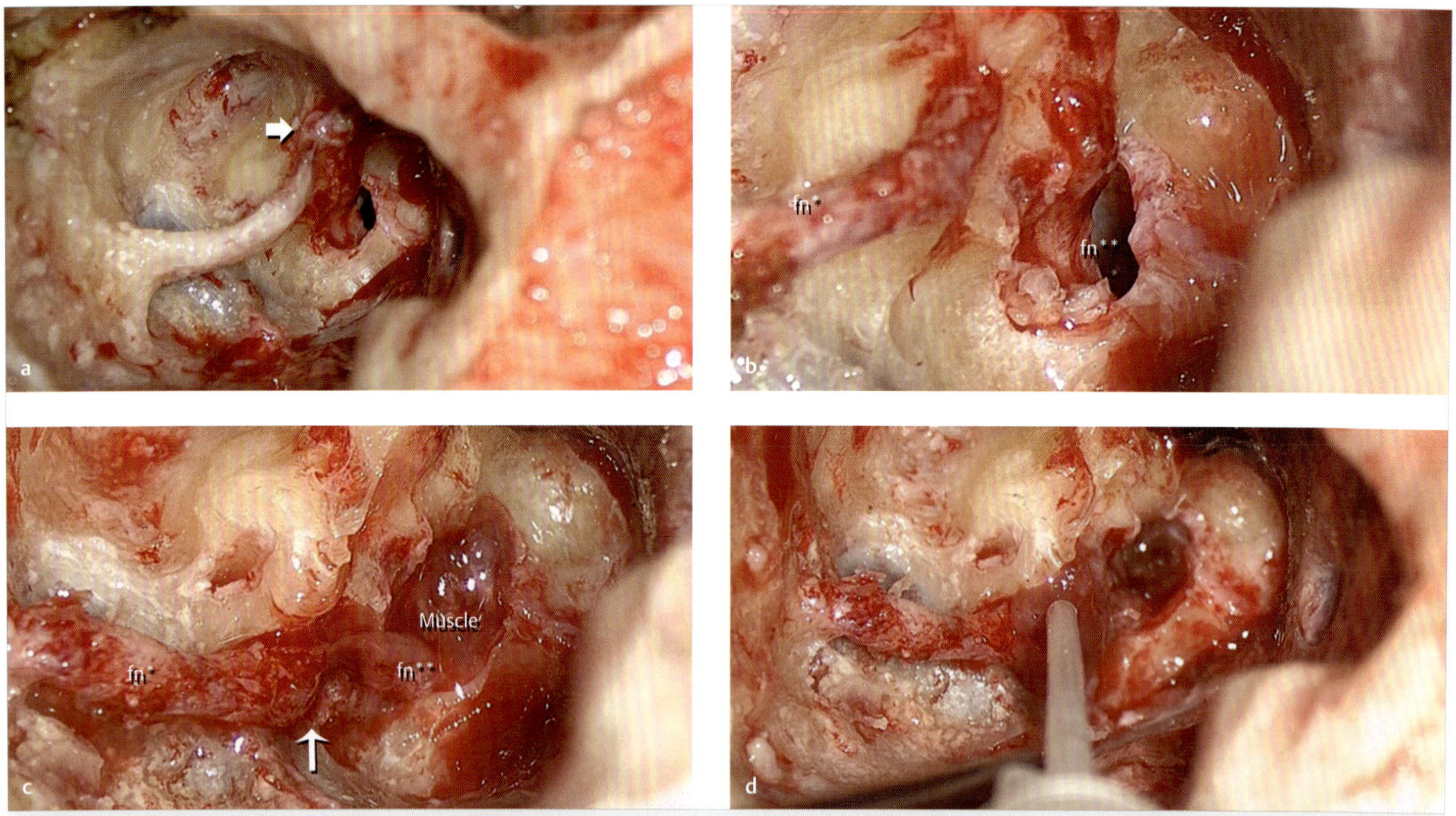

Fig. 14.2 Clinical Case 1, Left side: Transotic approach for a petrous apex cholesteatoma in subject with facial palsy. After cholesteatoma removal a facial nerve interruption between the tympanic segment of facial nerve and geniculate ganglion is seen (**[a]**: *white arrow*). The facial nerve is detected into the internal auditory canal (IAC) **(b)**. A mobilization of the distal and proximal stumps is performed in order to have an optimal approximation between the two stumps, performing an end-to-end anastomosis (**[c]**: *white arrow*). A piece of muscle is placed into the IAC in order to repair the defect and to fix the proximal stump. A piece of temporalis fascia is used to cover the connection between the two stumps of the facial nerve, and fibrin glue is used to reinforce the end-to-end anastomosis. *fn*: mastoid segment of facial nerve; fn**: facial nerve into the IAC.*

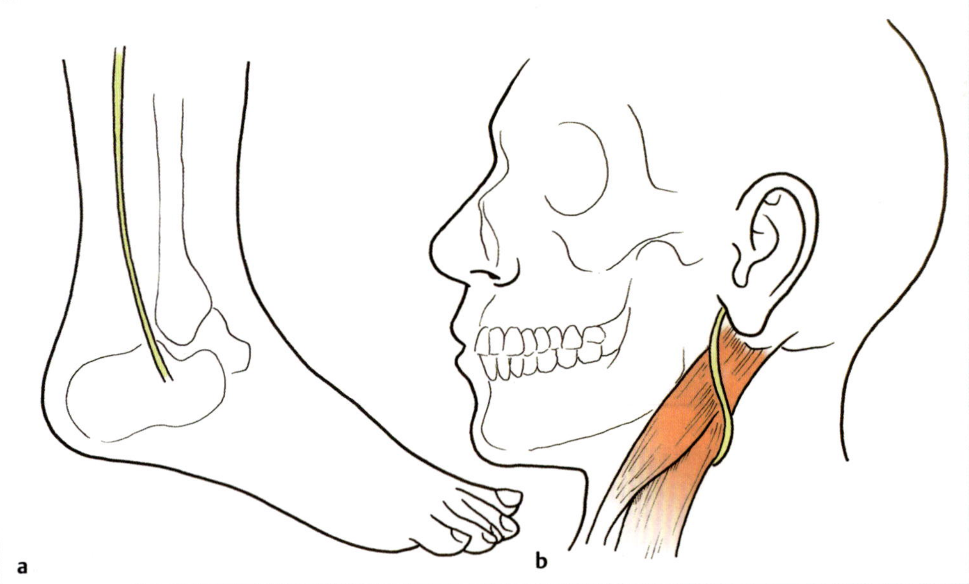

Fig. 14.3 **(a)** Sural nerve. **(b)** The great auricular nerve and the sural nerve.

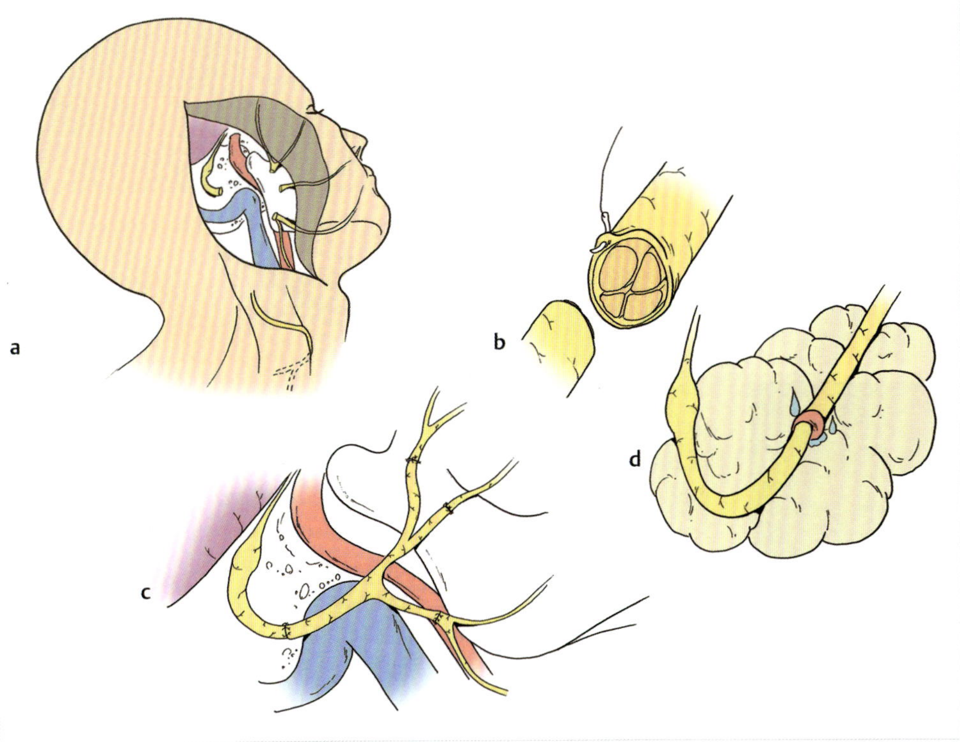

Fig. 14.4 Schematic drawing after infratemporal fossa for tumor removal. A large defect of the facial nerve involving the temporal bone and the parotid segments is noticed **(a)**. A cable graft anastomosis between the peripheral branches and the mastoid segment of facial nerve using the great auricular nerve is adopted **(b)**. An epineurial microsuture is performed **(c)**. The fibrin glue with a temporalis fascia is used to reinforce the anastomosis, and abdominal fat is used to fill the mastoid cavity, supporting the grafting, reducing the tension between the proximal and distal stumps **(d)**.

nerves with a similar caliber of facial nerve (▶ Fig. 14.3). The great auricular nerve has the advantages of proximity to the surgical field and up to 10 cm may be harvested. On the other hand, up to 40 cm of sural nerve can be harvested and it has richer neural fascicles. The main disadvantages are postoperative numbness in the ear or lateral foot respectively.

In both procedures, the stumps can be reapproximated using biological glue or epineurial microsutures. The former is particularly suitable for grafting as it is technically less complex and better applies to the cerebellopontine angle (CPA) structure's movements caused by cerebrospinal fluid (CSF) pulsation.

During the treatment of tumor involving the lateral skull base surgery, a facial nerve repair by interposition graft may be required. We can distinguish two situations:

- The facial nerve defect is in the temporal bone without involving the CPA.
- The facial nerve defect is in the CPA.

In case of large defect of the facial nerve in the temporal bone, a great auricular nerve graft should be used in order to recreate the continuity from the temporal bone in the proximal stump to the distal stump (since the peripheral branches of the facial nerve may be involved). Typical examples are a temporal bone paraganglioma with or without facial nerve invasion requiring the sacrifice of the nerve or a malignant tumor of the parotid gland involving the temporal bone requiring an infratemporal fossa approach with the sacrifice of the facial neve. In these cases, a long cable graft with ramification is necessary, especially if the defect of the nerve involves the mastoid and the parotid branches. A direct suture between the nerves to get the anastomosis is an optimal solution to fix the proximal and distal anastomoses. A piece of vein or temporalis fascia with fibrin glue should be used for covering the anastomosis so as to stabilize the nerve connection (▶ Fig. 14.4; see Clinical Case 2 and Clinical Case 3).

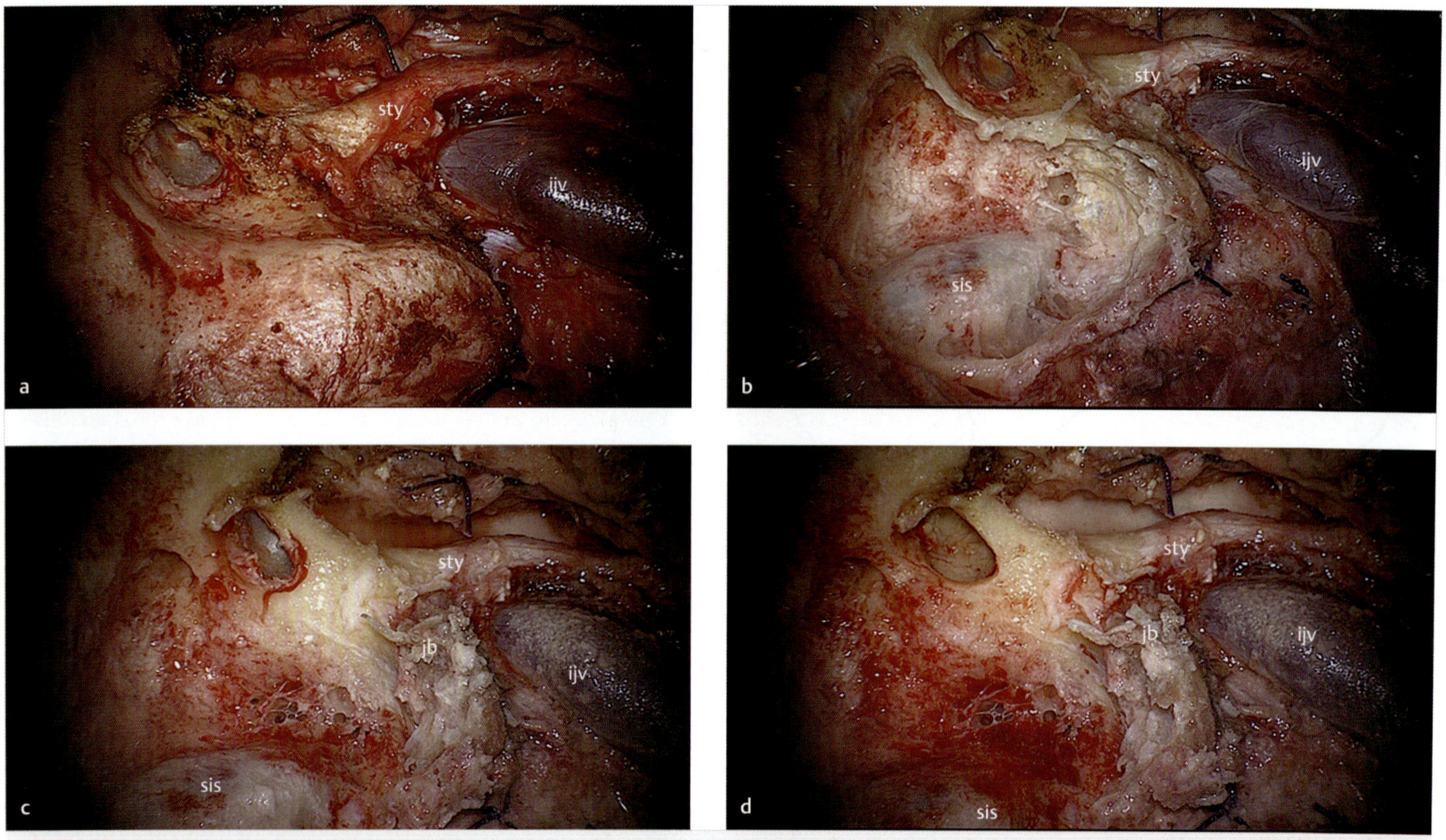

Fig. 14.5 Clinical Case 2, Right side: Infratemporal fossa approach for a malignant tumor of the parotid gland with infratemporal fossa extension. **(a)** A sacrifice of facial nerve into the stylomastoid foramen is done; a subtotal petrosectomy is started. **(b)** The mastoidectomy is performed and the mastoid tip is transected; the sigmoid sinus is noticed. **(c–d)** The jugular bulb is progressively skeletonized and the skin of the external auditory canal (EAC) with the eardrum is removed. *ijv: internal jugular vein; jb: jugular bulb; sis: sigmoid sinus; sty: styloid process.*

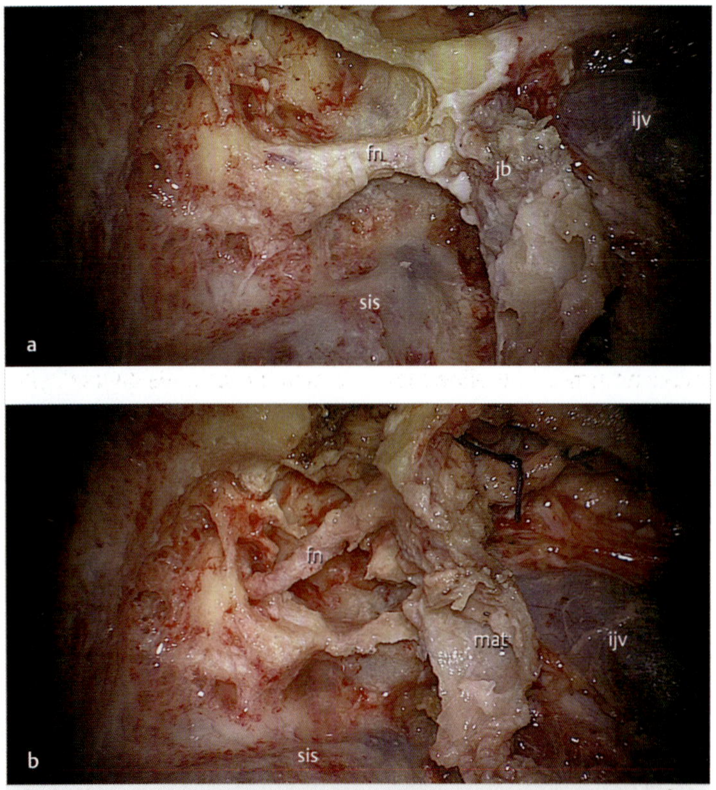

Fig. 14.6 Clinical Case 2, Right side: **(a)** The facial nerve is progressively isolated into the temporal bone from the styloid-mastoid foramen till the geniculate ganglion. **(b)** The mastoid tip is completely removed and the mastoid segment of facial nerve is mobilized. *fn: facial nerve; ijv: internal jugular vein; jb: jugular bulb; mat: mastoid tip; sis: sigmoid sinus.*

A sural graft is an optimal solution in case of large defect of the facial nerve in the CPA; it is really important to have the right length of the sural graft in order to avoid tension on the anastomosis. The graft shouldn't be in tension between the two stumps. A long S-shaped graft with the curved part resting over the trigeminal nerve may be useful in order to fix and stabilize the graft, avoiding tension between the anastomosis. A piece of temporalis fascia is placed and folded around the proximal anastomosis; a fibrin glue is used to reinforce the anastomosis. The distal anastomosis is placed in the internal auditory canal (IAC) wall and fixed using the fibrin glue; the dural layer of the IAC is used to cover the distal anastomosis (▶ Fig. 14.10).

14.1.4 Nerve Substitution

The most widely used nerve substitution technique is the hypoglossal-facial nerve anastomosis. The anastomosis can be either end-to-end or side-to-end (see ▶ Fig. 14.11 and Clinical Case 4, ▶ Fig. 14.12). During the end-to-end procedure, the facial nerve is sectioned just after the stylomastoid foramen and subsequently grafted to the hypoglossal nerve, which is transected under the digastric muscle intermediate tendon (▶ Fig. 14.11a, b). In this procedure the descending loop of hypoglossal nerve is grafted to the distal stump of the main trunk of hypoglossal nerve, avoiding emi-tongue atrophy. This surgical approach achieves relatively good outcomes, although inferior to direct grafting, and can be performed up to 2 years after the initial facial nerve injury. The main disadvantage is the residual emi-tongue paralysis. To avoid this collateral effect, the side-to-end technique was developed (▶ Fig. 14.11c, d). The facial nerve is identified backwards up until

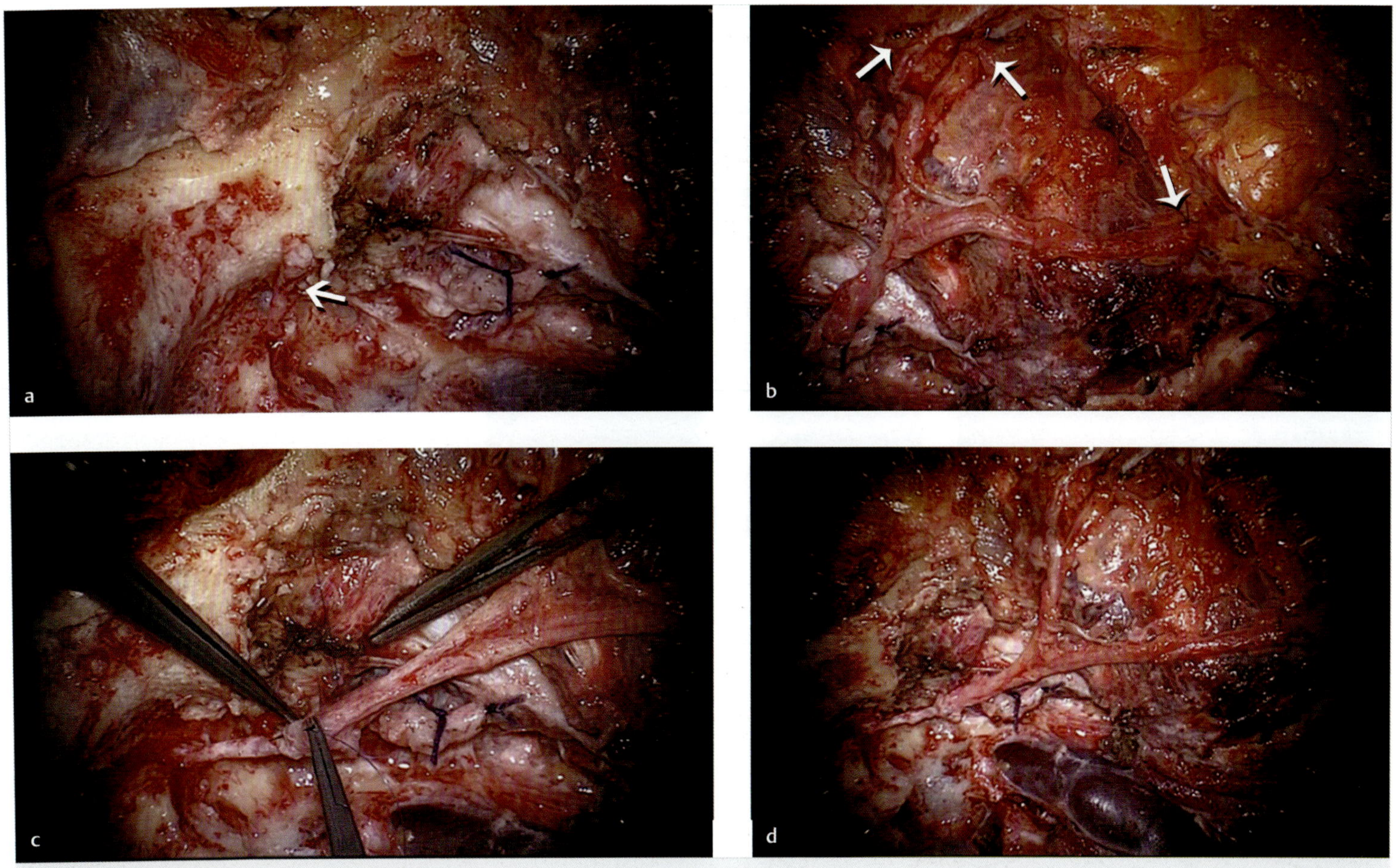

Fig. 14.7 Clinical Case 2, Right side: **(a)** The temporal bone facial nerve is mobilized until the geniculate ganglion (*white arrow*). **(b)** A great auricular nerve graft is used to connect the intratemporal facial nerve to the peripheral branches; a microsuture is performed between the cable graft and the peripheral branches of facial nerve (see the *white arrows*). **(c)** A microsuture is performed between the cable graft and the tympanic segment of the facial nerve. **(d)** A total reconstruction of the facial nerve by a cable graft is done.

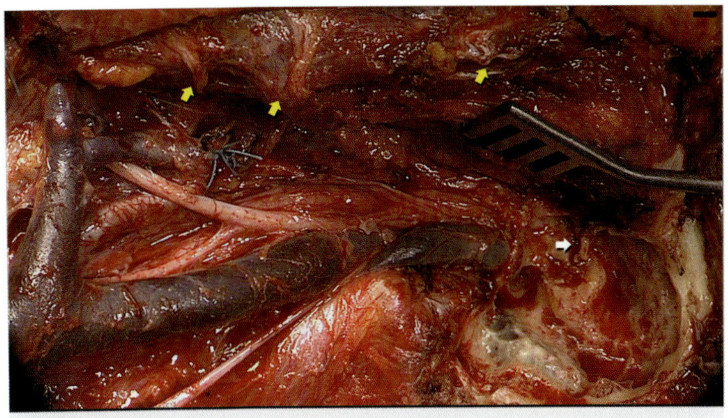

Fig. 14.8 Clinical Case 3, Left side: Surgical field after infratemporal fossa type A with sacrifice of facial nerve. Jugular foramen with the lower cranial nerve is widely exposed and the internal carotid artery (ICA) is preserved. A large interruption of facial nerve between the proximal stump (*white arrow* into the tympanic cavity) and the distal branches (*yellow arrows* into the parotid) of facial nerve is noticed.

the second genu, transected, and then sutured to the lateral surface of the hypoglossal nerve. In this manner, only a part of hypoglossal fibers is interrupted, so the remaining nerve still maintains its primary function. Side-to-end anastomosis provides fewer fibers for reinnervation. For this reason, it should be performed within 6 months of the injury in order to limit nervous fibrosis, thus increasing the chances of success.

A jump graft is a third option available if nerve substitution is chosen. By this approach the hypoglossal nerve is incised longitudinally and a great auricular nerve graft is then bridged between the hypoglossal nerve and the transected facial nerve.

14.1.5 Cross-Facial Nerve Graft

This procedure is suitable for those cases in which the main trunk of the facial nerve is damaged but distal branches remain viable. The principle used in this technique is the facial nerve's functional reserve, where there is an overlap in function among different nerve branches. This allows for several branches to be divided without impairing the normal function. A single or multiple branches of the injured facial nerve can be grafted to the undamaged contralateral nerve, using a sensory nerve graft to connect both ends (sural nerve is typically used due to its length) (see ▶ Fig. 14.13). At a pace of 1 mm per day, nervous fibers from the undamaged facial nerve will grow through the graft and repopulate the injured facial muscles. Therefore, recovery is slow and movement in the paralyzed emi-face will not develop for 9 to 12 months.

14.2 CSF Leak

A CSF leak is a pathological condition due to a defect in the dura or skull which creates an abnormal connection, or fistula, allowing for the body fluid to outflow. CSF leaks can be classified as traumatic (which cover for over 90% of cases), iatrogenic, and idiopathic.

The leak may occur from the external auditory canal (EAC) (otorrhea), nose (rhinorrhea), or directly from the site of trauma

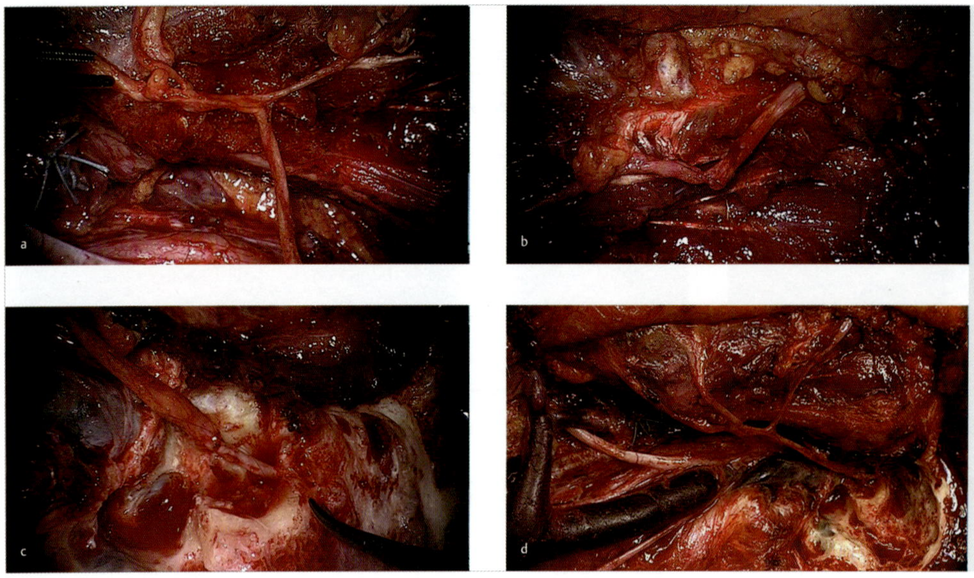

Fig. 14.9 Clinical Case 3, Left side: **(a)** A greater auricular nerve is used as cable graft to reconstruct the facial nerve defect. **(b)** A microsuture between the peripheral branches of the facial nerve and the cable graft is done. **(c)** A microsuture in between the proximal stump of facial nerve and the cable graft is performed. **(d)** A total reconstruction by a cable graft anastomosis is seen.

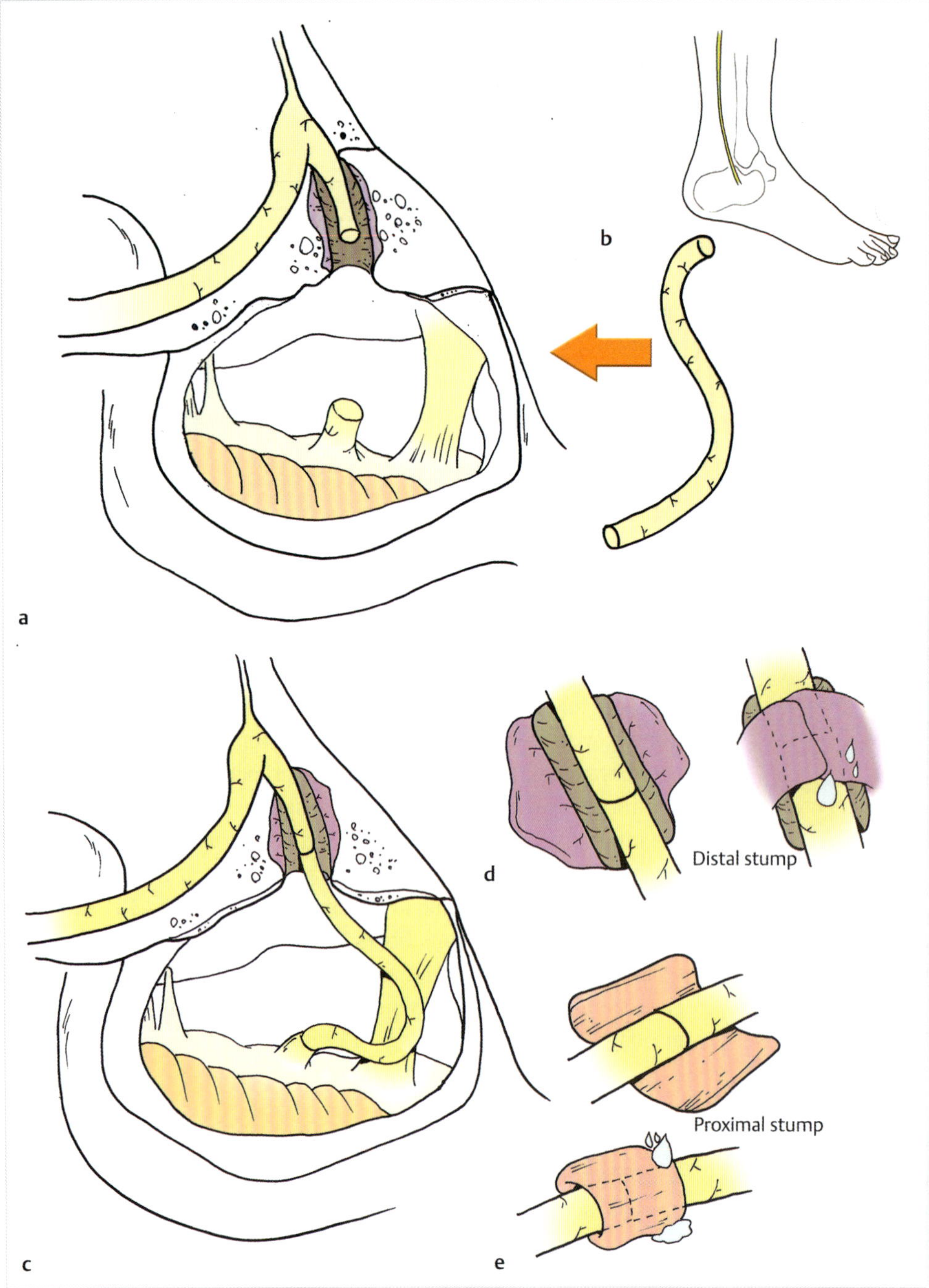

Fig. 14.10 Left ear: A large defect of facial nerve in the cerebellopontine angle (CPA) is seen **(a)**. In this case a sural nerve cable graft is harvested in order to repair the nerve defect **(b)**. The cable graft is placed in an S shape between the proximal and the distal stump of facial nerve with the curved portion resting on the trigeminal nerve in order to stabilize the graft in the CPA and avoiding tension between the cable graft and the nervous stumps **(c)**. The distal anastomosis is fixed using a fibrin glue and dural flap from the internal auditory canal (IAC) covering the nervous connection **(d)**. The proximal anastomosis is fixed using a temporalis fascia folding around the nervous connection and reinforced with fibrin glue **(e)**.

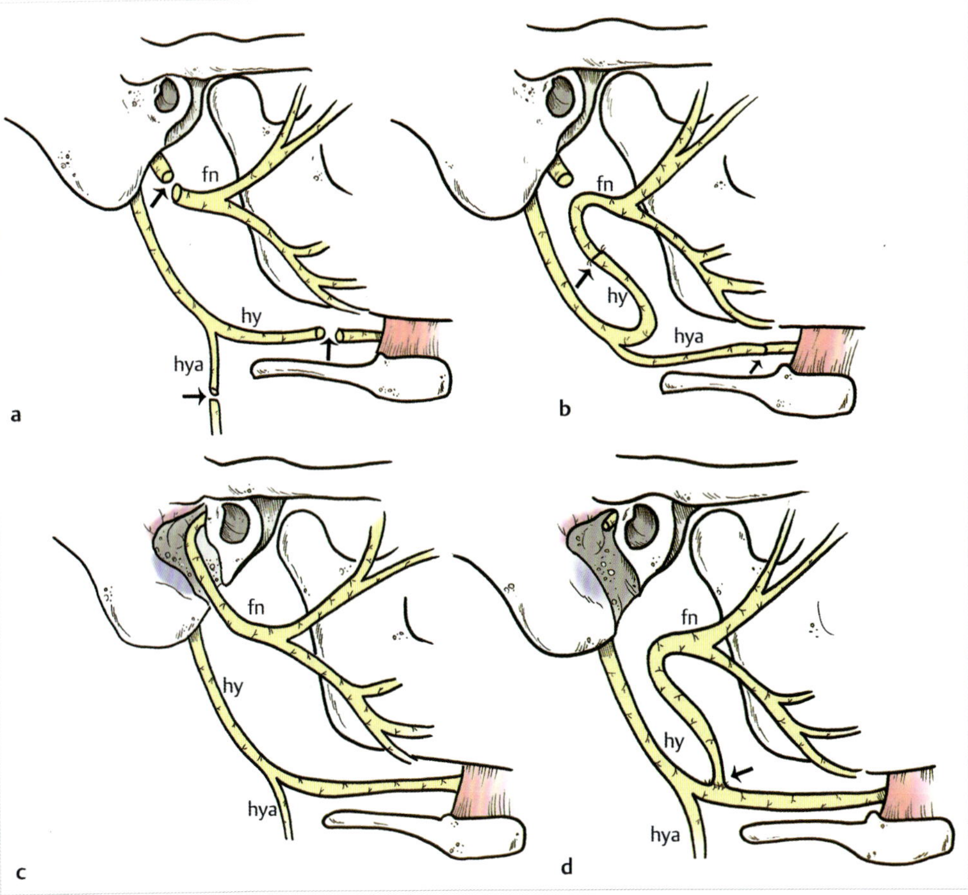

Fig. 14.11 Hypoglossal-facial anastomosis. End-to-end anastomosis **(a, b)**; side-to-end anastomosis **(c, d)**. *fn: facial nerve; hy: hypoglossal nerve; hya: ansa cervicalis of hypoglossal nerve.*

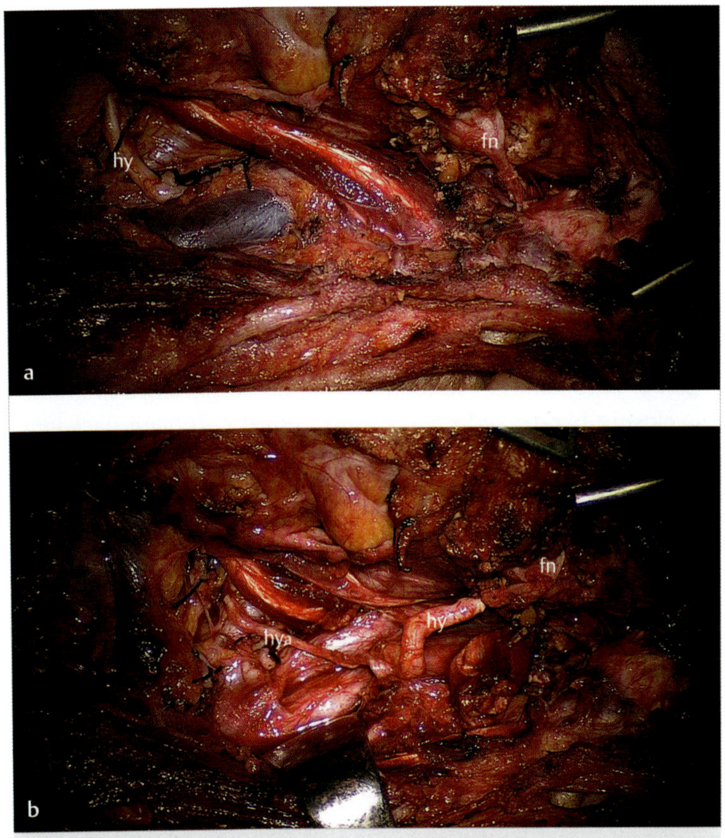

Fig. 14.12 (a, b) Clinical Case 4, Left side: End-to-end hypoglossal-facial anastomosis. *fn: facial nerve; hy: hypoglossal nerve; hya: ansa cervicalis of hypoglossal nerve.*

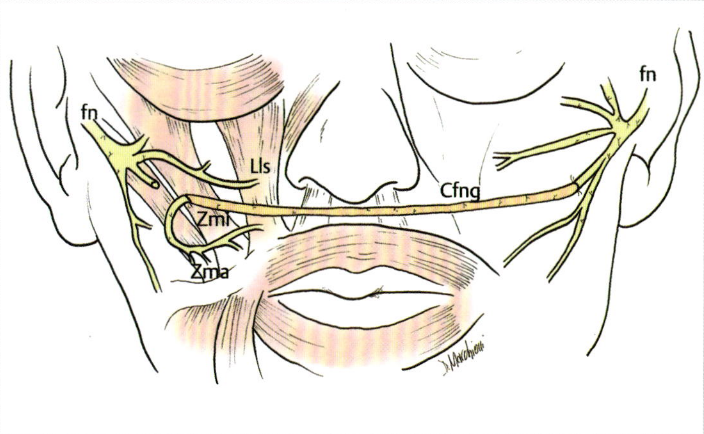

Fig. 14.13 Schematic drawing represents a cross-facial nerve graft from a buccal branch of the patient's nonparalyzed left side coapted in an end-to-end fashion to a buccal branch on the patient's paralyzed right side. *Cfng: cross facial nerve grafting; fn: facial nerve; Lls: levator labii superiorus muscle; Zma: Zygomaticus major muscle; Zmi: Zygomaticus minor muscle.*

or surgical wound. Even if the injury involves an otologic structure, CSF otorrhea is present only in case of an eardrum perforation or violation of the external ear canal. In the absence of such a defect, the fluid drains through the eustachian tube and presents as rhinorrhea. For this reason, otorrhea is far less common than otorhinorrhea and in most cases are a complication of acoustic neuroma and lateral skull base surgery. Regarding acoustic neuroma surgery, postoperative CSF leaks are the second most common complication, with an average of 10% leak rate reported in literature. While there is no significant difference between the type of surgical approach and the presence of CSF leak, the presentation of the leak itself can be different: rhinorrhea is most common in retrosigmoid and middle crania fossa approaches, while wound leak is more often a complication of translabyrinthine approach.

Rhinorrhea occurs via air cell tracts in the temporal bone. This event is more frequent in well-pneumatized bones. To avoid CSF leakage through the temporal pneumatization, it is crucial to carefully obliterate all the open air cells with bone wax or muscle plug at the end of surgical procedure. In case of retrosigmoid approach, a final endoscopic check of the temporal bone surface close to the IAC should be done in order to detect open cells around the meatus. In case of openings, a muscle plug with fibrin glue is used to obliterate these open cells. To prevent CSF leaks in the translabyrinthine approach, the eustachian tube must be obliterated with a piece of muscle; a careful obliteration of all the open cells is mandatory before closing the surgical field.

In transotic, transcochlear, and transpromontorial approaches, a blind sac closure of the EAC with eustachian tube obliteration by bone wax of muscle plug is performed; and all the open cells are sealed off by bony wax before sealing the surgical cavity with abdominal fat.

In case of failure of eustachian tube obliteration, the fat can be rapidly reabsorbed when it comes into contact with the air of the middle ear and a CSF leakage through the eustachian tube is expected.

The presence of an abnormal communication to the sterile subarachnoid space poses a great risk of infection for the patient. Acute meningitis is the initial symptom in about 30% of cases (*Streptococcus pneumoniae* followed by *Haemophilus influenzae* are the leading etiologic agents).

The main symptom of CSF leak is unilateral rhinorrhea, which can be continuous or intermittent as it collects in one of the paranasal sinuses and drains with changes of head position. CSF drainage can be elicited with a Valsalva maneuver or by performing the Queckenstedt-Stookey test (a manual compression of both jugular veins). Orthostatic headache and tinnitus are also often associated with CSF leaks. Other symptoms can help localize the drainage. For instance, anosmia is associated with a lesion in the anterior fossa and olfactory area; optic nerve deficits indicate an injury in the region of the tuberculum sellae/sphenoid sinus; unilateral conductive hearing loss is often present in case of otogenic spinal fluid leakage. However, it must be stressed that in most cases physical examination is unrevealing, especially in case of an intermittent CSF leak.

After a thorough medical history collection, work-up can include laboratory studies and multiple imaging techniques.

Beta-trace proteins and Beta2-Transferrin are proteins produced mainly in the central nervous system. Both assays are a highly specific (95–98 and 90–95% respectively), sensitive, and noninvasive procedures to identify the presence of CSF. A fast but highly unreliable test is the determination of glucose content with the use of glucose oxidase paper.

The gold standard imaging study is computed tomography (CT) scan with maximum 1 mm thick slice. Skull base defects can be easily demonstrated through this examination, although high-resolution CT scans might reveal small bone defects that do not leak. CT cisternography makes use of the injection of intrathecal contrast to determine the site of leakage. However, intermittent drainage might cause false-negative results. Magnetic resonance imaging (MRI) is only recommended as a first-line imaging modality if an encephalocele is suspected. MR cisternography uses T2-weighted imaging to highlight CSF, avoiding intrathecal injection of contrast. Scintiphotography with radioactive isotopes and injection of intrathecal fluorescein might be used in selected cases if previous analyses were inconclusive.

Because CSF leaks can lead to life-threatening complications, knowing when to treat a CSF leak conservatively or surgically is the most difficult part of management.

According to literature, up to 80% of CSF leaks due to lateral skull base surgery can be treated conservatively. This initial approach aims to ease the wound's natural healing process by lowering CSF pressure and reducing infections risk. Compressive dressing, bed rest while keeping the head raised at 30 to 40 degrees angle for 1 to 2 weeks, stool softeners, and strain avoidance are fundamental precautions to achieve a decrease of CSF pressure. Medication such as diuretics, carbon anhydrase inhibitors, and steroids can be given in order to reduce the production of spinal fluid. Persistent fistulas can be treated with CSF diversion. A lumbar drain (150 mL per day) kept for 3 to 5 days is the most common technique. The lumbar-peritoneal shunt is inserted into the subarachnoid space between two lumbar vertebrae, around the oblique muscles and into the peritoneal cavity where the body fluid is then absorbed. Yet, it must be noted that lumbar drains can increase the risk of pneumocephalus and meningitis.

Recurrent leaks must be treated surgically. In fact, surgical repair of iatrogenic CSF leakages is often required since spontaneous closure is rare and relapses are frequent. Though packaging of the middle ear and eustachian tube are standard procedures to avoid CSF drainage during lateral skull base surgery, formation of fistulas can still occur. The most used treatments to repair such defects include re-exploration of the wound, ventriculoperitoneal shunt placement, eustachian tube obliteration, mastoid obliteration, and middle fossa craniotomy with eustachian tube resection. The type of surgical approach is dictated by the location and cause of the fistula. Moreover, the original procedure and residual hearing must be considered to choose the most adequate treatment.

Dural tears and small defects can usually be repaired with watertight direct suture and adjuvant synthetic sealants or augmented closure by means of muscle tissue, fascial graft, or fat.

In case of preserved hearing, a mastoidectomy is usually performed. The bony labyrinth is skeletonized and air cell tracts are obliterated with bone wax and pâté. The antrum is then sealed and the mastoid is obliterated with fat.

Persistent rhinorrhea can be treated with a minimally invasive endoscopic endonasal eustachian tube obliteration.

Larger defects of the middle fossa floor (> 1 cm) are best addressed with a combined middle fossa–transmastoid approach and subsequent closure with bone (or other synthetic biocompatible materials if not available), fascia, and fibrin glue. In the case of encephaloceles, the brain tissue should be meticulously resected through bipolar electrocautery to prevent hemorrhage (see Clinical Case 5, ▶ Fig. 14.14).

14.3 Bleeding

Severe bleeding as a consequence of lateral skull base surgery is a rare but dreaded complication. Anatomical complexity, a narrow operating field, and the critical importance of nearby structures pose a further challenge for a correct management of emergency bleeding.

14.3.1 Intraoperative Bleeding

Major venous bleeding is usually caused by an accidental injury of the jugular bulb, sigmoid sinus, or emissary veins. In case of bleeding of emissary veins, a diamond bur without irrigation can be used to stop the blood loss. Smaller lesions to the sigmoid sinus and jugular bulb can be repaired easily with fibrin-coated collagen fleece or oxidized cellulose. Damage to the petrous sinus and temporal veins may cause venous insufficiency and thrombosis, both of which often lead to edema and ischemia of the temporal lobe. Major venous wounds might require the packing of the sigmoid sinus or the tympanic cavity in order to fully arrest the bleeding. The most significant draining vein of the temporal lobe is the inferior anastomotic vein (vein of Labbé). The vein of Labbé (VL) is the largest vein connecting the veins along the sylvian fissure with the transverse sinus. The accidental closure of Labbé vein is a rare and dangerous condition during lateral skull base approaches. It might be possible especially during transtentorial approaches and this complication can cause temporal lobe cerebral infarction, which results in an alteration in mental status and can lead to a coma and death.

Regarding arterial bleeding, one of the major concerns to lateral skull base surgeons is the lesion of internal carotid artery (ICA). The ICA is especially prone to damage during jugular paraganglioma surgery because of the close relationship between the tumor and the artery. The surgeon should sufficiently expose the artery during the procedure in order to allow enough room for instrumentation in case of bleeding. An ICA hemorrhage is a surgical emergency where urgent measures should include packing of the middle ear and stabilization of the circulation. Subsequent treatment varies according to the position and degree of injury. The use of angioplasty, ligation, muscle patches, and direct running sutures are reported in literature. After the bleeding has stopped, an angiographic evaluation is usually performed in order to check for possible aneurysms or dissections (see ▶ Fig. 14.15). Currently, treatment options for symptomatic and asymptomatic petrous ICA aneurysms include conservative management with serial imaging, endovascular ICA balloon occlusion, endovascular coil placement or stent-assisted coil insertion, placement of a flexible covered stent, or surgical trapping and revascularization with a high-flow bypass. The treatment should be tailored to the individual, depending on the condition of the patient and the nature of the lesion.

The complexity of the lateral skull base structures and their blood vessels can lead to major impairment of vital functions if

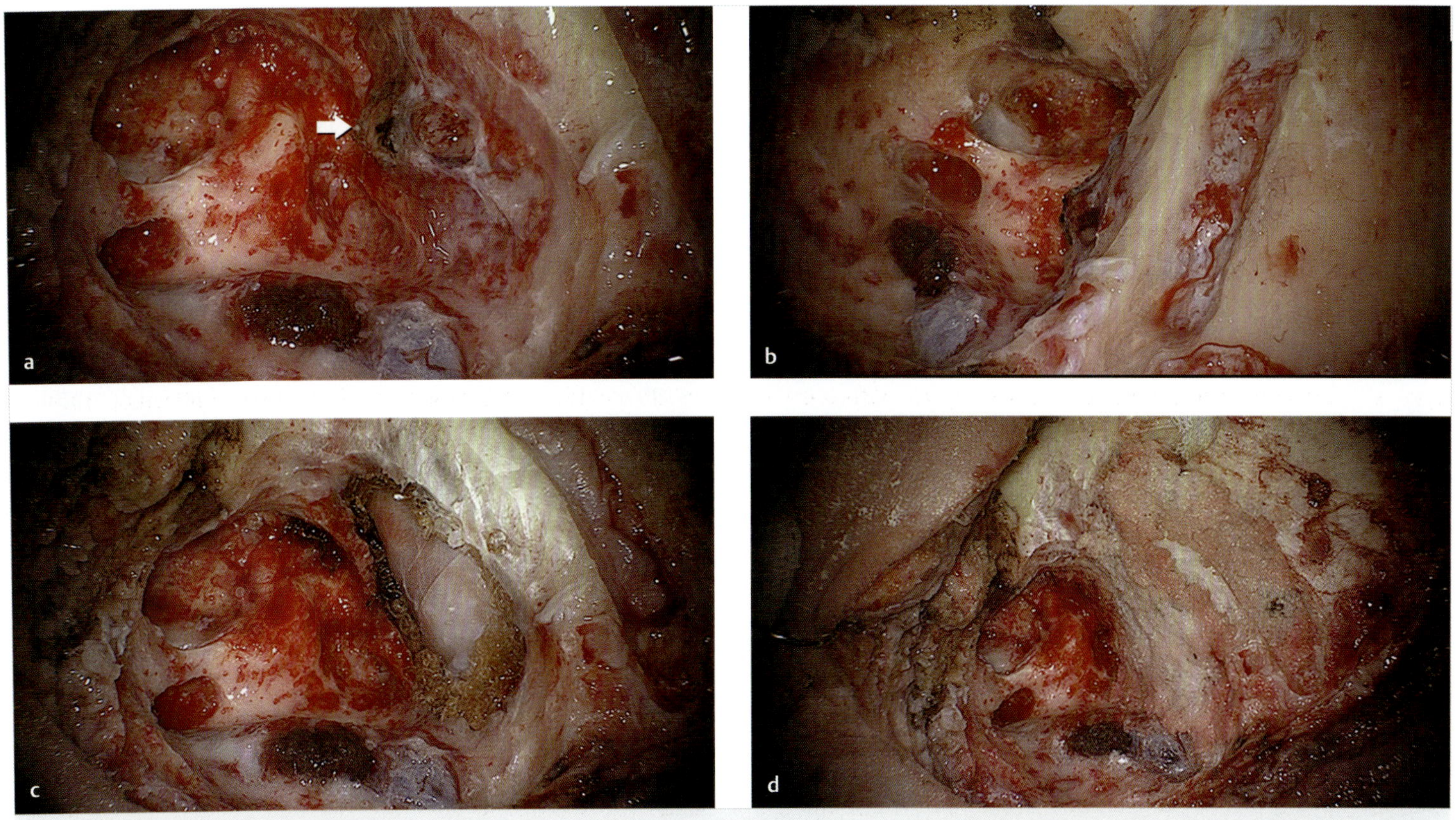

Fig. 14.14 Clinical Case 5, Left ear: **(a)** Encephaloceles of middle fossa, the brain tissue is resected. **(b)** A mini craniotomy is performed. **(c)** A Duragen is used in underlay through the craniotomy to repair the dural defect. **(d)** Bone paté with fibrin glue is also used to optimize the repair.

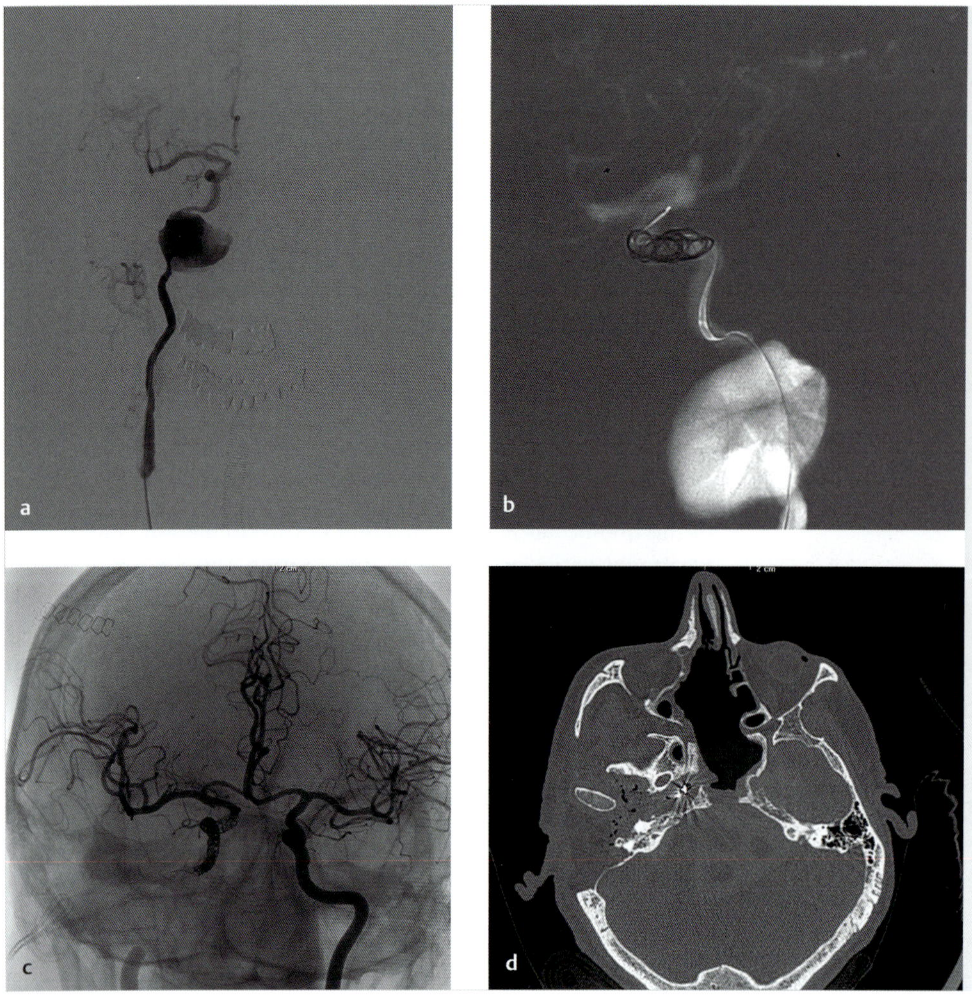

Fig. 14.15 Injury of intrapetrous internal carotid artery (ICA): Angiography shows aneurysm of intrapetrous ICA after injury during infratemporal fossa approach (a, b). After a well-tolerated occlusion balloon test to evaluate adequate collateral flow, an endovascular treatment with the occlusion of the vascularization of the aneurysm was performed (c, d).

damaged. For instance, arterial injury during vestibular schwannoma surgery could result in a brainstem stroke if the anterior inferior cerebellar artery or the perforating branches of the basilar artery are damaged. Damage to the anterior inferior cerebellar artery can provoke a pons infarction, which might cause hemiparesis and death. During surgery, in order to avoid arterial spasm, the surgeon should pay attention to avoid trauma of the artery for excessive manipulation or coagulation. In case of vasospasm a topical papaverine solution should be applied on the vascular structure.

All these examples further stress the importance of a detailed knowledge of the patient's anatomy.

14.3.2 Postoperative Bleeding

Postoperative intracranial bleeding represents one of the most dangerous situations in lateral skull base surgery. Control CT scans are usually recommended after lateral skull base surgery in order to show possible complications such as hematoma formation. Hematomas that require surgical revision are considered severe conditions. They are often caused by venous bleeding during subperiosteal plane preparation or small skin incisions that might be overlooked during the procedure due to limited view. Postoperative bleeding can result in a life-threatening situation due to the space-occupying effect on brain tissue. Blood clots are also thought to cause a blockage in CSF drainage pathways that might lead to hydrocephalus. Sudden headache, weakness, altered level of consciousness, movement impariment, nausea, vomiting, and hypoesthesia are symptoms associated with brain hemorrhage. It must be considered that such events may evolve within days after surgery. For this reason, successive radiological controls are advised if clinical signs and symptoms raise suspicion.

The usual manifestation of bleeding is an altered state of consciousness, with changing vital signs. For this reason, an early extubation of the patient after surgery is mandatory in order to check the vital signs with the patient awake, during the immediate postoperative time.

Since in the majority of cases, intracranial hematomas occur rapidly, in case of fast vital signs of deterioration, an immediate decompression should be performed, without waiting for a postoperative CT scan (see ▶ Fig. 14.16). In case of translabyrinthine, retrolabyrinthine, transpromontorial, transotic, and transcochlear approaches, a bedside decompression is easily achieved with wound opening and fat removal.

In case of retrosigmoid approach, a fast opening of the dura in the operating theater should be done in order to decompress the CPA. After hematoma removal the surgical field should be widely irrigated. Progressively raising the blood pressure is mandatory to carefully check the status of the hemostasis at the end of the revision surgery before closing the surgical cavity.

In case the patient's condition is stable but the diagnosis is doubtful, a CT scan should be immediately planned in order to detect any postoperative hematoma.

In case of limited and nonprogressive hematoma, a conservative treatment is suggested as the first choice, when performing a serial CT scans in the postoperative time.

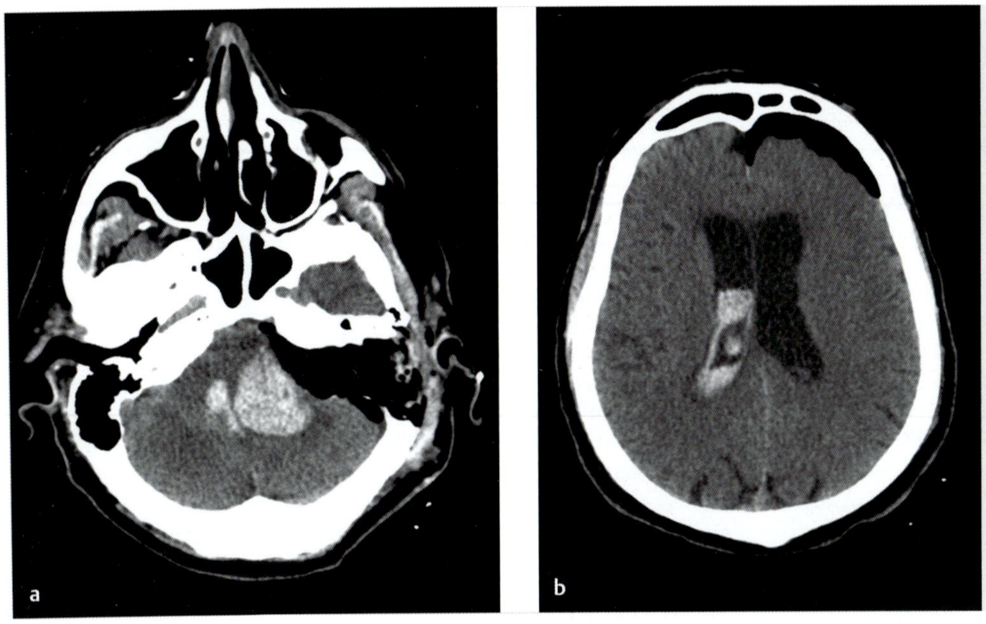

Fig. 14.16 **(a, b)** A postoperative cerebellar hematoma with ventricular involvement is seen in the computed tomography (CT) scan in axial view. This condition required an immediate revision surgery.

Suggested Readings

Anschuetz L, Bonali M, Guarino P, et al. Management of bleeding in exclusive endoscopic ear surgery: pilot clinical experience. Otolaryngol Head Neck Surg. 2017; 157(4):700–706

Bu Y, Chen M, Gao T, Wang X, Li X, Gao F. Mechanisms of hydrocephalus after intraventricular haemorrhage in adults. Stroke Vasc Neurol. 2016; 1(1):23–27

Chan JYK, Byrne PJ. Management of facial paralysis in the 21st century. Facial Plast Surg. 2011; 27(4):346–357

de Campora E, Marzetti F. La chirurgia oncologica della testa e del collo. 2nd ed. Elsevier; 2006

Fang Z, Tian R, Jia Y-T, Xu T-T, Liu Y. Treatment of cerebrospinal fluid leak after spine surgery. Chin J Traumatol/Zhonghua Chuang Shang Za Zhi. 2017; 20(2):81–83

Le C, Strong EB, Luu Q. Management of anterior skull base cerebrospinal fluid leaks. J Neurol Surg B Skull Base. 2016; 77(5):404–411

Lemonnier LA, Tessema B, Kuperan AB, et al. Managing cerebrospinal fluid rhinorrhea after lateral skull base surgery via endoscopic endonasal eustachian tube closure. Am J Rhinol Allergy. 2015; 29(3):207–210

Leonetti J, Anderson D, Marzo S, Moynihan G. Cerebrospinal fluid fistula after transtemporal skull base surgery. Otolaryngol Head Neck Surg. 2001; 124(5):511–514

Malik TH, Kelly G, Ahmed A, Saeed SR, Ramsden RT. A comparison of surgical techniques used in dynamic reanimation of the paralyzed face. Otol Neurotol. 2005; 26(2):284–291

May M, Schaitkin B. The Facial Nerve. 2nd ed. New York, NY: Thieme Medical Publishers; 2000

Nadol JB, McKenna MJ. Surgery of the Ear and Temporal Bone. Lippincott Williams & Wilkins; 2005

Paul P, Upadhyay K. Endoscopic endonasal repair of traumatic CSF rhinorrhea. The Indian Journal of Neurotrauma. 2010; 7(1):67–69

Presutti L, Mattioli F, Villari D, Marchioni D, Ghidini A. Trattamento endoscopico delle fistole rinoliquorali. In La Chirurgia Endoscopica dei Seni Paranasali e della Base Cranica. (19th ed., pp. 235–268). Quaderni Monografici di Aggiornamento A. O.O.I

Schick B, Dlugaiczyk J. Surgery of the ear and the lateral skull base: pitfalls and complications. GMS Curr Top Otorhinolaryngol Head Neck Surg. 2013; 12:Doc05

Index

Note: Page numbers set **bold** or *italic* indicate headings or figures, respectively.

G

H

I

J

K

L

M

N

O

U

V

W

X

Z